Berry & Kohn's

OPERATING ROOM TECHNIQUE

Berry & Kohn's OPERATING ROOM TECHNIQUE

**Nancymarie Howard Fortunato,
RN, BSN, BA, MEd, RNFA, CNOR, CPSN**

Perioperative Nursing,
Cleveland Clinic Foundation,
Cleveland, Ohio;
Perioperative Program Developer and Educator,
Lakeland Community College,
Mentor, Ohio;
RNFA Program Developer and Educator,
Educational Services for Professionals,
Ashtabula, Ohio;
Medical Research and Program Design,
Delphi Professional Services,
Wickliffe, Ohio

NINTH EDITION

with 448 illustrations

 Mosby

St. Louis Baltimore Boston Carlsbad Chicago Minneapolis New York Philadelphia Portland
London Milan Sydney Tokyo Toronto

Dedicated to Publishing Excellence

Editor-in-Chief: Sally Schrefer
Senior Editor: Loren Wilson
Developmental Editor: Nancy L. O'Brien
Project Manager: Deborah L. Vogel
Senior Production Editor: Jodi M. Willard
Designer: Bill Drone
Cover Designer: Mark Oberkrom

NINTH EDITION

NOTICE

Pharmacology is an ever-changing field. Standard safety precautions must be followed, but as new research and clinical experience broaden our knowledge, changes in treatment and drug therapy may become necessary or appropriate. Readers are advised to check the most current product information provided by the manufacturer of each drug to be administered to verify the recommended dose, the method and duration of administration, and contraindications. It is the responsibility of the appropriately licensed health care provider, relying on experience and knowledge of the patient, to determine dosages and the best treatment for each individual patient. Neither the publisher nor the editor assumes any liability for any injury and/or damage to persons or property arising from this publication.

Mosby, Inc.
A Harcourt Health Sciences Company
11830 Westline Industrial Drive
St. Louis, Missouri 63146

Printed in the United States of America

Library of Congress Cataloging in Publication Data

Fortunato, Nancymarie Howard.
   Berry & Kohn's operating room technique.—9th ed. / Nancymarie Howard Fortunato.
     p. ;   cm.
   Includes bibliographical references and index.
   ISBN 0-323-00968-9
    1. Operating room nursing.   I. Title: Berry and Kohn's operating room technique.   II.
Title: Operating room technique.   III. Atkinson, Lucy Jo. Berry & Kohn's operating room technique.
IV. Title.
   [DNLM: 1. Operating Room Nursing. 2. Operating Room Technicians. 3. Perioperative Care—
methods. WY 162 F745b 2000]
   RD32.3 .B4 2000
   617'.91—dc21   99-046828

99 00 01 02 03 TG/KPT 9 8 7 6 5 4 3 2 1

Dedicated to

Mary Louise Kohn

whose teachings brought forth this text, with love for perioperative caregivers.
She taught that the patient is the reason for our existence.
Her selflessness is an inspiration.

and

To the memory of
Edna Cornelia Berry

whose devotion to teaching was surpassed only by her devotion
to the care of surgical patients in the operating room.

Consultants

Ruth Bakst, RN, RNFA, CNOR
Perioperative Educator,
St. Luke's Medical Center,
Cleveland, Ohio;
Registered Nurse-Midwife,
Capetown, Africa

Patricia E. Chapek, RN, BA, CNOR
Chair, AORN Cardiothoracic Specialty Assembly;
Perioperative Nursing, Cardiac Department,
Cleveland Clinic Foundation,
Cleveland, Ohio

Greg Furness, ST
Surgical Technologist,
Cleveland Clinic Foundation,
Cleveland, Ohio

Mary Gilley, RN, MS, CNOR
Nurse Clinician,
Washington University Medical Center,
St. Louis, Missouri

Lesley Henderson, RN, MSN, CNOR, PhD Candidate
Educator,
Floyd College,
Rome, Georgia

Patti Houck, RN, RNFA, CNOR
Dr. Brian Davies, Inc.,
Akron, Ohio

Mary Lou Kubu, RN, BSN, CNOR
Perioperative Educator,
University Hospitals,
Cleveland, Ohio

Jim Laubert, RN, RNFA, CNOR
ENT Health Services, Inc.,
Middleberg Heights, Ohio

Janet Lewis, RN, MA, CNOR
Administrative Director, Surgical Services,
INTEGRIS Health,
Oklahoma City, Oklahoma

James Malson, RN, MSN, CRNA
Nurse Anesthetist,
Barberton Citizen's Hospital,
Barberton, Ohio

Maryann Mawhinney, RN, BSN, MEd, CNOR
Perioperative Nursing,
Holy Spirit Hospital,
Camp Hill, Pennsylvania

Vicki Moore, RN, MS, CNOR
Women's Health Nurse Practitioner,
Women for Women,
Dr. Michelle Martel,
Lynchburg, Virginia

Elizabeth Campbell Parsons, RN, MSN, CNOR
Clinical Coordinator, Perioperative Services,
Crawford Long Hospital of Emory University,
Atlanta, Georgia

Martin A. Phillips, III, RN, BSN, CNOR
Major, United States Army Nurse Corps,
Reserve Component 256th CSH,
Brookpark, Ohio;
Perioperative Nursing,
Hillcrest Hospital,
Mayfield Heights, Ohio

Marimargaret Reichert, RN, MA
President, Reichert Consulting,
Support Services to Healthcare Facilities and Medical
    Device Manufacturers,
Olmsted Falls, Ohio

M. Jane Rua, RN, BSN, JD
Attorney at Law,
Jeffries, Kube, Forrest, and Monteleone Company, LPA,
Cleveland, Ohio

Jill Thomas, RNC, LNHA, LNC
Wound Care and Long Term Care Consultant,
TST & Associates,
Bay Village, Ohio

Vanessa Vlack, RN, CNOR
Perioperative Nursing,
University Hospitals,
Cleveland, Ohio

Carolyn Volpicello, RN, MA, CNOR
Senior Staff Nurse,
St. Vincent Hospital and Medical Center,
New York, New York

Reviewers

Joyce M. Ackley, RN, CNOR
Clinical Educator—Cardiac, Thoracic, Vascular Surgery,
Memorial Medical Center,
Springfield, Illinois

Joanne D. Cimorelli, BS, RN, CNOR, CRNFA
RN First Assistant,
First Assistant Services,
Havertown, Pennsylvania,
Staff RN, Operating Room,
Presbyterian Medical Center of the University
 of Pennsylvania Health System,
Philadelphia, Pennsylvania

Carol A. deBlois, BSN, MA, CNOR
Coordinator of Perioperative Programs,
Bridgeport Hospital School of Nursing,
Bridgeport, Connecticut

Lee Ann Dobson, BSN, CNOR
Coordinator, Surgical Technology Program,
Carlow College,
Pittsburgh, Pennsylvania

Dorothy I. Donesky, BSN, MPH, RN, CNOR
Assistant Professor, Surgical Technology,
Loma Linda University,
Loma Linda, California

William Duffy, BSN, MJ, RN, CNOR
Director, Perioperative Services,
Evanston Northwestern Healthcare Corporation,
Chicago, Illinois

Susan Jane Fetzer, MBA, MSN, PhD, RN
Assistant Professor,
University of New Hampshire;
Staff Nurse, PACU,
Elliot Hospital,
Manchester, New Hampshire

Terri Grell, BSN, RN, CNOR
Surgical Technology Coordinator,
Kirkwood Community College,
Cedar Rapids, Iowa

Edith Hill, BSN, RN, CNOR
Perioperative Nurse Clinician,
The Genesee Hospital,
Rochester, New York

Roxanne Huckstep, AA, BS, RN, CNOR
Orthopaedic Specialist,
Riverside Regional Medical Center,
Newport News, Virginia

Patricia P. Kapsar, MBA, RN
Corporate Compliance Officer,
Bethesda Health Group, Inc.,
St. Louis, Missouri

Mary JB Larsen, BSN, RN, CNOR, RNFA
Operating Room Staff Nurse,
Huron Valley—Sinai Hospital,
Commerce Township, Michigan

Joanne Lester, MSN, RNC, OCN, CNP
Nurse Practitioner, Division of Surgical Oncology,
James Cancer Hospital & Solove Research Institute,
Columbus, Ohio

Lisa M. Loeffelholz, BS, MS
Assistant Professor, Microbiology/Biotechnology,
Kirkwood Community College,
Cedar Rapids, Iowa

Elizabeth Ness, BA, MSHA, CST
Surgical Technology Program Director,
Wayne County Community College,
Detroit, Michigan

Sharon L. Palestino, BSN, RN, CNOR, RNFA
Nursing Director, Orthopedics Operating Room,
Pennsylvania Hospital,
Philadelphia, Pennsylvania

Carolyn A. Parks, BN, RN, CNOR
Coordinator, Surgical Technology Program,
Penn Valley Community College,
Kansas City, Missouri

Regina Reilly, RN, CNOR, RNFA
Operating Room Staff Nurse and Surgical Assistant,
St. Mary Medical Center,
Langhorne, Pennsylvania

Wyveda Porter Rodriguez, PhD, RN, CNOR
Administrative Director,
Plaza Day Surgery Center,
Fort Worth, Texas;
Adjunct Assistant Professor,
University of Texas,
Arlington, Texas

Barbara J. Ryan, BA, BSN, RN, CNOR, RNFA
Operating Room,
Adirondack Medical Center,
Saranac Lake, New York

Christine E. Smith, MSN, RN, CNOR
Perioperative Clinical Specialist/Educator;
Faculty,
Delaware County Community College,
Media, Pennsylvania

Katie Steuer, BSN, RN, CNOR
Perioperative RN, Level III,
Dartmouth-Hitchcock Medical Center,
Lebanon, New Hampshire

Kay Swartzwelder, MSN, RN, CNOR
Director, Allied Health,
Collins Career Center,
Chesapeake, Ohio

Mary L. Sweeney, MN, RN, CNOR
Manager, Operating Room,
Harborview Medical Center,
Seattle, Washington

Teresa D. Vincent, RN, CNOR, CSPDT
Surgical Technology Program Director,
Madisonville Technical College,
Madisonville, Kentucky

Preface to the Ninth Edition

This time-honored text has its roots in the operating room (OR) orientation manual created by Mary Louise Kohn in the late 1940s while working as an OR educator at University Hospitals of Cleveland, Ohio. Her impeccable notes were a source of interest to many OR supervisors and educators who wanted to standardize their teaching techniques in accordance with Mary Louise's orientation tool. Many observers requested copies of her writings, and eventually the cost of providing copies became prohibitive. In 1951, at the request of her publisher and with the encouragement of her superiors, Mary Louise assembled her orientation material into a manuscript suitable for publication. She spent countless hours writing and revising material until the birth of her daughter. Her dedication to her family led her to seek assistance for this project from Edna Cornelia Berry, who became her willing partner and coauthor throughout the first four editions.

The first edition of *Introduction to Operating Room Technique* by Edna Cornelia Berry and Mary Louise Kohn was published in 1955. The first edition had the following goals:

- To explain the principles of sterile and aseptic technique
- To stress the necessity for their application in all surgical procedures
- To provide insight into the physiologic and psychologic impact of surgical intervention on each patient as a unique individual

Berry and Kohn's Operating Room Technique has been the perioperative text of choice for more than 45 years because it emphasizes the importance of the patient and his or her reliance on the perioperative caregiver. Every new edition of this classic perioperative text has addressed changing needs and evolving technologies while maintaining the fundamental focus that still remains valid after 45 years—the care of the surgical patient.

Berry and Kohn's Operating Room Technique is designed to meet the needs of educators, learners, and personnel who care for surgical or interventional patients in many diverse environments. Knowing the "why" of patient care is as important as knowing the "how." A strong emphasis is placed on understanding the rationale behind each patient care activity.

FEATURES OF THIS TEXT

- A focus on the physiologic, psychologic, and spiritual considerations of perioperative patients to provide guidelines and standards for planning and implementing comprehensive, individualized care.
- In-depth discussion of patients with special needs related to age or health status considerations, with an emphasis on the development of a plan of care tailored to the unique care parameters of all patients.
- Discussion of perioperative patient care for both inpatient and ambulatory procedures to highlight considerations based on the setting as well as the surgical procedure.
- Encouragement of the caregiver to identify and examine personal and professional development issues that influence the manner in which care is rendered.
- Emphasis on teamwork among perioperative caregivers to encourage cooperation in attaining positive patient care outcomes.
- Detailed information about the fundamentals of perioperative nursing and surgical technology roles. No other text provides step-by-step explanations for each basic technique. Pertinent historic perspectives are included in each section to provide information about the evolution of the topic being discussed.
- Building of knowledge in a logical sequence—from fundamental concepts to implementation during surgical intervention—to enable readers to apply theory to practice.

- Comprehensive coverage of a broad range of essential topics to provide a thorough understanding of fundamental principles and techniques and an understanding of their applications in various surgical procedures.

NEW TO THE NINTH EDITION

- This edition was reviewed, updated, and reorganized into 12 manageable sections. Educators and learners in both academic and clinical settings will find the arrangement user-friendly. The logical and sequential order of the subject matter will enable perioperative caregivers of all disciplines to review and sharpen their knowledge and skill levels. The carefully planned tables, boxes, and figures further clarify the textual content.
- Chapter objectives have been added to focus the learner's attention on important content to be mastered in each chapter.
- Androgogic and pedagogic learning principles have been defined for the benefit of the educator and the learner. All personnel in health care roles are involved with self-learning and patient education and should have knowledge of which method is appropriate.
- The use of computers as learning and clinical tools are included throughout the text. Internet search engines are described, and pertinent Web sites are incorporated throughout the specialty sections. The advantages and disadvantages of computerized documentation are described.
- Preoperative, intraoperative, and postoperative patient care chapters are clearly delineated and expanded to include points of interest for perioperative and perianesthesia caregivers.
- Material about the assessment and treatment of complications has been expanded into a new chapter, Potential Perioperative Complications.
- A new chapter entitled Microbiologic Considerations enables perioperative nurses, surgical technologists, and instrument processing personnel to better understand the transmission of and the human responses to infectious disease–causing microorganisms. New information about prion disease is included.
- Sterilization and disinfection practices and procedures have been divided into two chapters for clarity. These concepts have been separated to emphasize the differences between sterilization and the various levels of disinfection of patient care items and equipment.
- Patient care during anesthetic administration is divided into three chapters: General Anesthesia: Techniques and Agents, Local and Regional Anesthesia, and Physiologic Maintenance and Monitoring of the Perioperative Patient.
- Many new illustrations have been added to enhance the visual detail of basic perioperative principles and surgical anatomy.
- New boxes and tables serve to clarify and highlight information critical to perioperative practice.
- The most up-to-date current terms and AORN Standards, Recommended Practices, and Guidelines have been incorporated to reflect modern perioperative practice. The chapters have been updated to reflect AORN's name change, which was made in 1999 to reflect the contemporary membership. The organization is now officially named **AORN**. The descriptor attached after the written name is now "the Association of periOperative Registered Nurses."

ORGANIZATION

Section I is dedicated to the learner and the educator. The correlation of theory and practice is integral to the success of patient care in the perioperative environment. Professional and personal attributes of the caregiver are examined, with an emphasis on objectivity in the development of the plan of care. Legal and ethical issues are discussed.

Section II delineates the roles of the members of the health care team as both direct and indirect caregivers. Nonphysician first assistant roles and credentials (e.g., RNFA, SA, CST/CFA) are discussed.

Section III provides in-depth information on patient assessment and the development of an individualized plan of care, with the patient viewed as a unique individual. Special needs are identified by health condition and age. Geriatric and pediatric chapters are included.

Section IV examines the physical plant of the perioperative environment—both hospital-based and freestanding ambulatory facilities. Diagrams of perioperative suite designs are included. Care of the perioperative environment, occupational hazards, and safety issues are examined in depth.

Section V provides a dedicated chapter on microbiology and the importance of microbiologic control in the perioperative environment, with an emphasis on standard precautions. It delineates aseptic and sterile techniques in fundamental to intermediate aspects such as attire, scrubbing, gowning, and gloving. Separate chapters are provided regarding the sterilization and disinfection of surgical instrumentation and patient care supplies.

Section VI details the surgical instrumentation and equipment used during surgical procedures. Processing instrumentation and the safe use of specialized surgical equipment are presented.

Section VII discusses preoperative patient care and includes the family/significant other in the plan of care. Diagnostic and oncologic procedures are described.

Section VIII covers methods of anesthetic administration and the role of caregivers during this process. Physiologic patient monitoring and related complications are discussed in detail.

Section IX describes intraoperative patient care, including positioning, prepping, and draping. The interactive roles of the circulator and the scrub person are specified.

Section X focuses on the surgical site. Hemostasis and wound closure are discussed in detail. Wound assessment and healing throughout the perioperative care period is described. New boxes and illustrations reinforce these discussions.

Section XI presents an expanded view of postoperative patient care. The postanesthesia care unit is explained. The death of a patient is discussed, and the importance of legal evidence is stressed.

Section XII covers the surgical specialties. Each chapter includes the historic development of the specialty. Salient surgical anatomy is described and illustrated in line drawings for clarity.

PERIOPERATIVE EDUCATOR'S RESOURCE MANUAL

The *Perioperative Educator's Resource Manual* parallels the content of the main text and provides the perioperative educator with material that augments the lesson plan for each chapter. This manual includes study questions and answers, critical thinking activities, and suggested learning activities to help students apply newly gained knowledge.

Nancymarie Fortunato

Preface
to the First Edition

The material in this text is the outgrowth of the coauthors' experience in the operating room—one as instructor of students, the other as head nurse with some responsibility for instructing and guiding students. It is an adaptation of the instructor's teaching outline for which there have been many requests.

The aim of the book is to facilitate the nurse's study of aseptic technique and care of the patient in the operating room. Although this text is intended primarily for the student, the authors hope it may prove useful to the graduate nurse as well.

Since it is assumed that the student has studied pathological conditions necessitating surgical treatment, these conditions are not discussed. When applicable, and as a matter of emphasis, there is a reiteration of principles of sterile technique and safety factors for the patient. It is hoped this will aid in fixing the principles as patterns of thought and work.

While operative routines vary in different hospitals, underlying principles are the same. Consequently, basic principles are stressed and the authors have endeavored to keep the material as general as possible. Principles must be adapted to suit the situations found in individual hospitals. Specific linen, equipment, and procedures are mentioned merely to serve as a framework upon which to demonstrate principles or as samples for points of departure. However, the specific examples mentioned are workable procedures that have evolved. They are kept as uncomplicated as possible for student teaching and for use in the practical situation.

Instruments for operations are not listed and few are mentioned, because each hospital has its instrument lists, standardized for each case, to which students can refer.

Emphasis is placed upon meeting the psychological as well as the physical needs of the surgical patient. An endeavor is made where possible to correlate briefly the preoperative and postoperative care with the operative procedure, to give the student a complete concept of patient care.

The frequent use of the imperative mood is for the purpose of brevity, organization, and emphasis. Questions and assignments in each chapter are to aid the student in reviewing the material, in recalling pertinent facts, and in applying the principles to her specific situation.

Obviously, if the student starts scrubbing for cases with an older nurse after her first day or two in the operating room and if her operating-room theory is given concurrently with the practice, much of the material in this book will have been covered by individual instruction before class discussion.

The authors have attempted to maintain simplicity and brevity, and to present a concise outline for preliminary study. They suggest that the student supplement this material by reference reading.

The authors wish to express their grateful appreciation and thanks to those persons who by their interest and cooperation supported them:

To Miss Edythe Angell, Supervisor of the Operating Rooms at University Hospitals of Cleveland, for helpful suggestions during the preparation of the manuscript and for reading, critically, the entire manuscript. We are gratefully indebted to her because we have learned from her much of what appears in this text.

To Miss Janet McMahon, Educational Director, School of Anesthesia, University Hospitals of Cleveland, for valuable assistance in preparing Chapter 21. Also, to Dr. Edward Depp, Anesthesiologist, Euclid-Glenville Hospital, Cleveland, who offered suggestions on this chapter and reviewed it.

To Dr. C.C. Roe Jackson, of the faculty of Western Reserve University School of Medicine, for constructive criticism in reviewing Chapter 17. To Dr. Howard D. Kohn, also of the faculty, who has been most helpful in reading the manuscript and offering suggestions.

To Mrs. Geraldine Mink, Librarian, for her assistance; to Mrs. Leona Peck for her patience in typing the manuscript and for her helpful suggestions; to Miss Ruth Elmenthaler and Miss Margaret Sanderson of the operating-room staff for their assistance in making the photographs; and to Mrs. Anita Rogoff for drawing the illustrations.

Edna Cornelia Berry

Mary Louise Kohn

Cleveland, Ohio

Acknowledgments

To the librarians and library assistants at the Cleveland Clinic Foundation, Cleveland, Ohio

To the surgeons and anesthesia providers who answered many questions and provided information throughout this project

To my perioperative colleagues, who offered suggestions and support for revisions and updates to this edition

To my students, who continually keep me grounded in my roots as a bedside nurse

To Lucy Jo Atkinson, who taught me to pay close attention to detail and organizational structure of the written word

To Nancy Coon, my former editor; Loren Wilson, my current editor; Nancy O'Brien; and Jodi Willard for their patient assistance, guidance, and encouragement throughout the development and production of this ninth edition. The excitement and newness of utilizing electronic galleys for the first time required faith and confidence in my ability, which they freely gave.

And last, but not least:

To my loving family and friends, who have been there for me through the transitions of life

Contents

Berry & Kohn's

OPERATING ROOM TECHNIQUE

Section
I

Correlation of
Theory and Practice

Chapter 1

Introduction for the Learner

 Chapter Objectives

After studying this chapter, the learner will be able to:

- Identify three characteristics of adult learners.
- Name five educational resources available for the learner.
- Understand the difference between androgogy and pedagogy.
- Understand how adult learning principles apply to patient teaching.

The main focus of this chapter is to establish the framework for an in-depth study of perioperative patient care and to support the educational process of the learner. Consideration is given to the perioperative educator, who may not have had a formal education in the teaching of adult learners. Both learners and educators should understand that the same learning and teaching principles apply to patient education. Select terms commonly used throughout the text need to be understood as the basis for learning about and participating in the science and art of surgery, and these are listed in Box 1-1.

HISTORICAL BACKGROUND

Ancient Egyptian papyri chronicle the progress of medicine and surgery up to 1600 BC. Other influences on the historic development of surgery come from the Babylonian law, the Code of Hammurabi (1955-1913 BC). According to this law, if a patient died after a surgical procedure, retribution would be reflected on the surgeon in the form of amputation of his right hand. Ancient Persians had to perform successful procedures on three infidels before being pronounced as competent to practice surgery. Surgery was not considered a medical discipline until the era of the physician Claudius Galen (130-200 AD), who is considered the father of exper-

imental physiology. Despite his contributions, surgery remained a primitive practice and lacked a scientific base for the next 1200 years. Surgeons and barbers of thirteenth- and fourteenth-century England belonged to the same guild until 1540, when barbers agreed to confine their surgery practices to dentistry. These combined groups were dissolved in 1745, and by 1800 the Royal College of Surgeons of London was chartered.

CONTEMPORARY SURGERY

Health is both a personal and an economic asset. Optimal health is the best physiologic and psychologic condition an individual can experience. Disease is the failure of a person's body to adequately counteract undesired stimuli, invasive organisms, or stresses, with the result being disruption in the function or structure of an organ or body system. Other external forces, such as congenital anomalies, infection, or trauma, cause imbalances that interfere with optimal human health.

Surgical intervention is a common method of treating physiologic conditions. Many of the former contraindications to surgery related to patient age or condition have been eliminated. Because of better diagnostic and supportive services

Box 1-1   Terms Associated with Perioperative Education

androgogy   Teaching and learning processes for mature adult populations.

behavior   Actions or conduct indicative of a mental state or predisposition that is influenced by emotions, feelings, beliefs, values, morals, and ethics.

cognition   Process of knowing or perceiving, such as learning scientific principles and observing their application.

competency   Creative application of knowledge, skills, and interpersonal abilities in fulfilling functions to provide individualized patient care.

critical thinking   The mental process by which an individual solves problems.

disease   Failure of the adaptive mechanisms to counteract stimuli or stresses adequately, resulting in a disturbance in function or structure of any part, organ, or system of the body.

health, optimal   The best an individual can feel and function in a particular circumstance or with a disease process.

illness   A composite of many reactions or diseases.

knowledge   An organized body of factual information.

learning style   Individualized methods used by the learner to understand and retain new information. These may be visual, auditory, tactile, sensory, or performance-oriented behaviors.

objectives   Written in behavioral terms, statements that determine the expected outcomes of a behavior or process.

pedagogy   Teaching and learning processes for immature pediatric populations.

perioperative   Total surgical experience that encompasses preoperative, intraoperative, and postoperative phases of patient care.

psychomotor   Pertaining to physical demonstration of mental processes (i.e., applying cognitive learning).

skill   Application of knowledge into observable, measurable, and quantifiable performance.

surgery   Branch of medicine that encompasses preoperative, intraoperative, and postoperative care of patients. The work of a surgeon is both a science and an art.

surgical conscience   Awareness that develops from a knowledge base of the importance of strict adherence to principles of aseptic and sterile techniques.

surgical procedure   Invasive incision into body tissues or a minimally invasive entrance into a body cavity for either therapeutic or diagnostic purposes during which protective reflexes or self-care abilities are potentially compromised.

Table 1-1   Common Indications for Surgical Intervention

Surgical Intervention	Example
Diagnostics	Biopsy tissue sample
Repair	Closing of a hernia
Removal	Foreign body
Reconstruction	Creation of a new breast
Palliation	Relief of obstruction
Aesthetics	Facelift
Harvest	Autologous skin graft
Procurement	Donor organ
Transplant	Placement of a donor organ
Bypass/shunt	Vascular rerouting
Drainage/evacuation	Incision of abscess
Stabilization	Repair of a fracture
Parturition	Cesarean section
Termination	Abortion of a pregnancy
Staging	Checking of cancer progression
Extraction	Removal of a tooth
Exploration	Invasive examination
Diversion	Creation of a stoma for urine

As both a science and an art, surgery is the branch of medicine that encompasses preoperative preparation, intraoperative judgment and management, and postoperative care of patients. As a discipline, surgery combines total care of illness with an interventional (invasive or noninvasive) aspect of treatment. The purposes of surgical intervention include correction of defects, alteration of form, restoration of function after trauma, diagnosis and/or treatment of disease processes, palliation, or prolongation of life. A surgical procedure may be an invasive incision into body tissues or entrance into a body cavity or a noninvasive manipulation of a body structure. The technology of the modern age has elevated the practice of surgery to a more precise science. Improvements in patient care technology are attributed to the following:

- Surgical specialization
- Sophisticated diagnostic and imaging techniques
- Minimally invasive equipment
- Collaboration of caregivers and industry

The art of surgery encompasses the attitude of the entire surgical team, which should be one of concern, compassion, and empathy for the patient. Dedication to the safety and welfare of the patient is manifested by applying scientific knowledge and individualized care.

Patients have different reasons for undergoing a surgical procedure—relief from pain, restoration of form or function, prolongation of life, and prevention of complications. Common indications for surgical intervention are listed in Table 1-1.

Surgical procedures are performed in hospitals, in surgeons' offices, or in freestanding surgical facilities. Not all patients undergoing surgical intervention in a hospital are ad-

and drug therapies, many persons are now considered better candidates for surgery. In the 1930s, the English physician Lord Berkeley George Moynihan (1865-1936) said, "Surgery has been made safe for the patient; we must now make the patient safe for surgery." Surgery cannot be considered completely safe all of the time, and patient outcomes are not always predictable. Each patient and each procedure is unique. Perioperative caregivers should not become complacent with routines but should always be prepared for the unexpected.

mitted for an overnight stay. Outpatient procedures are safe for carefully selected patients. Although reference will be made to the hospital throughout this text, the practices and procedures described are applicable to many surgical care settings, including diagnostic and therapeutic facilities.

The types of procedures performed in a hospital or other health care facility vary according to the expertise of the surgeons, the community in which the facility is located, and the equipment available. Perioperative patient care is delivered at two levels: professional and technical. The purpose of this text is to provide a basis for learning the professional and technical patient care issues that support the surgical patient throughout the perioperative experience.

PERIOPERATIVE LEARNER

The learner in the perioperative environment may be a medical, nursing, or surgical technology student enrolled in a formalized educational program, or the learner may be a newly hired orientee. Medical students have a surgical rotation that includes participation in surgical procedures. They learn some of the basic principles of surgical technology and sterile technique to ensure the safety and welfare of patients.

Some nursing schools offer basic exposure to perioperative nursing either as part of the core curriculum or as an elective. After graduating from nursing school, the nurse needs further education before functioning as a perioperative professional. This education may take place in a postbasic/postgraduate perioperative nursing course offered by a community college or a hospital orientation program. Entry-level education for perioperative practice prepares nurses to be generalists. Most programs teach scrub and circulating roles. Specialization can follow after a period of time in professional practice.

Surgical technology programs focus primarily on scrubbing and instrumentation skill. Some programs offer circulating experiences under the supervision of a registered nurse. Most surgical technology programs provide scrub experiences in all specialties. After satisfactory completion of the program, many technologists are capable of functioning in the scrub role as a generalist or specialist. Advancing technology indicates the need for specialized competencies. Surgeons, perioperative nurses, and surgical technologists should continuously strive to learn new procedures and technologies.

Perioperative caregivers new to a particular practice setting should learn the specific performance expectations of that institution. All personnel go through an orientation process to familiarize themselves with the philosophy, goals, policies, procedures, role expectations, and physical facilities specific to that institution. Departmental orientation is specific to the area in which the caregiver will be employed.

All learners in the perioperative environment are adults and prefer not to be treated as children. This concept applies whether the caregiver is experienced or is a novice. Treating an adult learner like a child is counterproductive and becomes a barrier to learning. Regardless of the level of learning required, the general characteristics of the adult (andro-

Box 1-2	Characteristics of the Adult Learner as Compared to the Child Learner

Adult (Androgogy)	Child (Pedagogy)
Is self-directed	Is task oriented
Uses activities that follow transitions of maturity	Uses activities that follow stages of development
Uses intrinsic thought processes	Uses extrinsic thought processes
Uses problem-solving approach	Uses trial-and-error approach
Values self-esteem	Values self-esteem

gogic) learner as compared to the child (pedagogic) learner apply (Box 1-2). These concepts should also be applied to patient education programs.

Not everyone learns at the same speed or assimilates information in the same manner. Theoretical knowledge or a skill learned quickly by one individual may be difficult for another. Learning styles vary among individuals. Influencing factors include the following:

- Intelligence
- Cultural background
- Educational preparation
- Motivation to learn
- Personality characteristics
- Psychologic strengths or deficiencies
- Social skills, including communication skills
- Manual dexterity
- Physical senses
- Perceptual preferences and sensory partiality (e.g., visual vs. auditory)
- Environment

Each facility should define the role of the perioperative learner. Learners actually help prepare for, assist a qualified team member during, and clean up following surgical procedures, but they are not considered members of the staff compliment. Learners are not expected to assume responsibilities for which they are not fully prepared. Only through continued study and experience can individuals qualify as team members in the perioperative environment.

The learner is usually taught the scrub role functions early in the perioperative experience. (These functions are discussed in detail in Chapter 27 and throughout this text.) At first, an educator, preceptor, or other qualified staff member scrubs in, and gradually the learner is allowed to take over more of the work in the sterile field. One of the primary behavioral objectives is to gain knowledge and skill in sterile technique (Box 1-3), and performing the scrub role allows the repetition of working within the sterile field.

In addition to performing scrub functions, the learner should assist with circulating duties. The coordination of these two roles will become clear by learning standard

---

<table>
<tr><td>**Box 1-3**</td><td>**Behavioral Objectives for Perioperative Caregivers**</td></tr>
</table>

To identify the role and responsibility of each team member

To define current terminology associated with perioperative patient care

To compare and contrast knowledge of normal anatomy, physiology, and pathophysiology

To comprehend the interrelationships between physiologic, ethnocultural, and psychosocial factors that affect a patient's and his or her family's adaptation to the perioperative experience

To identify the procedures necessary to prepare each patient as an individual for the intended surgical procedure

To demonstrate the ability to select appropriate instrumentation, equipment, and supplies according to the individualized plan of care

To apply the principles of sterilization, disinfection, and aseptic and sterile techniques in the preparation and use of all materials used in the perioperative environment in order to prevent transmission of biologic contamination

To identify the potential environmental hazards to the patient and team

To understand the basic actions and uses of anesthetic agents, medications, fluid therapies, and electrolytes

To demonstrate knowledge and skill during the surgical procedure by anticipating the needs of the patient and the team

To understand the principles of wound management

To function as a team member by showing consideration for and cooperation with other perioperative caregivers

To communicate effectively with other patient care divisions within the facility

To develop the ability to perform safely and effectively during stressful situations

---

routines under supervision. Guidance and help from the clinical educator or experienced staff member helps the learner pull it all together. Surgeons and other staff members contribute to the learning process by supporting the efforts of the educator and the learner.

Personality traits in the learner, such as emotional stability, social skills, and psychologic characteristics, are continually assessed by the educator. An ill-tempered, moody, easily angered, and negative person can be very difficult to deal with as a future team member. The learner who does not possess assertive skills for dealing with stressful events cannot function effectively in a team environment. Subjective responses to all activities should remain on a professional level if the team is to function efficiently.

PERIOPERATIVE CLINICAL EDUCATOR

Experience in the perioperative clinical setting should be planned and supervised by an experienced perioperative educator. The term *educator* is used throughout this text to refer to the person responsible for planning, implementing, and evaluating the learner's experiences in the classroom and clinical perioperative setting. Other teaching personnel at the clinical site include preceptors and qualified registered nurses.

The learner takes an active role in the teaching/learning process. Behavioral objectives are determined by the educator and the learner; effective and organized educational experiences are then identified and coordinated with the perioperative team. The identified behavioral objectives should be attained through critical thinking exercises. Skill in questioning and encouragement in making discoveries allow the learner to use critical thinking as a learning tool. A structured curriculum uses written guidelines and relevant assignments for feedback to ensure that learning has occurred. Learner conferences should be held on a regular basis to discuss procedures and problems. Positive reinforcement helps the learner build confidence and competence. The educator should not punish a learner for making honest errors during supervised learning. Degradation and damage to self-esteem are barriers that do not facilitate learning. The learner should not be put in a position to perform any function for which he or she has not had adequate training or guided practice. The educator should maintain a list of procedures in which the learner has participated and for which his or her level of performance has been demonstrated.

Check-off sheets can be used to track experiential progress during the education process. Box 1-4 shows an example of a basic check-off sheet for the evaluation of skill in the scrub role. This sheet can be modified to apply to specialties as needed. The Association of Surgical Technologists (AST) and AORN, the Association of periOperative Registered Nurses, have developed skills checklists, and these are available through the organizations.

The educator should consider the impact on the learner who is seeing the perioperative environment for the first time. The operating room can appear cold, large, and overwhelming. A tour of the facility before beginning the program can help decrease the learner's anxiety.

Behavioral Objectives

Evaluation of the learner's progress is measured by how successfully the learner has met the behavioral objectives. Behavioral objectives should be identified and written in behavioral terms and based on standards of expected performance and accepted standards of patient care. Bloom's taxonomy provides a framework for structuring cognitive and affective learning. Therefore the concepts to be learned and the behavioral objectives to be met should form the foundation on which all perioperative caregivers build their practice. Each behavioral objective in Box 1-3 is measurable and can be evaluated by performance standards.

Box 1-4	Basic Example of a Check-Off Sheet for the Evaluation of Skills in the Scrub Role

Skill Performance Evaluation	Satisfactory	Needs Improvement	Comments
Wears OR attire properly:			
Dons personal protective gear			
Performs housekeeping duties:			
Before first procedure of day			
Between procedures			
After last procedure of day			
Sterile supplies:			
Plans and gathers supplies			
Checks integrity of package			
Checks sterility indicator			
Checks dates on perishables			
Places items on sterile surface:			
Opening wrapper(s)			
Heat sealed packages			
Bottle and vial dispensing			
Scrubs for setup and procedure:			
Hand scrubbing			
Gowns self correctly			
Gowns others			
Dons gloves:			
Closed method			
Open method			
Changes contaminated glove			
Gloves others			
Sterile setup:			
Drapes table and Mayo stand			
Positions items in the field			
Accountability:			
Labels solutions and drugs			
Practices safety			
Anticipates needs of surgeon:			
Coordinates with circulator			
Facilitates the first assistant			
Counts:			
Sponges			
Sharps			
Instruments			
Assembles instruments:			
Attaches knife blades on handles			
Loads or prepares suture			
Tests drills and devices			
Disassembles the table:			
Follows proper disposal of items			
Follows decontamination procedures			
Removes gown and gloves			

Elements of Effective Instruction

The organization of the material to be taught and the experiences to be assigned are further enhanced by the way the program is presented. The elements of effective instruction are summarized as follows:

1. Set clear and concise behavioral objectives that are measurable in performance terminology that describes knowledge, comprehension, application, analysis, understanding, and evaluation.
2. Establish a learning environment that is controlled by the educator.
3. Provide variation in presenting material. Videotapes and photographs can be alternated with lectures and hands-on practice. Handling instruments and supplies in a classroom is less intimidating than handling

them in the perioperative environment for the first time.

4. Encourage the exchange of questions and answers as an assessment tool. Learners often ask exactly what they need to know. The educator can determine areas of knowledge deficit.

5. Reinforce learning. After a skill has been taught, provide guided practice in the clinical laboratory before the task is actually performed in the perioperative environment. Provide positive support for desired behaviors. Self-assessment tools and performance evaluations provide feedback about the learner's progress.

6. Summarize the learner's accomplishments at regular intervals. Reviewing daily activities helps to reinforce the learning process by allowing the learner to associate the events of his or her experience with newly acquired knowledge.

The educator should work closely with the perioperative nurse manager. Classroom hours and clinical experience assignments are worked out together. The manager offers suggestions and coordination input for the benefit of the learner and staff members. The educator identifies areas of needed experience for the learner. An effort is made to confer and to coordinate any changes in the program with all personnel in the department. The educator and the manager collaborate with the assigned preceptors as needed. These strategies foster a friendly and cooperative relationship among learners, educators, management, and preceptor staff.

All perioperative staff members indirectly assist in teaching the learners within the guidelines of the structured learning experience. The learners gain knowledge by observing and working with members of the team. Everyone should be familiar with the level of the learners, the behavioral objectives, and the roles that staff members will be expected to assume with respect to teaching. Learners also should take the responsibility to update the staff about needed experience and their current level of achievement.

Hospitals or facilities offering the clinical perioperative setting for educational programs have policies and procedures that are adaptations of national standards. All personnel, including faculty members and learners, are expected to adhere to their content.

LEARNING RESOURCES

Books, journals, videos, slides, photographs, computers, and other audiovisual materials may supplement the lecture approach to perioperative education. Larger teaching institutions may have live closed-circuit television and interactive telecommunication systems that permit educators and learners to communicate from remote locations. Many audiovisual materials, such as videodiscs, audiotapes, and computer-assisted instruction, are self-contained units for self-study. A bibliography in a text such as this or at the conclusion of a journal article provides references to broaden the learner's

Box 1-5	Search Engines That Search Multiple Search Engines

www.metacrawler.com Returns search results from multiple search engines at one time

www.dogpile.com Searches multiple search engines on general topics and returns results

www.cen.uiuc.edu/exploring.html Internet Jumpstation that enables the user to search multiple search engines, including maps, addresses, and directories

database. Accessibility to current medical and scientific literature is without limit. Other sources include Web sites on the Internet and educational services that provide contact hours on-line.

The following are useful resources for acquiring and reinforcing knowledge:

1. *Library and literature file.* Books and current periodicals are available for the learner's reference in the medical library and learning centers at local colleges.

2. *Educational literature and videotapes* are available from surgical supply and instrument manufacturers. The literature that accompanies new equipment should be reviewed by all personnel who will be working with the item. In-services are usually provided by clinical staff associated with the industry. The purchasing agent is a good source for these types of references.

3. *Computer database information systems* are available in most facilities or through personal Internet access providers for researching topics of interest for self-study or for supplementing classroom presentations. Web browsers such as Netscape Navigator or Microsoft's Internet Explorer are easily downloaded for use in searching the World Wide Web (WWW). Search engines on the Internet (e.g., Infoseek, Yahoo, Lycos, Excite) are valuable tools for finding special interest groups and professional medical associations. Several helpful search engines are listed in Box 1-5. Most health-related organizations have a Web site full of information. AORN Online can be accessed via the Web site address **www.aorn.org.** AST has a Web site at **www.ast.org** that provides information about surgical technology. Terms associated with using the Internet are described in Box 1-6.

4. *Specialty on-line news groups* can be subscribed to through computerized on-line e-mail systems. Referred to as LISTSERV, these groups are communication tools for day-to-day discussions with others who have similar interests. They are available as daily e-mail entries or as a weekly digest. Perioperative nursing and nursing history LISTSERV lists are currently available for free subscription on the World Wide Web. Table 1-2 describes how to sign up for the perioperative LISTSERV.

Box 1-6	**Terms Associated with Computer and Internet Use**

address Series of letters and/or numbers that enables the user to locate a specific Web site or e-mail directory; also known as URLs (uniform resource locators).

bookmark An electronic marker selected by the user to record the address of a specific Web site for easy return.

browser Specialty software that enables the user to interact with or browse in Web sites. Examples include Internet Explorer and Netscape.

CuSeeMe Software program that enables visual and audio real-time communication via live digital camera connections through the computer.

download The transfer of information over the Internet between computers.

e-mail Communication between persons over the Internet through a service provider such as America Online.

file transfer protocol (FTP) Method of retrieving files between computers.

hypertext link Location on a Web site which, when clicked with the left mouse button, connects the user to another page in the site or to another Web site entirely.

hypertext markup language (HTML) Format for designing Web pages.

Internet relay chat (IRC) Real-time discussion over the Internet through a service provider.

Internet service provider (ISP) A company that provides a method of gaining access to the Internet for e-mail and entry to the World Wide Web. Examples include America Online (AOL) and Netcom.

LISTSERV Specialty communications through e-mail discussion group postings to a server. Messages between participants in a special interest group are sent back and forth in response to topic threads.

newsgroups Discussion groups that post messages on electronic bulletin boards; can be accessed through an Internet service provider.

search engine Service sites available on the Internet that enable a person to leaf through multiple pages on multiple Web sites to collect specific information on a select topic. Examples include Yahoo, AltaVista, Lycos, and Excite.

thread A specific topic line that is shared for several days through a newsgroup.

virus A harmful computer program that can enter a user's computer through a download or file transfer. Data can be destroyed or altered without the user being aware of the process. Care in accepting outside programs is recommended. Virus scanning software is commercially available to help protect computer systems. Updates are required on a periodic basis.

Web site A place on the World Wide Web that features a specific topic of interest. It may consist of several Web pages that can be accessed by clicking the left mouse button on a topic.

World Wide Web (WWW) Communication in text and graphic form that requires a computer, Internet service provider, and browser for access.

---

5. *Literary databases* are found on select Web sites and in most libraries. Examples of on-line literary databases include, but are not limited to, the following:
   a. *Cumulative Index to Nursing and Allied Health Literature (CINAHL)* is a widely used index for nursing and allied health. The database includes indexing by subject headings from virtually all English language nursing journals and allied health literature from January 1983, with bimonthly updates.
   b. *Medical Literature Analysis and Retrieval System On-Line (MEDLINE)* is a computer-based reference system available at most libraries in the United States and Canada. Many Web sites on the Internet offer free MEDLINE access. Biomedical journals, including nursing journals, are referenced. The file contains references dating from 1966 at the National Library of Medicine (**www.nih.gov**).
6. *Videotape library.* The Hospital Satellite Network (HSN) is a telecommunication service provided to hospitals in which subscribers can view videotape programs transmitted by satellite. Video Journal provides a new videotape program to subscribers every 2 months. These sources of audiovisual programs are available for purchase or rental.

TABLE 1-2	**How to Subscribe to Perioperative LISTSERV***

Area on the E-Mail Form	Type in This Information
Address line	listproc@u.washington.edu
Subject line	Leave subject line blank (AOL 3.0 users may need to type a period in this line; AOL 4.0 users should leave this line blank)
Message body	Subscribe Periop (type in your name) EXAMPLE: *Subscribe Periop Nancymarie Fortunato*

*Use e-mail to subscribe to the perioperative LISTSERV owned by Bob Baxter, RN, CNOR. After completion of the e-mail form, send it electronically like any other e-mail. Subscription confirmation should be received within 24 hours. Further questions can be answered by sending an e-mail to **bobaxter@sprynet.com**.

The array of health-related educational materials is endless. The Internet, which is accessible 24 hours a day, has opened many channels of information throughout the world. Many Web sites can be accessed in a bilingual mode, including Spanish, German, French, and Japanese. Some Web sites offer full-text articles that can be downloaded to a diskette or printed on a printer. The advancement of computer technology has made computer equipment small enough to fit in a briefcase and economical enough for the average household to own one computer and possibly two. When researching scientific data on the Internet, it is advisable to review more than one Web site to support the accuracy of the information. Caution is advised regarding providing personal information such as credit card numbers over the Internet; security may be an issue.

APPLICATION OF THEORY TO PRACTICE

Learning is a process of discovery and mastery of skills. Performance-based learning to function competently in an area such as the perioperative environment should take place on three levels: cognitive, psychomotor, and affective. The learner should understand the scientific principles (cognitive learning) underlying the technical skills (psychomotor learning) and should appreciate the necessity of adhering to these principles (affective learning). In simpler terms, the learner should know why to do what (cognitive), how (psychomotor), when, where, and by whom (affective). The learner should always have a rationale for each action. Learners and practicing perioperative caregivers should always know exactly why they are doing what they are doing—not just blindly perform tasks. This approach enables an intelligent modification of the plan of care in the event of an emergency or other untoward situation. In actual practice this knowledge may be critical for patient safety and the attainment of favorable outcomes.

Practice will give the learner an opportunity to apply his or her knowledge of the basic sciences. Theory becomes meaningful and valuable only when put to practical use. Some knowledge is gained through observation, but skills are learned through actual hands-on experience in applying the theory learned in the classroom or self-study laboratory.

In the perioperative environment, the learner observes living anatomy; its alteration by congenital deformities, disease, or injury; and its restoration or reconstruction. Perioperative experience enables the learner to be a more understanding, observant, and efficient person. In close teamwork with surgeons and anesthesia providers, the nurse and the surgical technologist participate in vital resuscitative measures and learn to care for anesthetized, unconscious, and/or critically ill patients. Learning to function in life-threatening situations is critical to the patient's welfare. In addition, the learner discovers that emergencies such as cardiac arrest are more easily prevented than treated. By learning how theory applies to clinical practice, he or she gains valuable experience that is applicable to any nursing

situation. The learner should strive to attain the following objectives:

1. Understand what surgical intervention means to a patient.
2. Recognize the importance of optimal physical and psychologic preoperative patient preparation.
3. Validate the need for constant patient observation intraoperatively.
4. Understand the cause of postoperative pain and/or complications.
5. Differentiate between seemingly innocuous occurrences and situations that, if left unrecognized and allowed to progress, lead to injury of the patient or a team member or damage to departmental equipment.
6. Cope with all situations in a calm, efficient manner and think clearly and act quickly in an emergency.
7. Attend to every detail, observe keenly, and anticipate the needs of the patient and team members.
8. Understand the importance of aseptic and sterile techniques and comprehensively and conscientiously apply knowledge to practice.

Above all, perioperative experience teaches that no surgical procedure is a minor event to the surgical patient! The only predictable element in the perioperative environment is the potential for an unpredictable occurrence. For practical use, hospitals may classify surgical procedures as major or minor, but in reality no such distinction exists. Every procedure has a deep personal meaning for each patient and his or her family, and the possibility of an unfavorable outcome can never be completely excluded. All perioperative procedures carry an element of inherent risk. A relatively safe procedure can rapidly become catastrophic, even fatal, if the patient:

- Is unknowingly allergic to a medication or anesthetic drug
- Develops uncontrollable bleeding
- Experiences cardiac arrest on the operating bed
- Goes into irreversible shock
- Succumbs to overwhelming postoperative infection

Although every precaution is taken to foresee and prevent adverse reactions, such reactions do occur on occasion. No matter how simple the procedure, an experienced, conscientious team member is always acutely aware of potential problems and gives undivided attention to the patient and procedure at all times.

During the learning experience, the learner will participate in or observe the preparation of supplies and equipment and learn their intended use. With practical experience, the learner will gain an appreciation for the precision of surgical instrumentation and equipment. Also, in helping to carry out a daily schedule of surgical procedures, the learner will become aware of the interdependence of the various departments within the facility and how they work together for the well-being of the patient. One of the most valuable learning experiences in the perioperative environment is the opportunity to see and become a part of real teamwork in action.

EXPECTED BEHAVIORS OF PERIOPERATIVE CAREGIVERS

Regardless of their respective roles, all perioperative caregivers are expected to be competent and humane. A patient's sense of security is grounded in how he or she perceives the behavior of the team as a whole. This leaves a lasting impression that patients associate with their experiences in the perioperative environment. The behavior of the team reveals self-confidence (or the lack of it), interest (or indifference), proficiency (or ineptness) and authority (or indecision). In addition to possessing technical knowledge and skill, personnel should display appropriate personal attributes and communication skills that inspire confidence and trust in patients and other team members.

Personal Attributes

Personal attributes are manifest in the attitudes displayed by an individual while performing his or her duties. These inherent characteristics contribute to interrelatedness of the team and the final outcome for the patient. Although these concepts are intrinsic to the individual and are certainly open to interpretation, the main premise remains focused on providing safe and efficient patient care through a team effort. Desirable personal attributes include, but are not limited to, the following:

- *Empathy.* Feeling persons can put themselves in another person's place and understand what that person is experiencing. As patient advocates, they convey compassion and a sense of personal worth. They do not let emotions indiscriminately obscure or override professional judgment or interfere with care.
- *Conscientiousness.* Persons with this quality do not compromise or sacrifice principles of self-accountability. A surgical conscience implies an awareness of the importance of strict application of knowledge and skill to ensure quality in practice. Team members should approach every procedure in the same way they would want to have it approached if it were being performed on themselves or their family members.
- *Efficiency and organization.* Persons who develop organized work habits are assured that the patients are properly prepared and the perioperative environment is ready with the required equipment in working order. They save time and energy by anticipating the needs of patients and team members. They are prepared for the unexpected. Efficiency provides reassurance and comfort to patients, surgeons, and the entire perioperative team.
- *Flexibility and adaptability.* Team members react quickly to changing circumstances in a calm and efficient manner and respond appropriately by altering the routine as necessary. Discriminating judgment prepares adaptable people to cope with all situations with professional decorum.

- *Sensitivity and perception.* Perceptive persons exhibit genuine interest and kindness in caring for patients and are sensitive to the special needs of the people in their environment. Perioperative team members should develop a sense of caring for each other as people and should try to understand the subjective aspects of working together in an often tense, fast-paced environment. Patience and kindness should be the prevailing attitudes of team members.
- *Understanding, reassuring, and supportive nature.* In a kind and emotionally controlled way, team members should allow others to express their feelings. This approach conveys to the patient the team's ability to relieve physical and emotional discomfort. Holding the patient's hand during the induction of anesthesia is one way of demonstrating support. A nonjudgmental stance while assisting a new team member to develop a new skill is very reassuring and leads to successful attainment of competency. Overt anger and hostility are not acceptable at any time in the perioperative environment.
- *Listening, observation, and communication skills.* People who listen and are attentive and observant will act effectively. Aware personnel will not underestimate the importance of communication in their relations with patients and colleagues.
- *Consideration.* Individuals who are considerate respect other people's rights and belief systems and do not automatically reject views different from their own. They convey to patients and colleagues an interest in them as unique persons and act accordingly. All personnel should be aware of ethnocultural differences and demonstrate respect for the personal value systems of others.
- *Informative and sincere approach.* Perioperative personnel should answer questions and share pertinent information for the mutual benefit of patients, families or significant others, and colleagues. Sharing information and forewarning can avoid problems. Caregivers should explain procedures and provide the rationale for these procedures before performing them. Reinforcement of the physician's explanations and orders supports the team effort.
- *Objectivity.* Objective individuals who are objective assemble factual data before making a judgment, and they view situations from all sides before taking action. Objectivity requires experience and self-discipline. This attribute does not exclude concern but neither is it based on personal, subjective feelings. Team members should remain sensitive to problems without imposing their own values or beliefs on others.
- *Impartial, nonjudgmental, open-minded approach.* Individuals who take this approach set aside value judgments when making decisions and do not permit their own values and attitudes to distort observations. They accept others as they are without attaching conditions to acceptance.
- *Versatility.* Persons who are versatile have a comprehensive knowledge of instrumentation and equipment. They

are familiar with numerous surgical procedures and the care required for many diverse patients. They approach each procedure as unique and individualized while also maintaining acceptable performance standards.

- *Analytical nature.* Persons who are analytical are competent in analyzing and correlating significant data about the procedure, the patient, and the needs of the team. They know the *why* as well as the *how* of surgical intervention. These persons are able to anticipate the unexpected and to prevent situations from developing into crises.
- *Creativity.* Creative individuals are innovative in devising effective methods to meet the individual needs of patients and colleagues by using available resources.
- *Humanistic approach.* Perioperative team members act in a humane way toward others. They consider the patient as a person, not as a surgical procedure. The perioperative team should not make the patient or colleagues the center of jokes and hurtful comments.
- *Sense of humor.* People with a sense of humor can maintain a balance for their own mental health through their perception of the ironies in life situations. Laughter can ease tension, but not at someone's expense or at an inappropriate time.
- *Manual and intellectual dexterity.* People with this quality have quick hands, sharp minds, and keen eyes.
- *Endurance.* Personnel with endurance are able to maximize their physical and emotional capacities and stamina. Perioperative personnel interact in a critical setting under stress, often for prolonged periods. Continual demands are made on them for keen observation, rapid judgment, and fast action. All personnel must be prepared for disaster and work rapidly, often under pressure, without sacrificing competency. Each team member is responsible for maintaining good health habits that enhance personal performance.
- *Intellectual eagerness and curiosity.* Perioperative team members have a responsibility to remain current in their knowledge. Documented proof of continuing education and demonstrated competence in performing functions are requirements of regulatory agencies.
- *Ethical manner.* Persons with this quality use ethical principles, moral values, and professional codes as the basis for making decisions and solving problems. Although personal values do influence behavior, they should not violate the legal or ethical rights of patients or the hospital. Personnel should always be honest and truthful. They should respect the equality of human rights and the dignity of others as human beings.

Communication Skills

Communication is the basis for the continuum of patient care and for teamwork among the staff. Relationships are established through communication. Therefore it is important for the perioperative caregiver to know and understand communication skills.

Communication is a process by which meanings are exchanged between individuals. It is necessary for successful interpersonal relations and serves to clarify actions. The process is cyclical, with each communicator influencing and being influenced by the other. Communication is both proactive and reactive, and both causative and purposive. In therapeutic communication the goals are patient-directed and patient-centered. Communication is effective only when the patient and caregivers understand one another. A capacity for sincerity and empathy is the most effective constituent of communication.

Principles of the Communication Process

Some principles of the communication process are as follows:

1. Communication incorporates the following:
   a. Sender (speaker, encoder)
   b. Message sent via a transmission channel (verbal, nonverbal)
   c. Receiver (listener, decoder)
2. The goals of communication are to inform, obtain information, release tension, and explore problems.
3. The following are channels of communication:
   a. Verbal words convey content of message through speaking and listening or writing and reading. For example, verbal communication through language is directed toward patient care by conferring about patient problems, teaching, and providing an interdisciplinary liaison on behalf of the patient.
   b. Nonverbal body language—including eye contact, facial expression, tone of voice, inflection of voice, gestures, posture, and body movements—convey feelings. Pictures, diagrams, and other visuals are other forms of nonverbal communication. Nonverbal communication provides clues to feelings and attitudes. Individuals often communicate through nonverbal channels without realizing it. Actions often speak louder than words. For example, touch is an effective means of communicating empathy when a patient is feeling sad, lonely, or isolated.
4. The sender puts thoughts into words or some other channel of communication and then transmits the idea in the form of a message to a receiver, who attempts to understand the thought. The mind decodes messages on the basis of previous experiences, prejudices, culture, moods, values, attitudes, feelings, and current motives.
5. Communication is facilitated by active listening. Listening involves physiologic, cognitive, and psychologic processes. Physiologically, sounds are heard. Cognitive ability interprets words and influences an individual's response to them. The psychologic state of mind and the relationship between sender and receiver affect communication interactions.
6. The setting for communication and the attitudes of those involved influence the degree of effectiveness.

An individual's emotional state affects listening. An anxious patient or learner may not hear, may misunderstand, or may draw erroneous conclusions.

7. Communication should be source-centered rather than message-centered. Unqualified statements are avoided.
8. The prerequisites of communication are knowing what you are going to say and to say what you mean. The speaker should verify or paraphrase until convinced that the receiver has the message.
9. A message can have variations of meanings:
   a. What the speaker means to say vs. what the speaker actually says
   b. What the receiver hears vs. what the receiver thinks he or she hears
   c. What the speaker says vs. what the receiver thinks the speaker said
10. For accurate interpretation of communication the sender should know the receiver's level of or capacity for understanding and use the appropriate language or channel.
11. There can be barriers to communication:
   a. Verbal: changing the subject, having a judgmental attitude (stating one's own opinion about a patient or situation), offering false or inappropriate reassurance, jumping to conclusions or taking things for granted, using medical facts or nursing knowledge inappropriately
   b. Nonverbal: showing a lack of trust or feeling, disinterest, rejection

Criteria for Determining the Success of Communication

1. *Feedback.* Let the sender know how you perceived the message so he or she knows if it was understood as intended. A breakdown in communication occurs when the idea of the receiver does not match the idea of the sender. Two people should have mutual understanding about the meaning of a message. Language should convey meaning.
2. *Appropriateness of reply.* Do not evaluate the receiver's comprehension solely on the basis of language. Nonverbal behavior should also be observed.
3. *Efficiency.* Is the sender overloading the listener? Is the listener's intrapersonal communication (i.e., silently talking to self or daydreaming) interfering with concentration on the message?
4. *Specific results.* Behavioral changes indicate that the goal is reached. Through communication the caregiver can influence behavior by encouraging the patient to express feelings or by redirecting the patient's actions toward more beneficial behavior.

Teamwork

A team is a group of two or more persons who recognize common goals and coordinate their efforts to achieve them.

Broadly defined, the health care team includes all personnel relating to the patient, those in direct patient contact, and those in other departments whose services are essential and contribute indirectly to patient care. Interdependence characterizes a team—without the other members, the goals cannot be met.

The team approach to patient care should be a coordinated effort that is performed with the cooperation of all caregivers. Team members should communicate and should have a shared division of duties to perform specified tasks as a unified body. The failure of any one member to perform his or her role can seriously impact the success of the entire team. Performing as a team requires that each member exert an effort to attain the common goals in a competent and safe manner. The actions of each team member are important. No one individual can accomplish the goal without the cooperation of the rest of the team.

Pride in one's work and in the team as a whole leads to personal satisfaction. High morale is facilitated by adequate staff orientation, staff participation in departmental decision making and problem solving, the receipt of deserved praise, the opportunity for continuing education, and motivation to reach and practice at the highest potential.

The common goal of the perioperative team is the effective delivery of care in a safe, efficient, and timely manner. To function efficiently, effective communication between team members is critical. Problems such as a break in aseptic or sterile technique must be identified and corrective actions taken. To fulfill expectations, team members must be aware of each other's needs for information. Efforts of other support services, such as radiology and pathology departments, must be coordinated with the needs of the surgeon.

Mutual respect is the foundation of teamwork. It is also a right. Respect is shown through collaboration, cooperation, and truthful communication. Verbal abuse, disruptive behavior, and harassment are out of place in the professional environment. Behavior that inhibits the performance of team members or threatens patient care should be factually documented and reported to superiors in the chain of command.

Teamwork requires the commitment and effort of team members to increase productivity, ensure quality performance, and participate in problem solving by communicating and cooperating with one another. A team approach is necessary for patient-centered care. Surgeons, assistants, anesthesia providers, patient care staff, and supporting services should coordinate their efforts. Each discipline contributes to successful outcomes of surgical intervention by working together as team. Several factors contribute to these successful outcomes:

1. Interdepartmental communication is important for mutual cooperation, consideration, and efficient collaboration.
   a. Patient care divisions and physicians share pertinent information concerning patients. Collected data are documented, thereby protecting the patient, the patient care personnel, and the facility.

b. Personnel work together in a congenial atmosphere with respect and appreciation for each other's unique skills and contributions. Team members benefit from the expertise of each other. Teamwork is at its finest in the perioperative environment.

c. Personnel are considerate of each other and of the patient.

(1) The surgeon should inform the team of any anticipated potential deviation from his or her regular routine for the scheduled procedure. An advance notice of changes can help avoid delays in obtaining needed equipment.

(2) The perioperative team promotes a quiet atmosphere to ensure the surgeon's uninterrupted concentration. Interruptions during the procedure can cause the team to lose concentration and jeopardize the safety of the patient or team members.

(3) The anesthesia provider and circulator assist each other with certain procedures such as medication administration and intubation.

2. Adequate preparation and familiarity with the surgeon's preferences and the surgical procedure to be performed are fundamental to teamwork. If the perioperative staff are unfamiliar with the routine and equipment, the patient or a team member may be at risk for injury. An adequately experienced and skilled team is essential for the effective performance of a safe, efficient procedure.

3. The patient has an unconditional right to the team's complete concentration and attention at all times. He or she is a unique individual who is completely dependent on the perioperative caregivers to work together as a team.

Although the ideologic differences of personnel may at times be a source of conflict, the care of the patient should be a priority over personality differences. Complex procedures, busy surgery schedules, or shortages of personnel should not interfere with the delivery of efficient, individualized patient care.

Clinical Competence

On the basis of experience and performance, patient care personnel can be categorized as novice, competent, proficient, or expert. The novice lacks experience but is expected to perform to the best of his or her ability with assistance. Most employers provide a formal orientation program for new patient care personnel. During this orientation period, the necessary knowledge, skills, and abilities should be developed to perform at a level of basic competency. As experience is gained, proficiency expands from a minimal competency to an advanced level of expertise. Competent practice requires critical thinking skills and decision-making ability. Statements of clinical competency are established by professional organizations such as AORN and AST. These guidelines are published by each professional organization and made available to practitioners of all disciplines.

REALITIES OF CLINICAL PRACTICE

When a formal educational experience is completed, a learner is eager to apply his or her skills and knowledge in an employment setting. A transition period from dependent learner to independent practitioner occurs. The realities of the work environment and the emotional and ethical dilemmas of some situations are experienced as basic competencies are developed. It can take 6 months to 1 year to feel confident as a functioning perioperative team member. Many facilities require personnel to take calls for emergencies after business hours.

Reality Shock

Each individual should learn the rules and accepted behaviors and assume responsibilities for personal behavior. Reality is a sense of actuality, a feeling that this is what the real world is all about. Reality shock sets in as the transition takes place from being a beginning learner to becoming an employed graduate professional nurse or surgical technologist. The familiar educator and peer learners are no longer present to give counsel, advice, and moral support. As caregivers attempt to adapt to new demands, they need to remember the following:

1. Learning does not end with basic education. It is an ongoing process throughout the caregiver's career.

2. All caregivers were once novices (although some may have forgotten those novice days). They have experienced the feelings and frustrations of being the newest staff member. The experienced caregiver should try to remember these feelings and offer encouragement to new personnel.

3. Patience is an asset while developing work habits and establishing working relationships. Expectations of self and of others should be realistic. Feelings of excitement and anticipation and the fear of failure or making mistakes are normal but should be expressed appropriately.

4. Applying the principles and techniques already learned will enable the caregiver to make sound judgments and appropriate decisions in the perioperative environment.

5. It is important to ask questions and acknowledge not knowing how to do something. Seeking help promotes professional growth.

Everyone wants and needs to become an accepted member of both social and work groups. The entire perioperative team, including the surgeon and anesthesia provider, is both a social group and a work group. Ambivalent feelings may arise on entering these groups. The pleasures of functioning as a team member may be offset by uncertainty about the ability to perform well. Initial goals will be task- and skill-oriented as learning focuses on policies, procedures, and routines. Eventually insecurity will be replaced with self-confidence. The display of confidence will increase trust, respect, and recognition from others as well as the personal satisfaction of accomplishment.

Dynamics of the Psychologic Climate

Learning to adapt to the variety of tasks and ever-changing demands in the perioperative environment is difficult. Some anxiety is to be expected, especially in situations in which feelings of insecurity are generated or a sense of intimidation pervades the environment. At times the demands of the job may seem to outweigh the personal resources of the caregiver. Confidence develops as skills are learned.

An understanding of expected performance is perhaps the most important element in the transition from basic learner to novice practitioner. The beginner should look for a support system, such as staff members who are willing to help bridge the gap. He or she should look for role models, those staff members who are emulated and respected for their clinical competence. The beginner should stick with the winners, those staff members who are reaping personal rewards and self-satisfaction from their work effort. The losers—staff members who have negative attitudes, complain, and do not make an effort to solve problems but instead create them—should be avoided.

Eustress vs. Distress

Physical and emotional stresses are part of daily life. Stress is the nonspecific reaction of the body, physiologically and/or psychologically, to any demand. The demand may be pleasant or unpleasant, conscious or unconscious. The intensity of the stressor will dictate adaptation. An individual's perception of a situation will influence the reaction to it.

Stress is not only an essential part of life but is also a useful stimulant. Positive stress, referred to as eustress, motivates an individual to be productive and efficient. It forces adaptation to the ever-present changes in the perioperative environment. The response should be quick (i.e., when a trauma victim arrives or a patient has a cardiac arrest). To expect the unexpected is part of perioperative patient care. Eustress fosters a sense of achievement, satisfaction, and self-confidence.

Stress that becomes overwhelming and uncomfortable is referred to as distress. In the perioperative environment, the behavior of others may be perceived as cause for distress. Policies, or a lack of them, can also be a source of distress if they are in conflict with the caregiver's expectations. Through adaptive mechanisms the caregiver can cope with the tensions, conflicts, and demands of the perioperative environment in either a collaborative or a nonproductive manner. Even though perceived as distress, some conflict is necessary to stimulate a change in work methods and solve organizational problems.

Patient care personnel may be distressed by the conduct of other team members. For example, it is uncomfortable to be harshly criticized by a surgeon. However, much that is said is not personally directed. Often the surgeon is reacting to his or her distress regarding unanticipated circumstances presented by the patient during the surgical procedure. The reactions of personnel will be influenced by their attitudes, mood, cultural and religious background, values and ethics, experiences, and concerns of the moment. Outbursts of anger are inappropriate at the operating bed at any time. However, constant frustration and inner conflict create the distresses that can lead to job dissatisfaction.

Stress Reduction

Assertive behavior is a useful tool for conflict resolution. Shared professional communication can keep the tension in the environment at a minimum. The caregiver should keep his or her composure at all times and maintain a professional and assertive (not aggressive) attitude. Personal conflicts between team members should be dealt with privately.

Humor can be an effective method of reducing anxiety. It should be used appropriately to defuse tension. Laughing at oneself helps to preserve self-esteem while learning from the experience.

At the end of the work shift, the caregiver should evaluate the events of the day, the emotions evoked, and how they were handled. What was done effectively? What coping skills may be needed to improve or enhance positive attitudes in the work environment and in interpersonal relations? Teamwork is essential in the perioperative environment, with every team member obligated to make a positive contribution.

Stress is a reality that need not create a sense of self-defeat. Regardless of the source of stress, the body responds, and the physiologic and psychologic effects can be subtle or intense. The determination of whether a stressor is good or bad depends on an individual's perception of the circumstances. Any event that creates a feeling of impending danger also creates the perception of loss of control. A major factor in stress management is maintaining control, which can be accomplished by learning to tune in to the balance between the body and the mind. The caregiver can learn to be prepared for life's difficulties by understanding how the perception of stress can affect decision making, self-expression, and subsistence in the world.

Listening to the Body

The caregiver should develop a sense for how the body signals exhaustion, hunger, illness, and/or physical pain. The body is a sensory barometer of the environmental effects on the caregiver, and ignoring physical signals decreases the ability of the body to manage stress. Going without sleep or skipping meals creates physical stress that can be avoided. Regular sleep and rest, exercise, adequate dietary practices, and routine health checkups provide a sound basis for care of the body.

Maintaining the Mind

Mental relaxation can help the caregiver to manage stress. Using meditation and mental imagery on a regular basis provides a break from stressful routines and allows the mind to fortify itself against the negative perceptions of a situation. Creating time to clear confusing thoughts and align productive thinking enables the body and the mind to support an emotional balance and a sense of well-being. This positive interaction can become an influence in a stressful situation and serve as an example to co-workers.

Bibliography

Beitz JM: Developing behavioral objectives for perioperative staff development, *AORN J* 64(1):87-95, 1996.

Beitz JM, Houck PM: Advanced perioperative nursing elective for baccalaureate students, *AORN J* 66(1):119-130, 1997.

Beyea SC, Nicoll LH: Accessing health care literature: what every perioperative nurse needs to know, *AORN J* 67(3):694-698, 1998.

Boegli E: Preceptorship: a gift that keeps on giving, *Surg Technol* 26(2):12-14, 1994.

Bower JO: Using patient simulators to train surgical team members, *AORN J* 65(4):805-808, 1997.

Brazen L, Roth RA: Using learning style preferences for perioperative clinical education, *AORN J* 61(1):189-195, 1995.

Bridges A, Thede LQ: Electronic education: nursing education resources on the world wide web, *Nurs Educ* 21(5):11-15, 1996.

Conger MM, Mezza I: Fostering critical thinking in nursing students in the clinical setting, *Nurs Educ* 21(3):11-15, 1996.

Donley DL: Promoting active learning in the classroom: an educator's challenge, *Surg Technol* 26(8):15, 24, 1994.

Grossman D, Taylor R: Cultural diversity on the unit, *Am J Nurs* 95(2):64-67, 1995.

Lessner MW et al: Orienting nursing students to cost-effective clinical practice, *Nurs Health Care* 15(9):458-462, 1994.

Marousky RT: Nurse's guide to the Internet: professional and personal benefits, *AORN J* 64(3):463-466, 468-469, 1996.

Masson L, Fain JA: Competency validation for cross-training in surgical services, *AORN J* 66(4):651-659, 1997.

Middlemiss MA, Van Neste-Kenny J: Curriculum revolution: reflective minds and empowering relationships, *Nurs Health Care* 15(7):350-353, 1994.

Modrcin MA et al: Perioperative nurses' guide to the library, *AORN J* 65(3):605-613, 1997.

National Committee on Education: *Preceptor guide for perioperative nursing practice,* Denver, 1993, Association of Operating Room Nurses.

Piatkowski CA: A surgical services learning needs assessment, *AORN J* 62(2):251-254, 1995.

Rae A, White K: Nurse's guide to the Internet: AORN on-line, *AORN J* 64(2):286-289,1996.

Ryer JC: *HealthNet,* New York, 1997, John Wiley & Sons.

Shuman J: Six ways to take this job and love it! *Am J Nurs* 94(6):59-63, 1994.

Sparks SM: The educational technology network, *Nurs Health Care* 15(3):134-141, 1994.

Strauss J: An OR nurse internship program that focuses on retention, *AORN J* 66(3):455-463, 1997.

Yoder ME: Preferred learning style and educational technology, *Nurs Health Care* 15(3):128-132, 1994.

Chapter 2

Foundations of Perioperative Patient Care

 Chapter Objectives

After studying this chapter, the learner will be able to:

- Identify the components of the nursing process.
- List two professional sources of patient care standards
- Describe how functional health patterns form the foundation of assessment.
- Discuss how human response patterns form the foundation of nursing diagnoses.

This chapter establishes the basis for perioperative patient care. The opening section gives a glimpse of historic patient care and progresses to modern perioperative practice. Select terms associated with professional patient care are defined in Box 2-1.

HISTORICAL BACKGROUND

Throughout history, practitioners of the healing arts have been both revered and feared. They have been depicted as magicians, holy men, and deities. As the population grew, so did the fascination with herbs and remedies. When a home-made concoction worked, it was considered divine intervention or magic; if it failed, it was considered evil. Without knowledge of the germ theory, mass epidemics that were uncured by local healers were considered suspect for demonic influence. Evil was thought to be the cause of all illness. During the Spanish Inquisition in the sixteenth century, a midwife who experienced complications with a complex childbirth was at risk for being accused of witchcraft or infant

sacrifice. More female healers than male healers were accused and executed during this dark era of patient care.

Nonphysician patient care is credited to the Greek physician Hippocrates (460-377 BC), the father of medicine. He instituted training for men who would administer the treatments and therapies prescribed by the physicians of the time. Although most care was rendered by family members, complex procedures were performed by these trained individuals. They were considered the first home caregivers. Aristotle (384-322 BC) was the son of a physician. He wrote *The Golden Cabinet of Secrets,* a collection of herbal remedies that included antispasmodics, astringents, sedatives, laxatives, and stimulants. This was a commonly used guide for medical care and was disseminated over the Middle East trade routes. Famous people such as Alexander the Great (356-323 BC), who was Aristotle's student, and Cleopatra (69-31 BC) used this herbal guide.

Traveling health care was started in the ninth and tenth centuries by military and religious groups, which primarily consisted of men. In 1050, 35 years before the first Crusade

(1085 AD), a hospital for the ill was dedicated in Jerusalem by the Knight Hospitallers of Saint John. Originally intended to be a religious order, the knights learned military skills to protect civilians on pilgrimages to the Holy Land.

Early nineteenth-century patient care gave rise to the clear separation of medicine and nursing. The profession of nursing was validated by Florence Nightingale (1820-1910), the first nursing theorist. Her concepts included the identification of the nurse as a skilled worker under the physician, who was the architect of medical treatment. She demonstrated that the environment and cleanliness ultimately affected the patient. Perioperative patient care is grounded in the control of the environment and the cleanliness of the devices therein. Box 2-2 lists several Internet addresses for further information on the history of patient care.

Box 2-1   Terms Associated with Professional Patient Care

accreditation   A method of professional evaluation and recognition of an institution for meeting educational, practice, and national standard parameters.

certification   A method of professional evaluation and recognition of an individual for meeting educational, practice, and national standard parameters.

credentials   Validation of professional recognition, such as licensure or certification.

licensure   Approval for practice granted by a governmental agency for a predetermined period of time, after which the approval process is repeated.

nursing diagnosis   Identification of patient problem, need, or health consideration, which may be actual or at risk; based on human response patterns according to NANDA.

nursing process   Organizational framework for planning patient care; this involves assessment, nursing diagnosis, outcome identification, planning, implementation, and evaluation of the plan.

outcome   The effect of an intervention.

profession   Vocation in a specialty requiring extensive education in liberal and scientific arts.

Box 2-2   Internet Sources of Patient Care History

web.bu.edu/SPECCOL/nursing.htm   History of Nursing Archives—Boston University

www.geocities.com/Athens/Forum/6011/   Men in American Nursing History

www.med.virginia.edu/nursing/centers/history.html   Center for Nursing Historical Inquiry—University of Virginia

www4.umdnj.edu/camlbweb/blacknurses.html   Black Nurses in History

www.aahn.org   American Association for the History of Nursing

In contemporary times, the patient care experience encompasses a broad scope of scientific yet humanistic activities. In perioperative patient care, the surgical procedure is the focal point. It is important that patients come to the perioperative environment optimally prepared—both physically and psychologically.

Both perioperative nurses and surgical technologists work toward a common objective—providing the safest possible care so that patients achieve favorable surgical outcomes. The professional perioperative nurse is responsible for the development of the patient-oriented plan of care, which is the creative application of the nursing process, scientific principles, judgment, skills, and interpersonal competencies.

PROFESSIONAL NURSING

The members of a profession must act responsibly in accord with their commitment to public trust and service. Simply stated, the word *profession* implies a combination and coordination of knowledge, skills, and ideals that are communicated through a highly specialized educational discipline. In this way, education sets the standards for practice. The following are characteristics of a profession:

- It defines its own purposes and code of ethics.
- It sets its own standards and conducts its own affairs and self-regulation; it has autonomy.
- Through research, it identifies and develops its own body of knowledge unique to its role.
- It requires critical thinking skills in clinical judgment, as well as problem-solving and decision-making skills in the application of knowledge.
- It engages in self-evaluation and peer review to control and alter its practices and accountabilities.

Professional nursing is dedicated to the promotion of optimal health for all human beings in their various environments. Nursing is both a humanistic art and an applied science. The art of professional nursing practice involves nursing diagnoses and the treatment of human responses to health and illness. The science behind the paradigm of nursing is based on theories about the nature of humankind, health, and disease. Nursing education prepares nurses to translate the art and science of nursing into relevant knowledge and skill. Professional nursing education is built on a solid base of general education in liberal arts, humanities, and natural and behavioral sciences.

Professional Perioperative Nursing

A wise physician once said that the physician's role is to cure sometimes, to relieve often, and to comfort always. The same can be said for the perioperative nurse, who embodies all that the word *nurse* has traditionally meant to a patient—provider of safety and comfort, supporter, and confidante. The patient's safety and welfare are entrusted to the operating room (OR) nurse from the moment of arrival in the perioperative environment until departure and the transfer of responsibility for care to another professional health care team member.

The perioperative nurse is a licensed registered nurse who is legally accountable for the delivery of care to patients in the perioperative environment, including interventions that assist the patient in a conscious or unconscious state. The primary emphasis of the nurse's responsibility is to the patient. The perioperative nurse identifies the physiologic, psychologic, and sociologic needs of the patient, develops and implements an individualized plan of care that coordinates interventions, and evaluates outcomes of the patient's perioperative experience. The nurse is accountable and responsible for patient care, whether accomplished personally or by another perioperative team member.

Patient-Nurse Relationship

To practice in a technologically complex environment, perioperative nurses must be flexible, and their skills must be diverse. Their roles incorporate both the technical and the behavioral components of professional nursing. Competent fulfillment of the perioperative nursing role is based on the knowledge and application of the principles of biologic, physiologic, behavioral, and social sciences. Perioperative nurses develop nursing diagnoses based on patients' problems, needs, and health status. This is essential information in the identification of expected outcomes and in the formulation of a perioperative plan of care.

The perioperative nurse shares a special humanized experience with the patient at a time of great stress and need in his or her life. This relationship encompasses feelings, attitudes, and behaviors, with mutual trust and understanding as vital components. Effective interaction encompasses concern for the unique personhood of both the patient and the nurse. The length of time spent with the patient is not as important as the quality of the interaction. The level of the interaction may directly affect the patient's perception of the delivery of care in the perioperative environment.

To achieve and maintain a viable cooperative relationship, the patient should be able to sense that the nurse unconditionally cares about his or her well-being. The nurse should remain aware that personal interaction is often predicated on culture, attitudes, beliefs, and past experiences. Knowledge of the impact of care on the patient's outcome enhances the attainment of the desired result.

Perioperative nursing care is a specialized combination of individualized and standardized care. Individualized care, the art of nursing, demonstrates genuine concern for the patient as a person and is not purely technical. Standardized care, the science of nursing, is derived from a body of scientific knowledge that has been developed through research and clinical practice. The perioperative nurse develops the plan of care through the use of the nursing process.

NURSING PROCESS

Perioperative patient care requires developing a plan of care and identifying expected outcomes through the nursing process (Box 2-3). The nursing process is a systematic approach to nursing practice using problem-solving techniques. This six-part process provides a systematic foundation for assessing the patient, establishing a nursing diagnosis,

---

Box 2-3 The Nursing Process

Assessment
Identify the actual or potential problems, needs, and health status considerations through appraisal of the physiologic, psychosocial, objective, subjective, cultural, and ethnic data related to the patient as an individual. Assessment is based on functional health patterns.
Document assessment data.

Nursing Diagnosis
Formulate prioritized actual or potential nursing diagnoses unique to the patient. Human response patterns guide the development of nursing diagnoses.

Identification of Outcomes
Develop measurable and attainable expected outcomes and mutual goals in collaboration with the patient, significant others, and other health care providers.
Identify realistic time frames in which fulfillment may be accomplished.

Planning
Establish and prioritize a working set of interventions for the actual problems, needs, and health status considerations.

Establish a contingency plan for the potential problems, needs, and health status considerations that may become actual during the course of the perioperative experience.
Include the patient's input for the construction of the individualized plan.
Document the plan of care in a retrievable manner.

Implementation
Share the plan with the perioperative team for continuity of care.
Activate the interventions in a systematic order of priority.
Discontinue any intervention that is ineffective.
Document the implementation of the interventions and their effectiveness.

Evaluation
Determine the effectiveness of the plan as the expected outcomes and mutual goals are met.
Reformulate the plan and implement new interventions as necessary.
Document the effectiveness of the plan of care in an ongoing, systematic manner.

identifying desired outcomes, planning interventions, implementing care, and evaluating the success of the plan. Human response patterns to health and illness are key elements in establishing a nursing diagnosis (Box 2-4).

Integration of the Nursing Process into Perioperative Patient Care

The six components of the nursing process are integrated into the three phases of the patient's perioperative experience: the preoperative phase, the interoperative phase, and the postoperative phase. Throughout the entire perioperative period, the patient is continually assessed, the plan of care is modified, implementation is effected, and the cycle is evaluated for the attainment of outcomes.

Preoperative Phase

The preoperative phase of the patient's surgical experience begins when the decision is made to undergo surgical intervention, and it ends when the patient is transferred to the OR bed. During this phase, the perioperative nurse performs the assessment, determines the nursing diagnoses, identifies potential outcomes, and develops a plan of care. The nurse assesses the patient to identify any actual or potential physiologic, psychosocial, and spiritual needs, problems, or other health status considerations. In collaboration with the patient and/or significant other, the nurse then determines the nursing diagnoses and identifies the expected outcomes of the perioperative experience. The perioperative nurse plans, prioritizes, and initiates the patient care necessary for the attainment of the desired outcomes.

Intraoperative Phase

The intraoperative phase begins with placement of the patient on the OR bed and continues until the patient is admitted to a postprocedural or postoperative area. Implementation of the plan and evaluation of care continues during this phase. The perioperative nurse either personally carries out the plan of care or supervises others in carrying out the plan with skill, safety, efficiency, and effectiveness. Modification of the plan may be necessary during the procedure.

Postoperative Phase

The postoperative phase begins with admission of the patient to a postprocedural or postanesthesia area, which may be a postanesthesia care unit (PACU) or an intensive care unit (ICU). Patients admitted to the facility on an ambulatory one-day-stay basis may return to the ambulatory unit. As indicated by the his or her condition, the patient will transfer from the immediate postoperative patient care division for progressive stages of self-care on a surgical unit before being discharged from the hospital. The postoperative phase ends when the surgeon discontinues follow-up care. Evaluation, the sixth component of nursing process, is completed during this phase.

STANDARDS OF PERIOPERATIVE CLINICAL PRACTICE

A standard is an authoritative statement established and published by a profession and by which the performance of practice can be measured. The standards of nursing practice establish parameters and competency levels against which the practice of the profession may be compared.

The ANA Standards of Clinical Nursing Practice reflect the nursing process and state the interventions to be performed. These standards are a description of a competent level of practice common to all nurses and form the foundation of all decision making in the provision of care to all patients. The interpretive statements that accompany each standard provide definitions of terms along with the interventions and guidelines necessary to achieve these standards. Criteria for the achievement of each standard are also stated and remain consistent with current nursing practice. Nursing practice is based on theory and is constantly evolving with the development of new technology and research. The standards are written in behavioral terms so nurses can measure to what degree each standard has been met.

The Standards of Perioperative Clinical Practice, originally published in 1981, were revised in 1992 by AORN, the Association of periOperative Registered Nurses.* The nursing activities inherent in each standard are incorporated in the nursing process during the three phases of surgical care.

Standard I: Assessment

The perioperative nurse collects patient health data. Data collection is continuous and ongoing. It may be gathered in the preoperative holding area, on the patient care unit, in the clinic, or by a telephone call to the patient at home. Information can be obtained from the patient's chart, by consultation with other members of the health care team (e.g., unit nurses, surgeon, anesthesia provider), through interviews with the patient and/or family or significant others, and by observation and physical assessment. Data collection is a progressive and orderly process of gathering meaningful information pertinent to the planned surgical intervention. It includes, but is not limited to, the following:

---

*In 1999 the AORN House of Delegates designated the name of their professional organization as AORN, the Association of periOperative Registered Nurses, to better describe the diverse roles of the professional nursing membership.

Box 2-4	**Human Response Patterns According to NANDA**	
Exchanging	Valuing	Perceiving
Communicating	Choosing	Knowing
Relating	Moving	Feeling

- Current medical diagnosis and therapy
- Diagnostic studies and laboratory test results
- Physical status and physiologic responses, including allergies and sensory or physical deficits
- Psychosocial status, including education level
- Spiritual needs, ethnic and cultural background, and lifestyle
- Previous responses to illness, hospitalization, and surgery
- Patient's understanding, perceptions, and expectations of the procedure

Pertinent data collected through physiologic and psychosocial assessment are documented. Box 2-5 lists the preoperative assessment parameters to be considered. The basic elements of a nursing assessment are described in the following sections.

Subjective Data

Subjective data include the patient's perceptions and expectations of the procedure and may be recorded in the form of a direct quote.

Objective Data

Objective data include the nurse's observations of the patient and the interpretation of baseline data.

Physiologic Assessment

The perioperative nurse performs a physical assessment of the patient. Techniques include inspection/observation, auscultation, percussion, palpation, and olfaction. The assessment of major body systems establishes the baseline health status of the patient. It provides a basis for planning appropriate patient care and also provides a database for postoperative evaluation.

The perioperative nurse should also be familiar with laboratory test norms so that critical deviations can be identified in all phases of perioperative care. Other important parameters for planning perioperative care include a knowledge of allergies, skin integrity, sensory or physical limitations, prosthetic devices, nutritional/metabolic status, and chronic illness. The routine use of medications can affect or interact with anesthetic medications and postoperative recovery. A patient who smokes and who will have general anesthesia needs to be taught coughing and deep breathing exercises. The patient who is dependent on alcohol or other drugs can suffer postoperative physiologic and psychologic manifestations of withdrawal. A chemically dependent person who is recovering from his or her addiction may refuse preoperative sedation and postoperative narcotics for pain.

Psychosocial Assessment

The perioperative nurse performs a psychosocial assessment. Illness makes a person vulnerable, and individuals vary in their ability to cope with stressful situations. Culture, religion, and socioeconomic factors have an impact on a patient's interpretation of illness and response to the interaction with the perioperative environment. Anticipatory apprehension, although normal to some degree, may diminish critical thinking and decision-making abilities. Stress may initiate an exaggerated response of normal coping mechanisms for self-protection. Establishing a preoperative psychosocial baseline facilitates prompt recognition of maladaptation to a perioperative event.

Documentation

Pertinent information should be recorded in the patient's chart for use by the perioperative team. Data collection forms the baseline for ongoing care in the perioperative environment. Computer programs can be used to establish a computerized patient database. The nurse enters the data obtained from physiologic and psychosocial assessments through physical examination, interview, and observation. The computer assigns the signs and symptoms—the defining characteristics—to nursing diagnostic categories. The related factors, expected outcomes, and nursing interventions may then be selected. A printed copy of the patient care plan is obtained for the patient's record. The nurse should review the printed copy and date and sign it for the permanent record.

Box 2-5 **Assessment Parameters That Are Monitored Throughout Perioperative Care**

Physiologic

Medical diagnosis
Surgical site and procedure
Results of diagnostic studies
Laboratory tests
Review of systems
Mobility, range of motion
Prosthetics (internal or external)
Sensory impairments
Allergies
Skin condition
Nutritional and metabolic status

Height and weight
Vital signs
Elimination pattern (e.g., continence)
Sleep, rest, exercise patterns
Medications
Substance abuse

Psychosocial

Cognition (e.g., mental status)
Cultural and religious beliefs
Perception of procedure
Expectations of care

Knowledge base (e.g., informed consent)
Readiness to learn
Ability to understand and retain teaching
Stress level (e.g., anxiety and fears)
Coping mechanisms
Support from family or significant others
Attitude and motivation (e.g., health management)
Affective responses (e.g., ability to express feelings)
Speech characteristics (e.g., language)
Nonverbal behavior

Standard II: Diagnosis

The perioperative nurse analyzes the assessment data in determining the nursing diagnoses. Nursing diagnoses are conclusions based on analysis and interpretation of the human response patterns revealed by the assessment data. These are concise written statements about a patient's actual or potential problems, needs, or health status considerations amenable to nursing intervention.

A medical diagnosis defines problems on the basis of a patient's pathologic condition(s). A nursing diagnosis identifies a patient's *response* to the condition(s). The North American Nursing Diagnosis Association (NANDA) has developed a list of nursing diagnoses. This list, known as a taxonomy, classifies human response patterns and standardizes the nomenclature for describing them. It includes definitions and defining characteristics for each diagnosis.

A nursing diagnosis has three components:

1. *Defining characteristics.* Human responses to altered body processes and other contributing factors describe the acuity of an actual or potential health status deviation. The nurse identifies the characteristics for which nursing interventions can legally be used to maintain current health status or to reduce, eliminate, or prevent its alteration. These interventions are based on human response patterns:
   a. *Problem.* Any health care condition that requires diagnostic, therapeutic, or educational action. Problems can be active (requiring immediate action) or inactive (having been solved). Problem-oriented medical records are built on this premise. An ongoing list is maintained in a database and is used throughout the managed care environment.
   b. *Need.* A lack of something essential for the maintenance of health that may be met through the plan of care. Needs may be actual (in existence at the time of assessment) or potential (anticipated to become actual during the length of stay [e.g., knowledge deficit]). Many of these needs are met through the intervention component of the plan of care.
   c. *Health status considerations.* A personal habit, lifestyle, or influencing agent that if uncontrolled can lead to a decline in physiologic or psychologic well-being (e.g., occupational hazards, exposure to chemical agent or smoke, or substance abuse).
2. *Signs (objective) and symptoms (subjective).* Data obtained during the assessment identify the defining characteristics of the patient's actual or potential health problems. The patient's functional health patterns are assessed (Box 2-6).
3. *Etiology/related factors.* The causes of problems may be related to physiologic, psychosocial, spiritual, environmental, or other factors contributing to the patient's health status. These causes define relevant risk factors to be considered in planning patient care.

Box 2-6	Gordon's Functional Health Patterns
Health perception/health management	Cognitive/perceptual
Nutritional/metabolic	Self-perception/self-concept
Elimination	Role/relationship
Activity/exercise	Sexuality/reproductive
Sleep/rest	Coping/stress tolerance
	Value/belief

Modified from Gordon M: *Manual of nursing diagnosis, 1997-1998,* St Louis, 1997, Mosby.

Documentation

Use of the NANDA terminology helps nurses establish standard communication when documenting nursing diagnoses. A common language facilitates continuity of patient care.

Standard III: Outcome Identification

The perioperative nurse identifies expected outcomes unique to the patient. Expected outcomes are the desired patient objectives following a surgical intervention; these outcomes occur within specified time frames and have specific criteria for evaluation. They direct patient care to modify or maintain the patient's baseline functional physical capabilities and behavioral patterns. The patient's rights and preferences are the cornerstones for expected outcomes. They should be realistic, attainable, and consistent with medical regimen and patient outcome standards for perioperative nursing. The results of care should be documented. In formulating expected outcomes as written statements, the perioperative nurse should consider, but not be limited to, the following:

- Absence of infection
- Maintenance of skin integrity
- Absence of adverse effects through proper application of safety measures
- Maintenance of fluid and electrolyte balance

Standard IV: Planning

The perioperative nurse develops a plan of care that prescribes interventions to attain the expected outcomes. Based on the assessment data, nursing diagnoses, and identified expected outcomes, the perioperative nurse devises a plan of care. The plan should include a provision for all phases of patient care in the perioperative environment. Key concepts to consider in planning perioperative patient care include, but are not limited to, the following:

- Participation of the patient and/or significant other in formulation of the plan
- Medical diagnosis and impact of surgical intervention on the patient's physiology
- Psychosocial and spiritual needs of the patient and his or her significant others
- Environmental safety, comfort, and well-being

- Provision of supplies, equipment, and technical expertise
- Current nursing practice

The plan of care should reflect current standards, facilitate the prescribed medical care, and work toward the attainment of desired outcomes. The scope of the plan is determined by assessment data. Any unusual data are considered for individualized patient care. Alternative options or interventions, not just routine procedures, are a necessary part of the plan. Regardless of format, the plan of care specifies the following:

- Patient care necessary to achieve expected outcomes
- Interventional priorities and sequence of care
- Availability of resources needed to implement the plan
- How, where, and by whom the care will be delivered
- Specific modifications for individualized aspects of care
- Methods for evaluating the effectiveness of the plan

Documentation

Standardized patient care plans may be developed for patient populations undergoing similar procedures, with space provided to note any unique or unusual patient assessment data. These care plans can be organized on preprinted forms to include the usual nursing diagnoses and expected outcomes and may include, but are not limited to, the following:

- Risk for knowledge deficit. . . . Patient will verbalize understanding.
- Risk for impaired skin integrity. . . . Patient's skin will remain intact.
- Risk for hypothermia. . . . Patient will remain normothermic.
- Risk for fluid imbalance. . . . Patient will maintain adequate fluid balance.
- Risk for injury. . . . Patient will not experience injurious event.

The format of the record may include checklists and spaces for specific patient data. This record accompanies the patient throughout the perioperative environment and serves as a guide for the perioperative team. Communication of the plan to all personnel involved in providing care to the patient is essential for continuity of care. The plan is modified as indicated by evaluation data.

Standard V: Implementation

The perioperative nurse implements the interventions identified in the plan of care. The plan of care is implemented throughout the perioperative care period. Scientific principles provide the basis for nursing interventions that are consistent with the plan for continuity of patient care in the perioperative environment. They are performed with safety, skill, efficiency, and effectiveness.

The patient's welfare and individual needs are paramount in every facet of activity and must not be compromised. Seemingly routine details are significant. For example, taking a defective instrument out of circulation may prevent injury

to the patient or team member. Checking the surgical lights before the procedure begins helps to ensure the vision of the surgeon in the surgical site. All preoperative preparations within the perioperative environment provide for the physical safety of the patient and team in an aseptic, controlled manner. The circulator also provides emotional support to the patient before transfer to the OR bed and during induction of anesthesia.

This text primarily focuses on interventions that perioperative nurses and surgical technologists perform to ensure achievement of expected patient outcomes. Implementation of safe and efficient patient care requires the application of technical and professional knowledge, sound clinical judgment, and a surgical conscience on the part of all team members. Nurses have a responsibility to monitor constantly the physical and psychologic responses of patients to care. They control environmental factors that affect outcomes of surgical intervention.

Documentation

All patient care interventions (both routine and individualized), observations of patient responses, and the resultant outcomes delineated in the patient care plan are documented as evidence of the care given. This written documentation becomes part of the patient's permanent record. The registered nurse circulator accountable for the patient's care is responsible for the documentation. The person completing the documentation should sign with his or her complete name and title. Interventions contributing to patient comfort and safety are identified. Activities other than direct patient care that are not recorded elsewhere and may affect patient outcomes are included (e.g., how tissue specimens were handled).

Writing nurse's notes or progress notes on the patient's chart or completing an accurate intraoperative observation checklist provides a profile of what has happened to the patient. The notes should contain what happened and why. Intraoperative records not only have legal value but are also valuable to the postoperative care team.

Standard VI: Evaluation

The perioperative nurse evaluates the patient's progress toward the attainment of outcomes. Evaluation is a continual process of reassessing the patient and his or her responses to implementation of the plan of care. Perioperative caregivers accommodate a variety of intense situations within a short time. The perioperative team is always on the alert and prepared to respond to the unexpected. The flexibility of the team is manifest in the quick modifications to the plan of care during emergency situations.

All components of the nursing process are performed concurrently during the intraoperative phase as changes occur in the patient's internal and external environments. The patient is observed during the surgical procedure and evaluated for responses to all interventions.

Determination of patient responses and the realization of expected outcomes can be verified by direct observation of and/or conversation with the patient. The perioperative nurse observes the patient's responses to interventions during the immediate preoperative and intraoperative phases of care in the perioperative environment. The perioperative nurse may accompany the patient to the PACU or postprocedural area to determine the level of attainment of expected outcomes. Ideally, the perioperative nurse visits the patient postoperatively on the patient care division or phones an ambulatory patient at home within 24 to 48 hours after discharge.

Documentation

The patient's permanent record should reflect the ongoing evaluation of perioperative nursing care and its outcomes. This includes a comparison of expected outcomes to the degree of outcome attainment as determined by the patient's responses to nursing interventions. Documentation provides legal evidence of results of the plan of care and revisions to the plan following reassessment of the patient.

Clinical Competency of the Perioperative Nurse

Using the framework of the nursing process, AORN published Competency Statements in Perioperative Nursing in 1986 and revised them in 1992. These broadly written statements of expected competencies can be used to develop position descriptions, to develop performance appraisals, and to organize orientation and staff development activities. They may serve as guidelines for the skills a nurse should reasonably expect to achieve in order to function as a perioperative nurse in the perioperative environment. These statements incorporate the many principles, procedures, and practices elaborated throughout this text for competent care of the surgical patient. They include competency to do the following:

1. Assess the physiologic health status of the patient.
2. Assess the psychosocial health status of the patient and family.
3. Formulate nursing diagnoses based on health status data.
4. Establish the patient's expected outcomes based on nursing diagnoses.
5. Develop a plan of care that identifies patient care interventions to achieve expected outcomes.
6. Implement patient care interventions according to the plan of care.
7. Evaluate the attainment of expected outcomes and effectiveness of patient care.
8. Participate in patient and family teaching.
9. Create and maintain a sterile field.
10. Provide equipment and supplies based on patient needs.
11. Perform sponge, sharps, and instrument counts.
12. Administer drugs and solutions as prescribed.
13. Physiologically monitor the patient during the surgical procedure and throughout the perioperative experience.
14. Monitor and control the environment.
15. Respect the patient's rights.
16. Demonstrate accountability.

SURGICAL TECHNOLOGY

The activities of registered professional nurses are supplemented and complemented by the services of allied technical health care personnel. The term *allied health care personnel* refers to individuals who have been trained in a health care–related science and have responsibility for the delivery of health care–related services but who are not graduates of schools of medicine, osteopathy, dentistry, podiatry, or nursing. Approximately two thirds of the health care work force is designated as allied health professionals. Educational preparation may be offered in colleges, vocational-technical schools, hospital-based programs, or military service schools. Technologists, technicians, and therapists in more than 130 occupational categories work collaboratively with and under the direction of physicians and registered nurses.

The surgical technologist, or ST, is a member of the direct patient care team and works intraoperatively with the surgeon, anesthesia provider, and registered nurse. This team is referred to as the perioperative team. The surgical technologist assists by preparing and handling supplies and equipment to maintain a safe and therapeutic surgical environment for the patient. The surgical technologist performs specific techniques and functions designed to exclude pathogenic microorganisms from the surgical wound.

A surgical technologist completes a 1- to 2-year intensive educational program. This program includes courses in anatomy and physiology, pathology, and microbiology as prerequisites to courses that involve the theory and application of technology during surgical procedures and for care of the perioperative environment. Other courses in the curriculum, such as pharmacology, help explain the underlying basis for the technical tasks to be performed. Courses in psychology, ethics, and interpersonal communication are fundamental to an appreciation of the humanities.

STANDARDS OF PRACTICE FOR SURGICAL TECHNOLOGISTS

The Association of Surgical Technologists (AST) has developed standards of practice that provide guidelines for the development of performance descriptions and performance evaluations. The quality of the surgical technologist's practice may be judged by these standards. The six authoritative statements that comprise the standards describe the scope of patient care and serve as a guide on which to base clinical practice.

Standard I

Teamwork is essential for perioperative patient care and is contingent on interpersonal skills. Communication is critical to the positive attainment of expected outcomes of care. All team members should work together for the common good of the patient. For the benefit of the patient and the delivery of quality care, interpersonal skills are demonstrated in all interactions with the health care team, the patient and family, superiors, and peers. Personal integrity and surgical conscience are integrated into every aspect of professional behavior.

Standard II

Preoperative planning and preparation for surgical intervention are individualized to meet the needs of each patient and his or her surgeon. The surgical technologist collaborates with the professional registered nurse in the collection of data for use in the preparation of equipment and supplies needed for the surgical procedure. The implementation of patient care identified in the plan of care is performed under the supervision of a professional registered nurse.

Standard III

The preparation of the perioperative environment and all supplies and equipment will ensure environmental safety for patients and personnel. The application of the plan of care includes wearing appropriate attire, anticipating the needs of the patient and perioperative team, maintaining a safe work area, observing aseptic technique, and following all policies and procedures of the institution.

Standard IV

Application of basic and current knowledge is necessary for a proficient performance of assigned functions. The surgical technologist should maintain a current knowledge base of procedures, equipment and supplies, emergency protocol for various situations, and changes in scientific technology pertinent to his or her performance description objectives. It is the responsibility of the surgical technologist to augment his or her knowledge base by studying recent literature, attending in-service and continuing education programs, and pursuing new learning experiences.

Standard V

Each patient's rights to privacy, dignity, safety, and comfort are respected and protected. Each member of the OR team has a moral and ethical duty to uphold strict observance of the patient's rights. The surgical technologist, like all members of the health care team, is expected to perform as a patient advocate in all situations. This is an accountability issue and should be part of each aspect of patient care.

Standard VI

Every patient is entitled to the same application of aseptic technique within the physical facilities. Implementation of the individualized plan of care for every patient includes the application of aseptic or sterile technique at all times by all members of the health care team. All patients are given the same dedication in their care.

Clinical Competency of the Surgical Technologist

The performance description developed by AST identifies performance objectives against which the surgical technologist may measure his or her level of competency. Adapted for this text are measurable competencies derived from the AST performance description for the surgical technologist. These objectives include competency to do the following:

1. Apply the principles of asepsis in a knowledgeable manner, assist in the sterilization and disinfection of equipment and supplies, maintain sterile technique at the sterile field, and assist with the terminal care of equipment and supplies after the surgical procedure is completed.
2. Identify emergency situations and institute corrective actions in a calm and efficient manner.
3. Maintain a current knowledge base and seek new learning experiences.
4. Provide a safe, efficient environment for the patient and the OR team.
5. Function in the role of patient advocate in support of the patient's rights, dignity, privacy, and best interest.
6. Perform within safe guidelines in the presence of the administration of anesthetic agents.
7. Maintain organizational skill and manual dexterity in the economy of time, motion, and supplies in a safe and efficient manner.
8. Demonstrate knowledge of anatomy and physiology and the recognition of pathologic deviations.
9. Perform in the role of surgical technologist in a professional manner at all times.
10. Perform as a team member for the common good of the patient and take responsibility for personal actions.

Scope of Practice

AST has identified three roles of the surgical technologist who has had specific education and job-related training: the scrub person, the circulator, and the first assistant. National certification examinations are available for qualified surgical technologists who meet specific eligibility criteria.

Scrub Person

The scrub person is a team member who is qualified to assemble supplies, prepare and maintain the sterile field, anticipate the needs of the sterile team during a surgical procedure, and provide a safe, efficient environment for the patient and team. On completion of the procedure, the scrub person is responsible for caring for the used equipment and supplies, disposing of contaminated articles in a safe manner, and assisting with patient care as indicated.

Circulating Surgical Technologist

Circulating duties are performed under the supervision of a professional registered nurse. Interventions performed are identified by the established plan of care developed by the professional registered nurse and are within the scope of educational preparation, supervised experience, and legal guidelines for surgical technologists.

Surgical Technologist First Assistant

First assisting duties may include exposure of the surgical site, hemostasis, and technical functions to assist the surgeon in carrying out a safe procedure with positive expected outcomes for the patient. This role is performed within the additional educational preparation, experience, and institutional guidelines for the surgical technologist first assistant.

CREDENTIALING

Credentialing refers to the processes of accreditation, licensure, and certification of institutions, agencies, and individuals. These processes establish quality, identity, protection, and control for the competency-based education and performance of professional and allied technical health care personnel. Credentialing also protects the public.

Accreditation

An accrediting body of a voluntary organization evaluates and sanctions an educational program or an institution as meeting predetermined standards and/or essential criteria. The National League for Nursing accredits schools of nursing. Surgical technology programs are accredited by the Commission on Accreditation of Health Education Programs (CAAHEP) in compliance with the Essentials for an Accredited Educational Program in Surgical Technology. The Joint Commission on Accreditation of Healthcare Organizations (JCAHO) accredits hospitals and ambulatory care centers. Other professional organizations offer accreditation for special interest groups.

Licensure

A license to practice is granted to professionals by a governmental agency, such as the state board of nursing or medicine. On completion of a formal academic education, nurses and physicians who successfully pass a state examination receive a license to practice in that state. To maintain this license, they must register with the state as required by law; hence the term *registered nurse*. Practical/vocational nurses also are licensed (LPN/LVN).

Most states grant a license by reciprocity or endorsement to applicants who wish to practice in their state but who took the examination in another state. Some states require licensure for some categories of allied health occupations, such as physical therapists. Surgical technologists and physician assistants are not currently licensed in any state.

Licensure is not offered on an indefinite basis. Applicants apply for renewal at specific time intervals determined by each state. Many states require proof of continuing education as a prerequisite for eligibility of relicensure.

Certification

A nongovernmental private organization can award a credential that attests to the competence or high level of knowledge of an individual who meets predetermined qualifications. Certification may be defined as documented validation of an individual's professional achievement of identified standards. To be certified is to demonstrate the attainment of more than minimal competency; it is a statement of certification-level knowledge. Certification is voluntary, whereas licensure is mandatory.

Certification is usually granted for a limited time. To retain this credential, an individual must complete the recertification process established by the certifying body. For recertification, some certifying organizations require a specified number of clinical hours, continuing education hours, a written examination, or a combination of these. Maintaining certification by going through this process demonstrates a high level of motivation and commitment.

Physicians, nurses, and allied health care personnel may be certified by their professional specialty association as being competent in knowledge and skills to practice. Applicants take an examination that tests knowledge in the area of specialization. Surgical technologists who successfully pass an examination attesting to their theoretical knowledge are certified by the Liaison Council on Certification (LCC), the certifying body for AST. These individuals become certified surgical technologists (CSTs). Similarly, a nurse anesthetist becomes a certified registered nurse anesthetist (CRNA) by passing the examination of the Council on Certification of Nurse Anesthetists.

Some nursing associations grant recognition of professional achievement and competence in current practice. A perioperative nurse who has been in clinical practice for 24 months and who has successfully passed an examination is certified by the Certification Board Perioperative Nursing (CBPN) as a certified perioperative nurse, which is designated as CNOR. Several nursing specialty organizations, such as the National Association of Orthopaedic Nurses (NAON) and the American Society of Plastic and Reconstructive Surgery Nurses (ASPRSN), offer certification examinations through their certifying bodies as an additional credentialing tool.

First Assistant Certification

A CNOR who has acquired additional knowledge and skill through structured, organized instruction and supervised practice may serve as a registered nurse first assistant (RNFA) under direct supervision of the surgeon. The RNFA should function solely as the first assistant and not perform the functions of a scrub person in combination with assisting duties. The role of the RNFA is recognized as being within the scope of nursing practice as an expanded role in all states. CBPN has developed a national certification examination for the RNFA who has attended a CBPN-approved RNFA program, has attained 2000 hours of first assisting experience during a period of 5 years, and can provide documentation of clinical competency. In the year 2000, a Bachelor of Science in Nursing (BSN) degree will be required for eligibility to become certified. After successfully passing the examination, a certified RNFA is entitled to use the acronym *CRNFA*. The CRNFA may recertify every 5 years by contact hours or by examination. Eligibility for recertification includes maintenance of CNOR status and documentation of active clinical practice as an RNFA with continued clinical competency for the 2-year period preceding the recertification date. For ease of processing, the certifications for CNOR and CRNFA were merged in January 1998 to allow recertification at the same intervals. The requirement for the combination recertification is 200 contact hours every 5 years; 100 of these hours must be RNFA specific.

A certified surgical technologist also may be trained to first assist. An associate's degree should be the minimal entry-level requirement for CSTs who enter a postgraduate first assisting program. For CSTs with at least 2 years of first assisting experience during the previous 4 years, a national certification examination is available from the Liaison Council on Certification for the Surgical Technologist (LCC-ST). After successfully passing this examination, the CST first assistant may use the acronym *CST/CFA*. At the time of original certification as a CFA, the CST portion of the certification is adjusted to be of the same time duration as the CFA portion of the certification. Both aspects of the certification will be adjusted for the same period of 6 years. Recertification as a CST/CFA is accomplished by providing documentation of practicing as a CST/CFA for 2 years of the 6-year certification period and by obtaining 100 continuing education credits in the categories defined by the LCC-ST. Another option is to document 2 years of practice as a first assistant within the 6-year period and take the certification examination again.

Bibliography

Allen GJ: Professionalism in the OR, *Surg Technol* 26(4):24-26, 1994.
American Nurses Association: *ANA standards of clinical nursing practice,* Washington, DC, 1991, The Association.
Association of Operating Room Nurses: *AORN standards, recommended practices, and guidelines,* Denver, 1998, The Association.
Association of Surgical Technologists: *AST job description: CST surgical assistant,* Englewood, Colo, 1990, The Association.
Association of Surgical Technologists: *Essentials and guidelines for an accredited educational program in surgical technology,* Englewood, Colo, 1992, The Association.
Association of Surgical Technologists: *Standards of practice,* Englewood, Colo, 1997, The Association.
Carpenito LJ: *Handbook of nursing diagnosis,* Philadelphia, 1993, JB Lippincott.
Demello AB, Pagragan CS: Development of professional excellence puts best foot forward, *AORN J* 67(1):214-228, 1998.
Dock LL, Stewart IM: *A short history of nursing,* ed 2, New York, 1929, GP Putnam's Sons.
Dunscombe A, Riall CT: Celebrating 40 years of progress in perioperative nursing techniques, *AORN J* 60(5):743-745, 747-748, 751-752, 1994.
Fujihara-Isozaki LF, Fahndrick J: Clinical pathways: a perioperative application, *AORN J* 67(2):376-390, 1998.
Gillette VA: Applying nursing theory to perioperative nursing practice, *AORN J* 64(2):261-269 1996.
Grundeman BJ, Fernsebner B: *Comprehensive perioperative nursing. Volume one: principles,* Boston, 1995, Jones & Bartlett.
Messina J: Development and implementation of a perioperative assistant training program, *AORN J* 66(5):890-904, 1997.
Nightingale F: *Notes on nursing: what it is, and what it is not,* New York, 1969, Dover Publications.
Null S et al: Development of a perioperative nursing diagnoses flow sheet, *AORN J* 61(3):547-557, 1995.
Proposed recommended practices for documentation of patient care in the perioperative practice setting, *AORN J* 61(3):616-621, 1995.
Roth RA: *Perioperative nursing core curriculum,* Philadelphia, 1995, WB Saunders.
Schramm CA, Hoshowsky VM: Developing competency-based perioperative orientation programs, *AORN J* 62(4):570-590, 1995.
Thompson S: The many roles of the perioperative nurse, *AORN J* 66(4):698-701, 1997.
Wieczorek P: Developing critical pathways for the operating room, *AORN J* 62(6):925-929, 1995.
Wurstner I, Koch F: Role redesign in perioperative settings, *AORN J* 61(5):834-844, 1995.

Chapter 3

Accountability and Professional Obligations

 Chapter Objectives

After studying this chapter, the learner will be able to:

- List three main aspects of accountability.
- Identify the purpose of informed consent.
- Discuss how work environment affects performance.
- Discuss how standardization influences patient care.

Nursing theorist Florence Nightingale (1820-1910) is credited with developing the environmental theory of patient care (Box 3-1). According to her theory, the caregiver is accountable for creating and maintaining the best possible environmental conditions to assist natural healing. She emphasized the need for prevention through education and teamwork. In her eyes, the team consisted of not only the caregivers but also the patient and family. She often approached her legislators with suggestions for bills and laws designed to protect patients and caregivers.

HISTORICAL BACKGROUND

Patient care has not always been provided by honorable, compassionate individuals. Until Florence Nightingale established standards of patient care and nursing education, the practice was haphazard and performed mostly by uneducated, untrained individuals. Not everyone had a family member to provide long-term care.

Churches ceased control of hospitals during the reformation of the eighteenth century. Free care associated with religious personnel was replaced with low-paid, uneducated workers. Most of the tasks were unpleasant and menial, and cleanliness was not a prime consideration. Hospitals became filthy dens of death. Low wages and abominable working conditions did not attract honest, educated people to the job. Those who could afford private treatment at home had a better chance of survival by avoiding cross-contamination with other patients.

John Howard, an English philanthropist, wrote a book entitled *Hospitals and Lazarettos,* which disclosed the deplorable nursing conditions in hospitals. Many patients were treated worse than prisoners. Personal possessions were stolen, and barbaric treatments resembled torture. Physicians wore bloody aprons during surgery and did not change or wash them between patients. Instruments were rarely even wiped clean between uses. Handwashing was considered unimportant. Decisions were made about treatments without consulting the

Box 3-1	Nightingale's Theory of Nursing	
Physical Environment	**Psychologic Environment**	**Social Environment**
Sanitation	Communication	Mortality data
Ventilation	Advice	Prevention of disease
Lighting	Variety	Education of caregiver
Noise	Scientific knowledge base	Nursing as distinct from medicine
Odors	Creativity	Accountability
Temperature	Spirituality	Responsibility

Box 3-2 Terms Associated with Accountability and Professional Obligations

accountability Answering for performance of a service or task.

advance directive Document that indicates wishes concerning health care and usually designates someone to make decisions if the patient is unable to do so for self.

advocacy Active support.

autonomy Self-government or independence.

consent Voluntary, autonomous permission to proceed with an agreed-on course of action.

obligation Duty or promise.

responsibility Social, moral, or legal duty.

rights Power or possession of privilege.

---

patient or family. During that dark era of patient care, few people accepted responsibility for the adequate performance of duties, and quality assurance was not a consideration. Undesired outcomes of care were commonly blamed on divine punishment.

ACCOUNTABILITY

Accountability means answering to someone for an obligatory action. As both learners and caregivers, perioperative nurses and surgical technologists are accountable to the following:

- Patients receiving services
- Employer
- Educational institution providing learning experiences
- Profession or vocation to uphold established standards of practice
- Self and other team members

A lack of accountability for behavior in the perioperative environment may result in patient injury or dissatisfaction with care. Health care providers have a legal and moral obligation to identify and correct situations that threaten a patient's safety and well-being. Most incidents that could endanger the patient and lead to legal actions can be prevented. Prevention focuses on the responsible performance of duty and continuous quality improvement. The provision of safe

care of the patient also protects caregivers and the health care facility from liability. It also upholds the reputation of the professions by maintaining the confidence of the consumer public. Failure of a caregiver to maintain accountability constitutes negligence. If negligence is established, any caregiver can be held liable for his or her own acts of omission or commission. Each person is responsible for his or her own negligent acts. Specific terms associated with accountability and professionalism are included in Box 3-2.

PROFESSIONAL OBLIGATIONS TO THE PATIENT

Inherent in professional practice is the duty to safeguard the well-being and rights of patients. The use of modern technology and the performance of surgical procedures places the patient at risk for harm. These factors also may present health care providers with ethical dilemmas that are complicated by legal issues. Respect for the patient's autonomy and the patient's right to make informed decisions about his or her own health care should be considered and balanced by the professional obligations of beneficence (the duty to benefit) and nonmaleficence (not to harm).

Patient's Rights

As a consumer, the patient purchases services to fulfill health care needs and is entitled to certain rights. Access to health care is recognized as a right, not a privilege, of every human being.

In the interest of "more effective patient care and greater satisfaction for the patient, his or her physician, and the hospital organization," the American Hospital Association adopted A Patient's Bill of Rights as a national policy statement. These rights are intended to be upheld by the hospital on behalf of its patients (Box 3-3).

General Consent

Most facilities require the patient or his or her legal guardian to sign a general consent form on admission. This form authorizes the attending physician and the hospital staff to render standard treatment or to perform miscellaneous procedures as the physician deems advisable. This general consent is relied on only for activities performed in routine care. Physicians and nurses should be knowledgeable about the statements on the form used in their facility.

Patients have the right to know what is being done to, for, and about them and their illnesses. For patients not wanting to know the details, their wish for only simple explanations or essential information should be respected.

Physician-Patient Relationship

The physician-patient relationship is a contractual one. Once a patient has been accepted for treatment, the physician has a duty to perform to the best of his or her ability. The physician

| Box 3-3 | **A Patient's Bill of Rights*** |

1. The patient has the right to considerate and respectful care.
2. The patient has the right to and is encouraged to obtain from physicians and other direct caregivers relevant, current, and understandable information concerning diagnosis, treatment, and prognosis.

   Except in emergencies when the patient lacks decision-making capacity and the need for treatment is urgent, the patient is entitled to the opportunity to discuss and request information related to the specific procedures and/or treatments, the risks involved, the possible length of recuperation, and the medically reasonable alternatives and their accompanying risks and benefits.

   Patients have the right to know the identity of physicians, nurses, and others involved in their care, as well as when those involved are students, residents, or other trainees. The patient also has the right to know the immediate and long-term financial implications of treatment choices, insofar as they are known.
3. The patient has the right to make decisions about the plan of care prior to and during the course of treatment and to refuse a recommended treatment or plan of care to the extent permitted by law and hospital policy and to be informed of the medical consequences of this action. In case of such refusal, the patient is entitled to other appropriate care and services that the hospital provides or transfer to another hospital. The hospital should notify patients of any policy that might affect patient choice within the institution.
4. The patient has the right to have an advance directive (such as a living will, health care proxy, or durable power of attorney for health care) concerning treatment or designating a surrogate decision maker with the expectation that the hospital will honor the intent of that directive to the extent permitted by law and hospital policy.

   Health care institutions should advise patients of their rights under state law and hospital policy to make informed medical choices, ask if the patient has an advance directive, and include that information in patient records. The patient has the right to timely information about hospital policy that may limit its ability to implement fully a legally valid advance directive.
5. The patient has the right to every consideration of privacy. Case discussion, consultation, examination, and treatment should be conducted so as to protect each patient's privacy.
6. The patient has the right to expect that all communications and records pertaining to his or her care will be treated as confidential by the hospital, except in cases such as suspected abuse and public health hazards when reporting is permitted or required by law. The patient has the right to expect that the hospital will emphasize the confidentiality of

this information when it releases it to any other parties entitled to review information in these records.
7. The patient has the right to review the records pertaining to his or her medical care and to have the information explained or interpreted as necessary, except when restricted by law.
8. The patient has the right to expect that, within its capacity and policies, a hospital will make reasonable response to the request of a patient for appropriate and medically indicated care and services. The hospital should provide evaluation, service, and/or referral as indicated by the urgency of the case. When medically appropriate and legally permissible, or when a patient has so requested, a patient may be transferred to another facility. The institution to which the patient is to be transferred should first have accepted the patient for transfer. The patient should also have the benefit of complete information and explanation concerning the need for, risks, benefits, and alternatives to such a transfer.
9. The patient has the right to ask and be informed of the existence of business relationships among the hospital, educational institutions, other health care providers, or payers that may influence the patient's treatment and care.
10. The patient has the right to consent to or decline to participate in proposed research studies or human experimentation affecting care and treatment or requiring direct patient involvement, and to have those studies fully explained prior to consent. A patient who declines to participate in research or experimentation is entitled to the most effective care that the hospital can otherwise provide.
11. The patient has the right to expect reasonable continuity of care when appropriate and to be informed by physicians and other caregivers of available and realistic patient care options when hospital care is no longer appropriate.
12. The patient has the right to be informed of hospital policies and practices that relate to patient care, treatment, and responsibilities. The patient has the right to be informed of available resources for resolving disputes, grievances, and conflicts, such as ethics committees, patient representatives, or other mechanisms available in the institution. The patient has the right to be informed of the hospital's charges for services and available payment methods.

Conclusion

Hospitals have many functions to perform, including the enhancement of health status, health promotion, and the prevention and treatment of injury and disease; the immediate and ongoing care and rehabilitation of patients; the education of health professionals, patients, and the community; and research. All these activities should be conducted with an overriding concern for the values and dignity of patients.

Reprinted with permission of the American Hospital Association, copyright 1992.

*These rights can be exercised on a patient's behalf by a designated surrogate or proxy decision maker if the patient lacks decision-making capacity, is legally incompetent, or is a minor.

should adequately explain—in clear, simple language—the nature, purpose, extent, potential hazards, and expected outcome of the procedure proposed, as well as other available options of therapy. Adequate translation should be provided for patients with a sensory, language, or cultural barrier. The patient usually wants to know about the anticipated duration of hospitalization, absence from work, and cost of the procedure. It should be the physician who informs the patient; this responsibility should not be delegated to a nurse or an assistant.

Immediately after the surgical procedure, the surgeon should speak to the patient's family or significant others about the procedure performed, the patient's condition, and the prognosis. On the rare occasion when a patient dies during the surgical procedure, the surgeon informs the family or next of kin. After surgery, the surgeon follows the patient's progress until discharge from his or her care or until a return to a referring physician is indicated. At this point the surgeon's duty to care for the patient is complete.

Second Opinion

If the surgeon or patient has doubts about the necessity of a procedure, another opinion should be sought from a qualified specialist in the appropriate field of surgery. Consultation is a common and desirable part of good surgical practice. A second opinion may be required by third-party payers (i.e., insurance carriers) or managed care services. This is particularly indicated if the surgical procedure involves extended disability. Hospital policy may require special consultation or consent for procedures resulting in reproductive sterilization or a pregnancy termination.

INFORMED CONSENT

Responsibility for Consent Before a Surgical Procedure

The surgeon is responsible for informing the patient about the risks, benefits, and possible complications of a proposed surgical procedure. The explanation should include a discussion of the removal and disposition of body parts, the potential for disfigurement or disability, and what the patient may expect in the postoperative period. The preoperative discussion also should include advice to the patient regarding diet, bathing, smoking, and other factors that might affect outcome and rehabilitation.

The surgeon has the ultimate responsibility for obtaining informed consent for the procedure and should document this activity in the appropriate place in the patient's permanent record. The patient or appropriate guardian may be required to sign this record in the presence of a witness. Failure to provide full disclosure of the risks of a procedure and alternative modes of therapy has led to successful negligence suits. The surgeon is liable for misrepresentations, whether by affirmative statement or by nondisclosure.

The consent document becomes a permanent part of the patient's medical record and accompanies him or her throughout the perioperative environment. When checking the patient's identity and chart on arrival in the OR, it is the duty of the circulator and the anesthesia provider to be certain of the following:

1. The consent is on the chart and is properly signed.
2. The information on the form is correct.

The anesthesia provider also has a responsibility to inform the patient of any potential for unfavorable reactions to any medication or anesthetic agent that may be given during the surgical procedure. The risks of anesthesia should be explained without causing the patient undue stress. The surgeon should also check the consent before an anesthetic is administered. If the surgeon intends or wants to perform a procedure not specified on the consent form, the circulator has the responsibility to inform the surgeon and/or proper administrative authority of the discrepancy.

Informed Consent for a Surgical Procedure

According to the American College of Surgeons, a reasonable approach to informed consent should involve answering the following patient questions:

1. What do you plan to do to me?
2. Why do you want to do this procedure?
3. Are there any alternatives to this plan?
4. What things should I worry about?
5. What are the greatest risks or the worst thing that could happen?

The patient has the right to waive an explanation of the nature and consequences of the procedure and has the right to refuse treatment. When a patient signs an agreement, consent is given for the specific procedure indicated on the form. Additional procedures should be listed and signed separately—not added after the patient has already signed the form.

An informed consent document specifically outlines each procedure to be performed and explains the risks and benefits of the procedure. A patient's consent is required for the following:

- Each surgical procedure to be performed, including secondary procedures such as incision and drainage
- Any procedure for which a general anesthetic is administered, such as examination of a child under anesthesia
- Procedures involving entrance into a body cavity, such as endoscopy
- Any hazardous therapy, such as irradiation or chemotherapy

The surgeon may be approved by the federal Food and Drug Administration (FDA) as a clinical investigator or by the Department of Health and Human Services (DHHS) as a researcher for the controlled experimental use of new drugs, chemical agents, or medical devices. Prior written consent based on an informed decision to participate in the research should be obtained from the patient. The surgeon completes an investigator's report that is returned to the supplier of the drug or device and eventually filed with the FDA (www.fda.gov). The patient is free to refuse or withdraw at any time from research carried out under the auspices of the DHHS. More information can be found on the DHHS Web site (www.os.dhhs.gov/).

Validity of Consent

The patient should personally sign the consent unless he or she is a minor, is unconscious or mentally incompetent, or is in a life-threatening situation. The next of kin, legal guardian, or other authorized person should sign for these patients. Explanations are given by the physician to the parent of a minor or to the legal guardian of an incompetent adult.

A consent document should contain the patient's name in full, the surgeon's name, the specific procedure to be performed, the signatures of the patient and authorized witness(es), and the date of signatures. A signed consent is legally regarded as valid for as long as the patient still consents to the same procedure. Institutional policy may vary.

The patient giving consent for treatment should be of legal age and mentally competent. Except in life-threatening, emergency situations, the patient should sign the consent form before premedication is given and before going to the operating room (OR) or other treatment area. The patient should be asked to sign at least 1 day before an elective surgical procedure. This may be done in the surgeon's office, hospital admitting office, or on the patient care unit, but it should be an informed consent that is freely given (without coercion). If the patient is:

- A minor, a parent or legal guardian should sign.
- An emancipated minor, married, or independently earning a living, he or she may sign.
- Illiterate, he or she may sign with an X, after which the witness writes, "Patient's mark." Because illiteracy implies the inability to read and write, the patient should indicate an understanding of a verbal explanation.
- Unconscious, a responsible relative or guardian should sign.
- Mentally incompetent, the legal guardian—who may be either an individual or an agency—should sign. A court of competent jurisdiction may legalize the procedure in the absence of the legal guardian. A spouse or responsible relative of legal age may sign for an adult or emancipated minor who is mentally incapacitated by alcohol or other chemical substances when the urgency of the procedure does not allow time to regain mental competence.

Consent documents vary. Policies related to informed consent are developed by the medical staff and governing body in accordance with legal requirements. All personnel involved in the care of patients should be familiar with these policies. All consent documents become a permanent part of the patient's medical record and accompany him or her throughout the perioperative environment.

Witnessing a Consent

A witness verifies that the consent was signed without coercion after the surgeon explained the details of the procedure. The patient's or guardian's signature should be witnessed by one or more authorized persons. The witnesses may be physicians, nurses, other facility employees, or family members as established by policy. Checking or witnessing the signature of the patient or other authorized person does not constitute validation of informed consent. The witness assumes no liability or responsibility for the patient's understanding. The witness signing a consent document attests only to the following:

- Identification of the patient or legal substitute
- Voluntary signature, without coercion
- Mental state of signatory (i.e., not sedated or confused) at the time of signing

Consent in Emergency Situations

In a life-threatening emergency, the consent to treat and stabilize is not essential. Although every effort should be made to obtain consent, the patient's physical condition takes precedence over a procedural permit. The patient's state of consciousness may prevent him or her from verbalizing or signing a permit for treatment. Permission for a lifesaving procedure, especially for a minor, may be accepted from a legal guardian or responsible relative by telephone, fax, or other written communication. If it is obtained by telephone, two nurses should monitor the call and sign the form, which is signed later by the parent or guardian on arrival at the facility.

Right to Refuse a Surgical Procedure

The patient should reconcile the advantages and disadvantages of the surgical intervention. Each patient is entitled to receive sufficient information from which to intelligently base a decision regarding whether or not to proceed. The patient has the right to decide what will or will not be done to him or her. Only after making this decision is the patient asked to sign a written consent for a surgical procedure.

The patient has a right to withdraw written consent at any time before the surgical procedure if his or her determination to do so is reached voluntarily and while in a rational state. The surgeon is notified and the patient is not taken into the OR. The surgeon should explain the medical consequences of refusing the surgical procedure. If therapeutically valid, alternative methods of medical management should be offered. The surgical procedure is postponed until the patient makes a final decision. The procedure may be canceled.

The surgeon should document the patient's refusal for surgical treatment. For legal protection, the surgeon should also obtain from the patient, parent, or legal guardian a written refusal for the procedure or other treatment. The physician is required to inform the patient of the consequences of refusing diagnostic tests or therapeutic procedures.

ADVANCE DIRECTIVES

The Patient Self-Determination Act enacted by the U.S. Congress in December 1991 ensures the patient of the opportunity to participate in decision making before a procedure. The law requires that patients be informed of their rights to make their own decisions regarding their health care. This Act applies to hospitals, nursing homes, home health care agencies, hospice programs, and health maintenance organizations (HMOs). It does not apply to freestanding ambulatory or office settings.

Each patient has the right to determine the care he or she wishes to receive and to participate in the selection of delivery methods. The caregiver has the obligation to respect the patient's wishes regarding his or her care. The patient is entitled to the right of self-determination in decision making and to be consulted in matters concerning his or her well-being. This right extends to the issue of refusing treatment. A hospital policy should provide for making the patient aware of his or her right of self-determination.

In many facilities, policies permit the patient to indicate his or her preferences for treatment in the event that he or she should become disabled or incoherent. This is a legal document called an advance directive. The term *advance directive* encompasses durable power of attorney and living wills. The living will concept allows the patient to refuse treatment or nonessential measures to prolong life in a hopeless situation. A durable power of attorney document designates the person authorized to make decisions in the event that the patient is incapacitated. It allows the wishes of the patient concerning his or her care needs to be met if he or she becomes impaired and cannot make decisions. The durable power of attorney does not apply to pediatric patients or to incompetent adults who are already under legal guardianship. These patients already have decision makers available to decide treatment options.

On admission to the facility, the patient is asked whether he or she has an advance directive or durable power of attorney. A federal regulation requires that the institution be aware of whether such a document exists and enact it in the event of impaired cognitive function of the patient. The perioperative team should be made aware of its existence. A copy, not the original, is placed in the patient's record. Advance directives may also indicate the patient's preferences concerning organ donation. The family may still be asked for consent before any procurement occurs after the patient's death. In some states, the family has the right to refuse procurement.

PATIENT ADVOCACY

A patient advocate recognizes the patient's and the family's need for information and assistance in coping with the surgical experience, regardless of the setting. As an advocate, the perioperative nurse can provide information discovered during patient assessment that identifies specific needs or health concerns that require action. Advance preparation can help the patient and family anticipate events. Assistance in cop-

ing acknowledges the anxieties and fears of the patient and family, regardless of how minimally invasive the procedure may seem. No procedure is minor to the patient! Each patient reacts differently. The patient senses some relief in knowing that the caregiver has taken the time to identify needs specific to his or her care. The patient advocate is a caregiver who does the following:

1. Establishes rapport with the patient, family, or significant other in a manner that conveys genuine concern and sincere caring
2. Encourages the patient and family or significant other to express feelings and to ask questions
3. Helps relieve anxiety and apprehension by providing factual information regarding what to expect
4. Helps the patient make informed decisions throughout the perioperative experience
5. Acts as a patient representative by communicating pertinent information to other team members
6. Oversees all activities throughout the perioperative experience to ensure the safety and welfare of the patient
7. Keeps the family informed of significant events throughout the perioperative experience
8. Protects the patient's rights by compliance with advance directives for care (living will, durable power of attorney, or both)

PROFESSIONAL OBLIGATIONS TO THE PERIOPERATIVE TEAM

Professional obligations may conflict with personal values. A perioperative nurse or surgical technologist has the right to refuse to participate in a specific procedure for religious or moral reasons, if these beliefs have been made known. These beliefs should be discussed as a condition of employment and noted in the employee's personnel file. From a legal standpoint, personal beliefs and values do not give nurses and surgical technologists the right to refuse to provide care to specific patients or in emergency situations. However, the refusal to accept an assignment on the basis of inadequate preparation or incompetence is not only a right but also a legal and ethical responsibility. Caregivers should not assume functions (e.g., first assisting) that cannot be performed competently without adequate education, supervision, and credentialing.

Work Assignments

The perioperative nurse manager is accountable for the appropriateness of work assignments and for the delegation of tasks to qualified personnel. The manager who assigns or delegates tasks can ultimately be held accountable for actions performed. Therefore the delegation of duties should be appropriate within the scope of nursing practice, and supervision should be adequate. Delegation implies directing a qualified, competent person to perform activities and tasks in a specific situation under the delegator's supervision. Supervision assumes appropriate guidance in the accomplishment of these duties, with periodic observation and evaluation of their performance and validation that the assignments were performed according to established standards of practice. Broadly interpreted, supervision includes provision of orientation, in-services and continuing education, policies and procedures, performance appraisal, and assistance as determined by qualifications and competencies. The nurse manager has a responsibility to determine the following:

1. The duties are those that a reasonable and prudent nurse manager would delegate either to licensed professional nurses or to unlicensed assistive personnel, based on state statutes and other regulations governing delegation of nursing practice.
2. The assigned person is qualified and can competently and safely perform tasks without compromising the patient's welfare.
3. The degree of supervision is appropriate to include observation and evaluation of performance.
4. The delegated duties were appropriately and completely performed.

The perioperative nurse or surgical technologist should be aware of his or her own competencies or limitations before assuming responsibility for duties in the circulator, scrub, or first assistant role. A current performance description should reflect duties for which employees are held accountable. Nurses should function within the limitations of the legal scope of nursing practice in their state.

Right to Refuse an Assignment

Caregivers should not assume responsibility for tasks or duties unless qualified or prepared to perform them. For example, the circulator can refuse an anesthesia provider's request to add anesthesia medications to an intravenous (IV) line. Professional and legal responsibilities and the patient's rights dictate that requests outside the performance description be reported to the nurse manager. The patient entrusts his or her well-being to others when undergoing a surgical intervention. Patient care personnel should act as patient advocates when a patient's rights are compromised.

Physician's Orders

The physician's orders should be understood and evaluated in relation to the patient's condition. If an order is difficult to understand, the caregiver should find out what is required before carrying it out. The patient should always be observed closely. A change in the patient's condition should be reported at once to the surgeon, anesthesia provider, or nurse manager. An order should not be carried out without checking or questioning it if it is not in the best interest of the patient. A patient's adverse reaction to a medication or an intervention of any type should be reported at once. The caregiver can be held liable for not reporting a patient's symptoms to the appropriate person in a timely manner. The adverse reaction may indicate a need for special medication or intervention. A delay in reporting may result in permanent or irreversible damage to the patient. In some cases, such as an allergic reaction, the delay could result in death.

Keeping the Nurse Manager Informed

The perioperative nurse manager is justifiably disconcerted if he or she learns from someone outside the perioperative environment about events that should have been communicated by the perioperative team. For the safety and welfare of patients and the efficient management of the perioperative environment, the nurse manager should learn through the proper channels what goes on in the department. He or she should be informed of the following:

- Any unexpected complication or change in the condition of a patient.
- Any injury to a patient or staff member.
- Any unusual incident, including noncompliance with policies or procedures by a surgeon, anesthesia provider, nurse, surgical technologist, or nursing assistant. Every member of the perioperative team has both a moral and a legal obligation to report a violation of accepted standards of patient care through appropriate administrative channels.
- Concerns about instruments, equipment, or other supplies. Broken instruments and equipment should be taken out of service and either repaired or replaced.
- Requests for unavailable equipment or for a change of procedure.
- Problems that can lead to conflict between team members or departments. The perioperative nurse manager will discuss with the respective manager any problems concerning another patient care unit or department.
- Any other problems that might impair efficiency within the perioperative environment. Advice should be sought and minor problems discussed before they develop into major incidents.

Impaired Team Member

Incompetence or dangerous performance for any reason cannot be tolerated anywhere in the facility. The impaired team member may be the surgeon, an assistant, the anesthesia provider, a nurse, or a surgical technologist. Evidence of a colleague's inability to function competently should be confronted both to ensure patient safety and to help the impaired colleague. Impairment is usually caused by dependency on a chemical substance such as drugs or alcohol. It is against the law to perform in the role of caregiver while under the influence of a chemical substance. Rendering patient care while under the influence of alcohol or a chemical substance is potentially hazardous to the patient and to the work of the team as a whole.

Team members are legally and morally obligated to prevent participation by a colleague who is impaired by alcohol or drugs or who is incompetent in any way. Legally, team members are accountable for what they know. The facility can be liable for not taking action on substantial information about the performance of an employee or physician. Signs and symptoms of impairment should be carefully and objectively documented with specific incidents. Most institutions have a form for documenting irregular events, and it is advisable to use this form for continuity of information and ease of flow through the chain of command.

Chemical dependency is a self-destructive behavior. Therefore the team members should be concerned not only for the patient but also for the impaired team member. Treatment programs are available to assist an impaired professional. After the documentation is carefully evaluated, the impaired professional is confronted by his or her superiors. He or she is given the opportunity to enter a treatment program, followed by a period of routine care after returning to the job. An impaired individual can be barred from practice by the state licensing board. A license to practice may be revoked or suspended for an act committed while impaired.

Working Conditions

The perioperative environment should be safe for both patients and personnel. Instruments and equipment should be used properly and maintained in good working condition. Broken instruments and malfunctioning equipment should be removed from the area, marked to prevent further use, and reported to the appropriate persons. The equipment should be sent for repair or replacement. The surgeon may need to be notified that a piece of equipment he or she routinely uses is unavailable.

The Occupational Safety and Health Act became public law in 1970. Under this law, the Department of Labor created the Occupational Safety and Health Administration (OSHA). The major purpose of OSHA is to ensure safe and healthful working conditions for employees. Both personnel and patients benefit when the frequency of work-related injuries and illnesses is reduced and when the facility is made as safe as possible. OSHA regulations and other personnel safety measures are discussed in detail in Chapter 13.

The perioperative environment is a high-risk area with respect to employee safety. Obvious hazards to the physical well-being of any employee should be brought to the attention of the nurse manager. If an employer fails to correct a condition that an employee believes is in violation of a safety or health standard, is physically harmful, or presents an imminent danger, the employee may request an inspection by an OSHA compliance officer.

Sexual Harassment

Members of the health care team have the right to work in an environment free from sexual hostility, coercion, and ha-

rassment. Accusations of sexual impropriety should be studied in terms of human behavior and how it is perceived by others. No two situations are alike. Feelings of harassment are very subjective and may be interpreted by others as insignificant. The caregiver who thinks that another person in the work environment is making sexual advances or uncomfortable innuendoes should document specific incidents by describing the event or the exchange of conversation and the circumstances surrounding the occurrence. The names of witnesses should be included in the report. Documentation should be processed through the chain of command. If the harassment involves a superior, the documentation may be given to the person at the next higher level above the accused offender. A copy of all reports should be retained in the caregiver's personal file at home.

According to Title VII of the Civil Rights Act of 1964 and the Equal Employment Opportunity Commission (EEOC) in 1980, sexual harassment is a barrier to employment. It is illegal and is prosecutable by law. No caregiver at any level of the chain of command should tolerate this type of behavior; no offender is exempt from prosecution. The employer may also be held responsible. This is particularly true when an employer is made aware of the situation but does nothing to remedy the problem.

IMPORTANCE OF STANDARDIZATION

Perioperative patient care personnel should be able to cope with all situations and to give patients the best of their skills and knowledge. Although the use of different techniques may achieve the same results, each hospital establishes policies and procedures for all personnel to follow based on standards, recommended practices, and guidelines developed by professional organizations. These written guidelines help prevent confusion and foster coordination of activities. Uniform procedures performed without deviation help personnel to develop skill and efficiency for the following reasons:

- The main purpose is to ensure the safety and welfare of the patient and personnel.
- It is easier for the perioperative educator and preceptors to teach learners consistent methods of patient care.
- Learning is easier if everyone performs procedures in the same way.
- Deviations show a need for evaluation of the procedures or the staff. Do the procedures need revision?
- Uniform procedures provide an efficient check during preparation for any surgical procedure.
- One person can take over for another at any time during the surgical procedure, if necessary, and know exactly where to find instruments and supplies.
- Routine procedures establish habits that increase speed in thought and action. Doing work in a certain way promotes a high level of proficiency.
- Knowing the standards allows intelligent decision making when a patient's condition requires modification of a routine.

All personnel involved in perioperative patient care should be thoroughly familiar not only with setups, policies, procedures, and surgeons' routines but also with equipment. Certain items and techniques for handling equipment are basic because comparable or identical equipment is used in all facilities. Efficiency is increased by knowledge of equipment and its use. Many items are used only during the surgical procedure; other items are returned to units with patients, and their use carries over to the care of patients there.

The following reference sources are useful in mastering and carrying out accepted procedures and techniques:

- *Standards of practice.* The nursing department establishes standards for appropriate patient care based on the standards developed by the American Nurses Association (ANA). Optimal standards of nursing practice guide the provision of patient care throughout the institution, and written policies and procedures reflect these standards. Institutional standards are based on standards established at national levels by the Joint Commission on Accreditation of Healthcare Organizations (JCAHO); AORN, the Association of periOperative Registered Nurses; the Association of Surgical Technologists (AST); ANA; other nursing organizations; and governmental agencies. Nurses should practice within the limitations of the Nurse Practice Act of the state in which they are licensed and practice. Copies of these documents are available for review from the nursing or hospital administration.
- *Hospital policy manual.* This manual contains basic and general administrative and patient care policies that apply to all hospital personnel. A copy is retained on each patient care unit and in all departments of the hospital.
- *Safety plan manual.* The potential hazards and identifiable situations that may cause injury to a caregiver or patient are described in the manual provided by the hospital safety committee. Plans for fire drills and evacuation routes are outlined.
- *Material safety data sheets (MSDSs).* These sheets describe chemicals used in the workplace and actions to take if they are spilled into the environment. Specific cleanup and disposal methods are outlined.
- *Disaster plan manual.* This manual outlines the plans for both internal and external disasters. An internal disaster is an event that happens within the facility (e.g., an explosion or a fire) and requires employee assistance for control of the situation and evacuation of personnel and patients. An external disaster is an event that happens outside the confines of the facility. An external disaster could be a natural phenomenon such as an earthquake or an accident such as a train wreck. Both events can cause injury to many people and require the activation of all services within the hospital in a short period. Personnel who are off duty will be called to work and assigned as needed.
- *Infection control manual.* This manual contains the policies and procedures designed to minimize the risk of infection and control the spread of disease within the health care facility. It includes state, local, federal, and professional standards for the protection of the patient and the caregiver.
- *Perioperative policy and procedure manual.* This manual, usually a hardcover ringed binder, contains the policies pertaining solely to the administration and operation of the perioperative environment. A copy is available for reference in the manager's office, at the control desk, or in both places. The primary purpose of the perioperative policy and procedure manual is to detail why and how procedures should be specifically performed within the perioperative environment. It includes both supportive procedures and procedures that involve direct perioperative patient care.
- *Orientation manual.* The orientation manual is designed to acquaint personnel with the environment, policies, and procedures specific to performance and the position descriptions of all personnel in the department.
- *Instrument book.* The instruments required for each surgical procedure may be listed in a separate book that is kept in the instrument room or processing area. Photographs or catalog illustrations help learners identify the vast number of instruments used.
- *Surgeon's preference cards/case cart sheet.* A preference card is maintained for each surgical procedure that each surgeon performs. The surgeon's specific preferences and any variance from the procedures in the procedure book are noted on these cards. The cards are revised as procedures and personal preferences for new technology change. A set of these cards is kept readily available in a central file or in a computer under the surgeon's name, and they are pulled for each day's surgical procedures. In preparing for each surgical procedure, nurses and surgical technologists consult both these cards and the procedure book. A surgical central supply department may use these cards to pack a case cart for each individual procedure. Figure 3-1 shows a sample case cart sheet using the surgeon's preference card.
- *Directories.* Alphabetic listings of the location of supplies and equipment are maintained for the instrument room, general workroom, sterile supply room, and general perioperative storage areas. Regardless of where the storage areas are located, personnel should know the location of supplies and equipment. Directories save time in trying to locate items.

CONTINUOUS QUALITY IMPROVEMENT (CQI)

Quality is a difficult concept to define, measure, and evaluate. Some elements of quality are listed in Box 3-4. Nursing research and experience have shown that quality cannot be ensured, only monitored and improved. JCAHO has adopted a definition of quality as "continual improvement" in patient care services to increase the probability of

Surgeon: Dr. Jay Finch	**Procedure:** D & C	**Patient:** Robin Byrd, age 34
Gloves: 8 nonallergic	**Prep:** Betadine kit	**Drapes:** Lithotomy pack
Positioning devices: Sling stirrups	**Suture:** None	**Sponges:** Raytec 4 × 4s

Instruments: D & C set
  Speculum
	Other supplies: 2 specimen cups
	  Sanitary napkin
	  Water-soluble
	  lubricant
		Have available: Vaginal packing
		  2 specimen sheets
		  Russell curette

Special requests: Prefers to send endocervical and endometrial specimens in separate containers for patients over the age of 50.		**Notes:** Remember to document the last menstrual period on the specimen sheet. Make sure that the result of the preoperative pregnancy test is on the chart.

Figure 3-1   Contents of computer-generated case cart procedure supply sheet. These sheets are generated at the time the procedure is scheduled using standardized surgeon's preference cards and patient-specific needs.

Box 3-4	**Elements of Quality**

Q *Quality* improvement as an ongoing process
U *Understanding* regulations, standards, policies, and procedures that provide guidelines for acceptable practices
A *Accountability* for one's own actions
L *Legal* rights of patients
I *Individualized* patient care
T *Technical* competency
Y *Your* surgical and ethical conscience

expected patient outcomes and to reduce the probability of undesired outcomes. Outcomes can be defined, monitored, and measured. Patient satisfaction is one outcome measurement that is critical in evaluating quality. Satisfied patients are more cooperative and receptive to therapy and teaching.

AORN has operationally defined quality perioperative patient care as "professional nursing practice that encompasses components of analysis and interpretation."* These components include providing patient care within an environment conducive to effectiveness and efficiency, meeting patient needs in a caring manner and in conformity with established standards, and achieving desired outcomes or reducing the probability of undesired outcomes as perceived by the patient through properly implemented practices. These components imply that quality care focuses on the service provided to meet the identified needs of the patient and on the process of performing the necessary tasks to ensure safety and efficiency.

*Operational definition of perioperative patient care quality, *AORN J* 49(5):1303-1305, 1989.

Each patient deserves the best possible care. Without the structure provided by the nursing process, health care services would be fragmented, and accountability for the quality of services rendered would be made difficult. Society demands the accountability of those who provide patient care services. Patients are protected by laws, standards, and recommended practices. Performance of care should comply with established policies and procedures of the hospital or ambulatory care facility and with professional standards of practice. Nurses should see that all patient care procedures and techniques are correctly executed with patient outcomes kept in mind.

Performance Improvement Studies

Most studies are designed to measure compliance with current policies and procedures and to identify the need for change in practice guidelines or the need for education of staff. Both strengths and weaknesses in performance are identified. Ultimately the purpose is to correct deficiencies and deviations from expected standards. Important aspects that impact the quality of patient care are identified, and a measurable indicator is established for each aspect. Data are collected either concurrently or retrospectively and are organized for evaluation. Data sources and methods of data collection should be appropriate for each indicator. Sample size and the frequency of data collection should be sufficient to identify trends or patterns in the delivery of care. A sample size of 5% of the monitored patient population selected for study or 25 patients or events, whichever is greater, is usually adequate to obtain reliable data.

Data are collected either concurrently or retrospectively. A concurrent study begins with a current manifestation and links this effect to occurrences at the same time (i.e., is related to care in progress). Formerly referred to as a process audit, this type of study focuses on a systematic series of actions that

Box 3-5	Sentinel Event Samples Identified by JCAHO

Reportable	Nonreportable
Any event that results in the loss of life or limb (death, paralysis, coma)	Any near miss
Suicide of a patient in an around-the-clock care setting	Full return of limb or bodily function by discharge or within 2 weeks of the initial loss of function
Infant abduction or discharge to the wrong family	Medication errors that do not result in death or the permanent loss of function
Rape	Any sentinel event that has not affected the recipient of care
Hemolytic transfusion reaction involving the administration of blood or blood products having major blood group incompatibilities	A death or injury that follows discharge against medical advice (AMA)
Surgery on the wrong patient or the wrong body part	Unsuccessful suicide attempts
Intrapartum maternal death not related to the birth process	Unintentionally retained foreign body without permanent loss of function
A perinatal death unrelated to a congenital condition in an infant weighing more than 2500 g	Minor hemolysis with no clinical sequelae
Assault, homicide, or other crime resulting in patient death or a major permanent loss of function	
A fall that results in death or major permanent loss of function as a direct result of the injuries sustained	

Data from www.aarc.org/sentinel_examples.html.

brings about an outcome. Through concurrent observation, the implementation component of the nursing process can be monitored during perioperative patient care to determine whether interventions are consistent with established standards for care and recommended practices. The interventions performed should protect the welfare and safety of the patient and should meet his or her identified physiologic and psychologic needs. The environment, including equipment or supplies used in the room, can also be evaluated at this time.

A retrospective study focuses on the end result of patient care or on a measurable change in the actual state of the patient's health as a result of care received. This evaluation of outcomes usually occurs through review of patient records. The study begins with a current manifestation and links this effect to some occurrence in the past (i.e., care previously given). Complications attributable to care in the perioperative environment may be identified (e.g., nerve palsy from poor positioning, infiltration of an IV infusion, or postoperative wound infection). The source of these complications may be difficult to identify unless every detail of actual care given and any unusual occurrences are recorded in the patient's record. Accurate and complete documentation is therefore essential for meaningful retrospective studies.

Any method that systematically monitors and evaluates the quality of patient care can enable perioperative nurses and surgical technologists to take corrective action for improvement of performance. Quality improvement studies also assist in the coordination of plans for patient care with surgeons, improve communications with other departments, identify needs for revision of policies and procedures, and reassess equipment, personnel, and other aspects of patient care.

Peer Review

Peer review differs from other quality improvement programs in that it looks at the strengths and weaknesses of an

individual practitioner's performance rather than appraises the quality of care rendered by a group of professionals to a group of patients. An associate with the same role expectations and performance description examines and evaluates the clinical practice of a peer. The individual is evaluated by written standards of performance, and the review should offer constructive criticism of the performance observed. Through this framework, caregivers gain feedback for personal improvement or confirmation of personal achievement related to their effectiveness of professional, technical, and interpersonal skills in providing patient care.

SENTINEL EVENTS AND PERFORMANCE IMPROVEMENT

Professional accountability requires professionals to monitor performance as it applies to patient outcomes. The identification of an undesired outcome may be the result of direct or indirect actions of the caregiver. Such an outcome is referred to as a sentinel event—an unexpected event that involves a risk for or the occurrence of death or serious physical or psychologic injury. Serious injury specifically includes loss of limb or function.* The term *sentinel* was selected to represent the concept because the seriousness of the event requires immediate investigation and response. These events significantly impact patient outcomes; they should be evaluated for root cause, and a plan to prevent its occurrence should be prepared.

In 1998 JCAHO developed and approved a list of sentinel events that should be voluntarily reported and other events that need not be reported (Box 3-5). The JCAHO publication

*www.jacho.org/sentinel/se_pp.htm, November 1998.

Conducting a Root Cause Analysis in Response to a Sentinel Event has been made available to institutions as a guideline for investigating the causes of sentinel events. The objective is to improve the system that has permitted the error to occur. Guidelines include a fill-in-the-blank questionnaire to help track the cause of the event.

The guidelines suggested by JCAHO allow each facility flexibility in determining the root causes for events specific to the environment. Using flowcharts, the facility can identify one or more of these root causes. Each facility is encouraged but not required to report sentinel events to JCAHO. Other sources, such as the patient, a family member, or the media, may generate the report. If JCAHO becomes aware of an event, the facility is required to perform a root cause analysis and action plan or other approved protocol within 45 days of the event.

Bibliography

Aoki Y et al: Significance of informed consent and truth-telling for quality of life in terminal cancer patients, *Radiol Med* 15(2):133-135, 1997.

Billick SB et al: Competency to consent to hospitalization in the medical patient, *J Am Acad Psychiatry Law* 25(2):191-196, 1997.

Brazell NE: The significance and application of informed consent, *AORN J* 65(2):377-386, 1997.

Capen K: Harassment issues should be dealt with before they become problems, *Can Med Assoc J* 156(11):1577-1579, 1997.

Dillman JM: Substance abuse in the perioperative setting, *AORN J* 62(1):111-112 , 1995.

Fortunato NM: Abusive behavior in the perioperative setting, *AORN J* 64(3):451-453, 1996.

Goldman RL, Ciesco E: Improving peer review: alternatives to unstructured judgments by a single reviewer, *Joint Comm J Qual Improv* 22(11):762-769, 1996.

Hohler S et al: OR dream team: a continuous quality improvement project, *AORN J* 65(6):494-499, 1997.

Hughes TL, Smith LL: Is your colleague chemically dependent? *Am J Nurs* 94(9):30-35, 1994.

Kaye J: Sexual harassment and hostile environments in the perioperative area, *AORN J* 63(2):443-448, 1996.

Kuhn JE: A nurse's right to refuse a patient care assignment, *AORN J* 62(3):412-416, 1995.

Mailhot CB: Culture and consent, *Nurs Manage* 28(3):48P, 1997.

Niles PA, Mattice BJ: The timing factor in the consent process, *J Transplant Coord* 6(2):84-87, 1996.

Owen S: The patient's right to know, *AORN J* 61(5):864-866, 1995.

Pape T: Legal and ethical considerations of informed consent, *AORN J* 65(6):1122-1127, 1997.

Paradies M et al: Root cause analysis for sentinel events, *Infect Control Today* 2(3):49-51, 1998.

Porter F: Key concepts in informed consent for perioperative nurses, *AORN J* 65(6):1105-1110, 1997.

Power KJ: The legal and ethical implications of consent to nursing procedures, *Br J Nurs* 6(15):885-888, 1997.

Rempusheski VF et al: Peer review by nursing research committees in hospitals, *Image J Nurs Sch* 28(1):51-53, 1996.

Robbins I et al: Sexual harassment in nursing, *J Adv Nurs* 25(1):163-169, 1997.

Roper KA, Russell G: The effect of peer review on professionalism, autonomy, and accountability, *J Nurs Staff Dev* 13(4):198-206, 1997.

Rotenberg VS: To inform or not to inform: a decision with psychobiological implication, *Med Law* 16(1):49-52, 1997.

Speigel AD, Springer CR: Babylonian medicine, managed care and Codex Hammutabi, circa 1700 BC, *J Community Health* 22(1):69-89, 1997.

Susser M: Health as a human right: an epidemiologist's perspective on the public health, *Am J Pub Health* 83(3):418-426, 1993.

Verheggan FW, van Wijmen FC: Myth and reality of informed consent in clinical trials, *Med Law* 16(1):53-69, 1997.

Williams L et al: Consent to treatment by minors attending accident and emergency departments: guidelines, *J Accid Emerg Med* 14(5):286-289, 1997.

Chapter 4

Legal and Ethical Issues

 Chapter Objectives

After studying this chapter, the learner will be able to:

- Define negligence as it applies to caregivers.
- Discuss the difference between a standard and recommended practice.
- Identify three potential events that could lead to a lawsuit.

Competent patient care is the best way to avoid the dilemma of a malpractice claim. Unfortunately, even under the best of circumstances a patient may suffer an injury and recover monetary damages as compensation. Understanding how a malpractice claim starts and how it proceeds is important in the effort to avoid the many pitfalls that can lead to being named in a lawsuit. Select terms associated with legal and ethical issues are found in Box 4-1.

HISTORICAL BACKGROUND

The Code of Hammurabi (1955-1913 BC) included penalties for physicians/surgeons who did not cure, a schedule of acceptable fees, and organization for the delivery of medical treatment. Punishments were specified for infractions of the code.

The first recorded medical malpractice suit was tried in England in 1374. The first one in the United States occurred in 1794. Throughout the nineteenth century and the early part of the twentieth century, litigation against physicians was quite uncommon and rarely affected nurses. Malpractice suits began to increase markedly in the 1970s as an increasing number of people sought health care services and became aware of their humanitarian and consumer rights.

LEGAL ISSUES

Any caregiver can be named in a lawsuit. Regardless of who is in charge of the team, each team member is responsible for his or her own actions. When one is giving care within the scope of practice and according to facility policy and procedure, the risk of being named in a malpractice or negligence suit is very limited. Honest mistakes can result in patient injury. If a suit is brought to court, a jury can evaluate a reasonable set of circumstances, facts, and testimony to render a verdict in favor of the caregiver. The plaintiff does not always win. If the verdict is found in favor of the plaintiff, the damages awarded may be for compensatory award.

Along with the development of consumerism, a movement that focuses on consumer rights, a well-informed American public has developed an increasingly litigious attitude, demanding compensation for bodily injuries or damages to personal property. The quality of health care in this country is assessed through the outcome of services rendered. If the outcome is unacceptable, patients tend to take grievances to court. The severity of an injury usually determines whether a claim of merit will arise, but other contributing factors include a breakdown of rapport between the patient and the health care team members and unrealistic expectations about the outcome of care.

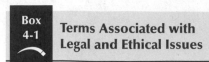

Box 4-1   Terms Associated with Legal and Ethical Issues

causation   Action directly or indirectly causing an injury.

damages   Compensation awarded to make restitution for an injury or a wrong.

defendant   Person named as the object of a lawsuit.

deposition   Statement given under oath that is a documentation of fact used in a court of law.

liability   Legally responsible for personal actions.

malpractice   Substandard delivery of care that results in harm.

negligence   Careless performance of duty.

plaintiff   Person who initiates a lawsuit.

tort   Wrong committed by one person against another; civil action.

Causes for litigation lie in patients' and their families' belief that physicians and/or health care organizations have not provided appropriate diagnosis, treatment, or results. Although the physician is professionally responsible for patient care, other patient care personnel act as part of the health care team, carrying responsibility for their own actions. Ancillary personnel and suppliers of equipment and drugs also are indirectly involved in treatment and may be held liable.

LIABILITY

To be liable is to be legally bound and responsible for personal actions that adversely affect another person. Every patient care provider should always carry out duties in accordance with standards and practice guidelines established by federal statutes, state practice acts, professional organizations, and regulatory agencies, as well as those that are common practice throughout the community. Deviation from these standards and practices that cause injury to a patient can result in liability for negligence or malpractice. For this type of civil suit to be successful for the plaintiff, he or she has to prove that negligent care or malpractice caused the injury.

Negligence is the failure to use the care or skills that any caregiver in the same or a similar situation would be expected to use. These acts of omission or commission that cause damage to a patient may give rise to tort action, which is a civil lawsuit.

Malpractice is any professional misconduct, unreasonable lack of skill or judgment, or illegal or immoral conduct. Malpractice and negligence claims usually are settled in a civil court, but, depending on the severity of the injury and the extent of the misconduct, they may be taken to criminal court. From the legal point of view of damages or fault, professional negligence usually is often synonymous with malpractice in a tort action. Factors contributing to a successful lawsuit on behalf of the plaintiff have been called the four *D's* of malpractice:

1. Duty to deliver a standard of care directly proportional to the degree of specialty training received

2. Deviation of that duty by omission or commission
3. Damage to a patient or personal property caused by the deviation from the standard of care
4. Direct cause of a personal injury or damage because of deviation of duty

Statutory laws (laws by legislation) and common laws (laws based on court decisions) differ from state to state. Courts differ at times in their interpretation of laws. Any caregiver who is in some manner thought to be responsible for injury to a patient may be sued. The nurse manager or clinical educator responsible for assigning duties to this individual may be included in the suit. Caregivers, such as nurses and technicians, are considered employees of the health care facility, and, if the court so rules, the facility is considered liable. The court may rule that a learner or an experienced practitioner is liable for his or her own acts. A learner may be held responsible in proportion to the amount and type of instruction received and judged by the standard of other learners in training. Any person giving patient care can be named as a defendant in a lawsuit. When in doubt about personal competency for a new or unfamiliar procedure, seek guidance from the clinical educator or immediate supervisor.

Medical care and professional liability have become institutional problems. The primary cause of professional liability claims is iatrogenic medical injury, an injury or other adverse outcome sustained by a patient as a result of treatment. Many incidents in the perioperative environment have been causes for a lawsuit.

Borrowed Servant Rule

In the past, the surgeon was considered the captain of the ship in the perioperative environment. If the surgeon had supervisory control and the right to give orders during the surgical procedure, then the operating room (OR) was like a ship and the surgeon like its captain. The captain, or master, was liable for the negligent acts of servants. Courts held that this doctrine, based on the master-servant relationship, was applicable by the mere presence of the surgeon. Once having entered the OR, the surgeon was considered to have complete control over other team members. Courts now recognize that the surgeon does not have complete control over the acts of the perioperative patient care team. The surgeon usually is not held responsible when a perioperative caregiver fails to carry out a routine procedure as expected. Courts have decided that certain procedures do not need to be supervised by the surgeon. According to the borrowed servant rule, the surgeon is liable for acts of team members only when he or she has the right to control and supervise the way in which a perioperative caregiver performs the task.

Independent Contractor

The employer may be held responsible for employees under the master-servant rule. However, the current trend is to hold an individual responsible for his or her own acts under the principle of the independent contractor. For example, a private scrub person, biomedical technologist, or first assistant may contract with several surgeons to provide services on a fee-for-service basis. These individuals are not directly employed by the facility but are usually credentialed by the medical staff department. Some questions may arise concerning the level of responsibility of the facility for credentialing someone who is accused of substandard practice. The facility will be named in the suit but may be dropped at a later date.

Doctrine of the Reasonable Man

A patient has the right to expect that all patient care personnel will use knowledge, skill, and judgment in performing duties that meet standards exercised by other reasonably prudent persons involved in similar circumstances.

Doctrine of *Res Ipsa Loquitor*

Translated from Latin, *res ipsa loquitor* means *the thing speaks for itself.* Under this doctrine, the courts allow the patient's injury to stand as inference of negligence. The defendant has to prove that he or she did not act negligently. Before this doctrine can be applied, three conditions must exist:

1. The type of injury would not ordinarily occur without a negligent act.
2. The injury was caused by the conduct or instrumentality within the exclusive control of the person or persons being sued.
3. The injured person could not have contributed to negligence or voluntarily assumed risk.

This doctrine applies to injuries sustained by the patient while in the perioperative environment, such as a retained foreign object (e.g., sponge, towel, needle, or other instrument), a fall, or a burn. The defendant must prove that a breach did not occur and that he or she was not negligent.

Doctrine of *Respondeat Superior*

An employer may be liable for an employee's negligent conduct under the *respondeat superior* master-servant employment relationship. This implies that the master will answer for the acts of a servant. If a patient is injured as a result of an employee's negligent act within the scope of that employment, the employer is responsible to the injured patient. The patient may name both the facility and the employee in a civil suit, but the employee may be dropped from the suit if he or she was following facility policy and procedure and acting within the appropriate scope of practice.

Doctrine of Corporate Negligence

Under the corporate negligence doctrine, the facility may be liable, not for the negligence of employees, but for its own negligence in failing to ensure that an acceptable level of care is provided. A hospital has a duty to provide services and is responsible for the following:

- Screening and verifying qualifications of staff members, including medical staff, according to standards established by the Joint Commission on Accreditation of Healthcare Organizations (JCAHO)
- Monitoring and reviewing performance and competency of staff members through established personnel appraisal and peer review procedures
- Maintaining a competent staff of physicians and other caregivers
- Revoking practice privileges of a physician and other caregivers when the administration knows or should have known that the individual is incompetent or impaired

Doctrine of Informed Consent

State statutes differ in their interpretation of the doctrine of informed consent, but all recognize the physician's duty to inform the patient of the risks, benefits, and alternatives of a procedure and to obtain consent before treatment. Failure to do so may be considered a breach of duty. A surgeon or anesthesia provider may be held liable for negligence if the patient can prove failure to disclose significant information that would have influenced a reasonable person's decision to consent. Informed consent is a protective act for the patient and the treating physician and should be documented appropriately. Informed consent is also discussed in Chapter 3 as a professional obligation.

Extension Doctrine

If the surgeon goes beyond the limits to which the patient consented, liability for assault and battery may be charged. This doctrine implies that the patient's explicit consent for a surgical procedure serves as an implicit consent for any or all procedures deemed necessary to cope with unpredictable situations that jeopardize the patient's health. By medical necessity and sound judgment, the surgeon may perform a different or an additional surgical procedure when unexpected conditions are encountered during the course of an authorized surgical procedure. The surgeon may extend the surgical procedure to correct or remove any abnormal or pathologic condition under the extension doctrine. The court will determine whether the patient consented to a specific procedure or generally to surgical treatment of a health problem.

Assault and Battery

In legal terms, assault is an unlawful threat to harm another physically. Battery is the carrying out of bodily harm, as by touching without authorization or consent. Lack of consent is an important aspect of an assault-and-battery charge. Consent must be given voluntarily with full understanding of implications. The purposes of a written, signed, and witnessed consent are to protect the surgeon, anesthesia provider, perioperative team members, and facility from claims of unauthorized procedures and to protect the patient from unsanctioned procedures.

Invasion of Privacy

The patient's right to privacy exists by statutory or common law. The patient's chart, medical record, videotapes, x-ray films, and photographs are considered confidential information for use by physicians and other health care personnel directly concerned with that patient's care. The patient should give written consent for videotaping or photographing his or her surgical procedure for medical education or research. The patient has the right to refuse photographic consent.

The patient has the right to expect that all communications and records pertaining to individualized care will be treated as confidential and will not be misused. This includes the right to privacy during interview, examination, and treatment. The surgery schedule bearing the names of the patients should not be posted in a location where the public or other patients can read it. Some patients, such as celebrities, may request to be admitted with an alias. Care is taken when identifying these patients so that they will not be confused with other patients and receive the wrong procedure. Community hospitals may be admitting persons from the surrounding neighborhood. The caregiver may be in a position to learn private information about a neighbor. Maintaining the confidentiality of patient information is imperative. Every health care worker has a moral obligation to hold in confidence any personal or family affairs learned from patients.

Patients who are part of a criminal investigation have rights. Victims and perpetrators both have the right of privacy and should not have information provided to the news media or other persons without express permission from the law enforcement agency in charge of the investigation. Information discovered by health care personnel during the course of care should be reported to the immediate supervisor in charge, who should in turn arrange for the information to be relayed to the authorities as soon as possible. Personnel are advised not to promise secrecy to a patient involved in some way with a suspected crime.

Abandonment

Abandonment consists of leaving the patient for any reason when the patient's condition is contingent on the presence of the caregiver. If the caregiver leaves the room knowing there is a potential need for care during his or her absence, even under the order of a physician, the caregiver is liable for his or her own actions.

In *Czubinsky v. Doctor's Hospital,* the surgeon ordered the circulating nurse to leave the room to help him start another procedure. During the circulating nurse's absence, the patient had a cardiac arrest. The only team members on hand were the anesthesia provider and the surgical technologist. At the trial the circulating nurse admitted to knowing that it was wrong to leave the patient, because of his condition, but left because of the surgeon's insistence. The expert witness testi-

fied that the circulator should not have been ordered away from the patient to work in another room. The court decided that if adequate help for resuscitation had been available in the OR during the patient's crisis, he would not have suffered permanent brain damage. According to the court, the circulating nurse had a duty to remain with the patient. This breach of duty resulted in permanent brain damage.

If an event necessitates leaving a patient, it is important to transfer care to another caregiver of equal status and function. In uncontrollable circumstances, the perioperative manager should be consulted immediately. The patient must not be left unattended. No one, not even a physician, may release a caregiver from a responsibility to a patient. A child or disoriented patient left alone or unguarded in a holding area, for example, may sustain injury by an electric shock from a nearby outlet or by some other hazard within reach. The circulator may be considered negligent by reason of abandonment for failure to monitor a patient in the OR. The circulator should be in attendance during induction of and emergence from anesthesia and throughout the surgical procedure to assist as needed.

Liability Insurance

Formerly it was thought that patients did not sue nurses and other patient care providers because they had no large assets. Unfortunately, this is no longer true. Increased autonomy increases the risk for liability. Perioperative nurses make independent nursing decisions based on their assessments, and they are able to carry out and/or delegate certain patient care interventions without a physician's order. No matter how careful the caregiver is, mistakes can happen. An unintentional wrong may cause injury to a patient. Most institutions carry insurance policies to cover incidents that result in harm to a patient when the event happens within the scope of institutional policies and procedures. In some instances the insurance may not adequately cover all of the expenses associated with a lawsuit.

The caregiver who accidentally caused the injury may be named in the suit as an individual or as a codefendant. The hospital liability may pay the lawyer's fees and damage awards but not lost wages incurred by deposition and court appearances. Carrying personal malpractice insurance protects against a possible discrepancy with the hospital's insurance coverage. A personal liability policy can be individualized to meet the practice of the insured. The policy costs are tax deductible, and the protection of personal assets and wages may well be worth the price of the coverage. Professional associations recommend individual professional liability insurance.

Liability Prevention for the Perioperative Team

Complex technologies, acuity of hospitalized patients' conditions, short-stay procedures, diverse roles of providers, staffing inadequacies, and other factors present challenges in managing risks of liability. Many surgeons restrict their practices to avoid patients who have complex diseases or who are at high risk of uncertain outcomes. Others practice defensive medicine, ordering tests principally to protect themselves against possible litigation. As lawyers have become increasingly sophisticated in representing injured patients, all health care providers need to take measures to protect themselves from litigation. A preventive strategy includes the following:

1. Become active within the professional organizations associated with setting the standards for practice. Most organizations provide up-to-date education and resources for improvement of practice. Have a voice in shaping the future of the profession.
2. Remain current with continuing education. Become certified.
3. Establish positive rapport with patients. Patients are less likely to sue if they perceive that they were treated with respect, dignity, and sincere concern. Patients expect information and good communication.
4. Comply with the legal statutes and standards of accrediting agencies, professional associations, and the health care facility.
5. Document assessments, interventions, and evaluations of patient care outcomes. Leave a paper trail that is easy to follow for the reconstruction of the event in question.
6. Prevent injuries by adhering to policies and procedures.
7. Control further insult or damage if an injury occurs by reporting problems and taking corrective action.
8. Maintain good communications with other team members.

In addition to these strategies, the institution or ambulatory care facility as the employer and the caregiver as the employee should take steps to avoid malpractice liability. A health care facility protects the patient, its personnel, and itself by maintaining good working conditions for a competent staff. Perioperative team members are hired after careful screening of educational preparation and licensure or certification credentials. The staff should be adequate in size, as well as properly trained and assigned. A continuous program of staff orientation and education should be provided. Policies and procedures are established in a manner consistent with standards for competent performance and patient safety.

DOCUMENTATION OF PATIENT CARE

Verbal communication between patients and health care providers does not constitute legal evidence in a court of law. Only the patient's medical records are legal evidence of care received or omitted. Entries by nurses and physicians in the record provide a history of the patient's clinical course and responses to treatment. The record identifies what occurred and what did not. It also serves as a means of communication between providers during the course of treatment for continuity of care. Deficiencies in the record can destroy the cred-

ibility of the record and of the providers. Policies and procedures should be in place for documentation. Each patient care facility is responsible for the following:

- Establishing, evaluating, and enforcing policies and procedures for patient care documentation
- Interpreting and outlining standards for care documentation in accordance with accreditation guidelines
- Protecting the privacy of patients by limiting unauthorized access and use of documented patient care data and reports
- Creating forms and charting formats for personnel to use in hard copy documentation
- Selecting protocol for computerized archives of patient care records and reports
- Providing a mechanism for retrieval of archived patient care records and reports for reference in a timely manner for routine or emergency care

The professional perioperative nursing role includes preoperative patient assessment and teaching, as well as postoperative evaluation of intraoperative care and reinforcement of preoperative teaching. All interactions with patients should be documented in the patient's chart, either in the nurses' notes or in the progress notes. The format for recording varies from institution to institution. Regardless of the format of the patient's record, all entries should be:

1. Documented on the appropriate form (code sheet, perioperative record, medication sheet, progress note). A scrap of paper without the patient's name stamped on it may get lost or discarded by accident.
2. Written legibly in ink without erasures. The charting procedure may be specific (e.g., all entries are to be made in black ink).
3. Stated factually. Documentation of objective data and services rendered should be very specific. Observations and actions should be stated definitively, objectively, and concisely. Record what is seen, heard, felt, or smelled (i.e., the facts without judgment or opinion). Write quotes of the patient's subjective expression.
4. Stated in understandable terminology. Abbreviations may be permissible only for very commonly accepted medical terms, such as T&A, D&C, OD, and TUR. Most institutions provide a standard list of their accepted medical abbreviations for charting purposes.
5. Dated (month, day, year), including the time (AM/PM) the note is written and the time action was performed as appropriate for significant events or changes in the patient's condition. Late entries are documented as per facility policy.
6. Signed with the full legal signature, title, and status of the writer.
7. Corrected if an error is made. The date, time, and initials of the person making a correction should be noted next to the correction. A single line should be drawn through incorrect information without obliterating it (the mistake should not be scribbled out or erased), and

the correct information should then be entered. White-out correction fluid is not acceptable.

Additional documentation in the patient's record should include the following:

- Execution of the physician's orders and the patient's responses
- Any teaching of the patient or family, including how he, she, or they indicated understanding
- Any unusual event, such as a fall, spontaneous change in condition, or injury
- Any and all visitors, especially physicians
- Any notification of physicians or supervisors

The perioperative nurse should be alert to signs that a patient does not clearly understand what is going to happen as a result of surgical intervention. This should be documented and brought to the attention of the surgeon. Significant observations should be recorded in the chart. For example, if a patient verbally withdraws consent for a surgical procedure or expresses a fear of death in the OR, the perioperative nurse is responsible for communicating this information to the surgeon and anesthesia provider, and for recording the patient's statement.

Standards for Patient Care Documentation

The standards for patient care documentation are established by the American Nurses Association (ANA) and JCAHO. The national standard of care requires that patient care documentation reflect the application of the nursing process (assessment, nursing diagnosis, outcome identification, planning, intervention, and evaluation) during the entire length of stay, according to ANA and JCAHO.

Individualized Documentation of the Nursing Process

Assessment

The assessment involves documented objective and subjective health conditions or attributes that are identified using several appropriate techniques. It involves the patient, significant others, and additional caregivers. This part of the nursing process is systematic and ongoing and includes the following:

- Physiologic data
- Psychologic data

Nursing Diagnosis

The nursing diagnosis is a documented defining characteristic of a problem, need, or other health consideration as identified by the North American Nursing Diagnosis Association (NANDA). These diagnoses are based on functional health patterns. This facilitates the identification of expected outcomes and the formulation of the plan of care. These diagnoses are derived from the assessment data and grouped in functional health patterns as described by Gordon. The 1989 NANDA taxonomy of Human Response Patterns sys-

tematically classifies the nursing diagnosis as the base upon which to organize assessment data into clearly defined patient-specific diagnoses. This provides individualization of care.

Gordon's Functional Health Patterns

- Health perception/health management. *Examples:* Risks for injury, health maintenance, compliance
- Nutritional/metabolic. *Examples:* Fluid volume, body requirement, temperature regulation, tissue perfusion, biologic process
- Elimination. *Examples:* Bowel, bladder, continence
- Activity/exercise. *Examples:* Behaviors, mobility
- Sleep/rest. *Examples:* Requirements, patterns
- Cognitive/perceptual. *Examples:* Confusion, verbalization, knowledge
- Self-perception/self-concept. *Examples:* Fear, anxiety, self-esteem
- Role/relationship. *Examples:* Communication, parenting, interaction
- Sexuality/reproductive. *Examples:* Dysfunction, sexual patterns, fertility
- Coping/stress tolerance. *Examples:* Adjustment, adaptation, self-harm
- Value/belief. *Examples:* Spirituality, ritual observance

NANDA Human Response Patterns

- Choosing: To select between alternatives
- Communicating: To transmit or impart thoughts and feelings
- Exchanging: To give and take in return
- Feeling: To consciously experience or sense
- Knowing: To recognize or acknowledge through cognitive activity
- Moving: To change body position, take action
- Perceiving: To apprehend with the mind
- Relating: To connect or link with a person or thing
- Valuing: To take concern with worth and usefulness

Outcome Identification

Outcome identification involves documented expected end results of patient care that are identified using nursing diagnoses. The outcomes are realistic, measurable, and established in collaboration with the patient, significant others, and other caregivers. Reasonable time elements are defined.

Plan

The plan is documented evidence of a course of action for patient care derived from assessment data, nursing diagnoses, and outcome identification. The plan of care is individualized, is based on current nursing practice, and provides for continuity of care.

Implementation

Implementation involves the documentation of activation of the plan of care. Interventions are safe, appropriate, and follow the plan of care.

Evaluation

Evaluation is the documentation of the attainment of expected outcomes, the effectiveness of the plan of care, the mode of intervention, and modification to the plan according to the patient's individualized requirements. Revision is demonstrated as a dynamic to validate changes in patient status.

Charting Modalities

Many ways of recording patient care information have been used over the years. Changes in technology have created more methods of recording patient care. For example:

- *Narrative charting.* Expository writing about significant events using third-person commentary, quotes, and standard abbreviations. Entries are sequential, timed, dated, and signed.
- *Block charting.* Short commentary on activity that resembles narrative charting covering a larger period of several hours or days. Entries are sequential, timed, dated, and signed.
- *Focus charting.* Specific documentation directed at a designated aspect of the patient's needs, status, or health considerations.
- *Subjective-objective (SOAP) charting.* Multidisciplinary approach to documenting care according to cues given by a patient with a specific set of signs and symptoms. This approach uses direct quotes and assessment data.
- *Problem-oriented charting.* Approach using a problem list as the working element from which care is planned. Working from the list, patient priorities are investigated, diagnosed, treated, minimized, solved, or remain ongoing. As problems are solved, they are stricken from the list.
- *Computer-generated charting.* Use of standardized care plans formulated in the computer and modified for the individual patient. The computer time and date stamps

the plan as it is printed for the hard copy record. This form of charting requires the caregiver's signature.
- *Computer software programs, check-off forms, and flow sheets.* Commonly used as shortcuts for record keeping. Unfortunately, it is easy to rely on the standardized data on these preprinted records and inadvertently omit potentially important individualized information.

Computerized Documentation

Many facilities have been using computers for patient admitting, billing, scheduling, and human resource information for several decades. Within the past 15 years patient data have been recorded and stored electronically at the division level. Personnel permitted to access this information are few in number and must log on using employee identification and passwords to enter the computer system. Passwords are changed at routine intervals. Retrievable data recorded and accumulated in these electronic files include patient care information, laboratory results, surgical reports, admission and discharge summaries, and many highly sensitive details about a patient's financial status. Nurses charged with the responsibility of accessing and contributing to computerized patient data should be aware that security and confidentiality must be protected. Maintaining the secrecy of passwords and logging off after use are common problems identified with unauthorized access. Some systems have a built-in log-off feature if the workstation is left idle for a prolonged period of time. If this happens, the user has to reenter the system by logging back on. Pros and cons of computerized documentation are listed in Box 4-2.

Perioperative Nurses' Notes

Specific care given in the perioperative environment should be documented on the patient's chart, not only for legal reasons, but also for the benefit of continuity of care. Most

Box 4-2	Pros and Cons of Computerized Documentation	

Pros	Cons
Useful for accumulation of data from many sources	Can be confusing for inexperienced users
Data retrieval is easier and efficient	Failure to log off can leave system available to unauthorized use
Information is legible and in standard terminology	Can be out of service for undetermined periods of time
Uses standardized formats, flow charts, and graphs	Needs periodic maintenance and software updates
Each entry and printing is time and date stamped	Backups of files are needed in case of failure
Can minimize error if physicians record orders online	Paper records must be kept when system is down
Data can be transferred between physician's office and care facility via fax	Impersonal interaction between patient and caregivers
Record updating is more timely and ongoing	Preoutlined care plans are less individualized
Can save time, space, and resources	Hardware and software can be costly to install
Easier to retrieve archived charts from previous admissions	Potential for breach of security if files are transferred on-line
Health care organizations with multiple remote sites can transfer patient data on-line	

facilities use a preprinted form with a standardized plan of care. Space is provided to add individualized patient needs and to document unusual interventions. Expected outcomes should be specified (e.g., that the patient is free from injury). The specific nursing interventions performed to achieve these outcomes and to protect the patient should be accurately and completely documented by the perioperative nurse. This information should include, but not be limited to, the following:

- Preoperative history, physical examination, laboratory reports, consent form, and other documents in the chart per institutional policy
- Patient identification and verification of the surgical site, informed consent, allergies, and NPO (nothing by mouth) status
- Significant intraoperative times, such as arrival in and departure from the OR, anesthesia start and finish, and incision and closure
- Patient's condition on transfer to and from the OR, as well as the method of transport to and from the OR, and by whom
- Level of consciousness or anxiety manifested by observable physical responses
- Patient position, and types of restraints and supports used for maintaining the patient's position on the OR bed and for protecting pressure areas, and by whom
- Personal property disposition, such as religious articles, hearing aid, eyeglasses, and dentures
- Skin condition and antimicrobials used for skin preparation, and by whom
- Location of electrosurgical dispersive electrode and monitoring devices
- Intravenous (IV) site, time started, type of needle or cannula, solutions administered IV (including blood products), and by whom
- Medication types and amounts (including local anesthetic agents), irrigating solutions used, and by whom
- Tourniquet cuff location, pressure, inflation duration, identification of unit, and applied by whom
- Estimated blood loss and urinary output, as appropriate
- Sponge, sharps, and instrument counts as correct or incorrect
- Surgical procedure performed, location of the incision, special equipment used (such as a laser), and prosthetic devices implanted, if applicable, including the manufacturer and lot/serial number
- Specimens and cultures sent to the laboratory
- Site and types of drains, catheters, and packing as applicable
- Wound classification
- Type of dressing applied
- Any unusual event or complication, and action performed
- All personnel in the room and their roles, including physicians, visitors, sales personnel, students, and others as applicable

Incident Report

An injury may occur to a patient or a caregiver during a surgical procedure. The injury may be caused by a lack of ordinary care, unintentional mishap, or equipment failure. When an accident or unusual incident occurs, whether or not it involves an injury, the factual details should be reported to the nurse manager and documented according to institutional policy. Details should be complete and accurate. They should be written as statements of facts without interpretation or opinion. For example, it should be stated that the area of the patient's skin under the inactive dispersive electrode of the electrosurgical unit was mottled and red when the electrode was removed, rather than that the patient's skin appeared burned by the dispersive electrode. The details of equipment used, including the serial number or asset tag identification of the generator and the lot number of the electrode, should be included. The action performed and care or treatment given as a result of accidental injury should be described. The equipment in question should be removed from service and tagged as out of order. The device should be inspected and approved for use according to institutional policy before it is returned to service.

Incident reports are completed per policy and retained by the risk management department. They should be reviewed as part of the overall institution and departmental quality improvement and risk management programs. Incident reports are considered work products and constitute privileged information. They may serve to refresh an individual's memory of events, however, for preparation of defense in a lawsuit. The fact that an incident report was completed should not be documented in the patient's permanent record. Examples of situations that require incident reporting are included in Box 4-3.

Benefits of Documentation to the Facility

There are many reasons for accurate documentation other than those for legal application. Some facilities use the data for strategic planning and growth of the organization. Bene-

---

Box 4-3	**Unusual Situations That Require Incident Reporting**

Falls or unexpectedly finding a patient, visitor, or other personnel lying on the floor
Injury to patient, visitor, or other personnel
Needle sticks
Any fire or smoke event
Possible theft or loss of an item
Malfunctioning equipment
Intruder or unauthorized personnel
Medication error
Medication reaction
Lost sponge or instrument during a procedure (incorrect count)
Object retained within patient

fits of accurate documentation to the facility include, but are not limited to, the following:

- Legal permanent record
- Billing and reimbursement
- Continuous quality improvement (CQI)
- Budget and financial planning
- Staffing ratios
- Research protocol
- Utilization review
- Risk management
- Patient acuity and census

STANDARDS OF CARE

A standard is an authoritative statement established by a professional organization or a regulatory agency. Standards established by professional organizations are broad in scope, relevant, attainable, and definitive. They outline for both the practitioner and the consumer/public what the quality of health care should be. They are the criteria used to evaluate competency in providing patient care. A standard of care is defined as those acts that a reasonably prudent person with comparable training and experience would perform under the same or similar circumstances. Professional standards delineate activities related to performance, quality improvement, continuing education, ethical behavior, and accountability.

Standards established by governmental regulatory agencies that are mandated by law are to be complied with. Those established by national professional associations are recognized norms. Although compliance may be voluntary, compliance should be attained. Perioperative standards of practice include professional and regulated standards.

Professional/Voluntary Standards

1. *Standards of Perioperative Nursing.* These standards, which originated as ANA standards of OR practice in 1975, were approved by ANA and by AORN, the Association of periOperative Registered Nurses, and published in 1981.
   a. *Standards of Perioperative Administrative Nursing Practice.* These are structural standards that provide a framework for establishing administrative practices.
   b. *Standards of Perioperative Clinical Practice.* These are process standards based on problem-solving techniques using principles and theories of biophysical and behavioral sciences. They describe how the nursing process is used.
   c. *Standards of Perioperative Professional Performance.* These are process standards that describe a competent level of behavior for the professional role of the perioperative nurse. The activities relate to quality practice performance appraisal, continuing education, collegial relations, ethical conduct, and use of resources and research.
   d. *Quality Improvement Standards for Perioperative Nursing.* These are process standards to assist in the development of quality improvement programs to monitor and evaluate the quality of patient care.
   e. *Patient Outcomes: Standards of Perioperative Care.* These are outcome standards that reflect desired observable patient outcomes during preoperative, intraoperative, and postoperative phases of the patient's surgical experience. They focus on common potential problems of patients undergoing surgical, diagnostic, or therapeutic intervention.

These five sets of standards for an optimal level of perioperative nursing practice are published in *AORN Standards and Recommended Practices for Perioperative Nursing.** The Operating Room Nurses Association of Canada has published *Recommended Standards for Operating Room Nursing Practice and Quality Assurance Audit.*

2. *Association of Surgical Technologists Standards of Practice.*† These are process standards that provide guidelines for safe and effective patient care in appropriate preoperative, intraoperative, and postoperative practice settings. They include interpersonal skills, environmental safety, and application of principles of surgical technology.
3. *JCAHO standards.* These standards, published in the *Accreditation Manual for Hospitals,*‡ are functional, performance-based standards that focus on actual clinical care provided directly to patients and on management of the health care organization providing services. They relate to efficiency, effectiveness, safety, and timeliness; to appropriateness, continuity, and availability of care; and to patient satisfaction. JCAHO evaluates compliance with these standards and reviews clinical outcomes of care provided as fundamental criteria for accreditation. Selective clinical indicators serve as outcome measurements for the processes of patient care.
4. *National Fire Protection Association (NFPA) standards.*§ These standards apply to environmental safety to reduce to the extent possible, hazards to patients and personnel.
5. *Association for the Advancement of Medical Instrumentation (AAMI) device standards.*¶ These standards provide industry with reference documents on accepted levels of device safety and performance and test methods to deter-

---

*Published by the Association of periOperative Registered Nurses, Inc., 2170 S. Parker Road, Suite 300, Denver, CO 80231-5711.
†Published by the Association of Surgical Technologists, Inc., 7108-C S. Alton Way, Englewood, CO 80112.
‡Published by the Joint Commission on Accreditation of Healthcare Organizations, 1 Renaissance Boulevard, Oakbrook Terrace, IL 60181.
§Copies of the NFPA standards are available from the National Fire Protection Association, 1 Batterymarch Park, Quincy, MA 02269.
¶Copies of the AAMI standards and recommended practices are available from the Association for the Advancement of Medical Instrumentation, 1901 N. Fort Meyer Drive, Suite 602, Arlington, VA 22209.

mine conformance. AAMI standards have also been established for sterilization, electrical safety, and patient monitoring for health care providers in relation to evaluation, maintenance, and use of medical devices and instrumentation.

6. *Clinically based risk-control standards.* These standards are written by medical specialty groups and professional liability underwriters. They establish appropriate benchmarks of acceptable practices and outcomes specifically for controlling liability losses. They may be incorporated into the health care facility's risk management program.

Regulatory Standards

1. *The 1965 Federal Medicare Act and all subsequent amendments to this Social Security Act.* This legislation incorporates the provision that institutions participating in Medicare must maintain the level of patient care recognized as the norm. Specific requirements are included.

2. *American National Standards Institute (ANSI) standards.* These standards concern exposures to toxic materials and safe use of equipment, such as lasers.

3. *Federal Food and Drug Administration (FDA) performance standards.* Federal Medical Device Amendments regulate the manufacture, labeling, sale, and use of implantable medical devices and many products used in or on patients. The FDA also controls treatment protocols for use of drugs. The manufacturer's lot number and product description of implanted devices should be attached to or included in the patient's chart.

4. *Agency for Health Care Policy and Research (AHCPR) clinical practice guidelines.* These standards include indicators for performance measurement. They are based on research and professional judgment regarding effectiveness and appropriateness of medical care, including safety, efficacy, and effectiveness of technology. This agency was created in provisions of the Consolidated Omnibus Budget Reconciliation Act of 1989. AORN has included perioperative interpretations of the AHCPR guidelines in the *AORN Standards, Recommended Practices, and Guidelines* publication.

5. *Occupational Safety and Health Administration (OSHA) standards.* These legally enforceable standards include permissible levels of toxic substances in the environment. Although explicitly developed to protect employees, patients receive secondary benefits from control of hazards in the environment.

RECOMMENDED PRACTICES

Recommended practices are optimum behavioral objectives for caregivers. They may not always be achievable, as standards are, because of limitations in a particular practice setting. Recommended practices state what ideally can be done.

AORN-recommended practices for perioperative nursing concern aseptic techniques and technical aspects of nursing practice directed toward providing safety in the perioperative environment. They are based on principles of microbiology, scientific literature, validated research, and experts' opinions. Although compliance is voluntary, individual commitment, professional conscience, and the practice setting should guide perioperative caregivers in using these recommended practices. They represent what is believed to be an optimal level of practice and are intended to be achievable.

Guidelines and recommended practices of other agencies, including AAMI, the Centers for Disease Control and Prevention (CDC), the National Institute for Occupational Safety and Health (NIOSH), and the Environmental Protection Agency (EPA), also are used for environmental, patient, and personnel safety.

Policies and Procedures

Policies and procedures reflect variations in institutional environments and clinical situations. They are established to protect employees, learners, and patients. They establish the facility's standard of care. Policies should be consistent with regulatory and professional standards of practice. Procedures define scope, purposes, and instructions to be carried out and by whom. They should be clearly written, current, dated, and reviewed periodically. Although policies and procedures vary from one institution to another, they provide guidelines for patient care and safety in that specific physical facility. Learning and following policies and procedures are protective measures against potentially litigious actions. Many hospitals document in the employee's personnel file that policies and procedures have been reviewed during orientation to the employment setting. Employees may be asked to sign a notation verifying knowledge of a new or revised policy or procedure after its introduction. Some policies and procedures apply to all employees; others refer to a specific department. Because of the potential legal implications, adherence to all policies and procedures is mandatory. Personnel are evaluated on their ability to follow policy and perform procedures correctly. The following examples should be included in the perioperative department manual. These procedures are incorporated into discussions in subsequent chapters.

Identification of the Patient

When a patient enters the facility, an identification wristband is put on the patient in the admitting area. To verify accuracy, the patient may be asked to spell his or her name and pronounce it. The circulator and anesthesia provider check the wristband with the patient and surgeon, the patient's chart, and the operating schedule. The surgeon should visit with the patient before an anesthetic is administered.

Protection of Personal Property

Personnel in preoperative areas are responsible for removing valuables and prostheses before patients go to the OR. The circulator is responsible for double-checking each patient and removing, as necessary, unnecessary items brought to the OR. Personal items such as religious medals, hearing aid(s), eyeglasses, dentures, or eye prostheses are commonly permitted to remain with the patient who is having local or regional anesthesia. The circulator should inform the anesthesia provider and the surgeon of their presence and document them on the patient's chart. Artificial extremities, undergarments, wigs, hairpins, wristwatches, and rings should be removed. Jewelry could get lost, or a ring might become stuck on the patient's finger as a result of postoperative swelling. In addition to the danger of losing or damaging these items, some could cause pressure areas on the anesthetized patient's body.

Any item that is removed should be placed in a rigid container and labeled with the patient's name and number. The patient's personal property should not be wrapped in a paper or linen towel that could inadvertently be discarded in a trash receptacle or laundry hamper. The container may be retained by the circulator during the surgical procedure and sent with the patient to the postoperative area. Alternatively, the circulator may immediately ask a nursing assistant to return the container to the patient care unit. This person should obtain a receipt for the patient's personal property from the person receiving it. The receipt is given to the circulator to put in the patient's chart along with a notation of the transaction in the nurses' notes. Patients value their property. A caregiver can be held liable for loss or damage to a patient's personal property.

Observation of the Patient

Unattended patients may fall from a stretcher or the OR bed. Falls are one of the most frequent causes of avoidable injuries. Side rails, restraints, and safety straps should be used to protect all patients, both children and adults. A small child could reach a tiny finger into an electrical socket. Patients should be observed at all times in the perioperative environment.

Positioning of the Patient

Care is taken when moving all patients to and from the OR bed. The patient should be positioned to ensure adequate exposure of the surgical site for the surgeon but not compromise any body system. Cardiopulmonary functioning should not be impaired. Adequate support of joints and limbs should be provided during movement into the desired position. The plan of care should include appropriate numbers of personnel for safe patient movement. Pressure areas should be adequately protected to prevent neurovascular damage. The surgeon determines the appropriate surgical position in consultation with the anesthesia provider. The circulator assists in positioning the patient. A stretcher is kept nearby at all times if a patient is placed in a prone position. In the event of an emergency, the patient will need to be placed in a supine position for emergency treatment such as cardiopulmonary resuscitation (CPR).

Many patients receive general anesthesia and are therefore unconscious. Constant vigilance is essential to safeguard patients who are unable to protect themselves. Liability on the part of the team would be difficult to dispute. Everyone in the perioperative environment has a duty to monitor and protect the patient at all times.

Aseptic Technique

Infection is a serious postoperative complication that may become life threatening for the patient. Perioperative patient care team members must know and apply the principles of asepsis and sterile technique at all times. Established procedures for aseptic technique, sterilization, and disinfection should be followed meticulously. An emergency situation in which asepsis becomes a secondary concern is a rare occurrence. Each team member should consider how personal preferences for care of self or a loved one should be applied to the care of patients.

Postoperative wound infection can originate in the OR from a break in technique by any team member. Inappropriate reuse of disposable items may be indefensible, as can use of an unsterile endoscope introduced into a body cavity. An unsterile scope can disrupt the mucous membrane and come in contact with the patient's vascular system. Strict asepsis and sterile technique prevent many postoperative complications. The following principle should be remembered: When in doubt about something's sterility, consider it unsterile. Hence the phrase, "When in doubt, throw it out."

Performance of Accurate Counts

The responsibility for accounting for all sponges, sharps, and instruments before the surgical procedure begins and at the time of closure rests with the circulator and scrub person. The surgeon and first assistant facilitate the count of the items on the surgical field before closure. If they have done their part in the count procedure and a sponge is left in the wound because of a miscount by the circulator, that caregiver may be held solely responsible. In such a case the surgeon, facility, and scrub person may be exonerated. Likewise, the scrub person may be deemed responsible for an incorrect count. Because accountability for sponges, sharps, and instruments is recognized as essential to safe practice and the standard of care, omission of appropriate counts or a facility's lack of established procedures for counting and accountability could result in a serious threat of liability. The circulator should document in writing the outcome of the final counts as correct or incorrect and any unusual incidents concerning them, including the need for an x-ray film to look for a lost item. If an x-ray film is taken, the name of the radiologist and his or her findings should also be documented.

Use of Equipment

All instruments, equipment, and appliances should be used and tested according to the recommendations and instructions of the manufacturer. Safety devices such as personal protective goggles or smoke evacuation apparatus should be employed as necessary. Electrical and laser equipment also should pass inspection by the biomedical engineering department and be tagged with a dated preventive maintenance sticker. Electrical equipment should be properly grounded to prevent electric shock and burns. Equipment or devices that are known or suspected to be faulty are not used. The facility should conduct appropriate training and competency reviews for the use of all equipment used in patient care. Personnel who set up and operate facility-owned equipment may be found negligent if a patient is injured. Great care is critical to prevent injury when using all equipment in the perioperative environment.

Prevention of Skin Injury

Skin injury may be caused by an electrical or thermal device, chemical agent, or mechanical pressure. Pressure necrosis is possible following any procedure, but especially procedures lasting more than 2 hours.

A burn may occur from the use of a hot instrument taken directly out of the autoclave, such as a mouth gag or a large retractor. The scrub person should immerse a hot instrument in a basin of cool, sterile water before handing it to the surgeon.

A patient may be burned during use of the electrosurgical unit (ESU). Inadequate skin contact or improper placement of the inactive dispersive electrode can cause an electrical burn. The tip of the ESU pencil tip or suction cautery probe remains hot after it is applied to tissues for hemostasis. Unintended burns may occur if the tip touches other body parts. Alcohol and other flammable solutions can be ignited, causing flash fires if the solutions are pooled under the patient or allowed to saturate drapes. A thermal burn also can occur from other types of electrical and laser equipment that is improperly used or maintained. The caregiver should be aware that the effects of some types of lasers on tissue are not readily visible until tissue necrosis takes place several days postoperatively.

Administration of Drugs

Any drug that the surgeon uses in the surgical site, such as an antibiotic or local anesthetic, is recorded by the circulator and by the surgeon in the perioperative note. The drug is checked by a registered nurse and the scrub person before it is transferred to the sterile field. The sterile medication container and syringes (if used) are labeled by the scrub person on the field. The scrub person frequently has more than one drug on the instrument table. Each is correctly labeled and administered appropriately. The scrub person repeats the name of the drug to the surgeon when passing it.

The standard of care indicates that a registered nurse is responsible for monitoring the cardiac and respiratory status of a patient receiving local anesthesia, with or without IV conscious sedation, if an anesthesia provider is not present. The nurse is expected to interpret the monitoring equipment, assess the patient, and initiate interventions promptly if the patient has an untoward reaction. Policies and procedures are delineated by each facility for care of the patient receiving local anesthesia.

Preparation of Specimens

With very few exceptions, tissue and objects removed from a patient are sent to the pathology department. The loss of a tissue biopsy specimen could necessitate a second surgical procedure to obtain another one. Incorrectly labeled specimens could result in a mistaken diagnosis, with possible critical implications for two patients. Also, the loss of a specimen could prevent determination of a diagnosis and sub-

sequent initiation of definitive therapy. The pathology report becomes part of the patient's permanent record as added documentation of the diagnosis.

Care for foreign bodies according to the policy of the facility. They may have legal significance and frequently are claimed by police, especially if the foreign body is a bullet or something implicated in a crime. These items are not to be left unattended at any time. A receipt from the person taking them protects personnel and the facility.

Patient Teaching

The patient and/or significant others need to be informed about treatment options and their roles in the process. The patient has the right to make decisions and to contribute to the development of the plan of care. The perioperative nurse can assist with preoperative teaching of deep-breathing exercises for postoperative recovery. Information should be provided verbally and in writing. The patient and/or significant others should respond appropriately in such a way as to signify understanding of the information. This is particularly important for ambulatory surgery patients who will go home under the care of others. Patient teaching and demonstration of understanding should be documented in the chart.

ETHICAL ISSUES

Some situations that arise in the perioperative environment may be contrary to personal morals, values, beliefs, or religion. Patient care personnel assume legal and ethical rights, duties, and obligations by virtue of employment and their relation with patients and other caregivers. Professional ethics are influenced externally by laws, policies, and societal codes. Personal ethics are influenced internally by life experiences, religious persuasion, and ethnocultural background. When faced with an ethical uncertainty, a caregiver needs to clarify the difference between personal and professional values, developing a personal philosophy of providing patient care. Caregivers should identify the situation at hand, acquire knowledge of laws and professional codes, and understand the ethical principles and values of others. After identifying these factors, the caregiver can make a rational decision in an ethical dilemma. The term *ethics* is explored in Box 4-4.

Professions have codes of conduct and documents that include value statements derived from moral concepts. The Code of Ethics of the Association of Surgical Technologists (AST) (Box 4-5) provides guidance for surgical technologists. Nurses may refer to the International Code of Nursing Ethics and to a code established by their own professional association, such as the ANA Code for Nurses (Box 4-6) or the Code of Ethics for Nursing of the Canadian Nurses Association. In the statement of the nature and scope of nursing practice titled *Nursing, a Social Policy Statement,* developed by the ANA Congress of Practice in 1980, nurses are committed to respect for human beings "unaltered by social, educational, economic, cultural, racial, religious or other specific attributes of human beings receiving care, including nature and duration of disease and illness." The ethics of a profession establish the role and scope of professional behavior and the nature of relationships with patients and colleagues.

Universal moral principles guide ethical decision making and activities in clinical practice. These include the following:

- *Autonomy.* Self-determination implies freedom of choice and ability to make decisions to determine one's own course of action. Decisions may be made in collaboration with others, based on reasonable and prudent information. Decisions should be acknowledged and respected by others.
- *Beneficence.* Duty to help others seek balance between what is good to do and what might produce harm to another or self.
- *Nonmaleficence.* Duty to do no harm.

Box 4-4 Ethical Behavior

E *Earnestness.* Take seriously responsibilities for which you are legally and morally accountable. Recognize the importance of decisions and the effect they will have on yourself and others.

T *Truthfulness.* State the facts. Autonomy includes being true to yourself. Also respect the rights of others who want and need to know the truth as the basis for self-determination or participation in decision making.

H *Honesty.* Express feelings openly. Honest relations foster effective communication and establish trust and confidence.

I *Integrity.* Adhere to your own values, but also to professional standards and codes, institutional policies and procedures, and societal and legal responsibilities. Know what interventions will be beneficial and what will cause harm.

C *Conscientiousness.* Evaluate the alternatives in making decisions and choosing interventions. Differentiate right from wrong, and act accordingly.

S *Sincerity.* Demonstrate a genuine concern and interest in the welfare of others, as well as in yourself. Sincerity builds confidence and self-esteem.

Box 4-5 Code of Ethics: Association of Surgical Technologists

1. To maintain the highest standards of professional conduct and patient care
2. To hold in confidence, with respect to patient's beliefs, all personal matters
3. To respect and protect the patient's legal and moral right to quality patient care
4. To not knowingly cause injury or any injustice to those entrusted to our care
5. To work with fellow technologists and other professional health groups to promote harmony and unity for better patient care
6. To always follow the principles of asepsis
7. To maintain a high degree of efficiency through continuing education
8. To maintain and practice surgical technology willingly, with pride and dignity
9. To report any unethical conduct or practice to the proper authority
10. To adhere to the Code of Ethics at all times in relationship to all members of the health care team

Adopted by Board of Directors, Association of Surgical Technologists, Englewood, Colo, 1985.

Box 4-6 Code for Nurses: American Nurses Association

1. The nurse provides services with respect for human dignity and the uniqueness of the patient, unrestricted by considerations of social or economic status, personal attributes, or the nature of health problems.
2. The nurse safeguards the client's right to privacy by judiciously protecting information of a confidential nature.
3. The nurse acts to safeguard the patient and the public when health care and safety are affected by incompetent, unethical, or illegal practice by any person.
4. The nurse assumes responsibility and accountability for individual nursing judgments and actions.
5. The nurse maintains competence in nursing.
6. The nurse exercises informed judgment and uses individual competency and qualifications as criteria in seeking consultation, accepting responsibilities, and delegating nursing activities.
7. The nurse participates in activities that contribute to the ongoing development of the profession's body of knowledge.
8. The nurse participates in the profession's efforts to implement and improve standards of nursing.
9. The nurse participates in the profession's efforts to establish and maintain conditions of employment conducive to high-quality patient care.
10. The nurse participates in the profession's effort to protect the public from misinformation and misrepresentation and to maintain the integrity of nursing.
11. The nurse collaborates with members of the health professions and other citizens in promoting community and national efforts to meet the health needs of the public.

From American Nurses Association: *Code for nurses with interpretive statements,* Washington, DC, 1985, The Association.

- *Justice.* Allocation of human, material, and technologic resources a person has a right to receive or claim (i.e., equality of care).
- *Veracity.* Devotion to truthfulness (i.e., to give accurate information).
- *Fidelity.* Quality of faithfulness, based on trust and honesty, that protects rights of individuals, such as dignity and privacy.
- *Confidentiality.* Respect for privileged information received from another person with disclosure only to appropriate others.

Values are operational beliefs an individual chooses as the basis for behavior. They may change over time. They may create conflicts when value systems are not compatible with the expectations of others. Values reflect ethics. Ethics refer to standards or principles of moral judgment and action. Ethics as a philosophy defines a systematic method of differentiating right from wrong within a specific belief system. Professional and societal codes and standards offer guidelines in this determination. Ethics and law are closely related. Legal doctrines often interpret ethical concepts.

The Bill of Rights of the Constitution of the United States establishes individual rights based on moral principles that respect human worth and dignity. The courts have upheld the right to individual autonomy in making health care decisions, as evidenced by rulings about such issues as abortion, the right to die, and living wills.

BIOETHICAL SITUATIONS

An ethical dilemma arises in the work situation when the choice between two or more alternatives creates a conflict between an individual's value system and moral obligation to the patient, to the family or significant others, to the physician, or to the employer and co-workers. Conflicts can be between rights, duties, and responsibilities.

Both legal and ethical considerations can cause conflicts. Legally, a patient has the right to choose among treatment alternatives or the right to refuse treatment. Philosophically, the patient's preference may be different from that of the health care provider. The primary responsibility to the patient is to ensure delivery of safe care. This includes use of appropriate and available technology, but only if this is the patient's choice, with informed consent freely given, or is known to be the patient's wish. Conversely, the patient and the caregiver may be forced to face court-ordered procedures or treatments. This may impose the need to assist in a surgical intervention such as a cesarean section on a woman who has moral or religious objections to this form of treatment, but who has been ordered by the court to have the procedure performed for the benefit of the unborn fetus. This example is extreme, but the courts are constantly working to define the rights of the unborn. In the issue of viability vs. possible death, the court usually supports measures necessary to sustain life. The caregiver who participates in a court-ordered procedure is protected by law, provided that the performance of his or her duties meets the standards of care.

Caregivers should decide for themselves the appropriate course of action when dealing with an ethical dilemma. By developing a personal philosophy and by understanding both professional and institutional philosophies, the caregiver may better answer many personal ethical questions, such as: When does life begin? When does it end? What is my perception of quality of life between conception and death? What is my role in health care? What are my moral rights in relation to my personal beliefs and values and those of others? Where are the dividing lines between a patient's personal rights to privacy and confidentiality and a legal or ethical duty of disclosure?

A few of the ethical dilemmas facing physicians and perioperative personnel are mentioned for personal consideration. It should also be noted that some of these issues are regulated by state statutes or federal court decisions. All caregivers should be familiar with statutes in the state in which they practice, particularly those regarding participation and the right to refrain on the basis of personal beliefs. The right to refuse to participate may be covered by a law, but not at the expense of a patient's safety and welfare. The patient cannot be harmed by acts of commission or omission.

Reproductive Sterilization

Voluntary reproductive sterilization as a contraceptive method may be contrary to the moral, ethical, or religious beliefs of a caregiver. Consent is required to perform reproductive sterilization. Some facilities require consent from a patient's spouse.

Abortion

Legalized abortion allows for induced termination of pregnancy. In the 1973 decision of *Roe v. Wade,* the U.S. Supreme Court ruled that any licensed physician can terminate pregnancy during the first trimester with the woman's consent. During the second trimester, the Court requires a state statute that regulates abortion on the basis of preservation and protection of maternal health. During the third trimester, legal abortion should consider meaningful life for the fetus outside the womb and endangerment to the mother's life and health.

Although by law physicians may perform abortions in health care facilities, many persons, individually and collectively, and institutions such as the Roman Catholic Church oppose abortion. Many persons believe that abortion is a form of active euthanasia because it takes the life of an innocent victim without consent. By selective abortion, one or more fertilized ova may be aborted so that others may mature properly in a multiple pregnancy, which is perhaps a result of fertility drugs.

In facilities where abortions and other reproductive procedures are performed, employees have the right to refrain from participation because of their moral, ethical, or religious beliefs, except in an emergency that threatens the life of the mother. These beliefs should be made known to the employer in writing. Some states have a protective statute for employees and employers regulating good-faith efforts to accommodate employees' beliefs. In other states, laws protect an employee from being forced by an employer to assist in abortions.

HIV and Other Infections

The prevalence of human immunodeficiency virus (HIV) infection, with or without acquired immunodeficiency syndrome (AIDS), has created a catastrophic health problem with many inherent emotional issues. Unlike other communicable diseases, HIV infection is a fatal illness with no known cure at this time, although some drug therapies may slow its progression. Its mode of transmission and methods of prevention are known. Therefore personal biases and prejudices should not discriminate against the infected patient. However, underlying attitudes about homosexuality and IV drug abuse may subconsciously influence the care of such patients. Are these patients any different from patients with hemophilia or persons who became infected through a contaminated blood transfusion? Should the infant with HIV be treated any differently than an infant with a congenital anomaly? Does the diagnosis make a difference to the health care provider and to the quality of care that the patient receives? Should it?

Knowing that HIV infection is transmitted by blood and body secretions, conscientious application of standard precautions for infection control should provide protection against occupational exposure to HIV, hepatitis, tuberculosis, and other communicable or resistant infections. The ANA Code for Nurses emphasizes that care is given regardless of the nature of health problems.

Other ethical questions concern screening and the reporting of test results vs. confidentiality. Do the same considerations apply to team members as to patients? What constitutes valid reasons for restricting or terminating employment on the basis of health status? This question has broader implications than just the issue of being seropositive for HIV. No state mandates by law that a health care worker can refuse to provide care for a patient with HIV infection. Risks vs. benefits to self, patients, and team members, plus potential litigation as a result of actions, should be evaluated in making ethical decisions. Confidentiality, privacy, and informed consent are human rights that should be protected, but the right to health care should be protected also.

Both AORN and AST have published statements encouraging health care facilities to provide policies and procedures to ensure the safety of patients and personnel. These organizations believe that providers have a right to know the HIV or other infectious status of patients, but that caregivers do not have the right to discriminate against HIV-positive patients. They should follow the CDC guidelines in caring for all patients to prevent transmission of infection.

Human Experimentation

Procedures still in developmental stages are performed in clinical research–oriented facilities with the patient's informed consent. Those willing to be pioneers in human experimentation have given, or will give, hope to many patients with poor prognoses. A caregiver should decide if he or she wants to participate in experimental surgery.

Quality of Life

Surgeons often must make critical decisions before or during surgical interventions regarding the quality of patients' lives following surgical procedures. Palliative procedures may relieve pain. Therapeutic procedures may be disfiguring. Life-support systems may sustain vital functions. Life-sustaining therapy may prolong the dying process. Many questions arise regarding care of terminally ill, severely debilitated or injured, and comatose patients. What will be the outcome in terms of mental or physical competence? When should cardiopulmonary resuscitation be initiated or discontinued? Physicians decide, but all team members are affected by the decisions.

How is euthanasia defined? Is mercy killing ethical, legal, or justified? Does the patient, family or guardian, physicians, or courts have the right to decide to abandon heroic measures to sustain life? The patient who is aware of the options and whose decision-making capacity is intact has the right of self-determination. OR personnel develop the plan of care guided by an advance directive.

Euthanasia

Euthanasia is derived from the Greek words meaning *good or merciful death.* Both active euthanasia and passive euthanasia are intentional acts that cause death, but the methods are different. An act of direct intervention that causes death is active euthanasia. Withholding or withdrawing life prolonging or life-sustaining measures is passive euthanasia. Death is caused by the underlying disease process, trauma, or physiologic dysfunction. This concept differs from physician-assisted suicide. Suicide involves the person causing his or her own demise.

The idea of euthanasia seems to violate traditional principles of medicine to preserve life, but our modern technologies can prolong life without preserving quality. Quality of life can be interpreted as life that has a meaningful value. Most human beings value having cognitive abilities, physical capabilities, or both, and living free of undue pain and suffering. This raises the ethical question of whether physicians should do what they technologically can do.

Right to Die

Courts have determined that patients have a constitutional right to privacy in choosing to die with dignity, or a common law right to withhold consent and refuse treatment. A mentally competent adult over the age of 18 can execute a living will, an advance directive, directing physicians and other health care providers not to use extraordinary measures to prolong life. Most physicians designate "extraordinary" measures as those that are optional, such as mechanical respiration, hydration, nutrition, medication, or a combination of these, and that sustain life. If it is the expressed wish of the patient, the physician writes do-not-resuscitate (DNR) orders. A living will relieves family members of decision making when the patient becomes terminally ill, incompetent, or comatose. No laws or court precedents deal specifically with the issue of DNR orders in the perioperative environment. Institutional policy should address this matter. Theoretically, a patient can attempt to sue for compensation for expenses under a negligence or battery charge. In general, courts are reluctant to hold health care workers liable for acts performed to maintain life. In *Anderson v. St. Francis,* defibrillation was performed despite a DNR order. The court found that sustaining life was not considered an injury and rejected the compensatory claim.

A patient who has a standing DNR order may require a procedure to decrease pain or palliate uncomfortable symptoms. Before going to the OR, the DNR order should be reaffirmed with the patient, guardian, or person who has durable power of attorney. The DNR order must be clarified before the patient goes to the OR. In an emergency, if there is doubt about the validity of the DNR order or a question concerning reconsideration of the order, the caregiver should participate in resuscitation. If there is any question about the patient changing his or her mind, a second chance may not be an option during an emergency situation. If the patient or legal guardian is specifically clear about upholding the DNR order in the OR, the team has the responsibility to follow the patient's wishes. A caregiver who has a moral objection to upholding a DNR order may request reassignment through the nurse manager of the department.

The issue of discontinuation of life-sustaining measures becomes more difficult in a comatose, mentally incompetent patient who has not executed an advance directive. Family members, in consultation with physicians, may request DNR orders. Caregivers are obligated to follow DNR orders.

Organ Donation and Transplantation

As a result of the Uniform Anatomical Gift Act of 1968, many adults carry cards stating that at death they wish to donate their body organs or parts for transplantation, therapy, medical research, or education. Most states include this information on a driver's license. If this legal authority is not available, some states have a required request law. In the event of legally defined brain death, the caregivers are required by this law to ask the family if they wish to allow organ retrieval for transplantation.

Transplant surgeons rely on the perioperative patient care teams who procure donor organs, eyes, bone, and skin. Organ transplantation has complicated the issue of time of death. Perfusion of oxygenated blood through tissues must be sustained by artificial means during procurement of vital organs with functional viability.

Legally, death has occurred when an individual has sustained either irreversible cessation of circulatory and respiratory functions or irreversible cessation of all functions of the entire brain, including the brainstem. Therefore the accepted definition of irreversible coma for potential donors includes unresponsiveness, no spontaneous movements of res-

piration, no reflexes, and a flat electroencephalogram. When brain death is determined by two physicians who are not part of the transplant team, the donor will be taken to the OR with artificial support systems functioning to perfuse organs. Some caregivers have moral questions about assisting with removal of viable organs from seemingly living bodies. At the conclusion of the procedure, when the last perfused organ is removed, cardiopulmonary support is discontinued and the anesthesia personnel leave the room. This is a difficult time for the remaining team who may still have the assignment of procuring nonperfused tissues, such as skin, bone, or eyes.

Perioperative caregivers who believe that donation of organs and body parts is a gift of love find it easier and ethically acceptable to participate in procurement procedures. Family members of donors have encouraged team members not to focus on their grief, but rather to focus on the gifts of life they are giving unselfishly to the recipients. This does not mean that the donor's family will not go through the grieving process. They will need support. Caregivers learn to cope with feelings associated with the procurement of donor organs in a manner similar to dealing with the sudden death of any patient in the perioperative environment.

Death and Dying

Intellectually, we know that death is inevitable. Death can be a difficult burden for caregivers to bear because our education, experience, and philosophy are dedicated to survival. Regardless of religious or cultural beliefs, death is a mystery, a passage from the known to the unknown. Perhaps, partially for this reason, the death of a patient in the OR is an unsettling experience, especially if it is unexpected.

One of the most difficult aspects of a death in the OR for the team members is the period after the actual event. The surgeon goes to inform the family. The assistants and anesthesia provider leave the room. Often the perioperative team is left alone with the patient's body. The patient should be prepared so that the family can view the body in an area adjoining the perioperative environment, where they can have privacy in expressing their feelings. The perioperative nurse may be expected to accompany the family and to lend support during the viewing. A chaplain or clergy should be called if desired by the family. Specific departmental policies should be developed to assist the caregiver with this difficult aspect of patient care. Coping strategies that can help team members may include the following:

1. Realize that everyone involved is part of a team effort.
2. Believe in a power greater than the skills of the team.
3. Share feelings with others. It is helpful for perioperative patient care team members to talk with each other about what happened. Encourage each other to share feelings associated with the loss. Crying is acceptable behavior.
4. Deal with the patient's death by identifying personally with the loss. Empathy is a positive emotion. Working through the grieving process brings a sense of closure to the relationship.

Some hospitals provide support groups to help staff members and bereaved families deal with death.

SURGICAL CONSCIENCE

The key elements of perioperative practice are caring, conscience, discipline, and technique. Optimal patient care requires an inherent surgical conscience, self-discipline, and the application of principles of asepsis and sterile technique. All are inseparably related.

The concept of a surgical conscience may simply be stated as a surgical Golden Rule: Do unto the patient as you would have others do unto you. The caregiver should consider each patient as himself or herself or as a loved one. Once an individual develops a surgical conscience, it remains inherent thereafter. Florence Nightingale summarized what is, in essence, its meaning when she said, "The nurse should keep a high sense of duty in her own mind, must aim at perfection in her care, and must be consistent always in herself."

A surgical conscience involves self-inspection coupled with moral obligation. Involving both scientific and intellectual honesty, it is self-regulation in practice according to a deep personal commitment to the highest values. It incorporates the caregiver's values and attitudes at a conscious level and monitors behavior and decision making in relation to those values. In short, a surgical conscience is the inner voice for conscientious practice of asepsis and sterile technique at all times. This conscientiousness applies to every activity and intervention, as well as to personal hygiene and health. An aseptic body image includes an awareness of body, hair, makeup, jewelry, fingernails, and attire. A team member with an infectious process, such as the flu, a cold, or an open skin lesion, clearly cannot work in the perioperative environment. Professional responsibility requires that patient safety is not compromised.

Correct practice of asepsis provides a foundation for development of a mature conscience—mastery of personal integrity and discipline. Development of this conscience incorporates knowledge of aseptic principles, perpetual attention to detail, and experience. All are facets of responsibility that involve trust. A surgical conscience does not permit a person to excuse an error but rather to admit and rectify one readily. It becomes so much an automatic part of the caregiver that he or she can see at a glance or instinctively know if a break in technique or violation of a principle has occurred. Conscience dictates that appropriate action be taken, whether the person is with others or is alone and unobserved.

A surgical conscience therefore is the foundation for the practice of strict aseptic and sterile techniques. Practice according to that conscience results in pride in oneself and in accomplishment, as well as an inner confidence that the patient is receiving quality care.

A very important aspect in assisting the development of a surgical conscience in others is communication skill. A team member should not be criticized for an error; that person should be given credit for admitting the error and should be helped to correct the violation. Fear of criticism is the primary deterrent in admission of fault. No one should be reluctant to admit a frank or questionable break in technique. However, any individual unmotivated to carry out expected practices as closely to perfection as possible has no place in the OR suite.

Bibliography

Au YK et al: Increasing OR efficiency with a specialty services manual, *AORN J* 64(1):96-104, 1996.
Beerman CM: The nurse's role in bioethics, *AORN J* 65(5):923-926, 1997.
Bird LJ: Computerization in the OR, *AORN J* 66(2):312-317, 1997.
Bogart JB et al: *Legal nurse consulting: principles and practice,* New York, 1998, CRC Press, Association of Legal Nurse Consultants.
Eckberg E: The continuing ethical dilemma of the do-not-resuscitate order, *AORN J* 67(4):783-790, 1998.
Fortunato NM et al: *Nursing law in Ohio,* Eau Claire, Wis, 1997, National Business Institute, Inc.
Gordon M: *Manual of nursing diagnosis, 1997-1998,* St Louis, 1997, Mosby.
Jacobson BS: Ethical dilemmas of do-not-resuscitate orders in surgery, *AORN J* 60(3):449-452, 1994.
Jordahl KA: Designing an OR procedure book for small health care facilities, *AORN J* 66(4):694-696, 1997.
Keffer MJ, Keffer HL: The do-not-resuscitate order, *AORN J* 59(3): 641-650, 1994.
McGraw KS: Should do-not-resuscitate orders be suspended during surgical procedures? *AORN J* 67(4):794-799, 1998.
Murphy EK: OR nursing law: are perioperative nurses borrowed servants? Are surgeons captains of the ship? *AORN J* 60(3):474-477, 1994.
Murphy EK: Types of legal claims brought against perioperative nurses, *AORN J* 65(5):972-973, 1997.
Murphy EK: Individual malpractice insurance decisions revisited, *AORN J* 67(6):1234-1236, 1998.
Onstott AT: Perioperative nursing care when sudden death occurs in the OR, *AORN J* 67(4):829-836, 1998.
Schroeter K: Perioperative nurses' involvement on nursing ethics committees, *AORN J* 64(4):588-596, 1996.
Steelman VM et al: Toward a standardized language to describe perioperative nursing, *AORN J* 60(5):786-795, 1994.
Zeil SE: Managing the risks of electronic health records, *AORN J* 68(2):281-283, 1998.
Zeil SE, Latham WH: Preparing to give testimony at a deposition and at a trial, *AORN J* 62(6):944-947, 1995.

Section II

The Perioperative Health Care Team

Chapter 5

The Perioperative Patient Care Team

 Chapter Objectives

After studying this chapter, the learner will be able to:

- Define the concept of the sterile team.
- Define the concept of the unsterile team.
- Describe the role of the circulator.
- Describe the role of the scrub person.
- Describe the role of the first assistant.

OPERATING ROOM TEAM

At no other time during the perioperative experience will the patient be so well attended as during the surgical procedure. The patient is surrounded by a surgeon, one or two assistants, a surgical technologist, an anesthesia provider, and a circulating nurse. These individuals, each with specific functions to perform, form the operating team. Throughout this text, this direct patient care team will be referred to as the operating room (OR) team. This team literally has the patient's life in its hands. The OR team is like a symphony orchestra, with each person an integral entity in unison and harmony with his or her colleagues for the successful accomplishment of the expected outcomes. Terms associated with members of the perioperative patient care team are defined in Box 5-1.

The OR team is subdivided according to the functions of its members:

1. The sterile team
   a. Surgeon
   b. Assistants to the surgeon
   c. Scrub person

2. The unsterile team
   a. Anesthesia provider
   b. Circulator
   c. Others. The OR team may also include biomedical technicians, radiology technicians, and others who may be needed to set up and operate specialized equipment or monitoring devices during the surgical procedure.

Sterile team members scrub (wash) their hands and arms, don a sterile gown and gloves, and enter the sterile field. The sterile field is the area of the OR that immediately surrounds and is specially prepared for the patient. To establish a sterile field, all items needed for the surgical procedure are sterilized (a process by which all living microorganisms are killed). After this process, the scrubbed and sterile team members function within this limited area and handle only sterile items.

Unsterile team members do not enter the sterile field; they function outside and around it. They assume responsibility for maintaining sterile technique during the surgical procedure, but they handle supplies and equipment that are not

61

Box 5-1   Terms Associated with Perioperative Team Members

anesthesia provider   Member of the unsterile team who administers anesthetics during the surgical procedure; may be a physician or a specially trained RN.

aseptic technique   Manipulation of sterile and unsterile items in the perioperative environment. Microbiologic principles are followed to minimize the risk for contamination.

assistant   Member of the sterile team who provides exposure and hemostasis during a surgical procedure; may be another physician or specifically trained personnel.

circulator   Member of the unsterile team who directs the activities of the OR during the procedure; should be a registered nurse.

scrub person   Member of the sterile team who passes instruments and facilitates the surgical procedure.

sterile team   Perioperative caregivers who provide direct care within the sterile field while wearing sterile OR attire.

sterile technique   Manipulation of sterile items within and around a sterile field.

surgeon   Physician who performs the surgical procedure.

unsterile team   Perioperative caregivers who provide direct care from the periphery of the sterile field while not wearing sterile attire.

considered sterile. Following the principles of aseptic technique, they keep the sterile team supplied, provide direct patient care, and handle other requirements that may arise during the surgical procedure.

STERILE TEAM MEMBERS

Surgeon

The surgeon must have the knowledge, skill, and judgment required to successfully perform the intended surgical procedure and any deviations necessitated by unforeseen difficulties. The American College of Surgeons (ACS) has stated the principles of patient care that dictate ethical surgical practice. Protection of the patient and quality care are preeminent in these principles. The surgeon's responsibilities include preoperative diagnosis and care, selection and performance of the surgical procedure, and postoperative management of care. The care of many surgical patients is so complex that considerably more than technical skill is required of a surgeon. The surgeon cannot predict that a surgical procedure will be simple and uncomplicated. The surgeon must be prepared for the unexpected by having knowledge of the fundamentals of the basic sciences and by having the ability to apply this knowledge to the diagnosis and management of the patient before, during, and after surgical intervention. The surgeon assumes full responsibility for all medical acts of judgment and for the management of the surgical patient.

A surgeon is a licensed physician (MD), osteopath (DO), oral surgeon (DDS or DMD), or podiatrist (DPM) who is specially trained and qualified by knowledge and experience to perform surgical procedures. After earning a bachelor's degree, all physicians complete the equivalent of 4 years of medical school. To become a surgeon, a physician completes at least 2 years of general surgical residency training before completing additional years of postgraduate education in a surgical specialty. The surgical residency provides the physician with education and experience in the preoperative evaluation, intraoperative treatment, and postoperative care of patients. Consultation and supervision are available from faculty and attending surgeons. By virtue of their postgraduate surgical education, most surgeons practice within a specific surgical specialty. Highly trained and qualified surgeons limit themselves to their specialty, except perhaps in emergency situations.

Qualification for surgical practice involves certification by a surgical specialty board approved by the American Board of Medical Specialists. Ten American specialty boards grant certification for surgical practice. All 10 boards governing the surgical specialties require at least 3 years of approved formal residency training, and most set the minimum at 4 or 5 years. Any physician who aspires to become a board-certified surgeon must meet these requirements.

Surgical procedures may be performed by physicians who do not meet the previously discussed criteria. These physicians include those who received an MD degree before 1968 and who have had surgical privileges for more than 5 years in a hospital approved by the Joint Commission on Accreditation of Healthcare Organizations (JCAHO), where most of their surgical practice is conducted; those who render surgical care in an emergency or in an area of limited population where a surgical specialist is not available; and those who by reason of education, training, and experience are eligible for but have not yet obtained certification.

A surgeon must become a member of the medical staff and be granted surgical privileges in each hospital in which he or she wishes to practice. Standards for admission to staff membership and the retention of that membership are clearly delineated in the bylaws formulated by the medical staff and are approved by the governing body of the hospital. The credentials committee has the primary responsibility for thoroughly investigating not only the training of an applicant but also his or her integrity, technical competence, and professional judgment. In making its recommendations, this committee can limit a surgeon's privileges as it sees fit, which ensures that each surgeon performs only those services for which he or she has been deemed competent.

Patients are entitled to protection and the assurance that a surgeon's surgical privileges are limited to those for which he or she has been trained and for which his or her competence has been demonstrated. The patient's choice of and confidence in a surgeon, as well as adherence to instructions and advice, are factors in the outcome of surgical intervention. A discerning patient will check the surgeon's qualifications before surgery.

A competent surgeon is a physician who realistically appreciates his or her own cognitive skills and personal characteristics and can intervene effectively in a patient's illness or injury. Appropriate clinical skills (e.g., data gathering, decision making, and problem solving) and appropriate personal characteristics (e.g., humanistic concern, accountability, and compassionate interpersonal behavior) are important attributes of a surgeon.

Assistants to the Surgeon

Under the direction of the operating surgeon, one or two assistants help to maintain visibility of the surgical site, control bleeding, close wounds, and apply dressings. The assistant handles tissues and uses instruments. The role of and need for an assistant will vary with the type of procedure or surgical specialty, the condition of the patient, and the type of surgical facility. In determining this need, the characteristics of the surgical procedure should be evaluated: anticipated blood loss, anesthesia time for the patient, fatigue factors affecting the OR team, and potential complications. For many simple procedures, it is unreasonable to insist that a second surgeon assist a competent surgeon. However, the assistance of another qualified surgeon is usually necessary for procedures requiring considerable judgment or technical skill and those requiring more than one sterile team. The hazards of a surgical procedure may depend more on the condition of the patient than on the complexity of the procedure itself. The surgeon should evaluate all factors to determine his or her need for assistance during the surgical procedure. The surgeon should be able to defend his or her decision if challenged or if not in compliance with medical staff bylaws.

Some surgical staffs classify surgical procedures as major or minor. If policy stipulates that a physician must assist on all major procedures, the surgeon should not be allowed to operate unless another qualified physician is present. Although a surgical procedure may be classified as minor, performing it without complications is sometimes technically difficult. In any surgical procedure that involves an unusual hazard to life, a qualified physician must be present and scrubbed as a first assistant. Determining what constitutes an unusual hazard depends on the conscience of the operating surgeon and is part of his or her responsibility to the patient.

First Assistant in Surgery

Ideally, the first assistant to the surgeon is a qualified surgeon or a resident in an accredited surgical education program. The first assistant should be capable of assuming responsibility for performing the procedure for the primary surgeon. The surgeon may request the assistance of an associate physician with whom a surgical practice is shared and to whom part of the patient's care may be delegated. Complex surgical procedures or multidisciplinary medical circumstances may require the services of an assistant who is proficient in another surgical specialty.

In hospitals with accredited postgraduate surgical residency training programs, a surgical resident usually acts as the first assistant. The resident is given increasing responsibilities under supervision as he or she develops skill and judgment. On completion of training, the resident is able to assume responsibility for continuity of surgical patient care. The staff surgeon in charge may delegate the performance of part of a surgical procedure to a resident assistant, provided the surgeon is an active participant throughout the essential part of the surgical procedure. The patient should be informed and give consent if a senior resident will be responsible for surgical treatment.

Specially trained nonmedical personnel such as oral surgeons and podiatrists perform or assist with surgical procedures in a hospital or ambulatory care facility only under the authority of the medical staff and the surgeon responsible for surgical services.

Nonphysician First Assistant

Nonphysician first assistants are required to complete a formal educational program for first assisting according to their practice discipline. Whether employed by a surgeon or a health care facility, practice privileges for nonphysician first assistants are based on verifiable credentials that attest to essential knowledge and skills.

Physicians Assistant The medical staff may approve privileges for a nonphysician allied health practitioner who is qualified by academic and clinical training to perform designated procedures in the OR and in other areas of surgical patient care. *Physicians assistant (PA)* is a generic term with two subcategories: the assistant to the primary care physician (PCA or PA-C [physician's clinical assistant]) and the assistant to the surgeon (SA or PSA [physician's surgical assistant]). The PA is required to have additional surgical training in order to first assist in surgery. Eligibility for appointment as an allied health nonphysician assistant for specified services is determined by the following criteria:

- Exercising judgment within areas of competence, with the physician member of the medical staff having the ultimate responsibility for patient care
- Participating directly in the management of patients under the supervision or direction of a member of the medical staff
- Recording reports and progress notes on patients' records and writing orders to the extent established by the medical staff
- Performing services in conformity with applicable provisions of medical staff bylaws, which may include obtaining medical histories and performing physical examinations

The SA performs duties under the direct supervision of a surgeon. The assistant may perform tasks delegated by the surgeon for the care of patients in any setting for which the surgeon assumes responsibility. The role of the SA cannot be rigidly defined because of variations in geographic, economic, and sociologic factors and state regulations of medical practices.

The responsibility an assistant may assume requires that, at the conclusion of formal education, he or she possess the knowledge, skills, and abilities necessary to provide services appropriate to the surgical setting. These services may include those of first assistant at the operating bed. After completion of a formal academic program, the PA and SA should attain national certification. The SA may be employed by the surgeon or the hospital but is required to receive credentialing from the medical staff. The medical staff bylaws delineate the practice privileges of the assistant within the hospital.

Registered Nurse First Assistant A certified perioperative nurse (CNOR) who has successfully completed an approved program based on the Core Curriculum for the Registered Nurse First Assistant of AORN, the Association of periOperative Registered Nurses, may seek a position as a registered nurse first assistant (RNFA) with a private surgeon, hospital, or clinic. The RNFA functions under the direct supervision of a surgeon. The RNFA functions solely as the first assistant and should not simultaneously perform the functions of a scrub nurse. The qualifications to function as a first assistant should include, but are not limited to, the following:

- Demonstrated competency in both scrub and circulator roles
- Knowledge and skill in applying the principles of aseptic and sterile techniques to ensure infection control
- Knowledge of surgical anatomy, physiology, fluid and electrolyte balance, acid-base regulation, clinical pathology, and wound healing as these factors relate to surgical procedures
- Comprehension of risk factors and potential intraoperative complications and knowledge of actions to minimize them
- Technical skill and manual dexterity in handling tissue, providing exposure, using instruments and devices, providing hemostasis, tying sutures and knots, and applying dressings
- Ability to recognize safety hazards and initiate appropriate preventive and corrective actions
- Ability to perform cooperatively and effectively with other team members
- Ability to perform effectively in stressful and emergency situations
- Certification in perioperative nursing
- Certification in cardiopulmonary resuscitation (basic cardiac life support or advanced life support)

The role of the RNFA is recognized in all states as being within the scope of nursing practice as an expanded role. Credentialing is controlled by individual state boards of nursing. Voluntary credentialing such as certification is attained by successfully passing a national examination. The Certification Boards, Inc. oversees the Certification Board Perioperative Nursing (CBPN) as it administers the examination. Suc-

cessful passage of the certification process entitles the RNFA to use the acronym *CRNFA* (certified RNFA). (See Chapter 2 for a description of eligibility for the certification of RNFAs.)

Surgical Technologist First Assistant A certified surgical technologist (CST) may also be trained to first assist. After successfully passing a national examination, the CST first assistant may use the acronym *CST/CFA*. (See Chapter 2 for a description of eligibility for the certification of CST/CFAs.)

Second Assistant to the Surgeon

Qualified nurses and surgical technologists may be used as second or third assistants for surgical procedures in which the surgeon deems their assistance is adequate and for which they have been trained. Second and third assistants are not involved in the actual performance of the procedure but primarily work with minimally invasive procedures, such as holding the endoscopic camera.

Immediately following graduation from medical school and before entering a postgraduate program in a surgical specialty, physicians complete at least 1 year of general surgical residency. Medical students also receive some exposure to the OR during their surgical clerkship. These general surgical residents and medical students usually function as second assistants in teaching institutions.

Scrub Person

The scrub person is a patient care staff member of the sterile team. The scrub role may be filled by a registered nurse (RN), a licensed practical/vocational nurse (LPN/LVN), or a surgical technologist (ST). The term *scrub person* is used throughout this text to designate this role and to elaborate on the specific technical and behavioral functions of the individual performing in this capacity.

The scrub person is responsible for maintaining the integrity, safety, and efficiency of the sterile field throughout the surgical procedure. Knowledge of and experience with aseptic and sterile techniques qualify the scrub person to prepare and arrange instruments and supplies and to facilitate the surgical procedure by providing the required sterile instruments and supplies. The scrub person must anticipate, plan for, and respond to the needs of the surgeon and other team members by constantly watching the sterile field. Manual dexterity and physical stamina are required. Other important assets include a stable temperament, an ability to work under pressure, a keen sense of responsibility, and a concern for accuracy in performing all duties.

Two scrub persons may join the team in teaching situations or during extremely complicated or hazardous surgical procedures. One scrub person may pass instruments and supplies to the surgeon while the other prepares the supplies.

An experienced preceptor may join the team to teach, guide, and assist the learner in functioning as a scrub person. When unexpected, unusual, or emergency situations arise, specific instructions and guidance are received from the surgeon or RN. The ST provides services and patient care under the supervision of an RN at all times.

Some facilities permit RNs or STs employed by surgeons to come into the OR to perform the scrub role for their employers. These private scrub persons should adhere to all hospital policies and procedures and to approved written guidelines for the functions they may fulfill.

UNSTERILE TEAM MEMBERS

Anesthesia Provider

Anesthesia and surgery are two distinct but inseparable disciplines; they are two parts of one entity. Adequate communication between the surgeon and the anesthesia provider is the patient's greatest safeguard. The anesthesia provider is an indispensable member of the OR team. Functioning as a guardian of the patient, the anesthesia provider should observe the principles of aseptic technique.

An anesthesiologist is an MD or DO, preferably certified by the American Board of Anesthesiology, who specializes in the art and science of administering anesthetics to produce various states of anesthesia. To become eligible for certification, physicians complete a 2-year anesthesia residency program. An anesthetist is a qualified RN, dentist, or physician who administers anesthetics. An anesthetist who administers a drug or gas works under the direct supervision of the anesthesiologist or the surgeon.

An RN is required to have a minimum of a bachelor's degree in nursing or science for entrance into a school of nurse anesthesia. To become a certified registered nurse anesthetist (CRNA), a graduate of an accredited nurse anesthesia program (a minimum of 2 years in length) must pass the certification examination of the Council on Certification of Nurse Anesthetists. Nurse anesthetists go through recertification every 2 years.

Throughout this text the term *anesthesia provider* is used to refer to the person responsible for inducing anesthesia, maintaining anesthesia at the required levels, and managing untoward reactions to anesthesia throughout the surgical procedure. Medically delegated functions of an anesthetic nature are performed under the overall supervision of a responsible physician or in accordance with individual written guidelines approved within the health care facility.*

Modern anesthesia is vastly superior to the anesthesia of previous years. The number of anesthetic agents available and the refinements of administration techniques have broadened its scope. A greater understanding of the pharmacologic action of anesthetic drugs has led to safer anesthesia. Choosing and applying appropriate agents and suitable techniques of administration, monitoring physiologic functions, maintaining fluid and electrolyte balance, and performing blood

replacements are essential responsibilities of anesthesia providers. They also share responsibility for minimizing the hazards of shock, electrocution, and fire. Appropriate precautions should be taken to ensure the safe administration of anesthetic agents. Anesthesia providers must be able to use and interpret correctly a wide variety of monitoring devices. They are responsible for overseeing the positioning and movement of patients. At no time is an anesthetized patient moved or positioned without the approval of the anesthesia provider.

Some anesthesia providers prefer to specialize in one area, such as cardiothoracic or obstetric anesthesia. The latter involves the simultaneous care of two lives. In some settings they participate in teaching and research as well as in clinical practice. Anesthesia providers are not confined to the OR, but this is their primary arena. In addition to providing pain relief to patients and optimal conditions for surgeons during surgical procedures, anesthesia providers oversee the postanesthesia care unit (PACU) until each patient has regained control of his or her vital functions. They also participate in the hospital's program of cardiopulmonary resuscitation as teachers and team members. They act as consultants or managers for problems of acute and chronic respiratory insufficiency that require inhalation therapy, as well as for a variety of other fluid, electrolyte, and metabolic disturbances that require intravenous therapy. In the intensive care unit or emergency department, their advice may be sought regarding the total care of unconscious, critically ill, or injured patients with acute circulatory disorders or neurologic deficits. Anesthesia providers also are integral staff members of pain therapy clinics.

Circulator

The primary circulator is preferably an RN. A qualified ST may assist with circulating duties under the supervision of a RN. The circulator plays a role that is vital to the smooth flow of events before, during, and after the surgical procedure. The patient's medical record is required to identify who provided circulating duties. Patients undergoing a surgical intervention experience both physical and psychosocial trauma. They enter an alien environment removed from personal contact with family and friends, and their physical and psychologic needs are great. Because most patients are unconscious or sedated, they are powerless and unable to make decisions concerning their welfare. At this critical time, patients need the professional judgment of others who function on their behalf, and these advocates should be within close physical and social proximity at all times. The circulator's role as the patient's advocate and protector is critical to the safety and welfare of the patient and extends throughout the entire perioperative environment.

The surgeon is in charge at the operating bed, but he or she relies on the circulator to monitor and coordinate all activities within the room and to manage the care required for each patient. The RN should be continuously knowledgeable about the status of the patient. To some extent, the circulator

---

*American Association of Nurse Anesthetists: *Guidelines for the practice of the certified registered nurse anesthetist,* Park Ridge, Ill, 1983, The Association.

controls the physical and emotional atmosphere in the room, which allows other team members to concentrate on tasks without distraction.

A qualified RN should be available at all times to respond to emergencies in the perioperative environment. "Available" has been interpreted by the Nurse Practice Acts to imply that an RN can supervise an unspecified number of contiguous rooms but should be immediately available to assist in each of these rooms uninterrupted; he or she can leave a room for short periods but can return immediately to supervise or assist as needed. However, the regulations in several states specify that one RN circulate in each room.

The circulating nurse is vital to the provision of care that includes, but is not limited to, the following:

1. Application of the nursing process in directing and coordinating all nursing interventions related to the care and support of the patient in the OR. Nursing diagnosis and decision-making skills are essential in assessing, planning, implementing, and evaluating the plan of care before, during, and after a surgical intervention. This is the professional perioperative role of the RN circulator.
2. Creation and maintenance of a safe and comfortable environment for the patient by implementing the principles of asepsis. The circulator demonstrates a strong sense of surgical conscience. Any break in technique by anyone in the room should be recognized and corrected instantly. Although sterile technique is the responsibility of everyone in the room, the circulator is on the alert to catch any breaks that others may not have seen. By standing farther away from the sterile field than others, the circulator is better able to observe the entire field and the sterile team members.
3. Provision of assistance to any member of the OR team in any manner for which the circulator is qualified. This role requires current knowledge of the legal implications of surgical intervention. The circulator knows the organization of the work and the relative importance of the factors involved in accomplishing it. An effective circulator ensures that the sterile team is supplied with every item necessary to perform the surgical procedure efficiently. The circulator must know all supplies, instruments, and equipment; be able to obtain them quickly; and guard against inadvertent hazards in their use and care. He or she must be competent to direct the scrub person.
4. Identification of any potential environmental danger or stressful situation involving the patient, other team members, or both. This role requires constant flexibility to meet the unexpected and to act in an efficient, rational manner at all times.
5. Maintenance of the communication link between events and team members in the sterile field and persons who are not in the OR but are concerned with the outcome of the surgical procedure. The latter includes the patient's family or significant other plus other personnel in the perioperative environment and in other departments of the hospital. The ability to recognize and effectively communicate situations involving the patient and/or other team members is a vital link in the continuity of patient care.
6. Direction of the activities of all learners. The circulator must have the supervisory capability and teaching skills necessary to ensure maintenance of a safe and therapeutic environment for the patient. Kindly given assistance builds up the learner's confidence. In this capacity the circulator acts as a supervisor, advisor, and teacher.

DEPENDENCE OF THE PATIENT ON THE QUALIFIED TEAM

The perioperative team works to promote the best interests of the patient every single minute. For the welfare and safety of the patient, the OR team must work efficiently as a functioning single unit. The members should be thoroughly familiar with procedures, setups, equipment, and policies and should be able to cope with the unpredictable. Their qualifications must be beyond reproach. They should have a high morale, mutual understanding, trust, cooperation, and consideration. Anyone who cannot function wholeheartedly as a qualified team member has no place in the OR.

All OR personnel should have the proven knowledge, skill, and ability to perform at an optimal level at all times. The validation of clinical competence is an important aspect of providing quality patient care. Once each member of the team has passed the novice stage, other criteria demonstrate and document the knowledge and skills gained through experience and continuing education. Aligning professionally with local, state, and nationally recognized organizations that establish the standards of practice provides an opportunity for growth. Certification may include completing a course of instruction and passing an examination. Other measurements of competence include performance evaluations in a clinical setting.

Bibliography

Association of Operating Room Nurses: *Core curriculum for the RN first assistant,* ed 2, Denver, 1994, The Association.

Association of Surgical Technologists: *Core curriculum for surgical technology,* ed 4, Englewood, Colo, 1996, The Association.

Association of Surgical Technologists: *Job analysis, surgical technologist,* Englewood, Colo, 1991, The Association.

Breakiron M: Professional collaboration includes recognition of every surgical team member's role, *AORN J* 66(5):905-906, 1997.

Forsythe L: RN first assistants increase access to quality surgical care in a rural setting, *AORN J* 65(1):45-46, 1997.

Hlozek CC et al: RN first assistants expand their perioperative role, *AORN J* 67(3):560-566, 1998.

National Certification Board, Perioperative Nursing: *A job analysis for the perioperative nurse,* Denver, 1992, The Board.

National Certification Board, Perioperative Nursing: *A job analysis for the RN first assistant,* Denver, 1992, The Board.

Poe D et al: Implementation of the RN first assistant role, *AORN J* 65(1):32-41, 1997.

Ponder KS: Opinion: the RN circulator, *AORN J* 60(3):459-462, 1994.

Rothrock JC: Ensure your role in the future of perioperative nursing, *AORN J* 66(1):144-145, 1997.

Chapter 6

Administration of Perioperative Patient Care Services

 Chapter Objectives

After studying this chapter, the learner will be able to:

- Define the role of the OR head nurse.
- Define the role of the OR educator.
- Describe the relationship between the perioperative environment and other patient care departments.

ESTABLISHING ADMINISTRATIVE ROLES

The perioperative patient care team surrounds the patient throughout the perioperative experience. This direct perioperative patient care team functions within the physical confines of the operating room (OR). This room is one part of the physical facilities that make up the total perioperative environment. Other areas in the perioperative environment include preadmission testing (PAT), the ambulatory services unit (ASU), and the postanesthesia care unit (PACU). Similarly, this team makes up only one part of the human activity directed toward the care of the surgical patient. Many other people function in an indirect relationship with the patient, contributing vital supporting services toward the common goal of ensuring a safe, comfortable, and effective perioperative environment. The relationship and duties of perioperative staff members will vary according to the size and extent of the physical facilities and the number of personnel employed. No person's job is insignificant. Each has important functions to perform, and each is responsible for assuming a part of the total workload. Terms associated with administration of perioperative patient care services are found in Box 6-1.

Perioperative Administrative Personnel

Personnel should know the direction of the entire organizational effort as a prerequisite for their successful functioning. Administrative personnel interpret hospital and departmental philosophy, objectives, policies, and procedures to the perioperative staff. These terms are defined as follows:

1. *Philosophy.* Statement of beliefs regarding patient care and the nature of perioperative nursing that clarifies the overall responsibilities to be fulfilled.
2. *Objectives.* Statements of specific goals and purposes to be accomplished during the course of action and definitions of criteria for acceptable performance.
3. *Policies.* Specific authoritative statements of governing principles or actions, within the context of the philosophy and objectives, that assist in decision making

Box 6-1 Terms Associated with the Administration of Perioperative Patient Care Services

administrator Person who directs or manages departmental affairs; may be a nurse or physician.

in-service education Departmental programs designed to introduce or demonstrate equipment, techniques, or procedures used in perioperative patient care.

manager Person who plans and executes directives passed down from administration.

materiels Supplies, such as reusable or disposable goods, ordered and maintained in stock for departmental use in patient care.

by providing guidelines for action to be taken or, in some situations, for what is not to be done.

   a. *Basic policies.* Statements of the principles of administration and its approach to functioning. Examples include disallowing smoking by anyone on facility premises.

   b. *General policies.* Guidelines of the principles dealing with everyday situations that affect all personnel within the hospital. Examples include requiring all personnel, regardless of role, to be certified in cardiopulmonary resuscitation (CPR).

   c. *Departmental policies.* Guidelines structured to meet the needs of a specific work unit (e.g., OR policies). Examples include dress codes for specific areas.

4. *Procedures.* Statements of task-oriented and skill-oriented actions to be taken in the implementation of policies.

Perioperative Nurse Manager

Some private hospitals and ambulatory care settings are supervised by a doctor of medicine or osteopathy. In larger accredited facilities a registered nurse (RN) is responsible for administration and supervision of all perioperative patient care services. The perioperative environment is a business unit and high-cost center of the hospital. It should be managed as a business to manage costs and maintain effectiveness. Therefore the title and functions of the perioperative nurse manager reflect the extent and complexity of the administrative responsibilities.

In larger hospitals the perioperative nurse manager may hold some variation of the title of director of perioperative services, or assistant vice president. Because of the magnitude of the administrative duties, actual supervision of personnel may be delegated to a line manager or charge nurse. In smaller hospitals, where administrative responsibilities are not as time-consuming, the perioperative nurse manager directly supervises personnel. In other situations one nurse may manage more than one clinical service, such as the OR, PACU, ASU, special procedures room, and/or central processing department. The term *perioperative nurse manager* is used throughout this text to designate the nurse who is re-

sponsible for coordinating patient care and related support services of the department.

The perioperative nurse manager should have general knowledge of nursing theory and practice, specialized knowledge of OR technique and management, and knowledge of business and financial management. The manager should possess leadership skills to supervise and direct patient care within the perioperative environment, according to established principles and professional standards. The main function of the manager is to provide leadership that promotes a cooperative team effort. To be a leader requires additional business skills and knowledge. These concern functions of management that include planning, organizing, staffing, directing, and controlling, plus the processes of problem solving, decision making, coordinating, and communicating.

The manager is responsible for the allocation and completion of work but does not do it all or make all of the decisions. Qualified personnel are employed, and they are delegated increasing responsibility as they develop competence in their work. The manager creates an organizational attitude that can function well in his or her absence.

The manager implements and enforces hospital and departmental policies and procedures. He or she also analyzes and evaluates continuously all patient care services rendered and, through participation in research, seeks to improve the quality of patient care given. The manager retains accountability for all related activities in the perioperative environmental. The scope of this accountability includes the following:

- Provision of competent staff and supportive services adequately prepared to achieve quality patient care objectives
- Delegation of responsibilities to professional nurses and assignment of duties to other patient care personnel
- Responsibility for evaluating the performance of all departmental personnel and for assessing and continuously improving the quality of care and services
- Provision of educational opportunities to increase knowledge and skills of all personnel
- Coordination of administrative duties to ensure proper functioning of staff
- Provision and fiscal control of materiels, supplies, and equipment
- Coordination of activities between the perioperative environment and other departments
- Creation of an atmosphere that fosters teamwork and provides job satisfaction for all staff members
- Identification of problems and resolution of them in a decisive, timely manner
- Initiation of data collection and analyses to develop effective systems and to monitor efficiency and productivity

Clinical Coordinator

An assistant nurse manager aids in administration and supervision of nursing service in the OR and is directly responsible to the perioperative nurse manager. This nurse acts as administrative head in the absence of the manager. The position usually does not exist in small hospitals. In large hospitals one or more clinical coordinators provide leadership to specific services and assist with the management of manpower and material resources.

Head Nurse

The head nurse functions in a line management position as a liaison between staff members and administrative personnel. In some hospitals the title of head nurse is given to the person whose position is comparable to that of a coordinator. In others, usually smaller hospitals, the perioperative nurse manager functions more or less in the capacity of a head nurse.

In large hospitals with many surgical specialty services, a head nurse may be responsible for the administration and direct supervision of patient care in a particular specialty service, such as ophthalmology, neurosurgery, cardiovascular surgery, or urology. With this structure there are several head nurses in the department. These head nurses should have the technical proficiency required for the specialty service for which they are responsible and should have sufficient managerial ability to plan for and administer effectively the patient care activities.

The duties of the head nurse include, but are not limited to, the following:

1. Planning for and supervising patient care activities within the OR suite or specific room(s) to which he or she is assigned
2. Coordinating patient care activities with the surgeons and anesthesia providers
3. Maintaining adequate supplies and equipment and providing for their economical use
4. Observing the performance of all staff members and providing feedback
5. Interpreting the policies and procedures adopted by the department and hospital administration
6. Informing the perioperative manager of needs and problems arising in the department and assisting with problem solving
7. Assisting with orientation of new staff members

Functions vary in different hospitals, but the position of head nurse, with its direct and continuous responsibility for both patients and staff, is an important one.

Perioperative In-Service Education Coordinator

Planned educational experiences are provided in the job setting to help staff members perform effectively and knowledgeably. Most hospitals have a staff development department or committee to plan, coordinate, and conduct educational and training programs.

A program is planned to ensure a thorough orientation for each new nursing service employee. All new personnel should become familiar with the philosophy, objectives, policies, and procedures of the hospital and nursing service. This general orientation program assists the new employee in adjusting to the organization and environment. It is coordinated with an orientation to the duties in the unit to which the employee is assigned.

The in-service coordinator may be a member of the staff development department, administrative staff, or both. This person is responsible for planning, scheduling, and coordinating the orientation of new staff. This includes review of policies and procedures, performance description, and standards specific to the perioperative environment. Based on an assessment of individual skills, the new employee is given guidance and supervision for a period of weeks to months until basic competencies are adequate to function independently. Head nurses, preceptors, and other experienced staff members assist with the orientation of new personnel.

In-service education programs should also be planned to keep the perioperative staff up to date on new techniques, equipment, and patient care practices. Programs focusing on fire prevention, electrical hazards, security measures, and resuscitation training are important to ensure personnel and patient safety. Professional and technical programs designed to develop specialized job knowledge, skills, and/or attitudes affecting patient care are planned and presented. The in-service coordinator is responsible for assessing the educational needs of staff members collectively and individually and then for planning, scheduling, coordinating, and evaluating in-service programs. This individual may also conduct some sessions.

Staff development programs, conducted on a continuous basis, enhance performance by maintaining job knowledge and clinical competence. In-service programs may be supplemented by other appropriate continuing education programs held outside the health care facility or presented by qualified persons representing industry.

Preceptor

The orientation process is facilitated by a one-to-one relationship between the new employee and an experienced staff member. The preceptor teaches, counsels, advises, and encourages the orientee until he or she can function independently. The preceptor is accountable for assessing the orientee's abilities, assigning activities accordingly, and assisting in carrying out duties safely. Learning needs can be assessed through interview, observation, and a skills checklist. To ensure consistency in teaching, the preceptor coordinates development of appropriate and measurable behavioral objectives for the orientee with the in-service coordinator, management staff, or both. The preceptor should evaluate performance and offer constructive feedback to build the orientee's self-confidence. To be effective, the preceptor should have an interest in teaching and should have acquired the necessary skills and experience with adult learners.

Perioperative Business Manager

Some hospitals employ a perioperative business manager, who sometimes has the title of unit manager. This person may report to the perioperative manager or directly to the hospital administrator. Lines of authority and responsibility between the business manager and the perioperative nurse manager should be clearly defined regardless of the organizational structure. The business manager directs the management of daily operational and indirect patient care functions in the perioperative environment.

Nonnursing administrative duties should include maintaining a clean, orderly, safe environment within the department for patients and personnel. This entails more than removing visible dust and dirt. A safe environment is one that is free of contamination, electrical and fire hazards, and negligence. Formulation of procedures is necessary. Personnel should be trained. However, inspection and follow-up are equally important. The business manager coordinates these efforts with the supporting service departments: housekeeping, maintenance, laundry, and materiels management. A business manager may prepare and administrate the department budget. Doing so may include maintaining inventories and evaluating supplies and equipment. If the hospital does not employ a business manager, the nurse manager or coordinator assumes responsibility for these duties.

Advanced Practice Nurse

Within any organization a formal structure of authority and responsibility exists. However, the evolution of technology and the acute illnesses of patients have changed the focus of functions for many nurses within the hospital organization. With experience, an advanced practice nurse (APN) can manage patient care and direct the activities of others. This practitioner may hold the title of perioperative nurse clinician, clinical nurse specialist (CNS), or APN. Although the term *practitioner* is used to describe any or all of these advanced roles, differentiation is made within the profession on the basis of formal academic education to include master's preparation.

In general, minimum preparation for this expanded role is a baccalaureate degree in nursing (BSN). The CNS, however, in an advanced role, has been defined as a graduate of a master's program in nursing (MSN) who is an expert in a clinical specialty, a role model for and consultant to professional nursing staff, and a teacher of patients and other personnel. He or she conducts research to validate nursing interventions. These skills can be used effectively for advanced practice in the perioperative environment. Many APNs are registered nurse first assistants (RNFAs), and those who have attained certification in this role are titled certified registered nurse first assistants (CRNFAs).

The APN is capable of exercising a high degree of discriminative judgment in planning, executing, and evaluating nursing care based on the assessed needs of patients having one or more common clinical manifestations. A practitioner may develop the plan of care for a group of orthopaedic patients, for example. This plan is coordinated for each patient with the surgeon, other professional nurses, and allied health care personnel who assist in the performance of functions related to the plan.

Clinical nursing interventions are not necessarily performed by the practitioner. The APN decides which nursing interventions can be performed by others and which he or she personally should do. These decisions are based on personal interaction with each patient and knowledge of the clinical condition. The practitioner exercises a degree of autonomy and independence within the clinical setting. Some state boards of nursing have permitted select APNs to have minimal prescriptive powers.

Because a practitioner has advanced academic preparation in theoretic knowledge and clinical experience in a particular clinical patient care setting and is an expert in nursing situations in that setting, qualified clinical coordinators may function as practitioners. In this role they assist in planning the total care for each surgical patient, coordinating nursing and supportive services and participating in the orientation, development, and evaluation of caregivers assigned to direct patient care functions in the perioperative environment. APNs who assess individual patient needs through personal patient interviews and physical examinations and who plan for individualized care in the perioperative environment truly function as perioperative nurse practitioners. They make decisions relative to direct and indirect patient care in the perioperative environment, using specialized judgments and skills. Problem solving and decision making are the heart of professional management and professional leadership.

The practitioner may work solely or primarily with the surgeons in a specific surgical specialty. Some APNs work as independent contractors with a surgical group as a qualifier for APN certification. This concept of nursing specialization coincides with the specialization of surgeons. With practice and formal or informal study, nurses develop expertise in planning and implementing care for patients with similar surgical problems. Skills and knowledge become highly specialized. Surgeons in that particular specialty rely on these nurses to supervise the care of their patients and to direct less experienced personnel on the perioperative team.

INTERDEPARTMENTAL RELATIONSHIPS

The perioperative environment is one of many departments within the total hospital organization. To provide continuity in patient care, many departments coordinate their efforts through the administration of the formal organizational structure of the hospital.

Every hospital has a governing body that appoints a chief executive officer (CEO), usually with the title of hospital administrator, to provide appropriate physical resources and personnel to meet the needs of patients. Administrative lines of authority, responsibility, and accountability are defined to establish the working relationships between departments and personnel (Figure 6-1).

A nurse executive, sometimes referred to as the vice president of patient care services or director of nursing services, reports to the hospital administrator. The perioperative nurse manager reports to the nurse executive if perioperative services are a division under management of the nursing service. In some facilities perioperative services are an independent unit not managed by the nursing service. The perioperative nurse manager then reports directly to the CEO, an

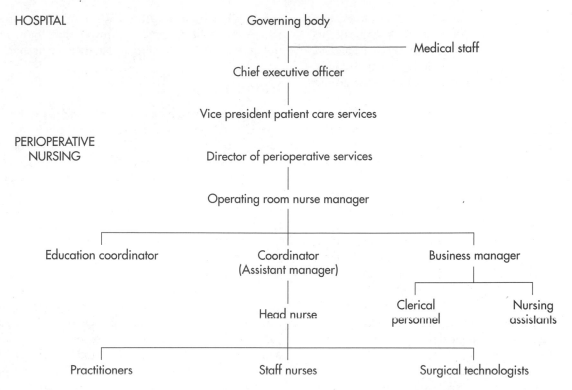

HOSPITAL

Governing body

Medical staff

Chief executive officer

Vice president patient care services

PERIOPERATIVE
NURSING

Director of perioperative services

Operating room nurse manager

Education coordinator

Coordinator
(Assistant manager)

Business manager

Head nurse

Clerical
personnel

Nursing
assistants

Practitioners

Staff nurses

Surgical technologists

Figure 6-1 Management structure. Administrative lines of authority, responsibility, and accountability are defined to establish working relationships between departments and personnel.

assistant administrator, or the chief of one of the medical services. Through either channel of administration, many activities in the perioperative environment are coordinated with other patient care units and departments within the facility.

Patient Care Units

Patients come to the OR directly from a short-stay or in-house patient care unit, an outpatient ambulatory care area, or the emergency department (ED). Channels of communication should be kept open between perioperative personnel and patient care personnel in other units. Coordination of preoperative preparation and transportation of patients prevents downtime in the perioperative environment. Many facilities use a checklist system to ensure adequate preparation of surgical patients in a timely manner. An RN or licensed practical/vocational nurse (LPN/LVN) signs or initials each item accomplished. By the time the patient leaves for the patient care unit, all of the preparations have been completed.

Emergency Department/Trauma Center

Victims of trauma and acutely ill patients often are seen initially in the hospital emergency department (ED). Cardiopulmonary resuscitative and other equipment is available to initiate prompt triage and treatment. Minor injuries usually can be treated in the ED. Some patients must be scheduled for an emergency surgical procedure, however. These patients may arrive in the OR before the results of all diagnostic tests are confirmed. Therefore communication between

OR, ED, laboratory, and x-ray personnel is vital to the success of surgical intervention. OR personnel should be advised of the nature of the injury or illness to prepare all needed equipment and obtain supplies for the emergency surgical procedure.

Designated regional trauma centers should have teams of surgeons, anesthesia providers, and perioperative personnel who are immediately available in the hospital 24 hours a day. A trauma nurse coordinator is administratively responsible for all personnel and activities to ensure comprehensive trauma care.

Labor and Delivery Suite/Obstetric Unit

The obstetric unit is divided into three separate areas: labor and delivery, postpartum care, and newborn nursery. Some labor and delivery areas have an OR for delivery by cesarean section (C-section). In other hospitals patients scheduled for either elective or emergency C-section are brought to the OR suite. In addition to supplies needed for the surgical procedure, adequate resuscitative equipment must be available for the newborn.

Intensive Care Unit

Because surgery has become more specialized and complex, specialized patient care facilities where concentrated treatment can bring the patient to a satisfactory recovery have become a necessity. This care is provided in an intensive care unit (ICU), which is open 24 hours a day, 7 days a week. It is staffed by highly trained and specialized RNs. Critically ill patients who need constant care for several days are admitted directly from the OR, PACU, ED, or other patient care unit. Each bedside is equipped with therapeutic and monitoring equipment.

Depending on the size of the facility and its specialty services, more than one specially designed and equipped surgical intensive care unit (SICU) may be provided. One ICU may admit only cardiovascular surgical patients (coronary care unit [CCU]), another may admit only pediatric patients (pediatric intensive care unit [PICU]), and another may admit only neurologic patients (neurologic intensive care unit [NICU]). In addition to SICUs, most hospitals also have a unit for nonsurgical (medical) patients (medical intensive care unit [MICU]). The increased efficiency that these units afford serves the best interests of both the facility and the patient. They create the most effective use of personnel and equipment and lower morbidity and mortality rates.

Movements of patients to and from the SICUs should be closely coordinated with the surgical schedule, the OR team, and the PACU personnel. If the surgeon or anesthesia provider anticipates that a patient will need intensive care postoperatively, an SICU bed is reserved at the same time the patient is scheduled for the surgical procedure. The appropriate SICU should be notified promptly when the surgeon determines that an unanticipated bed is needed. Sometimes the patient must wait in the OR or PACU for an available bed. Sometimes elective surgical procedures are postponed because sufficient SICU beds or staff are not available.

Radiology and Nuclear Medicine Departments

Frequently, personnel from the radiology (x-ray) and nuclear medicine (radiation therapy) departments assist with diagnostic or therapeutic procedures in the OR. For some procedures it may be necessary for perioperative personnel to go to the x-ray department to assist the surgeon during a procedure requiring sterile technique. Whenever a diagnostic procedure or surgical procedure is scheduled that will require use of x-ray equipment or a radioactive implant, all departments should be notified at least the day before. This facilitates the scheduling of personnel and workload in all departments.

Pharmacy

Many drugs are routinely stocked in the OR suite for the anesthesia providers' use, and some are kept for use by the surgeons during surgical procedures. These are obtained by requisition from the pharmacy. Narcotics are always kept under lock, and each dosage is recorded as dispensed.

The pharmacy is not an isolated department but an integral part of the hospital. Pharmacists are resource persons who convey drug information to physicians and nurses. They should be responsible for preparation of all admixtures, but often the mixing of medications is done by RNs in the pre-

operative holding area, OR, PACU, and SICU to expedite administration. The pharmacist is responsible for quality control of drug product services throughout the hospital.

Blood Bank

All hospitals have a blood transfusion service or blood bank. This is a highly technical service for collecting, testing, processing, and distributing blood products. If the hospital does not have its own blood bank, blood may be supplied from a regional blood center. Written policies and procedures for blood transfusion services must conform to the standards of the American Association of Blood Banks. These include criteria for accepting blood donors, laboratory testing of donors' and recipients' blood, and preparing and administering blood products for therapeutic purposes. Blood banks dispense whole blood, plasma, packed cells, or platelets only as they are needed.

If in advance of an elective surgical procedure the surgeon anticipates that blood loss replacement may be necessary, the patient may have his or her own blood (autologous) drawn and stored in the blood bank for autotransfusion, a blood replacement procedure. Blood bank technicians also may participate on autotransfusion teams for collection of patients' blood intraoperatively and postoperatively.

If autologous blood is not available or additional units of donor blood (homologous) are needed, a sample of the patient's blood is sent to the blood bank for type and crossmatch. In emergency situations this sample may be sent from the ED or the OR. The units of blood products ordered by the surgeon or anesthesia provider are prepared and labeled with the patient's name and blood data. Suspected or recognized adverse reactions to blood transfusion must be documented on the patient's chart and reported to the blood bank.

Pathology Department

The pathologist, a physician who specializes in the cause and effect of disease, may be on call at a few minutes' notice to examine tissue while the patient is anesthetized. This enables the surgeon to proceed immediately with a definitive surgical procedure if malignant tumor cells are found, without subjecting the patient to a second surgical procedure at a later time. A small laboratory may be located within the perioperative environment with equipment for microscopic tissue examination. This laboratory may be used for other tests and/or for taking photographs of tissue specimens removed from patients. Routinely, all tissue removed during a surgical procedure is sent to the pathology department for a minimum of gross examination.

Clinical Laboratory

Samples of blood, urine, or body fluids are taken to the clinical laboratory for analysis. Some analyses are routinely performed preoperatively. Others are done during a surgical procedure, such as blood gas analyses. Samples are obtained and immediately sent to the laboratory, or samples may be obtained during a surgical procedure for analysis later, such as a culture to determine the cause of an infection.

Biologic testing of sterile supplies is done routinely. The perioperative environment may be biologically tested when a contamination problem is suspected. The bacteriologist, who specializes in the study of microorganisms, may come into the OR suite to collect samples for testing, or samples may be collected and sent to the laboratory by OR personnel. The results provide a method for evaluating the effectiveness of procedures and the degree of adherence to environmental standards.

Medical Records Department

Clinical records include the admitting diagnosis, the patient's chief complaint, complete history and physical examination findings, the results of laboratory examinations, and the physicians' and nurses' care plans. Records should state the therapy employed, including surgical procedure(s), and include progress notes, consultation remarks, the patient's condition on discharge, or observations in case of death. A summary of the hospitalization experience should be complete. These records are signed by the physicians and nurses attending the patient.

The anesthesia record completed during the surgical procedure by the anesthesia provider also becomes part of the patient's record. The circulator should write pertinent remarks regarding the care rendered in the OR and the patient's response on the nurses' note sheet or the progress notes. Documentation is a responsibility of all professional team members implementing direct patient care.

Notes about the surgical procedure should be explicit, dictated promptly after completion of the procedure, and incorporated into the record of each surgical patient. For the surgeons' convenience, many hospitals have dictating machines or a phone hookup with the medical records department installed within the OR suite, usually located in the dressing room or lounge. Details of the preoperative and postoperative diagnosis and the surgical procedure itself may have medical and legal significance. It is the responsibility of the medical records department to transcribe the surgeon's dictation and to maintain the patient's chart after his or her discharge from the hospital. The patient's chart may be put on microfilm for storage.

Environmental/Housekeeping Services

Housekeeping functions are recognized as important preventive measures to eliminate microorganisms from the hospital environment. Each hospital establishes a routine for its particular needs. Usually the environmental/housekeeping services personnel and perioperative personnel share housekeeping duties in the perioperative environment. The amount of cleaning done by the perioperative personnel varies from one hospital to another. In many hospitals the members of the housekeeping department terminally clean all furniture,

flat surfaces, lights, and floors once a day at the end of the surgical schedule. In others they also clean the furniture and floors before the schedule starts and between each surgical procedure throughout the day. Whatever plan they follow, housekeeping personnel should have a storage area within the OR suite in which to keep their equipment and supplies. Equipment used for cleaning in the OR is not taken outside the suite.

The director of environmental/housekeeping services and the perioperative nurse manager plan the division of work. Personnel in each department should understand their responsibilities. The perioperative nurse manager checks the work of housekeeping personnel and keeps in touch with the director concerning their performance.

The director evaluates and chooses the proper solutions for effective cleaning, sets up a program and standard of performance for personnel, and sees that personnel are properly oriented and taught the appropriate procedures. This includes procedures for removal and disposal of trash and soiled laundry. Using a checklist helps to cover all areas to be cleaned and inspected on a routine basis, whether it is daily, weekly, or monthly. Weekly or monthly cleaning routines include walls and ceilings, in addition to the daily cleaning schedule within the perioperative environment.

The director impresses on the personnel the importance of the work and the part they play in enabling the perioperative personnel to carry out aseptic technique. The housekeeping personnel do indeed function as members of the team when working with the scrub persons and circulators between surgical procedures.

Maintenance Department

The maintenance department personnel work in close cooperation with the OR department by providing a continuous preventive maintenance program. This includes routine monitoring of ventilation and heating, electrical and lighting systems, emergency warning systems, and water supply. Humidity is recorded every hour in the maintenance department. All electrical equipment is checked monthly by maintenance department personnel. In addition, they regularly test the autonomous emergency power source and maintain a written record of inspection and performance.

The hospital water supply system should not be connected with other piping systems or with fixtures that could allow contamination of the water supply. The hot water supply and steam lines have temperature control devices and filters regulated by the maintenance department personnel. They are cleaned on a routine schedule, usually weekly, to prevent accumulation of mineral deposits.

Clinical Biomedical Engineering

Competent technical personnel should be available to every area of the hospital to ensure the safe operation of equipment. Nearly every surgical procedure uses some form of powered instrumentation. Because of the variety and complexity of the instrumentation currently in use, most hospitals have a clinical engineer and/or biomedical equipment technician on staff or available. This technical support group assists perioperative personnel in evaluating and selecting new equipment, in installing and operating it, and in maintaining it.

The clinical engineer is systems and applications oriented. This individual can compare different models and manufacturers' specifications and provide recommendations for purchase. The biomedical equipment technician is knowledgeable about the theory of operation, the underlying physiologic principles, and the practical, safe clinical applications of biomedical instrumentation. This individual can test, install, calibrate, inspect, service, and repair equipment. Every preventive service or repair is recorded in an instrument history file.

Materiels Management

In an effort to control escalating health care costs, many hospitals belong to contract buying groups. This concept has changed the nature of the purchasing function and the management of supplies. The organizational administrative structure varies, but the basic functions of materiels management are purchasing, processing, inventorying, maintaining proper function, and distributing supplies and equipment. Several departments are responsible for supplies.

Purchasing Department

The purchasing director coordinates the acquisition of supplies and equipment for the hospital. Standardization of products used throughout the hospital fosters quantity purchases, which provides leverage in negotiating prices with vendors. Items that are too expensive to stock in large quantities or that are used infrequently are ordered through the purchasing department as needed. In some hospitals this department is referred to as materiels management.

Central Storeroom

The purchasing director or materiels manager determines the supplies to be stocked for requisition by all of the departments of the hospital. Bulk inventories are received and warehoused in the central storeroom. Each department then requisitions supplies as needed, usually on a weekly basis.

Central Service

One area of the hospital is designed specifically for storing, processing, and distributing supplies and equipment used in patient care. This department may be referred to as central service or central supply; central processing; supply, processing, and distribution; or materiels management. The functional design and work flow patterns provide for separation of soiled and contaminated supplies from clean and sterile items. Supplies are replenished on the nursing units on a predetermined time schedule to maintain standard inventory levels. This may be done by central service, using an exchange cart system, in which a cart of fresh supplies is exchanged for the one in use. Control of patient charges for

supplies also may be coordinated by central service. Inventory control is computerized in most hospitals. Bar code technology on individual packages may facilitate patient charges and inventory management.

Sterile Processing

Supply needs in the OR are unique. Instruments, reusable products, and many other supplies must be decontaminated and cleaned after use and inspected, packaged, and sterilized before use. Two separated areas must be designated for these functions whether they are performed within the OR suite, in central service, or in a sterile processing department designed specifically for this purpose.

Hospitals built or renovated after the mid-1980s usually use a surgery case cart system. Personnel in sterile processing prepare individual carts with the required supplies and instruments for each scheduled surgical procedure. Instrument books and computerized surgeon's preference cards are routinely used to ensure that all the necessary supplies are included. Many of these are commercially prepared one-time-use items and devices that the patient will pay for. Lists for the patient charge items and the instruments provided are usually attached to the cart to assist personnel in appropriately accounting for all items. Each cart is transported to the assigned OR. After the surgical procedure, the cart with soiled supplies is returned to the decontamination area. Usually the decontamination and reprocessing of OR instruments and equipment are done in areas separated from supplies used in other hospital departments. This prevents mixing surgical instruments with those supplied to other units. The personnel assigned to the surgery case cart areas should be familiar with the supplies needed for each surgical procedure, how surgical instruments are used, and the proper method of cleaning and sterilizing each. Surgical technologists frequently are assigned to sterile processing because of their technical background.

Laundry Services

Many disposable, nonwoven fabrics are used. However, some woven fabrics are processed daily for use in the hospital, such as patient gowns, bedding, and towels. Hospitals that do not have laundry facilities as part of their physical plant use a commercial laundry service. An adequate inventory should be maintained for daily use. The manager of the laundry services assists in determining appropriate inventories and supervises the laundry processes. Reusable fabrics that must be sterilized before use are packaged and sterilized either in the laundry, central service, sterile processing department, or the OR suite, depending on where the sterilizing equipment is located.

Human Resources/Personnel Department

Careful selection of capable, highly motivated people contributes to efficiency and effectiveness. The human resources/personnel department helps to screen applicants.

Those seen as having potential for available positions are referred to the appropriate department head. Potential employees may be processed through the nursing service before an interview with the perioperative nurse manager is scheduled. The human resources/ personnel department assists in hiring and terminating all employees. This department also provides resources for employee assistance and assists with progressive discipline.

COORDINATION THROUGH COMMITTEES

A committee is a group of persons delegated to consider, investigate, take specific action, or report on a matter of mutual concern or interest. Many activities within the facility are coordinated by multidisciplinary committees.

Perioperative Committees
Operating Room Committee

The OR committee is a committee of the medical staff that is vital to the management of the perioperative environment. One surgeon is appointed chief or director of the department of surgery. In teaching hospitals a director is appointed chief of each specialty service (e.g., chief of orthopaedics). The anesthesia department also designates a director of that department. These individuals are responsible for professional practice and administrative activities within their respective departments. They should maintain continuing evaluation of the professional performance of all members of the medical staff who have been granted privileges in their specialty. They also serve as liaison representatives between the medical staff and hospital administration.

The chief of surgery, the chiefs or representatives of the specialty services, the chief of the anesthesia department, the perioperative nurse manager, the coordinator, and/or the OR business manager meet at regular intervals to review departmental activities. The hospital administrator and vice president of perioperative services may also be members of this committee or may be invited to attend meetings relevant to their concerns.

The OR committee formulates policies and procedures pertaining to utilization of facilities, schedule of surgical procedures, and maintenance of a safe environment. Evaluation of techniques and selection of new products may require review of reports from other departments or committees in addition to those prepared by perioperative personnel.

Because this committee determines policy and procedures for efficient functioning within the OR suite, persistent problems are brought before the committee, where recommendations for corrective action are made. For example, if temperature and humidity controls are not being effectively monitored or maintained, the committee may recommend to the hospital administration that procedures be reviewed and revised by the maintenance department or that new equipment be installed. If surgeons are repeatedly late in arriving, thus delaying the surgical schedule, stronger policy may be indicated for the control and better utilization of facilities. If a new product is purchased, a new procedure may need to be written to specify its use and care. Through data collection and a problem-solving approach to decision making, the OR committee seeks to improve the working relationships of all members of the OR team and the supportive services concerned with activities within the perioperative environment.

Policies and associated directives formulated and approved by the committee serve as guides for governing the actions of surgeons, anesthesia providers, and the patient care staff while in the perioperative environment. The perioperative nurse manager shares with the OR committee, hospital administration, and nursing service the responsibility for clarification, implementation, and day-to-day enforcement of approved policies and procedures.

Laser Safety Committee

The laser safety committee establishes policies and procedures, standards, documentation systems, and credentialing criteria for the use of lasers in the health care facility. The laser safety committee may also be responsible for the development of training and continuing education programs for physicians, nurses, and surgical technologists. This may be a subcommittee of the OR committee. Members should include, but are not limited to, the chief of surgery, the chief of anesthesia, physician representatives from each surgical specialty using the laser, the perioperative nurse manager, laser nurse specialists, a biomedical technician, and a representative of administration.

This committee may delegate safety surveillance duties to a laser safety officer (LSO) who is responsible for identifying problems and safety concerns with the use of lasers. The LSO may be a physician, nurse, or specially trained laser technician. The LSO is given the authority to stop any laser procedure if safety is in question.

Infection Control Committee

The infection control committee investigates hospital-acquired (nosocomial) infections and seeks to prevent or control them. Membership may vary but should include representatives of the medical staff, hospital administration, nursing service, and the epidemiologist or infection control coordinator. Representatives from other departments attend meetings when the agenda is relevant to their particular concerns.

The committee meets at least quarterly. Members form a defense against nosocomial infections by reviewing environmental factors and by determining whether the hospital is providing a safe environment for patient care. They review all infection reports and investigate nosocomial infections. Committee members also review policies and procedures and scrutinize the entire chain of asepsis in an effort to determine and then eliminate possible sources of infection.

This committee has the authority to approve changes necessary to eliminate any hazardous practices. Included in its jurisdiction is the education of personnel so that they can provide a high standard of patient care. A health care facility has a moral duty to provide a safe environment for its patients. The infection control committee aids the hospital in fulfilling this duty. Surveillance personnel assist in directing infection control policies, procedures, and practices.

Infection Control Coordinator

An infection surveillance, prevention, and control program uses the services of a key person and agent of the infection control committee—the infection control coordinator. Because this person is often an RN with special training in epidemiology, microbiology, statistics, and research methodology, he or she may be called an infection control nurse (ICN) or nurse epidemiologist. The infection control coordinator monitors the environment for infections. The ICN works in close collaboration with the infection control committee. The ICN's duties are as follows:

1. Promptly investigating outbreaks of disease or infection above expected levels.
2. Promptly identifying the origin and cause of outbreaks by epidemiologic study.
3. Acquiring, correlating, analyzing, and evaluating surveillance data and bacterial colony counts. This includes gathering information to compute and classify specific wound infection rates for all invasive procedures. Rates should be entered in the infection control committee record and be available to the department of surgery.
4. Tracking factors that contribute to infection problems.
5. Consulting with directors of critical areas, such as the OR. If an outbreak of postoperative infections occurs, the ICN confers with the OR nurse manager. They review the patients' intraoperative records to determine if the infected patients had the same procedure or same surgical team, or were operated on in the same room. They review antiseptic agents used for skin preparation, antibiotics used for wound irrigation, and other commonalities in patient care. If a patient develops signs and symptoms of infection within the immediate postoperative period, a causative factor in the OR is suspect.
6. Coordinating educational programs for personnel who influence infection control. The ICN is a consultant to all hospital personnel and a liaison officer in dissemination of information on infection control.
7. Assisting in employee health programs in regard to screening, immunizing, and monitoring the personal health of personnel.
8. Assisting in development and implementation of improved patient care procedures.
9. Comparing monthly statistics. There is cause for concern if the monthly reported surgical wound infection rate rises significantly. Reports and data can be helpful in evaluating aseptic practices if they are brought to the attention of personnel.
10. Reporting appropriate diseases to public health authorities.
11. Comparing products for effectiveness. The infection control committee approves disinfectants and antiseptics, for example, based on recommendations of the coordinator.
12. Obtaining information from surgeons about evidence of infection after discharge and conducting retrospective studies for statistical analysis.

In short, the infection control coordinator identifies problems, collects data to find the causes, investigates solutions, and makes recommendations for appropriate hospital policies and procedures to prevent infections. In evaluating infection problems, the ICN attempts to find a common denominator. This often leads to the source of the problem. For example, an outbreak of postoperative respiratory infections would lead to investigation of the cleaning and sterilizing of anesthesia equipment and respirators. Success of the control program depends in part on the information provided by a conscientious staff, including physicians.

Infection Control Program

An effective infection control program aims to reduce the incidence of infections and to control sources. Information collected through surveillance serves as a basis for corrective action. This information includes written records and reports of known or potential infections among patients and personnel.

Guidelines and standards for infection control and surveillance are published by the Joint Commission on the Accreditation of Healthcare Organizations in the *Accreditation Manual for Hospitals*. In general, these standards and guidelines include the following:

- Establishment of an effective hospital-wide program for surveillance, prevention, and control of infection
- Establishment of a multidisciplinary committee to oversee the program by reviewing surveillance reports and by approving policies, procedures, and actions to prevent and control infection
- Assignment of a qualified person(s) to be responsible for management of the infection surveillance, prevention, and control program
- Provision of written policies and procedures pertinent to infection surveillance, prevention, and control for all patient care departments and supporting services
- Provision of patient care support services that are adequately prepared to perform all required infection surveillance, prevention, and control functions

Surveillance

The Centers for Disease Control and Prevention (CDC), an agency of the Department of Health and Human Services, is the third largest section of the U.S. Public Health Service. Functioning on both national and international levels, its activities are multifaceted. It carries out a national surveillance of disease incidence and a program, including health education, in prevention of communicable diseases. Through liaison with state and local health departments, the CDC provides assistance and consultation to health care facilities for specific problem solving, analysis of surveillance data, or on-site investigation of serious outbreaks of infections. As part of its commitment to the prevention of nosocomial infections, the CDC furnishes information on how to structure an infection control program.

Performance Improvement Committee

Members of the performance improvement committee include representatives of both clinical and administrative personnel. This committee monitors routine activities, evaluates clinical outcomes, reviews incident reports, and conducts problem-focused studies in an effort to identify practices deemed substandard. Actual practices may be in violation of policy or not in compliance with accepted standards or governmental regulations. Noncompliance puts a hospital or ambulatory care facility at risk of legal liability. A productive and efficient committee will implement actions designed to eliminate real or potential problems, improve patient care, and reduce financial loss. Because of an emphasis on cost containment, review of utilization of facilities and risk management also may be concerns of this committee.

Many facilities employ a quality improvement coordinator and/or a risk manager to ensure implementation of committee decisions. The primary function of the person in this position is to assess actual practices and evaluate outcomes of patient care. The continuous quality improvement (CQI) coordinator may receive and respond to complaints about patient care or environmental hazards.

Each hospital department and patient care area may have its own quality improvement subcommittee. These unit-based committees monitor performance, identify ways to constructively solve competency problems, and seek opportunities for improvements in practices. Other interdepartmental subcommittees may focus on specific activities or problems requiring input from several disciplines. Reports from these subcommittees are reviewed by the CQI coordinator. Mutual problems are shared with the hospital committee.

Ethics Committee

A multidisciplinary ethics committee should represent the hospital and the community it serves. Representatives include physicians, nurses, social workers, patient relations liaisons, clergy, lawyers, bioethicists, and laypersons from the community. Their primary purpose is to educate the staff and the community regarding moral principles and processes of ethical decision making in the face of diverse issues that arise in the care of critically and terminally ill patients. They provide consultation to professional staff, patients, and families. This committee recommends policies and guidelines on such issues as informed consent, research protocols, and advance

directives. Perioperative nurses and surgical technologists often are confronted with social, ethical, and legal decisions concerning genetic and reproductive biology, organ transplantation, and death with dignity. The ethics committee can provide a forum for discussion of these issues. Some hospitals have a nursing bioethics committee in addition to the hospital committee. These committees provide education and consultation and develop policies and procedures. They are not decision-making bodies. They do not get involved in disciplinary matters.

Hospital Safety Committee

Representatives from administration, the nursing service, the medical staff, the engineering and maintenance departments, environmental/housekeeping services, the dietary department, and the safety director form the nucleus of the hospital safety committee. This group writes policies and procedures designed to enhance safety within the hospital and on hospital grounds. They exchange information with the infection control and quality improvement committees and conduct hazard surveillance programs. They meet at least every other month to investigate and evaluate reported incidents. Action is taken when a hazardous condition exists that could result in personal injury or damage to equipment or facilities.

Disaster Planning Committee

Health care facilities should have an organized plan for caring for mass casualties if a major disaster occurs. External disasters happen outside of the health care facility, such as an airplane crash or an event of nature (e.g., a flood or hurricane). Internal disasters, such as a fire or an explosion, happen inside the health care facility. Planning by the intrahospital committee includes consultation with local civil authorities and representatives of other medical agencies to establish an effective chain of command and to make appropriate jurisdictional provisions. This planning results in disaster-site triage to separate and distribute patients to ensure the most efficient use of available facilities and services.

External disaster drills are held at least twice a year to try out the plans developed by the committee, to seek to improve them, and to familiarize personnel with them. Plans for both types of disasters include the following:

- An information center within the hospital to facilitate a unified medical command and the movement of patients.
- A receiving area for the injured. Severely wounded casualties are given emergency care according to their needs and are sent at once to the OR or to other units as indicated or transferred to another facility. Ambulatory patients may be treated in the ED for slight injuries and sent home or admitted to the hospital as indicated.
- Special disaster medical records or tags that accompany patients at all times.

- A plan of organization of personnel. As soon as a hospital receives word of a disaster during the evening or night, several key persons are called. These in turn telephone others previously assigned to them, and these call still others, until the full staff has been notified. If the disaster occurs during the day, the full staff is usually on duty, although any off-duty personnel may be called. Other departments are alerted and come on duty as needed; these include personnel for the blood bank, laboratory, pharmacy, materiels management, x-ray department, and patient care units, including the OR, PACU, and ICU. If disposable drape packs are not in use, it may be necessary to alert some laundry personnel. Some key maintenance personnel should be available, especially electricians.
- Written departmental instructions for personnel. For the perioperative staff these may include sign-in procedures, checklists of duties, and patient scheduling procedures.

Personnel must know where to report, what to do, and where extra supplies are kept in case of an emergency. Extra supplies are stored in reserve in sufficient quantities to fill possible needs for a minimum of 1 week.

Bibliography

Abbott CA: Intraoperative nursing activities performed by surgical technologists, *AORN J* 60(3):382-393, 1994.

Advance practice nurse competency statement, *AORN J* 61(1):64-69, 1995.

Association of Operating Room Nurses: Standards of perioperative administrative practice. In *AORN standards and recommended practices for perioperative nursing,* Denver, 1995, The Association.

Buchanan LM: Therapeutic nursing intervention, knowledge development and outcome measures for advanced practice, *Nurs Health Care* 15(4):90-195, 1994.

Hylka SC et al: The role of advanced practice nurses in surgical services, *AORN J* 66(3):481-485, 1997.

Ladden C, Keane A: Perioperative nurse practitioners, *AORN J* 61(6):1067-1071, 1995.

Moss R, Thompson J: AORN sales course, *AORN J* 63(4):745-749, 1996.

Philosophy of perioperative nursing practice: definition of perioperative nurse; scope of perioperative nursing practice, *AORN J* 59(6):1188-1191, 1994.

Phippen ML, Applegeet C: Clinical issues: unlicensed assistive personnel in the perioperative setting, *AORN J* 60(3):455-457, 1994.

Zeil S: Spectators in the OR, *AORN J* 65(2):427-430, 1997.

Section

III

The Patient as a
Unique Individual

Chapter 7

The Patient: The Reason for Your Existence

 Chapter Objectives

After studying this chapter, the learner will be able to:

- Describe Maslow's hierarchy of needs.
- List the key elements of a patient-centered approach.
- Describe how the patient may perceive care.

HISTORICAL BACKGROUND

Patient care has changed throughout history. In 1922, medical texts by authors such as Morris King, M.D., included sections for nurses regarding patient care. Much of the information was relayed in the same manner as environmental theorist Florence Nightingale (1820-1910) directed in her classic text *Notes on Nursing: What It Is and What It Is Not.* Environmental influences included care of the sick room, attitudes and approaches of the caregiver, and housekeeping duties. Service and obedience to the physician was the most desired attribute. The uniform salary for patient care was four to five dollars per day.

Directories of nurses and persons providing patient care were available at pharmacies, physician's offices, and hospital nursing departments. Patient care in the home setting was available at a moment's notice. An emphasis was placed on how the nurse or caregiver was expected to behave and look. A preference for females between the ages of 25 to 30 showed clear sex bias.

Early texts examined the psyche of the patient, illustrating an understanding of the need for clear communication in the effort to gain trust. Early authors suggested that speaking in normal tones and keeping extraneous noise to a minimum would promote rapid recovery and wellness. They also suggested that an explanation of necessary tasks and an avoidance of sudden unexpected actions would foster cooperation during convalescence.

PATIENT-CENTERED CARE

The patient is the reason for the existence of the health care team. He or she looks to the perioperative team to fulfill his or her diverse needs during the preoperative, intraoperative, and postoperative phases of care (Figure 7-1). The patient is always the center of attention, not just when he or she is under the operating room (OR) spotlight. Terms associated with patient care are listed in Box 7-1.

Patient as an Individual

A patient may be defined as an individual recipient of health care services. Extremes of age (pediatric or geriatric) and

Figure 7-1 The OR from the patient's perspective.

Figure 7-2 Maslow's hierarchy of basic needs as related to surgical patient's needs during perioperative care.

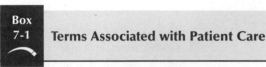

Box 7-1 Terms Associated with Patient Care

comorbid disease Illness associated with a combination of disease entities.

paradigm A model used as a foundation for a conceptual framework.

perception Using the senses, cognition, and awareness to evaluate the collective stimuli of the environment.

stress Internal perception of and response to stimuli in a positive or negative manner.

comorbid disease entities require individualization of the plan of care. To meet a patient's requirements and expectations effectively, personnel should have knowledge of his or her needs, problems, and health considerations. From a perioperative perspective, it is important to understand the impact a surgical procedure has on a patient's lifestyle.

Characteristics that individualize patients include, but are not limited to, the following:

- They are worthwhile and unique individuals.
- They respond psychosocially on the basis of their personal values, beliefs, and ethnocultural background.
- They have the capacity to adapt to both their internal and external environments.
- They have basic needs that must be met in order to maintain homeostasis.

Homeostasis is a consistent internal environment maintained by the patient's adaptive capabilities, and it has both a physiologic and a psychologic component. From a physiologic aspect, the patient's body strives to maintain equilibrium within normal limits through control mechanisms located in the endocrine glands and in the reticular formation in the brainstem. This stability depends partly on the structural integrity of the body, the adequacy of its functions, and environmental influences.

Psychologic homeostasis is based on emotional acceptance and a rational understanding of events that influence health and wellness. Fear and anxiety are common stressors that alter a patient's psychologic response to the health care system.

Patient's Basic Needs

Needs are factors that must be controlled or redirected to restore altered function. Nursing diagnoses are based on knowledge and understanding of a patient's needs and how to fulfill them. The surgical patient faces a threat to the needs identified by humanistic psychologist and motivational theorist Abraham Maslow (1908-1970): physical, security, psychosocial, emotional, and spiritual.

Hierarchy of Needs

In following Maslow's concept of a motivational hierarchy of needs to set priorities for care (Figure 7-2), the basic lower level or physiologic needs essential for survival must be met first. Satisfaction of the higher level needs for safety and security, belonging and acceptance, self-esteem, and self-actualization can then be met. Health care personnel should be concerned with a total picture of the patient's needs and consider all of them. In illness, needs can be influenced by factors

TABLE 7-1	Common Coping Mechanisms		
Mechanism	**Meaning**	**Objective Assessment**	**Example**
Denial	Rejects responsibility; unable or unwilling to accept the truth	Stammers; may or may not make eye contact; seems to be making excuses	"I do not have lung cancer."
Displacement	Shifts blame to a weaker substitute	Is submissive to power figures, but critical and oppressive to subordinates	"My doctor never tells me anything. The lab must be wrong."
Identification	Acts like an admired hero or villain	Shows outward signs of indecisiveness and low self-esteem	"My sister and I both feel ill. We both have the same disease, I'll bet."
Projection	Attributes unacceptable behavior to others	Acts suspicious of others; assumes a defensive posture	"The cigarette manufacturer enticed me to smoke."
Rationalization	Justifies behavior with plausible statements	May be defensive or smug; trying to save face; can become hostile	"I became ill only because cancer runs in my family."
Reaction formation	Acts differently than he or she feels inside	Is confused, irrational; has mood swings; may seem overly conscientious and moral	"These are not tears of sadness, they are tears of joy because I will be dead soon."
Regression	Reverts back to a more primitive state of being	May assume closed, fetal position; has crossed arms and legs; looks downward, cries; has prolonged silences	"I want my mother."
Repression	Blocks unacceptable thoughts and feelings	Has a blank stare, a questioning look; no in-depth discussions	"I don't remember what my diagnosis is. Why am I here?"

such as location of the pathologic condition, type of surgical procedure, and effectiveness of therapy. Also, priorities may change with changing situations. Preoperatively, anxiety and nutritional status are addressed. Intraoperatively, the team concentrates on the patient's physiologic needs for oxygen, circulation, and the prevention of shock and infection. Post-operatively, team members must prevent complications and encourage patient self-actualization. If the patient's needs are not met satisfactorily, undesirable consequences can occur.

Patient Reactions to Illness

To meet a patient's needs, the health care team should be sensitive to his or her feelings about the illness. A patient's reactions influence his or her behaviors and the staff's behavioral responses. An understanding of the patient's basic methods of coping will be helpful to the caregiver in developing the plan of care (Table 7-1).

Behavior

Health and human behavior are interdependent and often age dependent. Regardless of age, individuals with physiologic problems experience some emotional change that influences their behavior. Patients react to a new interpersonal environment according to their learned behavioral patterns. The following are basic facts about behavior:

- The perception of interaction within the environment creates individual differences in personality, behavior, and needs.
- A person's physical and psychosocial behavior is a response to stimuli in an attempt to maintain homeostasis.

- Behavior is complex. Behavioral acts have multiple causes in addition to a major precipitating one.
- A person functions on many levels simultaneously. Many factors determine an individual's response in a given situation.

Behavior should be evaluated in light of the person's specific situation and pertinent social forces such as family, culture, and environment. Patients respond to crises or personal threats in different ways. Some persons face suffering and surgical intervention with extreme courage, dignity, and fortitude. Others may revert to extreme fear or helplessness, even when faced with a relatively safe procedure. Overt behavior is not necessarily consistent with one's feelings but often reflects them most accurately. Patients often express frustration and fear behaviorally in an effort to cope with environmental stimuli.

Adaptation

In 1984, Sister Callista Roy proposed adaptation as a conceptual model for nursing. Any deviation from a person's normal daily pattern of living necessitates adaptation through innate or acquired defenses. Adaptation may involve physiologic or psychologic changes. Her paradigm as it applies to perioperative patient care includes the following:

1. The patient takes in stimuli and processes the information to produce a response.
   a. Effective adaptation is exhibited by a favorable response.
   b. Ineffective adaptation is exhibited by unfavorable response.

2. The environment around and inside the patient is constantly changing. The patient responds either favorably or unfavorably to each change.
3. The health status of the patient integrates the whole person as he or she adapts to changes in internal and external forces.
4. The process of nursing is a science, and the application of patient care is an art.

Both the mind and the body must adapt successfully in order for the patient to recover. Adaptation requires energy, ingenuity, and persistence. The adaptive process includes physiologic or psychologic changes that constitute an attempt to counteract stimuli so the individual can continue to function. If something interferes with this adaptation, the effects can be detrimental. Adaptation to illness includes the following three stages:

1. Transition from health: development of symptoms
2. Acceptance: coping and making decisions
3. Convalescence or resolution

Adaptation may be rapid or slow depending on the nature of the stimuli and on the patient's culture, learned responses, and developmental needs. Adaptations may be sensory, motor, or sensorimotor. The extent of adjustment required is contingent on the type of illness, the magnitude of disability, and the patient's personality.

Stress

Stress can be defined as a physical, chemical, or emotional factor that causes tension, and it may be a factor in disease causation. It is the result of a perceived threat and is manifested by changes in physiologic and psychosocial behavior. Stress tolerance depends on the individual and on the stressor—its intensity, duration, and type (either localized or generalized, such as pain).

Stressful factors can originate from within the individual or from the external environment. *Intrinsic* factors, or those that originate within a patient, include the following:

*   Hereditary or genetic factors, such as competency of the hormonal or enzymatic system.
*   Nature of the illness or disease process. This may be influenced by nutritional or immunologic status.
*   Severity of the illness or the presence of a stigma.
*   Previous personal experiences with illness. Chronic illness has a disruptive effect on lifestyle.
*   Age. Children feel threatened, whereas adolescents resent an interruption of activities and are painfully aware of body changes. Older people think about infirmity and death.
*   Intellectual capacity. Misconceptions can lead to a knowledge deficit about the disease. Impaired cognitive function creates an inability to understand or comprehend.
*   Disturbed sensorium. Hearing or sight loss intensifies a stressful experience.
*   General state of personal well-being.

Extrinsic factors originate from external sources and include the following:

*   Environment. The physical and social environment of the hospital is not the same as that of the home.
*   Family role and status. Expectations and authoritative relationships affect lifestyle, attitudes, and communications.
*   Economic or financial situation.
*   Religion. Beliefs influence attitudes and values toward life, illness, and death. For example, Jehovah's Witnesses will not permit transfusion of whole blood or blood components. Orthodox Jews must follow dietary laws in any environment. The fatalistic attitudes derived from some religious beliefs give a person little control over his or her environment and can render a patient passive and apathetic.
*   Cultural background, education, and social class. These factors are closely related to a patient's emotional responses and living habits. Significant elements such as food habits, daily living patterns, hygiene, family organization, child care, and orientation to the past, present, and future should be analyzed in relation to culture. An ethnic community is really a larger family. Roles taught by a cultural group influence the mores, beliefs, and social interactions of its members. Also, responses to pain may vary according to cultural or ethnic background. Some groups commonly show an exaggerated emotional response, whereas with other groups it is more appropriate to conceal suffering and feelings.
*   Social relationships. Family, significant others, and friends help satisfy the need for reassurance and provide a sense of being cared about.

Stress is both physiologic and psychologic. It can adversely affect appetite and bodily functions such as digestion, metabolism, and fluid and electrolyte balance. The secretion of adrenal cortical hormones delay wound healing and decrease resistance to infection. In addition, the patient's emotional needs come to the surface during times of markedly increased stress, which mobilizes defense mechanisms for flight or fight. The patient's ability to adapt depends in part on effective intervention.

Anticipatory apprehension, although normal to some degree, may diminish critical thinking and decision-making abilities and may initiate an exaggerated response. Patients feel vulnerable when threatened with the loss of body parts, bodily function, or life. The strangeness of the OR itself—its noises, odors, and equipment—represents a unfriendly environment.

Patient Perceptions of Care

Studies have shown that a patient's perception is based on expectations of high-level care. The patient's belief system defines what he or she considers to be good care. Perceptions of caring behaviors vary according to the degree of illness, type of procedure, level of cognition, and setting. Most patients believe that proficient and efficient perioperative care includes assistance with pain control, warmth, comfort, and a safe environment. The caregiver is also perceived as a patient advocate and a communication link with the family and/or significant others.

Research has revealed that preoperatively, a patient needs information about the surgical procedure, how it will be performed, and the type of anesthetic to be used. Intraoperatively, the patient assumes a passive role, entrusting his or her care to the perioperative team. Before administration of the anesthetic, the patient may be acutely aware of the surroundings and activities. Patients surveyed indicate that during this segment of intraoperative care they want to know what is happening as it takes place and desire reassurance from the circulator at his or her side. Patients expect the perioperative nurse to remain in close physical proximity and act promptly in an emergency. During and after the administration of the anesthetic, the patient places a strong sense of confidence in the team as a whole and has expectations of competence and efficiency. The professional nurse is considered a main source of protection during this period of vulnerability.

Postoperatively, the patient expects the perioperative nurse to monitor his or her condition closely and to provide pain relief as needed. In continuation of the passive role, the patient perceives the nurse as caring, protective, and efficient. Patients respond favorably to the following:

- Provision of privacy
- Sensitivity to the inconvenience of hospitalization
- Frequent family updates during the surgical procedure
- Attention to personal and special needs
- Friendliness
- Accurate and understandable information about tests and treatments

Family/Significant Others

A discussion of the patient would not be complete without specific mention of the patient's family or of others significant in his or her life. Illness often creates an emotional and financial burden on the family. They may experience considerable anxiety over the outcomes of surgery, the feelings of isolation, and the disruption of lifestyle.

Families need preoperative instruction in order to prepare for the postoperative outcomes and rehabilitation. They also need to be kept informed of the patient's progress during the surgical procedure and recovery period. Time passes more slowly during waiting periods, and family members may fear something has gone wrong if the wait is longer than anticipated. Some family members may prefer to wait at home or at work. The surgeon should contact a spouse, family, or significant other when the surgical procedure is over.

PATIENTS WITH SPECIAL NEEDS

The debilitated, chronically ill, or age-extreme patient has an increased difficulty in combating the stress of surgery and anesthetic agents. Other problems or health considerations that predispose the patient to intraoperative or postoperative complications include substance abuse or other serious subclinical conditions not revealed during the preoperative assessment.

Preoperative diagnostic and laboratory studies assist in establishing diagnoses and in pinpointing areas of deficiency. Surgical intervention is often postponed until a physiologic situation is improved or controlled (e.g., high blood pressure is lowered and cardiac dysrhythmias are corrected). Preoperative therapy may be indicated to control diabetes, reduce obesity, or treat infection to decrease the risk of complications.

Patients of various ages and stages of development have different needs, and the ways of meeting these needs will vary. A family-centered approach to care is valuable. Family cooperation is essential for communication with, interpretation for, and assistance with patients, particularly geriatric patients.

Patients with Sensory Impairments or Physical Challenges

Some patients come to the perioperative environment with conditions unrelated to the surgical problem. Sensory and physically challenged patients commonly have increased anxiety and require a highly individualized plan of care; these patients also have the potential for a problematic postoperative recovery.

Sensory Impairments

Communication is essential to assess adequately the needs of challenged patients and to care for them. Team members should know about and understand the patient's limitations. The patient has a right to know what will happen during the surgical experience and to participate in decisions about his or her care. The Rehabilitation Act of 1973 states that to receive federal funds, an agency "must provide, when necessary, appropriate auxiliary aids . . . to people with impaired sensory, manual or speaking skills to give them an equal opportunity to benefit from services." The complexities of each patient's situation should be evaluated and dealt with appropriately.

Language Barrier A language barrier can be a complex challenge. Anxiety increases in proportion to one's inability to communicate in a stress-producing situation. The inability to understand or to express oneself verbally is frustrating, and the patient's behavior may reflect his or her feelings of inadequacy or insecurity. Nonverbal body language through eye contact, pleasant facial expressions, and a gentle touch can comfort the patient who speaks a different language. Every effort should be made to obtain an interpreter to assist the patient and the health care team; many hospitals use interpreters for the ethnic groups within the community. Some patients are reluctant to share confidential medical information with a relative or friend. The interpreter should be trusted and accepted by the patient and should be sensitive to the needs of the surgeon and caregivers. The patient needs to be adequately informed before giving consent for a surgical procedure.

Hearing Impairment/Deafness

Hearing impairment varies from inner ear conduction changes that occur during the aging process and affect the distinction of some high-frequency consonant sounds to congenital profound sensorineural deafness. Conductive or sensorineural deafness may result from disease or injury to the ear at any age. The degree of impairment will determine whether the patient communicates through sign language, has a hearing-assistive cochlear implant, has a hearing aid, and/or reads lips. Written information is always helpful, provided the patient is literate. Pictograms work well with most patients. An interpreter can assist with patients who use sign language.

The following steps should be observed when communicating with a patient who has a hearing impairment:

1. Make sure the room is quiet and well lit, with minimal distractions.
2. Look directly at the patient. Speak clearly and slowly in a moderate tone of voice, with visible but not exaggerated lip movements. Facial expressions, touch, and body gestures can help communicate feelings and instructions.
3. Greet the patient without wearing a face mask, and attract the patient's attention before speaking.
4. Be sure the patient understands and responds appropriately to questions.
5. To help explain your actions, show the patient any equipment (e.g., a safety strap) before placing it on him or her.
6. Allow the patient to wear a hearing aid in the perioperative environment. If possible, try to know what type of device the patient uses and how to adjust the controls if it should start humming during the procedure.

Visual Impairment/Blindness

Like deafness, blindness can be a part of the aging process or a congenital anomaly. Cataracts is a common cause of the loss of visual acuity; this condition may be inherited but is more often associated with aging. Sight is also affected by the shape of the eye, other structural factors, and diseases and injuries.

Patients who are blind feel insecure in a strange environment; therefore the following steps should be observed when communicating with them:

1. Address the patient by name in moderate tones and introduce yourself.
2. Always speak to the patient before touching him or her. A gentle word followed by a gentle touch can comfort the patient.
3. To prevent a distressful reaction to unexpected noises or sensations, the patient should be told what is going to happen around him or her.
4. Guide the patient's hand will help him or her to feel secure, such as when he or she is being moved onto the operating bed.

A visually impaired patient should be permitted to wear eyeglasses in the perioperative environment as much as possible. If a general anesthetic is used, the glasses should be sent to the postanesthesia care unit (PACU) so they are available when the patient wakes up. Contact lenses must be removed before administration of a general anesthetic because they may dry on the cornea or become dislodged.

Physical Challenges

Patients who are physically challenged require a highly individualized plan of care. Physical problems such as contractures or pressure sores may make it difficult to position the patient on the operating bed. Creative supports and positioning aids are required, and additional assistance may be needed to move the patient safely. Exposure of the surgical site may be difficult to achieve.

Millions of people suffer from some form of arthritis. Children with juvenile rheumatoid arthritis have many systemic problems as a result of the disease process, which continues into adulthood. The onset of this autoimmune disease can occur at any age and can result in stiffness, swelling, and deformity of the joints of the hands, feet, and neck; inflammation of blood vessels; and tissue damage to organ systems. Joints need solid but padded support. Long-term treatment with nonsteroidal antiinflammatory drugs (NSAIDs) or corticosteroid therapy may affect bleeding intraoperatively and wound healing postoperatively.

Paralyzed patients, such as persons with spinal cord injury, are unable to move. Patients with lack of voluntary muscle control, such as persons with cerebral palsy, must be protected from falls or injuries during transport or transfer. These patients have decreased tactile sensitivity to heat and cold, so they must be protected from burns or hypothermia.

Impairments of Cognitive Function

Communicating with patients who have impaired cognitive function is sometimes difficult. Cognitive functions are based on intelligence and the ability to think, learn, remember, and solve problems. Explanations about procedures and the environment may seem confusing and frightening to these patients. Verbal communication should be attempted at the patient's level of understanding and response. Simple phrases and soft vocal tones can be reassuring. Cooperation during the surgical procedure may be hard to attain, and preoperative sedation may be necessary.

Patients with Alteration of Nutrition

Decreased intake and increased metabolic demands create nutritional problems in surgical patients. Drug therapy and procedural activities affect nutritional status; this should be taken into consideration when planning for a patient's nutritional needs. Table 7-2 describes the effects that certain drugs have on nutrition. The preoperative assessment may reveal risk factors associated with alterations of nutrition.

TABLE 7-2	Drugs That Interfere with Nutritional Status
Drug	**Effect on Nutrition**
Aluminum hydroxide	Binds with other nutrients, causing phosphate malabsorption
Aminoglycosides	Reduce carbohydrate metabolism
Amphetamines	Suppress appetite, causing weight loss
Antacids	Alter gastrointestinal pH
Anticholinergics	Decrease gastrointestinal motility, causing malabsorption
Antihistamines	Stimulate appetite and can cause weight gain
Antihypertensives	Decrease gastrointestinal motility, causing malabsorption
Antineoplastics	Impair nutrient absorption
Antirheumatoids	Impair nutrient absorption
Benzodiazepines	Stimulate appetite, causing weight gain
Cathartics	Cause calcium and phosphate loss
Chloramphenicol	Inhibits protein binding
Cytotoxic agents	Suppress appetite, causing weight loss
Immunosuppressives	Suppress appetite, causing weight loss
Isoniazid	Causes pyridoxine deficiency
Neomycin	Interferes with bile acids, causing iron, sugar, and triglyceride malabsorption
Phenobarbital	Causes vitamin D deficiency
Phenothiazines	Stimulate appetite, causing weight gain
Phenytoin	Causes osteomalacia
Steroids	Deplete sodium
Tricyclic antidepressants	Stimulate appetite, causing weight gain

Malnutrition

Malnutrition in the surgical patient is caused by an inadequate intake or use of calories and protein preoperatively and/or postoperatively. The discrepancy between the intake of essential nutrients and the body's demand for them creates a state of impaired functional ability and structural integrity. As a result of malnutrition, the patient may experience the following:

1. Poor tolerance of anesthetic agents
   a. Decreased metabolism of chemicals by the liver
   b. Inadequate excretion of toxins by the kidneys
   c. Unstable vital signs
2. Altered wound healing potential
   a. Decreased protein synthesis postoperatively
   b. Increased protein wasting and breakdown of skeletal muscle following severe traumatic injury
   c. Negative nitrogen balance with a serum albumin less than 3 g/dl and a blood urea nitrogen (BUN) less than 10 g/dl
3. Decreased serum electrolytes associated with anorexia, bulimia, alcoholism, and other chronic metabolic disturbances
   a. Hypokalemia (low potassium level)
   b. Hypomagnesemia (low magnesium level)
   c. Hypocalcemia (low calcium level)

Box 7-2	Factors That Increase a Patient's Risk for a Protein-Based Nutritional Deficit

Chronic illness	Sensory impairment	Immobility
Acute illness	Unconsciousness	Edentulousness
Stress	Polypharmacy	
Metabolic disease	Depression	

4. Increased susceptibility to infection from immunologic incompetence, with a total lymphocyte count less than 1500/mm^3
5. Sequential multisystem organ failure
   a. Dehydration
   b. Abnormalities in glucose regulation
   c. Abnormalities in clotting mechanisms
   d. Renal failure
   e. Cardiopulmonary failure
6. Increased risk of morbidity and mortality

Serum blood tests help determine nutritional status and include total proteins, albumin/globulin ratio, and BUN level. Body weight is also significant. The average adult patient needs a minimum of 1500 calories daily to prevent body protein catabolism. Hypermetabolic states can double that requirement to 3000 calories daily. If caloric intake is less than body requirements, protein is converted into carbohydrates for energy. Protein synthesis then becomes insufficient for restoration of body tissues. Box 7-2 describes patient conditions that place a patient at risk for protein deficiency and malnutrition.

Depleted reserves of essential elements must be replenished to replace tissue loss and expedite wound healing. Protein deficiency impairs collagen formation, thereby delaying the healing process. Water soluble vitamins C and B complex are important for tissue repair and nervous system function. The fat-soluble vitamins A, D, E, and K are important for neurovascular activities. The patient's depleted nutritional status lowers host resistance by impairing lymphocyte and neutrophil production. A definite relationship has been demonstrated between hypoproteinemia and proliferative postoperative infection.

Metabolism

Metabolism is the phenomenon of synthesizing foodstuffs into complex elements and complex substances into simple ones in the production of energy. It involves two opposing phases:

1. *Anabolism,* or constructive metabolism: the conversion of nutritive material into complex living matter; tissue construction
2. *Catabolism,* or destructive metabolism: the breaking down or dissolution by the body of complex compounds, often with the release of energy

Metabolic disorders such as diabetes and the stress response of traumatic injury can complicate the outcome of a surgical intervention. Hormonal responses to physical stress involve both anabolic and catabolic effects on the body, with catabolism being the predominant effect. The degree of metabolic reaction may depend greatly on the body's reserve of labile protein. The patient's preoperative nutritional state, the type and extent of the surgical procedure, and the effect of the surgical procedure on the patient's ability to digest and absorb nutrients affect immediate postoperative metabolism.

Catabolic responses are augmented by preoperative fasting, cathartic preparation, adrenocortical responses to tissue trauma during the procedure, blood loss, and alterations in fluid and electrolyte balance. Patients with burns, traumatic injury, absorptive disorders, or toxemia need careful nutritional replacement because they usually have a severe protein deficit. Hydration and renal function are closely observed and monitored in the perioperative environment.

Drugs also can have an adverse affect on metabolic balance. Broad-spectrum antibiotics limit a disease process, but in association with dietary inadequacy they can cause vitamin K deficiency in older patients by inhibiting the intestinal bacteria that produce that vitamin. Drug detoxification and/or excretion may be altered in patients with impaired kidney or liver function, leading to possible drug overdose.

Nutritional Supplements

Dietary management is used to correct metabolic and nutritional abnormalities before the surgical procedure. In some patients special nutritional supplements are indicated to build up or compensate for a permanent metabolic handicap. Successful therapy is indicated by weight gain, a rise in plasma albumin, and a positive nitrogen balance. A chemically defined elemental diet may be administered via the following routes:

- Oral intake
- Nasogastric tube
- Gastrostomy tube, with or without infusion pump
- Intravenous (IV) infusion of protein and dextrose through a peripheral vein
- Central venous cannulation for hyperalimentation

Hyperalimentation (Total Parenteral Nutrition)
Hyperalimentation, or total parenteral nutrition (TPN), is another method of fulfilling nutritional requirements. Essential nutrients are delivered directly into the bloodstream intravenously through a large central vein. This mode of therapy is used for patients with nutritional defects who fail to gain or maintain weight by other means and who are not amenable to oral intake or nasogastric intubation. For patients who require long-term nutritional assistance, TPN in coordination with other therapy provides the daily requirements necessary for metabolic function and protein synthesis.

BASIC SOLUTION   A concentrated hypertonic solution is used to provide 2500 to 3000 calories daily in a small volume. This solution usually consists of (1) glucose and fat emulsions to provide calories and (2) amino acids for protein synthesis. The physician orders the solution contents for each patient. A patient's specific needs for serum electrolytes de-

termine which essential elements, vitamins, and minerals are included.

Solutions are prepared in the pharmacy with strict aseptic technique under a laminar airflow hood. Because the solution is a medium for bacterial and fungal growth, it is stored at 39° F (4° C) until used and is warmed to room temperature before administration. Commercial TPN solutions are available. If used, they are modified to meet individual needs. Mixing additives poses a risk of contamination.

CENTRAL VENOUS CANNULATION   With central venous cannulation, a long-term large-bore catheter is surgically inserted through a large-diameter vein with high blood flow (e.g., the internal or external jugular, cephalic, or subclavian vein) into the superior vena cava or right atrium. A single-lumen, double-lumen, or triple-lumen catheter is used. These catheters are made of polymeric silicone with a polyester fiber cuff. Under C-arm fluoroscopy, the tip of the catheter is threaded into the vein through a venotomy to the desired position. The distal (external) end is brought through a subcutaneous tunnel with an exit point in the anterior chest wall. The polyester cuff anchors the catheter, and monofilament nylon sutures are used to maintain its position.

The Broviac catheter is slightly smaller (1 mm inside diameter) than the Hickman catheter (1.6 mm inside diameter). Therefore the Hickman catheter may be used intermittently for the infusion of pharmacologic or chemotherapeutic agents, antibiotics, and/or blood products or for the withdrawal of blood samples. A double-lumen catheter affords advantages of both: the Broviac port is used for continuous TPN, and the Hickman port is used for other needs.

INFUSION RATE   The pump-controlled infusion rate of the prescribed solution is calculated according to the amount of fluids ordered for a 24-hour period. Slow administration is necessary because bypassing the regulatory mechanism in the gastrointestinal tract and liver places an increased burden of elimination on the cells and kidneys. The flow rate is cautiously monitored because unstable blood glucose levels may result. The hypertonic TPN solution is viscous and has a high osmolarity that can cause massive cellular dehydration and congestive heart failure if rapidly infused. A decreased flow rate may result from a plugged filter or a change in body position.

PRECAUTIONS   Maintaining a closed IV system with minimal catheter manipulation is important. Leaks in external tubing can allow air to be sucked into the system during inspiration and result in an air embolus. Therefore all connections in the setup should be taped to prevent accidental separation. The patient is instructed to avoid touching the insertion site and to report any discomfort.

Strict asepsis is required for catheter insertion, maintenance, and infusion. The technique itself introduces a foreign body and exposes the circulation to a potentially dangerous external environment at a time when the patient can least afford complications. The possibility of sepsis is the greatest deterrent to hyperalimentation therapy.

There is risk for contamination every time the line is entered. Therefore a single-lumen central TPN line should be used only for the delivery of nutrition. It should not be used for piggyback IV setups such as the administration of blood constituents or medications, central venous pressure monitoring, or blood drawing for laboratory analysis. A multilumen catheter may be inserted for these purposes.

OTHER CONSIDERATIONS TPN is not a contraindication to ambulation. Long-term therapy can be accomplished at home with adequate professional instruction, supervision, assistance, and observance of strict aseptic technique. TPN is discontinued gradually to prevent rebound hypoglycemia and to permit adjustment to a lowered glucose level.

Patients with Diabetes

Diabetes mellitus is an endocrine disorder that affects glucose metabolism and the production of insulin in the beta cells of the pancreas. Insulin is a hormone that helps break down carbohydrates. If insulin is not produced in sufficient quantities or is of poor quality, carbohydrates are not metabolized and are excreted in the urine as glucose. Glucose molecules are large and damage the cellular structure of the renal tubules of the kidneys. Usually genetic in origin, diabetes mellitus can be triggered in predisposed individuals by environmental stress. Management of the surgical patient with diabetes depends on the type and control of the disorder, which will be one of three types:

1. *Type I: Insulin-dependent diabetes mellitus (IDDM).* The pancreas produces little or no insulin, thus necessitating regular administration of insulin by injection. Onset may be at any age but usually occurs in juveniles (adolescents aged 12 to 16) and adults up to age 40.
2. *Type II: Non–insulin-dependent diabetes mellitus (NIDDM).* The pancreas produces varying amounts of insulin. Onset may be at any age but usually occurs after age 40 in obese persons. Blood glucose levels are controlled by diet and the administration of oral antihypoglycemics.
3. *Diabetes mellitus associated with other conditions or syndromes.* Impaired glucose tolerance may be secondary to pancreatic or hormonal disease, drug or chemical toxicity, abnormal insulin receptors, or other genetic syndromes. The diabetes may be latent, asymptomatic, or borderline.

Stress caused by physical and emotional trauma, infection, or fever raises blood glucose levels and stimulates the pituitary and adrenal glands. The pituitary gland secretes adrenocorticotrophic hormone (ACTH), which stimulates the production of glucocorticoids. These glucocorticoids in turn increase gluconeogenesis, the formation of glucose by the liver from noncarbohydrate sources. The resultant extra glucose enters the bloodstream. Coincidentally, the adrenal glands secrete epinephrine, which accelerates the conversion of glycogen in the liver to glucose and also raises the level of blood sugar. More insulin is needed to metabolize this additional blood sugar. The primary goal in controlling diabetes is to maintain a stable internal environment, thereby averting a metabolic crisis. Extreme care must be taken to prevent the following:

1. Hyperglycemia and ketonuria
   a. A rise in blood glucose and ketones can precipitate severe fluid loss, causing dehydration and hyperkalemia from the release of potassium from cells.
   b. Some medications (e.g., cortisone) increase the level of blood sugar and antagonize the effect of insulin.
2. Ketoacidosis and acetonuria
   a. These conditions are caused by insulin insufficiency from natural causes or from a reduced or omitted insulin dosage.
   b. These conditions may result in coma and ultimately death if allowed to progress untreated.
3. Hypoglycemia and hypoglycemic shock
   a. These conditions are caused by too much insulin.
   b. They are of faster onset than ketoacidosis.
   c. Hypoglycemia is especially dangerous. It can occur during major surgical procedures because of the omission or delay of oral intake.
   d. These conditions can cause brain damage and put stress on the cardiovascular system.

Prevention of these states depends on the following:

- Physician's treatment of choice for diabetes
- Severity and type of disorder
- Existence of complicating conditions
- Type of surgical procedure

The preoperative assessment of patients with the potential for impaired glucose metabolism includes laboratory testing for fasting and postprandial blood glucose levels, urinalysis, complete blood count, BUN, and serum electrolyte determinations. A chest x-ray study and electrocardiogram are also advisable.

Common Complications

The balance between caloric intake and glucose metabolism is disrupted during the perioperative experience. Patients with NIDDM usually withstand a surgical intervention without crisis. Intraoperative metabolic control may be more difficult in patients with IDDM who have marked unpredictability and greater extremes in blood sugar levels. Lengthy major surgical procedures with extensive tissue trauma present the greatest challenge to regulation. Patients with diabetes are prone to the following:

- Dehydration and electrolyte imbalance.
- Infection.
- Inadequate circulation from neurovascular disease, causing deficient tissue perfusion.
- Hypertension.
- Hyperlipemia that affects both coronary and peripheral arteries. Peripheral edema can lead to gangrene.
- Delayed wound healing as a result of increased protein breakdown or compromised circulation. Glycogenesis,

the breakdown of glycogen to glucose in the liver, diverts protein from tissue regeneration.

- Neuropathy or nervous system disorders, which causes motor and sensory deficit.
- Nephropathy, which affects small blood vessels in the kidneys.
- Retinopathy, which affects small vessels in eyes, and blindness.
- Neuropathic skeletal disease. Severe bone destruction may cause neuropathic fractures.
- Neurogenic bladder, which causes incontinence. Urinary tract infections are common.

Diabetes causes many bodily changes that increase in frequency with duration of the disease. Physiologic dysfunctions, as listed in Table 7-3, make a person with diabetes a potentially high-risk patient.

Special Considerations

Scheduling elective surgical procedures early in the day for patients with diabetes minimizes the period during which oral intake is restricted. Assessment of these patients can minimize potential risks:

1. Capillary blood obtained by finger stick should be tested preoperatively for fasting serum glucose. The results provide baseline data to assess postoperative control.
2. The preoperative insulin dose may be reduced or eliminated to guard against hypoglycemia or insulin shock during the surgical procedure.
3. Continuous IV access is vital throughout the surgical procedure in case of a metabolic problem. An infusion of dextrose in water may be started to begin administering the daily carbohydrate requirement before the patient comes to the OR.
   a. Optional methods of management for patients who are insulin-dependent are determined by the severity of the disease, the preoperative control regimen, and the type of surgical procedure. Insulin may be added to the infusion or administered by subcutaneous injection. Amounts are determined by serum glucose levels.
   b. Adequate hydration must be maintained because a rising blood glucose level upsets osmotic equilibrium. Electrolytes may be added to maintain metabolic status.
   c. Fluid intake and output must be monitored to maintain hydration without fluid overload.
4. A metabolic crisis in an unconscious patient is difficult to detect. Therefore during long surgical procedures, blood glucose levels are monitored for hyperglycemia or hypoglycemia, and fractional urine specimens are monitored for ketones. Glucometers accurately measure capillary blood glucose levels. Monitoring is necessary to ascertain the patient's requirements for insulin, glucose, or both.

5. Nasogastric suction may cause acidosis, dehydration, or electrolyte imbalance.
6. Antiembolic stockings are usually worn by the patient during the surgical procedure and postoperatively as a precaution against thrombophlebitis and thromboembolism.
7. Skin integrity must be guarded to avoid sepsis.
   a. Strict aseptic and sterile techniques are extremely important to the infection-prone diabetic patient.

TABLE 7-3	Physiologic Dysfunctions in High-Risk Patients	
Diabetes Mellitus	**Obesity**	
Integumentary System		
Skin that may be dry, itchy	Hirsutism in women	
Loss of fat from adipose tissue	Excess subcuticular fat	
Injuries that heal slowly	Injuries that heal slowly	
Musculoskeletal System		
Neuropathic skeletal disease with bone destruction	Osteoarthritis	
Leg pain, neuropathy	Chronic back pain	
Muscular wasting	Strain on joints and ligaments	
	Joint pain	
	Diminished mobility	
Cardiovascular System		
Increased heart rate	Myocardial hypertrophy	
Predisposition to coronary artery disease	High blood pressure	
	Arteriosclerosis	
Predisposition to thrombophlebitis	Venous stasis	
	Varicose veins	
Peripheral edema		
Respiratory System		
Predisposition to infection	Shortness of breath	
	Decreased tidal volume	
	Decreased lung expansion	
Renal System		
Nephropathy	Vascular changes in kidneys	
Increased excretion		
Neurogenic bladder		
Gastrointestinal system		
Secretion of glucose by liver		
Neurologic System		
Neuropathy	Decreased intestinal mobility	
Sensory impairment	Predisposition to liver and biliary disease	
Retinopathy and blindness		
Endocrine System		
Poor or nonexistent insulin production	Predisposition to diabetes mellitus	
Poor metabolic control	Pituitary abnormalities	
Increased production of cortisol by adrenal glands under stress	Poor metabolic control	
	Dysfunctional uterine bleeding	
Electrolyte imbalance		

b. To protect bony prominences and to prevent pressure sores, foam padding or a gel mattress should be placed on the operating bed for surgical procedures expected to take more than 2 hours.
c. Hyposensitive tape is used to affix dressings.

Obese Patients

Obesity is prevalent in our society. It may be of one of two origins:

1. *Endocrine origin:* Usually associated with biliary, hepatic, or endocrine disease.
2. *Nonendocrine origin:* Usually associated with excessive caloric intake. It is referred to as morbid obesity when weight exceeds 100 pounds (45.4 kg) over the ideal weight.

Common Complications

Surgical patients who are 10% or more overweight have an increased incidence of morbidity and mortality caused by concomitant systemic diseases and physical problems. The degree of morbidity varies with the severity of the obese condition. The physiologic dysfunctions of obesity are listed in Table 7-3.

Obesity predisposes an individual to several conditions:

- Increased demand on the heart. Pulse rate, cardiac output, stroke volume, and blood volume increase to meet the metabolic demands of the adipose tissue (fat). Eventually this overload leads to myocardial hypertrophy (enlargement of the heart), and congestive heart failure may result. Coronary artery disease is also common.
- Hypertension (high blood pressure). Vascular changes in the kidneys are associated with hypertension and affect the elimination of protein wastes and the maintenance of fluid and electrolyte balance.
- Varicose veins and edema in the lower extremities. Poor venous return results from pressure on the pelvic veins and the vena cava. Venous stasis can ultimately contribute to thrombophlebitis and thromboembolism.
- Pulmonary function abnormalities. Hypoxemia, or inadequate oxygen in blood, may be associated with decreased tidal volume or poor gaseous exchange caused by excessive weight on the thoracic cavity. Patients who are obese are susceptible to postoperative pulmonary infection and pulmonary embolism.
- Diseases of the digestive system, such as liver or gallbladder disease.
- Osteoarthritis. This condition may limit mobility of the spine and joints.
- Diabetes mellitus.
- Malnutrition. Even though the obese patient is overweight, he or she may have a protein deficiency or other metabolic disturbance such as hyperlipidemia.

Special Considerations

The physical size of an obese patient presents problems for the OR and PACU teams. Safety precautions against injury, falls, and burns must be emphasized. Problems include the following:

1. Transporting and lifting the patient. Mechanical patient lifters are desirable. If these are not available, extra persons are needed to ensure safety in lifting.
   a. Stretchers and operating beds must be weight-appropriate and stabilized. Most operating beds cannot support more than 300 to 350 pounds. The manufacturer's instructions should be consulted. Tables should be tagged with clearly visible weight restrictions.
   b. In moving the patient from the stretcher to the operating bed, the wheels should be locked, and it should be suggested that the patient sit up. The back of the patient's gown should be untied, and the patient should be asked to feel for the far side of the bed so that he or she does not move too far and fall. Additional personnel should stand at the opposite side of the bed to prevent falls.
   c. Safety belts should be long enough to provide secure limitation of unwanted mobility. When the patient is supine, the belt is placed over the thighs 3 to 4 inches from the knees.
2. Keeping exposure to a minimum. Obese patients are often self-conscious.
3. Induction, intubation, and maintenance of anesthesia.
   a. On rare occasions, venous cutdown may be necessary to establish an IV line if peripheral veins are invisible.
   b. Mobility of the cervical spine to hyperextend the neck for intubation may be limited.
   c. Inefficient respiratory muscles, poor lung/chest wall compliance, and/or increased intraabdominal pressure in the supine position reduce ventilation capability.
   d. Inefficient ventilation lowers the concentration of gases entering the alveoli of the lungs, which prolongs induction time.
   e. Continuous uptake by adipose tissue requires higher concentrations of anesthetic agents to maintain anesthesia. Drug dosages must be calculated by body weight.
   f. The recovery period may be prolonged because adipose tissue retains fat-soluble agents and because the poor blood supply in this tissue eliminates agents slowly.
4. Positioning on the operating bed.
   a. Extra personnel may be necessary to assist with positioning.
   b. Massive tissue and pressure areas must be protected. Protuberances must be padded to prevent bruising and pressure injuries (Figure 7-3).

Figure 7-3 Positioning an obese patient for spinal surgery on an Andrews frame.

    c. Ventilation and circulation must be ensured.

    d. When an electrosurgical unit is used, the patient dispersive electrode is applied on a flat, dry, smooth surface and is not surrounded by overlapping skin folds because tissue could be burned.

5. Increased operating time due to mechanics of the surgical procedure.

    a. In an open procedure, the accessibility of deep organs (e.g., gallbladder) may be a problem.

    b. Large instrumentation may contribute to surgical trauma and postoperative pain.

6. Thromboembolic complications, which may occur because of venous stasis; erythrocytosis, which increases the viscosity of the blood; and a decrease in fibrinolytic activity. Anticoagulants such as subcutaneous heparin may be given prophylactically.

7. Delayed healing because of poor vascularity of adipose tissue. Obese patients have an increased incidence of postoperative wound infection and disruption.

    a. A sterile, closed drainage system is often used to drain accumulated fluid, thereby facilitating healing.

    b. It is harder to eliminate "dead space" in wound closure.

Chronic Comorbid Disease

Patients come to the OR for surgical procedures unrelated to a chronic cardiopulmonary or pulmonary disease. Even for unrelated surgeries, however, the presence of these conditions may present a high risk for physiologic complications.

Cardiovascular Disease

The surgeon is particularly concerned about hemostasis and the potential for hemorrhage in a patient who is taking an anticoagulant medication. A patient who takes aspirin prophylactically is instructed to discontinue its use for 2 weeks preoperatively.

    The anesthesia provider regulates the medications of patients who have an unstable blood pressure. Blood pressure is also monitored and maintained with appropriate medications in patients with a history of hypertension or hypotension. Tissue perfusion and oxygenation are critical to wound healing and are dependent on the circulatory status of the patient.

Pulmonary Disease

Any chronic condition that compromises pulmonary function presents a potential risk for a patient undergoing general inhalation anesthesia. Bronchoconstriction, edema, and excess mucus production cause uneven airway narrowing, creating a ventilation/perfusion mismatch. Severe hypoxemia, an abnormal deficiency of oxygen in arterial blood, can trigger life-threatening dysrhythmias and respiratory failure.

    Adequate ventilation is difficult in patients with asthma, chronic bronchitis, and pulmonary emphysema. Chronic obstructive pulmonary disease (COPD), which includes these conditions, is characterized by diminished inspiratory and expiratory capacity of the lungs. It is aggravated by cigarette smoking and air pollution. Smokers are advised to stop smoking at least 3 weeks preoperatively and are taught to use a spirometer. Deep breathing and coughing exercises may be helpful postoperatively. Mechanical ventilation with a respirator or intermittent positive pressure breathing (IPPB) apparatus may be necessary postoperatively to assist or control respiration. Patients who have trouble breathing are usually highly anxious and need emotional support.

Immunocompromised Patients

The immune system creates local barriers and inflammation to protect the body from invasion by pathogenic microorganisms and foreign bodies. Humoral and cell-mediated responses develop if these first-line defenses do not provide adequate protection. The humoral response produces antibodies to react with specific antigens. The cell-mediated response mobilizes tissue macrophages in the presence of a foreign body. Immunocompetence is the ability of the immune system to mobilize and deploy its antibodies and other responses to stimulation by an antigen. Immunocompetence may be threatened by a disease, a virus, or an immunosuppressive agent. Patients who are immunocompromised have a weakened or deficient immune response with a resultant decreased resistance to infection.

Immunosuppression

Immunosuppressive agents include corticosteroid hormones, which are given to prevent or reduce the inflammation caused by certain diseases. They are often prescribed for patients who have an autoimmune collagen disease (e.g., rheumatoid arthritis, systemic lupus erythematosus, and scleroderma) or an autoimmune hemolytic disorder (e.g., idiopathic thrombocytopenic purpura or acquired hemolytic anemia). They also are given to patients with adrenal insufficiency, as well as following organ transplantation to combat rejection. Antineoplastic cytotoxic agents for chemotherapy and radiation therapy, which are used to reduce malignant tumor cells, may also cause immunosuppression.

Common Complications The manifestations and clinical characteristics of the patient who is immunocompromised depend on the specific disease and the affected organ or system. For example, systemic lupus erythematosus can affect every organ system in the body. Adrenal insufficiency, as caused by Addison's disease, may be characterized by general debility. In contrast, organ transplantation or a malignant tumor may affect a single organ.

Special Considerations Many patients who are immunocompromised have skin rashes or lesions, painful joints, poor nutrition, and/or generalized malaise. They need physical and emotional support preoperatively. Aseptic and sterile techniques are important considerations for all surgical patients but are especially crucial for immunosuppressed and immunocompromised individuals, who are at high risk for developing a postoperative infection.

Acquired Immunodeficiency Syndrome

Patients with acquired immunodeficiency syndrome (AIDS) test positive for the human immunodeficiency virus (HIV) in serum and exhibit one or more signs and symptoms of an opportunistic disease, including pneumonia, fungal and/or parasitic infection(s), or malignant neoplasm. HIV can remain inactive and undetected in the body for many years before causing immunodeficient illness. During this time, no outward signs of HIV infection are noted, but it is possible for the patient to transmit the virus through blood, body fluids, or sexual contact. Both males and females, including infants and children, may be HIV-positive or diagnosed with AIDS. AIDS was once considered to be transmitted only through homosexual behavior among men, IV drug use, or tainted blood transfusions. It is now known that the virus is also transmitted through heterosexual contact, and an infected mother may transmit the virus to her fetus.

The diagnosis of an HIV infection is confirmed by at least two separate tests. One positive test is not a conclusive diagnosis and is usually repeated for clarity. Initial testing with the enzyme-linked immunosorbent assay (ELISA) is performed to detect the presence of HIV antibodies in the blood. The diagnosis is confirmed with either the Western blot test or the indirect immunofluorescence assay.

If a patient tests seropositive for HIV infection, it does not mean that he or she has AIDS. HIV invades and destroys T lymphocytes. During this process the patient's immune system is disabled. The normal T lymphocyte level is 1000/mm³; the severity of an HIV infection is measured by the level of T lymphocyte cells in the patient's blood. When the T-cell level decreases to between 200 to 500/mm³, the patient has seroconverted to an immunodeficient state and is considered to have AIDS. There is no known cure for HIV infection or AIDS. Some medications are available to delay seroconversion in HIV infection and to prolong the life of a patient who has seroconverted to AIDS. Pharmacologic therapy may in-

clude broad-spectrum antibiotics, antivirals, antidiarrheals, vitamins, and antineoplastics.

Common Complications A patient with HIV infection may complain of night sweats, unexplained fevers, dry cough, weakness, diarrhea, and swollen lymph glands. A patient who has seroconverted to AIDS may have multiple opportunistic infections and malignancies concurrently and generalized poor health. Extreme muscle and tissue wasting is common.

Many patients with AIDS have multiple external and internal lesions. The skin may have open wounds with infectious exudate and/or large swollen purple lesions associated with Kaposi's sarcoma (a malignant multifocal neoplasm of reticuloendothelial cells that spreads in the skin and metastasizes to the lymph nodes and viscera). Large, painful masses of lymph tissue may be present in the neck, axilla, and groin. Mechanical obstruction caused by Kaposi's lesions in the esophagus may prevent swallowing of food. Intestinal lesions may prevent the absorption of nutrients or cause bowel obstruction. Constant anorexia, nausea, vomiting, and diarrhea may prevent adequate intake by mouth. Nutritional supplementation by hyperalimentation may be indicated to meet a patient's high caloric needs.

AIDS causes the body to be susceptible to opportunistic infections because of the lowered resistance of the immune system. Opportunistic infections are caused by microorganisms that normally are nonpathogenic in a healthy individual. The mucous membranes of the mouth and genital areas may have herpesvirus lesions or white patches of candidiasis, a yeastlike fungus. Neurologically, the patient may have recurrent episodes of cryptococcal meningitis or toxoplasmosis, causing persistent motor dysfunction and mental changes.

The patient with AIDS experiences a continual cycle of acute and chronic respiratory infections. *Pneumocystis carinii* pneumonia (PCP) is the most common lung infection, followed by multiple-drug–resistant tuberculosis (MDR-TB). The patient may be in a perpetual state of respiratory distress. Central and peripheral cyanosis may be present. The respiratory effort expends high energy levels, causing the patient to deteriorate rapidly.

Special Considerations Patients with AIDS may be in poor physical condition depending on how the body systems have been affected. Most systems are eventually involved. The plan of care should incorporate the following considerations:

1. Moving the patient from the transport stretcher to the operating bed may require additional personnel for total lifting. The patient may not be able to move because of weakness or pain in the joints, muscle and tissue wasting, and superficial skin lesions.
2. Bony prominences, areas of decreased muscle mass, and devascularized tissue must be protected throughout the positioning process and surgical procedure. Blankets, restraints, monitoring devices, electrosurgi-

cal dispersive electrodes, drapes, instruments, and routine care devices may cause inadvertent harm to the patient despite the team's best efforts to protect the patient from injury.

3. IV line insertion, induction of anesthesia, and maintenance of the airway may be difficult. A suitable vein for infusion may be hard to identify because of former IV drug use or large areas of epidermal Kaposi's sarcoma. In extreme cases the only IV site may be a central venous catheter. Endotracheal intubation may be contraindicated because of potential hemorrhage from Kaposi's lesions in the trachea. Placement of an esophageal stethoscope or rectal temperature probe may rupture other internal Kaposi's lesions with the same result.

4. Postoperative wound healing is delayed or absent because of poor nutrition, decreased circulation, poor tissue integrity, and a continued immunodeficient condition.

Many patients with AIDS have been rejected by their families, especially if the virus was transmitted through a route not accepted or understood by family members. The diagnosis of AIDS may be the first time the family is made aware of the patient's alternative lifestyle. Psychologic support systems may consist of a small circle of friends who may also be infected with HIV or have AIDS.

Continual counseling should be emphasized in the discharge plan to include provisions for physiologic care and psychologic support. The patient, family, and significant other(s) should be educated about the potential routes of transmission, such as exposure to blood and body fluids through sexual contact or shared IV needles. The virus is also potentially transmissible through shared razors, toothbrushes, and tweezers because of the possibility of blood contamination. Dishes and eating utensils are considered safe when washed in hot soapy water, rinsed, and dried. Education should include learning about physical activities that do not pose a risk of transmission, such as hugging, shaking hands, and sitting in close proximity.

Confidentiality is a concern because of the nature of the routes by which HIV can be transmitted. It is an issue of the patient's right to privacy. Testing for HIV is not a routine preadmission laboratory procedure. If a patient is tested, the results should be placed in the appropriate section of the patient's chart with other laboratory results, not displayed on the front of the chart. Reporting of the results should be governed by institutional policy and treated in the same manner as all patient confidentiality issues. Dissemination of confidential patient information to inappropriate persons is a breach of duty to the patient's privacy and may be subject to legal action. Physicians and nurses may face disciplinary action, such as license suspension or revocation by the boards of medicine or nursing, as indicated.

Perioperative patient care personnel should provide care to all patients with equal professionalism, compassion, empathy, and positive regard despite any personal feelings about a patient's lifestyle or disease entity. Nonjudgmental care is essential for the psychologic wellness of patients with AIDS.

Catastrophic Illnesses

Although perioperative patient care personnel are most often involved with patients who have a favorable prognosis, they also care for patients of all ages who have a catastrophic illness and are having surgery to palliate or relieve a specific problem. The procedure may be palliative rather than curative. Included in this category are patients with:

- Malignancies who are severely debilitated and terminally ill
- Severe traumatic disabilities requiring lengthy hospitalization, such as following spinal cord injury or extensive burns
- End-stage renal disease, or patients waiting for an organ transplant

Maximum patient comfort and the relief of physiologic disturbances are primary concerns. All of these patients require highly individualized care. The manner in which patients are told the diagnosis and prognosis obviously has a great impact on their hope for recovery. Patients who have been thoroughly and considerately informed are easier to talk to, accept therapy more readily, and have greater trust in and communicate more openly with caregivers.

Each patient deals with such a diagnosis in his or her own way. Although it is not always so, many persons consider the diagnosis of cancer a death warrant and react accordingly. To be supportive, the caregiver should mentally review the Kübler-Ross stages of dying: denial, isolation, anger, bargaining, depression, and acceptance. (These stages do not always occur in this sequence.) Emphasis is placed on the present, with a focus on the patient's strengths and attributes and how best to use them. It is difficult to find hope when facing a radical, disfiguring procedure. Listening to the patient is particularly important.

Bibliography

Badger JM: Calming the anxious patient, *Am J Nurs* 94(5):46-50, 1994.
Borkgren MW, Gronkiewicz CA: Update your asthma care from hospital to home, *Am J Nurs* 95(1):26-34, 1995.
Deakins DA: Teaching elderly patients about diabetes, *Am J Nurs* 94(4):39-42, 1994.
Ekstrom I: Communicating with the deaf patient, *Plast Surg Nurs* 14(1):31-32, 1994.
Gusek A: 10 commonly asked questions about diabetes, *Am J Nurs* 94(2):19-20, 1994.
Kendrik JM, Powers PH: Perioperative care of the pregnant surgical patient, *AORN J* 60(2):205-216, 1994.

Chapter 8

Perioperative Pediatrics

 Chapter Objectives

After studying this chapter, the learner will be able to:

- Describe pediatric patient care in terms of developmental stages.
- Identify age-specific considerations in the care of pediatric patients.
- List several procedures that are performed on pediatric patients.

The surgical problems peculiar to children from birth to maturity are not limited to any one area of the body or to any one surgical specialty. Malformations and diseases affect all body parts and therefore may require the skills of any of the surgical specialists. However, pediatric surgery is a specialty in itself and is not adult surgery scaled down to infant or child size. Indications for surgery include congenital anomalies, acquired disease processes, and trauma. Many of these conditions are treatable or curable by surgical intervention. Additional information can be found at **www.pedisurg.com.**

INDICATIONS FOR SURGERY

Congenital Anomalies

A congenital anomaly is a deviation from normal structure or location in any organ or part of the body. It can alter function or appearance. Multiple anomalies may be present at birth. If an anomaly does not involve vital life functions, surgical intervention may be postponed until the results can be maximized and the risks of the surgical procedure are minimized by growth and development of body systems. If a newborn has a poor chance of survival without a surgical procedure, the risk is taken within hours or days after birth. Defects in the alimentary tract are the most common indication for an emergency surgical procedure during the newborn period, followed in frequency by cardiac and respiratory system defects. Mortality in the newborn is influenced by three uncontrollable factors: the multiplicity of anomalies, prematurity, and birth weight.

The presence of three or more physical anomalies is referred to as the *VACTERL* association or syndrome:

V Vertebral defect, such as spina bifida or myelomeningocele
A Anal malformation, such as imperforate anus
C Cardiac anomaly, such as patent ductus arteriosus or ventricular and atrial septal defects
T Tracheoesophageal fistula
E Esophageal atresia
R Renal anomaly, such as horseshoe kidney and renal dysplasia
L Limb defect, such as short radius syndrome or syndactylism

Acquired Disease Processes

Among acquired disease processes, appendicitis is the most common surgically corrected childhood disease. Malignant tumors occur in infants and children, but with minimal frequency when compared with occurrence rates for adults. Benign lesions are surgically excised, usually without further difficulty to the child.

Trauma

Accidental injury is the leading cause of death in children. The margin for error in diagnosis and treatment of a child is less than that for an adult with a similar injury. A child's blood volume is low compared with body size, and even a small loss of blood can be critical. Because the child's chest cavity is small, an abdominal or chest injury can be critical. Diagnosis is made quickly, and the patient is sent to the operating room (OR) if indicated. Examples of common injuries include blunt intestinal trauma caused by seat belt use on small children or head injuries caused by improper use of infant car seats. Other injuries that can occur, such as lacerations, fractures, or crushing injuries of hands and arms, may result in nerve, vessel, tendon, bone, and/or other soft tissue damage.

Skill is required in performing pediatric surgical procedures regardless of the indication for the procedure. Specialists in all fields develop these skills as a refinement of their specialties. Surgeons who perform pediatric surgery should have knowledge of the embryologic, psychologic, physiologic, and pathologic problems peculiar to the newborn, infant, and child. Knowledge has advanced pediatric surgery through the following:

- Recognition of differences between pediatric patients and adults.
- Accurate diagnosis and earlier treatment. This facilitates a more favorable outcome, especially in the fetus and preterm neonate. Neonatology is a growing subspecialty of pediatrics.
- Understanding of preoperative preparation of the patient and family.
- Availability of total parenteral nutrition (TPN) and other measures of supportive care for perioperative pediatric management.
- Advances in anesthesiology. These include new agents, perfection of techniques of administration, and an understanding of the responses of pediatric patients to anesthetic agents.
- Refinements in surgical procedures and instrumentation.
- Understanding of postoperative care. Larger facilities have neonatal and pediatric intensive care units.

CONSIDERATIONS IN PERIOPERATIVE PEDIATRICS

The nursing process is tailored to meet the unique needs of each pediatric patient. Assessment and nursing diagnosis are based on chronologic, psychologic, and physiologic factors specific to each patient. The plan of care should reflect consideration for age and reflect interventions modified according to the child's developmental stage as identified in Table 8-1. Developmental theorists emphasize that although the child has reached a certain age or physical size, psychologic growth is the key parameter by which communication is measured. Understanding individual differences enables the perioperative team to develop a positive rapport with the patient and family, which facilitates attainment of expected outcomes.

Not every patient of a particular age-group will meet standardized height and weight criteria; a child may be short or tall, or thin or heavy for his or her age. Although norms have been established by age-groups, the plan of care should reflect consideration for individual differences.

Chronologic Age

The chronologic age of the patient is a primary consideration in the development of the plan of care. An age-related baseline is a useful beginning for assessing pediatric patients effectively. Terminology used to categorize ages of pediatric patients includes the following:

1. Fetus: in utero
2. Newborn infant, referred to as a neonate
   a. Potentially viable: gestational age more than 24 weeks; birth weight more than 500 g and capable of sustaining life outside of the uterus (as defined by the World Health Organization)
   b. True preterm (premature): gestational age less than 37 weeks; birth weight 2500 g or less
   c. Large preterm (premature): gestational age less than 37 weeks; birth weight more than 2500 g
   d. Term neonate: gestational age 38 to 40 weeks; birth weight usually between 3402 and 3629 g (if less than 2500 g, the neonate is considered small for gestational age [SGA])
   e. Postterm (postmature): gestational age extended by more than 8 weeks
3. Neonatal period is first 28 days of extrauterine life
4. Infant: 28 days to 18 months
5. Toddler: 18 to 30 months
6. Preschool: 2½ to 5 years
7. School age: 6 to 12 years
8. Adolescent: 12 through 16 years

Pediatric Psychosocial Assessment

Assessment of psychologic development is based on age-related criteria (see Table 8-1) but includes assessment of individual differences. Comparison of established norms and assessment data is helpful in developing the plan of care. Environmental and parental influences can cause variance in affect, attitude, and social skills. Environmental influences on psychologic development include ethnic, cultural, and socioeconomic factors. The age of the patient may indicate his or her level of involvement with the environment. For example, an infant may have exposure only to immediate family members for external stimuli, but a preschool child may have experience with children in preschool and other children on a daily basis. Coping skills may or may not be developed, depending on the child's developmental stage.

Parenting practices may directly influence the way the patient responds to caregivers and the perioperative environ-

TABLE 8-1 Psychologic Developmental Stage Theories

Chronologic Age Ranges (Approximate)	Developmental Stage by Theorist			Characteristics of Psychologic Development
	Erikson	**Piaget**	**Loevinger**	
Birth-18 months	Trust vs. mistrust	Sensorimotor	Presocial	Learns to view self as being separate from the environment; begins to develop the concept of hope; learns to develop attachments to others; is dependent on caregiver for warmth, security, nourishment, nurturing, and stimulation; begins to use sounds and short words to communicate ideas; may view hospitalization as abandonment
19 months-3 years	Autonomy vs. shame/doubt	Preoperational	Symbiotic	Develops a two-way relationship with primary caregiver; suffers separation anxiety when isolated from established relationships; has short trials of independence; personality becomes introverted or extroverted; establishes a sense of will; uses sentences for communication; has fear of immediate threats; does not project thoughts beyond the present situation
4-6 years	Initiative vs. guilt	Preoperational	Impulsive	Asserts a separate identity; begins to have fear of real and imagined situations; senses peer acceptance and/or rejection; is concerned about disfigurement; may act out feelings; believes that every action has a purpose, either reward or punishment; learns to be self-protective; fears death or nonexistence; death is not always understood as being permanent; develops short-term self-control; uses compound sentences to communicate; mimics terminology used by fantasy characters
7-11 years	Industry vs. inferiority	Concrete operational	Conformist	Imitates actions and attitudes of peers and heroes; is aware of the differences of others and identifies with a particular social group; fears loss of self-control; understands the world in moderate detail; prefers honest explanations and reassurance of safety; does not want to be treated like a baby; strives for competency in daily tasks; can distinguish between fact and fantasy; has a greater understanding of death and its permanence; wants to be accepted as an individual; communicates well verbally and with basic writing skill
12-16 years	Identity vs. role confusion	Formal operational	Self-aware Conscientious	May change opinion in response to stereotypes; develops close personal relationships; understands values, rules, and ideals; begins to feel more important as an individual; fears alienation; body image is extremely important; is capable of abstract thought and reasoning; has a sense of aesthetic beauty; can merge sensory information and logic to derive a conclusion; prefers privacy and confidentiality; may question authority; is aware of opposite sex; may explore sexual activity; dreams about future lifestyle; wants to prove self-worth; globally communicates verbally and in writing
17 years-adulthood	Intimacy vs. isolation	Formal operational	Individualistic	Becomes aware of and accepts the interdependence of mankind; may feel some hostility toward authority; sometimes torn between the desire to be totally independent and dependent; seeks companionship of opposite sex; may be sexually active; refines interpersonal skills; demands privacy and confidentiality; plans for independent lifestyle as approach; refines verbal and written communication skill

ment. Pediatric patients respond differently in the presence of parents or guardians. Infants may be more cooperative if a parent is present. Conversely, an adolescent may want to demonstrate independence by asking the parent to leave the room. These actions may be completely opposite if the child has been abused or neglected. Lack of parental nurturing can cause a global deficit, including poor development of language and cognitive skills. Understanding the patient's level of psychologic development can help the caregiver communicate more effectively with the pediatric patient throughout the perioperative experience. Interaction should be according to his or her individual developmental level regardless of chronologic age.

Pediatric Physical Assessment

The physiologic assessment of pediatric patients is compared with national averages when establishing baseline norms. Physiologic development is influenced by genetics, nutrition, health status, and environmental factors. The physical assessment may reveal conditions that can adversely affect the outcome of a surgical procedure. Comparison of the patient's age, size, and psychologic development with established norms may enable the caregiver to assess for deficiencies in size or weight that may indicate a potential health problem. Unexplained marks or bruises may be a sign of abuse.

A small, frail child may have a congenital cardiac deformity or a malabsorption syndrome. Abuse or neglect may be manifested as a nutritional deficit. An extremely thin, malnourished adolescent may be intentionally bulimic or anorexic in response to a body image psychologic problem. An obese child may have an endocrine disease or a psychologic disturbance that causes overeating. These issues are important considerations because most dosages of medications given to pediatric patients are based on body weight in kilograms. Absorption and metabolism of medication will be influenced by the same physiologic parameters that govern nutritional status.

Metabolism and Nutritional Considerations

Infants have relatively greater nutritional requirements than do adults for minimizing loss of body protein. The resting metabolic rate of an infant is two to three times that of an adult, resulting in rapid metabolic imbalances in infants. The potential for complications increases proportionately with the duration of fluid restriction because infants are prone to hypovolemia and dehydration. Procedures performed on infants and toddlers should have priority on the surgical schedule so that these patients can return to a normal fluid and feeding routine as quickly as possible.

Infants may be given regular formula or a varied diet up to 6 hours before anesthesia and clear liquids, usually dextrose in water, up to 2 hours before the surgical procedure. A satisfactory state of hydration is thus maintained, and milk curds are absent from the stomach. Infants may be breastfed up to 4 hours before the surgical procedure. Breast milk has less or no curd and empties faster from the stomach than formula.

Infants should not miss more than one or two feedings. Oral intake is resumed promptly after the infant recovers from anesthesia.

Toddlers and preschool children may be permitted clear liquids up to 2 to 4 hours preoperatively. Intake of clear oral fluids in small amounts decreases the level of gastric acid contents by stimulating gastric emptying and diminishes the hunger-deprivation response.

Children over 5 years of age may have nothing by mouth (NPO) after midnight or 6 hours before induction of anesthesia. Exceptions may be necessary for children with fever, diabetes, or other special problems. For these children, clear liquids with supplemental glucose may be ordered to be given orally up to 2 hours preoperatively.

Older children may require slower progression of oral dietary intake postoperatively and are maintained with supplemental intravenous (IV) therapy that includes protein and vitamins. Vitamins K and C may be given to patients of any age-group.

Fluid and Electrolyte Balance Considerations

The newborn is not dehydrated and withstands major surgical procedures within the first 4 days of life without extensive fluid and electrolyte replacement. The renal system is easily overloaded by the administration of IV fluids. The newborn has a lower glomerular filtration rate and less efficient renal tubular function than does an adult. (Renal function improves during the first 2 months of life and approaches adult levels by age 2 years.) During the time of an average surgical procedure on a newborn, a total of 10 to 30 ml of fluid may be administered. Usually 5% dextrose in half-strength normal saline solution is infused.

Administration of excessive IV dextrose solution is avoided in infants younger than 1 year of age because they maintain lower glycogen stores. During physiologic stress the patient easily becomes hyperglycemic. Hyperglycemia acts as an osmotic diuretic, causing increased urinary output and dilutional hyponatremia. The increased urine volume can be a false indicator of renal and hemodynamic status. Seizures and neurologic damage may result. Seizures may be clinically undetected while the infant is under general anesthesia because the pharmacologic agents act as anticonvulsants.

Infants have a relatively larger body surface area–body mass ratio than do adults. When they become dehydrated, which can occur rapidly, bodily functions are disturbed, as is the acid-base balance. Plasma proteins differ in concentration from those of an adult. Fluid and electrolyte replacements are necessary. In children older than 1 year of age, isotonic solutions, such as normal saline or Ringer's lactate, are given IV per kilogram of body weight.

The hemoglobin level is lowest at 2 to 3 months of age (Table 8-2). The blood volume of the average newborn is 250 ml—approximately 75 to 80 ml/kg of body weight (Table 8-3). Significant blood loss requires replacement. Blood is typed and crossmatched in readiness. Although

TABLE 8-2	Pediatric Hematologic Value Ranges			
Age	**Hemoglobin (g/dl)**	**Hematocrit (%)**	**Leukocytes (mm³)**	**Platelets (mm³)**
Cord blood	13.7-20.1	45-65	9000-30,000	350
2 weeks	13.0-20.0	42-46	5000-21,000	260
3 months	9.5-14.5	31-41	6000-18,000	250
6 months-6 years	10.5-14.0	33-42	6000-15,000	250
7-12 years	11.0-16.0	34-40	4500-13,500	250

TABLE 8-3	Pediatric Blood Volume
Age	**Blood Volume (ml/kg)**
Newborn	75 to 80
6 weeks-2 years	75
2 years-puberty	72

Figure 8-1 Intraosseous infusion into tibia. Insertion site for needle placement is in anterior midline 1 to 3 cm below tibial tuberosity. Note that needle is perpendicular to medial surface and that tubing is secured on thigh.

blood loss is small in most cases, loss of 30 ml may represent 10% to 20% of circulating blood volume in an infant. The small margin of safety indicates the need for replacement of blood loss exceeding 10% of circulating blood volume. When replacement exceeds 50% of the estimated blood volume, sodium bicarbonate is infused to minimize metabolic acidosis.

Hypotension in an infant is not apparent until 50% of the circulating volume is lost. Hypotension is usually caused by myocardial depression from anesthetic agents, primarily inhalation anesthesia. The infant's myocardium has fewer contractile muscle fibers and more noncontractile connective tissue than is present in an older child or adult and therefore lacks myocardial force to maintain cardiac output. The cardiac output is dependent on the heart rate. Any decrease in heart rate directly affects blood pressure and body tissue perfusion.

IV infusions should be administered with the following precautions:

1. Dehydration is avoided. Therapy for metabolic acidosis, should it develop, is guided by measurement of pH, blood gases, and serum electrolytes.
2. Blood volume loss is measured as accurately as possible and promptly replaced. In an infant, rapid transfusion of blood may produce transient but severe metabolic acidosis because of citrate added as a preservative.
3. IV fluids and blood are infused through pediatric-size cannulated needles or catheters connected to drip chamber adapters and small solution containers. Umbilical vessels may be used for arterial or venous access in newborns less than 24 hours after birth. In extreme circumstances the umbilical vein can be accessed through a small infraumbilical incision and cannulated from inside the peritoneal cavity for rapid infusion. Scalp veins are used frequently on infants. If venous access cannot be quickly established, intraosseous infusion may be

indicated for fluid replacement (Figure 8-1). A cutdown on an extremity vein, usually the saphenous vein, may be necessary for toddlers and older children. An extremity should be splinted to immobilize it. A 250 ml solution drip chamber is used to help avoid the danger of overhydration. Adapters are set for accurate control of the desired flow rate.

Body Temperature Considerations

Temperature regulation is controlled in the anterior hypothalamus. Cooling causes vasoconstriction for the conservation of body heat. Extremes of cooling cause shivering that generates body heat and increases metabolic needs.

Newborns (especially preterm), infants, and children have wider average body temperature variations than do adults. Infants younger than 3 months do not have a shiver response. Body temperature in the newborn tends to range from as low as 97° to 100° F (36° to 37.7° C). Temperature begins to stabilize within this range 12 to 24 hours after birth if the environment is controlled. The relatively high rate of heat loss in proportion to heat production in the infant results from an incompletely developed thermoregulatory mechanism and from a body fat to lean mass ratio with only a thin layer of subcutaneous brown fat for insulation. Extensive superficial circulation also causes rapid dissipation of heat from the body. A hypothermic newborn or infant metabolizes anesthetic agents more slowly and is susceptible to postoperative respiratory depression and delayed emergence from anesthesia. The first sign of hypothermia in a child younger than 1 year of age is a heart rate below 100 beats per minute.

Oxygen consumption is at a minimum when abdominal skin temperature is 97° F (36° C). A room temperature 5° F (-15° C) cooler than that of abdominal skin produces a 50% increase in oxygen consumption, creating the hazard of acidosis. These factors account for the pediatric patient's susceptibility to environmental changes. The following can result in heat loss:

- *Evaporation.* When skin becomes wet, evaporative heat loss can occur. Excessive drapes can cause sweating. As sweat evaporates, it elicits a cooling effect.
- *Radiation.* When heat transfers from the body surface to the room atmosphere, radiation heat loss can result.
- *Conduction.* Placing the pediatric patient on a cold operating bed causes heat transfer from the patient's body to the surface of the bed.
- *Convection.* When air currents pass over skin, heat loss by convection results. Cold, wet diapers and blankets can cause heat loss by conduction.

Newborns, infants, and children are kept warm during the surgical procedure to minimize heat loss and to prevent hypothermia. Body temperature tends to decrease in the OR because of cooling from air-conditioning and open body cavities. Room temperature should be maintained as warm as 85° F (29° C). Continuous core body temperature monitoring should be performed (skin temperature sensors may be sufficient for short procedures). Other precautions should also be taken as follows:

1. A hyperthermia blanket or water mattress may be placed on the operating bed and warmed before the infant or child is laid on it. It is covered with a double thickness of fabric. The temperature is maintained at 95° to 100° F (35° to 37.7° C) to prevent skin burns and elevation of body temperature above the normal range. Excessive hyperthermia can cause dehydration and convulsions in the anesthetized patient.
2. A radiant heat lamp should be placed over the newborn to prevent heat loss through radiation. Warming lights with infrared bulbs may be used if a radiant warmer is not available. These lights should be about 27 inches (69 cm) from the infant to prevent burns; the distance should be measured. Plastic bubble wrap also provides insulation around the newborn to prevent heat loss by conduction but can cause heat loss by evaporation.
3. Wrapping the head (except the face) and extremities in plastic, such as plastic wrap, or Webril helps prevent heat loss in infants and small children. An aluminum warming suit or blanket may be used for toddlers and

older children. Forced-air warming blankets also are effective in maintaining core temperature.
4. Rectal, esophageal, axillary, or tympanic probes are used to measure core temperature. A probe placed into the rectum should not be inserted more than an inch (2 or 3 cm), because trauma to an infant through perforation of the rectum or colon can occur. Urinary catheters with thermistor probes may be useful if urinary catheterization is indicated.
5. Drapes should permit some evaporative heat loss to maintain equalization of body temperature. An excessive number of drapes, which can retain heat and put a weight on the body, are avoided. Combinations of paper, plastic, and cloth drapes may cause excessive fluid loss through diaphoresis and absorption into the drapes.
6. Solutions should be warm when applied to tissues to minimize heat loss by evaporation and conduction. The circulator should pour warm skin preparation solutions immediately before use. (Check the manufacturer's recommendations for warming solutions. Some iodine-based solutions become unstable when heated. The concentration of iodine increases when the fluid portion evaporates.) The scrub person dampens sponges in warm saline before handing them to the surgeon. Irrigant for urologic procedures should be warmed to body temperature.
7. Blood and IV solutions can be warmed before transfusion by running tubing through a blood and fluid warmer. Carbon dioxide for insufflation during laparoscopy can be warmed this way.
8. Blankets should be warmed to place over the patient immediately after dressings are applied and drapes are removed. The patient should be kept covered whenever possible before and after the surgical procedure to prevent chilling from the air-conditioning.

Indicators of Thermoregulatory Status   Hyperthermia (i.e., core temperature of the body over 104° F [40° C]) during the surgical procedure can be caused by fever, dehydration, decrease in sweating from atropine administration, excessive drapes, and drugs that disturb temperature regulation, such as general anesthetics and barbiturates. If the patient is febrile preoperatively, the surgical procedure may be delayed to allow reduction in temperature and to permit fluid administration. If an immediate surgical procedure is necessary and fever persists, anesthesia is induced and external cooling is employed. IV fluids may be given at room temperature instead of warmed during administration.

Signs of hypothermia include initial tachycardia and tachypnea. As chilling progresses, the pediatric patient becomes bradycardic with shallow respirations.

A sudden rise in temperature during the surgical procedure may indicate malignant hyperthermia. Immediate cooling with ice and cool fluids is necessary. More detailed information about malignant hyperthermia is described in Chapter 33.

Cardiopulmonary Status Considerations

The heart rate fluctuates widely among infants, toddlers, and preschool children and varies during activity vs. at rest (Table 8-4). Infants younger than 1 year of age tolerate a heart rate between 200 and 250 beats per minute without hemodynamic consequence. Heart rhythm disturbance is uncommon unless a cardiac anomaly is present. Cardiopulmonary complications manifest as respiratory compromise more frequently than as cardiac dysfunction. After age 5 years, cardiopulmonary response to stress resembles that of a young adult.

Cardiac and respiratory rates and sounds are continuously monitored in all age-groups by precordial or esophageal stethoscopy. Blood pressure, vital signs, electrocardiogram (ECG), and other parameters as indicated are also monitored throughout the surgical procedure (see Table 8-4). A pulse oximeter can be placed on the palm of the hand or on the midfoot of a newborn or small infant. Smaller patients suffer oxygen desaturation easily. A disadvantage of pulse oximetry is that it cannot detect instantaneous drops in oxygen saturation. It gives readouts of levels that have already occurred. Because of increased carboxyhemoglobin levels, it may be ineffective for patients who have had smoke inhalation or carbon monoxide poisoning. A pulse oximeter reading of 80% is clinically diagnostic of central cyanosis. Hypoxemia can cause bradycardia to decrease oxygen consumption of the myocardium.

Infants and toddlers are particularly susceptible to respiratory obstruction because of their anatomic structure. They are obligate nasal breathers. They have small nares, a relatively large tongue, lymphoid tissue present, and a small-diameter trachea, causing disproportionate narrowing of the airway. A cylindric thorax, poorly developed accessory respiratory muscles, and increased volume of abdominal contents limit diaphragmatic movement. The chest is more compliant and collapses easily.

TABLE 8-4	Pediatric Vital Sign Ranges		
Age	**Heart Rate/ Min**	**Respirations/ Min**	**Blood Pressure**
Newborn	100-170	30-60	40 systolic
Infant			
1 month	110-150	26-34	80/54
6 months	115-130	26-40	90/60
1 year	110-150	26-34	96/65
Toddler			
18-30 months	110-130	24-28	98/65
Preschool			
4 years	80-120	20-30	99/65
School-age			
6-9 years	70-115	20-30	100/60
10 years	70-110	18-26	110/60
Adolescent			
14 years	60-110	16-24	118/60

Pediatric Infection Risk Considerations

Newborns and infants are susceptible to nosocomial infection. Many preterm infants who have respiratory distress and circulatory problems survive because of advances in perinatal medicine. This has increased the population of high-risk and debilitated infants with reduced humoral and cellular defenses to infection. Aseptic technique is essential in handling neonates and all other pediatric patients.

An elective surgical procedure should be delayed in the presence of respiratory infection because of the risk of airway obstruction. Intubation of inflamed tissues may cause laryngeal edema. Coryza, inflammation of mucous membranes of the nose, is often a premonitory sign of an infectious respiratory disease.

Frequent use of antibiotics may lead to antibiotic resistance in some microorganisms. Many types of antibiotics are used to treat infection; however, it is advised that prevention by aseptic and sterile techniques is more beneficial to the patient.

Pediatric Pain Management Considerations

Infants and children are sensitive to pain. Their pain may be intense, but infants, toddlers, and preschool children are unable to describe its location and nature. School-age children may refer pain to a part of the body not involved in the disease process. Insecurity and fear in an older child may be more traumatic than the pain itself. Children should be observed for signs of pain (i.e., vocalizations, facial expressions, body movements, and physiologic parameters). Children also differ from adults in their response to pharmacologic agents; their tolerance to analgesic drugs is altered (Table 8-5).

PREOPERATIVE PSYCHOLOGIC PREPARATION OF PEDIATRIC PATIENTS

The pediatric surgical patient should be considered as a whole person with individual physical and psychosocial needs assessed in relation to the natural stages of development. Equally important are the adjustment and attitude of the parents toward the child, the illness, and the surgical experience. Parents' anxiety about the impending surgical procedure may be transferred to the child. Emotional support of both the patient and the parents, as well as parent and child teaching, are important aspects of preoperative preparation to help them cope. When an event is threatening, the patient changes cognitive and behavioral responses to deal with the specific demands of the situation. Most adults face stress with more control when fear of the unknown is eliminated. Therefore, parents need to be informed of events that will occur and to be taught how to care for their child preoperatively and postoperatively. If children are informed of sensations to be experienced, cognitive control of the event may occur. Children do not differ from adults in this respect. However, understanding varies with age.

TABLE 8-5	Pediatric Sedation and Pain Management		
Drug and Dosage		**Duration**	**Considerations in Administration**
Acetaminophen 10 mg/kg PO 20-25 mg/kg rectally		3-4 hours	Analgesia for minor procedures; antipyretic; absorption is delayed in infants, so dose should not be repeated for 6 hours; no effect on coagulopathy; no respiratory depression; may be combined with narcotic for major procedures
Codeine 0.5-1 mg/kg IM or PO		3-4 hours	Moderate pain relief; not given IV; can be given with acetaminophen
Diazepam 0.04-0.02 mg/kg IM or IV 0.12-0.8 mg/kg PO Not used for continuous infusion		1-3 hours 3-4 hours	Sedation and seizure control; can cause respiratory depression, jaundice, and vein irritation at IV site
Fentanyl Citrate 1-2 μg/kg IM or IV Continuous infusion: 0.5-2 μg/kg/hr PO lozenge is available		30-60 minutes	Excellent pain and anxiety relief; metabolized slowly in smaller children and infants; reversible with naloxone; short half-life; can cause respiratory depression, nausea, and vomiting; PO lozenge provides sedation but causes high incidence of preoperative nausea and vomiting
Hydromorphone Hydrochloride 1-4 mg per dose every 4 hr IM, IV, PO		4-5 hours	Not used for infants and young children; used for adolescents; side effects include CNS and respiratory depression, hypotension, bradycardia, increased intracranial pressure, and peripheral vascular dilation
Ibuprofen 5-10 mg/kg PO or rectally		3-4 hours	Can cause gastrointestinal bleeding; may affect platelet aggregation
Lorazepam 0.1 mg/kg IV		6-8 hours	Long half-life; sedation and seizure control; can cause respiratory depression, nausea, vomiting, and vein irritation at IV site; used for adolescents
Meperidine Hydrochloride 1-1.5 mg/kg IM, IV, or SQ Can be given PO, but less effective		3-4 hours	Excellent pain relief; reversible with naloxone; can cause respiratory depression, suppression of intestinal motility, and hypotension; may cause nausea and vomiting; not used in increased intracranial pressure; poor sedation; not a good premedicant
Midazolam Hydrochloride 0.1 mg/kg IV 0.08 mg/kg IM 0.5-0.75 mg/kg PO 0.3 mg/kg rectally in 5 ml normal saline Continuous infusion: 0.1 mg/kg/hr		30-60 minutes	Short half-life; may cause respiratory depression; excellent amnesic; sedation of choice for most pediatric patients
Morphine Sulfate 0.1-0.2 mg/kg IM, IV or SQ Not well absorbed PO Continuous infusion: 0.25-2 mg/kg/hr; average dose 0.06 mg/kg/hr		4-5 hours	Excellent pain relief; reversible with naloxone; can cause respiratory depression, suppression of intestinal motility, and hypotension; may cause nausea and vomiting; not a good premedicant
Pentobarbital 2-4 mg/kg IM, PO, or rectal		3-4 hours	Causes sedation and hypnosis; short-acting
Sufentanil Citrate 1-2 μg/kg IV Nasal spray		1-2 hours	Is 10 times more potent than fentanyl; very short half-life

PO, By mouth; *IM,* intramuscularly; *IV,* intravenously; *CNS,* central nervous system; *SQ,* subcutaneously.

The following are general considerations:

1. Psychologically it may be better for both the infant and the parents if a congenital anomaly is corrected as soon after birth as possible. The infant younger than 1 year of age will not remember the experience. Parents will gain confidence in learning to cope with a residual deformity as the infant learns to compensate for it. Fear of body mutilation or punishment may be of paramount importance to a preschool or young school-age child.

Children from 2 to 5 years of age have great sensitivity and a tenuous sense of reality. They live in a world of magic, monsters, and retribution, yet they are aggressive. School-age children, who have an enhanced sense of reality, value honesty and fairness. Their natural interest and curiosity aid communication. These children need reassurances and explanations in vocabulary compatible with their developmental level. Words should be chosen wisely. Negative connotations should be avoided, and the positive aspects should be stressed. The nurse should talk on the child's level about his or her interests and concerns.

Anxiety in the school-age child may be stimulated by remembrance of a previous experience. Many children undergo two or more staged surgical procedures before the deformity of a congenital anomaly or traumatic injury is cosmetically reconstructed or functionally restored. Familiarity with the nursing staff reassures the child. Ideally, the same circulator who was present for the first surgical procedure should visit preoperatively and be with the child during subsequent surgical procedures.

Fear of the unknown about general anesthesia may become exaggerated into extreme anxiety with fantasies of death. The school-age child and adolescent need facts and reassurances. General anesthesia should not be referred to as "putting you to sleep." The child may equate this phrase with the euthanasia of a former pet who never returned home. Instead the nurse should say, "You will sleep for a little while," or "You will take a nap." Tell the child about the "nice nurses" who will be in the "wake-up room after your nap." Parents should be encouraged to also display confidence and cheerfulness to avoid transmitting anxiety. Parents should be honest with their child but maintain a confident manner. The perioperative nurse should do the same. However, a school-age child should not be given information not asked for; questions should be answered, and misunderstandings should be corrected. The nurse should be especially alert to silent, stoic, noncommunicative children, many of whom have difficult induction and emergence from anesthesia. Children who have lost a sibling to death often fear hospitalization.

2. Some facilities hold parties for children and their parents before or after admission to explain routines and procedures before the surgical experience. At other facilities, personnel take children to the OR with their teddy bears so that they can see the different attire, lights, tables, anesthesia machine, and other equipment that might interest them. A child-size anesthesia mask becomes a toy that they are allowed to handle and place on the teddy bear. A clear plastic mask is less psychologically traumatic to a child than is an opaque, black rubber mask. An effective method of explaining procedures to children is to use the child's teddy bear and dress it as the child will look postoperatively. For example, a bandage is put on the bear if the child will have one postoperatively.

3. Separation from parent(s) or a trusted guardian is traumatic for infants over 6 months of age, toddlers, and preschool children. Infants require cuddling and bonding. Toddlers are only reaching the autonomy stage when hospitalization forces them into passive behavior, and thus their separation anxiety is greatest. Young children may fear strangers. The parent's presence is necessary for the toddler, and the parent should be encouraged to stay with the hospitalized child as much as possible. The child should be permitted to bring a toy or other security object to the OR suite if a parent cannot be present. Many anesthesia providers encourage parents to accompany an infant or child to the OR and to stay through induction if they wish to do so. The presence of a parent can significantly reduce anxiety and ease induction. Some facilities allow parents to accompany the child to the holding area but restrict entrance into the OR. Highly anxious parents who have difficulty coping with stress may cause an increase in the child's anxiety level.

4. Ambulatory surgery, if feasible, is an advantage because the child enters the facility an hour or two before the surgical procedure and returns home following recovery from anesthesia. This minimizes the trauma of separation.

5. A preoperative visit by a perioperative nurse should be planned to get to know the child, confirm appropriate consents, and provide emotional support to the family. Parents should be taught to provide postoperative care, especially before and after an ambulatory procedure. Verbal instructions may be supplemented with a videotape or storybook to reinforce understanding for both the child and the parents.

6. The patient should brought to the OR in a crib or on an appropriate-size cart by the perioperative nurse. Carrying him or her into the OR presents the risk for dropping or bumping the child.

PEDIATRIC ANESTHESIA

Pediatric anesthesia has become increasingly specialized as the many variables in the management of infants and children have become better understood. The anesthesia provider recognizes and respects the small margin for error and the uniqueness of the physiology and responses to drugs of pediatric patients. For example, the high metabolic rate of children causes rapid oxygen consumption. Changes occur rapidly in infants and children.

Preoperative Assessment by the Anesthesia Provider

A preoperative visit by the anesthesia provider to establish rapport and assess the patient is also a vital part of preparation of the pediatric patient. This visit is preferably made with the parents present so that the child will consider the anesthesia provider a trustworthy and caring friend. During physical assessment, special attention is given to the heart, lungs, and upper airways. Loose teeth are noted. Possible difficulties are anticipated. Preoperative care includes correction of dehydration, reduction of excessive fever, compensation for acidosis, and restoration of depleted blood volume. An American Society of Anesthesiologists (ASA) physical status classification is assigned to the pediatric patient. Consideration is given to the patient's age, developmental stage, psychologic characteristics, and past history to determine the patient's probable response to the anesthesia experience.

Premedication

Psychologic preparation of the child over 7 years of age can decrease the need for an anxiolytic (i.e., a sedative or minor tranquilizer to reduce anxiety). Crying greatly increases mucus in the respiratory tract. At the discretion of the anesthesia provider, premedication may be ordered to produce serenity. Some anesthesia providers prefer children to be well medicated; others favor minimal or no sedation. Infants younger than 1 year of age usually do not require premedication, but pacifiers with medication ports are commercially available for delivery of oral drugs. Premedication, which is tailored to the individual, varies considerably by age, weight, and health status. Preanesthetic sedation should allow the patient to be taken to the OR lightly asleep and should facilitate induction of anesthesia without awakening the child. It should also provide some analgesia during the recovery period.

Timing of administration is extremely important. To be effective, drugs should be given at least 45 to 60 minutes before the surgical procedure. The circulator should check with the anesthesia provider and the surgeon before sending for the patient. If ample time is not available for the appropriate effect of premedication, the anesthesia provider may prefer to omit the medication to avoid precipitation of psychologic trauma. Fast-acting drugs are available and may be useful for rapid sedation preoperatively. Narcotics, such as morphine sulfate and meperidine hydrochloride (Demerol), are rarely indicated for routine premedication in healthy pediatric patients.

No ideal premedicant exists, but the following drugs are commonly used (see also the comparison of sedatives in Table 8-5):

- Sufentanil citrate (Sufenta) given nasally (i.e., sprayed onto the nasal mucosa) facilitates separation from par-

ents by causing relaxation and drowsiness. The child becomes calm and cooperative.
- Fentanyl citrate (Sublimaze) can be incorporated into a lozenge or a flavored hard candy mounted on a stick (i.e., an anesthetic lollipop). When the child licks the candy, the drug is absorbed into the bloodstream through the oral mucosa and produces sedation for 30 to 60 minutes.
- Diazepam (Valium), 0.04 to 0.02 mg/kg administered intramuscularly (IM) or 0.12 to 0.8 mg/kg given orally (PO), causes relaxation for 3 to 4 hours. This drug has very few cardiovascular side effects.
- Midazolam hydrochloride (Versed), 0.08 mg/kg administered IM 15 minutes before induction, greatly reduces anxiety. Oral preparations also work well. This drug is also good for intravenous conscious sedation (IVCS) during endoscopy. Doses range between 0.2 and 0.3 mg/kg IV. Cardiovascular stability is good, and ventilation is not depressed.
- Scopolamine hydrobromide, 0.006 mg/kg, may be added to an IM injection of midazolam hydrochloride for further sedation and amnesic effect.
- Atropine sulfate, 0.01 to 0.02 mg/kg, may be administered IM, IV, or subcutaneously (SQ) to inhibit secretions, especially in a child with a severe airway problem, or to counteract bradycardia. Cardiac effects last about 1 hour. Dosage is decreased to 0.04 mg/kg for infants under 5 kg. It is not given in the presence of fever or glaucoma.
- Glycopyrrolate (Robinul), 0.004 to 0.01 mg/kg administered IM, lowers gastric acidity. It may be given as an alternative to atropine sulfate to reduce secretions. It is contraindicated in the presence of paralytic ileus, urinary tract obstruction, and glaucoma.

Anesthesia Equipment

Simple, lightweight anesthesia equipment is used. Disposable equipment is popular. Face masks, designed for minimal dead space, are available to closely fit a child's relatively flat face. Nonrebreathing circuits provide less resistance and valves for fresh flow of gas at higher flow rates relative to a child's metabolism and ventilation. To avoid hypothermia, anesthetic gases are warmed and humidified. Neonates are especially at risk for fluctuations in temperature regulation.

Induction

Induction is facilitated by a quiet atmosphere, a soft voice, and a reassuring touch. Children should be told what to expect without precipitating fear. The induction experience can be described as getting on a merry-go-round. Noises will seem louder. To avoid confusion, it is best for the child to listen to one person speak at this time. The circulator should remain at the patient's side, maintain a gentle touch, and be alert to the patient's needs and condition.

The following are considerations for anesthesia induction:

1. Restraints should be loose. Minimal pressure should be applied. If the patient is a newborn, infant, or toddler, restraint straps are omitted while the circulator holds the patient during induction. A toddler or preschool-age child is less frightened when holding onto someone's hands. Restraints can be applied after the patient is asleep.
2. A few drops of food extract of the child's choosing (e.g., mint, banana, or strawberry) can be placed in the face mask. This makes the anesthetic gas more acceptable and gives the patient a sense of control. The scent of anesthetic gas may be compared with the scent of special jet fuel used for airplanes or spaceships.
3. If the child is awake, crying, or struggling, apprehension during induction can be avoided by distraction and rapport. It is not easy to establish rapport with young children. Their cooperation may be solicited by counting out loud, singing the alphabet song, blowing up a balloon, taking a space trip, or discussing a favorite plaything or television character. The face mask can be held slightly above the face, permitting anesthetic gas to flow by gravity, and lowered gently as the child becomes drowsy. Some anesthesia providers permit the child to hold the mask.
4. Induction may be accompanied by regurgitation and aspiration of gastric contents in infants with pyloric stenosis, tracheoesophageal fistula, intestinal obstruction, or food in the stomach. The hazard is minimized by aspirating gastric contents with a sterile catheter before induction and leaving the tube in place for drainage during the surgical procedure. Rapid-sequence induction may also be used. This consists of thiopental sodium, muscle relaxant, and intubation with cricoid pressure (Sellick's maneuver) applied to close the esophagus and avoid silent regurgitation of food from the stomach. All trauma patients should be considered to have a full stomach.

Types of Induction

Inhalation   If asleep from premedication on arrival in the OR, the child can be anesthetized quickly. If the child is awake, induction may be initiated with inhalant anesthetic.

Nitrous oxide may increase peripheral vascular resistance if it is used to maintain general anesthesia for cardiovascular procedures. It may also increase the risk of air embolus because it combines with smaller air bubbles that may enter the system during repair of congenital heart defects. Potent inhalants are absorbed more rapidly in the presence of nitrous oxide and may cause myocardial depression and decrease cardiac output in very young children. Atropine may minimize this effect.

Rectal Induction   Given by enema, methohexital sodium (Brevital), 15 mg/kg of 1% solution, produces sleep in 6 to 8 minutes and lasts 45 to 60 minutes. This is a painless method used in the presence of parents for preschoolers or toddlers. The parent may hold the child. It is a good method for short diagnostic procedures. The anesthesia provider remains with the patient. Once the child is asleep, the anesthetic state may be maintained with an inhalant. Gentle assisted ventilation may be needed. This method is tolerated best in children under the age of 3 years.

Intravenous Infusion   IV infusion is often preferred for patients over 9 or 10 years of age. Induction with a small dosage of barbiturate or ketamine hydrochloride is rapid. Studies have shown that IV induction causes less psychologic trauma than inhalant methods. A mixture of lidocaine hydrochloride and prilocaine hydrochloride in a cream base is commercially available for application to the site to decrease pain associated with venipuncture.

Care is taken if the child has a central line. Infection or thrombosis may result. If the central line is used for anesthetic administration, all residual drug is flushed from the port so that none remains in the tubing after the procedure.

Ketamine hydrochloride, 1 to 2 mg/kg IV, is useful in a combative, burned, or hypovolemic patient. If given IM to a healthier child who weighs less than 10 kg, the usual dose is 5 to 10 mg/kg.

Epidural Block   A caudal epidural block may be used in combination with general anesthetic for orthopaedic, abdominal, or thoracic procedures.

Intubation

Airway obstruction in infants and children usually occurs early during anesthesia administration. When anesthesia deepens, airway insertion is essential after prior assisted ventilation. Assisted or controlled ventilation reduces the labor of breathing and therefore reduces metabolism. Placement of an endotracheal tube in the trachea of a newborn or infant differs from placement in a child or adolescent. Regardless of age, the airway must remain patent. Sterile equipment and gentle manipulation to avoid soft tissue injury are essential for intubating and suctioning. Other considerations include the following:

1. Endotracheal intubation is used by some anesthesia providers for all procedures in infants younger than 1 year of age. It is necessary for intraabdominal, intrathoracic, and neurosurgical procedures and for those about the head or neck areas, as well as for emergency procedures when contents of the stomach are uncertain. Intubation while the patient is awake may be used in neonates. A certain amount of jaw tightness (masseter muscle rigidity, trismus) is common in pediatric patients after the administration of succinylcholine, but this should be observed closely because it may also be a sign of malignant hyperthermia.
2. The size of the endotracheal tube is selected according to the width and length of the trachea. (See Table 8-6 for endotracheal tube sizes.) Endotracheal tubes for

children under 8 years of age are not cuffed. The tube allows for a slight space around the exterior circumference. Soft tissue at the narrowest level of the cricoid cartilage, located just below the vocal cords, forms a loose seal around the tube.

TABLE 8-6	Recommended Endotracheal Tube Sizes	

Age	Diameter (mm)
Preterm	2.5-3.0
Newborn	3.0
Newborn-6 months	3.5
6-12 months	3.5-4.0
12 months-2 years	4.0-4.5
3-4 years	4.5-5.0
5-6 years	5.0-5.5
7-8 years	5.5-6.0
9-10 years	6.0-6.5
11-12 years	6.5-7.0
13-14 years (and older)	7.0-7.5

3. The nasotracheal tube may inadvertently dislodge adenoid tissue and carry it into the trachea.

4. The head of a newborn or infant is elevated slightly and not hyperextended during placement of the endotracheal tube. A toddler also has a larger occiput and therefore needs little posterior extension of the head. A child with Down's syndrome is predisposed to instability of the odontoid articulation at the first cervical vertebra (C1) and is at risk of dislocation if the head is placed in extreme hyperextension.

5. A straight blade is usually used on the laryngoscope because the epiglottis must be raised to visualize the glottis during intubation (Figure 8-2). In an infant the epiglottis is long and stiff and projects posteriorly at an angle of 45 degrees above the glottis. The epiglottis of a toddler and a preschool child is short and easily traumatized.

6. Intubation and suctioning are preceded and followed by oxygen administration. If the process of introducing the endotracheal tube takes longer than 30 seconds, the patient should be ventilated with 100% oxygen before additional attempts at intubation ensue.

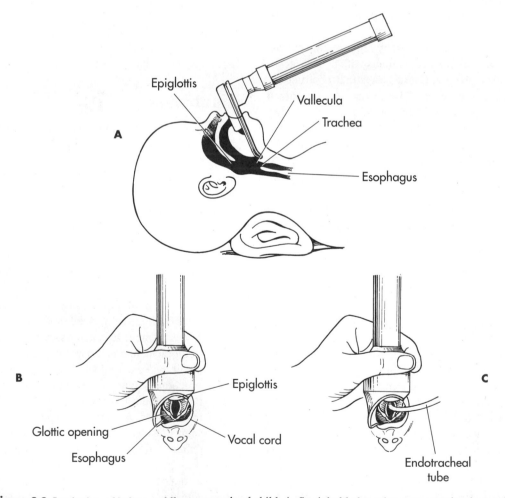

Figure 8-2 Intubation of infant, toddler, or preschool child. **A,** Straight blade on laryngoscope is advanced to vallecula, space between base of tongue and epiglottis. **B,** Gentle elevation of tip of blade lifts epiglottis to visualize glottic opening between vocal cords. **C,** Endotracheal tube is advanced below blade into trachea.

7. The length and diameter of the suction catheter should be considered when suctioning oropharyngeal secretions. An oversized catheter may perforate the oropharynx, trachea, bronchus, or esophagus.

8. The newborn's head is maintained in a neutral position, midway between full extension and full flexion, while an endotracheal tube is in place. The tip of the tube should be positioned in the midtrachea. The average distance between the vocal cords and the carina, where the trachea separates into two branches, is only 4 or 5 cm (about 2 inches) in a term neonate and much less in a preterm neonate. If the head shifts, the tube can slip up or down and lead to disastrous consequences.

Anesthetic Agents and Maintenance

The following characteristics of anesthetic agents and maintenance of anesthesia are considered:

1. Topical agents are not often used because of the hazard of overdose. Local anesthetic cream, EMLA, may be used to start an IV access point with minimal risk of toxicity.

2. Inhalation anesthesia, especially with halothane or sevoflurane, is popular. Nitrous oxide–oxygen-halothane is frequently used in combination with IV agents. Halothane and succinylcholine are contraindicated if there is a family history of malignant hyperthermia because they trigger the condition. Nitrous oxide is used with caution in patients with congenital cardiac defects, particularly in cyanotic conditions. Isoflurane (Forane) is irritating, necessitating slow and more difficult induction to prevent laryngospasm, but it offers the advantage of circulatory support. It is not useful in short procedures. Sevoflurane is less irritating to the airway and is comparable to halothane for induction. Emergence is smooth and rapid. Pain sensation may be immediate after arousal. Analgesia should be administered.

    Alveolar concentrations of inhaled anesthetics rise much more rapidly in pediatric patients than in adults because of relatively greater blood flow and smaller functional residual capacity. Children therefore have higher anesthetic requirements than do adults. To produce the same level of anesthesia, neonates require about 40% more halothane than do adults. Increased anesthetic requirement and more rapid induction can cause hypotension and reduced cardiac output in infants and children.

3. Ketamine provides sedation for preschool children during invasive diagnostic procedures. It is a short-acting general anesthetic for short procedures, such as burn debridement, tonsillectomy, or circumcision. Because it does not alter pharyngolaryngeal reflexes or skeletal tone, intubation is unnecessary. Cardiovascular and respiratory stimulation is minimal; ketamine may be useful in asthmatic and other poor-risk patients. It is contraindicated in the patient who has increased intracranial pressure. It is not advised for teenagers. Pre-

Agent	Maximum Pediatric Dose
Lidocaine hydrochloride	
Without epinephrine	4.5-5 mg/kg
With epinephrine (epinephrine should not exceed 10 μg/kg)	7-10 mg/kg
Bupivacaine hydrochloride	3 mg/kg
Tetracaine hydrochloride	2 mg/kg
Procaine hydrochloride	15 mg/kg
Chloroprocaine hydrochloride	15 mg/kg
Cocaine hydrochloride	1 mg/kg

TABLE 8-7 Local Anesthesia for Pediatric Patients

medication with diazepam counteracts possible emergence delirium.

4. Local anesthesia is commonly used as a supplement to light general anesthesia. Long-acting agents, such as bupivacaine hydrochloride (Marcaine), prolong postoperative analgesia, thus reducing or eliminating the need for narcotics (Table 8-7). Epinephrine added to bupivacaine enhances its duration to a greater extent in children than in adults. Large doses of epinephrine may interact with halothane and cause dysrhythmias. Doses of epinephrine up to 10 mg/kg are considered safe.

5. Epidural anesthesia can be administered for sensory blockade intraoperatively. The epidural catheter may be left in place for prolonged postoperative analgesia. A continuous infusion of narcotics provides uninterrupted pain management, as administered to adults to attenuate postoperative stress response.

6. Narcotics are used in situations similar to adult indications. Nitrous oxide–narcotic-relaxant provides stable anesthesia for the very ill patient. Fentanyl has minimal cardiovascular effect.

7. The critically ill neonate does not tolerate anesthesia well. Adequate ventilation and oxygenation are vital, but care is taken to avoid oxygen toxicity with resultant retrolental fibroplasia; neovascularization of the retina can produce blindness. Neonates and preterm infants under 34 weeks' gestational age and 1500 g or less body weight are at risk. Adequate blood-gas tension is ensured only by intraoperative invasive measurement.

8. Neuromuscular blockers are used judiciously. Infants younger than 1 year of age exhibit a lesser degree of blockade from succinylcholine than do older children. Bradycardia and an increase in intraocular tension are more conspicuous in infants. Response decreases with age. Dosage varies. A peripheral nerve stimulator should be used to assess blockade to avoid overdosage. Blockers seldom are required in infants because of their poorly developed abdominal musculature.

9. Consideration is given for postoperative analgesia. When halothane is reduced near the end of the surgical

procedure, a narcotic may be given. Regional or local infiltration will also provide relief of pain (e.g., following circumcision or cleft lip repair).

Emergence and Extubation

Airway problems are the most common concern on emergence from anesthesia and immediately postoperatively. At the conclusion of the surgical procedure, the oropharynx is suctioned. Some anesthesia providers also suction the stomach. All monitors are left in place until the patient is fully awake and extubated.

Reversal with a narcotic antagonist such as naloxone hydrochloride (Narcan) may be used to reverse narcosis but also has the effect of reversing analgesia. Pain sensation may result in restlessness. The usual dose is 0.01 to 0.1 mg/kg for infants and older children.

Extubation of an infant or child is preceded and followed by oxygen administration and performed either with the patient under deep anesthesia or on return of spontaneous respiration because laryngospasm is possible between these periods. Heart and breath sounds are monitored following extubation. If spasm occurs, oxygen is given by positive pressure. Airway obstruction, aspiration, and hypothermia are hazards of the recovery period. Children, particularly in the 2- to 5-year age-group, may develop hoarseness and a croupy cough following removal of an endotracheal tube. Racemic epinephrine (Vaponefrin) provides relief; 0.5 ml of 2.25% diluted in 3 ml of sterile water can be delivered through a face mask and nebulizer. Constant observation following extubation is required.

The patient should not be taken from the OR with a body temperature below 95° F (35° C). Below this crucial level, the risk of acidosis, hypoglycemia, bradycardia, hypotension, and apnea increases. This metabolic depression and delayed return of activity set the stage for possible sudden cardiac arrest. Dehydration and low humidity increase the viscosity of secretions. Pediatric patients require close watching for development of laryngeal edema, which is noted by croupy cough, sobbing inspiration, intercostal retraction, tachypnea, or tachycardia. Laryngeal edema greatly reduces the small diameter of the airway of an infant or toddler. Controlled humidity and oxygen are vital.

INTRAOPERATIVE PEDIATRIC PATIENT CARE CONSIDERATIONS

Basic principles of patient care and OR techniques used for adults apply to pediatric surgery. To differentiate this specialty from care of adult patients, a few points specific to pediatric surgery are mentioned as follows:

1. Hair is not removed with a depilatory or shaved, except for cranial procedures and as ordered by the surgeon for an adolescent.

2. Diagnostic studies may be done in the OR with the patient under local anesthesia before induction of general anesthesia for an open surgical procedure. An infant may be swaddled on a padded (papoose) board to restrain him or her from moving while x-ray films are taken and to permit easy change of position. A pacifier will help comfort and keep the infant quiet.

3. The patient is protected from injury. An infant or child should never be left alone anywhere in the perioperative environment, especially in the OR suite. Preparation for induction should be made before the child's arrival.
   a. Guard against a fall from a crib or stretcher. Side rails should remain up at all times. An overbed cage on a crib helps confine a toddler without restraint. Children are restrained at all times while on a stretcher or in a specially designed pediatric cart.
   b. Do not place a crib where the patient can reach an electrical outlet or near any article that can be picked up and cause injury.
   c. After the infant is asleep, pad wrists and ankles with several layers of sheet wadding. Restrain with Kerlix or roller gauze and pin straps to the sheet on the operating bed. Sheet wadding prevents possible abrasion of delicate skin by the restraint straps. Care is taken not to restrict circulation.
   d. Safety pins, open or closed, or other small objects are not left within reach of an infant or child.

4. Catheters as small as 8 French are available for use as needed in newborns and infants. A plain-tip or whistle-tip catheter is used for a stomach tube. An indwelling Foley catheter with a 3-ml balloon may be used for urinary drainage. Small, calibrated drainage containers are connected to permit accurate determination of output.

5. Positioning principles are essentially the same as those described for adults. Correspondingly smaller towel rolls, pillows, gel pads, and beanbags are used to protect pressure points and to stabilize anesthetized infants and children. The size of the child or adolescent determines the appropriate supports to maintain the desired position. A small towel roll at each side of the body takes the weight of drapes off the small body of an infant or keeps the patient in a lateral position.

6. A disposable drape sheet without a fenestration is often advantageous: the surgeon can cut an opening of the desired size to expose the site of intended incision. Small towels and nonpiercing towel clips are used with a laparotomy sheet if self-adhering and disposable drapes are not available. A standard opening 3 × 5 inches (7.6 × 12.7 cm) in a pediatric laparotomy sheet is frequently too large for a newborn or infant. Part of the fenestration may be covered with a towel.

7. Sponges are weighed while still wet; blood loss through suction is measured and estimated in the

drapes. The surgeon and anesthesia provider will determine if blood replacement is necessary, volume for volume, as it is lost.

8. Adhesive tape is abrasive to tender skin and should be avoided when possible. An adhesive spray or collodion is adequate over a small incision with a subcuticular closure and is especially desirable under diapers unless dressings are needed to absorb drainage. Care is taken that clothing or the blanket does not touch this substance until it is dry. Skin closure strips may be used instead of a liquid adhesive.

9. Dressings on the face or neck should be protected from vomitus and food particles, as well as from an infant's or toddler's hands. Elbows should be splinted when the patient potentially may disturb the incision, dressings, or a tube (Figure 8-3). This is particularly important following eye surgery or cleft lip or palate surgery, or when a tracheostomy tube is inserted.

10. A stockinette pulled over dressings on an extremity protects them from becoming dirty and helps keep them in place. This can be changed easily as needed, leaving the dressings in place.

Instrumentation

Gentleness and precision in handling small structures and fragile tissues are essential. Basic or standard instrument sets, sutures, needles, and other items used for surgical procedures on adults are duplicated in miniature to take care of infants and children in each surgical specialty. The perioperative nurse and surgical technologist should be informed about their patient and then use good judgment in preparing supplies for pediatric surgery. The following principles apply:

1. Size and weight are more critical factors than age in the selection of instruments, sutures, needles, and equipment.
2. Small instruments are used on the delicate tissues of a newborn, infant, or small child.
3. Hemostats should have fine points. A mosquito hemostat will clamp a superficial vessel but not a major artery.
4. Noncrushing vascular clamps permit occlusion of major blood vessels. They also can be placed across the intestine of a newborn or infant rather than a large, heavy intestinal clamp.
5. Lightweight instruments will not inhibit respiration. Instruments not in use on tissues are never laid on the patient, especially not on the chest. An instrument's weight could restrict respiration or circulation, or cause bruises. Return instruments to the Mayo stand or instrument table immediately after use.
6. Umbilical tape or vessel loops are used frequently to retract blood vessels and small structures, thereby giving the surgeon greater visibility in a small surgical site and eliminating the weight of retractors.
7. Needleholders have fine-pointed jaws to hold small, delicate needles.

Figure 8-3 Upper extremity restraint to splint elbow and hand of infant or toddler. Hand is pronated on armboard.

8. Surgical procedure on an adolescent will require adult-size instruments.
9. Scrub person closely watches the tissue being dissected and selects the instruments to hand to the surgeon accordingly.

COMMON SURGICAL PROCEDURES

General Surgery

Endoscopic Procedures

Gastroscopy, colonoscopy, and laparoscopy are performed for diagnosis of complaints of abdominal pain or symptoms of intestinal obstruction or inflammation. Procedures such as polypectomy, sphincterotomy, appendectomy, or insertion of a gastrostomy tube can be done in lieu of laparotomy. Endoscopic injection of sodium morrhuate is an alternative to a portosystemic shunt in children with bleeding esophageal varices.

Anastomosis Within the Alimentary Tract

Alimentary tract obstruction in a newborn or young infant is the most frequent cause for an emergency surgical procedure. The common sites of obstruction are in the esophagus, duodenum, ileum, colon, and anus. Atresia, an imperforation or closure of a normal opening, and stenosis, a constriction or narrowing, are the common causes of obstruction. The obstructive lesion is usually resected, and the viable segments of the viscera are anastomosed. A temporary gastrostomy, ileostomy, or colostomy may be necessary. Intestinal obstruction can develop in infants and children months to years after the newborn period from a predisposing or associated congenital anomaly or acquired disease process. Inflammatory diseases such as necrotizing enterocolitis, ulcerative colitis, Meckel's diverticulitis, or Crohn's disease, as well as other intestinal conditions such as Hirschsprung's disease or familial polyposis, require intestinal resection and anastomosis. An endorectal pull-through may be the procedure of choice to preserve the rectum.

Biliary Atresia   A form of intrauterine cholangitis that results in progressive fibrotic obliteration of bile ducts, biliary atresia may cause jaundice in the newborn. Excision of extrahepatic ducts or hilar dissection with a hepatic portoenterostomy procedure, such as portal hepatojejunostomy, is performed before the infant is 2 months old to relieve jaundice by improving bile drainage. If liver function becomes progressively impaired, liver transplantation may ultimately be necessary for survival.

Esophageal Atresia Esophageal atresia, with or without tracheoesophageal fistula, is an acute congenital anomaly characterized by esophageal obstruction, accumulation of secretions, gastric reflux, and respiratory complications. The goal of repair is to obtain an end-to-end esophageal anastomosis. The timing and technique to accomplish this goal depend on the specific type of anomaly, degree of prematurity, birth weight, and extent of other associated anomalies. Repair may be either primary or staged. Gastrostomy is performed initially to establish a conduit for feeding the newborn. Repair includes division of the tracheoesophageal fistula, if present, and anastomosis of the esophageal pouches. Submucosal myotomies and lengthening of the upper pouch permit primary anastomosis to establish alimentary tract continuity. This may be delayed to allow the esophagus to grow as the infant grows, so that the gap between the pouches shortens. A transthoracic or retrosternal interposition colon graft may be necessary for esophageal replacement if the gap between the proximal and distal segments is too large for a primary esophageal anastomosis. Usually an extrapleural approach is used for these procedures.

Imperforate Anus

If the anus remains closed (i.e., imperforate) during fetal development, the intestinal tract is opened surgically soon after birth. A posterior sagittal anorectoplasty or an abdominoperineal pull-through procedure may be done for primary management. Many children endure fecal incontinence or chronic constipation as they grow into their teens following these procedures in infancy. Various secondary procedures are performed, most frequently an endorectal pull-through procedure or gracilis muscle transplant for reconstruction of the rectal sphincter.

Pyloromyotomy

Pyloric stenosis is a congenital obstructive lesion in the pylorus of the stomach. The onset of symptoms usually occurs between the third and eighth weeks of life. The stenosis is relieved by pyloromyotomy. After cutting through serosa, muscle layers of the pylorus are divided.

Herniorrhaphy

Herniorrhaphy (i.e., hernia repair) is the most frequently performed elective surgical procedure in infants and children by general surgeons. Of the four types of hernias seen in pediatric patients, indirect inguinal hernia is the most common; it occurs much more frequently in male patients than in female patients and appears during the first 10 years of life. Female patients who have an inguinal hernia also may have a prolapsed ovary in the hernial sac. Although they are frequently seen, most umbilical hernias do not require surgical intervention. Hiatal (diaphragmatic) hernias and femoral hernias require surgical correction but are rarely acute problems in childhood. A hiatal hernia is a surgical emergency in the newborn if abdominal contents are in the chest, causing acute respiratory distress. Hernias in infants and children are caused by congenital weakness in the fascia, abdominal wall, or diaphragm.

Omphalocele

Failure of abdominal viscera to become encapsulated within the peritoneal cavity during fetal development results in herniation through a midline defect in the abdominal wall at the base of the umbilicus (i.e., omphalocele). Contents in the omphalocele sac are surgically reduced back into the peritoneal cavity. The method of closure depends on the extent of the defect. Skin may be closed primarily if the defect is small. More commonly, primary closure of the abdominal wall is facilitated by vigorous stretching of the wall and emptying of intestinal contents from the sac. Closure is performed without undue tension. Synthetic mesh or sheeting may be used. For large defects, closure of the abdominal wall usually is staged with implantation of a silicone silo or pneumatic prosthesis to reduce intestines at the first stage, followed by removal of the device and abdominal wall closure at the second stage. Similar techniques are used for closure of gastroschisis, a full-thickness abdominal wall defect lateral to and separate from the umbilicus, with herniation of abdominal viscera.

Appendectomy

Appendicitis, an acute inflammation of the appendix, is the most common cause for an abdominal surgical procedure in the school-age child. Gangrene or rupture may occur before diagnosis or surgical intervention. A questionable diagnosis may be confirmed by laparoscopy. Appendectomy may be performed by laparoscopy. Gasless laparoscopy using a planar lift device may be performed to avoid the use of carbon dioxide.

Splenectomy

Removal of the spleen may be indicated to correct hypersplenic disease, either congenital or acquired. Emergency splenectomy is necessary following rupture of the spleen, usually from blunt trauma. An attempt is made to salvage as much of the organ as possible to minimize future susceptibility to infection.

Urology

Pediatric urology concerns itself basically with the diagnosis and treatment of infections and congenital anomalies within the genitourinary tract. Some type of anomaly of the genitourinary system may be found in 10% to 15% of newborns. Secondary infections are frequently associated with congenital anomalies; chronic diseases are frequently associated with infections. The following surgical procedures include those most commonly performed by pediatric urologists.

Cystoscopy

Diagnostic evaluation and therapeutic removal of obstructions within the structures of the genitourinary tract may be performed through an infant- or child-size cystoscope. Cystoscopes from 9.5 through 16 French are used for infants and children. A size 3 French ureteral catheter can be introduced through the smallest-size cystoscope.

Nephrectomy, Nephrostomy, or Pyeloureteroplasty

Hydronephrosis, congenital or acquired, may necessitate surgical intervention. Nephrectomy is indicated only if severe disease is unilateral, with a contralateral kidney capable of life-sustaining function. More conservative nephrostomy or pyeloureteroplasty is indicated for bilateral or moderate to mild kidney disease.

Wilms' Tumor

Wilms' tumor is a malignant solid renal tumor that develops rapidly in a child usually under 5 years of age. Nephrectomy is necessary to resect the tumor. If the adrenal gland is intimately connected to the tumor in the upper pole of the kidney, the gland is resected en bloc with the renal mass. Vascular extension of the tumor into the suprahepatic vena cava may necessitate a cardiopulmonary bypass to ligate all tumor vessels. Ipsilateral periaortic lymph node dissection often is performed.

Neurogenic Bladder

Defective bladder function may be a result of a central nervous system lesion such as a myelomeningocele or spinal cord trauma. To preserve renal function and to achieve urinary continence in the presence of a neurogenic bladder, an enterocystoplasty may be performed. This procedure retains an intact urinary tract. An artificial urinary sphincter can be implanted to achieve dryness in the child who has sufficient dexterity to operate the pump.

Exstrophy of the Bladder

In exstrophy of the bladder, a congenital anomaly, the bladder herniates through the lower abdominal wall in the suprapubic region. Repair requires reconstruction of the lower abdominal wall and external genitalia, as well as provision for passage of urine. This can usually be accomplished in one surgical procedure on a female infant but requires two or more staged procedures in a male infant. A gastrocystoplasty may be the procedure of choice. If urinary continence cannot be established, urinary diversion through ureteral reimplantation may become necessary.

Ureteral Reimplantation

Repositioning of the ureters (i.e., ureteral reimplantation) may be performed to correct either congenital or acquired total urinary incontinence or vesicoureteral reflux.

Incontinence causes parents to seek help for an infant or child. Incontinence is usually not caused by a single factor. The urologist plans the procedure on the basis of an accurate assessment of anatomic and physiologic causes. Creation of a tubularized trigonal muscle, when reconstructed into a new bladder neck, acts as a sphincter to maintain continence. With ureters in the normal position, this muscular tube in the bladder wall cannot be constructed. Therefore the ureters are reimplanted superiorly into the bladder through a created tunnel. Care is taken that the ureters are not hooked or angled but follow a smooth curve into the bladder.

Vesicoureteral reflux is the most common reason for reimplanting ureters in pediatric patients. Chronic reflux, regurgitation of urine from the bladder into the ureters, can lead to pyelonephritis and hydronephrosis. Ureteral reimplantation may be required to prevent kidney damage. The objective of the surgical procedure is to position a segment of the ureters at a higher level within the bladder wall so that urine lies below orifices and intravesical pressure prevents reflux.

When ureters cannot be reimplanted in the bladder, a urinary diversion procedure may be necessary. Ureters are usually anastomosed to a nonrefluxing colon conduit.

Urethral Repair

The external opening (meatus) of the urethra may be displaced at birth. Hypospadias is an anomaly in the male in which the urethra terminates on the underside of the penis or on the perineum (Figure 8-4); in the female the urethra opens

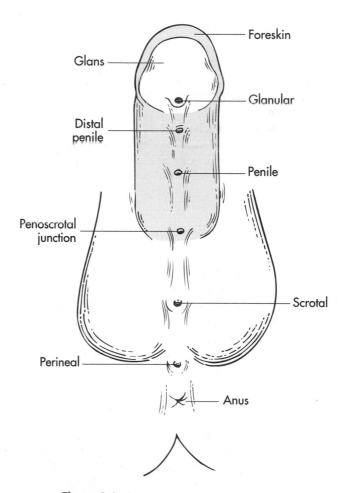

Figure 8-4 Meatal opening in hypospadias.

into the vagina. With epispadias in the male the urethra terminates on the dorsum of the penis; in the female it terminates above the clitoris. Multistage procedures are usually necessary to correct these anomalies. The goal is to center the meatus at the tip of the glans penis of the male. This may be accomplished in a one-stage procedure by a transverse island flap derived from prepuce or by a vertical-incision/horizontal-closure technique for distal coronal or subglandular hypospadias. This procedure is usually performed between ages 1 and 4 years.

Orchiopexy

One or both testicles that failed to descend during fetal development can be brought into the scrotum and stabilized with a traction suture until healing takes place. In the two-stage Torek's operation, the testicle and supporting structures are dissected free from the inguinal region. An adequate length of spermatic vessels is released to permit the testicle to reach the scrotal sac. After it is pulled down through the scrotum, the testicle is sutured to fascia of the thigh. At the second-stage procedure, 2 to 3 months later, the testicle is freed from the fascia and embedded into the scrotum.

If one or both testicles are absent, silicone prostheses may be inserted into the scrotum for cosmetic appearance. Psychologically for the child and parents, undescended testicles (cryptorchism) or absence (agenesis) of testicles is usually repaired at age 5 or 6 years, before the boy begins school.

Circumcision

Excision of the foreskin of the penis (circumcision) may be done to prevent phimosis, in which the foreskin becomes tightly wrapped around the tip of the glans penis, or to remove redundant foreskin. Circumcision is the most commonly performed pediatric surgical procedure. It should be done on newborns with the patient under local anesthesia. Circumcision, as an elective procedure, is contraindicated if an abnormality of the glans penis or urethral meatus is present. Urethral repair usually uses the foreskin as graft tissue.

Orthopaedic Surgery

Pediatric orthopaedic surgery is principally elective and reconstructive in nature to correct deformities of the musculoskeletal system. These deformities may be congenital, idiopathic, pathologic, or traumatic in origin. The extensiveness of the anomalies and functional disorders often involve prolonged immobilization and hospitalization. Many patients require a series of corrective procedures. Some of the conditions most commonly seen in the OR include those discussed in the following sections.

Fractures

Fractures that occur in infants and children generally are treated as they are in adults. Fixation devices are not well tolerated by children and often prevent uniting of the fracture. Closed reduction of long bone fractures is preferable.

Tendon Repair

Tendons may be lengthened, shortened, or transferred to correct congenital deformities of the hand or foot. Lacerated tendons are repaired to restore function. A tourniquet is used to control bleeding. The tourniquet cuff size should be appropriate for the size of the infant or child. Padding under the cuff is applied smoothly. Sheet wadding may be used under an infant cuff to protect delicate skin. The cuff should be tight but without restricting circulation before inflation. The time of inflation is closely watched to prevent ischemia. The surgeon may ask the circulator to release the pressure every 30 minutes on an infant or up to every 1 to 2 hours for an older child, depending on age. Tendon procedures are often lengthy.

Congenital Dislocated Hip

Displacement (dysplasia) of the femoral head from its normal position in the acetabulum can be present at birth, either unilaterally or bilaterally. If dysplasia is diagnosed early in infancy, closed reduction with immobilization usually corrects the dislocation without residual deformity. If dysplasia is not diagnosed until after the child has begun to walk, open reduction of the hip with an osteotomy to stabilize the joint may be necessary.

Leg Length Discrepancies

The epiphyseal cartilaginous growth lines progressively close as the child matures. Bones lengthen from the activity of the epiphyses. The absolute physiologic criterion for completion of childhood is when this cartilage becomes a part of bone. A discrepancy in activity of an epiphyseal line may retard or overstimulate growth of a bone in one extremity and not in its contralateral counterpart. When this occurs in one femur, legs become unequal in length. The orthopaedic surgeon may correct leg length discrepancies, usually in excess of 1 inch (2.5 cm), by epiphyseal arrest (i.e., stopping growth of the bone). This is done in the contralateral leg to let the shorter extremity catch up. The longer leg may be shortened by a closed intramedullary procedure. Under fluoroscopy, a reamer is inserted into the medullary canal of the femur through a small incision high on the hip. After the reamer widens the canal, a rotating saw is manipulated to cut a section from the bone. The bone ends are aligned and fixed with a flexible intramedullary rod.

Slipping of the upper femoral epiphysis causes displacement of the femoral head, which can occur as a result of traumatic injury or as a chronic disability usually seen in obese adolescents. Fusion of the epiphysis to the femoral neck may be necessary to prevent slipping and shortening of the leg.

Many limb deformities in children are a complex combination of angulation and shortening as a result of trauma, infection, metabolic bone disease, congenital deformity, and developmental problems. The Ilizarov external fixator technique provides an alternative treatment option. Thin, strong wires are transfixed through bones and attached to rings under tension. The rings, which encircle a leg or arm, are held firmly in place with threaded rods. Bolts on the rods are turned several times a day to pull cut ends of bone apart. Corticotomy, performed through a small skin incision after wires are inserted, preserves periosteal and endosteal blood supply to bone. This promotes rapid healing to regenerate new bone that fills in the gap.

Talipes Deformities

Combinations of various types of deformities of the foot, especially those of congenital origin, are referred to as *talipes* plus the medical term to describe whether the forefoot is inverted *(varus)* or everted *(valgus)* and whether the calcaneal tendon is shortened or lengthened.

Talipes varus, the condition known as clubfoot, is the most common of these deformities and may be unilateral or bilateral. The forefoot is inverted and rotated, accompanied by shortening of the calcaneal tendon and contracture of the plantar fascia. Conservative treatment by casting during infancy usually corrects a mild postural deformity before the infant bears weight on the foot. A wedge cast with turnbuckles may be applied to an older child to allow gradual manipulation. If conservative treatment is unsuccessful, an open surgical procedure may be necessary.

Talipes equinovarus, an idiopathic true clubfoot deformity, almost always requires surgical intervention for correction. In varying degrees, talipes equinovarus includes an incomplete dislocation (subluxation) of the talocalcaneonavicular joint with deformed talus and calcaneous bones, a shortened calcaneal tendon, and soft tissue contractures. As a result, the forefoot curls toward the heel (adduction, supination), the midfoot points downward (equinus), and the hindfoot turns inward (varus). The orthopaedic surgeon uses a sequential-release approach to obtain maximum correction of all contractures and realigns bones in the ankle joint. Pins are inserted, and the extremity is put in a cast to maintain alignment of the foot and ankle.

Scoliosis

Scoliosis is a lateral curvature and rotation of the spine, most frequently seen in rapidly growing school-age (over age 10) or adolescent females. Treatment depends on the degree and flexibility of the curvature, chronologic and skeletal age of the child, and preference of the surgeon. The child may be fitted with a Milwaukee brace, immobilized in a cast, or stretched by traction. As an alternative to these techniques, an electrical device may be applied with an underarm brace to stimulate muscle contraction on the convex side of the curvature. If untreated at an early stage, scoliosis produces secondary changes in vertebral bodies and in the rib cage. Spinal fusion is ultimately performed if the curvature has become severe (50% or more) or must be stabilized following corrections. Government-mandated screening programs in schools have reduced the need for surgical correction in many children.

The following procedures may be used for correction of scoliosis:

1. A wedge body jacket or Minerva jacket may be applied. Turnbuckles may be incorporated. Turnbuckles are adjustable metal rods placed along the edges of the wedge of the cast. Gradual opening of the turnbuckles by the surgeon as tolerated by the patient corrects the lateral curvature of the spine.

   A Sayre sling, an appliance used for head traction, is sometimes used when applying a body jacket to correct slight scoliosis. Traction is obtained by means of pulleys and a rope suspended from the ceiling or an arm of the fracture table.

2. Halo traction is used to stretch the spine in some patients in whom the spine is too rigid to be straightened in a cast. A metal band is applied to the skull by means of four pins inserted into the cortex of the skull. A Steinmann pin is inserted into the distal end of each femur. A traction bow is put on each pin. Weights, usually equal, are put on the halo and Steinmann pins and gradually increased as tolerated. When x-ray films show maximum correction, a spinal fusion is done. Traction may be continued until healing has taken place to the degree that there will be no loss of correction; a plaster jacket is then applied.

3. A Risser jacket is applied a few days preceding posterior spinal fusion to gain as much correction as possible. The orthopaedic table is used. Traction is applied by a chin strap, similar to a Sayre sling, and countertraction is applied by a pelvic girdle. The spine is straightened as much as possible, and the body and head are encased in plaster.

   Posterior spinal fusion may be performed as a two-stage procedure: vertebral body wedge resection at the first stage and insertion of Cotrel-Dubousset or Harrington rods with fusion at second stage. Bone fragments removed during the first stage may be saved for the second-stage fusion or sent to the bone bank. Rods and hooks are stainless steel; appropriate instruments are required to insert them. Two rods are inserted, one on either side of the curvature. These rods are secured to the spine and force it into a more nearly normal position. Implanted on the outside of the vertebral column, the rods apply a longitudinal force on the spine. The spine is then fused.

   The procedure may be done through a window in the Risser jacket, but usually the cast is bivalved and the patient lies in the anterior section. If the procedure is done through a window, an electric cast cutter should be at hand to bivalve the cast if the patient has any respiratory difficulties. After the procedure the bivalved posterior part is put in place and the jacket is fastened together by several rounds of plaster or by webbing straps with buckles. The patient is in the Risser jacket for a year. Progress is checked by x-ray films.

4. Segmental spinal fixation with Luque rods may be the procedure of choice to stabilize the spine following fusion. Two L-shaped rods are placed next to the spinous processes and held by wires threaded under the lamina of each vertebra to be fused. Transverse traction internally on each vertebra stabilizes the spine without the need for a postoperative cast.

5. Anterior spinal fusion through a transthoracic approach is performed as a one-stage procedure to correct severe curvatures in patients who have malformed vertebral bodies. With Dwyer instruments, titanium staples are fitted over vertebral bodies on the convex side of the curve. Each staple is held in place by two titanium screws. A multistrand titanium cable, threaded through the heads of the screws, is tightened to compress the vertebrae and straighten the curve. Staples and screws are secured the full extent of the curvature. A plaster body jacket may be applied after the procedure to immobilize the back until the fusion is healed. The patient is then ambulatory.

Ophthalmology

Congenital Obstruction of the Nasolacrimal Duct

An obstruction, usually at the lower end of the nasolacrimal duct that enters the inferior meatus of the nose, often results in dilation and infection of the lacrimal sac. Treatment consists of passing a malleable probe from the lid punctum through the nasolacrimal passages to push out the obstructing plug of tissue.

Oculoplastic Procedures on the Eyelids

Congenital malformations such as ptosis (drooping of the upper or lower eyelid) are corrected by extraocular procedures. Ptosis repair is indicated when the levator is inadequate. In the levator resection procedure, which shortens the muscle and gives a more physiologic result, the levator muscle may be approached through the skin (Berke's method) or the conjunctiva (Iliff's method). A fascial sling procedure to support the lid consists of attaching the upper lid margin to the frontalis muscle. Materials used include autogenous fascia from the thigh, homograft fascia, or synthetic nonabsorbable suture material. The Fasanella-Servat operation is a simpler procedure for obtaining only a small amount of lid elevation.

Extraocular Muscle Procedures

Surgical procedures on extraocular muscles to correct strabismus or squint are the third most commonly performed pediatric procedures between ages 6 months and 6 years. The trend is to correct the congenital type during infancy and the acquired type in preschool years. Patterns of using two eyes together are more flexible and adaptable in a young child. These procedures on extraocular muscles are done to correct muscle imbalance and promote coordination either by strengthening a weak muscle or by weakening an overactive one. The mechanical strength of a weak muscle can be increased by the following:

1. *Tucking.* A tuck is sutured in the muscle to shorten it, thereby increasing its effective power.
2. *Advancement.* The attachment point of the muscle is freed and reattached closer to the cornea, thereby increasing its leverage.

3. *Resection.* Part of the muscle is removed to shorten it, and cut ends are sutured together.

An overactive muscle can be weakened by the following:

1. *Tenotomy.* The point of attachment of the muscle is severed, and the muscle is dropped back, held by ligaments only.
2. *Recession.* The muscle is detached from the eyeball and reattached farther back to decrease its action.
3. *Myotomy.* The fibers of a section of the muscle are divided to diminish muscle action.
4. *Myectomy.* A section of the muscle belly is excised.
5. *Fadin procedure.* The muscle belly is sutured to the posterior sclera, thereby restricting muscle action considerably, producing a super-weakening effect.

Intraocular Procedures

Congenital Cataract Extraction   Under the operating microscope, with use of irrigation-aspiration and cutting instruments, the cataract and often the posterior capsule and a portion of the anterior vitreous are removed at one time. This procedure obtains a clear optical zone so that a contact lens can be fitted on the infant's eye within a few days postoperatively. The goal is to avoid intractable amblyopia (lazy eye) by correcting the defect during the first few weeks of life. An intraocular lens may be implanted. More commonly, epikeratophakia is performed to reshape the cornea or an epi lens is made from a donor cornea.

Goniotomy   Although congenital glaucoma is rare, early surgical intervention is urgent to prevent blindness. Goniotomy is a microsurgical procedure that involves dividing a congenital layer of abnormal tissue covering the drainage angle of the anterior chamber. It is performed by use of a special operative contact lens placed on the eye that permits visualization of the angle. An incision is made through an opening in the contact lens.

Otorhinolaryngology

Myringotomy

Secretory otitis media is the most common chronic condition of childhood. Fluid accumulates in the middle ear from eustachian tube obstruction. This condition is corrected by myringotomy, an incision in the tympanic membrane (eardrum) for drainage. Through aspiration of fluid and pus, pressure is released, pain is relieved, and hearing is restored and preserved. Myringotomy is done to prevent perforation of the eardrum and possible erosion of middle ear ossicles. When exudate is especially viscid, the patient has "glue ear" or mucoid otitis media.

Tympanostomy is commonly performed bilaterally in association with myringotomy. A self-cleaning plastic pressure-equalizing tube is placed through an incision in the tympanic membrane, bypassing the eustachian tube, to facilitate aeration of the middle ear space and to prevent reformation of serous otitis media. The tube usually extrudes spontaneously. Premature extrusion before normal eustachian tube function resumes may necessitate replacement of the tube.

Middle Ear Tympanoplasty

Congenital fused ossicles in the middle ear often are associated with stenosis or absence of an external auditory canal. Depending on the deformity, tympanoplasty may be performed with a temporalis fascia graft. If mobilization or ossiculoplasty is impossible, a total or partial ossicular prosthesis may be implanted to replace one or more ossicles. Congenital or acquired conductive deafness may be helped by tympanoplastic surgical techniques. Single-channel cochlear implants, approved for children, may be helpful for the profoundly deaf child.

Correction of Choanal Atresia

Newborns are obligate nose breathers and may die at birth if choanal atresia, congenital closure of nasal passages, is undiagnosed. They are unable to breathe and feed properly without an adequate nasal airway. Excision of bone or fibrous tissue blocking the posterior choanae usually is performed via a transseptal approach to create an opening into the nasopharynx. A CO_2 laser may be used to develop appropriate apertures.

Adenoidectomy

Abnormally enlarged lymphoid tissue or infected adenoids can obstruct breathing. A child usually is at least 2 years old before having adenoid tissue in the nasopharynx removed, but adenoidectomy can be done at an earlier age. Removal of adenoids can positively influence the outcome of otitis media with effusion in childhood. Adenoidectomy is usually done in conjunction with tonsillectomy.

Tonsillectomy

Tonsillectomy, the excision of hypertrophied or chronically infected tonsils, is not generally advised before the child is 3 years of age. General anesthesia is used for patients up to about 14 years of age. Tonsillectomy and adenoidectomy are frequently performed together, appearing on the surgical schedule as T&A. Sterile technique is carried out throughout the procedure. Precautions during the surgical procedure include control of bleeding and prevention of aspiration of blood or tissue.

Esophageal Dilation

Children, usually of preschool age, may ingest caustic agents that cause chemical burns of the mouth, lips, and pharynx and corrosive esophagitis. Long-term gradual esophageal dilation with balloon catheters or bougies may be necessary to restore adequate oral intake of food after the acute phase of traumatic injury. When all attempts at dilation fail, the esophagus is replaced. The most satisfactory source of esophageal replacement is the colon.

Laryngeal Papillomas

Recurrent respiratory papillomatosis is localized in the larynx of children. Laryngeal papillomas are benign, wartlike lesions caused by the human papillomavirus. Hoarseness is an early symptom; airway obstruction is a later, life-threatening sign. Ablation with the CO_2 laser, manipulated through the operating microscope, preserves underlying laryngeal muscles and ligaments while vaporizing papillomas located on vocal cords. Laser ablation is not a cure; recurrence often necessitates repeated procedures to maintain a patent airway.

Tracheal or Laryngeal Stenosis

Some accidental injuries result in a narrowing (i.e., stenosis) of the trachea or larynx. Of greater concern are the injuries that result from therapy for respiratory problems, especially in newborns. Prolonged endotracheal intubation can lead to injury from tubes that are too large for the lumen, are too long, or move too much. These injuries may require balloon dilation and/or endoscopic resection of the stenotic area. Most infants then require an intraluminal stent to maintain patency of their airways.

In the presence of severe circumferential intraluminal scarring with involvement of the cartilages, surgical reconstruction becomes necessary. Laryngotracheoplasty widens the stenosed cartilaginous framework of the airway in the midline anteriorly and posteriorly and reconstructs the mucosal lining. Free or composite rib cartilage grafts are taken with mucosal tissue of the perichondrium for lining the airway. A stent assembly with a tracheostomy tube supports the reconstructed airway during healing. It can then be removed and the tracheostomy closed.

Tracheotomy

Tracheotomy, incision into the trachea and insertion of a tracheostomy tube, is advisable in cases of severe inflammatory glottic diseases, when endotracheal intubation would be required for longer than 72 hours, and when respiratory support is necessary for longer than 24 to 48 hours to treat respiratory problems. Appropriate sizes and types of tracheostomy tubes for infants and children should be available. Tubes that are too large, too rigid, or too long, or that have an improper curve can produce ulceration and scarring at pressure points. Strictures that develop at the site of the tracheotomy may require resection to relieve airway obstruction after decannulation. Infants have a shorter neck and are prone to distal displacement of the tracheostomy tube from the intratracheal insertion point. Head motion will cause the tube to shift superiorly if it is not secured in position by ties.

Plastic and Reconstructive Surgery

With the exception of burns and other traumatic tissue injuries, most plastic and reconstructive surgery performed on infants and children is done to correct congenital anomalies. The most common of these surgeries include those discussed in the following sections.

Cleft Lip

Lack of fusion of the soft tissues of the upper lip creates a cleft or fissure. Cleft lips vary in degree from simple notching of the lip to extension into the floor of the nose. They may be unilateral or bilateral. The number of procedures required for correction depends on the severity of the deformity. Some plastic surgeons do a primary cheiloplasty, closure of the cleft lip, within the first few days after birth to facilitate feeding and to minimize psychologic trauma of parents. Surgeons who prefer to wait until the infant is older follow the "rule of 10s": 10 weeks, 10 g of hemoglobin, 10 pounds of body weight. Regardless of preferred timing, infiltration of a local anesthetic agent with epinephrine is usually the anesthetic of choice.

To relieve tension on the incision postoperatively, a Logan bow (a small, curved metal frame) may be applied over the area of the incision and held in place by narrow adhesive strips to splint the lip. Skin closure strips may be used. Arm or elbow restraints are used to prevent the infant from removing the bow or strips and injuring the repaired lip. These restraints are applied in the OR.

Cleft Palate

Failure of tissues of the palate to fuse creates a fissure through the roof of the mouth. Palatal clefts may be a defect only in the soft palate or may extend through both hard and soft palates into the nose and include the alveolar ridge of the maxilla. Cleft palate is often associated with cleft lip; however, the two deformities are closed separately. Palatoplasty, closure of the soft palate, is done before speech begins, to avoid speech defects. A mouth gag is used during the surgical procedure to permit access to the palate without obstructing the airway. General anesthesia is administered via an endotracheal tube. This may be supplemented by infiltration of a local anesthetic agent. When epinephrine is used by the surgeon to minimize bleeding, the anesthesia provider is informed.

In patients with bilateral and, frequently, unilateral clefts, an additional surgical procedure will be performed to elevate the tip of the nose and correct asymmetry before the child is 4 years of age.

Hemangioma

Hemangiomas are the most common of all human congenital anomalies. A hemangioma is a benign tumor (angioma) made up of blood vessels that may pigment or appear as a growth on the skin. All hemangiomas have abnormal patterns of hemodynamics, which is the effect of blood flow through tissues. Variations in vessel size distinguish the different types of these tumors. Argon or tunable dye laser or surgical excision in combination with a skin graft or pedicle flap repair are treatments of choice for intradermal capillary hemangiomas (port-wine stain). Cryosurgery, surgical excision, or steroid therapy may be used for some other cavernous-type tumors.

Otoplasty

Abnormally small or absent external ears can be reconstructed in several surgical stages. An autogenous rib cartilage graft with the perichondrium intact or a silicone or a porous polyethylene prosthesis is used for the supporting framework to produce an anatomic contour. Usually necessitated by microtia, a congenital anomaly, reconstruction of the external ear can follow traumatic injury with loss of all or part of the pinna. Free flaps of temporoparietal fascia are used to secure a prosthesis or may be used to cover a carved cartilage armature for secondary reconstruction.

Otoplasty procedures to correct protruding or excessively large ears are performed more frequently than are procedures for microtia. These procedures often are done on preschool-age children, usually boys, to prevent psychologic harm from teasing.

Syndactyly

Syndactyly is a congenital anomaly characterized by fusion of two or more fingers or toes. Webbing between fingers is the most common congenital hand deformity. Tissue holding digits together is cut to separate fingers. Separation of webbed digits almost always requires skin grafts to achieve good functional results.

Polydactyly

Polydactyly is a congenital anomaly characterized by the presence of more than the normal number of fingers or toes. A supernumerary digit may be alongside a thumb or little finger on one or both hands. Extra digits on the feet are less common. Skin and tissue resemble a rudimentary digit. Some supernumerary digits contain bone, ligament, and tendon. Excision is recommended at an early age. If the excised digit contains rudimentary bone, multistage procedures may be required to enhance function of the remaining digits of the affected extremity.

Neurosurgery

Children of all ages sustain head injuries with hematomas that must be evacuated. Although brain tumors occur in children, the more frequently performed pediatric neurosurgical procedures are related to correction of congenital anomalies.

Craniosynostosis

If one or more of the suture lines in the skull, normally open in infancy, fuses prematurely (craniosynostosis), the skull cannot expand during normal brain growth. A newborn with multiple-suture involvement may require surgical intervention because of increased intracranial pressure. Even fusion of a single suture puts a newborn at risk for altered cranial capacity and brain damage. The surgeon performs a craniectomy to remove the fused bone and to reopen the suture line(s). A strip of polyethylene or Silastic film may be inserted to cover bone edges on each side, or newly formed suture lines may be cauterized with Zenker's solution to prevent refusion. In an older infant or child, more extensive freeing of other bones may be necessary to achieve decompression of frontal lobes and orbital contents.

Craniofacial microsomia with severe facial asymmetry and the dysostosis of Apert's syndrome and Crouzon's disease also are associated with multiple skull and facial deformities. Craniofacial surgery, performed by a multidisciplinary team, involves repositioning and reshaping of skull and facial bones and a variety of soft tissue reconstructive techniques. Microplating systems may be used for rigid fixation of bones. The skull may provide a donor site without creating a deformity if bone grafts are required. Demineralized cadaver bone powder may be used to stimulate bone growth.

Encephalocele

Encephalocele is the herniation of brain and neural tissue through a defect in the skull. This is present at birth as a sac of tissue on the head. Usually these lesions can be removed 6 to 12 weeks after birth, unless the condition is complicated by hydrocephalus.

Hydrocephalus

Usually a congenital condition, hydrocephalus occurs when the passages between the ventricles are blocked and are dilated by accumulated cerebrospinal fluid. Failure of the absorptive mechanisms can also produce impairment in the normal circulation of cerebrospinal fluid, causing excess fluid to accumulate in the ventricles. Intracranial pressure thus created causes enlargement of the infant's head if the condition develops before fusion of cranial bones and often causes brain damage. Hydrocephalus may be diagnosed in utero by cephalocentesis, and a ventriculoamniotic shunt may be inserted to drain the ventricles. After birth, surgical treatment involves establishment of a mechanism for transporting excess fluid from the ventricles to maintain a close to normal intracranial pressure. This may be done by implantation of a shunt, which carries fluid from the lateral ventricle to the peritoneal cavity (ventriculoperitoneal shunt) or to the right atrium of the heart (ventriculoatrial shunt). Ventriculoatrial shunts are more commonly associated with infection, pleural effusion, and cardiac dysrhythmia. Other types of shunts are used, but less commonly, to bypass localized obstructions.

One end of the shunt catheter is put into the ventricle; the other end may connect to a one-way valve, which in turn is connected to the catheter that drains fluid distally from the head. An endoscopic technique may be used for catheter placement in the ventricle. Shunt malformation is usually caused by obstruction by the choroid plexus or debris. This complication can be reduced by positioning the shunt catheter tip opposite the foramen of Monro visually via a miniature fiberoptic pediatric neuroendoscope.

Catheters are made of silicone. An antithrombotic coating may be incorporated into the distal end. Some valves are regulated to open for drainage when predetermined pressure in the ventricle is reached. Other valves are designed as flushing devices to keep the distal catheter patent; the skin over the device is manually depressed to flush the system. For each patient the surgeon chooses the shunt mechanism that will be safest for the particular type of hydrocephalus being treated.

Follow-up minor revisions are sometimes necessary, generally because of growth of the child.

As an alternative to a shunt procedure, a ventriculostomy can relieve intracranial pressure. A rigid neuroendoscope is introduced into the third ventricle. The contact fiber of an Nd:YAG laser, inserted through the scope, blanches and perforates the floor of the third ventricle at several points to establish circulation of cerebrospinal fluid into the subarachnoid space.

Myelomeningocele

A saclike protrusion may bulge through a defect in a portion of the vertebral column that failed to fuse in fetal development. If the nerves of the spinal cord remain within the vertebral column and only the meninges protrude into the sac, the congenital anomaly is a meningocele. However, if the sac also contains a portion of the spinal cord, it is a myelomeningocele, with associated permanent nerve damage. The degree of impairment depends on the level and extent of the defect. Clubfeet, dislocated hips, hydrocephalus, neurogenic bladder, paralysis, and other congenital disorders often accompany a myelomeningocele. Each patient is evaluated and treated individually according to his or her needs. In general, it is best to delay the surgical procedure to repair a myelomeningocele until danger of development of hydrocephalus has passed or cerebrospinal fluid has been shunted. If the sac is covered with a thin membrane, meningitis (infection of meninges) is an imminent danger unless the defect is repaired soon after birth, usually within the first 48 hours, to close cutaneous, muscular, and dural defects.

Spina Bifida

Spina bifida, incomplete closure of the paired vertebral arches in the midline of the vertebral column, may occur without herniation of the meninges. A spina bifida may be covered by intact skin. Laminectomy may be indicated to repair the underlying defect.

Spastic Cerebral Palsy

Selective posterior rhizotomy can improve muscle tone and function of school-age children with spastic cerebral palsy. The procedure involves division of lumbar and sacral posterior nerve roots associated with an abnormal motor response as identified by nerve stimulation.

Thoracic Surgery

Aspiration of a foreign body can seriously compromise a child's respiratory status. Bronchoscopy may be necessary, with the child under general anesthesia, to remove the object. Bronchoscopy is also performed to diagnose tracheobronchial compression by an innominate artery, a vascular ring, or some other pathologic condition causing obstruction, stridor, or apnea. Thoracoscopy provides visualization of the chest wall and visceral pleura for diagnosis of diffuse or localized pulmonary disease. An intrathoracic biopsy can be obtained via a thoracoscope.

Pectus Excavatum

Pectus excavatum, a congenital malformation of the chest wall, is characterized by a pronounced funnel-shaped depression over the lower end of the sternum. Cardiopulmonary impairment can result from pectus excavatum. The deformity is corrected by resecting lower intercostal cartilages and substernal ligaments to free up the sternum. The sternum is elevated, and the cartilages are fitted to the sides of the sternum. The surgical procedure is done primarily for cosmetic purposes, but occasionally it is necessary to establish normal respiratory and circulatory function.

Cardiovascular Surgery

Congenital cardiovascular defects are the result of abnormal embryologic development of the heart or major vessels. During fetal life, blood bypasses the lungs through the foramen ovale and the ductus arteriosus to the placenta. From the placenta, the blood bypasses the liver through the ductus venosus. The right ventricle pumps 66% of the circulation, and the left ventricle pumps 34%. At birth the pulmonary ventilation is established, and the increasing pressure causes increased left atrial force that in turn causes the foramen ovale to close. The right atrial pressure drops, causing the blood flow to reverse. The ductus usually closes after 15 hours. Some neonates have a delay of 1 to 3 weeks for the complete closure of the ductus.

Most cardiovascular defects are diagnosed in infancy, often when symptoms of congestive heart failure develop within the first few days or months after birth. Corrective or palliative procedures are necessary to sustain or prolong the life of these infants. Many of these cardiovascular procedures are enhanced by or are made possible with the use of profound hypothermia and cardiopulmonary bypass. However, significant brain damage may be associated with a cardiovascular bypass in infants. Bypass perfusion time should not exceed 40 minutes between periods of temporary normal circulatory perfusion. Congenital defects in infants or children that are amenable to surgical intervention include the following.

Anomalous Venous Return

Failure of any one pulmonary vein or a combination of these veins to return blood to the left atrium precludes the full complement of oxygenated blood from entering the systemic circulation. The anomalous pulmonary vein or veins are transferred and anastomosed to the left atrium.

Coarctation of the Aorta

A coarctation is a narrowing or stricture in a vessel. This is one of the more common congenital cardiovascular defects, usually occurring in the aortic arch. It may cause hypertension in the upper extremities above the obstruction and hypotension in the lower extremities from slowed circulation below the coarctation. To correct the defect, the coarctation is resected and the aorta may be anastomosed end-to-end. An aortic patch graft may be necessary when the length of the coarctation prevents anastomosis. A subclavian flap angioplasty capable of growth in length and width, referred to as the Waldhausen procedure, is the surgical procedure of choice in infants.

Patent Ductus Arteriosus

During fetal life the ductus arteriosus carries blood from the pulmonary artery to the aorta to bypass the lungs. Normally this vessel closes in the first hours after birth to prevent recirculation of arterial blood through the body. If closure does not occur, blood flow may be reversed by aortic pressure, causing respiratory distress. Signs of patent ductus arteriosus (PDA) include widening pulse pressure and a characteristic murmur. The condition may be diagnosed by 1 month of age. Surgical intervention is indicated, in lieu of prolonged ventilatory support, to prevent development of chronic pulmonary changes. The PDA is clamped and ligated with ligating clips or suture.

Septal Defects

An open heart procedure with cardiopulmonary bypass is necessary to close abnormal openings in the walls (septa) separating the chambers within the heart.

Atrial Septal Defect   An opening in the septum between the right and left atria may be sufficiently large to allow oxygenated blood to shunt from left to right and return to the lungs. An atrial septal defect (ASD) can increase pulmonary blood flow, with resultant pulmonary hypertension, if the defect is not closed. Signs include acyanosis, thin body stature, and decreased tolerance to exercise. If the defect cannot be closed with sutures, a patch graft is inserted.

Ventricular Septal Defect   A ventricular septal defect (VSD) is usually located in the membranous portion of the septum between the right and left ventricles. It is the most common of the congenital heart anomalies. Signs include alternation between cyanosis and acyanosis. Patients with small defects are relatively asymptomatic, and repair may be unnecessary. Large defects with left-to-right shunting of oxygenated blood back to the lungs, thus increasing pulmonary hypertension, are closed. A patch graft may be required to close the defect.

Atrioventricular Canal Defect   An atrioventricular canal defect is present if the atrioventricular canal of connective tissue that normally divides the heart into four chambers has failed to develop. Deficiencies are present in the lower portion of the interatrial septum, upper portion of the interventricular septum, and tricuspid and mitral valves. The result is a large central canal that permits blood flow between any of the four chambers of the heart. A corrective procedure referred to as the Rastelli procedure involves repair of mitral and tricuspid valves and patch grafts to close septal defects. Creation of a competent mitral valve is of utmost importance to relieve pulmonary hypertension.

Tetralogy of Fallot

Tetralogy of Fallot is a combination of four defects:

1. VSD
2. Stenosis or atresia of the pulmonary valve and/or outflow tract into the pulmonary artery
3. Hypertrophy of the right ventricle
4. Dextroposition (displacement) of the aorta to the right so that it receives blood from both ventricles

Often referred to as "blue babies," infants with tetralogy of Fallot are cyanotic because insufficient oxygen circulates to body tissues. Total correction of the multiple anomalies is difficult. Assessment of the technical ease of correction is generally the dominant consideration. If cyanosis is severe, one of the following palliative shunt procedures may be performed during infancy to increase pulmonary blood flow:

1. *Blalock-Taussig procedure.* The right subclavian artery is anastomosed, end-to-side, with the corresponding pulmonary artery. Mixed arterial-venous blood from the aorta flows through the shunt to the pulmonary artery and into the lungs for oxygenation. A modification of this includes the use of a conduit graft, such as Gortex.
2. *Potts-Smith-Gibson procedure.* The descending aorta is anastomosed, side-to-side, with the left pulmonary artery. The shunt enlarges as the child grows, but it is more difficult to reconstruct than a Blalock shunt at a later time, when a corrective procedure is performed.
3. *Glenn procedure.* The superior vena cava is anastomosed with the right pulmonary artery. Modern versions are bidirectional, allowing flow to the right and left pulmonary arteries.
4. *Waterston procedure.* The ascending aorta is anastomosed with the right pulmonary artery. The anastomosis is placed on the posterior aspect of the aorta to provide perfusion to both pulmonary arteries.

With cardiopulmonary bypass and hypothermia, the VSD is closed with a patch graft that also corrects the abnormal communication between the right ventricle and the aorta. Then the obstruction to pulmonary blood flow is relieved. This may include enlarging the pulmonary valve and/or widening the outflow tract. Resection of obstructing cardiac muscle may be necessary with insertion of a prosthetic outflow patch. An aortic allograft containing the aortic valve with the septal leaflet of the mitral valve and the ascending aorta attached may be inserted. The septal leaflet of the mitral valve is used as a portion of the right ventricular outflow patch. All or part of the aortic valve and ascending aorta is used as a new conduit with the pulmonary artery or as a patch graft.

Transposition of the Great Vessels

In a transposition, the aorta arises from the right ventricle, and the pulmonary artery arises from the left ventricle. This creates essentially two separate circulatory systems—one systemic and the other pulmonary—but they are not inter- connected as in normal anatomy. Life depends on the presence or creation of associated defects to permit exchange of blood between the two systems. A palliative procedure, such as one of the following, is performed in the newborn to improve oxygenation and sustain life until the infant grows enough to tolerate a corrective procedure:

1. *Rashkind procedure.* In the cardiac catheterization laboratory, under fluoroscopy, a balloon catheter (deflated) is advanced into the right atrium, through the foramen ovale, and into left atrium. The balloon is inflated and pulled backward out of the left atria across the atrial septum to enlarge the foramen ovale, thus creating an ASD.
2. *Park procedure.* In the cardiac catheterization lab, under fluoroscopy, a catheter with a knife tip is passed through the right atria to enlarge the opening of the foramen ovale.
3. *Blalock-Hanlon procedure.* Atrial septectomy is done to create an ASD. A segment of the right atrium is excised.
4. *Pulmonary artery banding.* The pulmonary artery is constricted in the presence of a large VSD to prevent irreversible pulmonary vascular obstructive changes from developing.

A corrective procedure, such as one of the following, is usually performed when the child is between 18 and 36 months of age:

1. *Mustard procedure.* An intraatrial baffle made of pericardial tissue is sutured between the pulmonary veins and the mitral valve and between the mitral and tricuspid valves. The baffle directs systemic venous return into the left ventricle and lungs and allows pulmonary venous return to enter the right ventricle and aorta.
2. *Senning procedure.* Flaps of the intraatrial septum and right atrial wall form new venous channels to divert pulmonary venous blood flow. Any atrial and/or septal defects are closed.
3. *Jantene procedure.* The aorta and pulmonary artery are anatomically switched (i.e., transposed). This procedure is useful in infants with a VSD or a large PDA in addition to transposition of the great arteries.

Tricuspid Atresia

The absence (atresia) of a tricuspid valve between the right atrium and ventricle prevents normal blood flow through the chambers of the heart. Blood flows through an ASD, into an enlarged left ventricle, and through a small right ventricle to the pulmonary artery. Anastomosis of the superior vena cava with the right pulmonary artery or an aorticopulmonic artery shunt may be created as a palliative procedure to increase pulmonary blood flow in infancy. When the child is 3 or 4 years old, a corrective reconstructive Fontan procedure is performed. This procedure involves direct anastomosis of the pulmonary artery to the right atrium to create a connection between the pulmonary and systemic venous circulation.

Truncus Arteriosus

In truncus arteriosus a single artery carries blood directly from the heart (with a large associated VSD) to the coronary, pulmonary, and systemic circulatory systems. Initial palliative banding of the pulmonary arteries, as close to their origins off the truncus as possible, decreases pulmonary blood flow in an infant in congestive heart failure. At a later stage a corrective procedure can be performed to close the VSD and insert a conduit with an ascending aortic graft and aortic valve. Correction in infancy requires replacement of the conduit as the child grows.

Valvular Stenosis

Congenital aortic and/or pulmonary valve stenosis requires valvotomy, which is also referred to as the Brock procedure. An incision is made into the valve to open the narrowed or constrictive area obstructing blood flow.

POSTOPERATIVE PEDIATRIC PATIENT CARE

The patient is taken to a postanesthesia care unit (PACU) for observation. Larger facilities have a PACU specifically designed to accommodate phase I and II pediatric patients. Parents are usually permitted in the pediatric PACU. The patient usually finds comfort in parental presence.

The PACU nurse receives the postanesthesia report from the anesthesia provider and a postprocedural report from the perioperative nurse. Vital signs are taken and include temperature, pulse, respirations, and blood pressure. The objective signs found in the head-to-toe assessment are compared with preoperative baseline values. Cardiac monitoring and pulse oximetry is done. Physical assessment is performed and compared with other data obtained about the patient. Fluid intake and output is evaluated. The surgical site is inspected. Specific physician's orders pertaining to treatments and laboratory work are carried out.

The patient's recovery is evaluated at 5- to 15-minute intervals as the patient emerges from anesthesia to a more alert state. Each evaluation is documented in the patient's record per facility policy. The patient will be discharged from the PACU when he or she reaches specific physiologic parameters according to departmental policy. The anesthesia provider is responsible for the patient in the PACU and is responsible for his or her release criteria. The pediatric patient is not to be left unattended at any time.

The parents are instructed in postoperative home care and are informed about signs and symptoms that should be reported to the physician. The instructions should be given ver-bally and in writing with the appropriate emergency phone consult numbers included. Directions for prescription medications such as antibiotics or analgesics should be explained to the parents by the PACU nurse. Pediatric patients who are of an age of reason and understanding should be addressed directly and given the opportunity to ask questions.

Within 24 to 48 hours following discharge, a postoperative phone call should be made as a follow-up to care. Pertinent information should be exchanged about the care of the patient and progress in recovery. The caller should be qualified to answer questions about the procedure and the recovery phase. Patient and family satisfaction should be evaluated. Some facilities ask the parent to call in during the evening hours to give an update to the PACU nurse.

Bibliography

Andrews SE: Laser ablation of recurrent laryngeal papillomas in children, *AORN J* 61(3):532-544, 1995.

Barash PG et al: *Handbook of clinical anesthesia,* ed 3, Philadelphia, 1997, Lippincott-Raven.

Blesh P, Fisher ML: The impact of parental presence of parental anxiety and satisfaction, *AORN J* 63(4):761-768, 1996.

Davis JL, Klein RW: Perioperative care of the pediatric trauma patient, *AORN J* 60(4):561-570, 1994.

Derkay CS et al: Retrieving foreign bodies from upper aerodigestive tracts in children, *AORN J* 60(1):53-61, 1994.

Derkay CS et al: Pediatric tonsillectomy and adenoidectomy procedures, *AORN J* 62(6):887-902, 1995.

Ellerton M, Merriam C: Preparing children and families psychologically for day surgery, *J Adv Nurs* 19(6):1057-1062, 1994.

Fina DK: A chance to say goodbye, *Am J Nurs* 94(5):8-45, 1994.

Hay WW et al: *Current pediatric diagnosis and treatment,* Norwalk, Conn, 1995, Appleton & Lange.

Hendricks-Ferguson VL, Ortman MR: Selective dorsal rhizotomy to decrease spasticity in cerebral palsy, *AORN J* 61(3):514-525, 1995.

Holzman R: Outpatient anesthesia for children, *Curr Rev Nurs Anesth* 17(13):126-136, 1994.

Huddleston KR: Strabismus repair in the pediatric patient, *AORN J* 60(5): 754-760, 1994.

Kyzer SP, Stark SL: Congenital idiopathic clubfoot deformities, *AORN J* 61(3):492-506, 1995.

LaRosa-Nash PA et al: Implementing a parent-present induction program, *AORN J* 61(3):526-531, 1995.

Pierce LA: Safety and care of children during surgery, *Plast Surg Nurs* 14(2):99-100, 1994.

Schmidt K et al: How to apply the AHCPR's pediatric pain guideline, *Am J Nurs* 94(3):69-74, 1994.

Schweer L, Ose MB: Implementation of a regional pediatric trauma center, *AORN J* 61(3):558-571, 1995.

Steward DJ: *Manual of pediatric anesthesia,* ed 4, New York, 1995, Churchill Livingstone.

Thompson SW: *Emergency care of children,* Boston, 1990, Jones & Bartlett.

Williams EM et al: Neuroendoscopic laser-assisted ventriculostomy of the third ventricle, *AORN J* 61(2):345-359, 1995.

Wong DL: *Wong and Whaley's clinical manual of pediatric nursing,* ed 4, St Louis, 1996, Mosby.

Chapter 9

Perioperative Geriatrics

After studying this chapter, the learner will be able to:

- Discuss the theories of aging.
- Describe how comorbidity influences the care of geriatric patients.
- List the effects of aging on four body systems.
- Identify the effects of surgery on the geriatric patient.

PERSPECTIVES ON AGING

The process of aging is an orderly transformation of the body and mind that begins with birth and concludes with death. The term *geriatric* is taken from the Greek *yeros* (γερος), which means old. Persons over 65 years of age are often considered old or elderly. In actuality, a person with advanced age may maintain functional capabilities throughout his or her lifetime until adaptation to biologic, psychologic, and/or social influences is no longer sufficient to sustain the independent activities of daily living. The main influences on the aging process are genetics, environment, and lifestyle.

The medical discipline of geriatrics is related to the clinical implications of the physiology of aging and the diagnosis and treatment of diseases that affect older adults. Gerontology is the comprehensive scientific study of all aspects of the aging process, including the physiologic, psychologic, economic, and sociologic problems and considerations of the aging person. These factors are studied from the standpoint of the impact they have on the aging individual and the older population within society.

Data about the changes that occur as the result of natural processes and environmental exposure are inconclusive because the only data available are those derived from com-

parisons between existing generations. The experiences and exposures of these generations have been vastly different and widely influenced by the time period of the life span. No normal measurements are available on which to base the parameters of the aging process.

Life expectancy has increased steadily with major advancements in the study of disease processes, prevention, and treatment. The United States Department of Health and Human Services indicates that a person born in 1954 can expect to live to 68 years of age; a person born in 1988 can expect to live to 74 years of age. By the year 2030, 1 in every 10 persons will be older than 85 years of age, with only 41% of the population below the age of 35 years. The median age will be 40 years. This increase in life expectancy and decrease in mortality mean that the largest patient population will be geriatric patients—the fastest growing segment of the population.

As the life expectancy of the geriatric population increases, so does the incidence of comorbidity. Comorbidity is the existence of two or more disease processes in a single individual (e.g., coronary artery disease in a patient who has osteoporosis and may also be hypertensive and diabetic). It is the most common negative influence on the health status and functional ability of geriatric patients. A chronic condition affects recovery following surgical intervention, and many geriatric patients have multiple chronic or debilitating health problems. Comorbidity is also a major consideration in the attainment of expected outcomes; all medical diagnoses should be taken into account in the development of the plan of care.

Aging is viewed from many perspectives—some positive, some negative. The positive aspects involve respect for maturity and the wealth of knowledge gleaned from experiences. The negative aspects involve the debilitation, pervading weaknesses, and dependence that can occur during the closure of life. Philosophers tend to focus on the positive, inner peace derived from the wisdom acquired over many years. The view of aging adopted by an individual is based in part on the view of aging created by his or her cultural background. Geographic, financial, educational, and subjective influences shape the prototype of the older adult's place in society.

Cultural Considerations

Positive views of aging are found in many cultures that can trace their heritage back for many generations. Repetitious story telling and historical accounts support the cultural growth of an individual from youth to old age. Many cultures appreciate, honor, and respect their older members for their experience and maturity. Growing old with dignity is not feared or deemed repulsive. A positive view of aging may be observed in an individual who is a first-generation immigrant to a new land, because he or she may not have assimilated the value systems of the new environment. The individual may have retained many time-honored beliefs of his or her country of origin; the values are held dear and are deeply ingrained. Negative views of aging may be generated by cultures that are primarily youth-oriented. Most members of these societies are second- and third-generation descendants of immigrants. They have developed value systems that do not reflect their country of origin. In a close community, values are supported within the belief structure of the group as a whole.

A culture is a set of structured social behaviors and personal beliefs that enable an individual to respond to social situations and relationships within a close community. The foundation of human relationships in a culture is more than ethnicity or race. Specific cultural practices such as dietary habits, lifestyle, and hygiene should be of concern to the perioperative nurse. For example, a patient's physical condition may be a direct result of a traditional activity such as fasting. A geriatric patient who has been fasting may appear dehydrated, malnourished, or confused. This should be taken into consideration before the patient undergoes a surgical procedure. The psychologic assessment may reflect a high risk for an alteration in self-image because, although the patient may feel comfortable in his or her culture, he or she may have had a negative interaction with societal influences. For example, the media glorify young bodies and degrade the natural aging process, with advertisers using models that reflect the desirable aspects of youth and beauty. Cultural climate has a direct effect on the geriatric patient. The expected outcomes of the geriatric patient undergoing a surgical intervention will be influenced by his or her cultural views of aging and those of society as a whole.

Theories of Aging

Biologic, psychologic, and ethnocultural factors influence the manner in which an individual ages. The extrinsic influences surrounding the physical and psychosocial components depend on the interaction of the person with the environment and his or her view of health and wellness. Many older persons tend to optimistically overstate their actual health status and minimize or dismiss symptoms as age related. The intrinsic influences on the aging process are also interdependent, but to a less controllable degree. Certain inherited traits, such as pathologic conditions, are continued through the generations.

Each aged individual is unique and distinct. Perioperative nurses should understand the unique aspects of each geriatric patient before developing a perioperative plan of care. Generic care plans do not address the specific problems, needs, and health considerations of the individual. Understanding the theories of the aging process enables the perioperative nurse to provide care throughout the surgical experience in a way that will optimize the possible attainment of identified expected outcomes. The following theories explain aging as it is defined by science and research.

Wear and Tear Theory

The wear and tear theory suggests that the body loses its ability to keep pace with the maintenance of life processes. The sustenance of life suffers because the body begins to deteriorate in a natural, wearing-down process. The body continually tries to maintain homeostasis but degenerates over time because of cellular loss and destruction caused by interactions with the environment. During this process the body becomes increasingly vulnerable to injury and disease. If a disease state occurs, the body is less able to cope with normal homeostasis and even less able to tolerate the assault of illness. Eventually the body is unable to support life and ceases to function. Examples of wear and tear include, but are not limited to, the following:

- Prolonged exposure to the sun and other external sources can cause breakdown of the skin. Thinning of the skin makes bedridden or inactive persons vulnerable to pressure sores.
- Turbulent blood flow in the areas of bifurcation of blood vessels may cause rupture if the vessels are weakened by arteriosclerosis.
- The abuse of chemical substances and alcohol can damage liver and brain cells. Nicotine is responsible for many effects of smoking. Although these effects are self-induced rather than the result of natural wear and tear, they do affect health status.

Genetic Mutation Theory

Deoxyribonucleic acid (DNA) has been a target for age-related changes because it preserves the ongoing genetic message for the replication of cells and maintenance of the organism. DNA is a template, or coding mechanism, for the preservation of the life processes of cellular structures. Various agents damage DNA codes through physical, chemical, or biologic interactions. An alteration in the structure of DNA can cause the organism to change in a manner that is different from the original design. This alteration can occur within the cell itself or be caused by a force in the environment. Mutated DNA cannot perform the processes necessary for normal cell activities. A cell containing wrongly coded DNA will continue to replicate itself in the wrong patterns. It will not return to normal.

In the aging process, DNA may mutate for a variety of reasons and will continue to produce the wrong type of cells during replication. For example, skin cells may be deficient in collagen or in the elastic properties associated with supple tissue. As a result, the skin replication process may yield drier, less elastic skin. This is characteristic of the skin of an older person. In certain circumstances, the mutated DNA could cause tumor production or other pathologic conditions, such as skin cancers.

Major organ systems affected by these changes are the central nervous system, the musculoskeletal system, and the cardiovascular system. Other systems affected include the gastrointestinal, genitourinary, endocrine, and integumentary systems. Essentially, all body systems change during the aging process.

Viral Theory

Researchers have approached the concept that viruses may invade human cells and remain inactive until the body loses its ability to suppress them. This theory is closely linked to the genetic mutation theory because the virus can hide undetected in the DNA for many years. The replication process of the virus is similar to the replication of DNA. Some viruses are able to use genetic materials as a disguise to fool the body's immune system. The body does not recognize the virus as an invader or foreign substance.

The mechanism of viral activation is unknown but is very injurious to the body. Major target systems include the endocrine, nervous, and immune systems. The incubation period may be several decades. Because there is no proof of the viral theory, a treatment or cure is unknown.

Environmental Theory

Exposure to natural and synthetic elements in the environment may accelerate the aging process. Although climate is often blamed for an increased rate of aging, studies indicate that the natural flow of the aging process is comparable among different geographic regions. Tropical climates are cited most often as areas of premature aging. Studies of tropical populations show that aging is not accelerated by the temperature, although mortality in these areas *is* affected by poor nutrition, parasites, and tropical diseases. Both tropical and desert groups tested did not show any mean blood pressure elevations diagnostic of hypertension, arteriosclerosis, or coronary artery disease between the ages of 20 and 83 years. The most astounding finding was the absence of angina pectoris and sudden heart attack deaths. This may be partly a result of a physically strenuous lifestyle and a diet that is low in animal fat.

Extremes of climate do not seem to accelerate the aging process. Studies involving Eskimo populations have shown that, despite the difficult conditions of their lifestyles, blood pressure and cholesterol measurements do not vary significantly between the ages of 20 and 54 years. Mortality is affected by the harshness of the cold climate and the risk of physical injury or death associated with hunting and lifestyle practices.

Altitude has not been shown to accelerate the aging process. Studies performed among Peruvian Indians have shown stable blood pressures in a range lower than that of persons living at sea level. Ischemic heart disease is very low at higher altitudes. In several documented communities of mountain-dwelling people, many residents were over 100 years of age.

Ionizing radiation has been targeted as a cause of environmentally accelerated aging, but studies have not shown this to be true. Relevant evidence has shown that exposure to ionizing radiation does accelerate disease processes and pathologic conditions such as skin cancer, blood dyscrasias, and reproductive anomalies. Populations living in areas where nuclear tests frequently occurred have not shown signs of rapid aging when compared with control groups in nuclear-free areas. The most significant finding was an increase in leukemia and skin tumors.

Pollution causes many physiologic changes in the body. Chemicals in air, food, and water supplies have been shown to increase the incidence of health decline and disability. Exposure to pollutants throughout the life span dramatically shortens an individual's life expectancy through pathologic processes such as chronic lead poisoning and lung cancer.

Physical Factor Theory

Free radicals are being investigated as a potential cause of premature aging. Free radicals represent imbalances between the production and the elimination of unstable chemical compounds in the body. More research is needed to prove or disprove this theory.

Low-calorie diets do not alter the aging process in human beings. In populations studied for dietary habits, no increase in the life span is evident between control groups and groups who have a low caloric intake. The most remarkable factor is the lack of increase in body weight after 30 years of age. A low-calorie diet may range between 1800 and 2500 kilogram calories (kcal) per day depending on body size and gender. Notably, low-calorie diets are usually deficient in animal protein. Aged individuals who have low-calorie diets generally have lower blood pressure and lower serum cholesterol levels, with no significant change throughout the aging process. Subcutaneous fat deposits do not increase with age.

High-calorie diets that exceed 3200 kcal per day for men and 2200 kcal per day for women have the opposite effect on aging. An increase in caloric intake is accompanied by an increase in body mass that causes the individual to decrease body mobility. This is particularly evident in Euro-American populations, which often show a steady increase in weight up to the age of 60 years. Women in particular experience a thickening in fat deposits as they mature. Blood pressure and serum cholesterol levels steadily increase. The most significant elevations begin at age 50, with the development of coronary artery heart disease and atherosclerosis.

Animal fat content and excess calories are not the only considerations in the dietary aspect of aging and health. Vegetarians do not always follow a low-calorie pattern. They, too, can have a diet rich in fats, particularly if they consume saturated fats in the form of coconut oil. Salt is another consideration in the aging of the cardiovascular system. Diets high in sodium tend to increase circulating blood volume, thereby increasing systolic blood pressure. Studies have shown that an increase in systolic blood pressure significantly increases the risk of heart disease and stroke.

Exercise plays an important role in the health of the aging individual. Most populations studied have an exercise regimen linked to their activities of daily living. Persons in cultures characterized by many intrinsic diseases, parasites, malnutrition, poor hygiene, and harsh living conditions have remarkable physical fitness because of the amount of exercise they must perform to sustain life. Persons in affluent societies, in which the inhabitants are overfed and underexercised, do not enjoy good health in the same manner as the moderately fed and highly exercised residents of less advantaged societies.

As the body ages, the endocrine system declines, and the hormones responsible for the regulation of many interrelated body systems decrease in volume. Beta cells of the pancreas, thyroid, ovaries (in females), and testes (in males) exhibit less activity, which affects many other organ systems. For example:

- A decrease in estrogen production can increase the risk for osteoporosis and heart disease in women.
- A decrease in thyroid activity will decrease the basal metabolic rate and increase weight gain.
- A decrease in the efficiency of insulin production will decrease the efficiency of glucose metabolism.
- A decrease in testosterone production may decrease the libido in men.

Myths About Aging

Many misconceptions surround the process of aging. *Myths,* from the Greek *meethos* (μηθος), are stories created to explain the practices or beliefs of unknown origin regarding a person, place, or event. The creation of a myth about aging may be based on an isolated incident or a single observation and may not apply to all older adults. Some myths have a small basis in fact, but most are unfounded and have a harmful effect on social policy and interpersonal relationships.

Myths about the aging process may result in negative stereotypes, and a belief in negative stereotypes results in discrimination and improper treatment of the aging individual. Abnormal signs, symptoms, or behaviors exhibited by a geriatric patient usually indicate the presence of a pathologic process and should not be discounted as normal expectations of the aging process. Some of the negative myths about aging include the following:

- MYTH: Older adults are senile. TRUTH: If mental processes decline, it is usually the result of a contributing factor such as stroke, carotid insufficiency, or Alzheimer's disease.
- MYTH: Older adults do not engage in sexual behavior. TRUTH: Sexual desire remains throughout the life span. Sexual activity may decline because of decreased physical mobility, circulatory impairment, or the unavailability of a partner. Self-gratification may be the only outlet.
- MYTH: Older adults always decline in health after a surgical procedure. TRUTH: The identification of problems, needs, and health considerations during the assessment phase of the nursing process decreases the probability of unmet expected outcomes.

Myths and stereotypes must not be allowed to influence the assessment of geriatric patients. Every aspect of the physical, psychosocial, and ethnocultural data should be assessed as unique to each individual and not as a generic group expectation. Reaching the age of 65 years does not instantly transform individuals into being old and debilitated. As persons grow older, they may experience more developmental aging before they experience physical aging. Some persons become frail as they age, but this is not true of everyone. Age alone does not make individuals less productive members of society. By the twenty-first century, limitations and disabilities may be decreased because of scientific advances and a better understanding of the aging process and health promotion activities.

PERIOPERATIVE ASSESSMENT OF THE GERIATRIC PATIENT

The patient's ability to adapt to aging should be assessed by the perioperative nurse as part of the nursing process. With the exception of nursing diagnoses directly associated with the anticipated surgical procedure, specific nursing diagnoses should be associated with the patient's adaptation to the aging process. If positive adaptation has not been met, the risk is high for an augmentation of existing health conditions, such as a cardiovascular incident (e.g., stroke, myocardial infarction, or hypertensive crisis). Comorbidity is a leading cause of death among older adults. More than 73% of all geriatric patients have more than one medical diagnosis capable of causing death. Therefore recognizing potential problems in the attainment of expected outcomes is as important as identifying actual problems.

Geriatric patients may present to the perioperative environment for urgent or emergent surgery because of the clinical signs and symptoms associated with a life-threatening illness. Common urgent problems include intestinal obstruction, ruptured diverticula, and orthopaedic fractures. Vascular incidents such as ruptured aneurysm or bleeding from the gastrointestinal tract require immediate surgery. Sudden arterial occlusion that is unresponsive to chemical treatment is also considered emergent.

The postoperative phase of care is very important to the well-being of the geriatric patient. Maintaining or improving on the preoperative level of wellness should be considered a primary expected outcome. A preoperative functional assessment is the foundation of the plan of care. Baseline parameters vary to a high degree between individuals, and all patients do not age at the same rate. Some patients are *very young* at 70 years of age, and some are *very old*. The difference should be assessed, and optimal outcomes should be identified for each geriatric patient according to his or her level. Influences on the level of functioning include physical ability, psychosocial support and resources, and environmental interactions.

Functional Assessment

Functional assessment can serve multiple purposes. In the preoperative phase, the plan of care includes the patient's unique differences, family involvement, resources, and level of independence. Much of this data is obtained by observation, interview, and lifestyle questionnaires. The information may be obtained from the patient, family, or significant other.

Many aspects of the patient's unique nature are easily discerned during the preoperative interview. Adequate time should be allowed for the interview (at least 30 minutes) so the patient has time to reflect and respond. Reaction time slows with age. The nurse should listen for subtle modifications or inconsistencies in the patient's information regarding his or her health status. Sensory deficits should be considered, and the environment should be modified as needed during the interview. The nurse should establish rapport and have respect for the patient's dignity.

During the intraoperative phase, the functional assessment may allow for anticipation of needed supplies or additional help to accommodate the patient's needs. The patient's physical capabilities allow some independence in self-care. Patients tend to regress when they are not permitted to do things for themselves. A self-care deficit takes place when a patient feels the loss of independence while restrained on an operating bed. The freedom to assist with the transfer from the transport stretcher to the operating bed gives the patient a sense of participation in his or her own care. Maintaining a high level of self-esteem and value will enable the patient to prevent emotional regression or loss of control.

Activities of Daily Living

During the course of a normal day, an individual performs self-maintenance tasks and interacts with the environment. The ability to perform these activities of daily living is influenced by health status, emotions, mental clarity, and mobility. Limitations in performing these activities may be permanent or temporary, and many of the temporary limitations can be eliminated by medical or surgical treatment. The perioperative nurse should assess the activity level of the geriatric patient. Advance preparations may need to be considered before the patient can undergo a surgical procedure. Because of identified physical limitations, special positioning or additional padding may be needed in combination with some form of communication assistance at the time the surgical procedure is performed. The functional baseline is the patient's capacity to perform self-care (e.g., feeding, bathing, toileting). Any deviation from the baseline assessment in the postoperative phase should be recorded and reported to the patient's physician.

Functional Activities The activity patterns of geriatric patients reflect many aspects of their daily lives. Their ability to feed, bathe, and toilet themselves is one way to measure physical and psychologic wellness. Basic daily activities such as grooming and dressing may be indicators of the level of the patient's involvement with his or her own care. The range of self-care activities depends on various factors, such as whether the patient is active and mobile enough to shop for food and prepare meals or is living in assistive housing where these services are provided. The ability to provide self-care should be assessed preoperatively to evaluate the outcome in the postoperative phase (i.e., resumption of activity level).

Functional Capacity A basic assessment of physical strength and endurance will indicate whether the patient will be able to move from the transport stretcher to the operating bed. A patient who is weak or disabled by arthritis will need assistance or a total lift device. A patient who is visually impaired also may need assistance.

Communication through speech and hearing is vital to establishing the cognitive baseline. A hearing deficit or aphasia could be mistaken for a cognitive impairment. The patient who uses a hearing-assist device should be permitted to wear it to the operating room (OR) and, if possible, throughout the surgical procedure. It should be in place during the patient's emergence from anesthesia so he or she can hear requests to deep breathe or to move extremities.

The patient's sensory ability should be assessed. Tactile sensation dulls with age, and a patient's inability to feel external stimuli may lead to an inadvertent injury. Any sensory deficit, including a visual or hearing impairment, should be documented in the plan of care. The administration of a general anesthetic will alter the tactile assessment parameter during the intraoperative phase of care. As the patient emerges from anesthesia, the postanesthesia recovery nurses use the baseline assessment to measure the progress of the patient in the postoperative phase. Because of the interdependent aspects of the central nervous system with other vital physiologic systems, the evaluation of expected outcomes should include a sensory assessment.

Cognitive ability should also be assessed. The patient may be required to comprehend a command that is vital to the perioperative experience. A cognitive deficit may be of organic origin or result from a language barrier. Regardless of the reason, an inability to understand can cause anxiety for the patient and the caregiver. Alertness, short-term memory, capabilities to concentrate and problem solve, and motivation toward self-care are areas of cognition that influence the ability of the geriatric patient to adapt to illness and recovery. A patient who is cognitively impaired experiences disorientation and responds inappropriately to the environment. The impairment may be temporary but often is prolonged following anesthesia. Cognitive impairment may also be a permanent or chronic condition.

The patient's psychologic state should be assessed preoperatively because a change in mood or temperament may indicate an unexpected outcome caused by an injury or a physical problem resulting from the surgical procedure. Dementia, delirium, and emotional depression are common in older adults. Sudden withdrawal or a change in affect should be investigated promptly.

External Interactions

The manner in which an individual experiences illness depends on external forces and the number of barriers that may interfere with the attainment of outcomes. The nursing diagnoses may include a self-care deficit or an alteration in mobility status. These diagnoses factor significantly in the postoperative phase and should be taken into consideration and placed in the plan of care. The reaction of the patient to either one of these nursing diagnoses will depend on his or her interactions with the external environment, the availability of resources, and the presence of barriers.

Resources   The level of independence exercised by the geriatric patient may depend on the resources available. The type of housing may depend on self-care ability and financial security. In developing the plan of care, the perioperative nurse should consider how the patient will meet his or her postoperative needs at home. Will help be available, or will arrangements for a visiting nurse or a family caregiver be needed? The patient's possible need for transportation to and from the surgeon's office for postoperative checkups should be considered.

Barriers   The type of housing may be a problem for the postoperative geriatric patient. If he or she lives alone in a multilevel dwelling, going up and down stairs may pose a significant problem. The location of the bathroom or kitchen may complicate the self-care process. Financial constraints may limit the number of home health care visits by an independent agency. The unavailability of family members may necessitate planning for institutionalization, which may be temporary but may become permanent.

Psychosocial Assessment

Gathering data about a geriatric patient should begin with the assessment of how this individual views other aged people and his or her own progression through the aging process.

The assessment of a patient's self-concept may be an important indicator of a decline in the status of his or her psychologic health. A patient's views of health and normative activity are influenced by his or her culture and affect the attainment of outcomes. If the patient believes that older people are helpless, he or she may see the role of the aging process as one of helplessness. Although capable of many independent activities, this individual may adapt to an illness by becoming helpless. Even needing help for a temporary period may cause an older patient to believe that the condition is permanent. The perioperative nurse should be aware that the geriatric patient may experience a temporary period of helplessness. By establishing a functional baseline and stressing the temporary nature of postoperative recovery, the nurse can help the patient return to his or her routine.

The geriatric patient may feel rejected, unsupported, and worthless. Between 10% and 65% of geriatric patients experience depression and an alteration in self-image. The physical decline may be rapid when psychologic well-being is threatened. The perioperative nurse should be aware that the geriatric patient who is depressed and lonely needs additional emotional support throughout the surgical experience.

The perioperative nurse should be aware of his or her own subjective views of aging and cultural attitudes and should not allow personal feelings to influence the assessment process. The assessment of a geriatric patient should take into consideration the culture of origin, the cultural influence of the patient's current residence, and the patient's subjective perception of wellness and illness. Self-perception has a great influence on how well the geriatric patient adapts to aging. The nursing diagnoses should reflect the patient's adaptation, because adaptation will affect the attainment of the expected outcomes. The perioperative plan of care should reflect the need for ongoing evaluation by postoperative caregivers.

Adaptation to the Aging Process

Many adjustments should be made by an individual during the aging process. The adaptation to aging is unique for each individual and is influenced by physical condition, psychologic strengths and weaknesses, family and significant others, social support systems, financial resources, and functional ability. The geriatric patient develops a belief system about his or her life expectations primarily on the basis of subjective feelings. If the patient is in decline, the outlook is usually negative, based on how he or she feels at a particular period in time. If the patient is feeling well and able-bodied, the outlook is usually positive, which helps delay the patient's fear of declining health outside the expected parameters of aging.

The prevention of decline not related to normative aging is a key factor in the avoidance of health deficits. The patient who can postpone health problems caused by factors that include avoidable health considerations—accidents, poor nutrition, inactivity, depression, and the effects of loneliness, smoking, substance abuse, and obesity—will enjoy a higher quality of life in the later years.

Self-Perception of Health

The patient's view of his or her health plays an important role in his or her actual health status. If the patient perceives health as important, then preventive health maintenance should be a priority. The patient who feels well will perform the activities of daily living to the best of his or her ability. Minor interruptions in health status will not cause a major problem in the long-term prognosis of his or her return to baseline parameters.

Physical Assessment

The physical assessment of the geriatric patient begins with his or her general appearance. The perioperative nurse should first observe the patient from head to toe. The basic picture or image the patient creates can provide information about his or her health status. The patient should be assessed for posture, mobility, gait, rising or sitting, dexterity, body height and weight, body odors, psychologic affect, communication, and comprehension of surroundings. The perioperative nurse

should perform an assessment of the total patient by each body system. A summary of the physiologic changes associated with the normal aging process is provided in Table 9-1.

Any medications the patient takes on a routine or periodic basis should be listed on the chart, with their last dosages itemized. The patient should be encouraged to discuss all medications, including vitamins or topical ointments. Recreational drugs (e.g., street drugs, narcotics) should not be excluded from consideration just because the patient is older. Many medications can alter the results of blood work and the findings of the physical assessment. Drugs such as aspirin can alter blood tests for clotting times. Pain medications can alter sensorium. Smoking and alcohol use are important to assess because they can affect many body systems. All assessment data should be recorded in the chart. The perioperative nurse should read the physician's medical history and physical examination report and review laboratory reports to discern the medical diagnoses (Table 9-2). Any additional abnormal findings should be reported to the surgeon and the anesthesia provider.

TABLE 9-1	Physiologic Changes Associated with Normal Aging Processes in the Geriatric Patient	
Age-Related Factors	**Assessment Factors**
Integumentary System	
Decreased subcutaneous fat, decreased turgor (elasticity)	Thin, dry skin, wrinkles
Diminished sweat glands, dulled tactile sensation	Poor thermoregulation, heat and cold sensitivity
Thickened connective tissue	Keratosis (patchy overgrowths of dermis), warts, skin tags (especially on face and neck)
Increased fat deposits over abdomen and hips	Poor excretion of fat-soluble drugs
Diminished capillary blood flow, reduced vascularity, capillary fragility	Pressure sores, delayed wound healing, purpura or lentigo (liver spots), bruises
Dry mucous membranes, decreased salivation and secretions	Dry mouth and vagina
Musculoskeletal System	
Diminished protein synthesis in muscle cells, decreased muscle mass and tone	Muscle weakness, reduced strength, muscle wasting
Erosion of cartilage, thickened synovial fluid, fibrosed synovial membranes	Joint pain, swelling, stiffness, diminished range of motion
Diminished mobility, flexibility, and balance	Poor gait, poor posture, risk of falling
Increased porosity and demineralization of bone, thinning of intervertebral disks, decreased height	Ankylosing spondylosis, kyphosis, osteoporosis
Respiratory System	
Atrophied respiratory muscles, kyphosis or other postural changes, rib cage rigidity	Chest wall limitations
Reduced vital capacity	Dyspnea
Risk of pneumonia	Ineffective cough, and above respiratory factors
Cardiovascular System	
Decreased cardiac output and stroke volume	Chronic fatigue and dyspnea, orthostatic hypotension
Myocardial irritability and stiffness, decreased size of sinoatrial and atrioventricular nodes	Slow heart rate and circulation, dysrhythmias and murmurs
Increased vascular resistance, rigidity in arteries	Hypertension
Thickening and dilation of veins	Venous insufficiency, varicosities
Decline in renal blood flow	Edema in tissues

Continued

TABLE 9-1	Physiologic Changes Associated with Normal Aging Processes in the Geriatric Patient—cont'd

Age-Related Factors	Assessment Factors
Gastrointestinal System	
Decreased esophageal peristalsis, slowed emptying of stomach	Indigestion, frequent antacid use
Diminished saliva production, which slows breakdown of carbohydrates; reduced gastric secretion of hydrochloric acid, which impairs absorption of vitamins and minerals; hepatic insufficiency, which affects absorption of fats	Malnutrition
Loss of perineal and anal sphincter tone	Diarrhea, fecal incontinence
Decreased intestinal peristalsis, loss of abdominal muscle turgor, reduced mucosal secretions in intestines	Constipation, frequent laxative use
Endocrine System	
Reduced hormonal activity, decreased physical activity	Slowed basal metabolic rate, subnormal temperature
Slowed release of insulin from pancreas	Impaired glucose metabolism
Reduced thyroid hormone production	Dry skin, temperature intolerance, poor appetite, lethargy, memory lapse
Disturbed fluid and electrolyte balance	Hydration status
Genitourinary System	
Decreased renal blood flow, reduced number of glomeruli, reduced glomerular filtration rate, decreased excretory ability	Diminished renal function, risk of acid-base imbalance and drug toxicity
Loss of elasticity and muscle tone in ureters, bladder, and urethra	Urinary frequency, urgency, and nocturia
Decreased bladder muscle and sphincter tone, estrogen deficiency in female, enlarged prostate in male	Stress incontinence
Enlarged prostate in male	Urinary retention
Reduced testosterone, hypertrophied prostate, sclerosis of penile arteries and veins	Male: slow erection and ejaculation
Reduced estrogen; atrophied vulva, clitoris, and vagina	Female: sagging breasts, painful intercourse
Nervous System	
Decreased number of brain cells, reduced cerebral blood flow, reduced oxygen supply to brain	Cognitive deficits: delirium, temporary state of confusion, forgetfulness, disorientation, irritability, and/or insomnia; dementia, a permanent state of cognitive impairment
Decreased neurons	Paresthesia, akinesia, diminished pain perception
Diminished neurotransmitters, decreased neurons	Tremors, head nodding, or other repetitive movements
Degeneration of myelin sheath, which lessens motor neuron conduction	Slowed reflexes and reaction time
Reduced sound transmission as eardrum thickens, decreased hair cells and neurons, reduced blood supply to cochlea	Auditory impairment
Weakened lens muscles, hardening of lens, flattening of cornea, reduced blood supply (which leads to macular deterioration), increased rigidity of iris, reduced pupil size	Visual impairment: decreased acuity, poor perception of light and color, poor peripheral vision

Integumentary System

Establishing a preoperative baseline for the condition of the skin will facilitate evaluation of the expected outcome (i.e., no injury to the skin as a result of surgical intervention). Assessment of the integumentary system includes the skin, fingernails and toenails, and all hair patterns of the body, face, and scalp. The nurse should ask the patient if any skin changes have taken place within the past several months. The skin is inspected for color, temperature, sensation, texture, turgor, thickness, and amount of subcutaneous tissue. The geriatric patient has a decreased number of sweat glands and an increased sensitivity to external temperature. The patient may complain of skin dryness, itching, and flaking.

The surface of the body should be inspected for sores, ulcers, and moles that have exhibited change over time. The presence of broken or injured skin areas may indicate a pathologic condition such as skin cancer or diabetes. Skin rashes may indicate an allergy. Skin color can indicate liver disease or problems with other body systems (e.g., cardiovascular, respiratory). Bruises or abrasions may indicate a recent fall or possible elder abuse. Careful assessment of the

Text continued on p. 136

TABLE 9-2   Geriatric Laboratory Values in the Normal Aging Process

Laboratory Test	Reference Value for Patient Over Age 65	Clinical Implication of Increased Value	Clinical Implication of Decreased Value	Notes
Hematology				
Hemoglobin (slightly decreased in both genders; larger decrease in male)	M: 11.5-14.9 g/dl F: 11.7-13.8 g/dl	CHF, advanced COPD, dehydration, severe burns, polycythemia, high altitude	Anemia, cancer, chronic renal failure, fluid overload	Measures for anemia
Hematocrit (slight decrease in male)	M: 40%-50% F: 36%-46%	Dehydration, trauma, surgery, burns, polycythemia, diabetic acidosis, emphysema	Hemorrhage, anemia, leukemia, lymphoma, liver disease, kidney disease, malnutrition, lymphoma, collagen disease	Calculates red blood cell indices and hydration status
Red blood cells (RBCs) (number unchanged)	M: 4.6-6.0 million/μl F: 4.0-5.0 million/μl	Dehydration, polycythemia, high altitude, advanced COPD	Fluid overload, anemia, hemorrhage, chronic infection, leukemia, kidney disease	Abnormal clotting conditions may cause decreased count
Reticulocyte (unchanged with normal aging)	0.5%-1.5% of total RBC	Bone marrow response to anemia, incompatible transfusion, hemolytic anemia	Hypoplastic or pernicious anemia	Indicates number of immature RBCs
Mean corpuscular volume (MCV) (slightly increased in both sexes)	80-98 μm^3	Macrocytic anemia, chronic liver disease, anticonvulsant drugs, antimetabolites	Microcytic anemia, malignancy, rheumatoid arthritis, lead poisoning, irradiation	Helps differentiate among the anemias
Mean corpuscular hemoglobin (MCH) (unchanged)	27-31 pg	Macrocytic anemia	Microcytic or hypochromic anemia, iron deficiency	Helps differentiate among the anemias
Mean corpuscular hemoglobin concentration (MCHC) (unchanged)	32-36 g/dl	Spherocytosis	Hypochromic anemia, thalassemia	Helps differentiate among the anemias
Erythrocyte sedimentation rate (ESR) (increased in both sexes)	*Age 50-85* M: <20 mm/hr F: <30 mm/hr *> Age 85* M: <30 mm /hr F: <42 mm/hr	Acute MI, lupus, gout, rheumatoid arthritis, burns, surgery, bacterial infections, TB, some malignancies	Polycythemia, CHF, sickle cell anemia, degenerative arthritis, factor V deficiency, low plasma protein	Can be used to monitor inflammatory processes or occult conditions such as tuberculosis or tissue necrosis
White blood cells (WBCs) (number unchanged, but function decreases)	4500-10,000/cm^3	Acute infections, acute MI, tissue necrosis, parasites, stress, collagen disease	Hemopoietic disease, viral infection, lupus, alcoholism, rheumatoid arthritis	Determine whether production has decreased in the presence of organ system decline
Neutrophils (amount unchanged, but they become less effective)	Total 50%-70%	Acute infection, inflammatory disease, tissue damage, Hodgkin's disease	Bone marrow depression, viral disease, leukemia	Helps differentiate type of leukocytes
Lymphocytes (amount unchanged, but B and T cell functions decrease; increase in autoantibody production)	25%-35% (mean)	Acute viral infections, chronic bacterial infections, lymphocytic leukemia, Hodgkin's disease, multiple myeloma, adrenocortical hypofunction	Cancer, leukemia, MS, kidney disease, bone marrow depression, lupus, adrenocortical hyperfunction	Decreased level indicates immunosuppression; highest values measured at approximately 8:00 PM (2000 hr)

CHF, Congestive heart failure; *CNS,* central nervous system; *COPD,* chronic obstructive pulmonary disease; *DIC,* disseminated intravascular coagulopathy; *GI,* gastrointestinal; *IM,* intramuscular; *MI,* myocardial infarction; *MS,* multiple sclerosis, *TB,* tuberculosis.

| | **TABLE 9-2** | **Geriatric Laboratory Values in the Normal Aging Process—cont'd** | | |

Laboratory Test	Reference Value for Patient Over Age 65	Clinical Implication of Increased Value	Clinical Implication of Decreased Value	Notes
Monocytes (slight increase in both sexes)	4%-6% (mean)	Viral disease, parasites, cancer, monocytic leukemia, collagen disease	Lymphocytic leukemia, aplastic anemia	Value may peak at noon, 12:00 PM (1200 hr)
Eosinophils (unchanged)	1%-3% (mean)	Parasites, cancer, allergies, thrombophlebitis	Cushing's syndrome, stress, skin disease, burns, shock	Value may peak at midnight, 12:00 AM (0000 hr)
Basophils (unchanged)	0.4%-1.0% (mean)	Healing stage of infection/inflammation, leukemia	Stress, hypersensitivity reaction, hyperthyroidism	Measures this type of leukocyte
Platelets (unchanged)	150,000-400,000/μL	Hemorrhage, infection, malignancy, recent surgery, splenectomy, inflammatory disease, pulmonary emoblism, cirrhosis, TB, cardiac disease, pancreatitis, fracture	Bone marrow disease, defective thrombopoiesis caused by folic acid or B_{12} deficiency, immune disease, DIC, severe burns, massive blood transfusions, kidney or liver disease	If <100,000, bleeding is likely; <50,000, spontaneous bleeding can take place; <5,000 can be fatal. Many drugs can alter the results
Iron (decreases to 50%-75% of the normal young adult value by age 70)	M: 73-143 μg/dl F: 76-122 μg/dl	Pernicious hemolytic anemia, folic acid deficiency, liver damage, thalassemia, lead toxicity	Iron deficiency anemia, chronic blood loss, GI malignancy, peptic ulcer, rheumatoid arthritis, chronic renal failure	Helps differentiate cause of anemias
Total iron-binding capacity (TIBC) (decreases)	M: 291-387 μg/dl F: 293-355 μg/dl	Iron deficiency anemia, acute/chronic blood loss, polycythemia	Hemolytic anemias, sickle cell, renal failure, liver disease, rheumatoid arthritis, GI malignancy	Helps differentiate cause of anemias
Ferritin (unchanged, more sensitive indicator than serum iron value)	M: 20-300 ng/ml F: 20-120 ng/ml	Hemochromatosis, iron overload, acute or chronic infection, chronic renal failure, malignancies	Iron deficiency anemia, malnutrition, liver disease, nephrotic syndrome, malignancy	Reflects iron stores; recent transfusions can alter results
Transferrin (65-170 μg/dl are bound to iron; decreases with age)	250-390 μg/dl	Severe iron deficiency anemia	Liver damage, acute or chronic infection, cancer, anemia	Used to evaluate ability of blood to transport iron
Bilirubin	Indirect: 1.1 mg/dl Direct: <0.5 mg/dl	Indirect: liver damage, fasting. Direct: biliary duct obstruction. Direct and indirect: hemolysis, biliary obstruction causing liver damage		Helps determine liver function; breaks down in presence of light
Activated partial thromboplastin time (APPT) (unchanged by age)	Clot in 25-36 seconds	Presence of heparin or other anticoagulants		Monitors anticoagulant therapy; measures intrinsic coagulation (except factor VII and XIII)
Partial thromboplastin time (PTT)	60-85 seconds (Platelin test) 25-35 seconds (differs with method used to run test)			Less sensitive than APTT

CHF, Congestive heart failure; *CNS,* central nervous system; *COPD,* chronic obstructive pulmonary disease; *DIC,* disseminated intravascular coagulopathy; *GI,* gastrointestinal; *IM,* intramuscular; *MI,* myocardial infarction; *MS,* multiple sclerosis, *TB,* tuberculosis.

TABLE 9-2   Geriatric Laboratory Values in the Normal Aging Process—cont'd

Laboratory Test	Reference Value for Patient Over Age 65	Clinical Implication of Increased Value	Clinical Implication of Decreased Value	Notes
Prothrombin time (PT) (unaffected by age)	M: 9.6-11.8 seconds F: 9.5-11.3 seconds	Deficient fibrinogen, prothrombin, or factors V, VII, X; vitamin K deficiency; liver disease		Measures extrinsic coagulation factors
Glucose (increase 2 mg/dl per decade after age 35)	70-110 mg/dl	Diabetes mellitus, hyperadrenalism, stress, infection, burns, pancreatitis, thiazide use, recent surgery, acromegaly, pheochromocytoma	Alcoholism; malnutrition; physical exercise; hypoglycemia; stomach, liver, or lung cancer; hypothalamic lesions; hypoadrenalism; cirrhosis of liver	Two fasting blood sugar readings of ≥140 mg/dl confirms diabetes; hyperglycemia of aging may be caused by decreased insulin biosynthesis and changes in body composition associated with aging
Low-density lipoprotein (LDL)	<130 mg/dl, desirable 130-159 mg/dl, borderline	Increased risk for coronary artery disease		Condition is treated if value is >160 mg/dl, coronary artery disease, and two risk factors are present
High-density lipoprotein (HDL) (female may be higher than male until 70 years of age)	>35-40 mg/dl	Exercise, weight loss, alcohol intake	Coronary heart disease, diabetes, uremia, obesity, smoking, high-fat diet	Elevations desirable
Cholesterol (increased in male to age 50; decreased in female to age 50, then increases to age 70 and decreases again after age 70)	<200 mg/dl, desirable level	Uncontrolled diabetes, hypothyroidism, cirrhosis of liver, hyperlipidemia, nephrotic syndrome	Malabsorption, starvation, hyperthyroidism	Helps determine function of liver, nervous and cardiovascular systems, and metabolism
Triglycerides (values increase with age for female)	10-190 mg/dl 250-500 mg/dl, borderline risk	Biliary obstruction, diabetes, nephrotic syndrome, alcoholism	Malnutrition	In combination with increased cholesterol helps determine increased risk of coronary artery disease
Uric acid (male values are higher throughout life span, but female values elevate at age 40-50)	M: 2.6-9.2 mg/dl F: 1.9-8.5 mg/dl	Gout, alcoholism, metastasis, leukemia, glomerulonephritis, CHF, hemolytic anemia, polycythemia, psoriasis	Tubular acidosis, folic acid deficiency, burns, pernicious anemia	Thiazide diuretics can cause an increase in older adults
Blood urea nitrogen (BUN) (increases slightly with age)	M: 7.6-35.5 mg/dl F: 5.9-31.6 mg/dl	Acute MI, high protein intake, prerenal failure, renal disease, GI bleeding, sepsis, diabetes, high licorice ingestion, urinary tract obstruction	Low protein diet, severe liver damage, overhydration, malnutrition	May overestimate renal function in the elderly; should be interpreted in combination with creatinine to assess hydration status

Continued

TABLE 9-2	Geriatric Laboratory Values in the Normal Aging Process—cont'd

Laboratory Test	Reference Value for Patient Over Age 65	Clinical Implication of Increased Value	Clinical Implication of Decreased Value	Notes
Albumin (decreases with age because of decreased liver function by age 65)	M: 3.5-4.7 g/dl F: 3.7-4.6 g/dl	Multiple myeloma	Malnutrition, anemia, burns, liver disease, gallbladder disease, kidney disease, lupus, colitis, essential hypertension, metastasis	Less than 52%-68% of total protein may indicate kidney or liver disease
Total protein (slight decrease with age)	6.0-7.8 g/dl	Dehydration, vomiting, diarrhea, diabetes, acidosis, fulminating infection, leukemia, myeloma	Malnutrition, uncontrolled diabetes, malabsorption, GI disease, essential hypertension, blood dyscrasia	Used in diagnosis of liver and kidney disease
Creatinine (female values may be decreased due to lower muscle mass)	M: 0.8-1.2 mg/dl F: 0.6-0.9 mg/dl	High meat or fish intake, renal failure, shock, acute MI, lupus, cancer, diabetic nephropathy, acromegaly, large muscle mass	Decreased amounts not clinically significant	May increase with age and should be measured before giving prolonged administration of medication excreted by kidneys
Potassium (slight increase after age 60)	M: 3.7-5.6 mmol/L F: 3.5-5.3 mmol/L	Renal failure, hyperadrenalism, metabolic acidosis	Vomiting, diarrhea, laxative abuse, dehydration, starvation, stress, trauma, recent surgery, metabolic alkalosis, burns, hyperaldosteronism	Cardiac arrest can result if values are <2.5 or >7 mmol/L
Sodium	135-146 mmol/L	Excess sodium intake, inadequate fluid intake, diabetes insipidus, prolonged hyperventilation, impaired renal function, aldosteronism	Excess sodium loss by GI suctioning, prolonged sweating, diuretics, diarrhea, vomiting, adrenal insufficiency, burns, chronic renal insufficiency with acidosis	Assess with hydration status
Chloride	100-108 mEq/L	Severe dehydration, renal shutdown, hyperventilation, primary aldosteronism	Vomiting, gastric suctioning, intestinal fistula, CHF, edema	Hypochloremia may develop into tetany and depressed respirations; hyperchloremia may develop into rapid breathing, stupor, and coma
Calcium (age-related renal changes may decrease the baseline level)	8.0-10.2 mg/dl	Hyperparathyroidism, Paget's disease, metastasis, bone fractures, immobility, ingestion of calcium carbonate antacids, bone demineralization	Hypoparathyroidism, malabsorption, Cushing's syndrome, peritonitis, renal failure, obstructive jaundice	Hypercalcemia can cause stupor, coma, and cardiac arrest
Phosphate	2.5-4.5 mg/dl	Bone disease, acromegaly, intestinal obstruction, diabetic acidosis, renal failure	Alcoholism, diabetes, hyperalimentation, gram-negative bacteremia, alkalosis, acute gout, aspirin poisoning, prolonged diarrhea and vomiting	Measured to assess renal function and acid-base balance; evaluated in combination with serum calcium

CHF, Congestive heart failure; *CNS,* central nervous system; *COPD,* chronic obstructive pulmonary disease; *DIC,* disseminated intravascular coagulopathy; *GI,* gastrointestinal; *IM,* intramuscular; *MI,* myocardial infarction; *MS,* multiple sclerosis, *TB,* tuberculosis.

TABLE 9-2 **Geriatric Laboratory Values in the Normal Aging Process—cont'd**

Laboratory Test	Reference Value for Patient Over Age 65	Clinical Implication of Increased Value	Clinical Implication of Decreased Value	Notes
Lactic dehydrogenase (LDh)	M: 61-200 IU/ml F: 71-206 IU/ml	Acute MI, placement of intracardiac prosthetic valve, cardiac surgery, hepatitis, pernicious anemia, malignancy, pulmonary embolus, any hemolytic condition	Irradiation	Evaluated in combination with cardiac studies
Amylase	60-180 Somogyi units/ml	Acute pancreatitis, perforating peptic ulcer, upper GI surgery, acute alcohol poisoning, salivary gland disease, strangulated hernia, mesenteric thrombus, lung cancer	Pancreatic failure, liver damage, hepatitis	Results are more accurate in an early AM sample; helps differentiate acute pancreatitis from other cause of abdominal pain
Alkaline phosphatase (ALP) (increases in women after age 45)	M: 90-239 U/L F: 87-250 U/L	Healing fractures, bone tumors, liver disease, biliary obstruction	Vitamin D toxicity, hypothyroidism, pernicious anemia, malnutrition, vitamin C deficiency, magnesium deficiency	Usually performed in combination with other liver enzyme tests to assess liver condition
Creatinine kinase (CK) Creatinine phosphokinase (CPK)	18-392 IU/L M: 55-170 IU/L F: 30-135 IU/L	Hypokalemia, MI, postconvulsion status, carbon monoxide poisoning, malignancy, hyperthermia, embolism after defibrillation	Sedentary lifestyle	Immobility causes a low baseline and makes the diagnosis of acute MI difficult
CPK isoenzymes	CPK-MM 94%-100%	Continuous tremors, hypokalemia, skeletal muscle damage		Multiple IM injections can influence, as can strenuous exercise
	CPK-MB 0%-6%	Acute MI, hypokalemia, cardiac ischemia, cardiac surgery, muscular dystrophy, polymyositis		Rises 4-8 hours after MI, peaks in 18-24 hours and is present in 100% by 48 hours; returns to normal in 3-4 days
	CPK-BB 0%	Brain tissue injury, malignancy, shock, pulmonary infarction, renal failure, necrosis of large intestine, uremia, malignant hyperthermia		
Serum glutamic-oxaloacetic transaminase (SGOT); also known as asparate aminotransferase (AST)	8-20 IU/L	Acute MI, liver disease, trauma, IM injections, irradiation injury, pulmonary infarction		May falsely elevate after administration of opiates; progressively decreasing value indicates improvement of acute condition
Acid phosphatase	0-1.6 IU/L	Prostate cancer, Paget's disease, multiple myeloma	Decrease following an increase may indicate successful treatment of prostate cancer	Prostate manipulation 48 hours before test may alter the value

Continued

TABLE 9-2	Geriatric Laboratory Values in the Normal Aging Process—cont'd

Laboratory Test	Reference Value for Patient Over Age 65	Clinical Implication of Increased Value	Clinical Implication of Decreased Value	Notes
Serum glutamic-pyruvic transaminase (SGPT); also known as alanine amino-transferase (ALT) (in male, peaks at age 50, then decreases to lowest point after age 65)	M: 0-45 IU/L F: 20-37 IU/L	Hepatitis, mononucleosis, cholecystitis	Vitamin B_6 deficiency	Distinguish between hepatic and cardiac tissue damage
Prostate-specific antigen (PSA)	0.1-2.6 mg/ml	Prostatic cancer		Not present in all types of prostate cancer; prostate manipulation may alter results; cystoscopy or sigmoidoscopy may cause prostate manipulation
Triiodothyronine T_3 (decreases in male after age 60, decreases in female after age 70 or 80)	80-200 ng/dl	Hyperthyroidism, thyrotoxicosis, toxic thyroid adenoma	Severe trauma or illness, malnutrition	Measures level of thyroid function
Thyroxine T_4 (small decrease up to 25% with age)	4.5-11.5 µg/dl	Hyperthyroidism, viral hepatitis, myasthenia gravis	Hypothyroidism, strenuous exercise, renal failure, protein malnutrition	Measures level of thyroid function
Thyroid stimulating hormone (TSH) (increases in both genders after age 60)	2.54 µU/ml	Goiter, thyroiditis, iodine deficiency, neck irradiation, subtotal thyroidectomy	Hyperthyroidism, pituitary- or hypothalamic-related hypothyroidism	Measures level of thyroid function
Estrogen (male gradually increases, female markedly decreases)	M: 40-115 pg/ml F: <30 pg/ml	Ovarian cancer, adrenocortical tumor, some testicular tumors	Ovarian failure, pituitary insufficiency, psychogenic stress	Female sex hormone
Luteinizing hormone (LH)	M: 5-20 mIU/ml F: >75 mIU/ml	Ovarian failure	Hypothalamic or pituitary hypofunction, testicular tumors, testicular failure	May be evaluated in combination with other sex hormone levels to determine the effectiveness of replacement therapy
Follicle-stimulating hormone (FSH)	M: 10-15 mIU/ml F: 40-250 mIU/ml	Testicular failure, end-stage acromegaly, seminoma, ovarian failure	Anorexia nervosa, panhypopituitarism, hypothalamic lesions	May be evaluated in combination with other sex hormone levels to determine effectiveness of replacement therapy

CHF, Congestive heart failure; *CNS,* central nervous system; *COPD,* chronic obstructive pulmonary disease; *DIC,* disseminated intravascular coagulopathy; *GI,* gastrointestinal; *IM,* intramuscular; *MI,* myocardial infarction; *MS,* multiple sclerosis, *TB,* tuberculosis.

TABLE 9-2	Geriatric Laboratory Values in the Normal Aging Process—cont'd

Laboratory Test	Reference Value for Patient Over Age 65	Clinical Implication of Increased Value	Clinical Implication of Decreased Value	Notes
Prolactin (male increases, female may decrease slightly)	M: 1-20 ng/ml F: 1-20 ng/ml	Hypoglycemia, stress, postoperative pituitary surgery, dopamine depletion	Primary hypothyroidism, pituitary adenomas, lung or kidney tumors, increased estrogen levels	In the presence of pituitary tumor, value may exceed 100 ng/ml
Testosterone (male gradually decreases until age 70, then markedly drops; female decreases with age)	M: 3.9-7.9 ng/ml F: 0.21-0.37 ng/ml	Testicular tumors	Testicular failure, hypopituitarism	Male sex hormone
Total carbon dioxide (CO_2)	22-34 mEq/L	Metabolic alkalosis, respiratory acidosis	Metabolic acidosis, respiratory alkalosis	Consider the value in relation to pH and arterial blood gas values
Arterial pH (unchanged)	7.35-7.45	Respiratory or metabolic alkalosis	Respiratory or metabolic acidosis, narcotics	Acid-base level of the blood
Arterial oxygen (Pao_2) (gradual decrease)	75-100 mm Hg		Respiratory or cardiac disease	Measures the amount of oxygen (O_2) the lungs are delivering to the blood
Arterial carbon dioxide ($Paco_2$) (unchanged or may increase with age)	35-45 mm Hg	Impaired respiratory function, respiratory acidosis	Hyperventilation, respiratory alkalosis	Value compared in combination with bicarbonate (HCO_3) and pH to determine whether respiratory efforts are compensating for abnormal metabolic state
Oxygen (O_2) content	15%-23%		Impaired respiratory function	Measures the amount of O_2 carried by hemoglobin
Oxygen (O_2) saturation	94%-100%		Impaired respiratory function	Measures how much hemoglobin is carrying O_2
Bicarbonate content (HCO_3)	21-28 mEq/L	Metabolic alkalosis	Metabolic acidosis	Measures how the pH is influenced by metabolism
Urinalysis				
Bacteria	None	Urinary tract infection		10%-50% of all older adults have asymptomatic bacteriuria that returns after treatment and rarely causes renal damage or becomes a septic illness

Continued

		Clinical	Clinical	
	Reference Value	Implication of	Implication of	
	for Patient	Increased	Decreased	
Laboratory Test	**Over Age 65**	**Value**	**Value**	**Notes**
Bilirubin	None	Liver disease		Not a reliable moni-
Glucose	None	Diabetes, renal disease, thyroid disorders, liver disease, some CNS disorders, heavy metal poisoning, hyperalimentation		tor of glycemic status because the aged kidney has altered physical and reabsorptive properties
Ketones	None	Uncontrolled type I diabetes, starvation, metabolic complications of hyperalimentation		
pH	4.5-8.0	Alkalotic: urinary tract infection, metabolic or respiratory acidosis	Acidotic: renal tuberculosis, pyrexia, phenylketonuria, acidosis	
White blood cells (WBC)	0-4	Urinary tract or kidney infection		Treatment recommended only in the presence of additional symptoms
Red blood cells (RBC)	0-3	Urinary tract disease, renal failure		Increased amount indicates the need for further evaluation
Protein	0-1, not to exceed 150 mg/24 hr	Renal disease, CHF, diabetes		Common in older adults and can be caused by subclinical urinary tract infection
Specific gravity (lower maximum in older adults)	1.005-1.020	Dehydration, acute glomerulonephritis, shock, CHF, liver failure	Diabetes insipidus, fluid excess, tubular necrosis	Severe renal damage usually present if specific gravity does not change with changes in fluid intake

TABLE 9-2 Geriatric Laboratory Values in the Normal Aging Process—cont'd

CHF, Congestive heart failure; *CNS,* central nervous system; *COPD,* chronic obstructive pulmonary disease; *DIC,* disseminated intravascular coagulopathy; *GI,* gastrointestinal; *IM,* intramuscular; *MI,* myocardial infarction; *MS,* multiple sclerosis, *TB,* tuberculosis.

body surface can reveal pertinent data about the patient's health status, but differentiating normal from abnormal skin conditions may be difficult. Skin is often wrinkled as a result of changes in connective tissue. Pigmentation and skin tags can be normal lesions in the aging process.

The nails and nail beds of the fingers and toes should be observed for their presence or absence, texture, growth pattern, cleanliness, infection, and color. Clubbing and cyanosis of the fingertips and nail beds may indicate cardiovascular disease. Extreme overgrowth and deformity of the toenails may indicate decreased circulation to the feet and legs. An accumulation of soil and debris under the nails may indicate an inability to wash properly. Twisted and gnarled digits may

be painful to the touch, and this should be taken into consideration when planning positions for the surgical procedure. The nurse should be aware that even the surgical drapes may create enough pressure to cause discomfort.

Hair patterns on the scalp may show areas of thinning or loss. The nurse should note the condition of the hair, such as cleanliness, hair dye, and grooming. The condition of the hair may indicate the patient's level of interest or ability in performing self-care. A lack of care may be caused by inability or disinterest caused by depression. A patient who suffers from dementia may be unaware that the hair is dirty or uncombed.

Body hair patterns may be sparsely distributed in geriatric patients, with areas of thinning or absence. For this reason, hair removal from the surgical site is not routinely indicated. The extremities should be observed for the absence or patterns of hair growth or its absence. The lower legs may not have much hair because of circulatory changes. The color of the legs should be observed at this time; duskiness and mottling may indicate a problem with arterial blood flow, whereas ruddiness may indicate a venous blood flow problem. The shape and size of the lower leg should be checked for edema or ulceration. The condition of the extremities may have implications for positioning during the surgical procedure and may indicate the need for further systemic testing.

Musculoskeletal System

Assessment of the musculoskeletal system includes muscles, bones, posture, and gait. Muscle mass is usually decreased because muscle fibers atrophy, decrease in strength, and are fewer in number. Fibrous tissue replaces the lost mass. With less exercise and motion, the strength of the muscle is compromised. Tendons become hardened, and range of motion decreases. Muscle cramps are common.

The patient may report a decrease in height. This is caused by demineralization of the bones, kyphosis, and narrowing of disc spaces in the vertebral column. The long bones do not decrease in length but become thin and brittle (osteoporosis), especially in older women; 78% of all patients over 70 years of age have some degree of osteoporosis. Estrogen supplements after menopause may decrease the occurrence of brittle bones. However, fractures in the hips, vertebrae, wrists, and ends of long bones are common in older adults.

Assistance with moving or total lifting may be necessary to help the geriatric patient move from the transport stretcher to the operating bed for the surgical procedure. The plan of care should include lifting help or devices and adequate positioning supplies. Care must be taken not to injure bony structures that may be weakened by osteoporosis.

Ankylosing spondylosis, a chronic inflammatory disease characterized by the fixation or fusion of a vertebral joint, often causes age-related postures. The body of the geriatric patient assumes an altered shape with an increased forward thoracic curvature (kyphosis) and a flattening of the lumbar curvature. The patient may not be able to lie flat on the operating bed. Supine positioning may be painful unless the upper back and neck are supported. Fractures or subluxation of the cervical spine are possible if the ankylosed neck is allowed to fall back with the weight of the head. Twisting and forceful flexion can cause permanent damage to the vertebral column. Anteroposterior angles of the chest may be increased because of respiratory disease. Respiratory effort and chest excursion should be taken into consideration in planning positioning. In the preoperative assessment, the flexibility of the patient's spine and the presence of any deformity or associated disease should be noted. Flexion at the hip may be painful when the legs are maintained in a straight position. Placement of a safety belt over the thighs may exert counterpressure on the thighs, causing the legs to forcefully straighten against

the flattened lumbar curvature. Modified positioning may include a small pillow under the knees and thighs to allow the age-related flexion angle of the hips to assume a natural position. Care in the placement of a safety belt or other restraint should include circulatory checks throughout the surgical procedure.

The hands and feet may have painful deformities that should be considered when moving the patient to the operating bed and during positioning. Joints may be affected by arthritis, thickened synovium, and crystalloid formation in the synovial fluid. Arthritic joints are painful. The patient may have a long history of taking nonsteroidal antiinflammatory medications, corticosteroids, salicylates, and analgesics. The preoperative assessment should include an evaluation for the side effects associated with the long-term use of these medications. Gastrointestinal bleeding, prolonged clotting times, renal insufficiency, liver changes, loss of appetite, and alteration in mental status are common side effects and could adversely affect the desired outcomes of the surgical procedure.

The patient's center of gravity is altered by multiple changes in body shape. Postural imbalance caused by impaired mobility is often the cause of falls that result in fractures. Some geriatric patients limit attempts at ambulation because they fear the possibility of falling. The risk of falls is further increased by complicating conditions such as sedation, electrolyte imbalance, impaired vision, and altered proprioception (muscular stimulation). Orthostatic hypotension contributes to the potential for falling when the geriatric patient rises from a sitting position and experiences a sudden drop in blood pressure. A fall may be symptomatic of a health problem or a systemic illness.

Cardiopulmonary System

Assessment of the lungs, heart, and circulation provides a good source of information about the general health condition of the patient. The cardiovascular and respiratory systems are closely interrelated. To assess the lungs, the nurse should ask the patient to describe how his or her breathing is affected by exertion. The nurse can assess difficulty or inefficiency in breathing by observing the patient's physical activity, respiratory effort, chest shape, and lip color. The nurse should palpate the trachea to determine if it is in midline. A deviation to the right or left may indicate the presence of a tumor. Tracheal position is an important consideration in the maintenance of an airway during a surgical procedure. By listening to lung sounds with a stethoscope over the intercostal spaces, the nurse can refine the assessment to include specific sounds found in identified areas of each lobe. Percussion of the posterior chest wall tends to produce resonance except in very thin older adults, in whom tone is very hyperresonant. The normal sound is hollow and moderately loud, with a low pitch and long duration; the sound flattens over the rib bones. If the patient slumps forward and rounds the shoulders, the intercostal spaces widen for better percussion.

Establishment of a preoperative respiratory system baseline is important. Intraoperative breathing difficulties may be avoided by adapting a position to accommodate the needs of the patient. Postoperative problems may be diagnosed and treated more efficiently if the patient's original respiratory condition has been assessed. Lung disease may affect the ability to clear secretions from the bronchial tree by coughing. Pneumonia is a common postoperative complication in geriatric patients. Coughing and deep breathing exercises should be taught preoperatively.

The heart and systemic circulation are assessed as separate units and together as a system. The patient should be asked if he or she experiences dizziness, fainting, palpitations, or other abnormal subjective symptoms. The perioperative nurse should listen to heart sounds with a stethoscope. Dysrhythmias unrelated to heart disease are not uncommon in the geriatric patient, and many have systolic murmurs caused by aortic stenosis. The sinoatrial and atrioventricular nodes decrease in size with age, and signal interruption may occur. Clicks, murmurs, and abnormal sounds should be recorded in the assessment data.. The apical pulse should be counted and compared with the peripheral pulses of the radial, popliteal, posterior tibial, and dorsalis pedis arteries. A difference between the apical and the peripheral pulse may indicate an obstruction in a major artery. The jugular veins should be observed for distention. Veins in the lower extremities should be inspected for varicosities. Leg pain caused by circulatory impairment is common in older adults.

The carotid arteries should be auscultated with a stethoscope. Bruits and systolic murmurs, which are abnormal sounds, may indicate an evolving blockage. Dizziness or cognitive impairment may be caused by carotid insufficiency. Care must be taken not to exert pressure over the carotid area, because manipulation of a plaque could cause an embolus to break loose and travel to the brain. Sudden changes in mental status during a surgical procedure performed with a local anesthetic could be the result of an arterial occlusion caused by a plaque embolus.

The geriatric patient usually has decreased or slowed circulation to all areas of the body. This should be taken into consideration during the administration of local anesthetics, because absorption of the medication will take longer and the effects will be delayed. The surgical site should be tested for the effects of the anesthetic before the incision is made. Vasoconstrictive additives, such as epinephrine, may have an exaggerated effect. Postoperative dressings should not be applied too tightly because healing is affected by circulatory efficiency.

Blood pressure should be assessed in the sitting and lying positions, and both arms should be tested. Elevated systolic and diastolic blood pressures are a common finding in 40% of the geriatric patient population.

Assessment of laboratory blood values is important (see Table 9-2). Anemia is common among older adults and is often overlooked as a potential cause of cerebral ischemia. Both men (21%) and women (34%) have slight normal decreases in hemoglobin and hematocrit levels because the blood-forming mechanisms lose efficiency with age. In men, the decrease in androgen production may cause a noticeable decrease in hemoglobin. Extreme decreases in hemoglobin and hematocrit values are significant in the diagnosis of pathologic conditions in major organ systems, especially the gastrointestinal or genitourinary systems. Anemic conditions can also be caused by a nutritional deficit. In the absence of any other confirmed pathologic condition, hemoglobin or hematocrit levels below the lower limit of altitude-adjusted normal values (at sea level: hemoglobin 12 g/dl, hematocrit 35%) may signal anemia caused by malnutrition.

The white blood cells do not decrease in volume, but they do decrease in effectiveness. Inflammatory responses may be decreased or absent in the geriatric patient. This natural body response to injury may leave the patient more vulnerable to infection. The febrile response to infection may be diminished and therefore may not be a good indicator of a disease process. Older adults often have a subnormal baseline temperature.

Gastrointestinal System

Assessment of the gastrointestinal system should begin by observing for the visual signs of nutritional status, such as body weight, muscle wasting, bloating, and generalized weakness. Postoperative healing is profoundly affected by the ability of the cells to repair themselves. Both adequate nutrition and the ability to handle the necessary nutrients in the gastrointestinal system are essential for tissue restoration. Many socioeconomic, psychologic, and physiologic factors influence the nutritional status of the geriatric patient. Living on a fixed income may limit the amount of nutritious food a patient is able to purchase. An adequate diet should include at least 1 g of protein per kilogram of desirable body weight, with an emphasis on a decreased number of calories. The average daily caloric intake of an older woman should range between 1280 and 1900 calories; for an older man the average daily caloric intake should range between 1530 and 2300 calories. The perioperative nurse should keep in mind that actual caloric needs are unique for each patient and may vary in the presence of diabetes or other disease processes. A rapid weight gain or loss may indicate a serious pathologic condition. Dietary control should focus on the quality of food, not the quantity of food. Weight should be considered a vital sign in older adults and should be recorded in both pounds and kilograms. Many medications are prescribed according to body weight in kilograms.

Psychologically, the patient may feel that food does not taste right and may refuse to eat. Many psychologic reasons for malnutrition are rooted in a physiologic cause. The geriatric patient's appetite may be decreased because there are now fewer taste receptors in the mouth. The sense of smell may be diminished, or the patient's teeth may be in disrepair. Some patients are totally edentulous (toothless). The inability to taste, chew, and swallow discourages eating. Saliva production decreases and makes swallowing more difficult. Loose or missing teeth must be assessed because of the danger of aspirating a tooth during the surgical procedure. During the preoperative assessment, the perioperative nurse may find that a decreased ability to taste salty and sweet foods may cause the patient to increase the amount of salt and sugar in the diet. Increased salt intake may predispose the patient to congestive heart failure, and added sugar may cause an increase in unwanted body fat in proportion to muscle mass. The geriatric patient undergoing general anesthesia may receive stimulants and depressants; many of these are fat soluble. The fat-soluble drugs absorb faster but are excreted more slowly because of lower levels of intracellular fluid. Medications are unevenly distributed in the body, and the anticipated actions are unpredictable because fewer receptor sites react to the presence of the drug.

Digestion can be assessed by questioning the patient about food intake and the effects of the presence of food in the stomach. Older adults have decreased stomach motility, decreased gastric secretions, and slower stomach emptying time. The esophagus loses muscular tone and dilates slightly. Food may remain in the esophagus for longer periods of time. The perioperative nurse should ask the patient about the use of antacids and laxatives. Frequent use of antacids may indicate swallowing or stomach problems that should be investigated. Esophageal reflux in the presence of a hiatal hernia may need to be assessed preoperatively to prevent aspiration of gastric secretions. The inability to lie flat with food in the stomach may be the first symptom of a high-risk situation. Positioning and rapid-sequence induction of anesthesia may be a consideration. Cricoid pressure may be necessary for intubation and prevention of aspiration.

The geriatric patient may use laxatives to maintain bowel regularity. Constipation is caused by decreased motility, lowered intake of bulk and fluids, and inactivity. Oil-based laxatives can lead to malabsorption of the fat-soluble vitamins A, D, E, and K, which further impairs nutritional and general health status. The absorption of nutrients is impaired naturally in older adults as a process of aging because intestinal blood flow is reduced and the absorptive cells lining the intestines are decreased. Fiber is an important dietary additive but should be used with caution because it can cause bowel obstruction or diarrhea. Diarrhea in the geriatric patient causes a serious threat to well-being because it may lead to dehydration.

The minimum oral fluid intake should be 1500 ml daily. Some geriatric patients have limited fluid intake. A patient may fear incontinence, have altered sensorium and cognition, be unable to drink fluids independently, or have a decreased thirst sensation as part of the aging process. The serious nature of fluid balance in older adults is reflected in unstable electrolyte values and their direct impact on cardiac status. A preoperative assessment of hydration should be performed by the perioperative nurse. Signs of dehydration are dry tongue, sunken cheeks and eyes, severe loss of skin turgor, concentrated urine and, in some instances, mental confusion.

Blood tests may show a urea level above 60 mg/dl. A geriatric patient who is dehydrated should receive preoperative intravenous fluids to prevent complications.

Endocrine System

The endocrine system interfaces with all major systems of the body. The assessment of endocrine functioning is complicated by the normal age-related changes in other body systems. The endocrine system consists of the thyroid gland; the parathyroid gland; the pancreas; the adrenal, pituitary, and pineal glands; and the ovaries or testes.

Thyroid hormone production decreases by age 60 in men, whereas women experience decreased production by age 70. By 80 years of age, the thyroid gland reduces thyroid hormone production by 50%. The effects of this decreased production may be dry skin, memory lapse, temperature intolerance, lethargy, and appetite disturbance. Many signs and symptoms of thyroid disease may be confused with the normal aging process. Comorbidity may lead to abnormal laboratory test results in a patient with normal thyroid function.

Insulin is produced by the beta cells in the pancreas and affects the metabolism and storage of glucose. In healthy patients, glucose levels in the blood cause the pancreas to release insulin. The response of the pancreas is slowed in older adults, and the release of insulin may not be triggered by the same stimulus. Many geriatric patients are diabetic and have impaired glucose metabolism. Diabetes may be caused by deficient insulin production, insensitive insulin receptors, altered insulin release mechanisms, or inactivation of circulating insulin. An imbalance in blood glucose levels during the surgical procedure may predispose the patient to an unwanted outcome. Patients with diabetes often experience more postoperative infections and complications. Uncontrolled blood glucose metabolism has negative implications for all major body systems. Therefore ongoing assessment is important for the attainment of expected outcomes.

Genitourinary System

Assessment of the genitourinary system includes the bladder, urethra, ureters, kidneys, reproductive history, and genitalia. The first noticeable sign of a problem with the genitourinary system may be the odor of urine on clothing. The odor may be caused by lack of cleanliness but usually is caused by incontinence. More than 30% of the older population experiences some form of urinary incontinence, but many are reluctant to discuss this problem and may try to avoid it. The problem may stem from stress incontinence, confusion, neurologic disorders, urinary tract infection, or immobility that prevents the patient from getting to the bathroom quickly.

The geriatric patient may fear loss of bladder control during the surgical procedure. Previous bladder or prostate gland surgery may predispose a patient to involuntary urine release. The perioperative nurse should include this situation in the plan of care. The problem may be minimized during the surgical procedure if the patient has an opportunity to empty the bladder preoperatively. The nursing diagnoses should reflect not only urinary incontinence but also the associated anxiety level of the patient.

Assessment of the genital area should include observation of the perineum for redness and excoriation. The bladder should be palpated with the patient in the supine position. The presence of a distended bladder after the patient has voided may indicate urinary retention with an overflow condition. This condition should be checked preoperatively before the patient is catheterized in the OR. The urethra could be inadvertently traumatized if an obstruction (e.g., tumor or enlarged prostate gland) is present.

The kidneys decrease in effectiveness as a patient ages. By 50 years of age, renal blood flow and glomerular filtration rate decrease by as much as 50%. Although there may be no overt signs of a disease process, the perioperative nurse should be aware that the older patient is at increased risk for renal insufficiency and is highly susceptible to fluid overload, dehydration, or renal failure.

The perioperative nurse should make a baseline assessment of intake and output. During the surgical procedure, urinary output may be used to monitor the renal status of the patient. Renal impairment may delay the excretion of drugs by the kidneys and further complicate fluid balance. The urine should be assessed for color, concentration, the presence of particulate matter, and odor. Minimum urinary output during the procedure should be at least 30 ml/hr; more urine may be produced if the patient is taking diuretics or medications for blood pressure or cardiac control. Monitoring urinary output is difficult if the patient does not have an indwelling catheter or if he or she experiences urinary incontinence during the procedure. Postoperative care should include emptying the bladder to evaluate the expected outcome of adequate urinary output.

The reproductive assessment consists of the number of pregnancies a woman had during her childbearing years. Data about the method of birth should be included. Childbirth by cesarean section or a previous gynecologic surgery may indicate the possibility of pelvic adhesions that may be encountered if the planned surgical procedure includes entering the peritoneal cavity. Multiple vaginal births may cause uterine and bladder prolapse. The presence of a pessary for uterine elevation should be noted. The use of estrogen replacement therapy should be noted. The possibility of osteoporosis and heart disease is greater in older women who have not had estrogen replacement after menopause.

The breasts of both male and female patients should be palpated for masses. The male patient may exhibit gynecomastia, which is an increase of breast tissue caused by decreased production of testosterone. Previous mammograms should be available if breast surgery is planned. Any hormonal therapy should be noted in the assessment. If the breast is biopsied, the specimen may be tested for estrogen receptor sites. The loss of fibrous breast tissue in the woman is normal. The main palpable finding will be the terminal milk ducts, which feel like strands or spindles. Masses are not a common finding and should be investigated. Nulli-

parous women may be predisposed to breast cancer. Nipple discharge or retraction may indicate a serious condition. The breasts of the elderly woman may be pendulous and flaccid. Prepping and draping may be slightly more difficult because of sagging skin and lack of muscle tone.

In males, the genitalia may be diminished in size. The penis may be smaller, and the testes descend lower into the scrotum because the rugae are decreased or absent. Pubic hair may be sparse, pale, and coarse. The ability to achieve an erection may be decreased or absent, and the ability to ejaculate may be diminished. Orgasm may still be possible without the presence of an erection. The prostate may be enlarged, and the incidence of prostatic cancer increases with age. The male geriatric patient may experience embarrassment during a prostate examination, and all efforts should be made to preserve his dignity. Positioning for this examination may be difficult because of inflexible joints. The patient can be positioned in a lateral, modified jackknife or modified dorsal recumbent position. The presence of stool may hinder the palpation. Many prostate biopsies use transrectal ultrasound and needle aspiration and sampling of the gland. Rectal sphincter tone should be assessed in the patient who is undergoing a transrectal procedure. Anal tears, hemorrhoids, fissures, and defects in the musculature should be documented in the assessment data. Any stool present on the examiner's gloved finger should be tested for occult blood to establish the baseline, otherwise postoperative bleeding could be wrongly assessed as a problem caused by the surgical procedure. Baseline data may help to resolve the situation.

The female genitalia should be assessed both externally and internally. The patient should be placed supine in a modified lithotomy position. Spinal curvature or respiratory difficulty may prevent the patient from lying flat, and arthritic joints make lithotomy positioning a painful effort. Care should be exercised not to create embarrassment during the examination. The vulvar area should be inspected. The mons and labia will appear smaller and looser because of the loss of subcutaneous fat pads and the decrease in estrogen production. Lesions and discolorations should be noted. The skin of the perineum may be shiny, atrophic, and dry. The prepuce and clitoris may be atrophied, but orgasm is still possible. The vaginal opening may appear small, dry, and inelastic. A previous history of hysterectomy or oophorectomy should be obtained. The absence of the uterus or ovaries does not preclude examination of the vaginal vault. The anus should be inspected for tears, fissures, and hemorrhoids.

The internal assessment of the female genitalia includes a very gentle examination that involves insertion of a gloved, well-lubricated finger into the vagina. The vagina may feel shortened. The position of the bladder, rectum, and cervix should be ascertained. Protrusion of the bladder, rectum, or cervix may be present inasmuch as the patient experiences a loss of muscle tone with age. The abdomen is palpated as the uterus is carefully elevated. The uterus atrophies as part of the aging process; enlargement is caused by disease. The endometrium will still respond to the stimulation of hormonal therapy, causing uterine bleeding. The adnexa are identified, and no masses should be felt. The use of a smaller, prewarmed, well-lubricated speculum is usually necessary for visualization of the cervix and for obtaining a Papanicolaou (Pap) smear. Pediatric instrumentation may be needed. The vaginal lining will look thin, smooth, dry, and atrophied. Care is essential to prevent trauma when fingers or instruments are inserted into the vagina. Discharge and foul odors are abnormal and should be reported. Vaginal bleeding is a sign of a pathologic condition in the older woman.

Sexuality in older adults is an often overlooked and ignored reality. The activity between geriatric sex partners may vary in performance, but sexual pleasure is not abandoned because of advancing age. Intercourse may not take place in the same way as when the partners were young, but sexual contact and mutual gratification remains pleasurable. Many geriatric patients have been forced to deny their sexuality because of the loss of their sexual partner. Self-gratification may be practiced but is not openly discussed because of the personal nature of the act. The subject of sexuality should be approached gently, without jokes or condemnation. Dislocations of total hip joint prosthetics can occur during sexual intercourse. A surgical procedure that may alter sexual habits can be devastating. Empathy is critical to the patient's adjustment to a change of lifestyle. Counseling may be necessary to assist the patient and the sexual partner in expressing concerns. The perioperative nurse should be prepared to answer questions and listen to the patient as he or she expresses a sense of loss. The plan of care should reflect the nursing diagnosis of an alteration in sexuality and sexual expression.

Nervous System

Assessment of the nervous system includes the brain, spinal cord, peripheral nerves, and sensory organs. The nervous system is uniquely interdependent with every system of the body. Age-related changes in the brain consist of a decreased number of neurons, a decreased rate of impulse transmission, an increased reflex response time, and a decreased brain mass. The perioperative nurse should assess the geriatric patient and establish a baseline of neurologic function. Any deviation from baseline during the surgical procedure may indicate the presence of an additional or new pathologic condition involving the brain (e.g., stroke). Postoperatively, the ongoing assessment monitors the risk for a postprocedural deficit caused by medication or a pathologic condition.

The spinal cord and peripheral nerves are assessed together. During the functional assessment, the patient is observed ambulating, sitting, standing, maintaining posture, making intentional hand motions, and performing cooperative and purposeful actions such as writing. The perioperative nurse is able to observe for tremor, gait disturbance, shuffling of feet, unilateral weakness, or an alteration in mobility caused by a neurologic deficit. An assessment of the medications taken at home is important to determine the presence of transient nervous system side effects such as shaking and intention tremor. Smoking can cause a tempo-

rary decrease in cerebral blood flow, resulting in dizziness that may mimic a neurologic problem.

The sensory changes associated with aging involve decreased pressure and pain perception, difficulty differentiating between hot and cold, hearing loss, decreased visual acuity, and alterations in the senses of smell and taste and in spatial perception during locomotion. Preoperative assessment of tactile sensory conditions will enable the plan of care to reflect the need for protection of bony pressure points and for caution during the use of heat- or cold-producing equipment such as a hypothermia/hyperthermia mattress.

If a patient has sensory impairments such as a visual disturbance, a hearing loss, or altered spatial perception, he or she is at high risk for injury caused by falls. Patients with cataracts may be sensitive to the glare from bright OR lights. Allowing the patient to wear hearing aids and eyeglasses to the OR is beneficial to his or her adaptation to the surgical environment. Unexpected outcomes caused by sensory alteration can be prevented by developing a plan of care that considers the combined baseline abilities and sensory needs of the patient. For example, an assessment of hearing ability will dictate the need to facilitate communication.

INTRAOPERATIVE CONSIDERATIONS

Special precautions are indicated in caring for geriatric patients in the OR. The following factors should be taken into account:

- *Hypothermia.* Geriatric patients are at risk when their core body temperature falls below 96.8° F (36° C). A decreased basal metabolic rate, limited cardiovascular reserves, thinning of the skin, and reduced muscle mass affect the production and conservation of body heat. Measures must be taken to prevent inadvertent hypothermia caused by environmental factors. Precautionary measures include raising room temperature; using warm blankets and devices to circulate warmed air over body surfaces not included in the surgical site; warming anesthetic gases, solutions, and intravenous fluids; and covering the patient's head.
- *Positioning.* Patients should be lifted, not pulled, during transfer to and from the operating bed and during positioning on the operating bed. Skin is sensitive to abrasion because of decreased dermal thickness and turgor (elasticity). Joints may be stiff or painful due to calcification or degenerative osteoarthritis. Support of the back and neck prevents discomfort from osteoporosis, kyphosis, or rheumatoid arthritis. Padding and air supports protect pressure points and bony prominences. Circulation and respiration must not be further compromised. Decreased cardiac output, arteriosclerosis, venous stasis, reduced vital lung capacity, and reduced tissue oxygenation are characteristic changes in older adults.

- *Antiembolic measures.* Slow circulation and hypotension predispose older adults to thrombus formation and emboli. Antiembolic stockings or a sequential compression device on the legs helps decrease this risk.
- *Monitoring.* A decrease in renal circulation and excretory ability affects electrolyte balance and the excretion of drugs. Fluid and blood loss are not well tolerated, and hypovolemia can progress rapidly. Blood loss and urinary output must be monitored. Blood gases and electrolytes may need to be monitored depending on the type of surgical procedure and the patient's preoperative condition. The reaction to any anesthetic agents and drugs is closely monitored in all patients. Fluctuations in cardiac rate and rhythm may portend an impending crisis.

Anesthesia Considerations

Geriatric patients present a special challenge to the anesthesia provider. Physiologic function gradually deteriorates with age but not in a predictable manner or progression. The aging process is not a disease but a fundamental biologic alteration. In geriatric patients, disease is superimposed on senescent changes. The aged are more prone to multiple organ system failure. Changes in the central nervous system produce effects on other body systems.

Characteristics of some older adults include memory loss and confusion (which are exaggerated in an institutional environment), malnutrition, anemia, osteoporosis, low blood volume, poor liver or renal function, arteriosclerosis, diminished autonomic tone and reflexes, instability of circulation, and diabetes. Reactivity to stimuli decreases with advancing years. These patients therefore experience an altered response to stress, which is exemplified by a high pain threshold. They are more susceptible to the action of all drugs. Abnormal sleeping and breathing patterns, with the production of apnea by hyperventilation, are accentuated by opioids. These phenomena translate to a need for lower doses of anesthetics and of opioids for analgesia; the minimum anesthetic concentration required declines progressively with advanced age.

In older adults, oxygen masks may be difficult to fit because of the loss of teeth and/or bony substance in the jaw. Induction may be prolonged and ventilation made difficult because of chronic obstructive pulmonary disease or emphysema. With a rapid fall in blood pressure, patients are susceptible to hypoxia, stroke, renal failure, and the development of myocardial infarction. The problems of anesthetization are augmented because, with geriatric patients, surgical procedures tend to be major and take longer; many procedures pertain to malignant tumors, with additional surgery necessary.

A decrease in muscle mass, including the myocardium, with a corresponding increase in body fat takes place in the aging process; most anesthetics are fat soluble. Cardiac output and pulmonary capacity also diminish with age, with a decline in maximal oxygen uptake. In addition, anesthetics may reduce oxygen to the heart, kidneys, and brain, and geriatric patients are prone to hypotension, hypothermia, cerebral edema, and hypoxemia postoperatively. These fundamental physiologic changes necessitate a reduction of anesthetic dosages in geriatric patients.

Surgical mortality is higher in older adults than in the general population, especially if the surgery is an emergency procedure, which does not allow sufficient time for a thorough preoperative evaluation and preparation. Complications related to the cardiovascular system and cerebral circulation often are followed by respiratory problems, aspiration, and infection. Surgical morbidity can be reduced, however, by skillful anesthesia management.

POSTOPERATIVE CONSIDERATIONS

The health status of geriatric patients is compromised by the interaction of drugs and anesthetics and by the surgical procedure itself. The following must be monitored postoperatively:

- *Drug interactions.* Tolerance may be poor, and detoxification is slow. Drugs metabolize slowly in the liver and are excreted slowly by the kidneys. Fat-soluble drugs have a prolonged duration because they are absorbed by body fat, which increases with aging. Many anesthetic agents are fat soluble and are also myocardial and respiratory depressants. Narcotics and sedatives interact with anesthetics. Patients must be monitored for hypoxia, because oxygenation to the heart, kidneys, and brain will be less efficient. General anesthetics and some drugs cause transient mental dysfunction.
- *Aspiration.* Older adults may have difficulty swallowing because of dry mucous membranes, reduced salivation, and reduced esophageal peristalsis. Coughing is less productive because of muscular atrophy in the chest and rigidity of the rib cage. Patients must be watched for aspiration.
- *Infection.* Respiratory, urinary, or gastrointestinal tract infections may develop as a result of immunodeficiency. Pneumonia can be fatal. Poor dental hygiene may be the source of systemic infection. Healing is further delayed if an infection develops in a wound already compromised by a reduced vascular supply. The fever associated with infection in younger patients may not be as obvious in geriatric patients. Elevation of white blood cell count may be a better indicator.

Geriatric patients require a thorough preoperative assessment, an experienced anesthesia provider, considerate and knowledgeable patient care, meticulous aseptic and sterile techniques, and careful postoperative management. The patient and his or her family and/or significant others should be included in the development of the postoperative discharge plan. Planning should incorporate follow-up care with the surgeon.

Bibliography

Agency for Healthcare Policy and Research: Other patients with special needs: elderly patients, *Acute pain management,* pp 57-59, 1992, pub no 92-0032.

Bailes BK: Chronic alcohol abuse in elderly surgical patients, *AORN J* 65(5):963-970, 1997.

Branski SH: Delirium in hospitalized patients, *Am J Nurs* 98(4):16, 1998.

Ebersole P, Hess P: *Toward healthy aging: human needs and nursing response,* ed 5, St Louis, 1998, Mosby.

Hazen SE et al: General anesthesia and elderly surgical patients, *AORN J* 65(4):815-822, 1997.

Hoot-Martin JL et al: Interpreting laboratory values in elderly surgical patients, AORN J 65(3):621-626, 1997.

Horton R: The omnipresent still syndrome, *Lancet* 350(9085):1156, 1997.

Keough V, Letizia M: Perioperative care of elderly trauma patients, *AORN J* 63(5):932-937, 1996.

Moddeman GR: Barriers to pain management in elderly surgical patients, *AORN J* 61(6):1073-1075, 1995.

Mulley GP: Myths of aging, *Lancet* 350(9085):1160-1161, 1997.

Larsen PD et al: Assessment and management of sensory loss in elderly patients, *AORN J* 65(2):432-437, 1997.

Orem DE: *Nursing: concepts of practice,* ed 5, St Louis, 1995, Mosby.

Patterson C, Rosenthal C: Living a little more dangerously, *Lancet* 350(9085):1164-1165, 1997.

Province MA et al: The effects of exercise on falls in elderly patients: a preplanned meta-analysis of the FICIT Trials, *JAMA* 273(17):1341-1347, 1995.

Resnick NM, Marcantonio ER: How should clinical care of the aged differ? *Lancet* 350(9085):1157-1158, 1997.

St Pierre J: Functional decline in hospitalized elders: preventive nursing measures, *AACN* Clin Issues 9(1):109-118, 1998.

Staab AS: *Essentials of gerontological nursing: adaptation to the aging process,* ed 2, Philadelphia, 1996, Lippincott-Raven.

Tappen RM, Andre SP: Inadvertent hypothermia in elderly surgical patients, *AORN J* 63(3):639-644, 1996.

Theis SL, Merritt SL: A learning model to guide research and practice for teaching elder clients, *Nurs Health Care* 15(9):464-468, 1994.

Tinetti ME et al: Shared risk factors for falls, incontinence, and functional dependence: unifying the approach to geriatric syndromes, *JAMA* 273(17):1348-1353, 1995.

Valente SM: Recognizing depression in elderly patients, *Am J Nurs* 94(12):18-24, 1994.

van Weel C, Michels J: Dying, not old age, to blame for costs of health care, *Lancet* 350(9085):1159-1160, 1997.

Section
IV

The Perioperative Environment

Chapter 10

Physical Facilities

 Chapter Objectives

After studying this chapter, the learner will be able to:

- Identify specific areas within the OR suite wherein attire and behaviors affect the manner of care delivery.
- Discuss how environmental layout contributes to aseptic technique.
- Describe methods of environmental controls that contribute to an aseptic environment.

PHYSICAL LAYOUT OF THE OPERATING ROOM SUITE

Utilization of the physical facilities is important. The design of the perioperative environment offers a challenge to the planning team to optimize efficiency by creating realistic traffic and work flow patterns for patients, visitors, personnel, and supplies. The design should also allow for flexibility and future expansion. Architects consult surgeons and operating room (OR) administrative personnel before allocating space.

Planning and Design Team

The planning and design of the perioperative environment requires a multidisciplinary team, which may include the following:

- Department director
- Nurse manager
- Physicians (surgeon, anesthesia provider)
- Project manager (may be in-house personnel or a consultant)
- Information technologist

- Communications (telephone, intercom, emergency call)
- Support services (laboratory and x-ray)
- Infection control
- Architect

No one particular plan suits all hospitals; each is designed on an individual basis to meet projected specific future needs. The number of rooms required depends on the following:

- Number and length of the surgical procedures to be performed
- Type and distribution by specialties of the surgical staff and equipment for each
- Proportion of elective inpatient and emergency surgical procedures to ambulatory patient and minimally invasive procedures
- Scheduling policies related to the number of hours per day and days per week the suite will be in use and staffing needs
- Systems and procedures established for the efficient flow of patients, personnel, and supplies
- Consideration of volume changes and need for future expansion capabilities

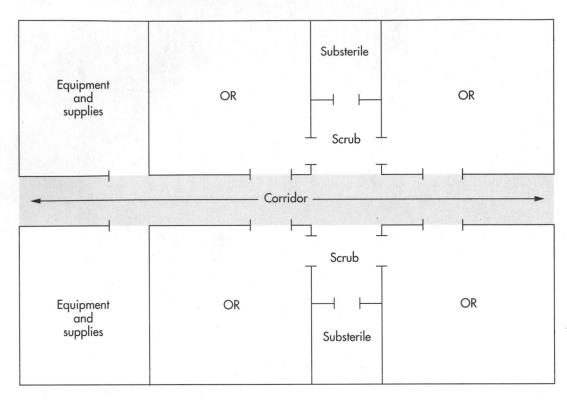

Figure 10-1 Central corridor, hotel style.

Location

The OR suite is usually located in an area accessible to the critical care surgical patient areas and the supporting service departments, the central service or sterile processing department, the pathology department, and the radiology department. The size of the hospital is a determining factor because it is impossible to locate every desirable unit or department immediately adjacent to the OR suite. A terminal location is necessary to prevent unrelated traffic from passing through the suite. A location on a top floor is not necessary for microbial control because all air is filtered to control dust. Traffic noises may be less evident above the ground floor. Artificial lighting is controllable, so that the need for daylight is not a factor; in fact, it may be a distraction during the use of video equipment and other procedures requiring a darkened environment. Many OR suites are underground or have solid walls without windows.

Principles in Design

The universal problem of environmental control to prevent wound infection exerts a great influence on the design of the OR suite. Clean and contaminated areas should be well differentiated. Architects follow two principles in planning the physical layout of an OR suite:

1. Exclusion of contamination from outside the suite with sensible traffic patterns within the suite
2. Separation of clean areas from contaminated areas within the suite

Physical planning of an OR suite, which separates clean from contaminated areas, makes it easier to carry out good aseptic technique. The clean area is often referred to as the restricted area.

Type of Design

Most OR suites are constructed according to a variation of one or more of four basic designs:

1. Central corridor, or hotel plan (Figure 10-1)
2. Central core, or clean core plan (Figure 10-2)
3. Combination central core and peripheral corridor, or racetrack plan (Figure 10-3)
4. Grouping, or cluster plan (Figure 10-4)

Each design has its advantages and disadvantages. Efficiency is affected if corridor distances are too long in proportion to other space, if illogical relationships exist between space and function, or if inadequate consideration was given to storage space, materiel handling, and personnel areas.

Space Allocation and Traffic Patterns

Space is allocated within the OR suite to provide for the work to be done, with consideration given to the efficiency with which it can be accomplished. The OR suite should be large enough to allow for correct technique yet small enough to minimize the movement of patients, personnel, and supplies. Provision must be made for traffic control. The type of design will predetermine traffic patterns. All persons—staff, patients,

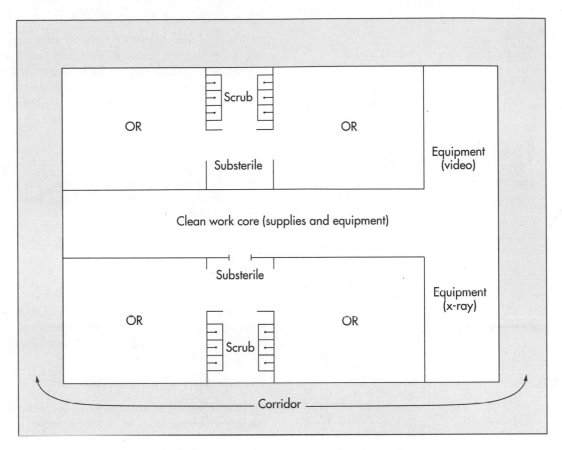

Figure 10-2   Central core, peripheral corridor style.

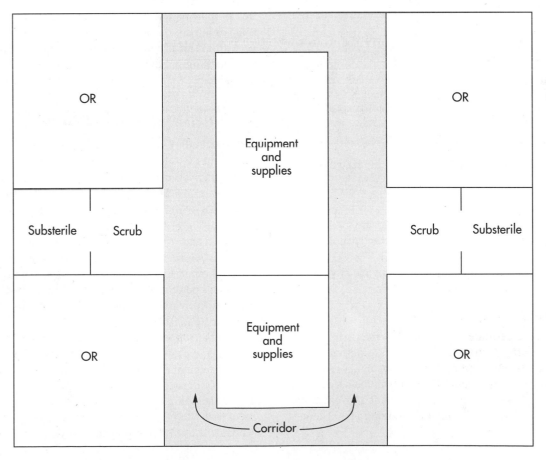

Figure 10-3   Central corridor, racetrack style.

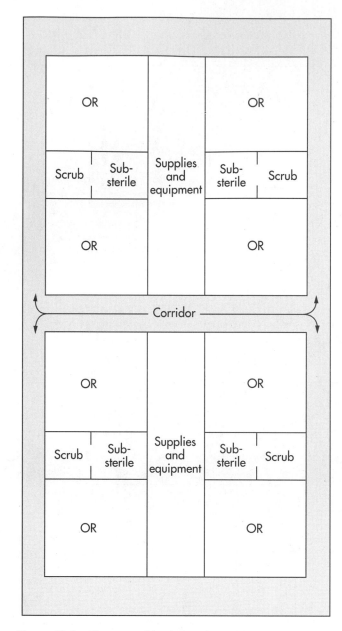

Figure 10-4 Cluster combination, peripheral and central corridor style.

and visitors—should follow the delineated patterns in appropriate attire. Signs should be posted that clearly indicate the attire and environmental controls required. The OR suite is divided into three areas that are designated by the physical activities performed in each area.

Unrestricted Area

Street clothes are permitted. A corridor on the periphery accommodates traffic from outside, including patients. This area is isolated by doors from the main hospital corridor or elevators and from other areas of the OR suite. It serves as an outside-to-inside access area (i.e., a vestibular/exchange area). Traffic, although not limited, is monitored at a central location.

Semirestricted Area

Traffic is limited to properly attired personnel. Body and head coverings are required. This area includes peripheral support areas and access corridors to the ORs. The patient may be transferred to a clean inside stretcher or wheelbase on entry to this area. The patient's hair must be covered. Traffic is limited to properly attired personnel.

Restricted Area

Masks are required to supplement OR attire. Sterile procedures are carried out in the OR. The area also includes scrub sink areas and substerile rooms or clean core area(s) where unwrapped supplies are sterilized.

VESTIBULAR/ EXCHANGE AREAS

Both patients and personnel enter the semirestricted and restricted areas of the OR suite through a vestibular or exchange area. This transition zone, inside the entrance to the OR suite, separates the OR corridors from the rest of the facility.

Preoperative Check-In Unit

If a remote same-day procedure unit is not available for admission of patients who arrive shortly before a surgical procedure, facilities must be provided within the unrestricted area of the OR suite for patients to change from street clothes into a gown. The area must ensure privacy. It may be compartmentalized with individual cubicles or be an open area with curtains. The decor should create a feeling of warmth and security. Lockers should be provided for safeguarding patients' clothes. Lavatory facilities must be available.

Preoperative Holding Area

A designated room or area should be available for patients to wait in the OR suite that shields them from potentially distressing sights and sounds. The corridor outside the OR is the least desirable area. The area should provide privacy. Individual cubicles are preferable to curtains. Hair removal and insertion of intravenous (IV) lines, indwelling urinary catheters, and/or gastric tubes may be done here. The anesthesia provider may insert invasive monitoring lines and give regional blocks. These procedures require good lighting. Each patient area is equipped with oxygen and suction, and devices for monitoring and cardiopulmonary resuscitation.

A nurse station within the area provides for medication storage and preparation and for interdepartmental and intradepartmental communication. Computer access to patient information, such as laboratory reports, and to patient care documentation facilitates completion of patients' records, if necessary. Coordination with persons managing the surgical schedule is essential to prevent delays.

Induction Room

Some hospitals have an induction room adjacent to each OR where the patient waits and is prepared preoperatively before administration of anesthesia. Invasive IV lines and/or regional anesthesia may be administered in this area.

Postanesthesia Care Unit

The postanesthesia care unit (PACU) may be outside the OR suite, or it may be adjacent to the suite so that it may be incorporated into the unrestricted area with access from both the semirestricted area and an outside corridor. In the latter design, the PACU becomes a vestibular area for the departure of patients.

Hospitals and ambulatory care facilities accommodate both patients and their families. A designated waiting area must be provided for families. This is most conveniently located outside the OR suite adjacent to the recovery area.

Dressing Rooms and Lounges

Dressing rooms must be provided for both men and women to change from street clothes into OR attire before entering the semirestricted area, and vice versa. Lockers are usually provided. Doors separate this area from lavatory facilities and adjacent lounges. Walls in the lounge areas should have an aesthetically pleasing color or combination of colors to foster a restful atmosphere. A window view of the outdoors is psychologically desirable. Dictating equipment and telephones should be available for surgeons in lounges or in an adjacent semirestricted area.

PERIPHERAL SUPPORT AREAS

Adequate space must be allocated to accommodate the needs of OR personnel and support services. The need for equipment, supply, utility rooms, and housekeeping determines support space requirements. Equipment and supply rooms should be decentralized, placing them near the appropriate ORs.

Central Control Desk

From a central control point, traffic in and out of the OR suite may be observed. This area usually is within the unrestricted area. The clerk-receptionist is located at the control desk to coordinate communications. A pass-through window may be used to stop unauthorized persons, to schedule surgical procedures with surgeons, or to receive drugs, blood, and various small supplies. A computerized pneumatic tube system within the hospital can speed the delivery of small items and paperwork, thus eliminating some messenger services, such as from the pharmacy to the control desk. Tissue specimens or blood samples also can be sent to the laboratory through some tube systems.

Computers may be located in the control area. Automated information systems and computers assist in financial management, statistical recording and analysis, scheduling of patients and personnel, materiels management, and other functions that evaluate the utilization of facilities. An integrated system interfaces with other hospital departments. It may have a modem that allows surgeons to schedule surgical procedures directly from their offices. Retrieval for review of patient records gives the perioperative nurse manager the opportunity to evaluate the patient care given and documented by nurses. Personnel records can be maintained. Other essential records can be stored in and retrieved from computer databases. The central processing unit for the OR computer system usually is located in or near the central administrative control area. A facsimile (fax) machine may be available for the electronic transfer of documents, records, and patient care orders between the OR and the surgeons' offices.

Security systems usually can be monitored from the central administrative control area. Alarms are incorporated into electrical and piped-in systems to alert personnel to the location of a system failure. A centralized emergency call system facilitates summoning help. Narcotics are kept locked up and can be signed out only by appropriate personnel. Access to exchange areas, offices, and storage areas may be limited during evening and night hours and on weekends. Doors may be locked. Some hospitals use alarm systems, television surveillance, and/or electronic metal detection devices to control intruders and to prevent vandalism. Computers and records must be secured to protect patients' confidentiality.

Offices

Offices for the administrative patient care personnel and the anesthesia department are best located with access to both unrestricted and semirestricted areas. These staff members frequently need to confer with outside persons and to be kept informed of activities within all areas of the suite.

Conference Room/Classroom

Ideally, a conference room or a classroom is located within the semirestricted area. This is used for patient care staff inservice educational programs and by the surgical staff for teaching. Closed-circuit television and/or videocassettes may also be available for self-study. The departmental reference library may be housed here.

Support Services

The size of the health care facility and the types of services provided determine whether laboratory and radiology equipment is needed within the OR suite.

Laboratory

A small laboratory where the pathologist can examine tissue specimens and perform frozen sections expedites the decisions that the surgeon must make during a surgical procedure when a diagnosis is questionable. A refrigerator for storing blood for transfusions also may be located in this room. Tissue specimens may be kept here before they are delivered to the pathology department.

Radiology Services

Special procedure rooms may be outfitted with x-ray and imaging equipment for diagnostic and invasive radiologic procedures or insertion of catheters, pacemakers, and other devices. The walls of these rooms contain lead shields to confine radiation. A darkroom for processing x-ray films usually is available within the OR suite if the volume of procedures warrants it or if the radiology department is not close by.

Work and Storage Areas

Clean and sterile supplies and equipment must be separated from soiled items and trash. If the OR suite has a clean core area, soiled materials should not be taken into this area. They should be taken to the decontamination area for processing and then storage, or to the disposal area. Work and storage areas must be provided for handling all types of supplies and equipment.

Anesthesia Work and Storage Areas

Space must be provided for the storage of anesthesia equipment and supplies. Gas tanks are stored in a well-ventilated area separated from other supplies. Nondisposable items must be thoroughly decontaminated and cleaned after use. A separate workroom usually is provided for care of anesthesia equipment. Dirty and clean supplies must be kept separated. The storage area includes space for drugs and anesthetic agents.

Housekeeping Storage Areas

Cleaning supplies and equipment need to be stored; the equipment used within the restricted area is kept separated from that used to clean the other areas. Therefore more than one storage area may be provided for housekeeping purposes, depending on the design and size of the OR suite. Sinks are provided, as well as shelves for supplies. Trash and soiled laundry receptacles should not be allowed to accumulate in the same room where clean supplies are kept; separate areas should be provided for these. Conveyors or designated elevators may be provided for prompt removal of bags of soiled laundry and trash from the suite.

Central Processing Area

Conveyors, dumbwaiters, or elevators connect the OR suite with a central processing area on another floor of the hospital. If efficient materiel flow can be accomplished, support functions can be removed from the OR suite. Effective communications and a reliable transportation system must be established. Some ORs send all of their instruments and supplies to the sterile processing department for cleaning, packaging, sterilizing, and storing. This system eliminates the need for some work and storage areas within the OR suite, but exchange areas must be provided for carts. The movement of clean and sterile supplies must be kept separate from that of contaminated items and waste by space and traffic patterns.

Case Cart System   Hospitals built or renovated after the mid-1960s provide facilities for a case cart system. Carts are prepared in a remote area and transported to the OR (Figure 10-5). Ideally, the processing department is located directly below or above the OR suite or immediately adjacent to it. Designated clean and contaminated elevators and dumbwaiters connect these respective areas in the two departments. Clean carts of supplies needed for each surgical procedure are delivered to the clean holding area in the OR suite. After use, the cart is taken to the contaminated holding area for return to the decontamination area. Carts may have open or closed shelves. The cart must be enclosed during transport. Some carts are designed to serve as the instrument table during the surgical procedure.

Each case cart should be large enough to hold the supplies, both sterile and nonsterile, for use during, and for cleanup after, one surgical procedure. These supplies are selected according to standard routines and the individual surgeon's preferences. For the system to be efficient, good communication must exist between the staff in the OR and the sterile processing departments. Surgeon's preference cards must be kept up to date. Inventory lists that are supplied with the carts may be used for patient charges and inventory control. A bar code or other computer label system may be used to facilitate these functions.

Utility Room

Some hospitals use a closed-cart system and take contaminated instruments to a central area outside the OR suite for cleanup. Some perform cleanup procedures in the substerile

Figure 10-5   Surgery case cart being loaded for transport to the OR.

room. Many, by virtue of the limitations of the physical facilities, bring the instruments to a utility room. This room contains a washer-sterilizer, sinks, cabinets, and all necessary aids for cleaning. If the washer-sterilizer is a pass-through unit, it opens also into the general workroom, which eliminates the task of physically moving instruments from one room to another.

General Workroom

The general work area should be as centrally located in the OR suite as possible to keep contamination to a minimum. The work area may be divided into a cleaning area and a preparation area. If instruments and equipment from the utility room are received from the pass-through washer-sterilizer into this room, an ultrasonic cleaner should be available here for cleaning instruments that the washer-sterilizer has not adequately cleaned. Otherwise, the ultrasonic cleaner may be in the utility room.

Instrument sets, basin sets, trays, and other supplies are wrapped for sterilization here. The preparation and sterilization of instrument trays and sets in a central room ensures control. This room also contains the stock supply of other items that are packaged for sterilization. The sterilizers that are used in this room may open also into the next room, the sterile supply room. This arrangement helps to eliminate the possibility of mixing sterile and nonsterile items.

Storage

Technology nearly tripled the need for storage space in the 1980s. Many older OR suites have inadequate facilities for storage of sterile supplies, instruments, and bulky equipment. Storage space should fit logically into the design of the suite.

Sterile Supply Room

Most hospitals keep a supply of sterile drapes, sponges, gloves, gowns, and other sterile items ready for use in a sterile supply room within the OR suite. As many shelves as possible should be freestanding from the walls, which permits supplies to be put into one side and removed from the other; thus older packages are always used first. However, small items must be contained in boxes or bins to prevent them from falling to the floor. Inventory levels should be large enough to prevent running out of supplies, yet overstocking of sterile supplies should be avoided. Storage should be arranged to facilitate stock rotation.

The sterile storage area should be adjacent to or as close as possible to the sterilizing area if sterilizing is done in the OR suite. Access to the sterile storage should be limited; it should be separated from high-traffic areas. Humidity should be controlled at 30% to 60%, and temperature should be 65° to 72° F (18° to 22° C). Ten air exchanges per hour are recommended.

Instrument Room

Most hospitals have a separate room or a section of the general workroom designated for storing nonsterile instruments.

The instrument room contains cupboards in which all clean and decontaminated instruments are stored when not in use. Instruments usually are segregated on shelves according to surgical specialty services.

Sets of basic instruments are usually cleaned, assembled, and sterilized after each use. Special instruments such as intestinal clamps, kidney forceps, and bone instruments may be stored after cleaning and decontamination. Sets are then made up according to each day's schedule of surgical procedures.

Storage Room

Some large portable equipment must also be stored in the OR suite, readily accessible for use. A storage room for this equipment, such as the orthopaedic table that may not be used daily, keeps equipment out of corridors when not in use. Lasers and video equipment can be damaged if inadvertently bumped by a passing stretcher in a corridor.

Scrub Room

An enclosed area for surgical scrubbing of hands and arms must be provided adjacent to each OR. Water spills on the floor are particularly hazardous if the scrub area is in a traffic corridor. An enclosed scrub room is a restricted area within the OR suite.

OPERATING ROOM

Each OR is a restricted area because of the need to maintain a controlled environment for sterile and aseptic techniques.

Size

The size of individual ORs varies. In the interest of economy and flexibility, it is desirable to have all ORs the same size, so that they can be used interchangeably to accommodate elective and emergency surgical procedures. Adequate size for a multipurpose procedure room for ambulatory surgery or endoscopy is at least 20 × 20 × 10 feet (6 × 6 × 3 meters), or 400 square feet (approximately 37 m²) of floor space. Larger rooms for cardiac or large procedures are 20 × 30 × 10 feet (600 square feet [approximately 60 m²]).

A room may be designed for a specialty service if use by that service will be high. The room must accommodate equipment, such as lasers, microscopes, or video equipment, that is either fixed (permanently installed) or portable (movable). Portable equipment may require more floor space—a minimum of 22 × 22 × 10 feet (484 square feet [approximately 45 m²]). A specialized room, such as one equipped for cardiopulmonary bypass or trauma, may require as much as 600 square feet (approximately 60 m²) of useful space.

Some rooms are designated for special procedures, such as gastrointestinal endoscopy, interventional radiologic studies, or the application of casts. Other rooms have adjacent areas used for specific purposes, such as visitor viewing galleries, or for installing special equipment, such as monitors.

Substerile Room

A group of two, three, or four ORs may be clustered around a central scrub area, work area, and a small substerile room. Only if the last-mentioned room is immediately adjacent to the OR and separated from the scrub area will it be considered the substerile room throughout this text.

A substerile room adjacent to the OR contains a sink, steam sterilizer, and/or washer-sterilizer. Although cleaning and sterilizing facilities are centralized, either inside or outside of the OR suite, a substerile room with this equipment offers the following advantages:

1. It saves time and steps. The circulator can do emergency cleaning and sterilization of items here. This reduces waiting time for the surgeon, reduces anesthesia time for the patient, and saves steps for the circulator. The circulator, or scrub person, if necessary, can lift sterile articles directly from the sterilizer onto the sterile instrument table without transporting them through a corridor or another area.
2. It reduces the need for a messenger service to obtain sterile instruments and allows the circulator to stay within the room.
3. It allows for better care of instruments and equipment that require special handling. Certain delicate or sensitive instruments, or perhaps a surgeon's personally owned set, usually are not sent out of the OR suite. Only the personnel directly responsible for their use and care handle them; the circulator and scrub person can clean them within the confines of the OR and this adjacent room.
4. The substerile room also usually contains a combination blanket and solution warmer, cabinets for storage, and perhaps a refrigerator for blood and medications. Specimen containers with labels may be conveniently stored in this room. Slips for charges or other records may be kept here. Individual hospitals may find it convenient to keep other items in this room to allow the circulator to remain in or immediately adjacent to the OR during the surgical procedure.

Doors

Ideally, sliding doors should be used in the OR. They eliminate the air currents caused by swinging doors. Microorganisms that have previously settled in the room are disturbed with each swing of the door. The microbial count is usually at its peak at the time of the skin incision because this follows disturbance of air by gowning, draping, movement of personnel, and opening and closing of doors. During the surgical procedure the microbial count rises every time doors swing open from either direction. Also, swinging doors may touch a sterile table or person. The risk of catching hands, equipment cords, or other supplies is increased.

Sliding doors should not recede into the wall but should be of the surface-sliding type. Fire regulations mandate that sliding doors for ORs be of the type that can be swung open if necessary. Doors do not remain open either during or between surgical procedures. Closed doors decrease the mixing of air within the OR with that in the corridors, which may contain higher microbial counts. Air pressure in the room also is disrupted if the doors remain open.

Ventilation

The OR ventilation system must ensure a controlled supply of filtered air. Air changes and circulation provide fresh air and prevent accumulation of anesthetic gases in the room. Concentration of gases is dependent solely on the proportion of pure air entering the air system to the air being recirculated through the system. Fifteen air exchanges per hour with three exchanges of fresh air are recommended for rooms with recirculated air. Some state building codes require 100% fresh air; others permit up to 80% recirculation of air. If air is recirculated, a gas scavenger system is mandatory to prevent the buildup of waste anesthetic gases. Various types of scavengers and evacuators are used to minimize air pollutants that are health risks for perioperative team members.

Ultraclean laminar airflow is installed in some ORs to provide up to 600 air exchanges per hour. This high-flow unidirectional air-blowing system is housed in a wall or ceiling enclosure. The airflow can be vertical or horizontal. The value of this system in reducing airborne contamination is inconclusive. Other types of filtered air-delivery systems that have a high rate of airflow are as effective in controlling airborne contamination. Filtration through high-efficiency particulate air (HEPA) filters can be 99.7% efficient in removing particles that are larger than 0.3 μm. These microbial filters in ducts filter the air, practically eliminating all dust particles. The ventilating system in the OR suite is separate from the hospital's general system and is to be cleaned, inspected, and maintained on a regular schedule.

Positive air pressures (0.005 inch [0.013 cm] of water pressure) of 10% in each OR is greater than that in corridors, scrub areas, and substerile rooms. Positive pressure forces air from the room. The inlet is at the ceiling. Air leaves through the outlets at floor level. If the reverse is true, air is drawn into the room around the doors and through open doors. Microorganisms in the air can enter the room unless positive pressure is maintained. Closed doors maintain this environment and prevent equalization of air pressure.

An air-conditioning system controls humidity. High relative humidity (weight of water vapor present) should be maintained between 50% and 60%. A relative humidity of not less than 50% to 55% is required. Moisture provides a relatively conductive medium, allowing static charge to leak to earth as fast as it is generated; sparks form more readily in atmospheres of low humidity.

Room temperature is maintained within a range of 68° to 75° F (20° to 24° C). A thermostat to control room temperature can be advantageous to meet patient needs: for example, the temperature can be increased to prevent development of hypothermia in pediatric, geriatric, or burn patients. Over-manipulation of controls can result in calibration problems. Controls should not be adjusted solely for the comfort of team members; patient normothermia is a strong consideration. Only the maintenance department can regulate temperature in some OR suites.

Even with controls of humidity and temperature, air-conditioning units may be a source of microorganisms that come through the filters. The filters are changed at regular intervals. Ducts must be cleaned regularly.

Floors

In the past, floors were conductive enough to dissipate static from equipment and personnel but not conductive enough to endanger personnel from shock or cause explosions from flammable anesthetic gases. Conductivity is not a prime concern in OR design because explosive anesthetic gases are no longer used. Flooring is available in many materials suitable for ORs, including asphalt tile, linoleum, and terrazzo. The most common flooring used today is seamless vinyl. These materials degrade with age and cleaning.

A variety of hard plastic, seamless materials are used for minor procedure room floors. The surface of all floors must not be porous but suitably hard for cleaning by the flooding, wet-vacuuming technique. Personnel fatigue may be related to the type of flooring, which can be too hard or too soft. Cushioned flooring is available.

Walls and Ceiling

Finishes of all surface materials should be hard, nonporous, fire resistant, waterproof, stain proof, seamless, nonreflective, and easy to clean. The ceiling should be a minimum of 10 feet (3 m) and may have acoustic, soundproof tiles. The height of the ceiling will depend on the amount and types of ceiling mounted equipment.

Wall paneling made of hard vinyl materials is easy to clean and maintain. Seams can be sealed by a plastic filler. Laminated polyester or smooth, painted plaster provides a seamless wall; epoxy paint has a tendency to flake or chip. Dust and microorganisms can collect between tiles because the mortar between them is not smooth. Most grout lines, including those made of latex, are porous enough to harbor microorganisms even after cleaning. Tiles can also crack and break. A material that is able to withstand considerable impact also may have some value in noise control. Stainless steel cuffs at collision corners help prevent damage.

Walls and ceilings often are used to mount devices, utilities, and equipment in an effort to reduce clutter on the floor. In addition to the overhead operating light, the ceiling may be used for mounting an anesthesia service core, operating microscope, cryosurgery device, x-ray tube and image intensifier, electronic monitor, closed-circuit television monitor and camera, and a variety of hooks, poles, and tubes. Demands for ceiling-mounted equipment are diversified. Suspended track mounts are not recommended because they engender fallout of dust-carrying microorganisms each time they are moved. If movable or track ceiling devices are installed, they should not be mounted directly over the operating bed but away from the center of the room and preferably recessed into the ceiling to minimize the possibility of dust accumulation and fallout.

Piped-In and Electrical Systems

Vacuum for suction, compressed air, oxygen, and/or nitrous oxide may be piped into the OR. The outlets may be located on the wall or suspended from the ceiling in either a fixed or retractable column. The anesthesia provider needs at least two outlets for oxygen and suction and one for nitrous oxide. To protect other rooms, the supply of oxygen and nitrous oxide to any room can be shut off at control panels in the corridor should trouble occur in a particular line. A panel light comes on, and a buzzer sounds in the room and in the maintenance department. The buzzer can be turned off, but the panel light stays on until the problem is corrected.

Electrical outlets must meet the requirements of the equipment that will be used. Some machines require 220-volt power lines; others operate on 110 volts. Permanently mounted fixtures, such as a clock and x-ray viewing boxes, can be recessed into walls and wired rather than plugged into outlets. Outlets suspended from the ceiling should have locking plugs to prevent accidental disconnection. Grounded wall outlets are installed above the 5-foot (1.5 m) level unless explosion-proof plugs are used. Electrical cords that extend down the wall and/or across the floor are hazardous. Straight or curved ceiling-mounted tracks are satisfactory for bringing piped-in gases, vacuums, and electrical outlets close to the operating bed. They eliminate the hazard of tripping over cords, but insulation materials around electrical power sources from mobile, ceiling-mounted tracks must be protected from repeated flexing to prevent cracks and damage to wires. Rigid or retractable ceiling service columns eliminate these hazards.

Multiple electrical outlets should be available from separate circuits. This minimizes the possibility of a blown fuse or a faulty circuit shutting off all electricity at a critical moment.

All personnel must be aware that the use of electricity introduces the hazards of electric shock, power failure, and fire. Faulty electrical equipment may cause a short circuit or the electrocution of patients or personnel. These hazards can be prevented by taking the following precautions:

1. Use only electrical equipment designed and approved for use in the OR. Equipment must have cords of adequate length and adequate current-carrying capacity to avoid overloading.
2. Test portable equipment immediately before use and ground correctly.
3. Discontinue use immediately and report any faulty electrical equipment.

Fire safety systems are installed throughout the hospital. All personnel must know the fire rules. They must be familiar with the location of the alarm box and the use of fire extinguishers.

Lighting

General illumination is furnished by ceiling lights. Most room lights are white fluorescent but may be incandescent. Recessed lights do not collect dust. Lighting should be evenly distributed throughout the room. The anesthesia provider must have sufficient light, at least 200 foot-candles, to adequately evaluate the patient's color.

To minimize eye fatigue, the ratio of intensity of general room lighting to that at the surgical site should not exceed 1:5, preferably 1:3. This contrast should be maintained in corridors and scrub areas, as well as in the room itself, so that the surgeon becomes accustomed to the light before entering the sterile field. Color and hue of the lights also should be consistent.

Illumination of the surgical site is dependent on the quality of light from an overhead source and the reflection from the drapes and tissues. White, glistening tissues need less light than dull, dark tissues. Light must be of such quality that the pathologic conditions are recognizable. The overhead operating light must:

1. Make an intense light, within a range of 2500 to 12,500 foot-candles (27,000 to 127,000 lux), into the incision without glare on the surface. It must give contrast to the depth and relationship of all anatomic structures. The light may be equipped with an intensity control. The surgeon will ask for more light when needed. A reserve light should be available.
2. Provide a diameter light pattern and focus appropriate for the size of the incision. An optical prism system has a fixed diameter and focus. Other types have adjustable controls mounted on the fixture. Most fixtures provide focused depth by refracting light to illuminate both the body cavity and the general operating field. The focal point is where illumination is greatest. It should avoid a dark center at the surgical site. A 10- to 12-inch (25 to 30 cm) depth of focus allows the intensity to be relatively equal at both the surface and depth of the incision. To avoid glare, a circular field of 20 inches (25 cm) in diameter provides a 2-inch (5-cm) zone of maximum intensity in the center of the field with 20% intensity at the periphery.
3. Be shadowless. Multiple light sources and/or reflectors decrease shadows. In some units the relationship is fixed; others have separately maneuverable sources to direct light beams from converging angles.
4. Produce the blue-white color of daylight. Color quality of normal or diseased tissues is maintained within a spectral energy range of 3500° to 6700° Kelvin (K). Most surgeons prefer a color temperature of about 5000° K, which approximates the white light of a cloudless sky at noon.
5. Be freely adjustable to any position or angle by either a vertical or horizontal range of motion. Most overhead operating lights are ceiling mounted on mobile fixtures. Some have dual lights or dual tracks with sources on each track. These are designed for both lights to be used simultaneously to provide adequate intensity and minimize shadows in a single incision. Many fixtures are adapted so that the surgeon can direct the beam by manipulating sterile handles attached to the lamp or by remote control at the sterile field. Automatic positioning facilitates adjustment, and braking mechanisms prevent drift (i.e., a movement away from the desired position). Fixtures should be manipulated as little as possible to minimize dispersion of dust over the sterile field.
6. Produce a minimum of heat to prevent injuring exposed tissues. Most overhead lights dissipate heat into the room, where it is cooled by the air-conditioning system. Halogen bulbs generate less heat than other types. Lamps should produce less than 25,000 μW/cm^2 of radiant energy. If multiple light sources are used, collectively they must not exceed this limit at a single site. Beyond this range, the radiant energy produced by infrared rays changes to heat at or near the surface of exposed tissues. A filter globe absorbs some infrared and heat waves over the lightbulb or by an infrared cylindric absorption filter of a prism optical system.
7. Be easily cleaned. Tracks recessed within the ceiling virtually eliminate dust accumulation. Suspension-mounted tracks or a centrally mounted fixture must have smooth surfaces that are easily accessible for cleaning.

An auxiliary light may be needed for a secondary surgical site. Some hospitals have portable explosion-proof lights. Others have satellite units that are part of the overhead lighting fixture. These should only be used for secondary sites unless the manufacturer states that the additional intensity is within safe radiant energy levels when used in conjunction with the main light source.

A source of light from a circuit separate from the usual supply must be available for use in case of power failure. This may require a separate emergency spotlight. It is best if the operating light is equipped so that an automatic switch can be made to the emergency source of lighting when the usual power fails.

Some surgeons prefer to work in a darkened room with only stark illumination of the surgical site. This is particularly true of surgeons working with endoscopic instruments and the operating microscope. If the room has windows, lightproof shades may be drawn to darken the room when this equipment is in use. Because of the hazard of dust fallout from shades, the windows may be painted in rooms where this equipment is routinely used. Even though the surgeon prefers the room darkened, the circulator or anesthesia provider must be able to see adequately to observe the patient's color and to monitor his or her condition. A grazing light over the floor can be installed.

Some surgeons wear a headlight designed to focus a light beam on a specific small area, usually in a recessed body cavity such as the nasopharynx. Fiberoptic headlights produce a cool light and reduce shadows. Both the surgeon and first assistant may wear a headlight. Alternatively, a light source that is an integral part of a sterile instrument, such as a lighted retractor or fiberoptic cable, may be used to illuminate deep cavities or tissues difficult to see with only the overhead operating light.

X-Ray Viewing Boxes

X-ray viewing boxes can be recessed into the wall. The viewing surface should accommodate standard-size films. The best location is in the line of vision of the surgeon standing at the operating bed. Lights for x-ray viewers should be of high intensity.

Clock

A time-elapsed clock, which incorporates a warning signal, is useful for indicating that one or more predetermined periods of time have passed. This may be used during surgical procedures for total arterial occlusion, when using perfusion techniques or a pneumatic tourniquet, or during cardiac arrest.

Cabinets or Carts

Each OR may be supplied with cabinets unless a cart system or pass-through entry is used. Supplies for the types of surgical procedures done in that room are stocked, or every OR may be stocked with a standard number and type of supplies. Having these supplies saves steps for the circulator and helps to eliminate traffic in and out of the OR. Glass shelves and sliding doors provide ease in finding and taking out items. Many cabinets are made of stainless steel or hard plastic. Wire shelving minimizes dust accumulation. Cabinets must be easy to clean. One cabinet in the room may have a pegboard at the back to hang items, such as table appliances.

Pass-through cabinets that circulate clean air through them while maintaining positive air room pressure allow transfer of supplies from outside the OR to inside it. They help ensure the rotation of supplies in storage or can be used only for passing supplies as needed from a clean center core. Some pass-through cabinets between the OR and a corridor accommodate supply carts directly from the sterile core, which are easily removable for restocking.

In lieu of or as an adjunct to cabinets, some hospitals stock carts with special sutures, instruments, drugs, and other items for some or all of the surgical specialties. The appropriate cart is brought to the room for a specific surgical procedure.

Furniture and Other Equipment

Stainless steel furniture is plain, durable, and easily cleaned. Each OR is equipped with the following:

- Operating bed with a mattress covered with an impervious surface, attachments for positioning the patient, and armboards.
- Instrument tables.
- Mayo stand. The Mayo stand is a frame with a removable rectangular stainless steel tray. The frame slides under the operating bed and over the sterile field. The tray serves to bring near the surgical field a supply of instruments that are used frequently during the surgical procedure.
- Small tables for gowns and gloves and/or the patient's preparation equipment.
- Ring stand for basin(s). This is optional because most ORs do not use splash basins.
- Anesthesia machine and table for anesthesia provider's equipment.
- Sitting stools and standing platforms.
- IV poles for IV solution bags.
- Suction canisters, preferably portable on a wheeled base.
- Laundry hamper frame.
- Kick buckets in wheeled bases.
- Wastebasket.
- Writing surface. This may be a wall-mounted, stainless steel desk or an area built into a cabinet for the circulator to document in the records.

Communication Systems

A communication system is a vital link to summon routine or emergency assistance or to relay information to and from the OR team. Many OR suites are equipped with telephones, intercoms, call-lights, video equipment, and computers. These communication systems may connect the OR with the clerk-receptionist's desk, the nurse manager's office, the holding area, the family waiting room, the PACU, the pathology and radiology departments, the blood bank, and the sterile processing department. These systems make instantaneous consultation possible through direct communication.

Voice Intercommunication System

Either monodirectional or bidirectional voice systems, via telephone or an intercommunication (intercom) system, are useful devices for the OR team but are potentially hazardous for the patient. Sounds are distorted to the patient in early stages of general anesthesia. Incoming calls over an intercom should not be permitted to disturb the patient at this time. Also, an awake patient should not receive traumatic information about a pathologic diagnosis (e.g., from a strange voice coming through an intercom speaker box after a biopsy has been performed). Installing any type of intercom equipment either in the adjacent substerile room or scrub area rather than in the OR helps to eliminate sounds that could disturb both the patient and the surgeon.

Call-Light System

In addition to or instead of a voice system, a call-light system can summon assistance from the anesthesia staff, pathologist, patient care staff, and/or housekeeping personnel. Activated in the OR by a foot- or hand-operated switch, a light alerts personnel at a central point in the suite or displays at several receiving points simultaneously.

Closed-Circuit Television

Television surveillance is an easy way for the nurse manager to keep abreast of activities in each OR. By means of a black-and-white or color video camera with a wide-angle lens mounted high in the corner of each OR, the manager may make rounds simply by switching from one room to another by pushing buttons at his or her desk and viewing a monitor in the office.

More commonly, television monitors serve a number of useful purposes for the surgeon in the OR. They are widely used for teaching surgical techniques. This keeps visitors out of the OR, which, in the interest of sterile technique, is advantageous. In addition, monitors provide a better view for more persons to see the surgical procedure from a remote area or through a microscope or endoscope. They can also be used for record keeping and documentation for legal purposes for the surgeon. Video recording is possible for this purpose.

As an aid to diagnosis, an audio-video hookup between the OR and the x-ray department permits x-ray films to be viewed on the television screen in the OR without having to be transported into the OR and mounted on viewing boxes. With such a hookup, the surgeon gains the advantage of remote interpretive consultation when it is desired.

A two-way audio-video system between the frozen-section laboratory and the OR enables the surgeon to examine the microscopic slide by video in consultation with the pathologist without leaving the operating bed. The pathologist can view the site of the pathologic lesion without entering the OR.

For these purposes the color television camera may be mounted over the operating bed in one of a number of ways. Usually it is attached to the stem of the operating light and outfitted with detachable sterilizable handles. An operating light with a television camera mounted in the center is available.

Video screens usually are adapted television sets and may be wall mounted or placed on floor stands that can be moved readily. All pieces of television equipment must be labeled to indicate that they comply with applicable electrical safety regulations for use in the OR. They also must be encased in nonporous materials that can be easily cleaned.

Computers

A computer terminal in each OR affords access to information and allows data input by the circulator. The type of hardware and software programs available dictates the capabilities of the automated information system. A keyboard, light pen, and/or bar code scanner may be used for input. The computer processes and stores information for retrieval on the viewing monitor and by printout from a central processing unit. The computer database helps the circulator to obtain and enter information that may include the following:

- Schedule, including the patient's name, surgeon, procedure, special or unusual equipment requirements, wound classification, elective or emergency procedure

- Preoperative patient assessment data, nursing diagnoses, expected outcomes, and plan of care
- Results of laboratory and diagnostic tests
- Surgeon's preference card with capability to update
- Inventory of supplies and equipment provided and used
- Charges for direct patient billing
- Intraoperative nursing interventions
- Timing parameters, including anesthesia, procedure, and room turnover
- Incident reports
- Postoperative care in the PACU

The computer terminal may be mounted on the wall or placed on a shelf or a portable table or cart. The computer keyboard can be moved so that the circulator can see the patient and the activities of the OR team while documenting intraoperative information, electronically, into the record. The computerized patient information that is generated in the OR may interface with the hospital-wide computer system.

Monitoring Equipment

Monitors and computers are designed to keep the OR team aware of the physiologic functions of the patient throughout the surgical procedure and to record patient data. The anesthesia provider or a perioperative nurse uses monitoring devices as an added means to ensure safety for the patient during the surgical procedure.

In some hospitals a central room may be set up to monitor all patients undergoing surgical procedures. More frequently, the monitors are housed in a room immediately adjacent to the OR, separated by a glass partition. These rooms are staffed by well-trained personnel who are familiar with the types of monitoring or computerized equipment in use. Documentation from computerized monitors becomes a part of the patient's medical record.

SPECIAL PROCEDURE ROOMS

Certain procedures or outpatient treatments may indicate the need for rooms designed for a specific purpose, such as cardiac catheterization, endoscopy, or cystoscopy. These rooms are designed with equipment for performing the specific interventional procedures, including specialized radiologic and monitoring devices. A radiologist and several endoscopists should be consulted when planning these types of facilities.

Cardiac Catheterization Room

Cardiac catheterization may be performed within the OR suite in a room equipped for fluoroscopy. Imaging screens are located near the head of the operating bed to allow the surgeon and the team to visualize the coronary arteries during the procedure. Monitors, suction, oxygen, and cardiopulmonary resuscitation equipment are available in this room for each cardiac catheterization procedure. The team must be alert for emergency situations, such as a perforated coronary artery, and be prepared for an emergency thoracotomy or transfer to an OR for an open procedure.

Endoscopy Room

Many OR suites have a designated room in which endoscopic procedures, such as bronchoscopy, are performed. Most are equipped for the use of lasers and electrosurgery. Some endoscopy rooms have x-ray and video capabilities. Some specialized equipment can be mounted from ceiling booms and is not portable between rooms.

Cystoscopy Room

A cystoscopy room may be available for a urologic endoscopic examination or procedure. Older cystoscopy rooms may be equipped with special floor drains for the disposal of fluids during the procedure. Modern styles have eliminated this drain for infection control reasons. Waste fluids are collected in special canisters and are disposed of like other biologically contaminated fluids. It is also equipped with x-ray and fluoroscopy machines because many procedures require the use of ra-

diopaque contrast media to visualize the kidneys, ureters, and bladder. Imaging screens are located in the room to allow the urologist to visualize the urologic structures during fluoroscopy. Some urologists use ultrasonic equipment, lasers, and electrosurgery to perform minimally invasive procedures.

Bibliography

American Institute of Architects Committee on Architecture for Health in conjunction with Department of Health and Human Services: *Guidelines for construction and equipment of hospital and medical facilities,* Washington, DC, 1997, AIA Press.

Centers for Disease Control and Prevention: *Guidelines for prevention of surgical wound infection,* Atlanta, 1998, The Centers.

Friberg B: Ultraclean laminar airflow ORs, *AORN J* 67(4):841-851, 1998.

Gregory MM: OR director, staff member input on OR architecture design, *AORN J* 66(6):1089-1091, 1997.

Groah L: *Perioperative nursing,* ed 3, Stamford, Conn, 1996, Appleton & Lange.

Johnson LC, Zeil SE: Environmental laws and the perioperative setting, *AORN J* 63(3):645-647, 1996.

Laufman H: *Hospital special care facilities: planning for user needs,* New York, Academic Press, 1981.

Streifel AJ: Hospital air quality monitoring for infection control, *Infect Control Today* 2(9):40, 42-43, 1998.

Chapter 11

Ambulatory Surgery

 Chapter Objectives

After studying this chapter, the learner will be able to:

- Compare the differences between hospital-based services and ambulatory surgery centers.
- Compare the flow of patient care between ambulatory status and full admission status.
- Identify eligibility criteria for ambulatory surgery patients.
- Compare the advantages and disadvantages of ambulatory surgery.
- Discuss the importance of postoperative teaching for ambulatory surgery patients.

Ambulatory surgery may be defined as surgical patient care performed under general, regional, or local anesthesia without overnight hospitalization. Some ambulatory facilities offer diagnostic testing and radiologic examinations, such as mammography.

HISTORICAL BACKGROUND

The concept of ambulatory surgery is not new but can be traced back to Egypt in 3000 BC. Simple surgical procedures have been performed in physicians' offices for years. The first ambulatory surgery facility was opened in 1970 in Arizona. The concept gained widespread acceptance and was endorsed by the American Medical Association (AMA). Ambulatory surgery became acceptable for both local and general anesthesia with select patients, and in 1973 guidelines provided by the American Society of Anesthesiologists strengthened the premise of same-day procedures.

In the early 1980s, changes in Medicare reimbursement policies motivated surgeons in all specialties to develop and refine surgical procedures for ambulatory settings. It was then that Medicare and Medicaid began to reimburse inpatient procedures from diagnosis-related group (DRG) codes while

continuing to reimburse at cost for approved outpatient or ambulatory procedures. For both patients and insurance providers, a cost savings is realized when the patient goes home after a short recovery period.

Shorter, less invasive surgical procedures that only minimally curtail physiologic functions and allow for rapid return to function are well suited to ambulatory surgery. The number of surgical procedures performed as ambulatory or outpatient procedures increases each year, with more than 11 million such procedures performed in 1990. Results of the 1995 National Survey of Ambulatory Surgery, which was conducted by the National Center for Health Statistics, showed that an estimated 29.4 million ambulatory surgical procedures were performed in hospitals and freestanding outpatient centers yearly (Table 11-1). More statistical information is available at the Web site for the Centers for Disease Control and Prevention (**www.cdc.gov**). The Web site of the Federated Ambulatory Surgery Association (**www.fasa.org**) lists pertinent historical events and the progress of the ambulatory surgery movement.

Other factors resulting in the increased use of ambulatory procedures are the development of improved fiberoptics and flexible endoscopes, regional anesthetic techniques, im-

161

TABLE 11-1	Procedures Performed in Ambulatory Settings by Body System	
Yearly Outpatient Surgical Procedures by Body System		**Surgeries Reported (in millions)**
Nervous system		0.98
Eyes		4.60
Ears		0.87
Nose, mouth		2.00
Respiratory system		0.34
Cardiovascular system		0.69
Digestive system		6.20
Urinary system		1.40
Female reproductive system		2.10
Musculoskeletal system		3.70
Integumentary system		2.80
TOTAL PROCEDURES		**28.30**

Data from the National Center for Health Statistics, Centers for Disease Control and Prevention, 1994. Retrieved on-line through FASTATS at **www.cdc.gov**.

Box 11-1

Terms Associated with Ambulatory Surgery

ambulatory care   Care delivered to a patient who is not confined to bed or in need of formal admission to a facility for a prolonged period of time.

monitoring   Clinical observation of a patient's condition and vital signs through continuous interpretation of vital signs, activities, and responses.

PAT center   Area of a facility designated for patient assessment and preadmission examination.

proved monitoring, and the development of short-acting preoperative medications, anesthetic agents, and narcotics. Changes in minimally invasive technologies have made many relatively complex surgical procedures amenable to ambulatory surgery. Ambulatory surgery is cost-effective, convenient, and efficient while remaining consistent with the same standards of care followed for hospitalized surgical patients. Patients have a right to expect comprehensive perioperative care from an ambulatory care facility. The risks, anxiety, and fears associated with a surgical procedure are not eliminated just because the setting is different or because advanced instrumentation is used. Terms pertaining to ambulatory surgical procedures are defined in Box 11-1.

AORN, the Association of periOperative Registered Nurses, has established a specialty assembly for nurses who practice in the ambulatory setting. A chairperson and council are selected by the assembly membership to serve 3-year terms. The Ambulatory Surgery Specialty Assembly publishes a quarterly newsletter in which to share information related to caring for same-day-surgery patients.

AMBULATORY SURGERY FACILITIES

Various terms are used to describe ambulatory care facilities, including outpatient surgery, same-day surgical unit, day surgery, or ambulatory surgery center. Conceptually, an ambulatory facility has the following:

- Preoperative testing and assessment area (PAT center)
- Admitting area
- Changing and dressing room with lockers and toilets
- Preoperative holding/preparation area
- Operating room (OR)
- Postanesthesia care unit (PACU) (or access to a PACU)
- Family waiting room

The decor of the ambulatory facility should be pleasing to enhance relaxation of the patient and family. Recliners are commonly available for postprocedural recovery. Many facilities have televisions with videocassette capability.

Priority patient parking areas should be conveniently located near the entrance to the facility, with parking spaces for disabled patients located nearest the entrance. Many hospital-based ambulatory facilities offer valet parking. The convenience of dropping off and picking up patients should considered in the design of the facility. Space requirements for parking areas are determined by the number and types of surgical procedures to be performed.

The location of an ambulatory surgery facility may vary. Examples of ambulatory surgery facilities include the following:

- *Hospital-based dedicated unit.* Patients come to a self-contained unit that is located within or attached to the hospital but physically separate from the inpatient OR suite.
- *Hospital-based integrated unit.* Ambulatory patients share the same OR suite and other hospital facilities with inpatients. The preoperative admission and holding area is shared. Ambulatory patients usually return to the same admission area for discharge after the procedure.
- *Hospital-affiliated satellite surgery center.* Patients come to an ambulatory surgery center that is owned and operated by a larger facility but geographically separate from it.
- *Freestanding ambulatory surgery center.* Patients come to a completely independent facility. Many of these facilities are owned and operated by physicians.
- *Office-based center.* Patients come to a physician's office that is equipped for surgery. Many private surgeons, dermatologists, periodontists, and podiatrists perform surgical procedures in their offices using a local anesthetic. This office-based center may accommodate one or more surgeons in the same specialty, or it may be a multiphysician, interdisciplinary clinic.

In addition to obtaining a state license and certificate of approval, an ambulatory care facility should comply with standards set by the Accreditation Association for Ambulatory Health Care (AAAHC) and the Joint Commission on Accreditation of Healthcare Organizations (JCAHO). Patient advocacy and consumer groups advise patients to select facilities carefully and to look for accreditation and credentialing by professional and governmental agencies. Accreditation and credentialing of a facility can be attained by, but is not limited to, the following:

- Compliance with structural standards
- Establishment of policies and procedures that support competent standards of care
- Appropriate credentialing of personnel
- Emergency preparedness
- Appropriateness of procedures performed at the facility

If complications develop (e.g., adverse reactions to an anesthetic), the patient may need to be admitted to a hospital for intensive care monitoring. Therefore freestanding ambulatory surgery centers and office-based centers need to have a patient transfer/admission agreement with a nearby hospital.

Freestanding recovery care centers have been developed to accommodate a 24- to 48-hour uncomplicated postanesthesia recovery period. Although they occur infrequently, the most common reasons for admission to a freestanding recovery care center or hospital after ambulatory surgery are pain, nausea and vomiting, urinary retention, and concern for wound integrity.

Approximately 65% of all surgical procedures are performed on an ambulatory basis safely and without complications. Some smaller facilities limit the use of ambulatory surgery to procedures that can be performed with local or regional block anesthetics. Facilities with PACU capability allow surgeons to perform procedures with the patient under general anesthesia. Although procedures performed in an ambulatory care facility are usually of short duration (15 to 90 minutes), the appropriate selection and evaluation of patients is essential. Nursing care and anesthesia management also are crucial factors in the experience of the ambulatory surgical patient.

THE AMBULATORY SURGICAL PATIENT

After a surgical procedure, many patients prefer to recuperate at home rather than in the hospital. These patients may be candidates for ambulatory surgery, depending on the nature and extent of the surgical procedure and on the patient's ability to follow instructions or to receive adequate care at home. Consideration is given to the duration and complexity of the surgical procedure, the risk of anesthesia, and the probability of postoperative complications. For select ambulatory surgery patients, arrangements for postoperative care can be made with a private home health agency. Several types of home/hotel-like facilities provide care for up to 72 hours after surgery. A hospital short-stay unit may provide postoperative care for observation and pain control for a 23-hour stay.

Patient Selection for Ambulatory Surgery

Patients are carefully screened before being considered safe candidates for ambulatory surgery. Criteria considered may include, but are not limited to, the following:

1. *General health status.* Acceptable patients are in class I, II, or stable III of the physical status classification of the American Society of Anesthesiologists (ASA). Patients are evaluated physically and emotionally to determine the possibility of complications during or after the surgical procedure. This evaluation includes a complete medical history, physical examination, and preanesthesia evaluation.
2. *Results of preoperative tests.* Patients may have tests on admission the morning of the surgical procedure, but preferably these tests are performed before the scheduled surgery date so the results can be evaluated. This prevents cancellation on the day of surgery if test results are unsatisfactory. Test results are placed on the chart that accompanies the patient to the OR. Preoperative tests may include the following:
   a. Complete blood count (CBC) and urinalysis—usually included in laboratory tests.
   b. Pregnancy test.
   c. Multichemistry profile for higher risk patients.
   d. Chest x-ray—may be required if clinically indicated.
   e. Electrocardiogram (ECG) may be required before general anesthesia for patients over 35 or 40 years of age.
3. *Willingness and psychologic acceptance by patient and family.* The patient should be willing and able to recuperate at home. Some patients lack adequate home care.

Each patient is individually assessed. Provision is made for competent care at home either by an agency or the patient's family. Compliance with preoperative and postoperative instructions by the patient and the availability of a responsible adult support person are essential factors. Other factors to consider when screening a patient for possible ambulatory surgery include the following:

- *Recovery period.* The surgeon should anticipate minimal or no postoperative complications. Patients in whom a prolonged period of nausea and vomiting is anticipated or in whom pain will not be relieved by oral analgesics are not ideal candidates for ambulatory surgery.
- *Reimbursement sources.* Most third-party payers prefer less costly ambulatory surgery whenever a procedure can be safely performed in this setting. Patient safety and quality of care depend on patient screening and support systems.

Preoperative Patient Instructions

Written instructions for both preoperative and postoperative care are given to the patient by the surgeon during an office visit or by the nurse during a preadmission visit to the ambulatory care facility. These instructions describe the admission, preoperative, intraoperative, recovery, and discharge procedures, and they should be written in a language the patient can understand. To protect both the surgeon and the facility, the patient should sign for receipt of these instructions and should sign that informed consent has been given for the intended surgical procedure. Instructions should include the following:

1. Preoperative instructions.
   a. Make an appointment for preadmission assessment and testing.
   b. Take nothing by mouth after midnight (or other specified hour) before admission unless ordered to do so by the surgeon. This includes medications, unless ordered.
   c. Perform any necessary physical preparation such as an enema or bathing with antimicrobial soap as ordered.
   d. Arrive at the facility by _____ AM/PM. (Time will depend on the scheduled time for the surgical procedure. A minimal wait at the facility helps to reduce preoperative anxiety. Patients are usually admitted at least 1 hour before the scheduled time of their surgical procedure.)
   e. Notify the surgeon immediately of a change in physical condition, such as a cold or fever.
   f. Wear loose and comfortable clothing, leave jewelry and valuables at home, and remove makeup and nail polish. (This may include the removal of acrylic fingernails for some procedures.)
2. Postoperative instructions.
   a. Arrange for a responsible adult support person to take you home. (After some procedures, the patient may not be permitted to drive or leave unattended.)
   b. Do not ingest alcoholic beverages, drive a car, cook, or operate machinery for 24 hours if a sedative or general anesthetic has been administered.
   c. Delay important decision making until full recovery is attained.
   d. Take medications only as prescribed, and maintain as regular a diet as tolerated.
   e. Shower or bathe daily unless instructed otherwise. This helps to relieve muscle tension and discomfort and keeps the wound clean.
   f. Call the surgeon if postoperative problems arise.
   g. Report to the nearest emergency department if your condition deteriorates.
   h. Keep follow-up appointment with the surgeon.

The patient should be reminded that the postoperative information will be reinforced and possibly updated at the time of discharge. The patient's level of understanding of the preoperative instructions and planned procedure is assessed by a telephone call from the perioperative nurse to the patient the day before surgery; at this time, the scheduled date and arrival time are also verified. The patient should be reassured that he or she will be given a written set of instructions before discharge from the facility.

INTRAOPERATIVE PATIENT CARE

Intraoperatively, the same precautions are observed by all team members as for any surgical procedure. These include strict adherence to the principles of aseptic and sterile techniques and other OR routines. Consideration for patient privacy and avoidance of embarrassment are essential.

The careful selection of patients, preoperative evaluation, and instructions help prevent complications from the anesthetic. Premedication, if given, is minimal. The surgical procedure should be less than 90 minutes in duration for general anesthesia and less than 3 hours for regional block. Local anesthesia or a regional block is preferable if appropriate. Spinal anesthesia is seldom used.

Cardiopulmonary resuscitation (CPR) equipment and nurses certified in CPR at a minimum level of basic cardiac life support (BCLS) should be available during the procedure (certification in advanced cardiac life support [ACLS] is preferred). Perioperative nurses specializing in the care of pediatric patients should have certification in pediatric advanced life support (PALS).

Patients who undergo general anesthesia or intravenous conscious sedation (IVCS) are scheduled for surgery early in the day; this allows for a maximum recovery time. Rapidly dissipating agents are administered, and various combinations of agents and drugs are used. Drugs associated with prolonged recovery are avoided unless there is a specific indication for their use. Doses of IV agents, such as narcotics and barbiturates, may be reduced to avoid delayed emergence. Newer technology, including Bispectral Analysis (BIS monitoring), allows the anesthesia provider to administer minimal amounts of an agent based on the patient's level of consciousness and sensorium. Anesthetic techniques should provide adequate depth of anesthesia but with minimal cardiorespiratory changes and side effects. Indications for endotracheal intubation are the same as for inpatients.

The patient who is undergoing local anesthesia is monitored continuously for any reaction to the medications and/or a change in physiologic status. If an anesthesia provider is not in attendance, a qualified perioperative nurse should be assigned to monitor the patient for behavioral and physiologic changes. This nurse should have a basic knowledge of the function and use of monitoring equipment and should not be assigned other duties while monitoring the patient's condition. This nurse measures and records the patient's vital signs before the injection of a local or regional block anesthetic or analgesic and every 15 minutes thereafter, monitors physiologic status according to written policy and procedure, and in-

Box 11-2	Monitoring Equipment Used for Local Anesthesia Patients

Electrocardiograph
Pulse oximeter
Blood pressure apparatus

Box 11-3	Discharge Criteria for Ambulatory Patients

Alert and oriented
Stable vital signs in comparison to baseline
No respiratory distress, hoarseness, or croupy cough
Able to void as appropriate
No dizziness or loss of sensorium
No nausea or vomiting
No active bleeding and no or minimal swelling or drainage on dressings
Able to tolerate oral fluids
No excessive pain that will not be alleviated with oral medications at home
Able to ambulate per developmental age or per physical limitations
Capable of self-care or accompanied by responsible adult
Appropriate mode of transportation

stitutes emergency measures if an adverse reaction occurs. This nurse should be responsible for interpreting, identifying, and reporting abnormal readings to the surgeon. Additional functions of this nurse may include starting oxygen, administering IV therapy, or giving medications when clinically indicated. Suggested intraoperative monitoring methods for patients undergoing local anesthesia are listed in Box 11-2.

The policies and procedures for monitoring patients undergoing local anesthesia should include patient risk criteria, the type of monitoring to be used, and interventions within the scope of nursing practice. All pertinent data and therapy are documented according to the policies of the facility.

The awake and alert patient needs to receive physical and emotional comfort throughout the surgical procedure. The field of vision may be small while the patient is draped, and tactile and other stimuli will come as a surprise if he or she is not forewarned. The patient should be told what is about to occur (e.g., "You will feel a needle sting"), what to expect (e.g., "You will have a burning sensation"), and what is expected of him or her (e.g., "Tell us if you feel pain"). The patient's questions should be answered truthfully and realistically. He or she should be reassured that appropriate amounts of the anesthetic will be administered as needed.

Conversation by team members should be appropriate and kept to a minimum. Hand signals between the surgeon and scrub person are more useful than a verbal request for instruments. However, the surgeon may request a No. 10 or 15 rather than a knife, or a Mayo or Metz rather than scissors. Strange noises should be explained to the patient (e.g., suction to remove an irrigating solution or the sound and odor of an electrosurgical unit [ESU]). Background music of the patient's choice may help to relax and distract him or her. Headsets are one option for this purpose and help to block out other noises. Although headsets can distract the patient from the ambient room noise, they can also distract the patient from following necessary directions during the procedure; therefore cautious use is suggested. Traffic in and out of the room should be kept to a minimum. A sign should be placed on the door to indicate the type of anesthesia being used (e.g., "Patient awake, local anesthesia").

POSTOPERATIVE CARE, DISCHARGE, AND FOLLOW-UP

Patients who have received a local anesthetic are returned to the ambulatory unit for a brief assessment and discharge. Patients who have undergone general anesthesia or IVCS or who need postoperative pain management are taken to the

PACU for a period of stabilization and observation. Medications may be given intravenously in small dosages; oral medications may cause nausea and vomiting that may prolong the length of stay. Routine orders may be established by policy for these analgesics and antiemetics.

Consciousness, rational behavior, and ambulation do not imply full recovery. Blood pressure and pulse rate may return to the normal range while residual myocardial depression continues. Patients may lapse back into sleep or drowsiness as the drugs used for general anesthesia are metabolized. Patients are under observation at all times in the PACU. Although a point scoring system is commonly used for establishing discharge criteria, this method should not be used to replace patient assessment data in determining suitability for discharge.

When all discharge criteria are met, patients are discharged on written order of the anesthesia provider and/or surgeon according to policy. Discharge criteria are listed in Box 11-3. Discharge is contingent on the patient's generalized condition. Vital signs are measured and compared to baseline, and the condition of the surgical site is documented. Patients who have questionable vital signs or an unstable physiology should be seen by a physician before discharge. Patients are not allowed to drive home if a general or regional anesthetic has been administered. The patient should leave the facility via an appropriate mode of transportation and accompanied by a responsible adult. Select patients who have undergone local anesthesia without sedation may be permitted to drive home if an order is written by the surgeon. The means of the patient's discharge should be documented.

Patient education is an essential element of ambulatory surgical care. Written discharge instructions are verbally reviewed with the patient and a responsible adult. The perioperative nurse should document how the patient or his or her representative signified understanding of the instruction. Some patients can verbalize or perform a return demonstration as confirmation. The patient is instructed when to arrange for a follow-up visit with the surgeon. Appropriate phone numbers for the surgeon, ambulatory center, and emergency help should be listed on the discharge instruction sheet. If problems occur after discharge, the patient is encouraged to contact the surgeon or ambulatory care facility.

Most complications occur within the first 48 hours of surgery. Therefore a registered nurse should call to check on the patient's progress and to reiterate postoperative instructions the following day, or at most within 2 days of discharge. The nurse reminds the patient to keep the follow-up appointment with the surgeon. Patients who plan to return to work within a day or two of surgery may be asked to phone the nurse themselves because they may not be home when the nurse makes routine calls during the day. Patient satisfaction can be surveyed using this method of postoperative contact.

PERIOPERATIVE DOCUMENTATION

The development, implementation, and evaluation of the plan of care should be documented in the patient's medical record. Documentation should include, but is not limited to, the following:

1. Preoperative care
   a. Preanesthetic evaluation by the anesthesia provider if a general, regional, or local anesthetic with sedation is to be given
   b. Nursing assessment data, nursing diagnoses, expected outcomes, plan of care, and preoperative teaching by the perioperative nurse
   c. Medical history and physical examination
   d. Laboratory reports and results of other tests
   e. Informed consent for the surgical procedure
2. Intraoperative care
   a. Anesthesia and medications administered
   b. Vital signs and intraoperative monitoring data
   c. Intraoperative implementation of the plan of care
   d. Surgical procedure note by the surgeon
   e. Any unexpected outcomes
3. Postoperative care
   a. Postanesthesia care, including monitoring of patient responses and medications
   b. Discharge instructions, including follow-up appointment with the surgeon and signs and/or symptoms of potential complications that require immediate medical attention
   c. Radiology, pathology, and any other medical reports
   d. Physical and psychologic status at the time of discharge
   e. Attainment of expected outcomes
   f. Mode of transport from the facility and destination, including relationship to the accompanying support person
4. Remote postoperative care
   a. Follow-up phone call within 24 to 48 hours to assess the patient's progress

   b. Follow-up phone call within 6 weeks to assess the patient's satisfaction with outcomes and services (for continuous quality improvement data)
   c. Patient follow up with the surgeon

ADVANTAGES AND DISADVANTAGES OF AMBULATORY SURGERY

Advantages

The development of rapid-acting anesthetics that have minimal prolonged side effects and the availability of short-acting narcotics (to control pain) and of antiemetics (to reduce nausea) allow the surgeon to perform many surgical procedures in an ambulatory care facility. The advantages of ambulatory surgery include the following:

1. It lowers costs for the patient and facility.
2. It returns the patient immediately to familiar surroundings that are less stressful than a hospital environment.
3. It reduces the period of the patient's dependency and lifestyle disruption.
4. It eliminates the psychologic trauma of hospitalization and separation from family or significant other, or from parents (for infants and children).
5. It frees inpatient hospital bed space for patients who require more extensive care without increasing hospital bed capacity.
6. It frees hospital staff and resources for the care of other patients.
7. It reduces the risk of nosocomial (hospital-acquired) infection that is inherent in hospitalization.

Disadvantages

Ambulatory surgery is not suitable for every patient. Although most patients who receive care in an ambulatory setting benefit from the experience, the following disadvantages have been identified:

1. Some patients have unrealistic expectations of their physical capabilities after surgery. They tend to feel fine until the anesthetic wears off. They may overextend the use of an anesthetized body part while still under the influence of a local anesthetic.
2. A patient's anxiety level may increase if not enough time is allotted for the preoperative preparation. This gives the patient the impression of being rushed through the system as if on a production line.
3. Unforeseen complications may arise in a patient who has never before received an anesthetic. A young child undergoing general anesthesia for an inguinal hernia repair may experience a metabolic crisis such as malignant hyperthermia (MH). Allergic responses to drugs and local anesthetics are potential adverse reactions.

4. The surgical procedure may reveal an unexpected secondary diagnosis that necessitates a more extensive procedure than anticipated or a second surgical procedure in an inpatient facility. Prolonged procedures increase the waiting period for patients scheduled to follow this unexpected extended procedure. The patient will need to be discharged at a later time, which may impose a hardship on the family (e.g., child or pet care).

5. Emergency transport to an inpatient facility may be necessary in the event of a surgical accident. For example, inadvertent penetration of a major artery or organ during a laparoscopic procedure may cause a life-threatening hemorrhage. Instrumentation, supplies, blood volume replacement, and blood salvage equipment may not be readily available at the freestanding ambulatory setting.

6. Time or space constraints may cause patients to feel they are being discharged too soon.

7. Patients may experience pain, nausea, vomiting, bleeding, swelling, and other complications that may necessitate overnight admission to the hospital for treatment and/or observation.

PERFORMANCE IMPROVEMENT FOR AMBULATORY SERVICES

Patient satisfaction is a key indicator of quality. Did the care received meet the patient's expectations? What are the patient's perceptions of care? In addition to the postdischarge telephone call, the patient may be asked to complete a questionnaire a week or more after discharge. Questions relate to the physical facilities, waiting periods, preoperative teaching, anesthesia or surgical complications, discharge instructions, and overall satisfaction with care. Supplemental questionnaires completed by surgeons are useful to obtain information for compiling statistics related to postoperative infections and complications (i.e., patient outcomes).

A continuous quality improvement program includes monitoring patient care and the environment, evaluating patient outcomes and services, and identifying and resolving problems. The program focuses on outcomes (i.e., results in accordance with standards for professional practice, ethical conduct, and legal requirements). Quality improvement in an ambulatory care facility must include an evaluation of policies and procedures regarding the appropriateness of patient selection, the surgical procedures performed, and the services provided.

Most patients who receive ambulatory surgery are satisfied with their care. Studies have shown that, if further surgery is indicated, most patients will choose to have the new procedure performed in an ambulatory setting. Lower incidents of postoperative complications have been documented, as well as lower costs of treatment for the patient. Preoperative teaching is beneficial in helping patients attain the expected outcomes. Careful patient evaluation and planning can make the ambulatory surgery a successful and positive experience for the patient, family, significant others, and caregivers.

Bibliography

Beatty AM et al: Relevance of oral intake and necessity to void as ambulatory surgical discharge criteria, *J Perianesth Nurs* 12(6):413-421, 1997.

Brumfield VC et al: Preoperative patient teaching in ambulatory surgery, *AORN J* 64(6):941, 943-946, 948, 1996.

Burden N: *Ambulatory surgical nursing,* Philadelphia, 1993, WB Saunders.

Cassidy J, Marley RA: Ambulatory surgery: preoperative assessment of the ambulatory patient, *J Perianesth Nurs* 11(5):334-343, 1996.

Centers for Disease Control and Prevention: FEDSTATS: ambulatory surgery in the United States, 1995, *Advance Data 296,* 1995.

Ferrara-Love R et al: Nonpharmacologic treatment of postoperative nausea, *J Perianesth Nurs* 11(6):378-383, 1996.

Gruendemann BJ: *Comprehensive perioperative nursing,* vol 1, Boston, 1995, Jones & Bartlett.

Hawshaw D: A day surgery patient follow-up survey, *Br J Nurs* 3(7):348-350, 1994.

Hylka SC: Comparative cost analysis of surgical procedures in an ambulatory eye center, *Nurs Econ* 12(1):51-55, 1994.

Ireland D: Legal issues in ambulatory surgery, *Nurs Clin North Am* 32(2):469-476, 1997.

Kleinpell RM: Improving telephone follow-up after ambulatory surgery, *J Perianesth Nurs* 12(5):336-340, 1997.

Lancaster KA: Care of the pediatric patient in ambulatory surgery, *Nurs Clin North Am* 32(2):441-455, 1997.

Lancaster KA: Patient teaching in ambulatory surgery, *Nurs Clin North Am* 32(2):417-427, 1997.

Mann A: A continuing postoperative complication: nausea and vomiting, *CRNA* 9(1):19-29, 1998.

Marley RA: Ambulatory surgery: postoperative nausea and vomiting, *J Perianesth Nurs* 11(3):147-161, 1996.

National Center for Health Statistics: *Quarterly fact sheet: monitoring health care in America, spotlight on ambulatory care in the US,* Hyattsville, Md, June 1997, US Department of Health and Human Services.

Oberle K et al: Follow-up of same day surgery patients: a study of patient concerns, *AORN J* 59(5):1016-1025, 1994.

Pandit UA, Pandit SK: Fasting before and after ambulatory surgery, *J Perianesth Nurs* 12(3):181-187, 1997.

Sherman DW: Developing quality assurance programs in ambulatory surgery, *Nurs Manage* 28(9):44-49, 1997.

Smith I, White PF: Anesthesia for ambulatory surgery, *Curr Rev Nurs Anesth* 16(20):171-180, 1994.

Spry C et al: Ambulatory surgery: RN staff in an ambulatory surgery center, *AORN J* 59(3):601-602, 1994.

Swan BA: A collaborative ambulatory preoperative evaluation model: implementation, implications, evaluation, *AORN J* 59(2):430-437, 1994.

Swan BA et al: Symptom distress and functional status changes during the first seven days after ambulatory surgery, *Anesth Analg* 86(4):739-745, 1998.

White PF, Smith I: Ambulatory anesthesia: past, present, and future, *Int Anesthesiol Clin* 32(3):1-16, 1994.

Zalewski DE: Fine-tuning preadmission surgical services, *Nurs Manage* 28(9):49, 51, 1997.

Chapter 12

Care of the Perioperative Environment

 Chapter Objectives

After studying this chapter, the learner will be able to:

- Describe how a room is prepared for the first case of the day.
- Describe how a room is cleaned between patients.
- Describe how a room is terminally cleaned at the end of the day.

HISTORICAL BACKGROUND

The perioperative environment has changed many times throughout history. In ancient times, the healer came to the patient's dwelling to perform the healing arts. The family would gather around to chant and pray to great spirits, and amulets, or charms, were displayed. Mysticism and ceremony played a big part in the treatment. Surgical procedures, such as trephining (drilling holes in the head) or bloodletting were performed to purge evil. Medicinal herbs and hallucinogenic compounds were often used to dull the senses during the procedure, which was performed with crude knives and stone instruments. Knowledge of human anatomy and physiology was limited. Archaeologic evidence has demonstrated that these patients lived through the procedures.

Later eras were witness to procedures performed in the patient's home. Formal hospitals had not been established. Physicians would engage public nurses and family members to prepare the room in the home. In some circumstances the procedure was performed on the kitchen table using instruments taken directly from the physician's black bag. These implements had not been washed since the previous use. Most were merely wiped clean by the nurse. Gloves and other surgical attire were not worn. Procedures performed were limited to the pain tolerance of the patient. Intraabdominal procedures were not performed, with the exception of cesarean sections for childbirth.

As anesthetic techniques improved and surgical procedures become somewhat safer, hospitals were the exclusive location of surgical suites. Hungarian obstetrician Ignaz Semmelweis (1816-1865) described the beginnings of the theory of infectious transfer between patients, and French bacteriologist Louis Pasteur (1822-1895) confirmed the existence of harmful microorganisms. This necessitated the need for a clean environment and clean practices.

169

ESTABLISHING THE PERIOPERATIVE ENVIRONMENT

The duties of the scrub person and circulator are many and varied as they prepare for the arrival of the patient in the operating room (OR). They are responsible for the cleanliness of the environment preoperatively, intraoperatively, and postoperatively so that the potential for contamination of the patient is kept to a minimum. They prepare and maintain the sterile field, work within it, and then break it down for terminal cleaning. These activities are performed in specific steps to minimize the risk of infection and maximize the use of time and supplies. Terms associated with preparation of the perioperative environment is found in Box 12-1.

Box 12-1   Terms Associated with Preparation of the Perioperative Environment

case cart   System of preselecting and delivering instruments and supplies to the perioperative environment. Some models include provision for the return of instruments and contaminated items to the appropriate decontamination area.
custom packs   Prepackaged disposable supplies prepared by the manufacturer or the distributor according to specific instructions and requests by a particular service at a facility.
terminal cleaning   Thorough cleaning and disinfection of the perioperative environment at the end of use.
turnover   Activity geared toward cleaning and preparation of the OR between cases for the next patient's arrival.

Preliminary Preparations

Preliminary preparations of the OR are completed by the circulator and scrub person before each patient enters the OR. Assistance is provided by environmental service personnel. It is a cooperative effort. Clean, organized surroundings are part of total patient care. A visual inspection of the room and its contents should be performed by the team before bringing in supplies for a case. Basic room contents should include the OR bed, anesthesia machine and supplies, electrosurgical unit (ESU), instrument table, preparation table, Mayo stand, suction apparatus, and receptacles for trash and reusable woven fabrics (Figure 12-1). Other tables or equipment are added as needed.

Before the First Surgical Procedure of the Day

The following housekeeping duties should be done before bringing supplies into the room for the first case of the day:

1. Remove unnecessary tables and equipment from the room. Arrange the appropriate furniture in an organized manner away from the traffic pattern.
2. Damp dust (with a facility-approved agent and lint-free cloth) the overhead operating light, furniture, flat surfaces, and all portable or mounted equipment with a disinfectant solution. Start at higher surfaces and work down to lower levels.
3. Damp dust the tops and rims of the sterilizer and/or washer-sterilizer and the countertops in the substerile room adjacent to the OR.

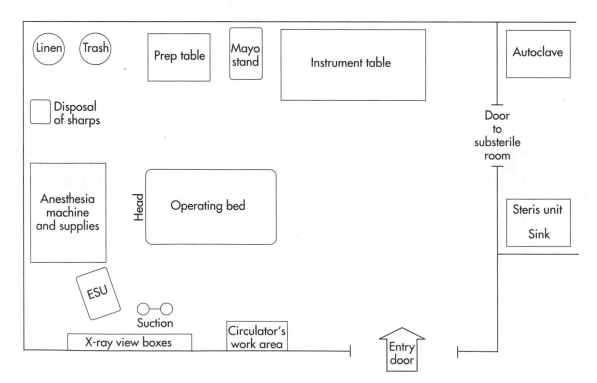

Figure 12-1   Layout of basic OR and substerile room. The traffic pattern from the doors should not interfere with the setup of the sterile tables or the transfer of the patient to the operating bed.

4. Visually inspect the room for dirt and debris. The floor may need to be damp mopped.

Setting Up the Room

1. A clean sheet, lift sheet, armboard covers, and restraining strap(s) should be on the operating bed. Put a pressure-reducing mattress or gel pads on the bed if needed to relieve pressure during a long procedure. A warming or cooling blanket may be needed to heat or cool the patient during a long procedure.

2. Position the operating bed under the overhead operating light fixture. Orient the head of the bed according to the type of procedure to be performed. Patient positioning for some procedures requires the anesthesia provider to be located at the patient's side instead of at the head of the bed.

3. Test the overhead operating light to check focus and intensity, and preposition it as much as possible. Do not leave the light turned on. The light should be positioned in relationship to the location of the surgeon at the operating bed and to that part of the patient's anatomy that will be encountered during the surgical procedure. The circulator should know how to change the lightbulb in case a bulb burns out during a procedure.

4. Connect and check the suction between the receptacle canisters and the wall outlet to be certain suction functions at maximum vacuum. Some facilities use in-line filters for specialized equipment. The filters are changed between cases. Gloves and personal protective equipment are worn to prevent contact with harmful microorganisms.

5. Place a waterproof laundry bag or antistatic plastic bag for disposal of reusable woven fabric items in the laundry hamper frame.

6. Place appropriately marked receptacles in the room for safe disposal of biohazardous items, such as sharps, disposable drapes, or other biologically contaminated materials.

7. Line each kick bucket and wastebasket with an impervious plastic liner with a cuff turned over the edge.

8. Arrange furniture with those pieces that will be draped to become part of the sterile field at least 18 inches (45 cm) away from walls or cabinets. They should be kept side by side, away from the laundry hamper, trash container, anesthesia equipment, doors, and paths of traffic.

9. If a case cart system is used, all or most of the needed supplies will be on the cart. These should be checked to ascertain that everything is there. Position the case cart near the instrument table. Obtain an appropriate set of sterile instruments. Place the sterile drape pack on the instrument table so that when opened, the wrapper will adequately drape the table and the drapes will be in their proper place (see Figure 12-2). Put a sterile basin set into the ring stand. If ring stands are not used in the facility, place the basin set on a preparation table.

10. Select the correct-size gloves and gowns for each member of the sterile team. Select the initial sutures to have ready for the surgeon. Open only those needed to begin the case, such as ties.

11. Collect additional instruments and supplies, according to the procedure book and the surgeon's preference card, from cabinets in the room or from another supply area within the OR suite.

12. Obtain special equipment, such as table appliances, pillows, or padding, needed to position and protect the patient.

13. Obtain appropriate patient monitoring equipment. Sequential compression devices may be indicated.

14. Obtain any specialized equipment that will be needed, such as an ESU, smoke evacuator, pneumatic tourniquet, laser, or operating microscope, and check/test for proper function. Have the appropriate attachments and adjunctive supplies in the room.

15. Gather protective devices such as x-ray protective gowns and/or lead screens and laser eyewear of the correct optical density as needed.

Opening Sterile Supplies

The doors to the room should be shut, and each team member present should be wearing appropriate OR attire. Before any sterile supplies are opened, the integrity of each package must be checked for tears and watermarks. If either are present, the package is unsafe to use. The process monitor should also be checked. Open packages as follows:

1. Remove tape from packages wrapped in woven fabric wrappers. The tape should be opened by breaking the seal on paper or nonwoven material. Removing tape strips from paper-wrapped items increases the risk of tearing the wrapper and exposing the contents to contamination. Check the chemical indicator to be certain the item has been exposed to a sterilization process.

2. Open the drape pack, instrument set, gown pack, and basin set so that the inside of each inner wrapper becomes the sterile table cover. With hands on the outside of the wrapper in a folded cuff, lift the wrapper toward yourself to avoid contaminating the contents of the pack. The area touched falls below table level, and the inside of the wrapper remains sterile. Do not reach over the inside of the sterile table cover or contents of the pack. Always lift the wrapper toward you (Figure 12-2).

   a. If packs or sets have sequential double wrappers, both layers are opened by the person opening supplies. The outer wrapper is considered the dust cover, and the inner wrapper the microbial barrier.

   b. Open other packages, such as sponges, gloves, and sutures, maintaining a sterile transfer to the appropriate sterile table. Touch only the outside of the outer wrapper. Avoid reaching over sterile contents and the sterile table. Enclose your hand in the wrapper to the extent possible.

   c. If small packages are sequentially double wrapped (i.e., a package inside a package), only the outer wrapper is removed. Usually the inner wrapper contains several smaller parts that may accidentally fall off the table when dispensed.

Figure 12-2 Opening sterile drape pack. Wrapper is lifted back while keeping hands on the outside. Hands are in folded cuff to avoid contaminating contents of pack. Area touched falls below unsterile table level; sterile inside of wrapper (now table cover) remains sterile.

    d. Instruments processed in rigid, closed container systems are opened by breaking the seal on the lid and raising it up and away from the tray. The inner basket of instruments is considered sterile, but the container itself is not. Sterile soft goods, sutures, and other individually wrapped items should not be opened into this pan because the edges are not considered sterile.

    e. If a sterile package is dropped, the item may be considered safe for immediate use only if it is enclosed in an impervious material and the integrity of the package is maintained. Dropped items wrapped in reusable woven fabric materials should not be transferred to the sterile table.

3. Open the gown and gloves for the scrub person on the Mayo stand or small table.

4. The circulator assists the anesthesia provider with patient care as the scrub person sets up the sterile field after scrubbing, gowning, and gloving.

Individual Patient Setups

Each patient has a right to individual supplies prepared just for him or her. Sterile supplies should not be opened until they are ready to be used. Tables should not be prepared and covered for use at a later time. The scrub person, working with an efficient circulator, should have time to set up the instrument table immediately before each surgical procedure.

    The practice of covering sterile setups is not in the best interest of the patient. Unless it is under constant surveillance, sterility of any setup cannot be guaranteed. Uncovering a sterile table is difficult and may compromise sterility. If a scheduled surgical procedure is delayed and a sterile setup has not been contaminated by the patient's presence in the room, the setup may remain open, under surveillance, by someone in the room with the doors closed. The setup should be used as close to the time of preparation as possible. Sterility is mainly event related, not time dependent.

    If a patient is taken into the OR and for some reason the surgical procedure is canceled before the procedure has begun, the tables should be torn down and the room cleaned as if the surgical procedure had taken place. The setup is considered potentially contaminated and may not be saved for another patient. Disposable items may be useful for the clinical educator in the department during orientation and education sessions.

Room Turnover Between Patients

Physical facilities influence the flow of supplies and equipment following the surgical procedure. However, basic principles of aseptic technique dictate the procedures to be carried out immediately after a surgical procedure is completed, to prepare the OR for the next patient. Every patient has the right to the same degree of safety in the environment. In addition, personnel working in the OR suite should be protected. Some patients have known pathogenic microorganisms; others have unknown infectious organisms. Therefore every patient should be considered a potential contaminant in the environment. Cleanup procedures should be rigidly followed to contain and confine contamination, known or unknown.

    The routine cleanup procedure can be accomplished expeditiously by the circulator and scrub person working cooperatively. While the circulator assists with the outer layer of dressing and prepares the patient for transport from the OR, the scrub person begins to dismantle the sterile field before removing gown and gloves. All instruments, supplies, and equipment should be decontaminated, disinfected, terminally sterilized, or contained for disposal as appropriate before being handled by other personnel.

    After a patient leaves the room, the immediate environment is cleaned and all surfaces are dried. Room cleanup between patients is directed at the prevention of cross-contamination. The cycle of contamination is from patient to environment and from environment to OR personnel and subsequent patients. Exposure to infectious waste is a hazard to all persons who encounter it. After each surgical procedure, the environment should be made safe for the next patient to follow in that room. Institutional policies and procedures for routine room cleanup should be designed to minimize the OR team's exposure to contamination during the cleaning process.

Room Turnover Activities by the Scrub Person

The patient should be thought of as the center, or focal point. The surrounding sterile field and all areas that have come in contact with blood or body fluids are considered contaminated. The primary principles of cleaning procedures are to confine and contain contamination and to physically remove microorganisms as quickly as possible. The sterile field is dismantled by the scrub person. A gown, gloves, a mask, protective eyewear, and a cap are worn for the procedure. Contaminated supplies, instruments, and basins are prepared by the scrub person and sent to the processing department for terminal cleaning and sterilization.

The following are also activities/responsibilities of the scrub person:

1. Remain sterile until the patient leaves the room. Push the Mayo stand and instrument table away from the operating bed as soon as the intermediate layer of the dressing is applied. Do not contaminate the table or Mayo stand until the patient has actually left the room.

2. Check drapes for towel clips, instruments, and other items. Be sure that no equipment is discarded with disposable drapes or sent to the laundry with reusable woven fabric drapes. Roll drapes off the patient to prevent airborne contamination; do not pull them off. Disposable drapes are placed in a plastic bag for disposal. Roll the wettest part of reusable woven fabric drapes into the center of the bag as far as possible to prevent liquid from soaking through the laundry bag, even though it is waterproof. Soiled drapes, whether disposable or reusable, should be handled as little as possible and with minimum agitation to prevent gross microbial contamination of air by dispersal of lint and debris.

3. Discard soiled sponges, other bloodied waste, and disposable items in appropriate impervious biohazardous waste receptacles.

4. Discard unused sponges, nonwoven drapes, and other nonbloody disposable waste into the trash.

5. Dispose of sharp items safely. Special care should be taken in handling all knife blades, surgical needles, and needles used for injection or aspiration. Remove the tip from the electrosurgical handle (pencil). Place these items in an appropriate rigid, puncture-resistant container for safe disposal to prevent injury and potential risk of contamination. The primary cause of accidental cuts and punctures to personnel, both within and outside of the OR, is disposal of surgical sharps at the end of the surgical procedure. Standardized systems designed specifically for safe handling and disposal of sharps prevent virtually all accidental cuts, punctures, and lacerations. Unused suture packets are discarded.

   Blades and needles should not be discarded loose in trash receptacles. These sharp items should be enclosed and secured for disposal in a sharps disposal container. A self-closing adhesive pad or box designed for this purpose is the safest device to use. A safe disposal procedure should be implemented and adhered to.

   a. Remove knife blades from handles. Point the blade toward the table, away from the field and other persons in the area so that if it breaks or slips, it will not fly across the room. Remove blades with a heavy instrument; never use fingers. Do not put knife handles in an instrument tray with blades left on them. Other instruments designed for replaceable cutting blades, such as dermatomes, should have blades removed; thereafter they may be handled with other instruments.

   b. Place reusable surgical needles, either on a needle rack or loose, into a perforated stainless steel box to be terminally cleaned and sterilized with the instruments. Check the suture towel or book to see that it is not discarded with needles in it.

   c. Burrs and drill bits should be disposed of in the same manner.

   d. Place reusable needles used for injection or aspiration in a perforated stainless steel box with surgical needles.

6. Remove blood, tissue, bone, and any other gross debris from instruments. All instruments, used and unused, must be cleaned, terminally sterilized, or undergo high-level disinfection before they are handled for definitive cleaning and sterilization and checked for proper functioning before reuse. Instruments should be presoaked and/or prerinsed before processing in a washer-sterilizer or decontaminator. Any biologic material remaining on instruments is more difficult to remove after they have been heat sterilized, because the material becomes baked on them. The biologic debris inhibits sterilization and disinfection processes.

7. Load the instrument washing tray with heavy instruments in the bottom. All hinged instruments are fully opened to expose maximum surface area, including box locks. Instruments designed to be disassembled are taken apart. Carefully space instruments to prevent contact of sharp edges or points with other instruments. Concave surfaces should be turned down. Load the tray into the case cart for return to the processing department.

8. Put glass syringes, medicine glasses, and other glassware, including those used by the anesthesia provider, into a separate tray. Syringes are separated. Check for disposable items and discard them in the trash without needles.

9. Suction detergent-disinfectant solution through the lumen of reusable suction tips. Thorough cleaning of the lumen is difficult to accomplish if biologic debris becomes dry. Disposable suction tips and tubing are recommended and are discarded with other infectious waste.

10. Invert small basins and solution cups over the instruments. Basins and trays too large for the washer-sterilizer or standard instrument sterilizer are put into plastic bags for transport to the decontamination area.

The Mayo tray may be included. Place these on the lower shelf of the case cart.

11. Dispose of solutions and suction bottle contents in a flushing hopper connected to a sanitary sewer. Personal protective equipment should be worn to protect from splashes. Disposable suction units simplify disposal. Commercial substances can be added to liquid in the disposable canister to solidify or gel contents for solid waste disposal. If disposable units are not used, decontaminate contents with disinfectant before hopper disposal. SafeCycle 40 (Steris Corporation, Mentor, Ohio) is a fluid waste management system that collects and holds up to 40,000 ml of fluid and bloody waste. It uses wall suction connections, collects suctioned material, and automatically disposes of it in the processing area without the need for exposure of personnel to the contaminated fluid. The unit self-cleans using sealed canisters of disinfectant.

    Wall suction units should be disconnected by the circulator to avoid contamination of the internal wall outlet. Rinse the container, plunger, and lid. Reusable glass suction containers are sterilized along with basins and trays.

12. Discard all used disposable table drapes in a plastic bag with used disposable patient drapes. All reusable woven fabric drapes from open packs should be laundered to replace moisture lost to the fabric by sterilization. Unused along with used reusable woven fabric drapes should be sent to the laundry.

13. Remove the gown before removing gloves. The circulator unfastens neck and back closures. Protect your arms and scrub clothes from the contaminated outside of the gown. Grasp the right shoulder of the gown with your left hand and, in pulling the gown off your arm, turn the sleeve inside out. Turn the outside of the gown away from your body with a flexed elbow. Then grasp your other shoulder with the other hand and remove the gown entirely, pulling it off inside out. Discard the gown in a laundry hamper if it is reusable or in a trash receptacle if it is disposable.

14. To remove gloves, use a glove-to-glove, then skin-to-skin technique to protect clean hands from the contaminated outside of gloves, which bear cells of the patient. Gloves are turned inside out as they are removed and are then discarded into a trash receptacle. Wash hands after removing gloves.

15. Make sure the case cart is covered with an impervious drape or closed before it is returned to the processing area.

Room Turnover Activities by the Team

After the patient leaves, the circulator is free to assist with cleanup of the room. Environmental service personnel may also be available to assist with cleaning. Regardless of which member of the team performs them, specific functions should be carried out to complete room cleanup. The following personnel and areas are considered contaminated during and after the surgical procedure:

- Members of the sterile team, until they have discarded their gowns, gloves, caps, masks, and shoe covers. These items remain in the contaminated area; scrub clothes are changed if they are wet or contaminated.
- All furniture, equipment, and the floor within and around the perimeter of the sterile field. If accidental spillage has occurred in other parts of the room, then these areas are also considered contaminated.
- All anesthesia equipment.
- Stretchers used to transport patients. These should be cleaned after each patient use.

Clean, but not sterile, gloves are worn to complete the room cleanup. The scrub person changes gloves after the sterile field is dismantled. Decontamination of the environment includes the following:

1. *Furniture.* Wash horizontal surfaces of all tables and equipment, including the anesthesia machine, with a disinfectant solution. Apply disinfectant from a squeeze-bottle dispenser and wipe with a clean cloth or a disposable wipe that is changed frequently. Spray bottles can cause particles to become aerosolized and should be avoided. All surfaces of mattress, pads, and screw connections of the operating bed are included. Mobile furniture can be pushed through disinfectant solution used for floor care to clean casters.

2. *Overhead operating light.* Overhead light reflectors should be wiped using a clean cloth that has been wetted with disinfectant solution specifically intended for this purpose. Commercial reflector cleaner prevents clouding of the surface that can cause dullness and glare. Lights and overhead tracks become contaminated quickly and present a possible hazard from fallout of microorganisms onto sterile surfaces or into wounds during surgical procedures. These should be cleaned on a daily basis.

3. *Anesthesia equipment.* All reusable anesthesia masks and tubing are cleaned and sterilized before reusing. Some of this equipment can be steam sterilized; if not, it may be sterilized by ethylene oxide gas and aerated before reuse. If this method is not available, items should be chemically sterilized according to the sterilant manufacturer's recommendations.

4. *Laundry.* After all cleaning procedures have been completed, cleaning cloths should be discarded or put in a laundry bag if they are not disposable. When all reusable woven fabric items, used and unused, have been placed inside the laundry bag, it is closed securely. To help protect laundry personnel, an alginate bag that dissolves in hot water may be used as the primary laundry bag or as a liner within a cloth bag. Reusable woven fabrics soiled with blood or body fluids are transported in leakproof bags.

5. *Trash.* All trash is collected in plastic or impervious bags, including disposable drapes, kick buckets, and

wastebasket liners. Bags should be sturdy to resist bursting or tearing during transport. Trash can be separated into infectious waste, noninfectious trash, and recyclable items. Separate receptacles should be available. Disposition of potentially infectious waste must comply with local, state, and/or federal regulations for contamination control measures. Appropriately labeled and color-coded leakproof bags for infectious waste and puncture-resistant containers for sharps should be used.

6. *Floors.* A perimeter of several feet in circumference of the surgical field is cleaned between cases. This perimeter expands in the direction of visible soilage. Wet vacuuming with a filter-diffuser exhaust cleaner is the method of choice for floor care in the OR. Machine cleaning is more effective than manual cleaning. If there is a great deal of suture material and gross soilage on the floor, wet-vacuum equipment may be used dry for the first treatment. The floor is then flooded, half of the room at a time, with a detergent-disinfectant solution. This solution may be dispensed from a pump spray or automatic spraying device attached to a central wet-vacuum equipment system. If portable equipment is used, a watering can may be used to flood the floor, although this method is slower and may wet the floor unevenly. Hot water may hasten the biocidal action of the disinfectant agent but may also soften tile adhesive. Room-temperature water requires at least a 5-minute contact time for effectiveness.

    Furniture is rolled across the flooded floor area to clean casters. The wet-vacuum pickup is used to pick up solution before furniture is repositioned. Standing platforms are considered part of the floor and may be flooded with solution to be picked up by wet vacuuming.

    The exterior of vacuum equipment and tubing is cleaned following each use, with special attention given to cleaning the rubber blade before the next use. If the hose is equipped with a brush attachment, this is washed and sterilized between uses.

    If wet-vacuum equipment is not available, freshly laundered, clean mops can be used. The floor can be flooded with detergent-disinfectant solution. One mop is used to apply solution, and one is used to take up solution. Following one-time use, mop heads are removed and placed in a laundry hamper with other contaminated reusable woven fabrics. Mop handles may be stored in the housekeeping storage area until they are needed again. Clean mops and disinfectant solution are used for each cleanup procedure.

7. *Walls.* If walls are splashed with blood or organic debris during the surgical procedure, those areas should be washed. Otherwise, walls are not considered contaminated and need not be washed between surgical procedures.

Cart System Cleanup

All reusable instruments, basins, supplies, and equipment, including suction bottles, are put on or inside the case cart. The cart is covered or closed and taken to the central decontamination area outside the OR suite for cleanup. A closed cart, especially if it has been used as the instrument table, is wiped off with a disinfectant solution before it is taken out of the room. A cart with contaminated supplies should be removed from the OR suite via the outer corridor if this is the design of the suite. If dumbwaiters or elevators are used, a separate one is provided for the contaminated cart. Clean and contaminated supplies are always kept separated.

The cart is designed to go through an automatic steam cart washer or a manual power wash for terminal cleaning after it is emptied and before it is restocked with clean and sterile supplies.

Getting the Room Ready for the Next Patient

The cleaning procedures described provide adequate decontamination and terminal sterilization following any surgical procedure. With a well-coordinated team, minimal turnover time between surgical procedures can be accomplished; in an average time of 15 to 20 minutes the room will be ready for the next patient. The turnover time includes cleaning up after one procedure and setting up for the next procedure. Additional equipment brought into the room for the next patient should be damp dusted before sterile supplies are opened.

Daily Terminal Cleaning
In the Operating Room

At completion of the day's schedule, each OR, whether or not it was used that day, should be terminally cleaned. Additional and more rigorous cleaning is done in all areas already discussed for cleanup between surgical procedures. At the end of the day's schedule, the following routine should be followed:

1. Furniture is thoroughly scrubbed, using mechanical friction in addition to chemical disinfection. Disinfectants are only adjuncts to good physical cleaning; "elbow grease" is probably the most important ingredient.
2. Casters and wheels should be cleaned and kept free of suture ends and debris. Equipment is available that automatically washes stretchers, tables, and platforms and then steam cleans and dries them within a matter of minutes.
3. Equipment, such as ESUs and lasers, should be cleaned with care so as not to saturate surfaces to the degree that disinfectant solution runs into the mechanism, causing malfunction and requiring repairs.
4. Ceiling- and wall-mounted fixtures and tracks are cleaned on all surfaces.
5. Kick buckets, laundry hamper frames, and other waste receptacles are cleaned and disinfected; these items are sterilized when feasible.
6. Floors are given a thorough wet-vacuum cleaning with wet-vacuum pickup used dry and then wet.
7. Walls and ceilings should be checked for soil spots and cleaned as necessary.

8. Cabinets and doors should be cleaned, especially around handles or push plates, where contamination is common.
9. Air-intake grills, ducts, and filter covers should be cleaned.

Outside the Operating Room

1. Countertops and sinks in the substerile room should be cleaned. The outer surface of the sterilizer, including the top, should be washed.
2. Scrub sinks and spray heads on faucets should undergo thorough cleaning daily. A mild abrasive on sinks removes the oily film residue left by scrub antiseptics. Spray heads, faucet aerators, or sprinklers should be removed and disassembled, if possible, for thorough cleaning and sterilization of parts. Contaminated faucet aerators and sprinklers can transfer organisms directly to hands or items washed under them. Scrub sinks should not be used for routine cleaning purposes.
3. Soap dispensers should be disassembled, cleaned, and terminally sterilized, if possible, before they are refilled with antiseptic solution. These dispensers can become reservoirs for microorganisms.
4. Walls around scrub sinks should receive daily attention. Spray and splash from scrubbing cause buildup of antiseptic soap film around the sink. This film should be removed.
5. Transportation and storage carts need to be cleaned with specific attention given to wheels and casters.
6. Cleaning equipment should be disassembled and cleaned before storage.

Weekly or Monthly Cleaning

A weekly or monthly cleaning routine is set up, in addition to the daily cleaning schedule, by the director of environmental/housekeeping services and the OR manager. Any routines for housekeeping are based on the physical construction of the department. However, if specific schedules are not established, some areas could be inadvertently missed. Areas to be considered are the following:

1. *Walls.* Walls should be cleaned when they become visibly soiled. If they are painted or tiled with wide porous grouting, these factors should be considered in planning cleaning routines. Washing walls in the OR and throughout the suite once a week is reasonable, but less frequent time intervals for cleaning may be acceptable if spot disinfection is performed on a daily basis. This requires adequate continuous supervision.
2. *Ceilings.* Ceilings may require regular special cleaning techniques because of mounted tracks and lighting fixtures. Specialized ceiling mounts for microscopes and booms for suspended equipment should be included in this plan. The types of fixtures are considered in planning cleaning routines.
3. *Floors.* Floors throughout the OR suite should be machine scrubbed periodically to remove accumulated deposits and films. Conductive flooring should never be waxed. Rounded corners and edges facilitate cleaning.
4. *Air-conditioning grills.* The exterior of air-conditioning grills should be vacuumed at least weekly. Additional cleaning is necessary when filters are checked and changed. Debris may be discharged into the room when the filter is changed. In-room air handlers are positive pressure. The filters should be changed on an off shift or on the weekend. The room should be terminally cleaned after changing the filters.
5. *Storage shelves.* Storage cabinets have been replaced in many OR suites by portable storage carts or pass-through shelving to a sterile core. Storage areas should be cleaned at least weekly or more often, if necessary, to control accumulation of dust, especially in sterile storage areas.
6. *Sterilizers.* All types of sterilizers should be cleaned regularly and tested as recommended by the manufacturer.
7. *Exchange/vestibular and peripheral support areas.* Walls, ceilings, floors, air-conditioning grills, lockers, cabinets, and furniture should be cleaned on a regular schedule.

CONSIDERATIONS FOR THE USE OF DISPOSABLE PRODUCTS

Disposable products can be useful in the OR. It is sometimes easier to discard a contaminated item after use than to clean and process it. The use of disposable products has become popular, but consideration of the logistics of using them includes determination of the benefits and/or consequences of their use. The production of disposable products often involves the use of natural resources and potential industrial damage to the earth's environment. Disposal of the contaminated item can pose similar problems. Many issues concerning economy, including labor costs, storage, delivery, and disposal, need to be evaluated on an individual basis. Economy may or may not be shown with the use of disposable products.

Pros and Cons of Disposable Products

A disposable product is used once with assurance of safety and effectiveness. It is not salvaged after use; it is discarded. The cost of adequately and safely processing supplies is high. This high cost has led to the purchase of many disposable supplies for one-time patient use. Some of these are patient-charge items (i.e., the cost of these items is added to the patient's bill). Use of patient-charge items requires specific and accurate record keeping. It also requires evaluation of the advantages and disadvantages of disposable products to justify the cost to the patient.

Advantages

1. When a sterile item is required, proper packaging and sterility must be assured. Sterility is guaranteed by reli-

able manufacturers as long as the integrity of their packages is maintained. Industry conforms to far more rigid standards of quality control than on-site conditions permit. All sterilized products are tested for sterility before they are distributed to purchasers.

2. Single-use items, such as urinary catheters, are aesthetically more acceptable to patients. More important, disposable products eliminate a potential source of cross-contamination.

3. Items such as needles and safety razors ensure more comfort for the patient because they are always new and sharp. Proper function is thus ensured.

4. Standardized service at reduced cost per unit may be provided. Sponges are precounted and sterilized, for example. Packs and trays become standardized and can be customized.

5. Loss and breakage in reprocessing reusable items are eliminated.

6. Labor costs of processing supplies are reduced, particularly in the tedious, meticulous cleaning and packaging of small items, such as needles and syringes.

7. The need for expensive mechanical cleaning equipment is reduced or eliminated.

8. Contaminated used items can be contained for safe disposal. Handling and processing are eliminated.

Disadvantages

1. Costly waste occurs if sterile items are contaminated or unnecessarily opened. Extreme care is needed in opening packages to maintain sterility. Handling should not compromise the integrity of wrappings. Even though sterility of products from reliable manufacturers can be assured, their handling and storing may pose a threat to the maintenance of this sterility.

2. Flexibility in complying with requests of individual physicians for special setups is compromised. No allowance is made for deviation from commercially supplied packs or trays unless customized kits are purchased. Procedures may need to be revised to conform to available items and sets.

3. If a defect is found in one package, it may extend throughout the total lot, requiring replacement of the total supply on hand.

4. The circulator may have to open an increased number of individually packaged items. Some disposable plastic products melt; they cannot be put into instrument sets before steam sterilization.

5. In the event of a disaster or a sudden increase in use, adequate inventory may not be readily available.

6. Potentially unstable products, such as some disposable trays containing medications, may carry an expiration date. Unless oldest products are used first, unnecessary costs are incurred if a product must be discarded because its time of reliability has expired. All dated products should be routinely checked for expiration.

7. Environmental ecology may be affected by incineration or disposal in landfills. Some medical waste is regulated by local and federal laws.

Other Considerations

Some other considerations regarding the use of disposable products include the following:

- *Direct labor costs.* Some hospitals have saved money by reducing their labor force through conversion to as many totally disposable systems as possible, such as intravenous therapy, drapes, and special procedure trays. In some geographic areas where efficient labor may be readily available at minimum wage, disposable products are more costly than labor. However, if professional personnel are being used for reprocessing supplies, use of disposable products will enable them to spend more time giving more care to patients and less time on "things."

- *Storage.* Proper and safe storage facilities should be provided. More storage space or more frequent deliveries may be required to maintain adequate inventories of disposable products.

- *Disposal.* Disposal may be an ecologic problem. Used items are taken to an incinerator, compactor, or other safe waste-disposal area. Waste should not be allowed to accumulate in the OR suite or in other hospital areas.

Reusing/Reprocessing Disposable Products

Manufacturers use extensive controls and testing procedures to ensure cleanliness, nontoxicity, nonpyrogenicity, biocompatibility, sterility, and function of disposable products. All items must be safe and effective for their intended patient uses. The manufacturer guarantees product stability and sterility for a single use only.

In this era of cost containment, salvage of undamaged disposable items may be attempted. The risks of salvaging items should be evaluated seriously. The health care facility assumes legal responsibility for items it chooses to reuse, reprocess, and resterilize. The manufacturer cannot be held liable for the efficacy of a disposable product or one intended for single use if the user chooses to reprocess it. The burden of liability rests with the processor.

Reuse

Reuse of a used disposable, single-use item requires cleaning, packaging, and sterilizing if it will be reused as a sterile item. Some products degrade with use. Many manufacturers have not tested their products for more than one use. To reuse a product, the product should be tested to validate patient safety.

Reprocessing

Repackaging and resterilizing unused sterile disposable items may be potentially hazardous. These are items that were opened and not needed, or they are clean but have been contaminated in some way (i.e., the original packaging is not intact). Many of these items are very expensive, and salvage seems to be an acceptable alternative. The manufacturer must provide written instructions for resterilization of unused but contaminated items by on-site personnel. Many of these items are heat sensitive. Services that rewrap and resterilize some types of clean, unused, and undamaged products are available. Such services must guarantee product stability and sterility.

Resterilization

Unopened sterile products may be combined so that only one sterile package or procedural tray needs to be opened rather than many single packages. Or an unsterile part of an item may need to be sterilized for use on the sterile field. The sterilization process must not alter the characteristics of any part of the product. Some products are labeled "do not resterilize." This instruction means that the product will be damaged in the process of resterilization. Manufacturer's recommendations should be followed.

Safety Considerations

Patient safety should be the prime concern in the decision to reuse, reprocess, or resterilize a disposable item. Several questions should be answered:

1. Is the item a noncritical/noninvasive device? Critical items, particularly those that will enter or be in contact with the bloodstream or mucous membranes, present the greatest risks of possible adverse effects. Cleaning of these items should not be attempted.
2. Is the item clean? Many porous materials cannot be thoroughly cleaned after use. If these are not adequately cleaned, microbial growth can predispose patients to infection. Lumens of catheters and tubing are especially difficult to clean. Biologic debris, which interferes with the sterilization process, must be mechanically removed, for example, with a brush that is capable of cleaning the entire length of a lumen.
3. Is the item nontoxic or nonpyrogenic after cleaning and reprocessing? Residues from some cleaning compounds and ethylene oxide gas are toxic. Water can contain pyrogens. Microorganisms can produce endotoxins and exotoxins. Aeration is required following ethylene oxide sterilization.
4. Is the item sterile? The sterilization method should be appropriate for materials in the item and in the packaging. The packaging material should allow penetration of the sterilant to all surfaces of the item and should prevent contamination during storage. Sterility should be verified by biologic testing for each type of product that is resterilized.
5. Is the integrity of the product maintained? Physical and/or chemical characteristics may be altered by cleaning agents, the cleaning process, or resterilization. Some materials deteriorate or become brittle, which can affect function.
6. Is the number of times an item has been reprocessed known and controlled? Although this is rare, a manufacturer's written instructions may include the number of times the product may safely be reused or sterilized. The user should ensure that this number is not exceeded. The manufacturer has no control after a product is purchased. If the item is not in its original package, it obviously has been reprocessed. Remember, disposable items are intended for single use only.
7. Is the item traceable? Reprocessing of implantable synthetic mesh or graft material should be controlled by lot numbers. The lot number on the product when first obtained from the manufacturer corresponds only with the processes at the point of controlled production. If the product is reprocessed on site, the lot number is no longer valid because the same controls are not in place for subsequent sterilization. Many variables can alter the safety of the product for reuse.

Unless the answers to these questions are yes, the item should not be reused. With or without written instructions from the manufacturer, the health care facility is liable for product stability and sterility of any item it processes and sterilizes.

Custom Packs

A custom pack is a preassembled collection of disposable supplies sterilized as a single unit. The components are specified by the user (i.e., the OR's specifications) for a particular procedure or specialty or a surgeon's preferences. These components are assembled and sterilized by a custom pack supplier or the manufacturer. A pack assembled by a manufacturer will have an assortment of products in a specific category, such as a kit of sutures, ligating clips, and skin staplers or a custom pack of disposable drapes. Many custom packs have approximately 100 diversified items needed for a specific type of surgical procedure, such as a pack for an open heart procedure. Care should be taken in handling packs because damage to or contamination of a custom pack may waste many sterile items.

The assembler sterilizes packs with either ethylene oxide gas or gamma radiation. All components of the pack must be compatible with the sterilization method. The assembler must adhere to government manufacturing regulations for testing to guarantee product stability and sterility and package integrity. Using custom packs may be cost-effective for the health care facility, and the following indirect savings are shared by the materiels management department and the OR:

1. Personnel time (labor costs) for handling supplies is reduced.
   a. It reduces turnover time between procedures by saving time spent gathering and opening supplies. The circulator has more time for direct patient care activities.
   b. It reduces setup time for the scrub person. Items can be prearranged in order of use and with components in proximity, such as suction tubing with a tip.
   c. It facilitates transport of supplies into storage or into a case cart system.
2. Storage space requirements are consolidated by storing supplies in bulk rather than individually.

3. Inventory control is facilitated.
   a. It simplifies listing of items in inventory. The supplier may maintain a computerized information system of usage and inventory levels.
   b. It reduces inventory. A minimal backup of supplies can be maintained.
   c. It reduces lost patient charges. The circulator can process one charge for the custom pack rather than itemizing items.
4. Standardization is encouraged by incorporating the basic items routinely used by surgeon(s) into custom packs. This helps to standardize preparations.
5. The infection rate may be decreased. The physical activity of opening supplies can disperse lint and dust into the air. Opening fewer packages decreases this potential environmental hazard.
6. Less environmental waste is generated by packaging material. Fewer disposable wrappers are used.

Many custom pack processors have addressed the problem of changes in surgeon's preferences by offering to supply the packs in small quantities. Changes are incorporated into new stock, thus decreasing the number of pack contents that may not be used. Some manufacturers will replace older or damaged packs for new stock. Evaluation of pack usefulness is ongoing and may change as the types and complexity of surgical procedures change.

Recycling

Many surgical supplies are recyclable. Recycling reduces not only the amount of waste in landfills or air pollution, but also the amount of virgin resources that are consumed. Paper wrappers and many plastic items that are noninfectious, nonregulated trash can and should be recycled. Recycling in the OR should be an integral part of the overall recycling program of the health care facility. Consideration of recycling potential can be part of the evaluation process in selecting products.

DRUG AND MEDICAL DEVICE LEGISLATION

In 1906 the U.S. government enacted the Pure Food and Drug Act, with the U.S. Department of Agriculture as the enforcing agency, to ensure the introduction of safe and sanitary foods to the public. The Food, Drug, and Cosmetic Act of 1938 extended regulation to include cosmetics and drugs and, to a minimal extent, medical devices. The Food and Drug Administration (FDA), within the Department of Agriculture, became the enforcing agency with authority to implement a preclearance mechanism requiring drug manufacturers to provide evidence of safety before a new drug could be sold. Sutures were classified as drugs.

The Kefauver-Harris Drug Amendments of 1962 added strength to the new drug clearance procedures. Drug manufacturers must prove to the FDA the effectiveness, as well as the safety, of drugs before making them commercially available. These amendments established a mechanism for clinical investigation to evaluate the efficacy of drugs. Depending on the nature of a drug, clinical studies often require several years before the FDA approves commercial sale of a product.

The Medical Device Amendments of 1976 gave the FDA regulatory control over medical devices. A medical device is defined as any instrument, apparatus, or other similar or related article, including any component, part, or accessory, promoted for a medical purpose that does not rely on chemical action to achieve its intended purpose. Under this definition sutures were reclassified as devices. All of the wound closure materials discussed in this chapter are classified as devices.

In 1988 the FDA reclassified many devices, including surgical attire, masks, gloves, and drapes, for control under FDA regulations. Medical devices are classified and receive FDA approval before they are marketed. They are classified into one of three classifications:

Class I devices are subject to general regulatory controls that ensure that they are as safe and effective as similar devices already being sold.
Class II devices must establish safety and effectiveness performance standards for a new type of product.
Class III devices are usually life-sustaining or life-supporting implants or external devices. The manufacturer must file for premarket approval before the device is tested clinically to substantiate effectiveness.

A mandatory reporting regulation was put into effect in 1984. This regulation requires manufacturers and importers to report to the FDA any death or serious injury to a patient as a result of the malfunction of a medical device. Through the Safe Medical Devices Act of 1990, health care facilities must report directly to the FDA and to the manufacturer the probability that a device caused or contributed to a patient's death, serious injury, or serious illness. Additional requirements for tracking certain permanently implantable devices became effective in 1993. Manufacturers are responsible for tracking devices from the manufacturing facility through the chain of distribution (purchasers) to the end users (patients). Health care facilities that implant and explant (remove) these devices must submit reports to manufacturers promptly after devices are received, implanted, and/or explanted. The manufacturer must be able to provide to the FDA the following specific information:

1. Device
   a. Lot, batch, model, and serial numbers or other identification used by the manufacturer
   b. Date(s) of receipt or acquisition within the chain of distribution
   c. Name(s) of person(s) or supplier from whom the device was received
2. Patient
   a. Date of implantation
   b. Name, address, and telephone number of the recipient patient

THE FDA MEDICAL PRODUCTS REPORTING PROGRAM

A. Patient information

1. Patient identifier | **2. Age at time of event:** or _____ **Date of birth:** | **3. Sex** ☐ female ☐ male | **4. Weight** _____ lbs or _____ kgs

In confidence

B. Adverse event or product problem

1. ☐ **Adverse event**   and/or   ☐ **Product problem** (e.g., defects/malfunctions)

2. Outcomes attributed to adverse event
(check all that apply)

☐ death _____ (mo/day/yr)
☐ life-threatening
☐ hospitalization – initial or prolonged

☐ disability
☐ congenital anomaly
☐ required intervention to prevent permanent impairment/damage
☐ other: _____

3. Date of event (mo/day/yr)

4. Date of this report (mo/day/yr)

5. Describe event or problem

6. Relevant tests/laboratory data, including dates

7. Other relevant history, including preexisting medical conditions (e.g., allergies, race, pregnancy, smoking and alcohol use, hepatic/renal dysfunction, etc.)

C. Suspect medication(s)

1. Name (give labeled strength & mfr/labeler, if known)
#1
#2

2. Dose, frequency & route used
#1
#2

3. Therapy dates (if unknown, give duration) from/to (or best estimate)
#1
#2

4. Diagnosis for use (indication)
#1
#2

5. Event abated after use stopped or dose reduced
#1 ☐ yes ☐ no ☐ doesn't apply
#2 ☐ yes ☐ no ☐ doesn't apply

6. Lot # (if known)
#1
#2

7. Exp. date (if known)
#1
#2

8. Event reappeared after reintroduction
#1 ☐ yes ☐ no ☐ doesn't apply
#2 ☐ yes ☐ no ☐ doesn't apply

9. NDC # (for product problems only)
–   –

10. Concomitant medical products and therapy dates (exclude treatment of event)

D. Suspect medical device

1. Brand name

2. Type of device

3. Manufacturer name & address

4. Operator of device
☐ health professional
☐ lay user/patient
☐ other: _____

5. Expiration date (mo/day/yr)

6.
model # _____
catalog # _____
serial # _____
lot # _____
other #

7. If implanted, give date (mo/day/yr)

8. If explanted, give date (mo/day/yr)

9. Device available for evaluation?   (Do not send to FDA)
☐ yes   ☐ no   ☐ returned to manufacturer on _____ (mo/day/yr)

10. Concomitant medical products and therapy dates (exclude treatment of event)

E. Reporter (see confidentiality section on back)

1. Name, address & phone #

2. Health professional?
☐ yes ☐ no

3. Occupation

4. Also reported to
☐ manufacturer
☐ user facility
☐ distributor

5. If you do NOT want your identity disclosed to the manufacturer, place an " X " in this box. ☐

FDA   **Mail to:** MEDWATCH
5600 Fishers Lane
Rockville, MD 20852-9787

or **FAX to:**
1-800-FDA-0178

FDA Form 3500 (6/93)   Submission of a report does not constitute an admission that medical personnel or the product caused or contributed to the event.

Figure 12-3   MEDWATCH reporting form. (Courtesy US Food and Drug Administration, Rockville, Md.)

c. Social Security number, if the patient's permission is obtained to release his or her Social Security number to the manufacturer
3. Physician(s) who prescribed, implanted, and/or explanted the device
4. End-of-life information about the device, as applicable
   a. Date of explantation
   b. Date of patient's death
   c. Date the device was returned to the distributor or manufacturer
   d. Date the device was permanently retired from use or disposed of

Also in 1993 the FDA began the voluntary MEDWATCH program to encourage physicians, nurses, pharmacists, and other heath care professionals to report adverse events and defects or problems with regulated drugs and devices. The purpose of MEDWATCH is to provide a nationwide standardized system for reporting to the FDA any medical device or drug suspected of causing a patient's death, life-threatening injury or illness, disability, prolonged hospitalization, congenital anomaly, and/or experience that required intervention to prevent permanent health impairment. The FDA provides a MEDWATCH reporting form (Figure 12-3). Examples of reportable problems include latex sensitivity, malfunction of drug infusion pumps, and failure of an alarm during malfunction of a ventilator.

Surgeons who implant or use medical devices, as well as nurses, surgical technologists, and others who handle them, must be adequately instructed in the proper care and handling of all devices to ensure patient safety. Most adverse events occur when devices are misused, are defective, or malfunction. However, an adverse patient reaction can occur when the device functions properly and is used appropriately. The FDA is responsible for investigating a report of an adverse event or product problem and for taking corrective action.

PRODUCT EVALUATION

The user of a product is best qualified to evaluate performance, safety, effectiveness, and efficiency. Before a decision is made to purchase or to standardize a particular item, a clinical evaluation should be conducted to solicit feedback from team members whose work will be affected by the product. This may involve the surgeons or anesthesia providers, as well as perioperative nurses and surgical technologists. Instruction should be provided on the correct use of the item before it is evaluated. Sales representatives may be permitted to assist in the trial of a product in the OR. While not providing direct patient care, they offer suggestions and consult with the users during the product trial.

To be valid, feedback should be an objective evaluation of function, quality, and use. Does it meet a need? Does it solve a problem? Is it cost-effective? Does it improve patient care? How does it compare with other brands? Several brands of the same product may be evaluated to select the most satisfactory one for the intended purpose and to standardize the inventory. Written evaluations are useful for the decision-making process after the trial period is over.

Many products are used only in the perioperative environment; others are also used in other patient care areas. Representatives from all user departments should assist the materiels manager in the selection of products. Most hospitals have a product evaluation committee for this purpose. A representative of the perioperative staff provides this committee with information regarding quality and effectiveness, based on feedback from user staff members.

Once a product has been purchased, the user assumes responsibility for its safety and its proper use for the purpose for which it is intended.

Bibliography

Abbott P: The best of both worlds . . . "reposables," *Todays Surg Nurse* 19(2):35-38, 1997.
Association of Operating Room Nurses: *AORN standards, recommended practices, and guidelines,* Denver, 1998, The Association.
Botsford J, Hixon SK: AORN Special Committee on Environmental Issues reports environmental survey results, *AORN J* 60(4):652-655, 1994.
Dascher FD, Dettenkofer M: Protecting the patient and the environment . . . new aspects and challenges in hospital infection control, *J Hosp Infect* 36(1):7-15, 1997.
French HM: Blueprint for reducing, reusing, recycling, *AORN J* 60(1):94-98, 1994.
Greaves J: Healthcare and the environment, *Br J Theatre Nurs* 4(3):14-16, 1994.
Raltz S et al: The impact of disposable equipment on room fee reimbursement for endoscopic retrograde cholangiopancreatography, *Gastroenterol Nurs* 17(1):14-16, 1994.
Richardson M: The standard guide to green nursing: 20 tips to protect the environment, *Nurs Stand* 8(18):50-52, 1994.
Rosenblatt WH et al: Recovery of unused operating room supplies for overseas orthopedic surgery, *Am J Orthop* 25(9):633-636, 1996.
Roth RA: *Perioperative nursing core curriculum,* Philadelphia, 1995, WB Saunders.
Spanton G: Reuse of disposables: is it worth the risk? *Can OR Nurs J* 15(4):28-30, 1997.
Weatherly KS et al: Product evaluation process: a systems approach to controlling health care costs, *AORN J* 59(2):489-498, 1994.
Willmer S et al: Reuse of single use items in minimal access surgery, *Br J Theatre Nurs* 7(3):11-13, 1997.

Chapter 13

Potential Sources of Injury to the Caregiver and the Patient

Chapter Objectives

After studying this chapter, the learner will be able to:

- Identify potential environmental sources of injury to patients and personnel in the perioperative environment.
- Discuss the prevention of injury through proper testing and use of equipment in the OR.
- Discuss the importance of fire and disaster drills.

The health care environment is laden with hazards for the caregiver and the patient. Therefore the health care facility should be made as safe as possible. Caregivers should make full and proper use of the safety and control measures established by facility policies and procedures. Failure to use equipment and devices in a safe manner places both the caregiver and the patient at risk for injury.

Safety goes hand in hand with knowledge, skill, and competency. Some equipment, such as lasers, x-rays, and chemical sterilizers, can cause long-range injury if personnel are lax in safety and protective practices. The education and training of personnel is essential to create an awareness of the potential hazards. No one should be permitted to use equipment until he or she has been properly instructed in its correct use and care. Each caregiver should use his or her own initiative to seek instruction when needed. Competency

in the use of equipment should be tested periodically because technology changes frequently, and the knowledge and skill associated with one piece of equipment may not apply to a newer model. In some instances the technology may become safer, but this is not always the case.

Potential hazards should be identified and safe practices established. Risk management service within the facility is charged with the responsibility of tracking issues of safety and potential injury. The recommendations that arise from these data are established to guide personnel in corrective actions. Patients and caregivers are never completely free from risks, but the risks can be minimized. Legally, safety refers to conditions that will not cause injury or harm to the employee, the patient, and other persons in the health care facility. Terms associated with environmental hazards are defined in Boxes 13-1 (radiation) and 13-2 (electricity).

Box 13-1 **Terms Associated with Radiation**

radiation Process of emitting radiant energy in the form of electromagnetic waves or atomic particles, or the combined process of emitting and transmitting radiant energy.

ionizing radiation Sufficient radiant energy to yield ions from the disintegration of the nuclei of unstable or radioactive elements. This radiation occurs naturally from cosmic rays, and these ions disrupt the electronic balance of atoms. Manmade x-rays and nuclear power are capable of modifying molecules within body cells as they pass through tissue. They can be mutagenic (i.e., cause mutations of DNA) in somatic body cells, predisposing a person to cancer, and in germ cells, predisposing a person to spontaneous abortion or congenital malformations.

nonionizing radiation Radiant energy that does not produce ions but can produce hyperthermic conditions that are harmful to the skin and eyes. With the possible exception of ultraviolet rays, wavelengths from electromagnetic spectrum do not alter DNA in body cells.

emissions Electromagnetic waves or atomic particles spontaneously given off by ionizing radioactive elements.

alpha particles Relatively large particles emitted from disintegrating radioactive atoms. These particles have dense ionization within short distances and are easily stopped by a thin sheet of paper.

beta particles Relatively small particles with greater penetration at a faster speed than alpha particles. They also are easily stopped.

gamma rays High-energy, short electromagnetic wavelengths emitted spontaneously from the nucleus of radioactive atoms. They have no mass but can be stopped by dense material such as lead.

x-rays High-energy electromagnetic waves capable of penetrating various thicknesses of solid substances and of affecting photographic plates. They are generated from high-velocity electrons only when a machine that produces them is turned on. They can be stopped by dense material such as lead or concrete.

sources Alpha or beta particles are emitted from different sources than those that generate gamma rays and x-rays. Sources used in the OR include the following:

fluoroscope Fluorescent light reproduces optical images of body structures identified by x-rays onto a luminescent screen. These images can be amplified with an image intensifier and projected onto a television monitor. Radiation exposure can be as much as 10 times greater during 1 minute of fluoroscopy than that of a single x-ray.

x-ray machine Fixed or portable generator projects x-rays through an enclosed tube directed at the patient. A focused beam passes through the patient to photographic film only when the generator is activated for single exposure.

radioactive implants Radioactive elements continuously emit alpha and beta particles and/or gamma rays. All radiation sources for therapeutic implantation are prepared by the nuclear medicine department. They require very special handling in the OR for the safety of both patients and personnel. Radionuclides, elements that have been bombarded in a nuclear reactor with radioactive particles, have primarily replaced the therapeutic use of radium and radon. Radionuclides emit radiation as they disintegrate.

external beam Gamma rays or x-rays are generated from orthovoltage (low) or megavoltage (high) linear accelerators or betatrons for preoperative, intraoperative, or postoperative radiation therapy.

measurements The intensity of radiation is expressed in different units of measurement:

roentgen (R) A measure of pairs of ions (charged particles) produced in air by gamma rays and x-rays; it is used in the calibration of radiation-producing sources.

radiation absorbed dose (rad) A unit of absorbed dose from all types of ionizing radiation, calculated as 100 units of energy per gram.

roentgen equivalent man (rem) A unit of equivalent dose derived by multiplying rads by quality factors for the relative biologic effects of a type of radiation. Rem is a measurement used in occupational monitoring: 1 rem = 1 R = 1 rad; 1 milliroentgen (mR) = 1/1000 rem.

sievert (Sv) An international unit of measure for equivalent dose, that is, an absorbed dose weighted by quality factor for the type of radiation: 1 Sv = 100 rem; 1 millisievert (mSv) = 1/1000 Sv = 100 mR.

curie Measures the radioactivity or number of spontaneous nuclear transformations per unit of time. It has no direct relationship to ionization, absorption, and dose equivalent.

half-life Time required for a radioactive element to lose 50% of its activity by disintegration, or the time required for the body to eliminate one half of the administered dose. Each radionuclide has its own half-life.

exposure Total quantity of radiation a body receives. This is cumulative over a lifetime.

latency period Period between exposure and the development of the effects of that exposure. Long-term effects of cumulative exposure may not be evident for as long as 20 years.

HISTORICAL BACKGROUND

Historically, the operating room (OR) has been a place full of hazards for both the patient and the caregiver. The primary dangers include but are not limited to fire, chemical exposure to anesthetic agents, and direct exposure to biologic material.

Concern about fire and explosions caused by anesthetic agents intensified in 1925 with the introduction of ethylene gas; the use of drop ether was already popular. In the following decade another highly flammable gas, cyclopropane, became popular. Proper ventilation systems and gas-scavenging systems for waste gases were either absent or highly inefficient. The potential hazard of static electricity causing combustion of flammable anesthetics has been minimized by elimination of the flammable agents. However, ignition from thermal devices continues to remain a fire hazard.

eee444ff44444f44fff4444fffffff4ff4fff4ffff44fff4ffffffffffffff

Box 13-2 Terms Associated with Electrical Safety

combustible Flammable substance capable of reacting with oxygen to burn if ignited.

conductive materials Not only those materials that are commonly considered as electrically conductive (e.g., metals), but also a class of materials that, when tested in accordance with NFPA standard 99C, have resistance to the passage of electricity not exceeding 1,000,000 ohms. Such materials are required where electrostatic interconnection is necessary.*

flammable Any gas or liquid, including oxygen, that will burn or is capable, when ignited, of maintaining combustion.

grounding Equipotential system of conductors that establishes a conducting connection—whether intentional or accidental—between an electrical circuit in equipment and the earth (or some other connecting body that serves in place of earth) to divert stray currents.

isolated power system Assembly of electrical devices that provides local isolated power, a single grounding point, and distinctive receptacles.

leakage current Any current not intended to be applied to a patient but that may be conveyed from exposed metal or other accessible parts of appliance to ground.*

line isolation monitor Instrument that continually checks the hazard current from an isolated circuit to the ground.*

macroshock Effect of large electric currents (milliamperes or larger) on the body.*

microshock Effect of small electric currents (as low as 10 microamperes) on the body.*

nonflammable anesthetic agents Inhalation agents that, because of their vapor pressure at a temperature of 98° F (37° C) and an atmospheric pressure of 760 mm Hg, cannot attain flammable concentrations when mixed with air, oxygen, or mixtures of oxygen and nitrous oxide.

path of least resistance Return path for current to ground with minimal resistance or through leakage current.

patient ground Terminal bus (a type of connection) that serves as a single focus for (1) grounding all electrical devices that serve a patient and are not connected by a power cord to a reference grounding point, and (2) grounding conductive furniture or equipment within the reach of any person who may touch patient.†

*From National Fire Protection Association: *NFPA 99C standard for medical gas,* Quincy, Mass, 1990, The Association.
†Modified from National Fire Protection Association: *NFPA 99C standard for medical gas,* Quincy, Mass, 1990, The Association.

Special conductive shoes or conductive shoe covers used to be worn by personnel in the OR to minimize the risk of fire caused by a spark of static electricity. On entering the suite, each person was required to stand on a conductivity testing device near the entrance to the department. At one time, undergarments made from synthetic fibers were discouraged in the OR because they were considered a potential source of static.

ENVIRONMENTAL HAZARDS

The perioperative environment poses many hazards for both patients and personnel. The potential for physical injury from electric shock, burns, fire, explosion, exposure to bloodborne pathogens, and inhalation of toxic substances is ever present. Therefore it is important that staff have knowledge of the hazards involved in equipment use, the causes of accidental injury, and the sources of health risks. All individuals have a personal responsibility to ensure a safe environment for themselves and others. Faulty equipment or improper usage increases the hazards of potential risk factors.

Classification of Hazards

Injuries can be caused by using faulty equipment, using equipment improperly, exposing oneself or others to toxic or irritating agents, or coming into contact with harmful agents. Hazards in the OR environment can be classified as follows:

- *Physical:* including back injury, fall, noise pollution, irradiation, electricity, and fire

- *Chemical:* including anesthetic gases, toxic fumes from gases and liquids, cytotoxic drugs, and cleaning agents
- *Biologic:* including the patient (as a host for or source of pathogenic microorganisms), infectious waste, cuts or needle-stick injuries, surgical plume, and latex sensitivity

Regulation of Hazards

Standards, guidelines, and recommended practices have been developed by many professional associations, such as AORN, the Association of periOperative Registered Nurses; and governmental agencies, such as the Department of Health and Human Services (DHHS). The policies and procedures of the health care facility should be developed and enforced in compliance with local, state, and federal regulations. Other agencies include, but are not limited to, the following:

- The American Conference of Governmental Industrial Hygienists (ACGIH) (**www.acgih.org**) sets standards for threshold limits for exposure to toxic materials.
- The American National Standards Institute (ANSI) (**www.ansi.org**) sets standards to limit exposures to devices that emit light or sound, such as lasers, ultraviolet light, and nonionizing radiation.
- The National Fire Protection Association (NFPA) (**www.nfpa.org**) sets standards for electrical codes and fire safety.
- The Joint Commission on Accreditation of Healthcare Organizations (JCAHO) (**www.jcaho.org**) establishes standards of patient care for accreditation.

Box 13-3	The Original Top Ten Occupational Hazards Identified by NIOSH, 1983

Occupational lung diseases
Musculoskeletal injuries
Occupational cancers
Amputations, fractures, eye loss, lacerations, traumatic death
Cardiovascular diseases
Reproductive disorders
Neurotoxic disorders
Noise-induced hearing loss
Dermatologic conditions
Psychologic disorders

Data from United States Department of Health and Human Services (www.dhhs.gov) and Centers for Disease Control and Prevention (www.cdc.gov).

- The Centers for Disease Control and Prevention (CDC) (**www.cdc.gov**) sets standards for infection control.
- The National Institute for Occupational Safety and Health (NIOSH) (**www.cdc.gov/niosh**) sets standards for ventilation systems and environmental protection in the workplace.
- The Environmental Protection Agency (EPA) (**www.epa.gov**) sets standards for the disposal of infectious and hazardous waste.
- The Food and Drug Administration (FDA) (**www.fda.gov**) sets standards and controls for the use of drugs, biologics, devices, and chemicals in patient care.
- The Center for Devices and Radiologic Health (CDRH) (**www.fda.gov/cdrh/**) sets standards for the management and monitoring of radiation in patient care.

In 1970 the Occupational Safety and Health Administration (OSHA) was created within the U.S. Department of Labor. Initially, OSHA adopted preexisting federal and national consensus standards and guidelines for environmental, patient, and personnel safety. Since its inception, OSHA has issued new standards and amended others, such as permissible exposure limits (PELs) to various occupational health and safety hazards. OSHA is authorized by law to enforce its standards, which may require employers to measure and monitor exposure to toxic or harmful agents, to notify employees of overexposure and provide medical consultation or care, and to maintain records of corrective actions. OSHA inspects health care facilities for compliance with standards. More information can be found at **www.osha.gov.**

The CDC oversees the activities of NIOSH. The research branch of NIOSH is the National Occupational Research Agenda (NORA). NORA has studied the earlier efforts of NIOSH to identify the top ten occupational hazards (Box 13-3). In its studies of work hazards, NORA found twenty-one actual occupational hazards. Several of these hazards have been grouped into a disease and injury category that can be compared to risks for health care workers and their patients (Box 13-4).

Box 13-4	Common Work-Related Health Conditions Identified by NORA, 1998

Acute and chronic airway disease
Select chronic disease
Chronic obstructive pulmonary disease
Contact dermatitis
Depression and anxiety
Fertility and pregnancy abnormalities
Hearing loss caused by noise and nonauditory exposures
Low back disorders
Molecular correlates of cancer
Musculoskeletal disorders of upper extremities
Occupational asthma
Occupational cancer
Occupational skin disease
Stress
Traumatic injuries

Data from United States Department of Health and Human Services (www.dhhs.gov) and Centers for Disease Control and Prevention (www.cdc.gov).

PHYSICAL HAZARDS AND SAFEGUARDS

The architectural design of the perioperative environment affects its overall efficiency and productivity. The physical facility is designed to control traffic patterns, decrease contamination, facilitate the handling of equipment and supplies, and provide a comfortable working environment.

Environmental Factors

Several factors contribute to providing a safe, comfortable working environment: temperature control, ventilation, lighting, color, and noise. Temperature control should provide physical comfort (i.e., it should not be too warm or too cool).

The ventilating system in the perioperative environment usually evacuates odors fairly quickly by exchanging air 15 times per hour, with 3 exchanges of fresh air. The ventilating system should help to remove toxic fumes and anesthetic gas waste. Perfume and other odors can cause nausea or respiratory congestion in sensitive persons. Heavy perfume can also have an annoying, lingering effect, and therefore persons in the perioperative environment should avoid wearing it.

Lighting should be adequate, but excessive glare causes fatigue. Illumination is the product of the light and the reflectance of the target. A bright, highly polished mirror finish on an instrument tends to reflect light and can restrict vision. Satin- or dull-finished instruments eliminate glare and lessen eyestrain. These instruments are made with varying degrees of dullness depending on the manufacturer. Lightly tinted or polarized eyewear may save sterile team members from visual fatigue but should not distort the color of tissues. For drapes and walls, soft, cool colors, especially blues and greens, are less reflective than white. Drapes with dark tones help to reduce the contrast between most tissues and the surrounding field.

Although attention is given to ventilation, lighting, and color, less attention is given to the design of the OR in terms of auditory effects. Some facilities have piped-in music in waiting areas. Music can be stimulating for personnel and relaxing for patients who are awaiting surgery or undergoing a surgical procedure under local anesthesia. The selection of music should be appropriate for the intended listener. Music with a low volume, moderate rhythm, and bright tone can motivate muscular activity and increase levels of efficiency of OR personnel. However, this type of music would not be conducive to relaxation for the patient who is awaiting surgery. On the other hand, music can be a distraction and an annoyance, especially for the anesthesia provider, who may depend on auscultation when monitoring the patient. Music should be turned off at the request of the patient, surgeon, or anesthesia provider.

Extreme noise from drills, fan motors in equipment, and other sources can be annoying and potentially dangerous to patients and personnel. The noise can become intense enough to increase blood pressure and to provoke peripheral vasoconstriction, dilation of the pupils, and other subtle physiologic effects. It can also interfere with necessary communication and thereby provoke irritation. The EPA recommends that noise levels in hospitals not exceed 45 decibels during daytime hours.

The OR should be as quiet as possible except for the essential sounds of communication between team members directly concerned with the patient's care. Any necessary talking should be done in a low voice. Counts or requests for supplies should be done quietly. Conversation unrelated to the surgical procedure is out of place. Even during the deep stages of anesthesia, a patient may perceive and remember noise that occurs during the surgical procedure. If a regional or local anesthetic is used, the patient can hear the conversation. Because patients interpret anything they hear in terms of themselves, all words should be guarded.

Major sources of noise in the OR involve paper, gloves, objects wheeled across the floor, instruments striking one another, monitors, and high-pitched power instruments, including suction. The scrub person should keep in mind the sources and the effects of this noise. The clattering of instruments should be avoided. Except while in actual use, suction tubing should be clamped or kinked. Paper wrappings should not be crushed. Monitors with audible signals should be placed as far away from the patient's ears as possible; continuous monitor beeps can also distract the surgeon and anesthesia provider. The circulator should keep the doors to the OR closed to shut out the noise of the corridors, of water running in the scrub room, or of the sterilizer operating in the substerile room.

Working in a pleasantly quiet environment is less fatiguing, produces fewer psychologic and physiologic adverse effects, and allows for greater efficiency on behalf of the patient.

Body Mechanics

Backache is a leading cause of work-related lost time and is second only to upper respiratory infections. Standing for prolonged periods, often in an awkward position, is a common cause of low back pain. Tiring body motions or an awkward or strained body posture should be avoided. Weight bearing on only one foot causes additional strain. When the feet are placed together while standing, constant muscular effort is required by the thigh muscles to maintain an erect posture. In contrast, when the feet are apart, the ligaments of the hips and knees support the body with less effort. Therefore maintaining a wide stance while standing at the operating bed for prolonged periods will be less fatiguing for the scrub person. While in a location to observe both the surgical procedure and the instrument table, the circulator can stand with the upper and lower extremities in a resting position. In this standing position the arms are clasped behind the back and the feet are in a wide stance.

Shoes should be considered for comfort and safety. Soft canvas or leather athletic shoes that tie or secure with Velcro provide adequate support for the foot. If running is required during an emergency, these shoes will be more secure than clog varieties with open backs.

The operating bed is adjusted to the best working height for the surgeon, which may not be the most comfortable position for the other members of the sterile team. Team members should be able to stand erect with their arms comfortably relaxed from the shoulders, without stooping, and they should not need to raise their hands above the level of their elbows for the majority of their work motions. Standing platforms (step stools) may be needed to elevate the scrub person and/or the assistant surgeon to a feasible working height. These platforms should be long enough and wide enough to allow a wide stance.

Correct posture while in the sitting position is equally important. The back is strongest when it is straight. When seated, team members should sit well back in the chair or on the stool with the body straight from hips to neck. They should lean forward from the hips, not from the shoulders or waist. This position puts the least strain on muscles, ligaments, and internal organs. Before and after the surgical procedure, the circulator and scrub person(s) should rest in a sitting position between periods of standing. If work is done in a sitting position, the stool or chair should be adjusted to the correct height for the working surface.

First assistants may develop carpal tunnel syndrome as a result of holding retractors in one position for prolonged periods. Carpal tunnel syndrome is a form of repetitive stress injury caused by tenosynovitis that places pressure on the median nerve of the hand. Consequently, the thumb, index, and ring fingers tingle and feel swollen. Self-retaining retractors help to relieve some of this strain.

Sprains and strains are common injuries sustained to the back, arms, or shoulders as a result of lifting patients or moving equipment. Several principles of body mechanics should be observed to minimize physical injury:

1. Keep the body as close as possible to the person or equipment to be lifted or moved while maintaining a straight back.
2. Lift with the large muscle groups of the legs and abdominal muscles, not the back.

3. Bend the knees to get body weight under the load, then straighten the legs to lift with the heels flat on the floor.
4. Lift with a slow, even motion, keeping pressure off the lumbar (lower back) area.
5. Push, do not pull, stretchers, tables, and heavy equipment on wheels or casters.
6. Use large body muscles to maneuver the base of portable equipment such as lasers or microscopes.
7. If standing for prolonged periods, stand in a wide stance with the heels apart so the ligaments of the hips and knees can support the body without effort.
8. Distribute weight evenly on both feet, but shift the body occasionally during prolonged periods of standing.
9. Sit with the back straight from the hips to the neck, and lean forward from the hips.
10. Align the head and neck with the body when standing or sitting, maintaining the lumbar curve.
11. Change position, stretch, or walk around occasionally if possible.
12. Pivot the entire body to avoid twisting at the waist.
13. Bend forward with hip flexion and hand support.
14. Avoid overhead reaching or overstretching; keep materials in the chest-to-knee range if possible; use platforms as appropriate.

A lifting frame or Davis roller helps to relieve the potential strain of moving unconscious or obese patients. Moving these patients alone can cause injury to the patient or the caregiver. Assistance is also needed to position patients on the operating bed. The physical therapy department or occupational health director can be a resource for teaching the patient care staff the proper techniques for lifting, bending, reaching, and pivoting.

Ionizing Radiation

Radiation cannot be seen or felt. Ionizing radiation produces positively and negatively charged particles that can change the electrical charge of some atoms and molecules in cells. These changes can alter enzymes, proteins, cell membranes, and genetic material. This can cause the death of cancer cells when radiation is used in therapeutic doses; however, exposure to radiation can also cause cancer, cataracts, bone marrow injury, burns, tissue necrosis, genetic mutations, spontaneous abortion, and congenital anomalies.

Perioperative patient care personnel may assist with invasive x-ray studies. If unprotected, they are exposed to scatter radiation from the patient during intraoperative procedures when x-rays are taken or when fluoroscopes and image intensifiers are used. Team members also are exposed during the implantation or removal of radioactive elements. Patients exposed to radioactivity for therapeutic purposes or by accident may emit radiation. The effect of radiation is directly related to the amount and length of time of exposure. Exposure is cumulative, and there is an extended latency period; the effects may not be evident for years. Therefore constant vigilance for personal safety is essential to avoid excessive exposure to ionizing radiation. Protection implies understanding the basic terms and adhering to strict policies and procedures. Box 13-1 defines terms associated with ionizing radiation.

Safety Considerations in the Use of Ionizing Radiation

Because of the adverse and cumulative effects of ionizing radiation on body tissues, safety precautions are taken to protect patients and personnel from the potential hazards. Box 13-5 lists safe radiation exposure limits according to the area of the body. If protective precautions are used, OR personnel rarely, if ever, exceed these safe limits.

Patient Safety A patient can be exposed to the primary beam of x-rays, the radioactivity of implants, and scatter radiation. Any exposure to radiation has biologic risks, and therefore the exposure should be as low as possible. To reduce the amount of radiation exposure, the following precautions should be taken:

1. The fluoroscope should be turned off when not in use. The patient is continuously exposed to radiation during fluoroscopy.
2. Every effort should be made to reconcile an incorrect sponge, sharp, or instrument count. An x-ray film should be made only as a last resort to locate a missing item.
3. Body areas should be shielded from scatter radiation or the focused beam whenever possible. A lead shield can be positioned between the patient and radiation source if it will not interfere with the sterile field or visualization for the x-ray study. The shield is placed before the patient is draped. A shadow shield connected to the x-ray tube may be a preferable alternative if a lead shield cannot be used.

 Box 13-5

Permissible Doses of Radiation as Established by the National Council on Radiation Protection and Measurements

Permissible doses of radiation are based on units of an equivalent dose quantity that express all radiations on a common scale for the purpose of calculating their biologic effects. The maximum permissible doses per year for occupationally exposed persons over 18 years of age varies by body parts:

- Whole body, including blood-forming organs, bone marrow, and gonads: 5 rem, 50 mSv
- Lenses of eyes: 15 rem, 150 mSv
- Other organs and tissues: 50 rem, 500 mSv
- Fetus in utero: 0.5 rem, 5 mSv; no more than 50 mR, 0.5 mSv in any 1 month of gestation during pregnancy

Exposure should not exceed 100 mR, 1 mSv per week.

a. Lymphatic tissue, the thyroid gland, and the bone marrow of the sternum are especially sensitive to radiation. Therefore a thyroid/sternal shield should be used during x-ray studies or fluoroscopy of the head, upper extremities, and chest.

b. To protect the testes or ovaries, a gonadal shield should be used during x-ray studies or fluoroscopy of the hips and thighs.

c. A lead shield should always be used to protect the fetus of a pregnant patient. Even low levels of scatter radiation may be harmful to the fetus. Therefore x-rays to the abdomen and pelvis are avoided, especially during the first trimester.

Intraoperative documentation should include the anatomic location of the direct x-rays or fluoroscopy, the type and location of radioactive implants, and shielding measures to protect the patient from scatter radiation.

Personnel Safety Safety precautions should be taken to protect team members from the potential hazards of ionizing radiation. Three key factors must always be remembered: time, distance, and shielding.

TIME Overexposure and unnecessary exposure should be avoided in all persons, and especially in those of childbearing age. Changes may occur in the reproductive cells as a result of radiation, leading to potential genetic defects. The following precautions should be used to limit the length of exposure to radiation:

1. Patient care personnel should rotate assignments on procedures that involve radiation.

2. Staff members may request relief from exposure during pregnancy. If this is not possible, a pregnant staff member should leave the room or be adequately shielded when x-ray studies are performed or fluoroscopy is used.

3. Radiation from an x-ray tube, fluoroscope, and image intensifier is present only as long as the machine is energized. These machines should be turned off when not in use.

4. Radioactive elements should remain in lead-lined containers until ready for implantation. They should be handled as quickly as possible, and always with special forceps, by trained personnel.

5. A patient who has received radioactive substances for diagnostic studies may emit up to 2 mR per hour. If possible, the surgical procedure should be delayed for at least 24 hours after the test.

6. Personnel should limit the time spent in close proximity to a patient who has had a diagnostic study with or an implantation of radioactive elements until disintegration reaches a low level.

7. Body tissues and fluids removed from patients with radioactive emissions should be contained quickly.

DISTANCE Automatic or manual collimators, which confine the x-ray beam to the precise size of the x-ray film or fluoroscopic screen, are required for all equipment. Most image intensifiers have a lead shield as part of the installation. A single-frame computerized recording device incorporated into the fluoroscopy system also helps to reduce exposure. Fluoroscopy produces more scatter radiation than do direct x-ray beams. Personnel should distance themselves as far as possible from the source of radiation, as demonstrated by the following procedures:

1. Unsterile team members who can safely do so should leave the room during each single x-ray exposure.

2. Holding devices should be used to maintain the position of the x-ray film and patient.

3. Sterile team members and others who cannot leave room should stand 6 feet (2 m) or more from the patient, if possible, and out of the direct beam during exposure. Team members should remember the inverse square law of distance: double the distance equals one fourth the intensity.

4. If possible, team members should stand behind or at a right angle to the beam on the side of the patient where the beam enters, not exits.

5. Lateral or oblique x-rays increase scatter radiation. Positioning the beam in a plane vertical to the pelvis or thighs helps to reduce scatter. For supine and upright x-rays, the beam should be directed at the floor or walls.

SHIELDING Lead that is at least 0.5 mm thick offers the most effective protection against gamma and x-rays to halt and absorb radiation scatter. Alpha and beta particles do not require shielding. The following guidelines for shielding should be observed:

1. The walls of rooms with fixed radiation equipment are usually lined with lead. Gamma rays can penetrate lead to a depth of 12 inches (30.7 cm). X-rays can be stopped with lead or thick concrete.

2. Portable lead screens should be available.

   a. Sterile team members and others who cannot leave the room should stand behind a screen while x-ray films are taken or while the patient is exposed to intraoperative radiation therapy. The screen(s) should be positioned behind a portable machine.

   b. When a lateral exposure is taken, the screen should be positioned behind the x-ray film cassette to absorb rays that penetrate through or scatter from the cassette.

   c. Persons preparing radioactive implants that emit gamma rays should do so from behind a lead screen that is up to 12 inches (30.7 cm) thick. A sterile drape can be put over the screen so the scrub person or other sterile team member can stand behind the screen and reach around it.

3. Lead aprons should be worn by sterile and unsterile team members.

   a. The lead apron is worn under the sterile gown.

   b. If the apron does not wrap around the body, team members should face the radiation source so the apron provides protection between the source and the body.

   c. To protect against beam and scatter radiation, team members should wear aprons during fluoroscopy and for lateral or oblique x-ray studies. Levels of scatter radiation are greater at lateral and oblique angles, and exposure time is prolonged during fluoroscopy.

   d. Lead aprons should be hung or laid flat when not in use. They should not be folded. Folding can crack the lead, making the shield ineffective.

4. Lead-impregnated rubber gloves can attenuate (reduce the intensity) of rays by 15% to 25%.

   a. Sterile gloves should be worn by sterile team members when the hands will be in direct exposure (e.g., during fluoroscopy), when injecting radioactive dyes or elements, and while handling radioactive implants.

   b. If it is necessary to hold a cassette in position for a single x-ray exposure, lead gloves should be worn.

   c. Lead gloves may be supplied sterile or sterilized by the appropriate method for reuse. The rubber should allow adequate aeration to avoid skin irritation of the wearer.

5. Lead thyroid/sternal collars or shields should be worn during fluoroscopy and exposure to oblique angle x-rays. Personnel within 6 feet (2 m) of the radiation source, including the anesthesia provider, risk exposure of the head and neck.

6. Leaded glasses may be worn to protect the eyes during fluoroscopy.

Lead shields should be tested routinely by the radiology department every 6 months or whenever damage is suspected. Defects may not be visually detected.

Monitoring Radiation Exposure

All personnel exposed to ionizing radiation with any frequency or during prolonged procedures should wear a monitoring device. The purpose of the device is to measure the total rems of accumulated exposure. Therefore the monitor is worn only by the person to whom it is issued and at all times of exposure for the designated period. Exposure data on the monitor are recorded for each individual either monthly or weekly, depending on the type of monitor.

Film badges are the most widely used monitors. These monitors contain small pieces of photographic film that are sensitive to different types of radiation: beta rays, gamma rays, and x-rays. Thermoluminescent badges and pocket dosimeters also are available. More than one monitor, of the same or a different type, may be worn.

Placement of the monitor is determined by which body parts are being monitored. The monitor should be consistently worn at the same area. A single monitor can be worn outside a lead apron at the level of the neck to measure exposure of head and neck, especially during fluoroscopy. Another monitor may be worn under the apron to measure exposure of the whole body and gonads.

Nonionizing Radiation

Radiant energy in the form of heat and/or light is emitted from radiowaves, microwaves, televisions, computers, radiant warmers, and light sources. For example, overhead operating lights produce heat. Fiberoptic light cables are cool, but the light transmitted is intense and can produce heat. Radiation from these sources is nonionizing (with the exception of ultraviolet lights, which can produce radiant energy in wavelengths and intensity sufficient to alter DNA in cells, burn tissue, and damage the eyes). Nonionizing radiation does not accumulate in the body and therefore does not require monitoring. Nonionizing radiation per se is not hazardous when properly controlled.

Lasers, one form of nonionizing radiation, concentrate very-high-energy light beams within a small circumference to produce intense heat. Laser is an acronym for *light amplification by stimulated emission of radiation.* Laser equipment should be used in accordance with established regulatory standards and guidelines and the manufacturer's instructions for laser safety. Lasers can vaporize, cut, or coagulate tissues directly exposed to the beams. They can cause thermal burns from indirect exposure. Fire, explosion, eye and skin exposure, and laser plume (smoke) also are potential hazards for patients and personnel. Safety measures should be taken.

Electricity

The appropriate use of electronic devices is a prime concern of health care providers and industry personnel who seek safer patient care. Underlying this concern is the rapidly expanding use of electronic equipment. The marketing and safety standards of medical electronic devices used in the perioperative environment are federally regulated. The standards and practices recommended by the Association for the Advancement of Medical Instrumentation (AAMI) are helpful to both manufacturers and users. Standards set by JCAHO should also be met for facility accreditation. Inadequately trained personnel or the malfunctions of devices such as electrosurgical units (ESUs), defibrillators, and x-ray machines are responsible for the fatalities and near-fatalities that occur. Terms associated with the principles of electricity are described in Box 13-2.

Parameters of Electricity

Electricity is the flow of electrons along a path. It consists of three basic parameters: voltage, resistance, and current.

Voltage   Voltage forces electrons to move through material in one direction and causes current to flow. It is measured in volts. The greater the number of volts, the more direct the path of the current.

Resistance   Resistance is the measurement of opposition to the flow of electrons through material. It is measured in ohms. Electricity flows easily through conductors (e.g., metals, carbon, water); flow is minimized by insulators (e.g., rubber, plastic, glass), which prevent the flow of electricity. The resistance of the human body is more similar to a conductor than an insulator.

Current Current is the rate of flow of electrons through a conductor. It is measured in amperes—the number of electrons passing a given point each second. Current flow is proportional to voltage and inversely proportional to resistance. The type of current may be one of two types:

1. *Direct current (DC),* as from a battery. This is a low-voltage current.
2. *Alternating current (AC),* as from a 110- or 220-volt line. This type of current has an alternating directional flow. AC is considered low voltage, but it is three times more powerful than low-voltage DC.

Grounding The grounding of all electrical equipment is essential for safety and the prevention of stray current leakage. Grounding systems are designed to discharge any harmful electricity directly to the ground without including the patient in the circuit. This prevents the inadvertent passage of electric current through the patient, thereby preventing shock or burn.

Electrical power is supplied through two wires—hot and neutral—which transmit current to the three-wire outlets in the building. The third wire is the ground wire. When the cord from an electrical device is plugged into an outlet, the hot and neutral wires deliver the current. The ground wire is attached to a copper pipe that is driven into the ground at the point where power enters the building. An electrical connection to the ground provides a means for current to flow through the ground wire (or any other conductive surface) to the ground rather than going to the neutral wire. The copper ground wire is used to prevent the metal housings of electrical equipment from becoming electrically "hot." The ground wire within the three-wire power plug and cord connects the equipment (instrument) housing to the ground contact in the receptacle (wall outlet). This provides a constantly available return path for current to the electrical source. When an instrument is grounded, leakage current returns through the ground wire to earth, causing no damage. However, if the ground path is absent or broken, leakage current will seek another path to ground. For example, if the insulation on wires is defective (e.g., broken or frayed cords or plugs), some current will leak or flow to other nearby conductors, such as the equipment housing.

Equipotential Grounding System Current flows between points only when a voltage difference exists between them. Therefore electric shock can be minimized by eliminating voltage differences. One system designed to do this is the equipotential grounding system, which maintains an equal potential or voltage between all conductive surfaces near the patient. To achieve equipotential grounding, all exposed conductive surfaces within 6 feet (2 m) of the patient are electrically connected to a single point that is itself connected by a copper conductor to the ground tie point at the electrical distribution center serving the area. Consequently, all exposed metal surfaces are electrically tied together and to the ground.

Isolation Power System Isolated power systems are used in hazardous locations such as ORs. An isolation transformer isolates the OR electrical circuits from grounded circuits in the power mains. Thus the isolated circuit does not include the ground in its pathway; the current seeks to flow only from one isolated line to the other. As a result, accidental grounding of persons in contact with the hot wire does not cause current to flow through the individual. A line isolation monitor checks the degree of isolation maintained by an isolated power system by continually measuring the resistance and capacitance between the two isolated lines and the ground. This measurement is called the hazard index. The monitor, a wall-mounted meter, has an alarm that is activated at the 2-milliampere level. This warning system indicates when inadvertent grounding of isolated circuits has occurred and alerts personnel to a dangerous situation. Because grounding can take place only when faulty equipment is plugged into ungrounded circuits, maximum safety is afforded by use of the isolation transformer. Ungrounded circuits fed through isolation transformers are required in OR and obstetric suites. Permanently installed overhead operating lights and receptacles in anesthetizing locations should be supplied by ungrounded electrical circuits.

The following steps should be taken in the event that the line isolation monitor alarm is activated during a surgical procedure:

1. Unplug the last piece of electrical equipment that was plugged into the power system.
2. Continue to unplug all equipment in the OR, including the anesthesia machine, to identify the faulty equipment. A battery-operated backup system may be needed.
3. Close the OR suite until a biomedical engineer can check for current leakage.

Electric Shock and Electrocution

Electrocution occurs when an individual becomes the component that closes a circuit through which a lethal current may flow. Lethal levels may be attained by currents through the intact body via the skin or by currents applied directly to the heart. Electric shock occurs when a current is large enough to stimulate the nervous system or large muscle masses (e.g., when the body becomes the connecting link between two points of an electrical system that are at different potentials). The physiologic effect of shock may range from a mere tingling sensation to tissue necrosis, ventricular fibrillation, or death. This effect is an electrical response of sensory cells, nerves, or muscles to electrical stimuli that originate either intrinsically (within the body) or extrinsically (outside the body). The severity of shock depends on the magnitude of the current flow and the path taken through the body. There are two types of shock: macroshock and microshock.

Macroshock   Macroshock occurs when current flows through a relatively large surface of skin. It usually results from inadvertent contact with moderately high voltage sources, expressed in milliamperes (1/1000 ampere). A current intensity of 1 to 5 milliamperes through the chest can cause severe burn at the point of contact. If the cardiac conduction system is involved, a current intensity of 50 to 100 milliamperes through the chest can cause ventricular fibrillation because the heartbeat is electrically controlled. Macroshock occurs through the trunk of the body, with the current following many paths; each path carries a fraction of the current. It may or may not be harmful depending on how much current flows through a susceptible heart along its path. Common sources of macroshock are electrical wiring failures that allow skin contact with a live wire or surface at full voltage. The victim, instrument, or surface should never be touched with bare hands in a case of shock. The power supply should be disconnected or an insulating material should be used to push the victim away from the source of electricity.

Microshock   Microshock occurs when current is applied to a very small contact area of skin. The development of medical techniques that permit the application of electrical impulses directly to the heart muscle has raised awareness of the extreme danger of microshock to an electrically sensitive patient. Cardiac microshock is a potential hazard of indwelling catheters filled with conductive fluid, probes inserted into the great vessels, and electrodes implanted around the heart. These devices multiply the potential for electrocution because they can be conductors of electricity. The external portion of a cardiac catheter generally consists of two parts: an inner conductor(s) of wires or conductive fluid and an outer insulating sheath. When there is a highly conductive pathway from outside the body to the great vessels and heart, small electric currents may cause ventricular fibrillation and cardiac arrest. When a shock has an internal route to the heart, it takes only one thousandth as much electricity to be fatal as when the shock is transmitted through the surface of the skin. Microshock occurs only if current from an exterior source flows through the cardiac catheter or conductor. Conductive intravascular catheters that disperse current at skin level diminish the risk of microshock. The most important precaution is to protect the exposed end of the cardiac conductor from contact with conductive surfaces, including the body. Rubber or plastic gloves should always be worn when handling the external end of a cardiac catheter or conductor.

Safeguards   Although the value of electronic devices is unquestionable, their use must not be allowed to cause electric shock or electrocution. Cardiac fibrillation and arrest may occur if a patient encounters an excess of accumulated small currents while connected to the ground through implanted electronic devices or by contact with other grounded objects, such as electrocardiograph (ECG) leads. Faulty electrical equipment may cause a short circuit or electric shock or can cause severe sparks that may be a source of ignition. The following safeguards should be used when working with electrical equipment:

1. Particular care should be used when operating high-voltage equipment such as x-ray machines, electrosurgical units, lasers, and electronic monitoring devices. These machines should be checked for frayed or broken power cords, properly functioning power switches, and grounding.
2. Power cables should not be stretched taut or across traffic lanes.
3. Liquids should never be placed on an electrical unit. A spill could cause an internal short circuit.
4. Electrosurgical and laser units may interfere with the operation of other equipment. Therefore they should be located on the operator's side of the table and as far as possible from the monitoring equipment. Preferably, these units are plugged into separate circuits to avoid overloading power lines. They should not be plugged into extension cords.
5. Equipment should be properly grounded to prevent small extraneous current leaks.
6. Machines should be turned off when plugging them into or unplugging them from the power receptacle and when attaching cords to the machine.
7. Power cords should be unplugged by pulling on the plugs, never the cords; this prevents breakage of wires.
8. All electrical equipment, including a surgeon's personal property, should be inspected by the biomedical engineering department before its initial use. Every piece must meet Underwriters Laboratories (UL) standards or other electrical safety requirements. All equipment should be inspected, preferably monthly but at least quarterly, and verified as safe for use. Equipment should be used according to the manufacturer's instructions.

Electrical and Thermal Burns

Monitors and all high-powered equipment are hazardous. Electrical energy is converted into thermal energy, and therefore the electricity supplied by a defective system may cause burns. The amount of heat produced depends on current density, contact time, and tissue resistance. As little as 300 milliamperes of current for 20 seconds can produce enough heat (113° F [45° C]) to burn intact skin. Current that is concentrated or has a high density at the point of contact can result in an electrical burn severe enough to require debridement.

Electrosurgical units generate high-frequency current. In these units, current flows to an active electrode that is used to cut or coagulate tissue. The patient is protected by using a dispersive electrode. This provides the high-frequency current present at the active electrode with a low-current density pathway back to the generator. Proper connections from the dispersive electrode to the patient and to the unit are essential to prevent burns. Burns can occur at the site of a dispersive electrode if it does not have adequate surface contact with skin or body tissue. Burns also can occur at the site of rings or other metal jewelry, ECG electrodes, or other low-resistance points from invasive monitor probes (e.g., temperature probes) if the current diverts to an alternate ground.

Conductive surfaces should be capable of providing a return path for current other than through the operating bed or its attachments. If the return circuit of high-frequency equipment is faulty, the ground circuit may be completed through inadvertent contact with metal parts or attachments of the operating bed. If the ground area is small, the current passing through the exposed area of skin contact will be relatively intense, causing a burn to the patient. For example, one such contact point may be the thigh touching the leg stirrup when the patient is in the lithotomy position.

Surface burns can occur when battery-operated equipment, such as a peripheral nerve stimulator, is used with external electrodes. Tetanic stimuli should be limited to 1 or 2 seconds.

Other potential sources of burns include malfunctioning controls on heat-generating devices that are in contact with the patient, such as radio-frequency diathermy or hypothermia/hyperthermia machines. Individual reactions to electrical hazards are influenced by factors such as the patient's nutritional state, the amount of body fat that acts as insulation, and the circulation in the body part in contact with the device.

Static Electricity

Static electricity consists of current of high voltage and low ampere. An electrostatic spark develops from friction and accumulates on physical objects. When two static-bearing objects come in contact, the one bearing the higher potential discharges to the one with the lower potential. Air is a nonconductor, but a high enough potential can overcome air resistance and jump the gap to a lower potential object. This causes an arc across air gaps, which are seen as spark(s) from the heat thus generated. These sparks can ignite flammable materials or gases.

Objects accumulate static in inverse proportion to their conductivity. A spark between two objects can occur only when an electrical path of good conductivity does not exist between them. Because earth has a zero potential, a charge is discharged to earth if it is brought into contact with earth directly or indirectly through a conductor. The aim is to provide adequate channels for the dissipation of static. Moderate conductivity has a tendency for the gradual spread of charge over both objects so they come to the same potential. The generation of static electricity cannot be prevented absolutely because its intrinsic origins are present at every interface. For static electricity to be a source of ignition, the following should be present:

- An effective means of static generation
- A means of accumulating the separate charges and maintaining a suitable difference of electrical potential

- A discharge of energy adequate to make a spark in an ignitable mixture

Fire and Explosion

Fire should be a matter of prime concern in the OR. Fires in an oxygen-enriched atmosphere (OEA) are fundamentally different in character than those occurring in normal atmosphere. The fire severity potential should be regarded as serious, with the potential for extensive damage and endangerment to lives of patients and personnel. The presence of flammable and combustible liquids, vapors, and gases in an OEA can result in the ultrarapid combustion of surrounding materials with explosive violence.

Anesthesia providers have discontinued the use of highly flammable anesthetic agents (e.g., cyclopropane and ether) in favor of halogenated agents. These noncombustible agents are mixed with air, oxygen, or nitrous oxide. Although oxygen and nitrous oxide are nonflammable gases, they do support and accelerate combustion. A fire or explosion is the result of a combination of three factors:

1. A flammable gas, vapor, or liquid (e.g., ethylene oxide, alcohol, ether, methane from the bowel, or collodion)
2. A source of ignition (e.g., laser or electrosurgery)
3. Oxygen (pure or in air) or some other substance that provides oxygen, such as nitrous oxide gas

Safeguards

Standards of the NFPA and AAMI are evaluated by JCAHO to safeguard against fire and explosion in anesthetizing locations. Requirements are less stringent where only nonflammable inhalation agents are used. For example, nonconductive flooring and footwear are acceptable when a nonexplosive anesthetic is used. The factors that can cause fire should be controlled.

Flammable Agents Spontaneous combustion can occur when flammable agents are exposed to an ignition source in the presence of oxygen. The following are safeguards to prevent spontaneous combustion:

1. Anesthesia machines, cylinders of compressed gas, and flammable liquid containers should be kept away from any source of heat and must not touch one another. A mixture of gases under high pressure is hazardous.
2. Oil or grease is not used on oxygen valves or on parts of anesthesia machines. Oil or grease should not contact any cylinders, including those containing ethylene oxide, compressed air, or nitrogen.
3. Flammable antiseptics and fat solvents are used for preoperative skin preparation before laser or electrosurgery. Vapors under drapes or pooled material on or around the skin can ignite.

Ignition Sources The minimum ignition temperatures of combustible materials in an OEA are lower than in air. The following list contains precautions to use when working with combustible materials:

1. Thermal devices and other heated objects can cause a fire or explosion.
   a. Precautions should be taken to prevent a laser beam, either directly or indirectly, from igniting drapes, sponges, and gowns or from melting an endotracheal tube.
   b. Electrosurgical units should not be used on the neck, trachea, nasopharynx, and adjacent areas if a flammable inhalation agent was used for the induction of anesthesia. Oxygen can cause a fire.
   c. Inadvertent activation of laser and electrosurgical units should be avoided. When not in use, handpieces should be placed in a holder on the sterile field, not left loose. Handpieces are hot after activation. Laser units should be on "stand-by" or turned off as appropriate.
   d. Beams from fiberoptic light carriers should not be directed onto a drape. Heat can build up until sufficient to produce burning or smoldering.
   e. Lights and sources of heat should be kept at least 4 feet (more than 1 m) away from the anesthesia machine and cylinders.
   f. Heat-generating equipment, such as the operating microscope and the projection lamp for fiberoptic lighting, must not be completely enclosed. Heat can build up under the covering.
   g. The hypothermia/hyperthermia machine should be at least 3 feet (1 m) away from the anesthesia machine, and both should be adequately grounded.
   h. Only approved photographic lighting equipment with suitable enclosures can be used. Strobe lamps are preferred.
2. An electrostatic (incendiary) spark can be an ignition source.
   a. The relative humidity (weight of water vapor present) in the perioperative environment should be maintained between 50% and 60%. Moisture provides a relatively conductive medium, therefore allowing static electricity to leak to earth as fast as it is generated. Sparks form more readily in low humidity.
   b. Explosion-proof electrical receptacles or locking plugs cannot be pulled apart accidentally. Grounding adapter plugs, multiple-outlet plugs, and extension cords are prohibited.
   c. Power cords should be rubber coated, and switches should be explosion proof. Electrical equipment should be plugged into the power receptacle before the anesthetic is administered and before the power switch is turned on.
   d. Motion should be minimal in the area around the anesthesia equipment and the patient's head. Friction on the reservoir bag should be avoided. Team members should watch that drapes do not touch the bag or cover the anesthesia machine.
   e. Patients are covered with cotton blankets. Woolen or synthetic blankets are prone to producing static electricity.
   f. The hair of patients, personnel, and visitors is covered to avoid static discharge.
   g. Antistatic outer garments are worn. Hose and undergarments in close contact with the skin may be made of synthetic material.
   h. Antistatic liners in kick buckets are handled with caution.
   i. Metals should not make contact with a force sufficient to produce percussion sparks.
   j. Anesthesia is discontinued as soon as possible if the ground monitoring system indicates a warning. Following completion of the surgical procedure, the room is not used until the electrical defect is corrected.

Fire Safety

All health care facilities have fire warning and safety systems. Staff members should be familiar with the location and operation of fire alarms and fire extinguishers and with evacuation routes and procedures. Fire drills are held quarterly. Personnel should know the uses of fire extinguishers, be able to distinguish among the three classes of them, and how to operate them:

Class A: pressurized water for combustibles such as paper, cloth, wood

Class B: carbon dioxide or dry chemical to smother flammable liquids, oil, gas

Class C: halon (bromochlorodifluoromethane halogenated compressed gas) to smother an electrical or laser fire without leaving a residue on equipment

When a fire extinguisher is used, the mnemonic *PASS* may aid in remembering how to operate the device:

P *Pull* the safety ring out of the handle.
A *Aim* the nozzle.
S *Squeeze* the handle.
S *Sweep* the spray over the base of the fire.

If fire should occur in the OR during a surgical procedure, the first concern is for the safety of the patient and personnel. To prevent explosion, the burning article is removed immediately from the proximity of the oxygen source and the anesthesia machine or outlet of piped-in gases. The fire on the field is smothered with wet towels, and burning drapes are removed from the patient. The shutoff valves for piped-in gases are turned off, and electrical power cords are unplugged. The mnemonic *RACE* may aid in preventing panic and should enable the team to act quickly in the event of fire anywhere within the perioperative environment:

R *Rescue* anyone who is in immediate danger.
A *Activate* the fire alarm.
C *Contain* the fire if possible.
E *Evacuate* the area.

The fire should be extinguished in the room, if possible, but the patient should be removed immediately from any danger. If the patient is anesthetized, he or she is evacuated on the operating bed. Anesthesia personnel should be assisted with life-support equipment, such as breathing bags and tubing. Team members should refer to the departmental policy and procedure manual for evacuation and safety protocols specific to the facility.

CHEMICAL HAZARDS AND SAFEGUARDS

Health care providers are exposed to many hazardous chemicals on a daily basis. The hazards of these chemicals include irritation of the eyes or mucous membranes, contact dermatitis or burns, toxicity that causes renal or liver disease, and exposure to carcinogens or mutagens. These or other effects may be immediate, delayed, or chronic. Hazardous chemicals in the workplace are controlled by government regulations, such as those of OSHA and EPA in the United States or those of the Control of Substances Hazardous to Health (COSHH) in Great Britain.

Chemicals should be labeled by the manufacturer with the identity of the agent(s) and appropriate warnings of hazards. The latter may be symbolic, that is, pictures added to words. Labels must not be removed or defaced. Employees should read the labels and understand procedures for safe handling and use. OSHA has incorporated *right-to-know* regulations in its standards. One part of this Hazard Communication Standard requires that employees have access to material safety data sheets (MSDSs) supplied by the manufacturer for each hazardous chemical in the workplace. A MSDS specifies the following:

- Composition and common names of the chemical
- Chemical and physical properties
- Known acute and chronic health effects, such as carcinogenic, mutagenic, or allergenic
- Exposure limits
- Protective measures
- Antidote or first-aid measures

OSHA standards are legally enforceable. Although not legally enforceable, NIOSH and ACGIH recommendations for exposure limits to hazardous gases and vapors in ambient air should be adopted for the safety of personnel.

Anesthetic Gases

Air-conditioning or ventilating systems help to prevent pockets of anesthetic gases in the OR, although concentrations around the anesthesia machine and the patient's head may not be remarkably reduced. Substantial amounts of gases can escape during surgical procedures. The patient's exhalations also can pollute the air in the OR and the postanesthesia care unit (PACU). Heavy gas can accumulate and channel along the floor as far as 50 feet (15 m). Confining agents by using a closed carbon dioxide absorption technique tends to restrict gases from getting into air streams.

Waste anesthetic gases are gases and vapors that escape from the anesthesia machine and its hoses and connections; from around the face mask on the patient; and from the patient's expirations. Although not conclusive, data indicate that personnel may incur health hazards if chronically exposed to waste anesthetic gas. Stress, long working hours, and other unknown related factors may contribute to this occupational risk. Possible health hazards include the risk of spontaneous abortion, congenital abnormalities in the offspring of male and female personnel, cancer, and hepatic and renal disease. Significant behavioral changes have been observed and include decreased perception, cognition, and manual dexterity. Personnel also may complain of fatigue or headache.

Studies of the retention of anesthetic agents in anesthesia providers following the administration of clinical anesthesia have demonstrated traces of gas in expired air for varying lengths of time—from 7 hours following nitrous oxide administration to 64 hours after halothane administration. It has been shown that high doses of nitrous oxide block the metabolism of vitamin B_{12}. Chronic exposure to trace levels of nitrous oxide may also lead to neurologic problems or neuropathy.

Because millions of inhalation anesthetics are administered annually, a substantial number of OR staff are occupationally exposed to these gases. OSHA enforces the NIOSH recommendations that room air not be contaminated by more than 0.5 parts per million (ppm) of halogenated agents per hour when used in combination with nitrous oxide or by more than 2 ppm per hour when used alone. Nitrous oxide should be controlled to less than 25 ppm during an 8-hour time-weighted exposure.

The consistently conscientious use of scavenging equipment and procedures is strongly recommended. Scavenging involves the removal of waste anesthetic gases, mainly by trapping them at the site of overflow on the breathing circuit; this is followed by disposal to the outside atmosphere, where the gases are safely diluted. The rate of removal of gases by the disposal system depends on the rate at which fresh air enters the OR and the patterns taken by air currents as they circulate through the room.

The proper use of scavenging equipment can reduce exposure to trace concentrations of gas by 90% to 95%. Personnel exposure should be reduced to the lowest practicable limits by reducing waste gas to the most technically feasible level. A waste-gas control program to ensure the continuing purity of environmental air includes the following measures:

1. Good work practices of anesthesia providers. The major source of waste gas in the OR is the intentional outflow of gases from the anesthesia breathing system. The quantity of gases discharged varies depending on the type of breathing system, the gas-flow rate, and gas concentration.
2. Use of a well-designed, well-maintained scavenging system. Inexpensive, practical, and effective exhaust systems are available. The gas evacuation system

should be attached to every anesthesia machine and ventilator to scavenge excess gases directly into a vacuum line with a minimum flow rate of 440 ppm.

3. Use of proper anesthesia technique.
   a. Different techniques of administration result in different exposure levels. Some leakage is uncontrollable.
   b. All components of the breathing system should fit well. Masks should fit facial contours to ensure a good seal. An oral or nasal airway may reduce the escape of gas from around the mask.
   c. Liquid halogenated agents should not be spilled. The gas flow should not be turned on until the mask is in place or the patient is intubated and the endotracheal tube is connected to the breathing circuit.
   d. Masks, tubing, reservoir bags, and endotracheal tubes should be inspected after each cleaning for leaks, holes, and abnormalities. Disposable equipment is preferable to recycled equipment.

4. Proper maintenance of anesthesia equipment through the following measures:
   a. Daily routine checking of anesthesia machines for leaks. NIOSH recommends that the total leak rate of each machine not exceed 100 ml/min at 30 cm of water pressure. Leaks can be detected with a gas analyzer or bubble test.
   b. Periodic preventive maintenance of all machines and fittings by a manufacturer's representative every 6 months, with in-house monitoring at least quarterly.

5. Maintenance of a high flow rate of fresh air into the air-conditioning system through engineering control procedures. A good ventilating system (preferably not a recirculating one) is also important in the PACU. The ventilation system should comply with the minimum requirements of 20 air changes per hour.

6. Use of an OR atmospheric monitoring program to record trace anesthetic levels and to determine the effectiveness of the previous measures. Specialized monitoring equipment, such as an infrared analyzer, is the only way to detect leaks. Dosimeters are available for each individual to wear to indicate exposure.

Sterilizing Agents

The chemical agents used to sterilize heat-sensitive items can be toxic or can vaporize to emit noxious fumes that are irritating to the eyes and nasal passages, even at low levels of exposure.

Ethylene Oxide

Ethylene oxide (EO) is used in a gaseous form for sterilization and is known to be a mutagen and carcinogen. The residual products can be toxic if there is direct contact with the skin or if the gas is inhaled. Exposure can cause dizziness, nausea, and vomiting. Ethylene glycol and ethylene chlorohydrin are by-products of a reaction with moisture, such as on the hands. All porous items sterilized with EO should be

aerated to dissipate the gas. The PELs for EO are 5 ppm for a short-term exposure of 15 minutes and 1 ppm time-weighted average (TWA) over 8 hours.

Formaldehyde

Formaldehyde may be used in a gaseous or liquid form. The vapors are toxic to the respiratory tract. Formaldehyde is a potent allergen, mutagen, and carcinogen, and it can cause liver toxicity. The PEL is 1 ppm TWA (NIOSH recommendation) to 3 ppm TWA (OSHA standard) over 8 hours.

Glutaraldehyde

Glutaraldehyde is the least toxic of the three sterilizing agents, but the fumes from the liquid form may be irritating to the eyes, nose, and throat. Contact dermatitis has been reported. The PEL is 0.2 ppm per exposure. Glutaraldehyde should be used only in a closed container and in a well-ventilated area. A dosimeter is available to determine the airborne concentration of fumes.

Disinfectants

Some of the disinfectants used to clean or decontaminate equipment and furniture can be irritating to the skin and eyes. Gloves and goggles should be worn when using these chemicals, and the agents should be used in proper dilution. The fumes from some agents can irritate the nasal passages. OSHA has set exposure limits for the following disinfectants:

- Isopropyl alcohol: 400 ppm TWA
- Phenol: 5 ppm TWA
- Sodium hypochlorite: 1 ppm per exposure

Methyl Methacrylate

Commonly referred to as bone cement, methyl methacrylate is a mixture of liquid and powder polymers. It should be mixed at the sterile field just before use. The vapors released during mixing are irritating to the eyes and can damage soft contact lenses. The vapors are also irritating to the respiratory tract, and they can cause drowsiness. Methyl methacrylate may be a mutagen, a carcinogen, or toxic to the liver. The liquid solvent can cause corneal burns if it splashes into the eyes. It also can diffuse through latex gloves to cause an allergic dermatitis; gloves that are impermeable to this solvent are available. A scavenging system should be used to collect the vapors during mixing and to exhaust it to the outside air or absorb it through activated charcoal. The PEL for methyl methacrylate has been established at 100 ppm TWA.

Drugs and Other Chemicals

Antineoplastic cytotoxic drugs used for chemotherapy can be hazardous, as can laser dyes and other pharmaceuticals. All chemical agents should be prepared and administered to minimize unnecessary exposures for both patients and personnel. Chemicals should be combined or mixed with diluents only when this is known to be a safe practice, as specified by the manufacturer.

Safe Handling of Cytotoxic Agents

Antineoplastic cytotoxic agents have carcinogenic and mutagenic properties, and most can cause local and/or allergic reactions. Personnel should avoid inadvertent direct contact with skin or eyes, inhalation, and ingestion during handling. Written precautions and procedures for handling, preparing, administering, and disposing of cytotoxic agents should be followed. Basic guidelines for the use of cytotoxic agents include the following:

1. Protect self from skin and respiratory contact. Preferably, prepare agents under a vertical laminar flow hood. Whether or not a containment hood is available, wear thick gloves, a mask, eye protection, and a gown.
2. Wash hands after handling cytotoxic agents and all items that have been in contact with them, including those used for administration.
3. Place all cytotoxic waste in sealed, leakproof bags or containers. Incineration is recommended for all materials used in preparing and administering cytotoxic agents.

BIOLOGIC HAZARDS AND SAFEGUARDS

The transmission of infection and disease within the health care facility is a concern of both consumers and providers. Biologic hazards do exist in the environment, and every effort should be made by health care providers to protect their patients and themselves. Universal precautions are a necessity (i.e., treating all body fluids and materials as infectious). Employers must ensure that the appropriate protective equipment is available and that employees are trained to wear and use it.

Infectious Waste

Infectious medical waste is an environmental concern both within and outside the health care facility. The EPA defines infectious waste as waste capable of causing an infectious disease. It contains pathogens with enough virulence and quantity that exposure to them could result in an infectious disease in a susceptible host. The disposal of potentially infectious waste generated in health care facilities is regulated by governmental mandates. Although regulated medical waste refers to the portion of waste that has the potential to transmit infectious disease, a uniform definition of what constitutes regulated medical waste has not been universally adopted. Factors that should be considered in deciding if something is infectious waste include the following:

• The presence of pathogenic organisms in sufficient numbers to be capable of causing infection in living beings. Many microorganisms are incapable of causing infection.

• The presence of a portal of entry into a susceptible host. A cut, needle stick, puncture wound, or skin lesion provides a portal of entry, but not all living beings are susceptible hosts to infectious diseases.

These two factors permit the regulation of medical waste that poses a risk to public health and the environment and creates aesthetic concerns for the public. Potentially infectious waste is considered to be blood and blood products, pathologic waste, microbiologic waste, and contaminated sharps. This includes items contaminated by blood, such as sponges, drapes, gowns, and gloves. These items should be segregated from general waste, such as wrappers.

Infectious waste is placed in leakproof containers or bags strong enough to maintain integrity during transport, and these bags should be closed and either labeled or color coded. For example, red bags may be used to differentiate infectious waste. Needles and sharps should be put in puncture-resistant containers. If the outside of the container is contaminated, double bagging is necessary for safe handling during transport to the disposal area. Waste can be steam sterilized or decontaminated with microwaves before compaction and disposal in a landfill, or it can be incinerated. Federal, state, or local regulations should be followed for disposal.

Biohazards

All patients are potential sources of infection. OSHA defines occupational exposure as reasonably anticipated skin, eye, mucous membrane, or parenteral contact with blood or other potentially infectious materials during the course of duty. This contact includes blood, tissues and organs, and all body fluids. Careful handling of and adequate protection from potentially contaminated equipment also is important. Handwashing is a must after every patient contact or glove removal. Personal exposure should be a concern of all team members.

To be in compliance with OSHA standards, every health care facility must develop a written exposure control plan that includes procedures for evaluating an incident and for determining when exposure has occurred. Engineering controls include safety devices or equipment designed to minimize or eliminate a biohazard. Likewise, restrictions or changes in work practices should ensure the safety of all patients and personnel in the environment. For example, food must not be stored in the same refrigerator as blood products or specimens. Eating and drinking are prohibited in areas where contact with blood or other potentially hazardous material is possible. Eating should never be allowed in the OR during a surgical procedure.

Blood-Borne Disease

A penetrating injury (e.g., a needle stick or cut) or a splash (e.g., into the eye or onto mucous membranes) with fluid contaminated with blood or body fluids must not be ignored. Hepatitis, human immunodeficiency viruses, and other blood-borne pathogens can be transmitted through breaks in the skin or contact with mucous membranes. The hepatitis B vaccine is recommended for all high-risk health care workers. If exposure to blood or body fluid occurs, the following procedures should occur:

1. Stop activity immediately and step back from the point of contamination.
2. Squeeze the skin around the needle stick or cut to expel blood and contaminants.
3. Cleanse the puncture site or flush the eye with cool water.
4. Report the incident and seek medical attention promptly.
5. Follow the particular protocol established by the facility for follow-up.

If a needle stick is involved, most facilities will draw a baseline blood sample from the patient and the injured caregiver. Periodic blood samples are drawn over a period of months to make sure results remain clear. Caregivers who have been contaminated by a high-risk patient or a patient known to have hepatitis B or HIV-positive patient should be treated with the appropriate drugs and followed by the employee health department.* Additional information about postexposure prophylaxis and guidelines for treatment can be found at a Web site maintained by the CDC: **www.cdc.gov/epo/mmwr/preview/mmwrhtml/00052722.htm.**

Surgical Plume

Plume is generated by the thermal destruction of tissue or bone. Blood-borne pathogens, mutagens, carcinogens, and other toxic substances can be aerosolized by lasers, electrosurgery, and powered surgical instruments. Masks capable of filtering particles at least as small as 0.1 μm are recommended to prevent inhalation. Face shields, goggles, or eyeglasses with side shields should be worn to protect the eyes.

A smoke evacuator should be used to suction laser and electrosurgical plumes. The evacuator has a filtration system that incorporates a prefilter to trap particles, an ultralow penetrating air filter for particles in the 0.1 μm range, and a charcoal filter to absorb odor and hydrocarbons. The nozzle should be held close to the surgical site. Wall suction is not recommended for smoke evacuation because an in-line filter is necessary to avoid clogging the system. OR personnel can change the filters in some evacuators, whereas others require maintenance by the biomedical technician. Filters are contaminated with biohazardous material and should be disposed of in the same manner as items contaminated with blood and body fluids. Gloves, masks, and protective eyewear should be worn when changing filters because the connecting couplers have been contaminated with plume and the material may be released into the air when the connection is disengaged.

---

*CDC Personnel Health Guideline: Postexposure prophylaxis for percutaneous or permucosal exposure, 26(3):298-313, 1998.

Reproductive Hazards
Male Reproductive Health Implications

Chemical, radiologic, and physical exposures can cause abnormalities in sperm numbers, shapes, and motility. The reaction experienced by an individual will depend on the agent, duration of exposure, and other health status considerations. Chemicals such as ethylene varieties can accumulate in the epididymis, seminal vesicles, or prostate, causing decreased sperm production and decreased ability to fertilize an ova. Some chemicals can affect the man's ability to perform sexually either because of impotence or decreased libido. Chromosomal DNA can be affected, because sperm are produced every 72 days and are stored in the epididymis for 15 to 25 days, where they mature and begin to swim. These changes can cause fetal abnormality if fertilization does take place.

According to NORA, more than 1000 workplace chemicals can cause reproductive effects in animals. Many chemicals have never been tested and also may be implicated in birth defects. More information is available at **www.cdc.gov/niosh/malrepro.html.**

Female Reproductive Health Implications

Excessive exposure to ionizing radiation, waste anesthetic gases, and ethylene oxide during pregnancy may cause a spontaneous abortion or a congenital fetal anomaly. Pregnant employees may be more susceptible to fatigue from standing for prolonged periods, lifting heavy items, and eating and taking breaks at irregular intervals. Exposure to infectious diseases also is a hazard. The health care facility should have a policy for pregnant employees, which may include transferring a pregnant employee from a hazardous area such as the OR. For the safety of the fetus, assignments should limit exposures whenever possible. For example, a pregnant woman should not assist with the implantation of radioactive elements.

An employee who is pregnant is personally responsible for her own welfare and for the safety of her fetus. Immunizations should be current, especially for hepatitis B and rubella, and she should follow the safeguards described in this chapter to limit her exposures to the lowest possible levels. Ultimately, the employee should decide for herself whether or not she wishes to continue working in the perioperative environment.

Latex Sensitivity/Allergy

Many items used in the OR, such as surgical gloves, catheters, drains, medication vial stoppers, tubing, anesthesia breathing circuits, endotracheal tubes, breathing bags, and syringe plungers, contain natural latex (Table 13-1). Some synthetic products are referred to as latex but do not contain the protein that causes reaction. Natural latex is manufactured from the milky sap *(Hevea brasiliensis)* obtained from rubber trees. A water-soluble protein in natural latex contains an antigen that can cause a potentially fatal allergic response. Two types of responses have been identi-

TABLE 13-1	Care of the Latex-Sensitive Patient

Commonly Used Latex Products	Latex-Free Alternatives	Patient Teaching	Considerations
Anesthesia breathing circuit, endotracheal tube, breathing bag	Disposable plastic breathing circuits and endotracheal tubes	NA (not applicable)	Dispose of used equipment.
Bite blocks for oral surgery	Dental rolls, rolled gauze squares, silicone blocks	NA	Avoid using counted radiopaque sponges.
Catheters, enema tips, and drains	Silicone catheters and drains	Instruct patient to report irritation or discomfort in area of drain or catheter.	Patients rarely have silicone sensitivity; check product for content in manufacturer's enclosed literature.
ECG leads, dispersive electrodes, pulse oximeter leads	Nonlatex gel pads	Instruct patient to report irritation at application site.	Patient may have sensitivity to conductive gel; may need to use water-soluble lubricant.
Elastic bandages, antiembolism stockings	White cotton bandages	Instruct patient to report any sensory changes in bandaged part, such as tingling, pain, or loss of sensation.	Nonelastic bandages or stockings may restrict movement and have less expansion properties; circulation may become impaired if applied too tightly.
Elastic and adhesive tape	Plastic, paper, or silk tape	Instruct patient to report irritation around or under area of tape.	Some patients have sensitivity to adhesive rather than tape backing.
Elastic bands on surgical caps, shoe covers, urinary catheter leg bags, plastic pants, disposable diaper	Cloth towel or paper caps with ties to cover hair; cloth hook and loop leg bands, cloth diapers	Instruct patient to report irritation around hairline or leg(s).	Cloth diapers will not be impervious to leaks; cloth hook and loop bands may impair circulation to leg.
Embolectomy catheters	Silicone catheters	NA	Check composition of entire catheter and balloon.
Hypothermia/hyperthermia blanket, hot water bottle, heating pad, mattress cover	Disposable plastic warming blankets and pads	Instruct patient to report irritation or discomfort.	Observe for temperature control of device to avoid skin injury.
Latex gloves, finger cots	Plastic or other nonlatex gloves	Instruct patient that utility gloves used at home may contain latex.	Use nonlatex sterile gloves; vinyl utility gloves for nonsterile activities.
Positioning devices, such as eggcrates, donuts, wedges, rolls	Rolled blankets and towels	NA	Roll blankets around larger objects, such as plastic water bags, for more height.
Rubber shods	Silicone catheter or plastic tubes	NA	Should be radiopaque; plastic shods are not as pliable.
Syringe plungers in plastic syringes	Glass syringes	Instruct patient that plungers in plastic syringes used for self-administered injectable medications contain latex.	Air-powered autoinjector device or implantable medication dispensing mechanism are options at home.
Tubing as on blood pressure cuffs and endoscopic insufflators	Disposable plastic tubing and cuff covers	NA	Wrap limb with cotton sheet wadding to avoid contact.

fied: local and systemic. Local reactions are less severe and occur when latex comes in contact with the skin, causing skin rash, itching, redness, and burning. A patient may have a systemic reaction when a latex product comes in contact with the mucous membranes, serosa, or peritoneum during a surgical procedure. This reaction is more severe, causing anaphylactic shock or death. The signs of severe anaphylaxis are hypotension, tachycardia, bronchospasm, and generalized erythema.

FDA studies have shown that 6% to 7% of patient care personnel and surgeons are sensitive to natural latex rubber. Health care personnel who are frequently exposed to latex products can become sensitized. Several items used in the OR contain latex but are not identified as having latex as a product content (e.g., the elastic bands on caps and shoe covers or mattress and pillow covers). The manufacturer should be consulted to determine whether a product in use contains latex and whether a latex-free substitute is available. Latex proteins can contaminate the starch on prepowdered gloves, thus providing a potential route of airborne exposure to allergens during donning. Sterile surgical nonlatex gloves are available commercially but are more expensive. They should be used only when an allergy is confirmed or is highly suspected in the user or in a patient receiving care.

Testing procedures are available for the detection of a latex allergy. Testing all personnel and patients would be a costly endeavor, but testing persons suspected of having a latex sensitivity should be considered. Patients should be asked preoperatively if they have a known sensitivity (i.e., a history of a reaction after handling a toy balloon or wearing rubber gloves). Children with spina bifida, persons with constant latex exposure, and persons with multiple allergies are known to be prone to latex allergy. Allergies to certain foods, such as avocados, potatoes, bananas, tomatoes, chestnuts, kiwi fruit, and papaya, may be implicated in natural latex allergies per NIOSH.

RISK MANAGEMENT

The perioperative environment is a high-risk environment. The risks can be minimized by adhering to the many safeguards discussed in this chapter. An effective risk management program continuously seeks to provide working conditions that will not jeopardize the health and safety of employees. Such a program has at least four key elements:

1. Administration.
   a. Regulations, recommendations, guidelines, and laws should be enforced to prevent disastrous consequences of occupational hazards.
   b. Policies and procedures should be written, reviewed periodically, and updated as appropriate. All employees should have access to them.
   c. Protective attire and safety equipment should be made available to employees, as appropriate.
   d. Monitoring devices should be used in all hazardous locations as recommended by regulatory agencies.
   e. Employee health services should be provided for immunizations and in the event of injury.
2. Prevention.
   a. Regular in-service programs should be conducted to keep employees informed about hazards and safeguards.
   b. Employees should be taught how to use and care for new equipment before it is put into service.
   c. Employees must know the location and use of emergency equipment, such as fire extinguishers and shut-off valves.
   d. Employees must wear protective attire, as appropriate.
   e. Routine preventive maintenance should be provided for all potentially hazardous equipment.
3. Correction.
   a. Faulty or malfunctioning equipment should be taken out of service immediately.
   b. Any injury should be reported, with medical attention sought as soon as possible.
   c. Unsafe conditions should be reported.
4. Documentation.
   a. Records of preemployment medical examinations and periodic examinations for the surveillance and early detection of disease should be maintained for each employee. These records should be retained in a permanent file after termination of employment in case there is a future health problem.
   b. New employees may be given a letter explaining the occupational risks at the time of employment.
   c. Incident reports regarding injuries to personnel and patients should be filed with the administration of the facility.

The prevention of injuries is vital to maintaining a safe environment. It is everyone's responsibility.

Bibliography

Addington C: All the right moves: a program to reduce back injuries for OR nurses, *AORN J* 59(2):483-488, 1994.
Ball K: Surgical smoke: is it safe to breathe? *Todays Surg Nurse* 18(5):16-21, 1996.
Beezhold DH et al: The transfer of protein allergens from latex gloves, *AORN J* 59(3):605-613, 1994.
Black LA, Presson AC: Hazardous drugs, *Occup Med* 12(4):669-685, 1997.
Bloodborne infections: a practical guide to OSHA compliance, Arlington, Tex, 1992, Johnson & Johnson Medical.
Chang WP et al: Exposure of anesthesiologists to nitrous oxide during pediatric anesthesia, *Ind Health* 35(1):112-118, 1997.
Department of Health and Human Services (NIOSH): *Guidelines for protecting the safety and health of health care workers,* pub no 88-119, Washington, DC, 1988, US Government Printing Office.
Fiedler MA, Biddle C: Review of chemical, medication, and anesthesia toxicity in the OR, *AORN J* 67(2):398, 401-406, 409-411, 1998.
Francis MC et al: Exclusion of noninfectious medical waste from the contaminated waste stream, *Infect Control Hosp Epidemiol* 18(9):656-658, 1997.
Garb JR, Dockery CA: Reducing employee back injuries in the perioperative setting, *AORN J* 61(6):1046-1052, 1995.
Hall JE et al: Environmental monitoring during gaseous induction with sevoflurane, *Br J Anaesth* 79(3):342-345, 1997.
Halstead MA: Fire drill in the operating room: role playing as a learning tool, *AORN J* 58(4):697-706, 1993.
Harris HR: Anesthetic gas: danger in the OR, *Surg Technol* 26(10):14-15, 1994.
Jessiman DR: Education bridges the gap between manufacturers and patients, *Todays Surg Nurse* 19(2):39-43, 1997.
Klein BR, editor: *Health care facilities handbook,* ed 4, Quincy, Mass, 1993, National Fire Protection Association.
LaMontagne AD, Kelsey KT: Evaluating OSHA's ethylene oxide standard: employer exposure–monitoring activities in Massachusetts hospitals from 1985 through 1993, *Am J Public Health* 87(7):1119-1125, 1997.

Mace SR et al: Latex allergy in operating room nurses, *Ann Allergy Asthma Immunol* 80(3):252-256, 1998.

Melman CT, DiPasquale TG: Radiation exposure to the orthopaedic team during fluoroscopy: "How far is far enough?" *J Orthop Trauma* 11(6):392-398, 1997.

Paradies M et al: Root cause analysis for sentinel events, *Infect Control Today* 2(3):49-51, 1998.

PlumeFacts buyers' guide for ultimate plume protection, PlumeFacts, 1995, AORN Congress Edition.

Prado C et al: Biological monitoring of occupational exposure to isoflurane by measurement of isoflurane exhaled breath, *J Appl Toxicol* 17(3):179-183, 1997.

Register K: Mesa Lutheran adjusts to a new fluid waste management system, *Infect Control Today* 2(6):38, 1998.

Regulated medical waste definition and treatment: a collaborative document, *AORN J* 59(6):1176-1183, 1994.

Regulations, the law, standards, what is the real status? *PlumeFacts* 4(3):1-4, 1994.

Reis JG: Latex sensitivity, *AORN J* 59(3):615-621, 1994.

Schaefer JA: Respiratory protection in the health care setting, *Occup Med* 12(4):641-654, 1997.

Suruda A: Health effects of anesthetic gases, *Occup Med* 12(4):627-634, 1997.

Thompson JW et al: Fire in the operating room during tracheostomy, *South Med J* 91(3):243-247, 1998.

Ulmer B: Occupational safety and health administration acts on guidelines for electrosurgical smoke, *AORN J* 67(6):1244-1245, 1998.

Zaza S et al: Latex sensitivity among perioperative nurses, *AORN J* 60(5):806-812, 1994.

Section

V

Surgical Asepsis
and Sterile Technique

Chapter 14

Microbiologic Considerations

 Chapter Objectives

After studying this chapter, the learner will be able to:

- Understand the differences between microorganisms.
- Describe the natural lines of defense of the human body.
- Identify several favorable living characteristics of microorganisms.
- Describe how disease is spread.

Because of the prevalence of community-acquired infections and the potential for development of nosocomial infection (acquired during the course of health care), careful attention to the creation and maintenance of a safe and therapeutic environment is mandatory. Knowledge of causative microorganisms, including their modes of transmission, life cycles, and methods of control, is the basis of prevention of infection. The Centers for Disease Control and Prevention (CDC) has issued guidelines for prevention of transmission of infections. Whether at a surgical site or systemic in the body, infection can lead to sepsis, which is a serious and potentially fatal postoperative complication.

The development of passive and active immunization and antibiotic therapy had revolutionary effects on surgical practice. Nevertheless, the ideal state of infection-free surgical procedures is not always a reality. Infections at the surgical site and systemic infections continue to occur. The key to control lies in understanding microbiologic principles. The intent of this chapter is to introduce microbiologic concepts and give the reader a basic understanding of microorganisms. Terms pertinent to the understanding of microbiology in the perioperative environment are defined in Box 14-1.

HISTORICAL BACKGROUND

Approximately 5 million microorganisms live in the Earth's many habitats. Each type of microorganism has specific features that distinguish it from the rest. The mechanism and rationale for grouping and categorizing microorganisms was originally described in 1763 by Swedish naturalist Carolus Linnaeus (1707-1778) and refined by French scientists Antoine Laurent de Jussieu (1748-1836) (plants) and Georges Leopold Culvier (1769-1832) (animals). Contributions made by German biologist Ernst Haeckel (1834-1919) (bacteria) and American scientist Robert H. Whittaker (1924-1980) (fungi) further refined the study of microbiology.

As techniques and instrumentation became more refined, American biologist Herbert Copeland (1902-1968) (protozoa) reclassified all known microorganisms and segregated nucleated and nonnucleated microorganisms into separate kingdoms. Scientific classification of organisms currently identifies five kingdoms: animals, plants, fungi, Monera (bacteria), and Protista (algae, protozoa, and parasitic organisms). Similarities, physical structure, and relationships, as well as differences and independent life cycles, define how each microorganism is assigned to its

Box 14-1   Terms Associated with Microbiology

aerobe   Microorganism that requires air or the presence of oxygen for maintenance of life.

anaerobe   Microorganism that grows best in an oxygen-free environment or one that cannot tolerate oxygen (e.g., *Clostridium* species that causes gas gangrene).

antibiotics   Substances, natural or synthetic, that inhibit growth of or destroy microorganisms. Used as therapeutic agents against infectious diseases; some are selective for a specific organism; some are broad-spectrum antibiotics.

antimicrobial agent   Chemical or pharmaceutical agent that destroys or inhibits growth of microorganisms.

cross-contamination   Transmission of microorganisms from patient to patient and from inanimate objects to patients and vice versa.

epidemiology   Study of occurrence and distribution of disease; the sum of all factors controlling the presence or absence of a disease.

flora   Bacteria and fungi normally inhabiting the body, often delineated as resident or transient.

infection   Invasion of the body by pathogenic microorganisms and the reaction of tissues to their presence and to toxins generated by the organisms.

    community-acquired infection   Infectious disease process that developed or was incubating before the patient entered the health care facility.

    nosocomial infection   Hospital-associated or acquired infection not present when the patient was admitted to the health care facility. Infection may occur at the surgical site or as a complication unrelated to the surgical site.

superinfection   Secondary subsequent infection caused by a different microorganism that develops during or following antibiotic therapy.

microorganisms   Living organisms, invisible to the naked eye, including bacteria, fungi, viruses, protozoa, yeasts, and molds (synonym, *microbe;* adjective, *microbial*).

opportunists   Microorganisms that do not normally invade tissue but are capable of causing infection or disease if introduced into the body mechanically through injury, such as tetanus bacillus, or when resistance of the host may be lowered, as by HIV infection.

pathogenic   Producing or capable of producing disease.

sepsis   Severe toxic febrile state resulting from infection with pyogenic microorganisms, with or without associated septicemia. Septicemia is a clinical syndrome characterized by significant invasion of microorganisms from a focus of infection in tissues into the bloodstream. Microorganisms may multiply in the blood. Infection of bacterial origin carried through the bloodstream is sometimes referred to as bacteremia.

standard precautions (formerly referred to as universal precautions)   Procedures followed to protect personnel from contact with blood and body fluids of all patients.

---

kingdom. Further identification includes subdivisions within each group.

The study of microorganisms has led to many lifesaving advantages. Vaccines have been developed to prevent many communicable diseases. The first of these was developed by Edward Jenner (1749-1823), an English physician. In 1796 he inoculated a child with a cowpox vaccine to prevent smallpox. Subsequently, vaccines and antitoxins have been developed to provide passive immunity against such infectious diseases as diphtheria, rubella, and poliomyelitis. Although they have been nearly eradicated, these and other infectious diseases still occur, sometimes in epidemic proportions.

MICROORGANISMS: NONPATHOGENS VS. PATHOGENS

Specific numbers of microorganisms with plantlike or animal-like characteristics are considered nonpathogenic in the human body. Nonpathogenic microorganisms do not pose a particular threat to health. Natural resident flora can be found in the reproductive tract secretions, gastrointestinal tract, nasopharyngeal mucus, respiratory passages, and any superficial ductal opening, such as sweat and oil glands. These flora have specific roles in their natural location. Some resident intestinal flora aid in the synthesis of vitamins but can cause an infection if they are relocated to a skin wound.

The term *infection* is used when nonresident flora invade a susceptible area. The term *superinfection* is used when resident flora are out of balance and the increased number cause a pathogenic condition. If the count of microbial colonies increases above normal or the colonies grow in an area where they are not usually found, an infection results and the microorganisms are considered pathogenic. They can invade healthy tissue through some power of their own or can injure tissue by producing a toxin. Pathogenic microorganisms can cause sepsis—a severe toxic febrile state—or death.

Body fluids in a healthy state, such as urine and cerebrospinal fluid, do not normally contain microorganisms. Other fluids that under normal circumstances do not contain microorganisms include blood, peritoneal fluid, synovial fluid, amniotic fluid, tears, semen, and breast milk. Since microorganisms are not visible on gross inspection, exposure to any body substance should be considered contaminated and treated accordingly.

Identification of Microorganisms

Microorganisms, with the exception of viruses, have intracellular DNA. The DNA is either enclosed in a nuclear membrane (eukaryotic) or loose in the cytoplasm (prokaryotic). Bacteria and blue-green algae are the only prokaryotic microorganisms. Bacteria remain in a primitive state unchanged by evolution. All other microorganisms are eukaryotic and have changed many times on an evolutionary scale.

Specimens and/or cultures of tissues or body fluids may be sent to the microbiology laboratory for identification. Treatment is prescribed according to the type of microorganism present in the body. Accurate identification of the microorganism is critical to the selection of the appropriate therapy. Criteria used by laboratory personnel to identify the type of microorganism include the following:

- Cell morphology
- Mobility or motility
- Presence or absence of spores
- Native pigment
- Gram's stain reaction
- Growth factors (optimal growth conditions, speed of replication/reproduction, and how it grows in various media)
- How it colonizes
- Antibody detection in the host
- Metabolism and atmosphere requirements
- Biochemical activity (endotoxin or exotoxin)
- Sensitivity to exogenous chemicals or substances

The type of substance taken from the body may be a clue as to the type of microorganism.

Viability of Microorganisms

Any microorganism can become a pathogen. When transferred from one place to another, they pass through a dormant, or lag, phase of about 5 hours or longer. Then each organism divides itself about every 20 minutes.

The key element to preventing pathogenic disease is to understand the microorganism's mode of transmission, life cycle, and favorable living conditions. Box 14-2 describes the favorable living conditions associated with the proliferation of pathogens. Interference with the viability and survival of pathogenic microorganisms can prevent infection.

Natural Lines of Defense

The human body is remarkable in its ability to protect itself by intact barriers, membranes, and bacteriostatic secretions. Three lines of defense are particularly important for prevention of disease. The *first line of defense* involves generalized good health and incorporates natural biochemical, mechanical, and anatomic protection through the following:

- *Skin.* Stratified epithelium contains sweat (sudoriferous) and oil (sebaceous) glands, which are bactericidal. Natural flora inhibit each other. The epithelium must remain intact to afford protection. Desquamation and low pH impede bacterial colonization.

> **Box 14-2** **Favorable Living Conditions of Microorganisms**
>
> Can live with or without oxygen; some require no special gaseous environment.
> Can live with or without moisture; some can completely dry out and be reconstituted.
> Can live with or without light; some like complete darkness.
> Can live in a neutral or alkaline pH; most will die in an acidic environment.
> Can live with or without warmth; some can grow in the freezer compartment of the refrigerator.
> Can get nourishment from a living host or decayed matter; some can absorb nutrients from the environment.

- *Mucous membranes.* An effective barrier when intact, these line all natural body orifices except the ears, which secrete cerumen (earwax). Mucous membranes have bactericidal properties and are slightly acidic pH.
- *Reflexes.* Examples include vomiting, gagging, and blinking.
- *Sneeze.* Mucociliary escalator of the respiratory tree moves mucus and debris from the respiratory tract.
- *Genitourinary/reproductive tracts.* Immunoglobulin (IgA), found in mucus, and enzymes are produced; these have a slightly acidic pH.
- *Eyes.* Enzymes and IgA protect the conjunctiva and structures of the eye.
- *Cellular level.* Interferon is naturally formed in the cell to fight against viral attack.
- *Stomach acid.* Acid kills most pathogens.
- *Muscular closure of orifices.* Muscular closure provides a mechanical barrier against orifices such as the cervix and sphincters.

The *second line of defense* involves the collaborative effort of several body systems to prevent the proliferation of pathogenic microorganisms. These provide secondary protection if the microorganism breaks through the first line of defense. The second line of defense includes the following:

- *Inflammatory response.* This can be localized or systemic; biochemical, mechanical, and anatomic activity fights invading microorganisms and lays the groundwork for healing.
- *Antibody production.* Production is stimulated by the presence of an antigen. Some antibodies can be replicated for future exposures to the same microorganism.
- *Temperature elevation.* This can be localized or systemic. Some microorganisms are destroyed or repelled by heat.

The *third line of defense* can be acquired naturally or induced therapeutically. The third line of defense requires actual exposure to the pathogen in some form during which temporary or quasi-permanent resistance is attained. Methods include the following:

- *Passive immunity.* A "preformed" immunoglobulin (antibody) is introduced into the body. No memory for replication of the protective antibodies remains in the body.
- *Active immunity.* The body has the ability to develop a memory for production of antibodies in response to specific antigens. Live, dead, or attenuated microorganisms trigger the response. Some exposures require a booster injection to spark the memory and maintain immunity.

Spread of Infection

Pathogenic microorganisms initially invade and aggregate in a body system or at a localized site, such as an abscess. The proliferation of infectious material is easily supported by the warmth, chemical composition, moisture, and other components of the body. Local spread is supported by the surface of the wound, necrosis of tissue, diminished inflammatory response, and absence of anatomic barriers. Other pathways of infection include any body orifice, duct, or lumen of a broken vessel. Veins are particularly vulnerable because they are often associated with venous sinuses and have low pressure. The central nervous system (CNS) shares a similar risk for infection because the cerebrospinal fluid is under lowered pressure and has components that are rich in nutrients. As microbial colonies increase in number, infection may be carried through the body in the lymphatic system and may eventually become blood-borne. Major organ systems can become involved and can result in multisystem organ failure and death. Any body fluid or substance is a potential carrier of pathogens (Box 14-3).

According to the CDC, 2 million patients acquire nosocomial infections.* Approximately 77,000 of these patients die of sepsis associated with these infections. Annually, it costs more than 4 billion dollars to treat nosocomial infection. Knowledge of how the cycle of spreading infection works is the most important element of prevention. Considerations include the following:

- Identifying the reservoir of the pathogen
- Identifying the portal of exit of the pathogen from the reservoir
- Identifying how pathogens are transmitted
- Identifying the portal of entry into a susceptible host
- Identifying the invasion of the susceptible host

Infectious Process

Clinically, infection is the product of the introduction, metabolic activities, and pathophysiologic effects of microorganisms in living tissue. It can develop in the surgical patient as

---

*Nosocomial infection, 1996, www.cdc.gov.

Box 14-3	Body Fluids and Substances That May Transmit Pathogens
Blood	Amniotic fluid
Semen	Tears
Vaginal secretions	Nasal secretions
Breast milk	Respiratory secretions
Feces	Peritoneal fluid
Urine	Pericardial fluid
Cerebrospinal fluid	Cerumen
Unfixed tissue specimen	Sebum
Synovial fluid	Smegma
Vitreous humor	Bile
Aqueous humor	Any open wound
Saliva	Any exudate or transudate

a preoperative complication following an injury or as a postoperative complication.

An infection may begin at the surgical site between the fourth and eighth postoperative day. Infection, usually bacterial in origin, develops as a diffuse, inflammatory process, known as cellulitis and characterized by pain, redness, and swelling. This inflammatory response is the body's initial line of defense directed toward localization and containment of the infecting organism. Red blood cells, leukocytes, and macrophages infiltrate the area, with pus formation (suppuration) often following. An abscess forms as a result of tissue liquefaction with pus formation, supported by bacterial proteolytic enzymes that break down protein and aid in the spread of infection. Fibrolysin, for example, an enzyme produced by hemolytic streptococcus, may dissolve fibrin and delay surgical site healing. The body attempts to wall off an abscess by means of a membrane that produces surrounding induration (hardened tissue) and heat. Localized pus should be drained promptly.

If localization is inadequate and does not contain the infectious process, spreading and extension occur, causing regional infection. Microorganisms and their metabolic products are carried from the primary invasion site into the lymphatic system, spreading along anatomic planes, causing lymphangitis. Failure of the lymph nodes to hold the infection results in uncontrolled cellulitis. Subsequently, regional and/or systemic infection may develop, characterized by chills, fever, and signs of toxicity. Septic emboli may enter the circulatory system from septic thrombophlebitis of regional veins communicating with local infections. These emboli and pathogenic microorganisms in the blood seed invasive infection and abscess formation in remote tissues.

Sepsis elevates the patient's metabolic rate 30% to 40% above average, imposing additional stress on the vital systems. For example, cardiac output is about 60% above normal resting value. The body's defenses and ability to meet the stress govern whether the infectious process progresses to septic shock. Multiple infection sites, the presence of shock, and inappropriate antibiotic therapy result in a poor prognosis. Obviously, the key to avoiding infection is prevention,

| TABLE 14-1 | Transmission of Pathogenic Microorganisms That Can Cause Infection in Susceptible Host |

PATHOGEN →	TRANSMISSION TO →		SUSCEPTIBLE HOST → Factors for Survival	INFECTION →
Types	**Sources/Vectors**		**of Pathogen**	**Virulence**
Bacteria		⎡ Skin	Moisture	Primary invader
Aerobic	Airborne ⎯	⎢ Hair	Food	Opportunist
Microaerophilic		⎣ Air	Proper temperature	Toxin
Anaerobic			Time	Exotoxin
			↓	Endotoxin
Fungus	Droplet	Nasopharynx		Heterogenous effect
Yeast		⎡ Fomites/inanimate objects	Dormant (lag) phase or spores	Cytotoxic
Virus	Contact ⎯	⎢ Break in technique	↓	Enzyme effect
		⎣ Person-to-person contact	Reproduction	Clotting effect

but if an infection begins, the next most important step is to identify the microorganism and treat it appropriately. More than one microorganism may be present; therefore treatment is highly individualized.

The ultimate resolution of infection depends on immunologic and inflammatory responses capable of overcoming the infectious process. This is associated with drainage and removal of foreign material, including debris of bacteria and cells, lysis (disintegration) of microorganisms, resorption of pus, and sloughing of necrotic tissue. Healing then ensues.

Who Is at Risk for Exposure?

Perioperative personnel who provide direct and indirect patient care are at risk for exposure to potentially harmful microorganisms. Wearing personal protective equipment (PPE), such as gowns, gloves, and eyewear, decreases the risk but does not eliminate it. The risk of exposure is proportionate to the proximity to the patient in the OR. The closer to the surgical field (source of blood and/or body substance), the higher the risk. The surgeon, assistants, and scrub person have a higher risk by role and proximity. They share an increased incidence of needle sticks and puncture wounds. The circulator, environmental services personnel, and instrument processors are also at increased risk for body substance exposure because of specimen handling, cleaning processes, and other contaminants in the environment.

Exposure rates to blood and body substances for OR personnel have been reported as 10 per 100 procedures. Sharps were responsible for 3 of 100 exposures reported. Of glove tears reported, 93% were in single-gloved caregivers. Approximately 63% of glove tears in a single-gloved individual revealed a blood exposure. In 20% of double-gloved individuals who had a glove puncture, only 6% had evidence of inner-glove puncture. In 74% of injuries with sharps, the injuries were self-inflicted by carelessness.

The patient is also at risk. If a needle stick occurs, the needle may come in contact with the patient after penetrating the caregiver, thereby exposing the patient. Some patients have health conditions that predispose them to vulnerability for infection. Considerations related to higher risk include immunosuppression, an immature immune system (preterm and term infants), radiation therapy, burns, diabetes, nutritional depletion, smoking, chemotherapy for cancer, older patients, steroid use, sickle cell disease, alcoholism, liver and kidney disease, and preexisting infection being treated with antibiotic therapy (superinfection/opportunistic infection may ensue) (Table 14-1).

TYPES OF PATHOGENIC MICROORGANISMS

Infections may be caused by one or several combinations of microorganisms. In this chapter, each of the five main types of microorganisms is described according to structure, life cycle, and mode of transmission; examples of each type of microorganism are provided (Table 14-2). Common methods for destruction of microorganisms are discussed in Chapters 17 and 18.

Protozoa

Although microscopic, protozoa are relatively large. They grasp and ingest food particles and are motile. Protozoa have many diverse pathogenic mechanisms, although most types are not harmful to healthy humans. Protozoa become pathogenic as a result of opportunistic infection. Each species has a distinct reproductive cycle. Some parasitic protozoa reproduce only in a living host, such as in a female mosquito of the genus *Anopheles* (e.g., *Plasmodium malariae*). Other species of protozoa living free in watery environments split by binary fission to form two daughter cells. Cryptosporidiosis (*Cryptosporidium parvum* from calves) and toxoplasmosis (*Toxoplasma gondii* from domestic cats) are examples of parasitic diseases that currently cause diseases in humans living in contemporary cities.

Characteristics

1. *Structure.* Protozoa are animal-like parasites that are single-celled microorganisms without a morphologically distinct cell wall. They are eukaryotic with chromosomes and aerobic.

TABLE 14-2	Common Pathogens in OR Environment, Using Mnemonic *Search Every Source To Provide Safe Care For Health*		
Micro-organism	**Usual Environment**	**Mode of Transmission**	
Staphylococci	Skin, hair Upper respiratory tract	Direct contact Airborne	
Escherichia coli	Intestinal tract Urinary tract	Feces, urine Direct contact	
Streptococci	Oronasopharynx Skin, perianal	Airborne Direct contact	
Mycobacterium tuberculosis	Respiratory tract Urinary tract	Airborne, droplet Direct contact	
Pseudomonas	Urinary tract Intestinal tract Water	Direct contact Urine, feces Water	
Serratia marcescens	Urinary tract Respiratory tract	Direct contact Water	
Clostridium	Intestinal tract	Direct contact	
Fungi	Dust, soil Inanimate objects	Airborne Direct contact	
Hepatitis virus	Blood Body fluids	Blood-borne Direct contact	

2. *Life cycle.* Protozoa reproduce sexually (in a sanguineous host) or by binary fission (free in nature). They are capable of walling off and resist drying out by becoming cystic. They can be reactivated by moisture and prefer to live in a watery environment. Larger and more complex than bacteria, they ingest decaying organic matter. They have some diffusion through the cell membrane.
3. *Transmission.* Contact is through ingestion of a cyst in soil or water, the fecal-oral route, or a bug bite. Dissemination is commonly blood-borne directly to major organs. There may be direct contact with the organism through mucus secretions from the genitourinary tract.

Protozoan Disease Examples

1. Blood-borne protozoa passed by insect vectors include *P. malariae, Trypanosoma rhodesiense* (African sleeping sickness), and *Trypanosoma cruzi* (South American: Chagas' disease).
2. A localized parasitic infestation passed by the sandfly is leishmaniasis (nonhealing skin lesions).
3. Intestinal protozoa acquired free in nature include *Giardia lamblia* (enteritis), which is commonly misdiagnosed because symptoms mimic colitis.
4. Genitourinary protozoa include *Trichomonas vaginalis.* Vulvovaginitis or urethritis can be transmitted through sexual contact or fomites.
5. Amebic dysentery protozoa include *Sarcodinia* and *Entamoeba* species.

Fungi

More than 100,000 species of fungi have been identified. Not all fungi are pathogenic (causing mycosis). A *Penicillium* variety is used to make the antibiotic penicillin and to give flavor to Roquefort cheese. The blue color of the cheese is caused by collections of spores.

The body responds to tissue invasion by a fungus with an inflammatory response. Respiratory responses include hypersensitivity reaction to fungal antigens. According to statistics compiled by the CDC, the number of nosocomial fungal (mycotic) infections doubled between 1980 and 1990.

Characteristics

1. *Structure.* Fungi are plantlike structures that lack chlorophyll and therefore are unable to photosynthesize. True fungi are nonmotile. Fungi are eukaryotic and range in size from microscopic to large mushroom forms. Yeast species are single celled but cling together with like cells. Fungi are aerobic. Molds are multicellular and reproduce by airborne spores that can be inhaled.
2. *Life cycle.* Molds can reproduce sexually and asexually by forming spore sacs referred to as budding (such as in yeasts). A parasitic saprophyte that thrives in a dark, damp, aerobic, warm environment, a fungus lives on decaying material. It can produce toxins referred to as aflatoxins and mycotoxins, found in moldy foodstuffs.
3. *Transmission.* Infection can be transmitted by spores in direct contact with the respiratory system, nonintact skin, or mucous membranes.

Fungal Disease Examples

1. Respiratory fungal diseases include aspergillosis *(Aspergillus fumigatus)*, histoplasmosis (*Histoplasma capsulatum,* commonly found in bat and bird excreta), cryptococcosis (*Cryptococcus neoformans,* found in pigeon excreta), and pneumocystis pneumonia (*Pneumocystis carinii,* which was originally thought to be a protozoan; DNA and RNA studies showed it was a red yeast fungus possibly carried on dogs).
2. Mucous membrane fungal diseases include thrush and vaginitis *(Candida albicans).*
3. Cutaneous fungal diseases include athlete's foot and tinea.

Viruses

A virus is not an independent cell unit and is not capable of autonomous metabolism. It is an obligate intracellular parasite that is confined to living in a host cell, such as a somatic cell, or a bacterium. As a bacteriophage, a virus can attach itself to a bacterium and create an opening. While still attached, the nucleic acid of the viral capsule enters the bacteria. The empty capsule remains attached to the bacteria. Once the virus is inside the host cell, regardless of the cell type, it uses the cell's genetic contents and metabolic machinery for replication. New viruses are passed out the cell membrane, and they in turn attach to other cells to repeat the replication process. Some viruses engorge the cell, causing it to rupture, thus dispersing the virus into the host's body.

During viral infection, the host cell reacts to invasion by producing an inflammatory response, antibodies, and interferon to slow the progression of viral replication. Some cellular immunity is developed (e.g., in mumps and chickenpox). Some viruses can attach to nerve cells and undergo activation, deactivation, and reactivation cycles, such as in herpes simplex types I and II (herpes simplex virus). Some of the nerve cells destroyed by viral invasion include motor neurons, which when damaged cannot be repaired or replaced, such as in polio. Until the discovery of viruses as a separate entity by Dmitri Iwanowski (1864-1920) in 1892, viruses were identified only by the diseases they caused. Martinus Beijerinick (1851-1931) made significant contributions to scientific knowledge by expanding the knowledge of viruses. The virus species can usually be identified by the specific alterations in structure and function effected in the host cell as seen under electron microscopy. Other diagnostics include detection of viral antigen, nucleic acid, or antiviral antibody in the serum.

Characteristics

1. *Structure.* Viruses are composed of a protein capsule but have no true cellular components other than nucleic acid. They are categorized by the morphologic core structure of their nucleic material—either DNA or RNA (not both)—and the presence or absence of an envelope. They can mutate. Viruses are extremely small and are visible only by electron microscope.
2. *Life cycle.* A virus must have a living biologic host cell. The virus enters a host cell and uses the host's genetic and other cellular protein material for replication.
3. *Transmission.* Infection can be transmitted through blood and body fluids of animals and humans. Some viruses can be transmitted by insect bites, such as ticks or mosquitoes; other viruses are transmitted by the fecal-oral route. Direct contact of virus with nonintact skin or mucous membranes can allow entry.

Viral Disease Examples

Hepatitis Infection   Viruses can produce several types of acute and chronic inflammation of the liver. The pathogens causing viral hepatitis create an occupational hazard to health care providers. A patient may be in an acute stage of the infection but more commonly is an unknown carrier of one and occasionally two of the viruses that can cause hepatitis.

HEPATITIS A   Hepatitis A virus (HAV) infection is an acute illness that is usually brief but can last for several months. It is spread by oral ingestion of contaminated water and food, especially shellfish, and by fecal contaminants. It is most infectious during the 2 weeks before the onset of symptoms and until after the first week of jaundice. The incubation period is 14 to 90 days, with an average of 28 days. Immune globulin may be effective if given within 2 weeks of exposure. HAV infection is the most common type of viral hepatitis and causes critical disease if it occurs in combination with other types of hepatitis. HAV infection as a single entity is not a major nosocomial problem because it does not have a chronic carrier state. It is usually self-limiting and does not typically cause chronic liver damage. A vaccine is available for areas where HAV is endemic.

HEPATITIS B   Hepatitis B virus (HBV) infection is a major nosocomial problem. Carriers are a main source of cross-infection. Hepatitis B surface antigen is the carrier state of HBV. This can be harbored for prolonged periods of up to 15 years and has been found in practically all body fluids of infected persons. It is transmitted percutaneously or permucosally by blood, saliva, semen, and other body fluids. It is not found in feces or urine, according to the U.S. Department of Health and Human Services. The incubation period is 60 to 90 days before mild to severe symptoms become apparent. Chronic hepatitis, cirrhosis, or liver carcinoma may develop. A liver transplant may be necessary.

Serologic tests are used to diagnose infection, detect carriers, and monitor high-risk persons. Patients who have undiagnosed hepatitis, who fail to reveal they have chronic hepatitis, or who are asymptomatic carriers can transmit the virus to health care providers. Perioperative, emergency department, blood bank, laboratory, and hemodialysis unit personnel are especially at risk. HBV surface antigen is easily transmitted by direct contact with blood and body fluids via a needle stick or break in the skin, such as a minor cut or hangnail, or via a splash into the mucosa of the eye, nose, or mouth. HBV can be transmitted by fomites, through sexual intercourse, and from an infected mother to a neonate during birth.

Preexposure immunization over a period of 6 months through a series of three injections of 10 µg (1 ml) of recombinant vaccine against HBV is recommended for all persons at risk. The injections are given in the deltoid muscle because injection in the gluteal muscle has been shown to not produce immunity. After exposure, such as following an accidental needle stick, both the vaccine and hepatitis B immune globulin are given. Since 1991 the Occupational Safety and Health Administration (OSHA) has mandated that health care facilities make these immunizations available to personnel. The series may need to be repeated in 7 years if the titer falls below a detectable level in the serum.

HEPATITIS C   Hepatitis C virus (HCV) is a blood-borne RNA virus. Recipients of multiple transfusions or chronic hemodialysis, intravenous drug users, and health care workers are at risk. Persons with acute HCV infection are asymptomatic but have a higher mortality if they are simultaneously exposed to HAV. A screening test detects the presence of antibodies in the blood. Incubation varies from 2 weeks to 6 months. The infection may progress insidiously in a carrier for as long as 25 years. Immediate HCV postexposure treatment consists of immune globulin injections. Persons who become infected with HCV have a 40% to 60% chance of becoming chronic carriers and may be treated with interferon and ribavirin. Newer treatments approved by the FDA in 1998 include Rebetron (combined interferon A and ribavirin) injections for 6 months. Women should avoid pregnancy while taking this drug.

HCV infection can precipitate chronic hepatitis, cirrhosis, and liver cancer. A liver transplant may be needed. Mortality rates associated with HCV infection exceed 10,000 deaths per year. This form of hepatitis may surpass HIV infection in the number of new cases reported each year. An estimated 4 million persons in the United States have HCV infection. There is no cure, although 15% recover without lasting effects.

HEPATITIS D Hepatitis D virus (HDV) infection coexists with HBV infection or superinfects an HBV carrier. A defective RNA virus, HDV requires HBV for its survival and replication in both acute and chronic forms. HDV infection is communicable during all phases of active infection. It can lead to necrotizing liver disease and death. The majority of patients developing this complication of HBV infection are intravenous drug abusers who used contaminated needles. Immunization against HBV will also prevent hepatitis D.

HEPATITIS E Hepatitis E virus (HEV) infection is common in Asia, Africa, and Mexico. The incubation period is 15 to 64 days, with an average of 25 to 42 days in different epidemics. The characteristics of HEV are similar to those of HAV, and there are no specific serologic tests for HEV at this time. HEV infection is spread via the fecal-oral route through contaminated water or food or from poor sanitation conditions. Current immunoglobulins do not provide protection. HEV infection has no known chronic carrier state, and full recovery in infected persons can usually be expected. The best protection is proper handwashing.

HEPATITIS G Hepatitis G virus (HGV) infection is rare (2000 cases diagnosed per year). Most infected persons have no clear symptoms. It is transmitted by infected blood, and exposure to HCV increases mortality associated with the disease.

Herpes Infection

Related DNA viruses that form eosinophilic intranuclear inclusion bodies are collectively called herpesviruses. The viral infections they cause may be acute and highly contagious, or they may remain latent for many years even if antibodies are in circulation.

HERPES SIMPLEX INFECTION Herpes simplex virus (HSV) is the pathogen of herpes simplex infections. These cutaneous infections may cause localized eruptions, similar to blisters, on the border of the lips or external nares, in the mouth, or in the genital or anal region. Transmission is by direct contact with vesicle fluid from lesions or with saliva. The infection may be transmitted to the neonate during passage through an infected birth canal. HSV also can cause cutaneous eczema, acute stomatitis, keratoconjunctivitis, acute retinal necrosis, and meningoencephalitis. Herpes simplex infections are common in HIV-infected and other immunocompromised patients.

Patients who have a history of HSV infection may be treated with oral acyclovir preoperatively to prevent an outbreak in the surgical wound. This prophylaxis is particularly important for patients who are having facial procedures, such as a chemical peel or face-lift.

HERPETIC WHITLOW Herpetic whitlow, a herpesvirus infection of the fingers, is transmitted by direct contact with oral secretions from a person with active herpesvirus or from an asymptomatic carrier. Entry of the virus into the host is via a cut or break in the skin or in nail folds. Herpetic whitlow is an occupational hazard to nurses, physicians, dentists, and anesthesia providers.

Cytomegalovirus Infection

Cytomegalovirus (CMV) may infect salivary glands or viscera, causing enlargement of cells. Transmission can be by direct contact with body fluids, secretions, and excretions. CMV infection usually is asymptomatic in a healthy person, but it is an opportunistic pathogen in immunosuppressed patients with HIV infection or AIDS. Lymphadenopathy, enteritis, and pneumonitis may persist. Chorioretinitis and blindness may result in the end stage of infection. CMV infection may also be associated with hepatitis. CMV may infect arterial smooth muscle cells, stimulating them to proliferate, which can contribute to the formation of atherosclerotic plaque. CMV is the most common cause of congenital viral infection; it may be transmitted from an asymptomatic mother during pregnancy. A CMV-infected infant may develop neurologic problems. Latent CMV may become reactivated following organ transplantation. The incidence of primary and reactivated CMV infection is fairly high after renal, cardiac, and bone marrow transplantation.

Human Papillomavirus Infection

Condylomas (venereal warts) are caused by the human papillomavirus (HPV) and are transmitted through vaginal, anal, or oral-genital sexual contact. The infectious process appears as accumulations of warts over the perineal and/or anogenital surface. HPV infection in women can lead to cervical carcinoma. Over 200 varieties have been identified. Some subtypes have been associated with an increased incidence of cervical cancer. Not all of them are visible or pigmented. Some patients are infected simultaneously with multiple varieties.

Treatment for venereal warts includes cryotherapy with liquid nitrogen, electrosurgical removal, CO_2 laser ablation, chemical peel with trichloroacetic acid (TCA), and/or topical application of medication (podophyllum 10% to 25% in a benzoin tincture, podofilox 0.5% solution or gel, or imiquimod 5.0% cream). Patients with wart accumulations of 0.5 to 1 cm^2 respond to topical applications. Patients with larger areas greater than 10 cm^2 may require staged surgical intervention.

Some infections are extensive, and the treatment may leave the patient with chronic reflexive neurologic pain, such as vulvodynia. Patients should be advised that their sexual partners also need to be evaluated for venereal warts. Most of the topical medications have not been approved for safe use during pregnancy.

Human Immunodeficiency Virus Infection

The human immunodeficiency virus (HIV) clearly represents a worldwide threat to public health that is unprecedented in modern times. Since this virus was introduced into the United States in the late 1970s, the resultant infection has spread at an alarming rate via contaminated blood and infected persons. Clinical problems in patients with seropositive sera began appearing in 1978. Because of its effect on the immune system and its unknown origin when first reported in 1981, this infection became known as acquired immunodeficiency syndrome (AIDS). In 1983, researchers at the Institut Pasteur in Paris isolated the lymphadenopathy-associated virus (LAV). In 1984 a similar retrovirus called human T-cell lymphotropic virus type III (HTLV-III) was reported by the National Institutes of Health in Bethesda, Maryland. Since 1986, LAV and HTLV retroviruses causing AIDS or related illnesses have been known collectively as HIV.

Retroviruses synthesize DNA from RNA, a reversal of the usual process. As a result of this reversal process, there is a high rate of mutation, making resistance to antiviral drugs a major problem. Normally when a virus enters the body, helper T lymphocytes (T cells) release proteins that activate the immune system to produce antibodies against the virus and macrophages to attack the virus. HIV is different from other viruses in that it attacks the cell membrane of these white blood cells. When the virus penetrates the T-cell membrane, the viral RNA and enzyme are released into the T-cell cytoplasm and converted into DNA. This newly formed DNA penetrates the T-cell nucleus, causing replication of the HIV virus. The cell dies, and the virus is released into the bloodstream to attack other helper T lymphocytes and macrophages, thus compromising the immune system.

HIV can live and reproduce in macrophages without stimulating the production of antibodies because the viral composition resembles the host cell. HIV will survive in blood and any body fluid that contains white blood cells. The primary routes of transmission are through sexual intercourse and by direct contact with blood and blood products. HIV may be transmitted to the fetus by the blood of an infected mother or to the neonate via breast milk. HIV is not transmitted by casual contact with an infected person. The virus is relatively fragile and easily destroyed outside the body.

After exposure, antibodies may not be identified through serologic testing for 6 to 12 weeks, and detection can be delayed for up to 18 months or longer. Enzyme immunoassays (EIAs) and the Western blot analysis are used to test for the presence of antibodies. Blood banks test donor blood for HIV antibodies. Transplant donors also are tested.. Blood screening for HIV has been routine in the United States since 1985, thus decreasing the potential for transmission by blood transfusion. Seropositive blood is destroyed, and the donor is notified.

The incubation period before symptoms of infection develop ranges from 6 months to 5 years or longer. Persons in whom the antibody is identified are considered infected and infective. They are classified by physical findings.

ACUTE INFECTION   The acute stage of HIV infection lasts 2 to 3 weeks. Symptoms may be specific to an opportunistic infection or disease, but marked fatigue, prolonged diarrhea, weight loss, dry cough, enlarged lymph nodes, fever, and night sweats are striking features. Infections are primarily viral, mycobacterial, and fungal in origin. Oral candidiasis lesions (thrush) may be the first observable symptom. *Pneumocystis carinii* pneumonia, an unusual lung infection caused by a fungal parasite, is quite common. Other common infections are CMV, HSV, cryptococcosis, and *Mycobacterium avium-intracellulare* complex disease. The patient may survive one infection only to succumb to another. Prophylactic drug therapy aims to prevent or delay the onset of infections. Malignancies and lymphomas also may develop.

Acquired Immunodeficiency Syndrome
As the HIV infection progresses, the cell-mediated immune system is irreversibly compromised. As concentration of the virus gradually increases, the patient becomes symptomatic for clinical manifestations of AIDS. Clinical diagnosis of AIDS requires a positive test for HIV antibodies, any one of the specified opportunistic infections, and a lowered T-cell count. AIDS is not a well-defined disease but rather a state of immune dysfunction. AIDS causes persistent destruction of the helper T lymphocytes (white blood cells that stimulate production of antibodies), resulting in profound immunosuppression (diminished resistance to infection and disease). The acronym *AIDS* helps to define the disease process:

A *Acquired:* HIV has passed from one person to another by blood or body fluid in direct cell-to-cell contact; infection is not hereditary except through transplacental transfer from an infected mother to a fetus.

I *Immune:* The normal defense system protects the body against certain diseases and opportunistic infections; immunity depends on the production of antibodies.

D *Deficiency:* The immune system becomes compromised (i.e., immunosuppressed against opportunists); the host is unable to protect the person with no previous history of immunodeficiency against opportunists.

S *Syndrome:* A group of symptoms or laboratory evidence indicates the presence of a particular disease, abnormality, or infection; seroconversion is positive for HIV antibodies.

P. carinii pneumonia is the most common opportunistic respiratory infection. *M. avium-intracellulare* complex, the most common AIDS-related bacterial infection, is a leading cause of the wasting syndrome (i.e., loss of body fat and weight). Kaposi's sarcoma, a vascular tumor, is the most common malignancy. HPV and HSV infection may be present. Neurologic disease may cause dementia. Lymphomas and opportunistic infections of the brain, spinal cord, and peripheral nerves are not uncommon.

ASYMPTOMATIC INFECTION   The patient may be completely asymptomatic of infection but tests seropositive for HIV antibodies, which confirms the presence of virus in the body.

PERSISTENT GENERALIZED LYMPHADENOPATHY   Swelling or enlargement of lymph nodes suggests cellular immune dysfunction. Prolonged infection with HIV may occur without the formation of HIV antibodies.

HIV-Related Clinical Manifestations   Originally referred to as AIDS-related complexes, a variety of health conditions suggest an impaired immune system. The patient who does not have one of the specific opportunistic infections but is seropositive for HIV antibodies does not technically have AIDS. An infectious disease, such as tuberculosis, and some cancers may be a result of a deteriorating immune system. AIDS may develop within a year of seroconversion.

A patient may be infected but may not yet test positive. Health care providers who have a valid reason to be concerned that they may have been infected may request to be tested. Few health care providers seroconvert from a single needle stick or splash of blood on mucous membranes. Handling all needles and sharp instruments carefully and using barriers to avoid direct contact with blood and body fluids are the best measures to prevent work-related transmission of HIV. An HIV inhibitor such as zidovudine may be given immediately after exposure. A vaccine has not been developed for immunization. Antiviral agents interfere with the life cycle of the virus. Immune-modulating agents stimulate function of the suppressed immune system.

Infectious Conditions Related to Viruses: Transmissible Spongiform Encephalopathy

Transmissible spongiform encephalopathy (TSE) is a family of diseases that cause fatal neurologic disorders. Infection is through an unconventional route. A neurologic cellular protein referred to as a prion causes the disease. Exposure to a prion through direct contact with neurologic tissue, incidental inoculation with neurologic matter, implantation through contaminated instrumentation, and possibly a genetic autosomal dominant predisposition are theorized sources. Ingestion of food contaminated with neurologic material, such as cerebrospinal fluid, is also considered a possible route of transmission. Although a virus has not been identified, a viral source has not been ruled out. Forms of TSE that affect humans and animals include the following:

- Creutzfeldt-Jakob disease (CJD)—human
- New-variant Creutzfeldt-Jakob disease (nvCJD)—human, with possible link to bovine spongiform encephalopathy
- Bovine spongiform encephalopathy (BSE)—cattle
- Scrapie—sheep

Creutzfeldt-Jakob Disease   Although rare, CJD is a progressive, fatal disease characterized by dementia, myoclonus (muscle spasms), and multifocal neurologic symptoms. Initial infection produces no inflammatory response but clearly destroys neurons. It was first described in 1920 by German psychiatrists Hans Gerhard Creutzfeldt and Alphonse Maria Jakob. Thought to be associated with genetic factors that influence susceptibility to the formation of abnormal neurologic protein, the condition may be dormant

for more than 30 years before the onset of symptoms. The disease then progresses rapidly, leading to coma and death, usually within 2 years of onset. CJD is not the same as nvCJD or BSE. Diagnosis is made on the basis of a characteristic electroencephalogram (EEG) and brain biopsy positive for protein prion accumulation with neuron destruction. Autopsies of the brains of patients with suspected Alzheimer's disease revealed that 13% had undiagnosed CJD, and the tissue sampled resembled that of other TSE-infected mammals.

CJD is particularly virulent, and the prions are resistant to destruction by heat, chemicals, radiation, freezing, drying, and organic detergents. The prions are most susceptible to soaking in sodium hydroxide for 1 hour. Instruments should be steam sterilized for 1 hour in a gravity displacement sterilizer at 270° F (134° C) or for 18 minutes in a prevacuum sterilizer (longer than normal cycles) at 274° F (134° C) before routine cleaning. Sterilization of tissue that has been fixed with formalin is impossible.

Standard precautions for prevention of blood-borne exposure must be strictly observed, although a blood-borne source has not been identified. Suction canister contents and used cleaning solutions should not be disposed of in the sanitary sewer system. All biologic material should be disposed of according to facility policy and procedure. Approximately 85% of CJD cases have an unexplained origin. Contaminated neurologic tissue sources include dural grafts, corneal transplants, and human growth hormone. There is no treatment or cure.

New-Variant Creutzfeldt-Jakob Disease   First described in Great Britain in 1996, nvCJD is a distinct entity from CJD in that it resembles a human variant of BSE. Human illness has been demonstrated after ingestion of beef contaminated with CNS tissue from BSE-contaminated cattle.

Postexposure Prophylaxis for Transmissible Spongiform Encephalopathy   Any percutaneous exposure to known or suspected TSE-infected CNS tissue should be irrigated with 0.5% sodium hypochlorite. Skin exposure requires a thorough hand scrub with sodium hydroxide. Mucous membrane exposure should be followed by cleansing with soap and water. More information about CJD can be found at the following Web sites:

- **www.cjd.ed.ac.uk/**
- **www.cdc.gov/ncidod/diseases/cjd/qa96bse.htm**

Bacteria

Bacteria are essential to human life. We are dependent on many of their metabolic processes. Many antibiotics are derived from bacteria, such as erythromycin, Chloromycetin, and kanamycin. Some photosynthesizing types convert carbon dioxide to water and oxygen. More than 5000 species of bacteria have been named, and many more exist unidentified. Most of the morphologic differences in bacteria are found in metabolism, chemical composition, or resultant effect on the host. Bacteria can survive in diverse environments. For example, *Thermoplasma acidophilum* is found in the hot springs of Yellowstone Park and is capable of living in a 140° F (60° C) environment with an acidic pH of 1 to 2. Unfortunately, many varieties of bacteria are pathogenic or are capable of becoming pathogenic.

Characteristics

1. *Structure.* Bacteria are microscopic single-celled structures (1 to 10 μm). Two billion bacteria can be contained in a single drop of water. Bacteria have DNA but no formal nucleus (prokaryotic) and no membrane-bound organelles.
   a. Cocci are round. Examples include strains of staphylococcus and streptococcus. Diseases include impetigo and gonorrhea.
   b. Bacilli are rod shaped, and some can form spores. They are the most common type of bacteria. Examples include *Escherichia, Proteus,* and *Pseudomonas* species.
   c. Spirochetes are spiral shaped. Disease examples include syphilis, leptospirosis, and Lyme disease.
   d. Pleomorphs can change shape from rod to round, making positive identification difficult. Diseases include mycoplasmal infection, typhus, rickettsial infection, chlamydia, psittacosis, and Rocky Mountain spotted fever. *Rickettsia* and *Chlamydia* organisms must live in a host cell. They are intracellular parasites.
2. *Life cycle.* Bacteria can be aerobic, anaerobic, facultative, or microaerophilic. They can reproduce asexually by binary fission (split into equal halves). Some studies have shown that some genes may be transferred between bacterial species during viral infection.
3. *Transmission.* Infection is transmitted by direct contact or through animal or insect bites.
4. Some bacteria are encapsulated, which is a defense mechanism against phagocytic activity of leukocytes. These bacteria may be ingested by white blood cells, but instead of being killed and digested, they remain within the phagocyte for a time and are then extruded in a viable condition. The presence of a capsule is associated with virulence among pathogenic bacteria.

Differentiation of Bacterial Types A universal way to determine the differences in bacteria is to stain the cell. Danish physician Christian Gram (1853-1938) developed a method of applying a solution of crystal violet and iodine (gentian violet) to the cell wall followed by exposure to 95% alcohol and acetone. Gram-positive bacteria retain a stain of dark purple-blue. Gram-negative bacteria retain only a stain of light pink after the rinsing process. Gram's stain is also used to identify nonbacterial substances such as trophocysts (helminth eggs) and larvae.

Endospores Endospores are the resting, protective stage of about 150 species of gram-positive rod-shaped bacilli. Gram-negative bacilli do not form endospores. Select bacilli are capable of producing one endospore in response to an environmental threat, such as extreme heat or chemicals. When conditions suitable for bacterial growth are reestablished, the endospore reverts back to its original cellular structure for active vegetative growth and reproduction.

In the vegetative, or active growth state, spore-forming bacilli are no more difficult to kill than non–spore-forming bacteria. Most other microorganisms are killed easily by the processes of sterilization and disinfection, but bacterial spores are not. Examples of heat- and chemical-resistant spores include *Bacillus* and *Clostridium* species. Nonpathogenic varieties of the *Bacillus* spore-forming microorganisms are used in sterilizers to test for efficacy (e.g., *Bacillus subtilis*). Other examples of potentially fatal diseases caused by spore-forming bacilli include anthrax, tetanus, gas gangrene, and botulism.

Bacterial Toxicity

Pathogenic microorganisms produce substances that adversely affect the host locally and/or systemically on invasion. Toxic substances affecting tissues, cells, and possibly enzyme systems diffuse from the microbial cells. The cellular substance of a wide variety of organisms is toxic also. In addition, harmful effects may be produced indirectly by activation of tissue enzymes by bacteria. Such toxic substances include the following:

1. *Exotoxins.* These classic bacterial toxins are the most potent toxins known. As little as 7 ounces (200 ml) of crystalline botulism type A toxin is said to be able to kill the world's entire population. Exotoxins appear to be proteins, are denatured by heat, and are destroyed by proteolytic enzymes, which break down protein. These bacteria are typically gram-positive and form spores. Examples of diseases include tuberculosis, clostridial infection, diphtheria, anthrax, and leprosy.
2. *Endotoxins.* These toxins are contained within the cell wall of bacteria and are released when the cell wall is broken. They are heat stable and are not digested by proteolytic enzymes. On parenteral inoculation they cause a rise in body temperature and are known as bacterial pyrogens. They increase capillary permeability with the resultant production of local hemorrhage. Although they cause injury to body cells at the site of infection, endotoxins more importantly cause serious, often lethal, effects by dissemination and widespread injury to many tissues throughout the body. Endotoxic shock may occur in bacteremia caused by gram-negative bacteria. Examples of diseases include typhoid, shigellosis infection, and the plague. Microorganisms include *Escherichia coli, Salmonella,* and *Pseudomonas.*

3. *Heterogeneous substances.* Microorganisms also form a variety of other heterogeneous (dissimilar) toxic substances, which may contribute to the disease process directly or facilitate the establishment of foci of infection. Toxins, which diffuse from the intact microbial cell, have the following various effects:

   a. Cytotoxic effect (leukocidin) destroys white blood cells (e.g., causing leukopenia, or reduction of leukocytes below normal).

   b. Kinase effect interferes with the clotting mechanism of blood.

   c. Enzymatic effect causes bacterial hemolysins to dissolve red blood cells or fibrin, thereby inhibiting clot formation. Coagulase, an enzymatic substance of bacterial origin, is causally related to thrombus formation. Coagulase-positive staphylococcus, *B. subtilis, E. coli,* and *Serratia marcescens* accelerate clotting of blood and induce intravascular clotting.

Toxic Shock Syndrome   Toxic shock syndrome (TSS) is an acute condition caused by exotoxins secreted by strains of *Staphylococcus aureus.* The pathogen can invade any part of the body. TSS is characterized by fever over 102° F (38.9° C), hypotension, erythematous rash, and injury to multiple organ systems. Diagnosis is based on the presence of abnormal clinical and laboratory findings. Prompt supportive treatment and antibiotic therapy are crucial. Desquamation, peeling of skin (usually from the palms of the hands and soles of the feet), occurs 1 to 2 weeks after onset. Recovery is usually complete, but TSS is potentially fatal if untreated. It can originate from a surgical wound, burn, postpartum infection, or septic abortion infected or colonized with the implicated toxin. TSS can afflict any age-group of either sex.

Septic Shock   Septic shock is a state of widely disseminated infection, often borne in the bloodstream (i.e., septicemia). Early septic shock may begin with fever, restlessness, sudden unexplained hypotension, a cloudy sensorium, hypoxia, tachycardia, rapid breathing, and/or oliguria. One or more of these symptoms may be present. Toxic or metabolic by-products increase capillary permeability, permitting loss of circulating fluid into the interstitial fluid. Endotoxins released by bacteria promote vasodilation and hypotension.

Septic shock is most frequently produced by gram-negative bacteria. As shock progresses, the patient develops cold clammy skin, sharply diminished urinary output, respiratory insufficiency, cardiac decompensation, disseminated intravascular coagulation, and metabolic acidosis. The high-risk category comprises patients with severe infection (e.g., peritonitis), trauma, burns, impaired immunologic status, diabetes mellitus, or extreme age, as well as patients who have undergone an extensive invasive procedure.

Treatment consists of control of the infectious process, early administration of antibiotics, fluid-volume replacement, and oxygen. Diuretics, sodium bicarbonate, vasoconstrictors, vasodilators, inotropic agents, or heparin may also be indicated. Corticosteroids may be used, but their use is controversial. A monoclonal antibody may be administered to reduce endotoxins.

Bacterial Disease Examples

Tuberculosis   Tuberculosis (TB) is caused by the acid-fast gram-positive bacterium *Mycobacterium tuberculosis.* Tubercle bacilli usually infect the lungs (pulmonary TB), but they may be present in joints, kidneys, ovaries, or other organs. Acute miliary tuberculosis may be seen in an abdominal procedure as generalized peritonitis. TB is an opportunistic organism. Individuals at high risk include persons immunosuppressed from HIV infection, corticosteroid therapy, chemotherapy, or malnutrition. Persons with diabetes mellitus, cirrhosis, alcoholism, silicosis or other lung disease, or prolonged contact with an actively infected person are also at risk. The tubercle bacillus can remain dormant, encased in a hard shell, for years after exposure. Because the bacillus may become airborne by droplets from the respiratory tract, the disease must be monitored and controlled to prevent cross-infection. Unsuspected active cases and inactive carriers represent a particular hazard. Patients with acute disease are isolated and placed on respiratory secretion precautions for approximately 2 weeks following initiation of treatment.

Therapy is long term, usually 6 to 12 months of drug therapy. Isoniazid (INH) and rifampin most effectively kill reactive bacilli and prevent reactivation. Pyrazinamide, ethambutol, and streptomycin also may be used for multidrug therapy; some other drugs that are less effective and have more side effects may be indicated. *M. tuberculosis* mutates and may become resistant to a single-drug or multidrug therapy regimen. Multidrug-resistant tuberculosis (MDR-TB) can be fatal, especially in HIV-infected persons.

The following is recommended in the care of surgical patients who have active TB:

1. Postpone elective surgical procedures, if possible, until the patient shows a response to drug therapy (i.e., is no longer infectious as confirmed by a negative sputum smear).

2. Use disposable anesthesia equipment to the extent possible. Reusable equipment must be sterilized or undergo high-level disinfection immediately after use. A bacterial filter on the endotracheal tube or at the expiratory side of the breathing circuit may be useful in reducing the risk of contamination of anesthesia equipment or the discharge of tubercle bacilli into ambient air.

3. Use respiratory isolation precautions for patients with positive sputum. This includes putting a mask on the patient during transport to the operating room (OR). The transporter also wears a TB-filtering mask. OR team members should wear face-fitting masks that filter particles of 1 μm at a 95% efficiency level (i.e., a disposable high-efficiency particulate air [HEPA] filtered mask, valveless dust-mist respirator, or dust-fume-mist filtered respirator). Powered respirator masks equipped with HEPA filters may be worn during high-risk pro-

cedures such as bronchoscopy, endotracheal intubation, and tracheal suctioning.

4. Perform the surgical procedure at a time when other patients and a minimum number of staff members are present in the OR suite (i.e., at the end of the day's schedule, if possible). Keep OR doors closed and traffic to a minimum.
5. Sterilize critical items (i.e., those entering the bloodstream or body cavity); semicritical items (i.e., those in contact with mucous membranes only) may be sterilized or undergo high-level disinfection with a tuberculocide.
6. Move the patient into an isolation room that has negative pressure ventilation with a local exhaust and HEPA air filtration and/or ultraviolet radiation lamps.
7. Screen high-risk patients and test personnel at least annually. Testing includes a chest x-ray film and skin test. Exposed personnel should be retested every 6 months.

TB is the number one fatal infectious disease in the world. In many facilities yearly TB testing of all OR personnel is mandatory. The most accurate test is the Mantoux test, which is administered by injecting 0.1 ml of purified protein derivative (PPD) of tubercle bacillus subcutaneously in the forearm to form a small wheal under the skin. The site is examined in 24 to 72 hours. Redness, itching, and induration of 8 to 10 mm at the site of injection are considered a positive or a significant reaction. Further testing and chest x-ray films may be performed before treatment can begin. Reaction of less than 8 mm at the site of injection is considered an insignificant or negative reading, and no further action is needed.

Sexually Transmitted Diseases Any sexually active person who has multiple partners is at risk for acquiring a sexually transmitted disease. In addition to those previously discussed (HBV, HIV, and HSV infections), gonorrhea, syphilis, and chlamydia are transmitted by sexual contact. Transmission can also occur from contact with secretions containing the causative organism, such as those a health care provider might encounter through a cut or broken skin.

GONORRHEA *Neisseria gonorrhoeae* most often infects the genitourinary tract, but it may infect the rectum, pharynx, or conjunctiva. Burning, itching, and pain around the vaginal or urethral orifice with purulent discharge are characteristic symptoms. If untreated, the infection can spread to cause inflammation within the peritoneal cavity and septicemia. Disseminated infection is more common in women than in men. Gonorrhea is treated with penicillinase-inhibiting antibiotics. Generally, patients should be treated simultaneously for presumptive chlamydial infections.

As a prophylactic measure, a one-time instillation of silver nitrate, erythromycin 0.5% ophthalmic ointment, or tetracycline 1% ophthalmic ointment may be administered within 1 hour after birth to protect the neonate against potential contamination by vaginal secretions of an infected mother. Single-use tubes or ampules are preferable to multiple-use tubes to prevent cross-contamination between newborns. A newborn with a known gonorrheal infection will need further antibiotic treatment.

SYPHILIS Routine screening for syphilis in hospitalized patients and couples applying for marriage licenses is a thing of the past. However, the incidence of syphilis is on the increase again. *Treponema pallidum* is a blood-borne spirochete that may infect any organ system. Syphilis is characterized by distinct stages of effects over a period of years if it is untreated by antibiotics. Congenital syphilis results from prenatal infection unless the infected mother is treated within the first 4 months of pregnancy.

In the first stage (primary syphilis) a lesion on the skin or mucous membrane, most commonly around the anogenital region, quickly forms a chancre. This is a painless ulceration that exudes fluid laden with spirochetes. The chancre heals spontaneously within 40 days. During the second stage (secondary syphilis), spirochetes migrate from the chancre throughout the bloodstream. The disease can remain contagious for as long as 2 years during this stage. The third stage (tertiary syphilis) may not develop for many years. When it does, secondary lesions may damage or destroy tissues and body structures, including the heart and CNS with ensuing mental disability or death.

CHLAMYDIA Chlamydial infection is caused by *Chlamydia trachomatis* (bacteria). It is the most prevalent sexually transmitted disease, more common than gonorrhea and syphilis. It is transmitted only by person-to-person contact. It occurs more often in men than in women but is more frequently asymptomatic in women than in men. Chlamydia can cause epithelial tissue inflammation, ulceration and scarring of the urethra and rectum, and damage to reproductive organs. Pelvic inflammatory disease (PID) is a serious complication in women. Asymptomatic salpingitis is a major cause of tubal infertility or ectopic pregnancy. Exposure of infants to *C. trachomatis* in the birth canal can cause neonatal conjunctivitis and pneumonia.

Helminths

Adult helminths (worms) are not true microorganisms but are considered parasites in humans and animals. Most adult worms are visible to the naked eye, but the eggs and larvae are microscopic. Symptoms are increased as the number of worms increases. The host responds by increasing immunoglobulin IgE and macrophage levels in the blood to fight the invasion. The eggs and larvae are very irritating to tissues, causing intense granulomatous inflammation.

Large volumes of invading worms can cause mechanical obstruction of lumens, such as in the gastrointestinal tract, or tunnel-through organs, such as the heart or lungs. Many intestinal varieties cause nutritional and/or hematologic depletion of the host. If a worm dies while in the host's tissue, it becomes encased in inflammatory exudate. Helminths may be found in populations living in rural farm lands with feces in the soil or in immigrant communities. Young children may acquire pinworms through fecal-oral ingestion in day care or school settings.

Characteristics

1. *Structure.* Morphologically more complex than protozoa, helminths can be round and tubular (nematodes), flat (cestodes), or flat and large (trematodes).
2. *Life cycle.* Helminths are hermaphrodites. Eggs are laid in a host and are passed through excreta. Eggs hatch, becoming larvae and reentering a host by penetration or introduction through a vector. Larvae mature in the host, becoming adults capable of self-reproduction. They can become blood- and lymph-borne.
3. *Transmission.* Introduced by insect bites, some can self-penetrate host tissues and skin, and some are acquired by ingesting undercooked flesh from an infected animal or shellfish. Fecal-oral route transmission of eggs and/or larvae is common. Wading in contaminated water permits penetration of skin by active larvae.

Helminth Disease Examples

1. Nematode diseases include intestinal pinworms and hookworms, and trichinosis in skeletal muscle of pigs. Filarial worms cause filariasis (elephantiasis), which is transmitted by fly or mosquito bites and becomes blood-borne.
2. Cestode diseases include intestinal tapeworms.
3. Trematode diseases include blood-borne flukes.

ANTIMICROBIAL THERAPY

Antimicrobial drugs or agents are a prominent part of the surgeon's armamentarium. They are adjuvants to, not substitutes for, strict adherence to aseptic and sterile principles and careful surgical technique.

Antibiotics

Antibiotics act by killing (bactericidal) or inhibiting the growth (bacteriostatic) of bacteria. To be effective, the bacteria must be sensitive to the activity of the antibiotic. Some antibiotics are broad spectrum and attack many aerobic and anaerobic bacteria; others selectively destroy specific species. Antibiotics do not affect viruses and many fungi and yeasts.

The penicillins, cephalosporins, aminoglycosides, and carbapenems are the common categories of antibiotics. The penicillins include natural penicillin G and synthetic or semisynthetic derivatives. Some are rendered inactive by penicillinase, an enzyme secreted by certain bacteria that antagonizes the action of penicillin (e.g., *Staphylococcus aureus*). Several synthetic penicillins are resistant to penicillinase. Cephalosporins also are resistant to penicillinase, but cross-sensitivity may develop between them and the penicillins. They have a broad spectrum of effectiveness and low toxicity. Aminoglycosides are effective against gram-negative organisms (e.g., *Pseudomonas, Serratia,* and *Escherichia* species), but they are ototoxic and nephrotoxic in a dose-related manner. Aminoglycosides (acids) precipitate when mixed with heparin and are incompatible with some cephalosporins and penicillins (bases). They should be given at separate times or through separate lines. Adverse effects, such as respiratory arrest, may occur with concurrent use of aminoglycosides and neuromuscular blockers or anesthetic agents. Among the carbapenems, the newest group of antibiotics, imipenem/cilastatin sodium has the broadest aerobic and anaerobic activity of any antibiotic. It is particularly effective against intraabdominal sepsis, with minimal side effects of nausea and vomiting, and susceptible organisms in the respiratory and urinary tracts.

The incidence of allergic reactions to penicillin is relatively high. Patients should be questioned about allergies before any drug is administered and closely watched for signs of toxicity as evidenced by skin rash, gastrointestinal disturbance, renal disorder, fever, or blood dyscrasia.

The efficacy of antibiotics is greatly reduced when multiple organisms are involved in an infection. Sufficient risk warrants their use, however. Antibiotics are given as follows:

1. Therapeutically to eliminate sensitive viable organisms during a clinical course of infection and in grossly contaminated and traumatic wounds. The choice of antibiotic and the duration of therapy should be determined by clinical factors (i.e., pathogen, severity and site of infection, and clinical response). A broad-spectrum drug may be given while awaiting results of cultures and sensitivity tests.
2. Prophylactically to prevent the development of infection. Prophylaxis implies that the microorganism is attacked by the antimicrobial agent when it harbors in tissue before colonization takes place. A prophylactic antibiotic is given before surgical intervention, bacterial invasion, or clinically evident infection. These agents are effective as supplements to host defense mechanisms in selected patients. Antibiotic prophylaxis is recommended as follows:
   a. For procedures associated with brief exposure to possible infection; evidence indicates that antibiotics can reduce infection (e.g., cystoscopy following cystitis).
   b. For procedures not frequently associated with infection, but when occurrence would have disastrous or life-threatening consequences (e.g., clean wounds, or insertion of a prosthetic implant such as a heart valve, vascular graft, or total joint replacement).
   c. For procedures associated with a high risk of infection. Organisms are predictable and susceptible to antibiotics (e.g., clean-contaminated wounds such as a biliary tract with obstruction or transection of the colon).

The probability of infection is determined in the first few hours after bacterial invasion, when capillary permeability and host response are at a peak immediately after bacterial contamination. Therefore timing and duration of drug administration are crucial. To be effective, the prophylactic antibiotic must be present in adequate concentration in tissues at the time of wound creation or contamination. Selection of the appropriate drug and early use are pertinent factors. The antibiotic regimen is governed by the site of the surgical procedure, potential pathogens to be found, and the patient's history of drug sensitivities. Drugs may be given preoperatively and/or intraoperatively and possibly for a short period postoperatively. The CDC recommends the following:

1. Except for cesarean section, parenteral antibiotic prophylaxis should be started within 2 hours before a surgical procedure to produce a therapeutic level during the surgical procedure and should not be continued for more than 48 hours. A 12-hour limit is desirable for most types of wounds. Parenteral use for more than 24 hours increases the risk of antibiotic toxicity and development of resistant strains of bacteria or superinfection and does not further reduce the risk of infection.
2. For cesarean section, prophylaxis usually is given intraoperatively after the umbilical cord is clamped.
3. Oral, absorbable prophylactic antibiotics should not be used to supplement or extend parenteral prophylaxis. They should be limited to 24 hours before the surgical procedure when used prophylactically in colorectal operations.
4. Topical antimicrobial products used in the wound should be limited to agents that will not cause serious local or systemic side effects.

Resistance to Antibiotic Therapy

Antibiotic resistance is a serious problem. A drastic change in the pattern of life-threatening infections has occurred since the advent of broad-spectrum antibiotics and penicillinase-resistant penicillins. Gram-negative bacilli, both aerobic and anaerobic, deeply concern clinicians because the incidence of infections by bacteria of supposedly low virulence (e.g., *Serratia* organisms), is increasing. These microorganisms are capable of causing deep, latent infections, rapidly colonize, and are transferred among individuals by hands or equipment. Many of these organisms develop plasmid-mediated resistance to antibiotics. This means that a bacterium carrying genetic particles (plasmids) that allow it to replicate will not be affected by the antibiotic (i.e., will be resistant to it).

Methicillin-Resistant Staphylococcus aureus

Methicillin-resistant *S. aureus* (MRSA) is not plasmid mediated. However, it is resistant not just to methicillin, a penicillin, but to other categories of antibiotics as well. This resistance has probably developed as a result of overuse of these broad-spectrum agents. Clinically, MRSA poses an important nosocomial problem, whether by infection of patients or colonization in health care workers. Vancomycin, a highly toxic antimicrobial drug, seems to be effective against MRSA.

Vancomycin-Resistant Enterococci

Vancomycin-resistant enterococci (VRE) have flourished since 1989. Studies have shown that VRE genes can be passed on to other gram-positive cocci, such as vancomycin-resistant *Streptococcus pneumoniae* and *S. aureus* (VRSA). Cases of VRSA have been reported in Japan. The CDC is currently compiling statistics on gram-positive vancomycin resistance. Previous treatment with vancomycin or multiantimicrobial therapies increases the risk for VRE. The greatest routes for spread of VRE are the hands of caregivers and contaminated equipment. According to the CDC, prevention of VRE includes, but is not limited to, the following:

- Education of the staff
- Prevention of transmission by isolating known colonized or infected patients
- Early detection of colonization or infection with VRE
- Screening of all enterococci isolated from blood and body substances (except urine) for vancomycin resistance
- Prudent use of vancomycin

Approved antimicrobial agents have been shown to be effective for the cleaning and disinfection of medical devices and environmental surfaces used in the care of antibiotic-resistant patients. The CDC has not issued time lines for periods of isolation for VRE-infected patients, but three successive negative cultures, 1 or more weeks apart, is one possible guideline that has been used by some institutions.*

Antifungal and Antiviral Drugs

Fungal and viral infections can be problematic. Topical antifungal drugs usually control fungus. *Candida albicans,* for example, can lead to a fatal opportunistic systemic infection. Candicidin is a specific fungicide for this organism.

Viruses are not usually a risk to a healthy patient undergoing an elective procedure. Hepatitis and HIV present a unique challenge because they are a potential threat to the caregiver. Knowledge of the medication and the disease it treats may be involved in perioperative patient education. Dosages will vary. Examples of available antiviral agents include, but are not limited to, the following:

- Ribavirin for respiratory syncytial virus infection
- Zidovudine/dideoxyinosine for HIV infection
- Ganciclovir for CMV infection
- Acyclovir/famciclovir/valacyclovir for HSV infection
- Rimantadine/amantadine for influenza
- Didanosine for retrovirus infection
- Lamivudine for retrovirus infection
- Stavudine for retrovirus infection

Guidelines for preventing the spread of vancomycin-resistant microorganisms, 1997, www.cdc.gov.

Bibliography

Brown P et al: Creutzfeldt-Jakob disease in a husband and wife, *Neurology* 50(3):684-688, 1998.

Castellani RJ et al: Biopsy diagnosis of Creutzfeldt-Jakob disease by Western blot: a case report, *Hum Pathol* 28(5):623-626, 1997.

Department of Health and Human Services: Draft guideline for the prevention of surgical site infection, part III, *Fed Register* 63(116):33168-33179, 1998.

Hanley PE et al: Tuberculosis makes a comeback, *AORN J* 63(4):705-715, 1996.

Hsiao KK: From prion diseases to Alzheimer's disease, *J Neural Transms Suppl* 49:135-144, 1997.

Manuelidi L: Decontamination of Creutzfeldt-Jakob disease and other transmission agents, *J Neurovirol* 3(1):62-65, 1997.

Michels M et al: When is sick too sick to work? *Infect Control Today* 2(5):94-97, 1998.

Pugliese G: Handling bloodborne exposure, *Infect Control Today* 2(6):40-44, 1998.

Ronk LL: Surgical patients with multi-resistant bacteria, *AORN J* 61(6): 1023, 1025, 1027, 1030, 1032, 1033-1034, 1995.

Schonberger LB: New variant Creutzfeldt-Jakob disease and bovine spongiform encephalopathy, *Infect Dis Clin North Am* 12(1):111-121, 1998.

Sharbaugh RJ: A brief overview of nosocomial infection in acute care facilities, *Infect Control Today* 2(5):22, 24, 28, 1998.

Sternbach G et al: From Creutzfeldt-Jakob disease to the mad cow epidemic, *J Emerg Med* 15(5):701-705, 1997.

Thompson J: AORN's multisite clinical study of bloodborne exposures in OR personnel, *AORN J* 63(2):428-430, 433, 1996.

Weber T, Aguzzi A: The spectrum of transmissible spongiform encephalopathies, *Int Virol* 40(2-3):198-212, 1997.

Chapter 15

Principles of Asepsis and Sterile Technique

 Chapter Objectives

After studying this chapter, the learner will be able to:

- Define aseptic technique.
- Define sterile technique.
- Describe the transmission of microorganisms.
- List several principles of standard precautions (formerly known as universal precautions).

Aseptic and sterile techniques are based on sound scientific principles and are carried out primarily to prevent the transmission of microorganisms that can cause infection (Box 15-1). Microorganisms are invisible but are present in the air and on animate and inanimate objects. To prevent infection, all possible measures are taken to create and maintain an aseptic environment for the patient. Infection that is acquired during the course of health care is known as a nosocomial infection. Such an infection may occur in the postoperative wound or as a complication unrelated to the surgical site. A postoperative infection is a very serious, potentially fatal complication that may result from a single break in sterile technique. Therefore the basis of prevention is the knowledge of causative agents and their control, as well as the principles of aseptic and sterile techniques. To effectively apply the principles of asepsis, environmental control, and sterile techniques discussed in this chapter, the meaning of terms related to aseptic technique must first be understood (Box 15-2).

Asepsis literally means *without infection,* and it implies the absence of microorganisms that cause infection. It is impossible to exclude all microorganisms from the environment, but for the safety of both patients and personnel, every effort is made to minimize and control these microorganisms. The methods by which microbial contamination is prevented in the environment are referred to as *aseptic techniques.* These practices are the key to the containment of microorganisms.

Sterile technique refers to creating and working within the sterile field. To protect the patient during invasive procedures, microorganisms in the sterile field are kept to an irreducible minimum. The patient is at risk for infection any time tissues are interrupted or instrumentation is introduced into the vascular system. Sterile items should be used to prevent the introduction of pathogens into the patient's body.

HISTORICAL BACKGROUND

In ancient times demons and evil spirits were thought to be the cause of pestilence and infection. The strange methods used to drive them away were replaced with purification by fire. Heat is still used today as one means of destroying microorganisms.

Not until Ignaz Semmelweis (1818-1865) advocated the value of handwashing and Louis Pasteur (1822-1895) taught his germ theory did physicians begin to study the cause of infections and the means of controlling them. Robert Koch (1843-1910), who isolated the tubercle bacillus, advocated

Transmission-Based Precautions for the Prevention of Pathogenic Microorganisms as Proposed by the Centers for Disease Control and Prevention

Airborne

The use of special air-handlers and ventilation and respiratory protection is recommended for susceptible persons. Contaminated air currents can settle on or be inhaled by susceptible persons.

Particles smaller than 5 μm may carry airborne droplet nuclei. Examples of airborne diseases include varicella, tuberculosis, and rubeola.

Droplet

A distance of more than 3 feet from the source patient is recommended. Masks should be worn by those closer than 3 feet and should be worn by the source patient during transport.

Droplet particles are larger than 5 μm and are disseminated during coughs, sneezes, and talking. Droplets do not travel over 3 feet and are not suspended in the air.

Examples of droplet diseases include diphtheria, mumps, pertussis, and influenza.

Contact

The use of gloves when coming in contact with items contaminated with blood or body substances is recommended.

Gowns are recommended if there is a potential for contamination of clothing.

Cleaning and disinfecting patient care equipment after use protects other patients.

Data from United States Department of Health and Human Services (www.dhhs.gov) and Centers for Disease Control and Prevention (www.cdc.gov).

Terms Associated with Aseptic Technique

aerosol   Dispersion of fine mist, droplets, or particulate matter into air (v.t.: *aerosolize,* to become airborne).

antisepsis   Prevention of sepsis by the exclusion, destruction, or inhibition of growth or multiplication of microorganisms from body tissues and fluids.

antiseptics   Inorganic chemical compounds that combat sepsis by inhibiting the growth of microorganisms without necessarily killing them. They are used on skin and tissue to arrest the growth of endogenous microorganisms (resident flora), and they must not destroy tissue.

asepsis   Absence of microorganisms that cause disease; freedom from infection; exclusion of microorganisms (adj.: *aseptic,* without infection).

aseptic body image   An awareness of body, hair, makeup, clothes, jewelry, fingernails, and attire. Team members must be aware of their proximity to areas that are considered sterile vs. those that are contaminated.

aseptic technique   Methods by which contamination with microorganisms is prevented (alternate term: *aseptic practice,* to maintain asepsis).

barrier   Material used to reduce or inhibit the migration or transmission of microorganisms in the environment. Barriers include attire of personnel, drapes over furniture and patients, packaging of supplies, and filters in ventilating system.

carrier   Person who has potentially pathogenic microorganisms on or in his or her body and disperses them into the environment.

contaminated   Soiled or infected by microorganisms.

cross-contamination   Transmission of microorganisms from patient to patient and from inanimate objects to patients and vice versa.

decontamination   Cleaning and disinfecting or sterilizing processes carried out to make contaminated items safe to handle.

disease   Specific entity that is the sum total of numerous characteristics of one or more pathologic processes; failure of the body's adaptive mechanisms to counteract adequately the stress to which it is subjected, resulting in a disturbance in the function or structure of any part, organ, or system of the body.

fomite   Inanimate object that may be contaminated with infectious organisms and serves to transmit disease.

isolation   Special precautions taken to prevent the transmission of microorganisms from specific body substances.

pathogenic   Producing or capable of producing disease.

pathogenic microorganisms   Microorganisms that cause infectious disease. They can invade healthy tissue through some power of their own or can injure tissue by a toxin they produce.

sepsis   Severe toxic febrile state resulting from infection with pyogenic microorganisms, with or without associated septicemia.

spatial relationships   An awareness of sterile, unsterile, clean, and contaminated areas and their proximity to each. This would include the height of scrubbed team members in relation to each other and the sterile field. The circulator must be aware of his or her closeness to the sterile field and of the appropriate means to control environmental contaminants.

standard precautions   Procedures followed to protect personnel from contact with the blood and body fluids of all patients (formerly referred to as universal precautions).

sterile   Free of microorganisms, including all spores.

sterile field   Area around the site of incision into tissue or introduction of an instrument into a body orifice that has been prepared for the use of sterile supplies and equipment. This area includes all furniture covered with sterile drapes and all personnel who are properly attired.

sterile technique   Methods by which contamination with microorganisms is prevented to maintain sterility throughout the surgical procedure.

surgically clean   Mechanically cleaned but unsterile. Items are rendered surgically clean by the use of chemical, physical, or mechanical means that markedly reduce the number of microorganisms on them.

terminal sterilization and disinfection   Procedures carried out for the destruction of pathogens at the end of the surgical procedure in the OR or in other areas of patient contact (i.e., PACU, ICU, nursing unit).

unsterile   Inanimate object that has not been subjected to a sterilization process; the outside wrapping of a package containing a sterile item; a person who has not prepared to enter the sterile field (syn.: *nonsterile*).

the use of bichloride of mercury as an antiseptic. These events triggered interest in antisepsis.

Pasteur's work was pursued by Joseph Lister (1827-1912), the English surgeon who became known as the father of modern surgery. Because the relationship between bacteria and infection was now known, he searched for a chemical that could combat bacteria and surgical infections. He was the first to use a carbolic solution on dressings, which reduced the mortality of his patients to some degree. Lister believed infections were airborne. In 1865 he started to use carbolic spray in the operating room (OR). He then used it in the wound, on articles in contact with the wound, and on the hands of the surgical team. The result was a notable decrease in mortality, but the carbolic solution caused wound necrosis and skin irritation in both patients and team members. The solution also had an anticoagulant effect, which made hemostasis difficult. Not all surgeons were convinced of the value of surgical antiseptics. It was not until 1879, at a medical meeting in Amsterdam, that Lister's antiseptic principles of surgery were truly accepted by the medical profession.

German surgeons played a role in the transition from antisepsis to asepsis. Gustav Neuber (1850-1932) introduced mercuric chloride in 1886 to clean his apron, and he advocated scrubbing the furniture with disinfectant and wearing gowns, boots, and caps. He eventually sterilized everything that came in contact with wounds. The first steam sterilizer was introduced in Germany in 1886. Surgeons began to accept that all things coming into contact with a wound should be sterile. Aseptic technique evolved through the refinement of surgical technique, the use of a controlled environment, precise housekeeping methods, and aseptic precautions to protect patients and personnel from infection.

TRANSMISSION OF MICROORGANISMS

People remain the major source of microorganisms in the environment. Everything on or around a human being is contaminated by the body in some way. The action and interaction of personnel and patients also contribute to the prevalence and dispersion of organisms.

There are many sources of contamination in the OR environment. Transmission-based precautions should be implemented in the perioperative environment and in any area with the potential to transmit potentially pathogenic microorganisms. Transmission-based precautions are described in Box 15-1. Perioperative personnel are primarily concerned with protecting the environment of the OR suite, because surgical procedures should be performed under optimal aseptic conditions. Two areas are most critical for the introduction and spread of microorganisms:

1. Semirestricted areas
2. Restricted areas

Most microbes grow in a warm, moist host, but some aerobic bacteria, yeasts, and fungi can remain viable in the air and on inanimate objects. Microbiologic considerations and specific microorganisms are described in Chapter 14. The physical sources of contamination are described in the following sections.

Skin

The skin of patients, OR team members, and visitors constitutes a microbiologic hazard. Sebaceous (oil) and sudoriferous (sweat) glands contain abundant resident microbial flora, many of which have the potential to become pathogenic if colonized in greater than average numbers or if colonized on a weakened host. In an average individual, an estimated 4000 to 10,000 viable contaminated particles are shed by the skin each minute. Some disperse up to 30,000 particles per minute; these individuals are referred to as *shedders*. Shedders are densely populated with virulent organisms, such as *Staphylococcus aureus,* and shed contaminated skin cells into the environment. Patients who are shedders have a much higher incidence of infection at the surgical site. On all individuals, the major areas of microbial shedding include the head, neck, axillae, hands, groin, perineum, legs, and feet. Cosmetic detritus and body powders are also laden with potential pathogens. Microbial shedding is contained effectively by appropriate antiseptic cleansing and maximum skin coverage.

The following are key points for all personnel entering the OR:

1. Bathe daily with soap that contains an antibacterial agent. This can reduce shedding.
2. Wash hands before entering the OR suite and after every patient contact to prevent infection and cross-infection. This handwashing technique involves a vigorous rubbing together of all surfaces of well-lathered, soapy hands, followed by rinsing them under a stream of water.
3. Don clean OR attire for each entry into the OR suite. Long sleeves are worn by unsterile team members.
4. Cover any cuts and abrasions. Open wounds on the skin are portals for infection, and infected wounds can disseminate microorganisms.
5. Wear gloves when handling blood, body fluids, or tissue specimens, and wash hands after removing sterile and unsterile gloves.

Hair

Hair is a gross contaminant and a major source of staphylococci. The extent to which the microbial population is attracted to and shed from hair is directly related to the length and cleanliness of the hair. Hair follicles and filaments harbor resident and transient floras. Hair can become a mechanical irritant in wound healing and cause a foreign body tissue reaction. Hair should be shampooed frequently. Caps or hoods are worn to cover hair completely, including facial hair. Hair should be contained at all times in semirestricted and restricted environments.

Nasopharynx

Organisms forcibly expelled by talking, coughing, or sneezing give rise to bacteria-laden dust and lint as droplets settle on surfaces and skin. Persons known as *carriers* harbor many organisms, most notably group A streptococci and *S. aureus,* without experiencing the harmful physical effects of infection. Surgeons and anesthesia providers may be carriers more so than other caregivers because of their intimate contact with patients' respiratory tracts. Shedders and/or carriers may be identified through nasopharyngeal culturing. Some departments, such as obstetrics and the newborn nursery, may require routine periodic cultures as a condition of employment. When multiple patients develop the same or similar postoperative infections, infection control teams at the facility actively seek the source of the infection.

Masks are worn in all restricted areas to cover the nose and mouth and should be changed after caring for each patient. Coughing and sneezing explode droplets into the environment, and therefore persons with a respiratory infection should not be permitted in the OR suite. Talking should be kept to a minimum.

Fomites

Contaminated particles are present in the dust that rests on inanimate objects such as furniture, OR surfaces (walls, floors, cabinet shelves), equipment, supplies, and fabrics. Covert contamination may result from improper handling of equipment such as anesthesia apparatus or intravenous (IV) lines and fluids. Contamination also may result from the administration of unsterile medications or the use of unsterile water to rinse sterile items. Any unsterile item placed within the sterile field causes contamination and increases the risk of infection.

In maintaining a sterile environment, the following key points should be considered:

1. Prompt decontamination of used equipment and reusable supplies.
2. Prompt disinfection of OR surfaces (e.g., disinfecting furniture and floors, disposing of waste and laundry).
3. Separation of clean and soiled items. Sterile storage areas are physically separated from decontamination areas.
4. Proper packaging and storing of supplies. External shipping cartons should be removed before bringing supplies beyond the unrestricted area in the OR suite.
5. Placement of dust covers over sterile items during transport and while in prolonged storage.

Air

The perioperative environment contains thousands of particles per cubic foot of air. During a long surgical procedure, the particle count can rise to more than one million particles per cubic foot. Air and dust are vehicles for transporting particles laded with microorganisms. Heat rises, and therefore the lights and other heat-generating equipment of the OR produce convective upcurrents. Airborne contamination can be generated by personnel; every movement increases the potential for infection of the surgical site. Particulates that become airborne can settle on an open wound. Between 80% and 90% of the microbial contaminations found in an open surgical site come from ambient (room) air.

Microorganisms have an affinity for horizontal surfaces, of which the floor is the largest. From the floor, microorganisms are projected into the air. Endogenous flora from the patient's skin, oropharynx, tracheobronchial tree, and gastrointestinal tract, as well as exogenous flora, are also significant. Microorganisms from patients or carriers settle on equipment and flat surfaces and then become airborne. Airborne particles increase significantly during the activity before incision and after wound closure. Relief personnel create significant air currents. The potential for draft increases each time the door to the OR opens and closes.

An effective ventilation system is essential to prevent patients and personnel from breathing potentially contaminated air, which can predispose them to infection.

Human Error

Although air is a vehicle for the transmission of microorganisms, direct person-to-person contact is the most common route of transmission. Human error is an exogenous source of contamination, and it is not to be underestimated. Failure to follow the principles and applications of sterile and aseptic techniques places the patient and personnel at risk—a risk that could be prevented. Errors should be readily admitted and corrected.

Cross-Infection

Every patient in the OR should be considered to be a potential source of infection. Standard precautions (formerly referred to as universal precautions) and routine aseptic techniques are observed whether or not a patient is known to have an infectious condition. Care, caution, and conscientiousness on the part of all team members is essential at all times. Thorough handwashing after every patient contact is important.

SOURCES OF INFECTION

The incidence and types of infections that occur in surgical patients may be the result of a preexisting localized infectious process, a systemic communicable disease, or an acquired perioperative complication.

Community-Acquired Infection

Community-acquired infections are natural disease processes that developed or were incubating before a patient's admission to the hospital or ambulatory care facility.

Communicable Infection

Systemic bacterial, viral, or fungal infections may be transmitted from one person to another. A detailed discussion of these infections can be found in Chapter 14.

Spontaneous Infection

Examples of localized infections that require surgical diagnosis and/or treatment for management or that occur as adjuvants to medical therapy include acute appendicitis, cholecystitis, or bowel perforation with peritonitis. Therapy consists of identification of the infection site and causative microorganism, excision or drainage, prevention of further contamination, and augmentation of host resistance.

Nosocomial Infection

The term *nosocomial* is derived from the Greek word for nurse, *nosokomia* (νοσοκομια). An infection is considered hospital-associated or acquired (i.e., nosocomial) during the course of health care if it was neither present nor incubating when the patient was admitted.

Approximately 35% of all nosocomial infections develop in surgical patients. They may occur as complications of surgical or other procedures performed on uninfected patients. They may also occur as complicating infections in organs unrelated to the surgical procedure that occur with or as a result of postoperative care. The majority of nosocomial infections are related to instrumentation of the urinary and respiratory tracts. Wound infection is the second most common infection. The following are examples of nosocomial infections:

- Urinary tract or respiratory tract infection, or infected pressure or stasis ulcers
- Cellulitis or abscess formation related to the surgical procedure (e.g., intraabdominal abscess following a gastrointestinal procedure)
- Thrombophlebitis or peritonitis, both of which are regional extensions of postoperative or posttraumatic infections
- Liver, lung, or visceral abscess following the surgical procedure often performed for penetrating injuries or malignant metastases
- Bacteremia or septicemia, the postoperative systemic infections that result from dissemination of microorganisms into the bloodstream from a distributing focus

Exogenous

An exogenous nosocomial infection is acquired from sources outside the body, such as personnel or the environment. Cross-contamination occurs when organisms are transferred to the patient from another individual or inanimate object.

Endogenous

An endogenous infection develops from sources within the body. Most postoperative wound infections result from seeding by endogenous microorganisms. Disruption of the balance between potentially pathogenic organisms and host defenses permits the invasion of microorganisms for which the patient is the primary reservoir. For example, abdominal sepsis may result from enteric flora if the intestine is perforated or transected.

ASEPTIC TECHNIQUE AND ENVIRONMENTAL CONTROLS

Control of the environment is a necessary part of overall infection prevention. The inanimate and animate environment of the OR suite presents a risk for the transmission of microorganisms. The aim of a microbiologically controlled environment is to keep contamination to a minimum.

AORN, the Association of periOperative Registered Nurses, has developed standards and recommended practices for achieving the optimal level of technical and aseptic practices in the care of perioperative patients. These guidelines are intended to give direction and information for the formulation of institutional policies. Individual hospital policies and procedures reflect variations in the physical environment and/or in clinical situations, which determine the degree to which these recommended practices can be implemented. All health care facilities should incorporate into their policies and procedures the recommendations for infection control from the Centers for Disease Control and Prevention (CDC), as well as the regulations for the prevention of exposure to bloodborne pathogens from the Occupational Safety and Health Administration (OSHA).

The perioperative environment is designed both to optimize function and safety and to protect patients from sources of contamination. The OR suite includes specific areas for traffic, support systems, administration, communication, and storage as described in Chapter 10. Traffic patterns are designed to flow smoothly and to prevent backtrack and crossover traffic. Clean and soiled activities, areas, personnel, and sterile and unsterile supplies should be distinctly separated.

Aseptic barriers such as sterile gowns and gloves protect sterile areas, isolate surgical sites from infectious contaminants, and keep the number of microorganisms to a minimum. To slow or prevent the transfer of organisms, these barriers must be impervious to the passage of such microorganisms under ordinary operating conditions. Procedures are established to provide barriers against the migration of microorganisms from any potential source of microbial contamination.

Environmental Services/Housekeeping

Housekeeping practices that use the most effective supplies, techniques, and equipment available are a most important aspect of infection control. Good housekeeping techniques should reduce microbial flora by approximately 90%. Housekeeping procedures include cleaning and disinfecting the perioperative environment, handling soiled laundry, and disposing of solid waste. Disinfectants are used in combination with thorough mechanical cleaning. These procedures are performed by environmental service personnel under supervision and are carried out according to established practices, policies, and schedules as described in Chapter 12. Of primary concern are locations that by design or construction are difficult to clean (e.g., lavatories and work rooms) and areas that may be touched by patients or personnel.

Any equipment or procedure requiring water in its operation can support microbial growth, especially if the water is not changed frequently or if the sinks are not cleaned. Unsterile water, the universal solvent and transporter, can support, maintain, and protect almost every contaminant produced by human beings. Water especially supports the growth of gram-negative bacilli, including *Serratia* and *Pseudomonas* microorganisms. Airborne particles produced during hand scrubs can contaminate the area around the scrub sink. Disinfectants reduce the contamination potential of unsterile cleaning water.

The following housekeeping points are especially relevant to infection control and the prevention of cross-infection and are listed to emphasize the importance of aseptic environmental control:

1. The faucet head should be of a type that does not hold water and should be removed for terminal sterilization. Containers for antimicrobial handwashing agents should be cleaned and terminally sterilized before refilling.
2. No surface should remain wet, which would support microbial growth.
3. Organic debris should be promptly removed from walls and other surfaces with a disinfectant to prevent drying and airborne contamination.
4. Lights should be cleaned after every procedure. Overhead tracks should be cleaned at least twice daily: before the first scheduled surgical procedure and on completion of the day's schedule.
5. The entrance to the OR suite and the floors in corridors and rooms should be cleaned with a wet-vacuum system. Dry debris is first removed with a dry vacuum; the floor is then sprayed with a detergent-disinfectant solution and wet-vacuumed.
6. Housekeeping equipment should be cleaned and dried for storage. Moisture and darkness are conducive to microbial growth.
7. Disposable trash should be separated into infectious and noninfectious waste and put in impervious receptacles.
8. Service elevators rather than chutes should be used to remove soiled laundry and waste/trash from the OR suite. Chutes become grossly contaminated with airborne particles and are a fire hazard.
9. Waste should be contained at the source of origin to prevent aerosol generation during handling. Contaminated waste is decontaminated and/or sterilized before compaction or disposal in the general environment. Incineration is the most effective means of waste disposal, especially of infectious wastes. However, health care facilities must comply with local, state, and federal regulations for contamination control and waste disposal.
10. Adequate time must be allowed between patients for proper terminal disinfection of the OR. A patient must not be assigned to an inadequately cleaned OR, which could be a source of a surgical site infection.
11. All areas and equipment throughout the perioperative environment should be cleaned on a regular basis as defined by institutional policy. These areas include the grills, vents, and filters of the air-conditioning system; storage shelves and cabinets; lighting fixtures; walls; and other areas in offices, lounges, dressing rooms, storage areas, workrooms, and corridors. Handles of cabinets and push plates of doors should be cleaned several times daily.

Control of Airborne Contamination

Air currents and movement in the OR should be kept to a minimum to prevent airborne contamination. Viable microorganisms from the air settle on horizontal surfaces. Proper cleaning of these surfaces helps to control this contamination. The ventilating system and efforts to minimize air turbulence and contaminants also are important factors.

Air-Conditioning System

When properly designed, installed, and maintained, a conventional air-conditioning system effectively reduces the number of airborne organisms by removing dust and aerosol particles. Air contaminated by dust and lint is removed as fresh, clean outside air is supplied. Recirculation of filtered air at a minimum rate of 20 volume exchanges per hour, at least four of which are fresh air, is considered safe and economical. However, fire codes in some states require 100% outside fresh air. All air, whether recirculated or fresh, is filtered before entering the OR. The system uses high-efficiency particulate air (HEPA) filters to reduce the number of particles larger than 0.5 μm to 1 to 5 per cubic foot. The dilution principle is used: Air enters from a ceiling vent, is diluted, and passes out through vents at floor level. Filters are located downstream from the air-processing equipment so microorganisms will not be drawn into the room. The system maintains a positive pressure if the doors to the room remain closed.

Ultraclean Air System

Often referred to as laminar airflow, a special air-handling system for the filtration, dilution, and distribution of air may be installed in one or more ORs. High-risk procedures such as total joint replacement, cardiac surgery, or organ transplantation are performed in this environment. Laminar airflow is a controlled, unidirectional, positive pressure stream of air. From a ceiling diffuser, clean air flows downward at a high velocity, progressively decreasing as it flows radially outward. The controlled airstream entraps particulate matter and microorganisms. The flow returns to the system and passes through a prefilter to remove gross particles. It then passes through a HEPA filter that traps and eliminates more than 99% of all particles larger than 0.3 μm, including virtually all bacteria and most viruses. A rate of 100 to 400 air changes per hour is possible; most systems deliver approximately 240.

To complete the laminar airflow system, sterile team members wear a total body exhaust gown, which resembles a spacesuit and covers the entire body. Air is piped into the headpiece and removed through filtered tubes. The hood or helmet is equipped for hearing and speaking. Negative pressure is maintained under the gown by a vacuum hose. The system provides body cooling for the wearer.

Laminar airflow with a total body exhaust system reliably reduces bacterial contamination at the wound site. Although an ultraclean air system provides microbe-free air (no more than one organism per cubic foot) with minimal air turbulence, it is not a substitute for meticulous surgical technique. The decrease in particle count does not significantly reduce the rate of infection at the surgical site. It is an adjunct to controlling airborne contamination.

Doors

The doors to the OR should be kept closed except as necessary for passage of the patient and personnel or supplies and equipment. If the door is left open, the positive air pressure in the room equalizes with the negative air pressure in the hallway. Disrupted pressurization mixes the clean air of the OR with the corridor air, which has a higher microbial count. Cabinet doors should remain closed.

Traffic and Movement

Traffic in and out of the OR is kept to a minimum. Only essential personnel should be allowed inside the OR. The amount of activity in the room increases as the number of people present increases. This in turn increases the potential for contamination as a result of the shedding and air turbulence that carries microbes to the wound. Movement in the OR should be reduced to a minimum.

Lint

Agents are added to the final rinse during laundering to minimize the lint that results from the friction of woven fibers against each other. Disintegrated paper from disposable products is another source of lint on fabrics. Therefore paper products should not be discarded in the same receptacle as soiled reusable woven fabrics.

Isolation Precautions

The isolation of patients by diagnosis or body substance is related to the mode of transmission of pathogenic microorganisms (i.e., air, droplet, and contact). Isolation precautions and guidelines are discussed in detail in hospital procedure books and in the CDC Guideline for Isolation Precautions in Hospitals. There are different methods of isolation technique:

- Category-specific isolation precautions for patients with suspected or confirmed communicable disease transmitted either by droplets via the airborne route (e.g., pulmonary tuberculosis) or by enteric excretions, drainage, or secretions
- Disease-specific isolation precautions for contact with patients known to be infected with specific pathogens
- Body substance isolation incorporating standard precautions for contact with all body substances of all patients, regardless of the diagnosis (all patients are considered contaminated)
- Protective isolation for immunosuppressed patients

The purpose of these precautions is to prevent the transmission of pathogenic microorganisms. Isolation and barrier techniques protect both personnel and other patients. Each hospital may incorporate into its procedures whichever methods are most appropriate for its particular needs and patient population.

The perioperative staff should be informed that a patient requires isolation precautions before that patient comes to the OR. A sticker on the patient's chart indicates the type of hospital isolation. For most patients the same precautions apply in the OR as on the unit, and a common sense approach is used. In all types of isolation the most important control measure is thorough handwashing before and after close patient contact; after handling contaminated objects, body fluids, or excretions; and between patients. Isolation techniques must not be implemented in a way that causes the patient to feel victimized. The patient should be educated to accept the regimen.

STANDARD PRECAUTIONS

As established by the CDC and enforced by OSHA, standard precautions (formerly referred to as universal precautions) protect health care workers from contact with blood and body fluids of all patients. Standard precautions include considerations for the following:

- All body fluids
- Handwashing
- Barrier clothing
- Handling of used patient care equipment and linen
- Occupational exposure to blood-borne pathogens
- Patient placement

Recommendations for standard precautions have been modified to reflect routes of transmission.* The format for the CDC's identification of routes of transmission includes *airborne, droplet,* and *contact* precautions. The potential for becoming infected through skin exposure depends on colonization, duration of contact, the presence of skin lesions on the

---

*Centers for Disease Control and Prevention, 1997. www.cdc.gov.

hands, and immune status. Standard precautions supplement other recommended practices for environmental controls and are the minimum precautions for all invasive procedures. An invasive procedure involves any entry into body tissues or cavities in any procedural environment. Standard precautions are in effect for any procedure during which bleeding occurs or for which the potential for bleeding or exposure to body substances exists. Standard precautions involves the following:

1. *Protective barriers and personal protective equipment.* Appropriate barriers, such as personal protective equipment (PPE), prevent contact of the skin and mucous membranes with blood and body substances. PPE and other barrier materials must prevent blood and other fluids from passing through or reaching the wearer's clothing or body. The type of PPE used depends on the task and the degree of anticipated exposure. Examples include gloves, eyewear, gowns, hair covers, and masks.
   a. Gloves reduce contamination of hands. Intact gloves, both sterile and unsterile, are used. Latex, vinyl, and other materials are used in the manufacturing of these gloves. Care is taken to avoid natural rubber latex (NRL) when either the patient or the caregiver has a latex sensitivity. Vinyl may be more permeable to some viruses than latex.
      (1) Sterile gloves are worn for procedures that involve the invasion of body tissues when a sterile field is created. Double gloving does not prevent puncture wounds but may be appropriate for procedures in which the risk of glove tears is high.

      With double gloving, the exterior glove has a mechanical squeegee effect on a sharp object as it punctures its surface. The innermost glove further squeegees material from the sharp object, which reduces the potential numbers of microorganisms that come in contact with the wearer. Sterile glove liners may provide protection from skin cuts. Double gloving also may substantially reduce the risk of exposure from the seepage of blood and fluid through gloves onto hands during long procedures or in the presence of voluminous blood loss.
      (2) Unsterile latex or vinyl examination gloves are worn for procedures that do not require a sterile field, such as handling specimens, placentas, newborns, and contaminated items (e.g., sponges).
      (3) General-purpose utility gloves are worn for cleaning instruments and for decontaminating and housekeeping procedures involving potential blood contact. These heavy duty gloves may be decontaminated and reused.
      (4) Gloves are changed after every contact with patients or contaminated items. Latex and vinyl gloves are discarded.

(5) The hands are washed immediately after glove removal. All gloves have microscopic holes and may be permeable to certain substances or microorganisms. The mechanical and chemical actions of handwashing significantly decrease the risk associated with the permeability of glove materials.
   b. Masks protect personnel from aerosols and patients from droplets. They are worn for all invasive procedures. The mask should be changed immediately if grossly contaminated by a splash of blood or body fluid.
   c. Eyewear with side shields or full face shields protect the mucous membranes of the eyes, nose, or mouth. They are worn for procedures in which blood, bone chips, amniotic fluid, or the aerosol of other body fluids may splash or be projected into the eyes. Goggles with enclosed sides and chin-length face shields offer better protection than eyeglasses.
   d. Gowns or aprons made of fluid-resistant material protect the wearer from a splash with blood and body fluids. A plastic apron may be worn under a woven fabric gown. Impervious gowns offer better protection. Disposable impervious gowns are preferred.
   e. Shoe covers or boots protect the wearer when gross contamination on the floor can be anticipated. Grossly soiled shoe covers or knee-high disposable boots are removed before the wearer leaves the room.
2. *Prevention of puncture injuries.* Needles, knife blades, and sharp instruments present a potential hazard for the handler and user. Skin may be punctured or cut if caution is not taken. Specific recommendations for handling disposable surgical needles, syringes and needles, and knife blades (collectively referred to as *sharps)* include the following:
   a. Do not manipulate sharps by hand. Use an instrument to attach the blade to the knife handle. Arm the needle directly from the suture packet when possible. Do not bend or break an injection needle. Pass needles in a needleholder. Sharp instruments and needles may be passed on a tray or magnetic mat for a *hands-free technique* rather than from hand to hand. Remove instruments from the surgical field after use, and return them to the Mayo stand or instrument table promptly.
   b. Do not recap used injection needles except with a recapping safety device.
   c. Do not remove the needle from a disposable syringe after use.
   d. Place all used blades and needles in a puncture-resistant container.
3. *Management of puncture injuries.* If a glove is torn or punctured, remove the puncturing sharp or instrument from the sterile field immediately, and change the glove promptly.

If the skin is punctured or cut, remove both gloves immediately. If both gloves are not removed, the risk of introducing microorganisms from the remaining contaminated glove is increased. Squeeze the skin to release blood. Wash out contaminants under running water with an antiseptic, then irrigate the wound with a virucidal disinfectant such as an iodophor, bleach, or peroxide. Report the incident immediately, and document all actions on the appropriate form. Baseline testing may be necessary for the punctured individual and the patient.

4. *Oral procedures.* Although transmission by saliva is unlikely, contact with blood-contaminated saliva and gingival fluid is expected during dental and surgical procedures in the oropharyngeal cavity. Mouth protection, ambu bags, and/or other ventilation devices should be available for emergency airway resuscitation. Respiratory secretions coughed up during endotracheal procedures are often infectious.

5. *Care of specimens.* All specimens of blood, body fluids, and tissues should be contained to prevent leaking during transport to the laboratory. The outside of the container should be clean. The circulator, while wearing gloves, needs to disinfect the outside of a culture tube handed from the sterile field or a container if it has been contaminated. Care is taken not to get blood and body fluids on the pathology slip.

6. *Decontamination.* All instruments are thoroughly cleaned before sterilization or high-level disinfection. The surfaces of furniture and floors are cleaned and decontaminated with a detergent-disinfectant. Blood or body fluids that have spilled on the floor during a procedure should be wiped up immediately and the area decontaminated. Gloves, masks, and eyewear are worn for cleaning procedures.

7. *Laundry.* Soiled woven fabrics should be handled as little as possible and are transported to the laundry in leakproof bags. All laundry is considered contaminated and should be handled by only gloved hands. Laundry should be washed in water at 160° F (71.1° C) or higher with 50 to 150 parts per million (ppm) of chlorine bleach. Temperatures lower than 160° F (71.1° C) can be used for washing laundry if the appropriate antimicrobial detergent is used. Commercial dry cleaning uses chemicals that reduce the transmission of pathogens.

8. *Waste.* Blood and suctioned fluids may be safely poured down a drain that is connected to a sanitary sewer. A solidifying agent can be added to disposable suction containers to disinfect the produce and convert it into solid waste. Trash is disposed of by incineration or sent to a sanitary landfill in sealed containers as required by local ordinances or state regulations. Trash bags must be leakproof and of sufficient thickness and strength to ensure integrity during transport. For disposal purposes, waste may be differentiated as either infectious or noninfectious. Bags are either color coded (e.g., red for infectious waste) or labeled as biohazard.

9. *Handwashing.* Thorough handwashing with an approved antimicrobial agent following every contact with a patient, contaminated items, or suspected contamination protects both the patient and personnel, and it cannot be overemphasized.

10. *Avoid touching mucous membranes.* Eating and/or drinking are prohibited in any area where there is a risk of exposure. Applying lip balm or cosmetics or adjusting contact lenses in the perioperative environment significantly increases the risk of exposure. Hand-to-mouth and hand-to-eye contact can contribute to microbial transmission.

11. *Prophylaxis.* Perioperative personnel are encouraged to know their HIV and HBV (human immunodeficiency virus and hepatitis B virus) antibody status. The disclosure of a positive status to the appropriate facility is recommended.* Personnel who participate in invasive procedures are at risk for blood-borne exposure and should have an HBV immunization. Experts disagree about the need for booster injections after 7 years in order to maintain the antibody titer.

For their own protection and for the safety of patients, all health care providers should be familiar with policies and procedures and must understand the need for standard precautions. A health care provider should report a blood or body fluid exposure as defined by policy. The surgeon and first assistant usually are at greatest risk. Similarly, a patient should be informed of any incident in which he or she is exposed to the blood of a health care provider.

APPLICATION OF STERILE TECHNIQUE

Sterile technique prevents the transfer of microorganisms into body tissues during invasive procedures. Freshly incised or traumatized tissue can become infected easily, regardless of the area of the body. Intact skin and mucous membranes are the body's first line of defense against infection, but a portal for microorganisms is created if the integrity of the skin is interrupted. Depending on their intended purpose and body contact, the items and equipment for patient care are classified into the following categories according to the level of sterility necessary for safe use:

- *Critical.* Any item entering the body tissues underlying the skin and mucous membranes must be sterile (i.e., free of microorganisms, including spores). These items are handled to maintain sterility.

---

*Association of Operating Room Nurses: *AORN revised statement on the patient and health care workers with bloodborne diseases including human immunodeficiency virus (HIV),* Denver, 1987 (revision 1997), The Association.

- *Semicritical.* Sterility is less critical for items that come into contact with intact skin or mucous membranes. These items are surgically clean (i.e., mechanically cleaned and disinfected to reduce microorganisms but unsterile). Some items are disinfected immediately before use and are handled to prevent contamination before use. Other items are terminally sterilized, but sterility is not maintained during use.
- *Noncritical.* Items that will come into contact with only intact skin or mucous membranes in an area remote from the surgical site may be cleaned, terminally disinfected, and stored unsterile between patient uses.

Surgical procedures are performed under sterile conditions; contamination with microorganisms is prevented to maintain sterility throughout the procedure. A sterile field is created around the site of incision into tissues or the site of introduction of sterile instruments into a body orifice. Conversely, all material and equipment used during a surgical procedure are terminally decontaminated and sterilized after use with the assumption that every patient is a potential source of infection for other persons.

It is essential that all members of the perioperative team know the common sources and mechanisms of contamination by microorganisms in the perioperative environment. Sterile technique is the particular responsibility of everyone caring for the patient in the OR. All members of the OR team must be vigilant in safeguarding the sterility of the sterile field. Any contamination must be remedied immediately.

PRINCIPLES OF STERILE TECHNIQUE

Sterile technique is the basis of modern surgery. The patient is the center of the sterile field, which includes the personnel wearing sterile attire and the areas of the patient, operating bed, and furniture that are covered with sterile drapes. Strict adherence to the recommended practices of sterile technique reflects the surgical conscience of the perioperative team and is mandatory for the safety of the patient and personnel in the environment. The principles of sterile technique are applied under the following conditions:

- In preparation for an invasive procedure by sterilization of necessary materials and supplies
- In preparation of the sterile team to handle sterile supplies and intimately contact the surgical site by scrubbing, gowning, and gloving
- In the creation and maintenance of the sterile field, including skin preparation and draping of the patient
- In the maintenance of asepsis throughout the surgical procedure
- In terminal sterilization and disinfection at the conclusion of the surgical procedure

If these principles are understood, the need for their application becomes obvious.

Only Sterile Items Are Used Within the Sterile Field

Items such as drapes, sponges, or basins may be obtained from a stock supply of sterile packages. Other items, such as instruments, may be sterilized immediately before the surgical procedure and taken directly from the sterilizer to the sterile tables. Every person who dispenses a sterile article must be sure of its sterility and of its remaining sterile until used. Proper packaging, sterilizing, delivery to the field, and handling should provide such assurance. If there is any doubt about the sterility of any item, it should be considered not sterile. Items that could be or are known to be contaminated, such as in the following situations, must not be transferred to the sterile field:

- If a sterilized package is found in a contaminated area (e.g., the general unsterile workroom).
- If uncertain about the actual timing or operation of the sterilizer. Items processed in a suspect load are considered unsterile.
- If an unsterile person comes into close contact with a sterile table and vice versa.
- If a sterile table or unwrapped sterile items are not under constant observation.
- If the integrity of the packaging material is not intact.
- If a sterile package wrapped in a material other than plastic or another moisture-resistant barrier becomes damp or wet. Humidity in the storage area or moisture on hands may seep into the package.
- If a sterile package wrapped in a pervious woven material drops to the floor or other area of questionable cleanliness. These materials allow the implosion of air into the package. A dropped package is considered contaminated. If the wrapper is impervious and the area of contact is dry, the item may be transferred to the sterile field. Packages that have been dropped on the floor should not be put back into sterile storage.

Sterile Persons Are Gowned and Gloved

Gowns are considered sterile only from the chest to the level of the sterile field in the front, and from two inches above the elbows to the cuffs on the sleeves. When wearing a gown, only the area that can be seen in front down to the level of the sterile field should be considered sterile. Usually this does not extend below waist level. The following practices are observed:

1. Self-gowning and gloving should be done from a separate sterile surface to avoid dripping water onto sterile supplies or a sterile table.
2. The stockinette cuffs of the gown are enclosed beneath sterile gloves. The stockinette is absorbent and retains moisture, and therefore this part of the gown does not provide a microbial barrier. The cuffs are areas of friction and can cause microbial contamination.

3. Sterile persons keep their hands in sight at all times and at or above waist level or the level of the sterile field (Figure 15-1).
4. Hands are kept away from the face, and the elbows are kept close to the sides. The hands are never folded under the arms because of perspiration in the axillary region. The neckline, shoulders, and back also may become contaminated with perspiration. The back of the gown is not under constant observation and therefore must be considered contaminated.
5. Sterile persons are aware of the height of team members in relation to each other and the sterile field. Changing levels at the sterile field is avoided. The gown is considered sterile only down to the highest level of the sterile tables. If a sterile person must stand on a platform to reach the surgical site, the standing platform should be positioned before this person steps up to the draped area. Sterile persons should sit only when the entire procedure will be performed at this level. If one person on the team sits, the entire team should be seated.

Tables Are Sterile Only at Table Level

The result is the following:

1. Only the top of a sterile, draped table is considered sterile. The edges and sides of the drape extending below table level are considered unsterile.
2. Anything falling or extending over the table edge, such as a piece of suture, is unsterile. The scrub person does not touch the part hanging below table level.
3. When unfolding a sterile drape, the part that drops below the table surface is not brought back up to table level. Once placed, the drape is not moved or shifted.

4. Cords, tubing, and other materials are secured on the sterile field with a nonperforating clip to prevent them from sliding over the table edge.

Sterile Persons Touch Only Sterile Items or Areas; Unsterile Persons Touch Only Unsterile Items or Areas

For example:

1. Sterile team members maintain contact with the sterile field by means of sterile gowns and gloves.
2. The unsterile circulator does not directly contact the sterile field.
3. Supplies are brought to sterile team members by the circulator, who opens the wrappers on sterile packages. The circulator ensures a sterile transfer to the sterile field. Only sterile items touch sterile surfaces.

Unsterile Persons Avoid Reaching Over the Sterile Field; Sterile Persons Avoid Leaning Over an Unsterile Area

For example:

1. The unsterile circulator never reaches over a sterile field to transfer sterile items.
2. The circulator holds only the lip of the bottle over the basin when pouring solution into a sterile basin in order to avoid reaching over a sterile area (Figure 15-2).
3. The scrub person sets basins or glasses to be filled at the edge of the sterile table; the circulator stands near this edge of the table to fill them.

Figure 15-1 Sterile persons keep hands in sight at or above waist or level of sterile field. Gowns are considered sterile only in front from chest to level of sterile field, and the sleeves from above elbows to cuffs.

Figure 15-2 Circulator pouring sterile solution into sterile basin. Note that only lip of bottle is over the basin. Unsterile person avoids reaching over sterile field.

4. The circulator stands at a distance from the sterile field to adjust the light over it; this prevents microbial fall-out over the field. Sterile light handles are preferred for manipulation of the surgical lights.
5. The surgeon turns away from the sterile field to have perspiration removed from the brow.
6. The scrub person drapes an unsterile table toward self first to protect the gown. Gloved hands are protected by cuffing a drape over them (Figure 15-3).
7. The scrub person stands back from the unsterile table when draping it in order to avoid leaning over an unsterile area (Figures 15-4 to 15-6).

The Edges of Anything That Encloses Sterile Contents Are Considered Unsterile

The boundaries between sterile and unsterile areas are not always rigidly defined (e.g., the edges of wrappers on sterile packages and the caps on solution bottles). The following precautions should be taken:

1. When opening sterile packages, a margin of safety is always maintained. The inside of a wrapper is considered sterile to within 1 inch of the edges. The circulator opens the top flap away from self, then turns the sides under. The ends of the flaps are secured in the hand so they do not dangle loosely. The last flap is pulled toward the person opening the package, thereby exposing the package contents away from the unsterile hand.
2. Sterile persons lift contents from packages by reaching down and lifting them straight up, holding their elbows high.
3. The flaps on peel-open packages should be pulled back, not torn, to expose the sterile contents. The contents should not be permitted to slide over the edges.

The inner edge of the heat seal is considered the line of demarcation between sterile and unsterile. The sterile item should be presented to the scrub person. Flipping can cause air turbulence and the item may miss its mark and fall to an unsterile area.

Figure 15-4   Draping large unsterile table. Scrub person holds the sterile fan-folded table drape high and drops it on the center of the table, standing back from the table to protect gown.

Figure 15-5   Scrub person unfolding sterile table drape. Scrub person stands back from unsterile table and unfolds drape first toward self. Note that hands are inside sterile cover to protect them.

Figure 15-6   Scrub person continuing to unfold sterile table drape. Hands are inside sterile cover for protection. Scrub person may now move closer to the table since the first part of unfolded drape now protects gown.

Figure 15-3   Sterile scrub person draping a small table. Sterile persons avoid reaching over unsterile field. The scrub person therefore drapes unsterile table first toward self, then away. Gown is protected by distance, and hands are protected by cuffing drape over them.

4. If a sterile wrapper is used as a table cover, it should amply cover the entire table surface. Only the interior and surface level of the cover are considered sterile.

5. After a sterile bottle is opened, the contents are either used or discarded. The cap cannot be replaced without contaminating the pouring edges.

6. Steam reaches only the area within the gasket of a sterilizer. Instrument trays should not touch the edge of the sterilizer outside the gasket.

The Sterile Field Is Created as Close as Possible to the Time of Use

The degree of contamination is proportionate to the length of time that sterile items are exposed to the environment. Precautions must be taken as follows:

1. Sterile tables are set up just before the surgical procedure.
2. It is virtually impossible to uncover a table of sterile contents without contamination. Covering sterile tables for later use is not recommended.
3. A covered table is not under observation at all times.

Sterile Areas Are Continuously Kept in View

Inadvertent contamination of sterile areas must be readily visible. To ensure this principle, the following steps must be taken:

1. Sterile persons face sterile areas.
2. Someone must remain in the room to maintain vigilance when sterile packs are opened in a room or a sterile field is set up. Sterility cannot be ensured without direct observation. An unguarded sterile field should be considered contaminated.

Sterile Persons Keep Well Within the Sterile Area

Sterile persons allow a wide margin of safety when passing unsterile areas and observe the following rules:

1. Sterile persons stand back at a safe distance from the operating bed when draping the patient.
2. Sterile persons pass each other back to back at a 360-degree turn (Figure 15-7).
3. Sterile persons turn their backs to an unsterile person or area when passing.
4. Sterile persons face a sterile area to pass it.
5. Sterile persons ask an unsterile individual to step aside rather than risk contamination.
6. Sterile persons stay within the sterile field. They do not walk around or go outside the room.
7. Movement within and around a sterile area is kept to a minimum to avoid contamination of sterile items or persons.

Figure 15-7 Sequence of one sterile person going around another. They pass each other back to back, keeping well within the sterile area and allowing a margin of safety between them.

Sterile Persons Keep Contact with Sterile Areas to a Minimum

The following rules are observed:

1. Sterile persons do not lean on sterile tables or on the draped patient.
2. Sitting or leaning against an unsterile surface is a break in technique. If the sterile team sits to operate, they do so without proximity to unsterile areas.

Unsterile Persons Avoid Sterile Areas

Unsterile persons maintain an awareness of sterile, unsterile, clean, and contaminated areas and their proximity to each. They must be aware of their closeness to the sterile field. A wide margin of safety must be maintained when passing sterile areas by observing the following rules:

1. Unsterile persons maintain a distance of at least 1 foot (30 cm) from any area of the sterile field.
2. Unsterile persons face and observe a sterile area when passing it to be sure they do not touch it.
3. Unsterile persons never walk between two sterile areas (e.g., between sterile instrument tables).
4. The circulator restricts to a minimum all activity near the sterile field.

Destruction of the Integrity of Microbial Barriers Results in Contamination

The integrity of a sterile package or sterile drape is destroyed by perforation, puncture, or strike-through. Strike-through is the soaking of moisture through unsterile layers to sterile layers or vice versa. Ideal barrier materials are resistant to abrasion and impervious to permeation by the fluids or dust that transport microorganisms. The integrity of a sterile package and the appearance of the process monitor must be checked for sterility just before opening.

To ensure sterility, the following precautions must be taken:

1. Sterile packages are laid on dry surfaces.
2. If a sterile package wrapped in absorbent material becomes damp or wet, it is resterilized or discarded. The package is considered unsterile if any part of it comes in contact with moisture.
3. Drapes are placed on a dry field.
4. If solution soaks through a sterile drape to an unsterile area, the wet area is covered with impervious sterile drapes or towels.
5. Packages wrapped in woven fabric or paper are permitted to cool after being removed from the sterilizer and before being placed on a cold surface; this prevents steam condensation and the resultant contamination.
6. Sterile items are stored in clean, dry areas.

7. Sterile packages are handled with clean, dry hands.
8. Undue pressure on sterile packs is avoided to prevent forcing sterile air out and pulling unsterile air into the pack.

Microorganisms Must Be Kept to an Irreducible Minimum

Sterile technique in the surgical site is an ideal to be approached; it is not absolute. All microorganisms cannot be eliminated, but this does not obviate the necessity for strict sterile technique. There is general agreement about the following:

1. *Skin cannot be sterilized.* Skin is a potential source of contamination in every invasive procedure. Inherent body defenses usually can overcome the relatively few organisms remaining after preparation of the patient's skin. Organisms on the face, neck, hair, hands, and arms of the OR team are a hazard. All possible means are used to prevent the entrance of microorganisms into the wound. Preventive measures include the following:
   a. Mechanical washing and chemical antisepsis is used to remove transient and resident floras from the skin around the surgical site of the patient and from the hands and arms of sterile team members.
   b. Gowning and gloving of the OR team is accomplished without contamination of the sterile exterior of gowns and gloves.
   c. Sterile gloved hands do not directly touch the skin and then touch deeper tissues. Instruments used in contact with skin are discarded and not reused.
   d. If a glove is torn or punctured by a needle or instrument, it is changed immediately. The needle or instrument is discarded from the sterile field.
   e. A sterile dressing should be applied before the drapes are removed to reduce the risk of the incision being touched by contaminated hands or objects.
2. *Some areas cannot be scrubbed.* When the surgical site includes the mouth, nose, throat, or anus, the number of microorganisms present is great. Various parts of the body, such as the gastrointestinal tract and vagina, usually are resistant to infection by the floras that normally inhabit these parts. However, the following steps may be taken to reduce the number of microorganisms in these areas and prevent them from scattering:
   a. The surgeon makes an effort to use a sponge only once, then discards it.
   b. The gastrointestinal tract (especially the colon) is contaminated, and measures are used to prevent spreading this contamination.
3. *Infected areas are grossly contaminated.* The team avoids disseminating the contamination.
4. *Air is contaminated by dust, droplets, and shedding.* The following environmental control measures are used:
   a. Drapes placed over the anesthesia screen or attached to IV poles at the head of the bed separate the anesthesia area from the sterile field.

b. Movement around the sterile field is kept to a minimum to avoid air turbulence.

c. To avoid the dispersion of lint and dust, drapes are not flipped, fanned, or shaken.

d. Talking is kept to a minimum in the OR. Moisture droplets are expelled with force into the mask during the process of articulating words.

e. OR attire is worn properly: the mask covers the nose and mouth, the hair is completely covered, and body covers are close fitting. Unsterile persons wear long sleeves with knitted cuffs.

NO COMPROMISE OF STERILITY

There is no compromise with sterility. In clinical practice an item is considered either sterile or unsterile. Team members should always be as certain of sterility as possible. That certainty rests on the fact that the necessary conditions have been met and that all factors in the sterilization process have been observed. Obviously it is impossible to prove that every package is free from bacteria, but a single break in technique can compromise the life of a patient. OR personnel must maintain the high standards of sterile technique they know are essential. Every individual is accountable for his or her own role in infection control.

Bibliography

Allen G, Josephson A: Meeting infection control standards in the OR, *AORN J* 62(4):595-596, 599-602, 1995.

Association of Operating Room Nurses: *AORN standards, recommended practices, and guidelines,* Denver, 1998, The Association.

Birckbichler JW: Microbial reduction on linen, *Infect Control Today* 2(8):12, 16-18, 1998.

Department of Health and Human Services Centers for Disease Control and Prevention: *Guideline for isolation precautions in hospitals;* www.cdc.org.

National Institute for Occupational Safety and Health: *NIOSH recommended guidelines: personal respiratory protection of workers in healthcare facilities potentially exposed to tuberculosis,* Cincinnati, 1992, The Institute.

Otero RB: Prevention of disease transmission in a healthcare setting, *Infect Control Today* 2(7):30-38, 1998.

Patterson P: Hepatitis proves a greater threat than HIV, *OR Manager* 10(4):1, 6, 1994.

Patterson P: Programs to help prevent TB transmission in the OR, *OR Manager* 11(2):14-15, 1995.

Rathkowski PL: Traffic control, *AORN J* 59(2):439-448, 1994.

Ronk LL, Girard NJ: Risk perception, universal precautions compliance: a descriptive study of nurses who circulate, *AORN J* 59(1):253-266, 1994.

Wagner WM et al: Designing an infection control program to protect us from ourselves, *Infect Control Today* 2(8):51-52, 1998.

Chapter 16

Attire, Surgical Scrub, Gowning, and Gloving

 Chapter Objectives

After studying this chapter, the learner will be able to:

- Identify the components of appropriate OR attire.
- List specific components of protective attire.
- Describe the sterile parameters of the surgical gown.

HISTORICAL BACKGROUND

The evolution of special operating room (OR) attire as an adjunct to asepsis paralleled the development of aseptic and sterile techniques in the latter half of the nineteenth century. Many surgeons of that time continued to perform surgical procedures while wearing street clothes under pus- and blood-encrusted aprons despite the expansion of germ theory knowledge.

One of the earliest mentions of specific OR attire appeared in a nurse's training handbook that advised the nurse to bathe before a surgical procedure, to take a carbolic bath before laparotomy, and to wear long sleeves and a clean apron for the surgical procedure. As late as 1900, the surgeon often relied on the nurse to have the necessary instruments in an apron pocket. Although the apron has long since given way to the present scrub attire, long sleeves are again recommended for anesthesia providers and circulators to reduce the shedding of microorganisms and to protect them from contact with body substances.

The first use of caps and sterile gowns occurred in Germany while English surgeon Joseph Lister's (1827-1912) principles of antiseptic surgery were still being debated. In some ORs bacteria-laden, infection-causing woolen suits and Prince Albert coats were replaced by OR garb made of sterilizable material that lessened the introduction of pathogenic microorganisms into the wound. The use of sterile gowns antedated the routine use of caps, gloves, and masks, although in 1883 Gustav Neuber (1850-1932) insisted that team members wear caps also.

Emphasis on personal cleanliness expedited acceptance of special OR attire, but these standards were not rigidly practiced in all hospitals. Various styles of turbans and shower cap–style head coverings were worn from about 1908 to the 1930s, when hair was generally acknowledged to be an attraction for and shedder of bacteria.

In a 1900 photograph, the team was operating in short surgical gowns and rubber gloves but without caps or masks. Charles Mayo and his team were photographed in 1913 operating in surgical gowns, caps, and masks. The onlookers, however, wore only white coats over street attire. Another photo showed the surgeon in a gown, cap, gloves, and a mask below his nose; the instrument nurse in a gown and head cover but no mask; and the anesthetist and other nurses in gowns but regular nurses' caps. Universal standards of attire did not exist at that time.

In 1897 American surgeon William Halsted (1852-1922), chief of surgery at Johns Hopkins, designed a semicircular instrument table to separate himself, in sterile gown and gloves, from observers in street clothes who watched him operate.

Rubber surgical gloves were introduced, not to protect the patient but to protect the wearer's hands from the harsh, irritating antiseptic solutions and hand soaks of the 1870s and 1880s. Their use was not popularized until the 1890s, when Halsted's nurse complained of dermatitis. One of his assistants began to wear gloves routinely for surgical procedures in 1896, although Halsted himself is known for popularizing the use of gloves to protect patients from the bacteria of ungloved hands. Johann von Mikulicz (1850-1905), a pioneering Romanian surgeon, advocated the wearing of cotton gloves in 1896 also, but these were soon found to lack the qualities of impermeable rubber gloves for infection control. Disposable latex gloves, introduced about 1958, were a welcome innovation that saved countless hours of daily glove reprocessing, repairing, and sterilizing.

Gauze masks were advocated by Mikulicz in 1897, when the droplet theory of infection was demonstrated. However, it was not until 1926, when wound infections yielded the same organisms as found in the noses and throats of surgeons and nurses, that masks became obligatory. Although gauze masks were routinely worn, their efficiency decreased rapidly during wearing from saturation with saliva. Often the nose was not properly covered.

In 1924 one of the first OR nursing texts described the attire of the OR nurses: the circulator wore an OR cap, but no mask, and a gown with a pocket for a pad and pencil; the scrub nurse wore both a mask and a gown. By the 1930s and 1940s, scrub dresses began to replace nurses' regular uniforms, heretofore worn under the sterile gown. Observers in the OR were gowned, capped, and masked. In the 1960s, full skirts were replaced by close-fitting scrub dresses and pantsuits that reduced the hazard of brushing against a sterile table when near or passing by it.

In 1950, as restrictions became more rigid, OR personnel were required to change shoes when entering the OR suite and to wear only those shoes when within the suite. Shoe covers became popular both as a method of keeping the shoes clean and for preventing dissemination of soil from the shoes.

OPERATING ROOM ATTIRE

Terms associated with attire, scrubbing, gowning, and gloving for a surgical procedure are listed in Box 16-1.

Box 16-1   **Terms Associated with Attire, Scrubbing, Gowning, and Gloving**

antimicrobial agent   Antiseptic soap or cleanser used for cleaning the skin of patients and caregivers that has a fast-acting, broad-spectrum action to reduce the count of microorganisms before a surgical procedure.
barrier   Physical or mechanical obstacle between a person and a hazardous substance or microorganism.
personal protective equipment   Eyewear, masks, hair cover, shoe covers, gown, apron, and/or gloves worn to prevent airborne, droplet, or contact-based transmission of potentially hazardous substances or microorganisms.
scrub suit   Attire intended for wear in the OR.
subungual   Under the fingernails.
surgical hand scrub   Process by which the hands and arms of the team are rendered clean by mechanical and chemical action before a surgical procedure.

Purpose

Sebaceous and sweat glands in and around hair follicles over the entire surface of the body contain microorganisms that are continually shed into the environment. The purpose of OR attire is to provide effective barriers that prevent the dissemination of microorganisms to the patient and protect personnel from blood and body substances of patients. OR attire has been shown to reduce microbial shedding from over 10,000 particles per minute to 3000, or from 50,000 microorganisms per cubic foot to 500, and to prevent contamination of the surgical wound and sterile field by direct contact.

Definition

OR attire consists of body covers, such as a two-piece pantsuit, head cover, mask, and shoe covers, as appropriate. Each has an appropriate purpose to combat sources of contamination exogenous (external) to the patient. A sterile gown and gloves are added to this basic attire for scrubbed sterile team members. Proper attire is a part of aseptic environmental control that also protects personnel against exposure to communicable diseases and hazardous materials. Eyewear and other protective attire are worn by personnel as appropriate for anticipated exposure to biologic contaminants.

Dress Code

The OR should have specific written policies and procedures for proper attire to be worn within the semirestricted and restricted areas of the OR suite. The dress code should include aspects of personal hygiene important to environmental control. Protocol is strictly monitored so that everyone conforms to established policy, such as the following:

1. Dressing rooms located in the unrestricted area adjacent to the semirestricted area of the OR suite are

reached through the outer corridor. Street clothes are not worn beyond the unrestricted area.

2. Only approved, clean, and/or freshly laundered attire intended for use in the OR is worn within the semirestricted and restricted areas. This policy applies to everyone entering the OR suite, both professional and nonprofessional personnel and visitors.

   a. Clean, fresh attire is donned each time on arrival in the OR suite and as necessary at other times if the attire becomes wet or grossly soiled. Blood-stained or soiled attire, including shoe covers, is not only unattractive, but can also be a source of cross-infection. Soiled attire is not worn outside the OR suite.

   b. An adequate supply of clean attire should always be available. Attire is laundered daily, only in the hospital's laundry facilities. It should not be taken home for laundering. If it were taken home, the risk for contamination of family members might be increased if clothing were contaminated with resistant microorganisms (e.g., those causing Creutzfeldt-Jakob disease or tuberculosis [TB]).

   c. Masks should be changed between patients.

3. OR attire should not be worn outside the OR suite. This protects the OR environment from microorganisms inherent in the outside environment and protects the outside from contamination normally associated with the OR. Before leaving the OR suite, everyone should change to street clothes.

   a. On occasion, such as for lunch breaks, a single-use cover gown or coverall may be worn over OR attire outside the suite. The practice of cover gowns is not encouraged. If used, the gown is discarded, if disposable, or put in a laundry hamper after wearing. Some hospitals provide laboratory coats. These are completely buttoned and worn only once.

   b. A clean, fresh scrub suit should be put on after return for reentry to the suite.

   c. OR attire should not be hung or put in a locker for wearing a second time. It should be discarded in the trash or put in a laundry hamper after one use, as appropriate.

4. Impeccable personal hygiene is emphasized.

   a. A person with an acute infection, such as a cold or sore throat, should not be permitted within the OR suite. Persons with cuts, burns, or skin lesions should not scrub or handle sterile supplies because serum, a bacterial medium, may seep from the eroded area. An open skin lesion may be a portal of entry for cutaneous contact with blood-borne pathogens.

   b. Sterile team members who are known carriers of pathogenic microorganisms should routinely bathe and scrub with an appropriate skin antiseptic agent and shampoo their hair daily. Some carriers should be treated with appropriate antibiotics until nasopharyngeal culture findings are negative.

   c. Fingernails should be kept short (i.e., should not extend past the fingertips). Routine manicures prevent cracked cuticles and hangnails. Subungual areas harbor the majority of microorganisms on hands. Fresh nail polish on short, healthy nails may not alter the microbial count on fingernails. Polish may seal crevices. However, damaged nails and chipped or peeling polish may provide a harbor for microorganisms. Studies have shown that artificial nails and other enhancers harbor organisms, especially fungi and gram-negative bacilli. These are prohibited from wear in the OR.

   d. Jewelry, including rings and watches, should be removed before entering semirestricted and restricted areas. Organisms may be harbored under rings, thus preventing effective handwashing. Necklaces or chains can grate on the skin, increasing desquamation. They might break and fall into a wound or contaminate a sterile field. Pierced-ear studs should be confined within the head cover. Dangling earrings are inappropriate in the OR.

   e. Facial makeup should be minimal.

   f. Eyeglasses should be wiped with a cleaning solution before each surgical procedure.

   g. External apparel that does not serve a functional purpose should not be worn.

   h. Hands are washed frequently and thoroughly. Washing before and after using the restroom can reduce the risk of self-contamination. Using hand cream regularly helps prevent chapped, dry skin. Bacteriostatic varieties may help to reduce microbial counts on the skin.

5. Comfortable, supportive shoes should be worn to minimize fatigue and for personal safety. Shoes should have enclosed toes and heels; clogs and sandals should not be worn because they may not provide a safe surface to the feet for fast walking or running during an emergency. Cloth shoes do not offer protection against spilled fluids or sharp items that may be dropped or kicked. Shoes are cleaned frequently, whether or not shoe covers are worn.

Components of Attire

Each item of OR attire is a specific means for containment of, or protection against, the potential sources of environmental contamination, including skin, hair, and nasopharyngeal flora and microorganisms in air, blood, and body substances. Scrub suits and head covers are worn by all personnel in the semirestricted areas of the OR suite. Masks are also worn in the restricted areas. Additional items, such as protective eyewear, gloves, and shoe covers, are worn during a surgical procedure and for protection during hazardous exposure.

Body Cover

Everyone dons attire intended for use within a semirestricted or restricted area (e.g., scrub suit). A variety of scrub suits, either two-piece pantsuits or one-piece coveralls, are available in either a solid color or an attractive print. All should fit the body snugly. Pantsuits confine organisms shed from the perineal region and legs more effectively than dresses; 90% of bacterial dissemination originates from the perineum. Panty hose do not contain this shedding and may in fact increase it by constant friction.

Shirt and waistline drawstrings are tucked inside pants to avoid their touching sterile areas. Microorganisms multiply more rapidly beneath a covered area. A tunic top that fits snugly may be worn on the outside of pants. The scrub suit should be changed as soon as possible whenever it becomes wet or visibly soiled.

Persons who will not be sterile team members should wear long-sleeved jackets over a scrub suit. The sleeves help contain shedding from axillae and arms and help to protect from biologic contamination caused by splashes. The jacket should be closed to prevent a bellows effect and the possibility of brushing against the sterile field during movement.

A one-piece coverall with or without an attached hood and shoe covers are convenient garb for a visitor whose presence in the OR will be brief (e.g., the pathologist).

Head Cover

Since hair is a gross contaminant, a cap or hood is put on before the scrub suit to protect the garment from contamination by hair. All facial and head hair is completely covered in the semirestricted and restricted areas. Various types of lightweight caps, helmets, and hoods are available. Most of them are made of disposable, lint-free, nonporous, nonwoven fabrics. If hair is long, a shower cap–style hat or hood is worn to cover the neck area. Headgear should fit well so that it confines and prevents escape of any hair. Hair should not be combed while one is wearing a scrub suit. Persons with a scalp infection should be excluded from the OR and treated. Hair is also a source of electrostatic spark.

Shoe Covers

Shoe covers may be worn in the semirestricted and restricted areas. Knee-high impervious styles will protect the wearer from spills into or onto shoes during procedures wherein extensive fluid irrigation and/or blood loss can be anticipated. Some surgeons wear plastic or rubber boots. The legs of scrub pants are tucked into boots.

Studies have not shown a significant correlation between footwear and wound infection. However, the flow of traffic is one critical factor in airborne dispersal of microbes from the floor. Unprotected street shoes can increase floor contamination. Shoes restricted to wear in the OR suite or shoe covers over shoes are preferable in reducing microbial transfer from the outside into the OR suite. Protective gloves should be worn to change shoe covers whenever they become wet, soiled, or torn. Shoe covers can inadvertently become soiled and harbor microorganisms. They should be removed before entering the dressing room area and must be removed before leaving the OR suite.

Mask

A mask is worn in the restricted area to contain and filter droplets containing microorganisms expelled from the mouth and nasopharynx during breathing, talking, sneezing, and coughing. Some tight-fitting masks also effectively reduce exposure to submicron particles by filtration of inhaled air. Many masks filter about 99% of particulate matter larger than 5 μm in diameter, but only about 45% to 60% of particles 0.3 μm in diameter. Aerosolized particles and viruses dispersed in laser and electrosurgical plume or by power instruments may be this small. Masks provide some protection to the sterile team members from blood-borne pathogens that may splash or spray toward the nose or mouth.

Reusable cotton masks are obsolete; they filter ineffectively as soon as they become moist. Contemporary disposable masks of soft, clothlike material in very fine synthetic fiber materials fulfill the following essential criteria:

1. They are at least 95% efficient in filtering microbes from droplet particles in exhalations and also filter inhalations. A fluid-resistant mask is advantageous.
2. They are cool, comfortable, and nonobstructive to respiration.
3. They are nonirritating to the skin. Disposable masks are made of polypropylene, polyester, or rayon fibers. Some have fiberglass filters. If a person is sensitive to one type, he or she should try another brand.

Some experts believe that masks should be worn to protect team members rather than to protect patients from moisture droplets. However, current practice recommendations of AORN, the Association of periOperative Registered Nurses, are that masks be worn at all times in the restricted area of the OR suite—where sterile supplies will be opened and scrubbed persons may be present—including areas where scrub sinks are located. Masks should always be worn in the OR itself whether or not a surgical procedure is in progress. Masks are worn on entering the room before, during, and after the surgical procedure (i.e., during setup and cleanup). This includes terminal cleaning at the end of the day and restocking of supplies. The policy in some OR suites may be less restrictive. The institution's written policy should be followed by all team members, departmental staff, and visitors.

To be effective, a mask filters inhalations and exhalations. Therefore it is worn over both the nose and the mouth. To be effective, air must pass only through the filtering system; thus the mask needs to conform to facial contours to prevent leakage of expired air. Venting, the drawing of air back and forth, can occur along the sides, top, and bottom of the mask. Wearing two masks is not recommended because the extra thickness can cause venting from the effort to breathe through it. Ejected droplets should not escape the filter action.

Masks are designed with pleats or are conical, like a cup, for a close fit, but improper application can negate their efficiency. The strings should be tied tightly, if this is the method of securing the mask, to prevent the strings from coming loose during the surgical procedure. The upper strings are tied at the back of the head; the lower strings are tied behind the neck (Figure 16-1). The strings are never crossed over the head because this distorts the contours of the mask along the cheeks. Masks have an exterior pliable metallic strip that can be bent to contour the mask over the bridge of the nose. A close-fitting mask or a small strip of nonallergenic tape over the nosepiece also helps to avoid steaming of eyeglasses. To prevent cross-infection, masks should:

1. Be handled only by the strings, thereby keeping the facial area of a fresh mask clean and the hands uncontaminated by a soiled mask. Do not handle the mask excessively.
2. Never be lowered to hang loosely around the neck, be placed on top of the cap, or be put in a pocket. Avoid disseminating microorganisms.
3. Be promptly discarded into the proper receptacle on removal. Remask with a fresh mask between patients.
4. Be changed frequently. Do not permit the mask to become wet. Talking should be kept to a minimum.

If a sneeze is eminent, one should step back away from the field and sneeze directly into the mask without turning the head sideways. Expelled air will be forced out the sides of the mask and directly into the sterile field through the vent if the head is sideways. The purpose of the mask is to filter air through the filtration material. Ideally, stepping away from the field and turning the head 180 degrees with the back of the head to the field may minimize exposure of the field. It may be necessary to remove the gown, gloves, and mask. The hands should be washed with antimicrobial soap before and after cleaning the nose and applying a new mask. The hands should be rescrubbed before donning a sterile gown and gloves.

Personal Protective Equipment

Personnel should be protected from hazardous conditions in the semirestricted and restricted areas. Depending on the exposure that will be encountered, protective attire should be

Figure 16-1 Mask covers nose and mouth and conforms to facial contours. Upper strings are tied at back of head; lower strings are tied behind neck.

worn. The type and characteristics of this attire depend on the task and degree of exposure anticipated. Protective attire does not allow blood or other potentially injurious materials to reach the inner clothing, skin, or eyes. Other considerations concerning protective attire are as follows:

1. Aprons
   a. A decontamination apron worn over the scrub suit protects against liquids and cleaning agents during cleaning procedures. It should be a full-front barrier.
   b. Fluid-proof aprons are worn by sterile team members under permeable reusable sterile gowns when extensive blood loss or irrigation is anticipated. They should be lightweight and full front.
   c. Lead aprons worn under sterile gowns protect against radiation exposure during procedures performed under fluoroscopy or image intensification or when personnel are exposed to radioactive implants.
2. Eyewear
   a. Eyewear or a face shield is worn whenever a risk exists of blood or body substances from the patient splashing into the eyes of sterile team members. Bone chips and splatter can be projected from bone-cutting instruments. Several styles of goggles and eyeglasses with top and side shields fit securely against the face. Antifog goggles fit over prescription eyeglasses. A combination surgical mask with a visor eye shield or a chin-length face shield are other options. Care is taken that the lower edge of the face shield does not touch the front of the gown.
   b. Laser eyewear should be worn for eye protection from laser beams. Lenses of the proper optical density for each type of laser should be available and worn.
   c. Protective eyewear, preferably a face shield, should be worn by personnel handling or washing instruments when this activity could result in a splash, spray, or splatter to the eyes or face.
   d. Eyewear or a face shield that becomes contaminated should be decontaminated or discarded promptly.
3. Gloves
   a. Nonsterile latex or vinyl gloves are worn to handle any material or items contaminated by blood and body substances. Gloves should be worn only during the period of contact, not continuously. Clean objects and sterile packages should not be handled with contaminated gloves.
   b. Sterile gloves are worn by sterile team members and for all invasive procedures. Liners may be worn under gloves to protect the hands from cuts.
   c. Lead gloves may be needed for protection from radiation exposure. The surgeon may wear latex gloves impregnated with lead for procedures performed under fluoroscopy.

d. Thick gloves should be worn for skin protection from ethylene oxide exposure if sterilized packages must be handled before aeration.

e. Utility gloves are worn for cleaning and housekeeping duties. Sterile and nonsterile single-use disposable latex and vinyl gloves are discarded after use. They should not be washed and reused. Soaps and surfactants decrease the surface tension of the gloves and increase the risk of wicking through micro holes in the gloves. Hands are washed after removing gloves.

Gown

A sterile gown is worn over the scrub suit to permit the wearer to come within the sterile field. It prevents intercontamination between the wearer and the field and differentiates sterile (scrubbed) from nonsterile (unscrubbed) team members. The gown should provide a protective barrier from strike-through (i.e., migration of microorganisms from the skin and scrub suit of the wearer to the sterile field and the patient, and penetration of blood and body substances from the patient to the scrub suit and skin of the wearer).

Both reusable and disposable gowns, in a variety of styles, are in use. Although the entire gown is sterilized, the back is not considered sterile, nor is any area below the level of the sterile field, once the gown is donned. Wraparound sterile gowns that provide coverage to the back by a generous overlap are recommended. These gowns are secured at the neck and waist before the sterile flap is brought over the back and secured by ties at the side or front. A sterile vest put on over the gown covers any exposed back area of scrub attire but does not render the back sterile. The cuffs of gowns are knitted stockinette to snugly fit wrists. Sterile gloves cover the cuffs of the gown.

Gowns should be resistant to penetration by fluids and blood and should be comfortable without producing excessive heat buildup. Most single-use disposable gowns are made of spun-laced fiber or nonwoven, moisture-repellent materials. Some of these are reinforced with plastic on the forearms and front. Reusable gowns should be made of a densely woven material. Loosely woven, 140-thread-count, all-carded cotton muslin or similar-quality permeable material is not a barrier to microbial migration. Some 180-thread-count cotton gowns have insets of 270-thread-count fluid-resistant fabric or plastic film to reinforce the sleeves from the cuffs to the elbows, and the front from the midchest to below the waist. Pima cotton with a 270- to 280-thread count per square inch treated with a moisture-repellent finish is an acceptable woven textile. Some reusable gowns are a cotton-polyester blend. Tightly woven 100% polyester gowns are impervious to moisture. Seams of the gowns should be constructed to prevent penetration of fluids.

Sterile team members may not need a reinforced barrier gown for every procedure; the scrub person usually can safely wear a single-layer impervious gown. The surgeon and first assistant are at greatest risks during procedures within the abdominal or chest cavity, when blood loss will be more than 200 ml, or when the time will exceed 2 hours. The amount of blood and fluid on the outside of the gown is a critical factor in strike-through by wicking. Blood-borne pathogens can penetrate fabric without visible strike-through. The forearms are the most frequently contaminated areas. Therefore the surgeon and first assistant should wear a gown with at least reinforced or plastic-coated sleeves for these procedures.

Woven textile gowns withstand about 75 launderings and sterilizing cycles before appreciable deterioration of the finish occurs. Monitoring the number of uses is necessary to remove the gown from use at the sterile field when it is no longer an effective barrier. Also, an additional rinse cycle may be required in the laundering process to remove residual detergent that could adversely affect the fabric. Mechanical damage from sharp instruments or snags will destroy the integrity of the gown, jeopardizing its purpose. The gown should be changed if it is punctured or torn during the surgical procedure. Textile gowns can be patched only with heat-applied vulcanized mending fabrics.

All woven and some nonwoven gowns are not flame retardant. Fire-resistant gowns should be worn for laser surgery and preferably when electrosurgery is used.

Special attire often is worn with ultraclean laminar airflow systems. A body exhaust gown envelops the wearer from the top of the head to within about 16 inches (40 cm) of the floor. If a gown that fits closely at the neck is used, a rigid face mask or helmet should be worn. With both types of gowns, an exhaust system is attached for body cooling and airflow. Powered coolant vests for wear under scrub attire are commercially available.

Gloves

Sterile gloves complete the attire for sterile team members. They are worn to permit the wearer to handle sterile supplies and tissues of the surgical wound. Surgical gloves are made of natural rubber latex, synthetic rubber, thermoplastic elastomers, neoprene, vinyl, or polyethylene. Disposable latex gloves are worn most frequently. Latex is a polymeric membrane of natural rubber with an infinite number of holes between lattices. However, it is a better barrier than vinyl, which may allow permeation of blood and fluids over prolonged exposure. Latex gloves of varying thickness, with a minimum of 0.1 mm, can be chosen to meet the needs of the surgeon for tactile sensation. Latex contains protein antigen and is cured with agents that may cause an allergic dermatitis or systemic anaphylaxis. Hypoallergenic milled gloves that do not contain these sensitizers are available. Latex gloves labeled "hypoallergenic" do not always prevent reaction in a highly sensitive person. Several varieties of synthetic nonlatex sterile gloves (e.g., those made of neoprene) are available commercially. Sterile team members should not wear latex gloves if the patient has a known latex sensitivity or allergy.

Gloves are packaged in pairs with an everted cuff on each to protect the outside of the sterile glove during donning. The inner paper wrap of the disposable glove package protects the sterility of the gloves when they are removed from the outer wrap. Glove packages are generally the peel-apart type. Before opening, the package should be inspected for damage or wetness, which indicates contamination. When the inner paper is unfolded, the wearer finds the right glove to the right, and the left glove to the left, palm sides up (Figure 16-2).

Both inner and outer surfaces may be prelubricated with an absorbable dry cornstarch powder before the sterilization process to facilitate donning and to prevent adhesion of the glove surfaces. During donning, this powder is aerosolized into the room air and affects persons other than the wearer, including the patient. Although considered absorbable and inert in tissue, the powder may cause serious complications, such as starch granulomas, adhesions, or peritonitis if it is introduced into wounds. Consequently, it is important to remove the powder from the outside of the gloves after donning them. They may be thoroughly wiped with a sterile damp towel or rinsed with sterile saline. Immersion in a splash basin should be avoided because the powder clumps and accumulates on the surface of the water and redeposits on the surface of the glove. Latex protein allergens can adhere to powder, thus providing another potential route of exposure or sensitization if the powder is aerosolized during a rinsing process. Latex coated on the inside with a hydrogel lubricant allows smooth donning of gloves without the hazard of glove powder.

Surgeons frequently puncture their gloves, most often on the index finger of the nondominant hand. Glove puncture and minute holes in gloves are hazardous to both patients and team members. Seepage under the glove poses a threat to a team member if his or her skin is not intact. The risk of blood contamination of the fingers increases the longer the glove is worn. If a sterile glove is punctured or torn, it should be changed immediately to prevent escape of microorganisms from the wearer's skin and seepage of blood and body substances from the patient into the glove. Microbial colonization may be minimized if latex gloves are impregnated with an antiseptic, and gloves with puncture indicators are commercially available. High-molecular-weight polyethylene gloves resist punctures and tears.

Some surgeons and team members prefer to double glove (wear two pairs of sterile gloves). The inside glove should be a half size larger than the outside glove. This reduces hand constriction caused by multiple layers of tight gloves.

Some sterile team members wear sterile glove liners for protection from scalpel cuts or instrument tears. These do not protect the hands from punctures, such as needle sticks. Liners are usually worn between two pairs of sterile surgical gloves, usually a half size larger than usual so that they will not constrict circulation. The liners may be made of polymer fibers or a metal mesh. Some are disposable; others may be sterilized with steam or ethylene oxide.

Petrolatum-based lotions or lubricants should not be used on the hands before donning latex gloves. Hydrocarbons will penetrate latex, causing a change in its physical characteristics, including tear resistance.

Criteria for Operating Room Attire

Attire should be:

1. An effective barrier to microorganisms. Both reusable woven and disposable nonwoven materials are used. The design and composition should minimize microbial shedding.
2. Made of closely woven material void of dangerous electrostatic properties. The garment should meet National Fire Protection Association Standards (NFPA-56A), including resistance to flame.
   a. Undergarments of synthetic material such as nylon are permissible when in close contact with the skin, such as hosiery.
   b. Nylon and other static spark–producing materials are forbidden as outer garments.
3. Resistant to blood, aqueous fluids, and abrasion to prevent penetration by microorganisms.
4. Designed for maximal skin coverage.
5. Hypoallergenic, cool, and comfortable.
6. Nongenerative of lint. Lint can increase the particle count of contaminants in the OR.
7. Made of a pliable material to permit freedom of movement for the practice of sterile technique.
8. Able to transmit heat and water vapor to protect the wearer.
9. Colored to reduce glare under lights. Various types of clothes in colorful prints that fulfill the necessary criteria are both attractive and functional.
10. Easy to don and remove.

SURGICAL SCRUB

Definition

The surgical scrub is the process of removing as many microorganisms as possible from the hands and arms by mechanical washing and chemical antisepsis before participating in a surgical procedure. The surgical scrub is done just

Figure 16-2 Gloves on unfolded open wrapper, right glove to right, and left glove to left, palm sides up.

before gowning and gloving for each surgical procedure. Despite the mechanical action and the chemical antimicrobial component of the scrub process, skin is never rendered sterile.

Microbiology of the Skin

The skin is inhabited by the following organisms:

- Transient organisms acquired by direct contact. Usually loosely attached to the skin surface, they are almost completely removed by thorough washing with soap or detergent and water.
- Resident organisms below the skin surface in hair follicles and in sebaceous and sweat glands. They are more adherent and therefore more resistant to removal. Their growth is inhibited by the chemical phase of the surgical scrub. Resident skin flora represent the microorganisms present in the hospital environment. They are predominantly gram-negative microorganisms, but some are coagulase-positive staphylococci. Prolonged exposure of skin to contaminants yields a more pathogenic resident population (i.e., capable of causing infection).

In freeing the skin of as many microorganisms as possible, two processes are used:

1. *Mechanical.* The process removes soil and transient organisms with friction.
2. *Chemical.* The process reduces resident flora and inactivates microorganisms with an antimicrobial or antiseptic agent (i.e., an inorganic chemical compound that inhibits growth of microorganisms without necessarily killing them).

Purpose

The purpose of the surgical scrub is to remove soil, debris, natural skin oils, hand lotions, and transient microorganisms from the hands and forearms of sterile team members. More specifically, the purposes are as follows:

- To decrease the number of resident microorganisms on skin to an irreducible minimum
- To keep the population of microorganisms minimal during the surgical procedure by suppression of growth
- To reduce the hazard of microbial contamination of the surgical wound by skin flora

Scrub Sink

Adequate scrubbing and handwashing facilities should be provided for all operating team members. The scrub room is adjacent to the OR for safety and convenience. Individually enclosed scrub sinks with automatic sensor controls or foot- or knee-operated faucets are preferred to eliminate the hazard of contaminating the hands after cleansing.

The sink should be deep and wide enough to prevent splash. Aerated faucets prevent splatter. A sterile gown can-

not be donned over damp scrub attire without resultant contamination. Reusable woven gowns may be particularly vulnerable to strike-through of moisture after repeated washings.

Scrub sinks should be used only for scrubbing or handwashing. They should not be used to clean or rinse contaminated instruments or equipment.

Equipment

Sterilized reusable scrub brushes or disposable sponges may be used. Single-use disposable products may be a brush-sponge combination and are preferred. Some are impregnated with antiseptic-detergent agents. Disposable products are individually packaged. If reusable brushes are taken from the dispenser in which they were sterilized, each brush should be removed without contaminating the others. Brushes may be wrapped to provide sterile individual packages. The brush should not cause skin abrasion. The scrubbing solution is dispensed onto the brush or sponge by a foot pedal from a container attached or adjacent to the sink. Six drops (about 2 to 3 ml) of solution is sufficient to generate a lather for the scrub procedure. Waste of antiseptic solution should be avoided.

Debris should be removed from the subungual area under the nail of each finger. Plastic single-use, disposable nail-cleaning products are available. Reusable nail cleaners are terminally cleaned and sterilized between uses. Orangewood sticks are not used to clean under the fingernails because the wood may splinter and harbor *Pseudomonas* organisms.

Antimicrobial Scrub Agents

Various antimicrobial (antiseptic) detergents are used for the surgical scrub. The following are characteristics of the scrub agent:

- Broad-spectrum antimicrobial
- Fast acting and effective
- Nonirritating and nonsensitizing
- Prolonged acting (i.e., leaves an antimicrobial residue on the skin to temporarily prevent growth of microorganisms)
- Independent of cumulative action

Although the action of the agent is important in relation to its efficacy, mechanical friction and effort while scrubbing are equally important. Frequent scrubbing with the same agent tends to inhibit reestablishment of resident flora. Some agents have more residual effect than others. Variables in effectiveness of the scrub are mechanical factors, chemical factors, and individual differences in skin flora. More than one agent usually is available in the scrub room for personnel who are allergic or sensitive to a particular agent.

Antiseptic and antimicrobial skin scrub products are chosen from among those approved by the Food and Drug Administration (FDA) for surgical hand scrubs. Each product has a specific antimicrobial agent. Antiseptics alter the physical or chemical properties of the cell membrane of microorganisms, thus destroying or inhibiting cellular function.

Chlorhexidine Gluconate

A 4% aqueous concentration of chlorhexidine gluconate in a soap base or 0.5% in alcohol exerts an antimicrobial effect against gram-positive and gram-negative, fungal, and viral microorganisms. It reacts poorly against TB microorganisms. Residues tend to accumulate on the skin with repeated use and produce a prolonged effect. This agent produces effective, intermediate action and cumulative reductions of resident and transient flora. The residual effect is maintained for more than 6 hours. Chlorhexidine gluconate is rarely irritating to the skin, but it is highly ototoxic and irritating if splashed in the eye. It can cause permanent corneal damage. Caution should be observed when scrubbing with this agent.

The alcohol-based chlorhexidine preparation is effective if the hands are bathed in the solution for 20 to 30 seconds after mechanical cleansing.

Iodophors

A povidone-iodine complex in detergent fulfills the criteria for an effective surgical scrub. It is available in concentrations of 10%, 7.5%, 2%, and 0.5%. Iodophors are intermediate-acting antimicrobial agents against gram-positive and gram-negative, TB, fungal, and viral microorganisms. Iodophors have minimal residual effect, but this is not sustained for a prolonged period (over 6 hours). Iodophors can be irritating to the skin. Persons allergic to iodine should not scrub with these agents.

Triclosan

A solution of 1% triclosan is a nontoxic, nonirritating intermediate antimicrobial agent that inhibits growth of a wide range of gram-positive and gram-negative, and TB microorganisms. Triclosan does not work as well against fungi. Antiviral action is unknown. It develops a prolonged cumulative suppressive action when used routinely. The agent is blended with lanolin cholesterols and petrolatum into a creamy, mild detergent. It may be used by personnel sensitive to other antiseptics, although it can be absorbed through intact skin. Triclosan is less effective than chlorhexidine gluconate and iodophors.

Alcohol

Ethyl or isopropyl alcohol (60% to 90%) is rapidly antimicrobial against all microorganisms. It is volatile and does not have residual activity. It is nontoxic but has a drying effect on skin. Alcohol preparations, usually in a foam, contain emollients to minimize drying. If other agents cannot be used because of skin sensitivity, mechanical cleansing with soap to remove transient organisms may be followed by cleansing with an alcohol-based skin cleanser.

Hexachlorophene

In concentrations up to 3%, this agent is most effective after buildup of cumulative suppressive action. The action is slow, but effective, against most gram-positive bacteria; it has poor action against all other microorganisms. Its high potential for neurotoxicity makes it unsuitable for routine use. Hexachlorophene is available by prescription only.

Parachlorometaxylenol

Used in a concentration of 1% to 3.75%, this agent does not substantially reduce microorganisms immediately. It does not produce sustained residual activity. Its antimicrobial activity can be altered significantly by the composition of the antiseptic product. Efficacy data should be reviewed before these products are used for surgical scrubs.

Preparation for the Surgical Scrub
General Preparations

1. The skin and nails should be kept clean and in good condition, and the cuticles should be uncut. If hand lotion is used to protect the skin, a non–oil-based product is recommended.
2. Fingernails should not reach beyond the fingertip to avoid glove puncture.
3. Fingernail polish should not be chipped or cracked. Freshly applied polish may be worn if permitted by facility policy.
4. Artificial devices should not cover natural fingernails.
5. All jewelry should be removed from the fingers, wrists, and neck. Jewelry harbors microorganisms.

Preparations Immediately Before the Scrub

1. Inspect the hands for cuts and abrasions. Skin integrity of the hands and forearms should be intact (i.e., without open lesions or cracked skin).
2. Be sure all hair is covered by headgear. Pierced-ear studs should be contained by the head cover. They are a potential foreign body in the surgical wound.
3. Adjust the disposable mask snugly and comfortably over the nose and mouth.
4. Clean eyeglasses if worn. Adjust protective eyewear or the face shield comfortably in relation to the mask.
5. Adjust water to a comfortable temperature.

Surgical Scrub Procedure

The length of the surgical scrub varies, as does the scrub procedure. Variations may depend on the frequency of scrubbing, the agent used, and the method. A vigorous 5-minute scrub with a reliable agent may be as effective as a 10-minute scrub done with less mechanical action. Prolonged scrubbing raises resident microbes from deep dermal layers and is therefore counterproductive. Care should be taken not to abrade the skin during the scrub process. Denuded areas allow the entry of microorganisms. Too short a scrub may be equally ineffectual.

Everyone should scrub according to a standardized written procedure. The time required may be based on the manufacturer's recommendations for the agent used and documentation of the product's efficacy in the scientific literature. A copy of the procedure should be posted in every scrub room.

Subsequent scrubs should follow the same procedure as the initial scrub of the day. When gloves are removed at the end of the surgical procedure, the hands are contaminated and should be immediately washed. Resident microorganisms multiply rapidly in the warm, moist environment under the gloves. Hands should be washed as soon as the gloves are removed, but they will become contaminated as soon as contact is made with any inanimate items.

Methodology of Scrubbing

The surgical scrub procedure may be either the timed method or the counted brush-stroke method. If properly executed, they are both effective, and each exposes all surfaces of the hands and forearms to mechanical cleansing and chemical antisepsis. One should think of the fingers, hands, and arms as having four sides or surfaces. Both methods follow an anatomic pattern of scrubbing: the four surfaces of each finger, beginning with the thumb and moving from one finger to the next, down the outer edge of the fifth finger, over the dorsal (back) surface of the hand, then the palmar (palm) surface of the hand, or vice versa, from the small finger to the thumb, over the wrists and up the arm, in thirds, ending 2 inches (5 cm) above the elbow. Since the hands are in most direct contact with the sterile field, all steps of the scrub procedure begin with the hands and end with the elbows.

During and after scrubbing, keep the hands higher than the elbows to allow water to flow from the cleanest area, the hands, to the marginal area of the upper arms.

Timed Method
The fingers, hands, and arms are scrubbed by allotting a prescribed amount of time to each anatomic area or each step of the procedure.

FIVE-MINUTE SCRUB
1. Wet the hands and forearms.
2. Apply 6 drops (2 to 3 ml) of antiseptic agent from the dispenser to the hands.
3. Wash the hands and arms thoroughly to 2 inches (5 cm) above the elbows, several times. Rinse thoroughly under running water with the hands upward, allowing water to drip from the flexed elbows.
4. Take a sterile brush or sponge (from a package or dispenser) and apply an antiseptic agent (if it is not impregnated in the brush). Scrub each individual finger, including the nails, and the hands, a half minute for each hand.
5. Hold the brush in one hand and both hands under running water, and clean under the fingernails with a metal or disposable plastic nail cleaner. Discard the cleaner after use.
6. Again scrub each individual finger, including the nails, and the hands with the brush, a half minute for each hand, maintaining lather.
7. Rinse the hands and brush, and discard the brush or sponge.
8. Reapply the antimicrobial agent and wash the hands and arms, applying friction to the elbows, for 3 minutes. Interlace the fingers to clean between them.
9. Rinse the hands and arms as before.

Counted Brush-Stroke Method
A prescribed number of brush strokes, applied lengthwise of the brush or sponge, is used for each surface of the fingers, hands, and arms. A short prescrub wash loosens surface debris and transient organisms. Scrubbing by brush or sponge removes resident flora.

The procedure is as follows:

1. Wet the hands and arms.
2. Wash the hands and arms thoroughly to 2 inches (5 cm) above the elbow with an antiseptic agent.
3. With the hands held under running water, clean under the fingernails carefully with a metal or disposable plastic nail cleaner. Discard the cleaner after use.
4. Rinse the hands and arms thoroughly under running water, keeping the hands up and allowing water to drip from the elbows.
5. Take a sterile brush or sponge from a dispenser or package. Apply an antiseptic agent to the brush or sponge (if not previously impregnated).
6. Scrub the nails of one hand 30 strokes, all sides of each finger 20 strokes, the back of the hand 20 strokes, the palm of the hand 20 strokes, and the arms 20 strokes for each third of the arm, to 2 inches (5 cm) above the elbow.
7. Repeat step 6 for the other hand and arm.
8. Rinse the hands and arms thoroughly.

GOWNING AND GLOVING

The sterile gown is put on immediately after the surgical scrub. The sterile gloves are put on immediately after gowning.

Purpose

A sterile gown and gloves are worn to exclude skin as a possible contaminant and to create a barrier between the sterile and nonsterile areas.

General Considerations

1. The scrub person gowns and gloves himself or herself and then may gown and glove the surgeon and assistants.
2. Gown packages preferably are opened on a separate table from other packages to avoid any chance of contamination from dripping water.
3. Avoid splashing water on scrub attire during the surgical scrub because moisture may contaminate the sterile gown.

Drying the Hands and Arms

After scrubbing, the hands and arms should be thoroughly dried before the sterile gown is donned to prevent contamination of the gown by strike-through of organisms from wet skin.

The gown package for the scrub person contains one sterile gown, folded before sterilization, with the inside out so that the bare scrubbed hands will not contaminate the sterile outside of the gown. A reusable or disposable towel for drying the hands is placed on top of the gown during packaging. The hands are dried as follows:

1. Reach down to the opened sterile package and pick up the towel. Be careful not to drip water onto the pack. Be sure no one is within arm's reach (Figure 16-3).
2. Open the towel full-length, holding one end away from the nonsterile scrub attire (Figure 16-4). Bend slightly forward to avoid letting the towel touch the attire.
3. Dry both hands thoroughly but independently. To dry one arm, hold the towel in the opposite hand and, using an oscillating motion of the arm, draw the towel up to the elbow.
4. Carefully reverse the towel, still holding it away from the body. Dry the opposite arm on the unused (now uppermost) end of the towel.

Gowning and Gloving Techniques

Sterile gloves may be put on in two ways: by the closed gloving technique or by the open gloving technique. If it is done properly, gloves can be put on safely either way. The method of gloving determines how the gown is donned.

Closed Glove Technique

The closed gloving method is preferred except when changing a glove during a surgical procedure or when donning gloves for procedures not requiring gowns. Properly executed, the closed gloving method affords assurance against contamination when gloving oneself, because no bare skin is exposed in the process.

Gowning for the Closed Glove Technique

1. Reach down to the sterile package and lift the folded gown directly upward (Figure 16-5).
2. Step back away from the table into an unobstructed area to provide a wide margin of safety while gowning.
3. Holding the folded gown, carefully locate the neckline.

Figure 16-4 Scrub person, holding towel away from body, dries only scrubbed areas, starting with hands. He or she avoids contaminating hands on areas proximal to elbows, then discards towel.

Figure 16-3 Scrub person preparing to gown removes hand towel on top of gown from opened package.

Figure 16-5 Scrub person, picking up gown below neck edge, lifts it directly upward and steps away to avoid touching edge of wrapper. Note that sterile inside of wrapper covers table. Gown is folded inside out.

4. Holding the inside front of the gown just below the neckline with both hands, let the gown unfold, keeping the inside of the gown toward the body. Do not touch the outside of the gown with bare hands.

5. Holding the hands at shoulder level, slip both arms into the armholes simultaneously (Figure 16-6).

6. The circulator brings the gown over the shoulders by reaching inside to the shoulder and arm seams. The gown is pulled on, leaving the cuffs of the sleeves extended over the hands. The back of the gown is securely tied or fastened at the neck and waist, touching the outside of the gown at the line of ties or fasteners in the back only (Figures 16-7 and 16-8).

Figure 16-6 Scrub person, putting on gown, gently shakes out folds, then slips arms into sleeves without touching sterile outside of gown with bare hands.

If the gown is wraparound style, the sterile flap to cover the back is not touched until the person has gowned and gloved. A sterile gown may be wrapped around in various ways:

1. With gloved hands, release the fastener or untie the ties at the front or side of the gown. Hand the tie on the right to a sterile team member who remains stationary. Allowing a margin of safety, turn around to the left, thereby completely covering the back with the extended flap of the gown. Accept the tie from the assistant and secure the ties at the left side of the gown.

2. If you are the first person to gown and glove and other sterile team members are not available to assist, snap a sterile instrument such as an Allis forceps (never a hemostat or clamp for hemostasis) to the tie on the right. Carefully hand the instrument to the circulator. While he or she remains stationary, turn to the left, thereby covering the back. Take the tie in hand. The circulator then releases and places the instrument aside; it is considered contaminated. Tie the ties at the left side.

3. Some disposable gowns have the end of one tie covered by a disposable strip. Hand the strip to the circulator, taking care to protect the hands. Turn around toward the opposite side, thereby closing the gown. Grasp the tie at a distance from the end. The circulator pulls the strip, releasing it from the still-sterile end of the tie, and discards it. Tie the ties at the front or side of the gown as indicated.

If the top of the gown drops downward inadvertently, discard the gown as contaminated. Never reverse a sterile gown or drape if the wrong end is dropped toward the floor.

Gloving by the Closed Glove Technique

1. Using the left hand and keeping it within the cuff of the left sleeve, pick up the right glove from the inner wrap of the glove package by grasping the folded cuff.

Figure 16-7 Circulator, pulling gown on for closed gloving technique, reaches inside gown to sleeve seams and pulls gown on, leaving cuffs of sleeves extended over hands.

Figure 16-8 Circulator completes pulling on scrub person's gown, secures ties on inside of back, and closes fastener at neck.

2. Extend the right forearm with the palm upward. Place the palm of the glove against the palm of the right hand, grasping in the right hand the top edge of the cuff, above the palm. In correct position, glove fingers are pointing toward you and the thumb of the glove is to the right. The thumb side of the glove is down (Figure 16-9).

3. Grasp the back of the cuff in the left hand and turn it over the end of the right sleeve and hand. The cuff of the glove is now over the stockinette cuff of the gown, with the hand still inside the sleeve (Figures 16-10 and 16-11).

4. Grasp the top of the right glove and underlying gown sleeve with the covered left hand. Pull the glove on

over the extended right fingers until it completely covers the stockinette cuff (Figure 16-12).

5. Glove the left hand in the same manner, reversing hands. Use the gloved right hand to pull on the left glove (Figures 16-13 to 16-15).

Open Glove Technique

The open gloving technique is used for changing a glove or the gown and gloves during a surgical procedure. It also is used when only sterile gloves are worn, as for intravenous cutdown or administration of spinal anesthesia, or in the emergency department when donning sterile gloves, as for suturing lacerations.

Figure 16-9 For closed gloving technique, using left hand and keeping it within cuff of sleeve, gowned scrub person picks up right glove. Palm of glove is placed against palm of right hand, grasping top edge of glove cuff above palm.

Figure 16-11 Cuff of glove is now over stockinette cuff of sleeve, with hand still inside sleeve.

Figure 16-10 Back of cuff is grasped in left hand and turned over right sleeve and hand.

Figure 16-12 Top of right glove and underlying sleeve of gown are grasped with left hand. By pulling sleeve up, glove is pulled onto hand.

Figure 16-13 Using gloved right hand, left glove is picked up and placed with palm of glove against palm of left hand. Back of cuff is grasped above palm in right hand and turned over left sleeve and hand.

Figure 16-15 Top of left glove and underlying gown sleeve are grasped with right hand, and sleeve is pulled up, pulling glove onto hand.

Figure 16-14 Cuff of left glove is now over stockinette cuff of sleeve, with hand still inside sleeve.

Figure 16-16 Circulator fastens back of scrub person's gown for open gloving technique. Note that hands extend through stockinette cuffs.

Gowning for the Open Glove Technique

1. Reach down to the sterile package and lift the folded gown directly upward.
2. Step back away from the table into a clear area to provide a wide margin of safety while gowning.
3. Holding the folded gown, carefully locate the neckline.
4. Holding the inside front of the gown just below the neckline with both hands, let the gown unfold, keeping the inside of the gown toward the body.
5. Holding the hands at shoulder level, slip them into the armholes simultaneously without touching the sterile exterior of the gown with bare hands.
6. The circulator reaches inside the gown to the sleeve seams and pulls the sleeves over the hands to the

wrists. Then the back of the gown is securely closed at the neck and waist with ties or fasteners, touching the outside of the gown at the line of ties or fasteners in the back only (Figure 16-16).

Gloving by the Open Glove Technique

This method of gloving uses a skin-to-skin, glove-to-glove technique. The hand, although scrubbed, is not sterile and must not contact the exterior of the sterile gloves. The everted cuff on the gloves exposes the inner surfaces. The first glove is put on with the skin-to-skin technique, bare hand to inside cuff. The sterile fingers of that gloved hand then may touch the sterile exterior of the second glove (i.e., glove-to-glove technique).

Figure 16-17 Scrub person gloving right hand with open gloving technique. With left hand, person grasps right glove on folded-back cuff and lifts it directly up and away from wrapper. Right hand is inserted in glove. Note that left hand touches only cuff or inside of glove, which is skin-to-skin technique.

Figure 16-19 As cuff of left glove is pulled up over cuff of sleeve, gloved fingers of right hand touch only outside of left glove, near wrist. If stockinette is not tight, a pleat is folded and held with right thumb while pulling glove over cuff. Contact with exposed skin would contaminate right glove. (A pleat cannot be held if regloving because cuff is contaminated.)

Figure 16-18 Picking up left glove, scrub person lifts glove from wrapper by slipping gloved right fingers under protective cuff, using glove-to-glove technique. Bare hand does not touch outside of glove.

Figure 16-20 With completely gloved left hand, left fingers are inserted under folded-back cuff of right glove and glove cuff is pulled up over right sleeve cuff, using glove-to-glove technique.

The procedure is as follows:

1. With the left hand, grasp the cuff of the right glove on the fold. Pick up the glove and step back from the table. Look behind you before moving.
2. Insert the right hand into the glove and pull it on, leaving the cuff turned well down over the hand (Figure 16-17).
3. Slip the fingers of the gloved right hand under the everted cuff of the left glove. Pick up the glove and step back (Figure 16-18).

4. Insert the hand into the left glove and pull it on, leaving the cuff turned down over the hand.
5. With the fingers of the right hand, pull the cuff of the left glove over the cuff of the left sleeve. If the stockinette is not tight, fold a pleat, holding it with the right thumb while pulling the glove over the cuff. Avoid touching the bare wrist (Figure 16-19).
6. Repeat step 5 for the right cuff, using the left hand, and thereby completely gloving the right hand (Figure 16-20).

Gowning Another Person

A team member in sterile gown and gloves may assist the surgeon or another team member in gowning and gloving by taking the following steps:

1. Open the hand towel and lay it on the surgeon's hand, being careful not to touch the hand.
2. Unfold the gown carefully, holding it at the neckline.
3. Keeping your hands on the outside of the gown under a protective cuff of the neck and shoulder area, offer the inside of the gown to the surgeon. He or she slips the arms into the sleeves.
4. Release the gown. The surgeon holds arms outstretched while the circulator pulls the gown onto the shoulders and adjusts the sleeves so that the cuffs are properly placed. In doing so, only the inside of the gown is touched at the seams.

Gloving Another Person

1. Pick up the right glove and grasp it firmly with the fingers under the everted cuff. Hold the palm of the glove toward the surgeon.
2. Stretch the cuff sufficiently for the surgeon to introduce the hand. Avoid touching the hand by holding your thumbs out (Figure 16-21).
3. Exert upward pressure as the surgeon plunges the hand into the glove.
4. Unfold the everted glove cuff over the cuff of the sleeve.
5. Repeat for the left hand.
6. If a sterile vest is needed, hold it for the surgeon to slip the hands into the armholes. Be careful not to contaminate the gloves at the neck level. If the gown is a wraparound, assist the surgeon. Remember that the back of the gown is not considered sterile even if a sterile vest is worn.

Changing Gowns During the Surgical Procedure

Occasionally a contaminated gown must be changed during a surgical procedure. The circulator unfastens the neck and waist. Grasped at the shoulders, the gown is pulled off inside out. The gown is always removed first. The gloves are removed using a glove-to-glove and then skin-to-skin technique. If only the sleeve is contaminated, a sterile sleeve may be put on over the contaminated one.

Changing Gloves During the Surgical Procedure

If a glove becomes contaminated for any reason during a surgical procedure, it must be changed immediately. If stepping away immediately is not feasible, the contaminated hand

Figure 16-21   In gloving surgeon or another person, scrub person holds glove with palm toward him or her. Scrub person keeps thumbs extended outward to avoid being touched by bare hands of person donning gloves.

should be held away from the sterile area. The glove is changed as follows:

1. Turn away from the sterile field.
2. Extend the contaminated hand to the circulator who, wearing protective gloves, grasps the outside of the glove cuff about 2 inches (5 cm) below the top of the glove and pulls the glove off inside out.
3. Preferably, a sterile team member gloves another. If this is not possible, step aside and glove the hand, using the open gloving technique.

The closed gloving technique cannot be used for a glove change during a surgical procedure without contamination of the new glove by the sleeve of the gown or without contamination of the hand by the cuff of the gown. The contaminated cuff may not be pulled down over the hand. If the closed method is used, both gloves and the gown are removed and another sterile gown is donned before the gloves. The scrub person should change his or her own gloves before gowning and gloving another team member.

Removing the Gown and Gloves

The gown is always removed before the gloves at the end of the surgical procedure.

Removing the Gown

The circulator unfastens the neck and back closures of a reusable gown so that the wearer does not contaminate his or her scrub suit or damage the closures. If wearing a wraparound gown, the wearer unfastens the waist closure in front. The wearer may unhook Velcro or snap closures on a disposable gown by himself or herself. The gown is always removed inside out to protect the arms and scrub suit from the contaminated outside of the gown. The gown is removed as follows:

A   **B**   **C**

Figure 16-22   Sequence of scrub person removing soiled gown at end of surgical procedure. Clean arms and scrub suit are protected from contaminated outside of gown. **A,** With gloves on, cuffs of gown are loosened and shaken down over wrists. Then right shoulder of gown (unfastened or untied) is grasped with left hand. **B,** In pulling gown off arms, arm of gown is turned away from body with flexed elbow. **C,** Other shoulder is grasped with other hand, and gown is removed entirely by pulling it off inside out and keeping arms clean.

1. Grasp the right shoulder of the loosened gown with the left hand and pull the gown downward from the shoulder and off the right arm, turning the sleeve inside out (Figure 16-22, *A*).
2. Turn the outside of the gown away from the body with flexed elbows (Figure 16-22, *B*).
3. Grasp the left shoulder with the right hand and remove the gown entirely, pulling it off inside out (Figure 16-22, *C*).
4. Discard the gown in a laundry hamper or in a trash receptacle (if disposable).

Removing the Gloves

The cuffs of the gloves usually turn down as the gown is pulled off the arms. A glove-to-glove, then skin-to-skin technique is used to protect the clean hands from the contaminated outside of the gloves, which bear cells of the patient (Figure 16-23). The gloves are removed as follows:

1. Grasp the cuff of the left glove with the gloved fingers of the right hand and pull it off inside out.
2. Slip the ungloved fingers of the left hand under the cuff of the right glove and slip it off inside out.
3. Discard the gloves in a trash receptacle.
4. Wash hands.

A   **B**

Figure 16-23   Sequence of scrub person removing soiled gloves at end of surgical procedure. First, glove-to-glove technique **(A)**, then skin-to-skin technique **(B)** is used to protect "clean" hands from contaminated outside of gloves, which bear cells of patient. Gloves are turned inside out for removal.

Bibliography

Association of Operating Room Nurses: *AORN standards, recommended practices, and guidelines,* Denver, 1998, The Association.

Babb JR et al: Risk of airborne transmission in an operating theatre containing four ultraclean air units, *J Hosp Infect Control* 31(3):159-168, 1995.

Baur X et al: Can a threshold limit value for natural rubber latex be defined? *J Allergy Clin Dermatol* 101(1):24-27, 1998.

Berridge DC et al: A randomized controlled trial of double- versus single-gloving in vascular surgery, *J R Coll Surg* 43(1):9-10, 1998.

Breeze W: It is time to standardize surgical hand scrubs? *AORN J* 60(2):294-295, 1994.

Deshmukh N et al: A comparison of 5-minute povidone-iodine scrub and 1-minute povidone-iodine scrub followed by alcohol foam, *Mil Med* 163(3):145-147, 1998.

Edlich RF, Watkins FH: Glove powder: facts and fiction, *Surg Serv Manage* 3(2):47-50, 1997.

Faoagali J et al: Comparison of the immediate, residual, and cumulative antibacterial effects of Novaderm, Novascrub, Betadine Surgical Scrub, Hibiclens, and liquid soap, *Am J Infect Control* 23(6):337-343, 1995.

Fisher MD et al: Ease of donning commercially available powder-free surgical gloves, *J Biomed Mater Res* 33(4):291-295, 1996.

Herscovici D Jr et al: Comparison of cloth gloves used in orthopaedic surgery: a clinical and experimental evaluation, *J Orthop Trauma* 12(2):106-110, 1998.

Korniewicz DM, Rabussay DP: Surgical glove failures in clinical practice settings, *AORN J* 66(4):660-668, 671, 673, 1997.

Loeb MB et al: A randomized trial of surgical scrubbing with a brush compared to antiseptic soap alone, *Am J Infect Control* 25(1):11-15, 1997.

Lundburg M et al: Latex allergy from glove powder—an unintended risk with the switch from talc to corn starch? *Allergy* 52(12):1222-1228, 1997.

Marin-Bertolin S et al: Does double gloving protect surgical staff from skin contamination during plastic surgery? *Plast Reconstr Surg* 99(4):956-960, 1997.

Mathias JM: Is it time to shorten the five-minute scrub? *OR Manager* 10(4):1, 9, 12, 1994.

Newsom SW, Shaw P: Airborne particles from latex gloves in the hospital environment, *Eur J Surg* (579):31-33, 1997.

Paulson DS: Comparative evaluation of five surgical hand scrub preparations, *AORN J* 60(2):246-256, 1994.

Poon C et al: Studies of the surgical scrub, *Aust N Z J Surg* 68(1):65-67, 1998.

Rabussay D, Korniewicz DM: The risks and challenges of surgical glove failure, *AORN J* 66(5):867-872, 874, 876-877, 1997.

Rikimaru T et al: Bacterial activities of povidone-iodine against mycobacterium, *Dermatology* 195(2):104-106, 1997.

Roth R: *Perioperative core nursing curriculum,* Denver, 1995, Association of Operating Room Nurses.

Salisbury DM et al: The effect of rings on microbial load of healthcare workers' hands, *Am J Infect Control* 25(1):25-27, 1997.

Sharma JB et al: Blood splashes to the masks and goggles during caesarean section, *Br J Obstet Gynecol* 104(12):1405-1406, 1997.

Steelman V: Is it really necessary to go powder free? *Infect Control Today* 2(5):29-30, 1998.

Sullivan KM et al: The right glove for the right job, *Infect Control Today* 2(7):20, 22, 24, 26, 28, 1998.

Truscott WM: Examination glove selection criteria and infection control, *Infect Control Today* 2(5):40-42, 44, 46, 48, 52, 54-56, 1998.

Wheelock SM, Lookinland S: Effect of surgical hand scrub time on subsequent bacterial growth, *AORN J* 65(6):1087-1092, 1094-1098, 1997.

Woods JA et al: Surgical glove lubricants: from toxicity to opportunity, *J Emerg Med* 15(2):209-220, 1997.

Wynd CA et al: Bacterial carriage on the fingernails of OR nurses, *AORN J* 60(5):796-805, 1994.

Zinner NL: How safe are your gloves? *AORN J* 59(4):876-882, 1994.

Chapter 17

Sterilization

 Chapter Objectives

After studying this chapter, the learner will be able to:

- Define the term *sterilization*.
- List three methods of sterilization.
- Describe the process for preparing an item for sterilization.
- Identify the primary hazards associated with each type of sterilization.
- Discuss monitoring the sterilization process.

Pathogenic microorganisms, as well as those that do not normally invade healthy tissue, are capable of causing infection if introduced mechanically into the body. Standardized procedures that are based on accepted principles and practices are necessary for the sterilization or disinfection of all supplies and equipment used for patient care in the perioperative environment. Following established protocols for instrument processing helps to minimize the patient's risk for infection of the surgical site. The terms associated with sterilization are defined in Box 17-1.

HISTORICAL BACKGROUND

By the end of the nineteenth century, the concepts of Semmelweis, Pasteur, Lister, Nightingale, Neuber, and others were established to control the OR environment. Surgeons had moved out of the front parlors and into hospitals. Disinfectants were used to clean furniture, floors, and walls. Antiseptic solution or green soap was used to clean the skin of patients and members of the perioperative team. The team wore gowns and gloves.

Heat-resistant bacteria were demonstrated in 1876. In the 1880s, sterilization by boiling was introduced. Everything used during a surgical procedure was boiled, including linens, dressings, and gowns. Around 1886, the German surgeon Ernst von Bergmann (1863-1907) and his associates introduced the steam sterilizer, which was a great improvement over his previous method of soaking surgical supplies in bichloride of mercury. Surgeons soon learned that steam under pressure was necessary to raise the temperature sufficiently to kill heat-resistant microorganisms and spores. Vacuum-type pressure sterilizers and dry heat sterilizers followed.

Used as a fumigant for insects in the early twentieth century, ethylene oxide was recognized as an antibacterial agent around 1929, when it was used to sterilize imported spices. It has been used as a sterilizing agent in industry and in hospitals since the 1940s. Sterilization by irradiation has since been developed and is used for the sterilization of commercially prepared surgical supplies.

Chemical sterilants began with carbolic sprays and mercurial compounds. Although not the method of choice, these products underwent many changes to improve their safety and efficacy. Instruments that could not be heat sterilized posed a problem for the surgeon. Glutaraldehyde, introduced in 1963, was the first chemical solution approved by the

---

Box 17-1 **Terms Associated with Sterilization**

sterilization Processes by which all pathogenic and non-pathogenic microorganisms, including spores, are killed. This term refers only to a process capable of destroying all forms of microbial life, including spores. The sterilizer is a piece of equipment used to attain either physical or chemical sterilization. The agent used must be capable of killing all forms of microorganisms.

terminal sterilization and disinfection Procedures carried out for the destruction of pathogens at the end of the surgical procedure in the OR or in other areas of patient contact (i.e., PACU, ICU, patient care unit).

wicking Passage of fluids through a material by passive action. Also referred to as capillary action or strike-through.

Environmental Protection Agency (EPA) as a sterilant for heat-sensitive instruments.

STERILIZATION VS. DISINFECTION

A sterile item has been exposed to a sterilization process to render it free of all living microorganisms, including spores. As long as sterility is maintained, this process renders items safe for contact with nonintact tissue and for exposure to the vascular system without the transmission of infection. The sterilization process should provide the highest level of assurance that an item can be expected to be free of known viable pathogenic and nonpathogenic microorganisms, including spores. For items and materials that cannot be sterilized, disinfectants are used to kill as many microorganisms in the environment as possible. (Disinfection is described in Chapter 18.)

STERILIZATION

Bacterial spores are the most resistant of all living organisms because of their capacity to withstand external destructive agents. Although the physical or chemical process by which all pathogenic and nonpathogenic microorganisms (including spores) are destroyed is not absolute, supplies and equipment are considered sterile when all parameters have been met during a sterilization process.

Reliability Parameters for Sterilization

Two types of parameters are considered for the reliability of sterilizing methods: product-associated parameters and process-associated parameters.

Product-Associated Parameters

1. *Bioburden:* the degree of contamination with microorganisms and organic debris
2. *Bioresistance:* factors such as heat and/or moisture sensitivities and product stability

3. *Biostate:* the nutritional, physical, and/or reproductive phase of microorganisms
4. *Bioshielding:* characteristics of the packaging materials
5. *Density:* factors affecting penetration and evacuation of the agent

Process-Associated Parameters

1. Temperature
2. Humidity/moisture/hydration
3. Time
4. Purity of the agent and air, and the residual effects or residues
5. Saturation/penetration
6. Capacity of the sterilizer and the position of items within the chamber

Methods of Sterilization

Reliable sterilization depends on the contact of the sterilizing agent with all surfaces of the item to be sterilized. Selection of the agent used to achieve sterility depends primarily on the nature of the item to be sterilized. The time required to kill spores in the available equipment then becomes critical. Sterilization processes are either physical or chemical, and each method has its advantages and disadvantages. The following are available sterilizing agents (sterilants):

1. Thermal (physical)
   a. Steam under pressure/moist heat
   b. Hot air/dry heat
2. Chemical
   a. Ethylene oxide gas
   b. Formaldehyde gas and solution
   c. Hydrogen peroxide plasma/vapor
   d. Ozone gas
   e. Acetic acid solution
   f. Glutaraldehyde solution
   g. Peracetic acid 0.2% solution
3. Radiation (physical)
   a. Microwave (nonionizing)
   b. X-ray (ionizing)

Sterilization Cycle

The time required to achieve sterilization is referred to as the process cycle, which includes the following:

- Heat up and/or penetration of the agent
- Kill time (i.e., exposure to the agent)
- Safety factor for bioburden
- Evacuation or dissipation of the agent

Monitoring the Sterilization Cycle

To ensure that instruments and supplies are sterile when used, it is essential that the sterilization process be monitored. The general considerations are mentioned in the following sections. Specific tests are discussed later in this chapter with each method of sterilization.

Administrative Monitoring

Work practices are supervised. Written policies and procedures are strictly followed by all personnel responsible for sterilizing and handling sterile supplies. If sterility cannot be achieved or maintained, the system has failed. Policies and procedures pertain to the following:

1. Decontaminating, terminally sterilizing, and cleaning all reusable items; disposing of disposable items in the appropriate manner
2. Packaging and labeling items
3. Loading and unloading the sterilizer
4. Operating the sterilizer
5. Monitoring and maintaining the records of each cycle
6. Adhering to safety precautions and preventive maintenance protocol
7. Storing sterile items
8. Handling sterile items ready for use
9. Making a sterile transfer to a sterile field at the point of use
10. Tracking and recalling items if an item in a particular load is not safe for use

Mechanical Indicators

Sterilizers have gauges, thermometers, timers, recorders, and/or other devices that monitor their functions. Most sterilizers have automatic controls and locking devices, and some have alarm systems that are activated if the sterilizer fails to operate correctly. Records are reviewed and maintained for each cycle. Test packs or special diagnostics are run at least daily, as appropriate for the type of sterilizer, to monitor the functions of each sterilizer. Such tests can identify processing errors.

The manufacturer of the sterilizer provides a manual for the comprehensive care and maintenance of the sterilizing device. Reliable operation is dependent on the following:

- Routine maintenance that consists of daily inspections and scheduled cleanings per the manufacturer's recommendation. All gaskets, gauges, graph pens, drain screens, paper rolls, ink cartridges, and charting devices should be repaired or replaced by qualified personnel as needed.
- Preventive maintenance (PM) that includes periodic calibration, lubrication, and function checks by qualified personnel on a scheduled basis. Each PM should be documented.

Chemical Indicators

External indicator tape, labels, or paper strips should be clearly visible on the outside of every package to differentiate between sterilized and unsterilized items. The indicator helps to monitor the physical conditions within the sterilizer to alert personnel to malfunctions, human errors in packaging, or improper loading of the sterilizer.

An internal indicator may be placed inside a package in a position most likely to be difficult for the sterilant to penetrate (Table 17-1). If a chemical reaction of the indicator does not show the expected results, the item should not be used. Indicators do not establish the sterility of an item; they indicate only that process parameters have been met.

Biologic Indicators

Positive assurance that sterilization conditions have been achieved can be obtained only through a biologic control test. A biologic indicator is a preparation of living spores that are resistant to the sterilizing agent. The preparation may be supplied in a self-contained system (e.g., dry spore strips) or in sealed vials or ampules of spores in suspension. To perform the test, a biologic unit that has been exposed to the sterilant and an unprocessed biologic unit (control) from the same lot number are incubated for the same period of time. If sterilization has occurred, the processed biologic unit will not grow any microorganisms. The unprocessed biologic control unit will grow microorganisms and display a change in color. If the unprocessed biologic unit fails to grow microorganisms, its spores have been inactivated. In such a case, the processed unit also may have been inactive before processing; thus the biologic test is rendered invalid. The entire load is considered unsterile when either the test indicator or the control is in question. Test indicators and controls should be interpreted by qualified personnel.

Each sterilization process requires biologic testing at regular intervals. Consecutive biologic monitors should be run each time the sterilizer is calibrated, repaired, or relocated. Biologic testing involves incubation according to the manufacturer's recommendations. The bacterial spores used for biologic monitoring and testing intervals include the following:

- *Bacillus stearothermophilus* at 131° to 140° F (55° to 60° C) tests steam under pressure daily and with each load of implantables.
- *Bacillus subtilis* at 95° to 98.6° F (35° to 37° C) tests dry heat and ethylene oxide with every load.
- *B. subtilis* testing is performed daily for low temperature hydrogen peroxide plasma.
- Peracetic acid sterilizers are tested according to the manufacturer's recommendations.

A rapid readout biologic indicator specifically for monitoring a high-speed pressure steam sterilizer with a gravity displacement cycle is based on the fluorometric detection of a *B. stearothermophilus*–bound enzyme, rather than on spore growth. The enzyme becomes fluorescent yellow within 60 minutes as the spores are killed.

Biologic indicators need to conform with the testing standards of the United States Pharmacopeia (USP). A control test is performed at least weekly in each sterilizer (see Table 17-1). Many hospitals monitor on a daily basis; others test each cycle. Every load of implantable devices is monitored, and the implant should not be used until negative test results are known. All test results are filed in a permanent record for each sterilizer.

TABLE 17-1	**Guidelines for the Use of Chemical and Biologic Indicators***				
AAMI	**AHA**	**AORN**	**CDC**	**JCAHO**	

Chemical

Purpose: to indicate items exposed to the sterilization process; to monitor one or more sterilization parameters; to detect failures in packaging, loading, or sterilizer function. Indicators do *not* verify sterility.

Placement

AAMI	AHA	AORN	CDC	JCAHO
External: On all packages except if internal indicator is visible *Internal:* In center or area least accessible to sterilant within each package	With each package; can be used inside or on outside	*External:* Visible on every package *Internal:* Inside each package	*External:* Attached to each package *Internal:* Inside large pack	With each package, no designation to inside or outside

Biologic

Purpose: to document efficacy of sterilization process by killing resistant spores; to ensure that all process parameters are met; to detect nonsterilizing conditions in sterilizer.

Steam

AAMI	AHA	AORN	CDC	JCAHO
Frequency: At least weekly, preferably daily *Placement:* Positioned in cold point in test pack, normally bottom front of sterilizer	*Frequency:* Once a day	*Frequency:* At least once a week, preferably daily, and with each load of implantables	*Frequency:* At least once a week, and with each load of implantables	*Frequency:* At least weekly (daily is recommended), or with each load if sterilization activities are performed less frequently or if load contains implantable or intravascular material

Ethylene oxide

AAMI	AHA	AORN	CDC	JCAHO
Frequency: Every load *Placement:* Inside pack in geometric center of load	*Frequency:* Every load	*Frequency:* Every load	*Frequency:* At least once a week, and with each load of implantables	*Frequency:* At least weekly (daily is recommended), or with each load if sterilization activities are performed less frequently or if load contains implantable or intravascular material

*All organizations require that indicators be used routinely.
AAMI, Association for the Advancement of Medical Instrumentation; *AHA,* American Hospital Association, *Guidelines for the Hospital Central Service Department; AORN,* Association of periOperative Registered Nurses; *CDC,* Centers for Disease Control and Prevention; *JCAHO,* Joint Commission on Accreditation of Healthcare Organizations.

Packaging Items for Sterilization
Packaging Considerations

The packaging materials for all methods of sterilization should do the following:

1. Permit penetration of the sterilizing agent to achieve sterilization of all items in the package.
2. Allow the release of the sterilizing agent at the end of the exposure period and allow adequate drying or aerating.
3. Withstand the physical conditions of the sterilizing process.
4. Maintain integrity of the package at varying atmospheric and humidity levels. In dry climates or at high altitudes, some packaging materials are susceptible to rupture during sterilization or dry out and crack in storage.
5. Provide an impermeable barrier to microorganisms, dust particles, and moisture after sterilization. Items must remain sterile from the time they are removed from the sterilizer until they are used.
6. Cover items completely and easily and fasten securely with tape or a heat seal that cannot be resealed after opening. Seal integrity should be tamperproof. A margin of at least 1 inch (2.5 cm) is considered a standard for safety on all sealed packages. Pins, staples, paper clips, or other penetrating objects must never be used to seal packages, because these cannot be removed without destroying the integrity of the package and contaminating the contents. Scissors

should not be used to cut off the end of a package. Contents cannot be drawn out over this cut end because the contents would be contaminated by the edge of the packaging material. For the same reason, packages are never torn open below a seal.

7. Resist tears and punctures in handling. If accidental tears and holes do occur, they must be visible.
8. Permit identification of the contents and evidence of exposure to a sterilizing agent. Chemical indicator tapes or strips on the outside of packages change color during exposure to a sterilization process. They do not indicate sterility, only that the package has been sufficiently exposed to a given parameter to change the color of the indicator. Indicators show that all parameters have been met.
9. Be free of toxic ingredients and nonfast dyes.
10. Be lint free or low linting.
11. Protect the contents from physical damage.
12. Permit easy removal of the contents with transfer to the sterile field without contamination or delamination (separation into layers).
13. Be economical.

Packages should be wrapped far enough away from sterile storage areas so that mixing sterile and nonsterile packages is not possible. Nonsterile cabinets should be labeled conspicuously. A procedure for sending items to and receiving items from the sterilizer should be set up so that sterile and nonsterile packages can never be confused en route. This procedure must be understood by everyone.

Packages may be wrapped with nonwoven or woven materials sequentially in two layers. Double-thickness wrapping in one layer without using the sequential method is also acceptable. The wrappers can be stitched around the edges or bonded/fused together. Aseptic presentation to the sterile field is the prime consideration. Each facility should determine which method and material is best suited to the clinical environment.

Items are enclosed with all corners of the wrapper folded in. Either a square or an envelope fold may be used (Figures 17-1 and 17-2). After an item is wrapped in one wrapper, the package is wrapped in the second wrapper. A cuff turned back on the first fold of each wrapper provides a margin of safety to prevent contamination when opening after sterilization. Packages can be fastened securely with pressure-sensitive chemical indicator tape.

Packaging Materials and Methods

Packaging materials must be compatible with the sterilization process. The following materials may be safely used to wrap items for steam sterilization because they permit steam penetration, adequate air removal, and adequate drying.

Woven Fabrics Reusable woven fabrics are commonly referred to as muslin or linen. When no other alternative is available, a 140-thread-count carded 100% cotton muslin is used. Steam sterilizer cycles are based on a time-temperature profile of 140-thread-count muslin. This type of fabric is not moisture resistant and is used in a double thickness. Two pieces are sewn together on the edges only, with a blind hem and without cross-stitching, so the wrapper is free of holes. This wrapper should withstand between 50 and 75 launderings before becoming too worn to be a microbial barrier. A laundering mark-off system is helpful to monitor the number of times a wrapper has been used. The manufacturer should provide information about the number of launderings and sterilization cycles the wrapper can withstand.

Before resterilization, woven fabrics are laundered to rehydrate them. The moisture content of the woven material affects steam penetration and prevents superheating during the sterilization process. The fabric should be stored at a room temperature of 64° to 72° F (18° to 22° C) and in a relative humidity of 35% to 70%. Before use, the woven fabric is inspected for holes and patched with vulcanized patches if necessary. Fabric may create free-floating lint in the OR.

Nonwoven Fabrics Nonwoven fabrics are a combination of cellulose and rayon with strands of nylon randomly oriented through it, or they are a combination of other natural and synthetic fibers bonded by a method other than weaving. These fabrics have the flexibility and handling qualities of woven materials and are available in several weights. Lightweight is used in four thicknesses; medium weight is the most economical for wrapping items in two thicknesses; and heavy-duty weight is used when a single wrap is used for wrapping supplies for sterilization. Packages are wrapped in the same manner as with woven fabrics. Nonwoven fabrics provide an excellent barrier against microorganisms and moisture during storage after sterilization. They are disposable and virtually lint free. Some manufacturers provide a recycling service for nonwoven wrappers.

Peel Packs or Pouches Pouches and tubes made of a combination of paper on one side and clear plastic film on the other are satisfactory for wrapping single instruments, odd-shaped items, and small items. For sterile presentation, a peel-open seal may be preformed on one end. The open end is either heat sealed or closed with indicator tape after the item is inserted. All air is expressed from the package before sealing. Self-sealing pouches with adhesive flaps that do not require heat sealing are also available.

The sequential packaging of supplies in a smaller pouch into a larger pouch is not routinely necessary. However, this method may be useful for keeping multiple small items together, such as a set of bone screws. The aseptic presentation of tiny parts to the sterile field without dropping items on the floor can be accomplished with sequential packaging. The manufacturer's instructions should be consulted if sequential peel pouches will be used.

Sealants and Labeling Chemical indicator tape is used to seal packages such as peel pouches and wrapped items. Steam-sensitive tape resembles tan-colored masking tape and reveals dark stripes when exposed to steam steriliz-

1. Place items assembled for pack in center of two sheets of wrapping material.

2. Fan fold open end away from you over items. Cuff top layer.

3. Repeat same procedure with end toward you, lining up cuff directly on top of first cuff.

4. Miter left end and fold neatly up and over top of pack.

5. Repeat with right side of pack.

6. Repeat step 2.

7. Repeat step 3.

8. Repeat step 4.

9. Repeat step 5 and securely affix with pressure-sensitive indicator tape over end.

Figure 17-1 Square fold for wrapping item for sterilization. Single-layer heavy wrap may be applied in this manner. (Modified from the Association for the Advancement of Medical Instrumentation: *Good hospital practice: steam sterilization and sterility assurance; ANSI/AAMI ST46-1993,* Arlington, Va, 1993, American National Standards Institute.)

1. Place two wrappers on flat surface with one point toward you. Place item to be wrapped in center of wrapper with its length parallel to you.

2. Fold corner nearest you over item until it is completely covered. Fold corner back toward you 2 to 3 inches.

3. Fold left side of wrapper over and parallel to item. Fold end of corner back 2 to 3 inches.

4. Repeat with right side. Lap center folds at least one-half inch.

5. Tuck in side edges of remaining corner to eliminate any direct opening to item. Bring top corner down to bottom edges and tuck in, leaving point for opening.

6. Repeat step 2.

7. Repeat step 3.

8. Repeat step 4.

9. Bring point of wrapper completely around package and seal with appropriate tape.

Figure 17-2 Envelope fold for wrapping item for sterilization. Single-layer heavy wrap may be applied in this manner. (Modified from the Association for the Advancement of Medical Instrumentation: *Good hospital practice: steam sterilization and sterility assurance; ANSI/AAMI ST46-1993,* Arlington, Va, 1993, American National Standards Institute.)

ing conditions. Gas-sensitive tape is light green and reveals dark stripes after exposure to gas sterilizing conditions. Peel pouches are usually heat sealed and have an indicator area or dot that changes color in response to steam or gas exposure. They may be sealed with steam or gas-sensitive tape. These sealants are not indicators of sterility but are a visual means by which to validate exposure to sterilant conditions.

The sealing tape on the outside of the package should be labeled with a dark marker that is resistant to moisture, bleeding through, or smearing. Preprinted labels may be used instead. The date of processing and a load number should be attached to each package. These forms of identification are helpful in tracking and locating items that have been processed in batches. A recall of items may be necessary if the sterility of a particular load is in doubt.

Rigid Closed Containers   A metal or plastic rigid closed container system may be used for sterilizing instruments singly or in sets. A stainless steel mesh or perforated basket lined with foam porous padding nests in the rigid container. The lid is affixed to the container base by metal snap locks. Plastic break-away shrink bands secure the flip locks and act as chemical external indicators by changing color. The body of the container is labeled with the contents. A load-identifying label is affixed to the container before processing.

Most styles of closed containers have single-use unidirectional air filters in the lid and bottom. These filters are changed each time the container is processed. The closed container is placed into the steam sterilizer so the steam can penetrate through the bottom and lid. The processing temperature and time should be established by the manufacturer of the closed container system.

After the sterilization process is complete, the container is placed on a firm dry surface adjacent to the sterile table. The circulator breaks the shrink band seal by flipping the locks and then lifts the lid toward himself or herself. The outer rigid container is not considered sterile. The scrub person carefully reaches into the container without touching it and grasps the handles of the sterile inner basket, lifting it straight up and out. The sterile basket containing the instruments can be placed on the sterile back table. Sterile supplies are not to be opened into the rigid container because the edges are not considered sterile.

THERMAL STERILIZATION

Heat is a dependable physical agent for the destruction of all forms of microbial life, including spores. It may be used moist or dry. The most reliable and commonly used method of sterilization is steam under pressure.

Steam Under Pressure: Moist Heat Sterilization

Heat destroys microorganisms, and this process is hastened by the addition of moisture. Steam in itself is inadequate for sterilization. Pressure that is greater than atmospheric pressure is necessary to increase the temperature of steam for the thermal destruction of microbial life. Moist heat in the form of steam under pressure causes the denaturation and coagulation of protein or the enzyme-protein system within cells.

Direct saturated steam contact is the basis of the steam sterilization process. For a specified time and at a required temperature, the steam must penetrate every fiber and reach every surface of the items to be sterilized. When steam enters the sterilizer chamber under pressure, it condenses on contact with cold items. This condensation liberates heat, simultaneously heating and wetting all items in the load and thereby providing the two requisites: moisture and heat. This sterilization process is spoken of in terms of degrees of temperature and time of exposure, not in terms of pounds of pressure. Pressure increases the boiling temperature of water but in itself has no significant effect on microorganisms or steam penetration.

Exposure time depends on the size and contents of the load and the temperature within the sterilizer. At the end of the cycle, revaporation of water condensate must effectively dry contents of the load to maintain sterility; the water is dried from the sterilized pack or item.

The vegetative forms of most microorganisms are killed in a few minutes at temperatures ranging from 130° to 150° F (54° to 65° C); however, certain bacterial spores will withstand a temperature of 240° F (115° C) for more than 3 hours. No living thing can survive direct exposure to saturated steam at 250° F (121° C) for longer than 15 minutes. As the temperature of the steam is increased, the time of exposure may be decreased. A minimum temperature-time relationship is maintained throughout all portions of the load to accomplish effective sterilization. Prions (pronounced *preeons*) such as Creutzfeldt-Jacob Disease (CJD) are not a living plant, animal, or virus. They are infectious protein material and must be steam sterilized for a minimum of 1 hour at 270° F (132° C) after soaking in sodium hydroxide at room temperature for 1 hour. If a prevacuum sterilizer is used, the item can be processed for 18 minutes at 274° F (134° C) after the 1-hour exposure to sodium hydroxide.

Advantages of Steam Sterilization

1. Steam sterilization is the easiest, safest, and surest method of on-site sterilization. Heat- and moisture-stable items that can be steam sterilized without damage should be processed with this method.
2. Steam is the fastest method; its total time cycle is the shortest.
3. Steam is the least expensive and most easily supplied agent. It is piped in from the facility's boiler room. An automatic, electrically powered steam generator can be mounted beneath the sterilizer for emergency standby when steam pressure is low.
4. Most sterilizers have automatic controls and recording devices that eliminate the human factor from the sterilization process as much as possible when operated and cared for according to the recommendations of the manufacturer.
5. Steam leaves no harmful residue. Many items such as stainless steel instruments withstand repeated processing without damage.

Disadvantages of Steam Sterilization

1. Precautions must be used in preparing and packaging items, loading and operating the sterilizer, and drying the load.
2. Items need to be clean, free of grease and oil, and not sensitive to heat.
3. Steam must have direct contact with all areas of an item. It must be able to penetrate packaging material, but the material must be able to maintain sterility.
4. The timing of the cycle is adjusted for differences in materials and sizes of loads; these variables are subject to human error.
5. Steam may not be pure. Steam purity refers to the amount of solid, liquid, or vapor contamination in steam. Impurities can cause wet or stained packs and stained instruments.

Types of Steam Sterilizers

Sterilizers that are designed to use steam under pressure are often referred to as autoclaves to distinguish them from sterilizers that use other agents. Personnel charged with the responsibility of operating steam sterilizers must fully understand the principles and operation of each type. They must be aware of the problems that cause malfunction, which includes attaining the sterilization temperature and maintaining it for the required period of time, trapped air, and dirty traps.

Gravity Displacement Sterilizer The metal construction of the gravity displacement sterilizer contains two shells (either round or rectangular) that form a jacket and a chamber. Steam fills the jacket that surrounds the chamber. After the door is tightly closed, steam enters the chamber at the back, near the top, and is deflected upward. Air is more than twice as heavy as steam. Thus by gravity, air goes to the bottom and steam floats on top. Steam, entering under pressure and remaining above the air, displaces air downward (both in the chamber and in the wrapped items) and forces it out through a discharge outlet at the bottom front. The air passes through a filtering screen to a waste line. A thermometer located at this outlet below the screen measures the temperature in the chamber. When steam has filled the chamber, it begins to flow past the thermometer (Figure 17-3). The timing of the sterilizing period starts only when the thermometer reaches the desired temperature.

When air is trapped in the chamber or in wrapped items, the killing power of steam is decreased in direct proportion to the amount of air present. Because the vital discharge of air from the load always occurs in a downward direction, never sideways, all supplies are prepared and arranged to present the least possible resistance to the passage of steam downward through the load from the top of the chamber. Air and steam discharge lines are kept free of dirt, sediment, and lint.

Figure 17-3 Schematic cross section of steam-under-pressure sterilizer. Steam enters at top of chamber to displace air or enters after air is withdrawn by vacuum. Air and steam are evacuated at bottom of chamber. Temperature of steam is measured in air-steam drain line near vent.

Many gravity displacement steam sterilizers operate on a standard cycle of 250° to 254° F (121° to 123° C) at a pressure of 15 to 17 pounds per square inch (psi). The size and contents of the chamber determine the exposure period; the minimum exposure time is 15 minutes. Exposure time may vary if a closed sterilization container system is used. Some air-powered instruments may require longer exposure periods at different temperatures. The manufacturer's instructions included with the instrumentation should be consulted for the recommended times and settings for steam sterilization.

Prevacuum Sterilizer In this high-vacuum sterilizer, air is almost completely evacuated from the chamber before the sterilizing steam is admitted. This is accomplished to the desired degree of vacuum by means of a pump and a steam-injector system. A prevacuum period of 8 to 10 minutes effectively removes the air to minimize the steam penetration time. The steam injector preconditions the load and helps eliminate air from the packages. As a result, the sterilizing steam almost instantly penetrates to the center of the packages when admitted to the chamber, because the air has been vacuum-pumped out. If the items in the load are easily penetrable and the sterilizer is functioning properly, there is no demonstrable time difference between complete steam penetration of large or small, tight or loose packages. Therefore the maximum capacity of the sterilizer can be used. A postvacuum cycle draws moisture from the load to shorten the drying time. The Bowie-Dick test is performed daily to ensure that the air vacuum pump is functioning properly.

Temperatures in the prevacuum sterilizer are controlled at 270° to 276° F (132° to 135.5° C) at a pressure of 27 psi. Some prevacuum sterilizers with computer-controlled pulsing air evacuation systems reach temperatures between 275° and 285° F (135° and 141° C). All items are exposed to a temperature of at least 270° F (132° C) for a minimum of 4 minutes. A complete cycle takes approximately 15 to 30 minutes, depending on sterilizer capacity.

Flash/High-Speed Pressure Sterilizer A flash/high-speed pressure sterilizer may have either a gravity displacement or a prevacuum cycle; the gravity displacement cycle is the most common. The flash/high-speed pressure sterilizer operates at a pressure of 27 psi at sea level (or a maximum of 22 psi at 5000 feet above sea level) to increase the temperature in the chamber to between 270° and 275° F (132° and 135° C). The minimum exposure time at this temperature is 3 minutes for unwrapped nonporous, uncomplicated stainless steel items without lumens. When porous items or instruments with instrument marking tape or lumens are included in the load, timing is increased to 4 minutes or longer in a prevacuum sterilizer and to 10 minutes or longer in a gravity displacement sterilizer. With these cycles, the entire time for starting, sterilizing, and opening the sterilizer is a minimum of 6 to 7 minutes. Steam should be maintained in the jacket at all times.

Flash sterilizers should not be used for routine sterilization of complete instrument sets. Flash sterilization in a high-speed pressure sterilizer should be used only in urgent, un-

planned, or emergency situations (e.g., individual items inadvertently dropped or forgotten) for which no alternative method exists. Specially designed surgical suites with in-room sterilizers may provide an acceptable form of flash sterilization. Items to be permanently implanted in the body are not flash sterilized for immediate use unless the results of biologic monitoring are immediately available. Sterility is not ensured without the results of biologic test indicators.

Container systems are available for flash sterilization to protect items during transfer from the sterilizer to the sterile field. The manufacturer of the container should provide scientific evidence of its suitability for the sterilizer in use.

A high-speed pressure sterilizer used for the flash sterilization of unwrapped instruments is physically located in or immediately adjacent to the OR (e.g., the substerile room). A sterile transfer is made from the sterilizer to the sterile field. Transferring the sterilized item to the sterile field without contaminating it is difficult. The following methods may be used for transporting the sterilized instrument to the sterile field:

1. If the OR is connected to the substerile room containing the sterilizer, the sterile scrub person may enter the substerile room, retrieve the sterilized item, and return to the sterile field. The sterile scrub person takes great care not to contaminate his or her gown or gloves in the process. The scrub person uses sterile towels for protection from contact burns from the hot tray.
2. The circulator may use a special open flash-sterilization tray with a detachable handle. With this method, the tray is sterilized with the instrument inside. The inside of the tray is considered sterile. The outside surface is considered contaminated and is not placed in direct contact with the sterile field. When the cycle is complete, the circulator attaches the nonsterile handle to the outside front of the tray and carries it to the scrub person, who in turn retrieves the sterile item without touching the edges of the tray.

   Closed varieties are commercially available that allow an item to be flash sterilized in a covered container. The outside is considered contaminated, but the inside is considered sterile. The circulator removes the lid toward self, touching only the edges. The scrub person reaches inside to remove the sterile item.

Precautions

With all types of steam sterilizers, the following precautions are taken to ensure safe operation:

1. Turn on the valve for steam in the jacket before use. Steam may be kept in the jacket throughout the day. (It may be turned off at the end of the surgical schedule if departmental policy indicates this practice.) The jacket maintains heat, so do not touch the inside of the chamber when loading. Check the sterilizer; not all of them have a steam jacket.
2. Never put heat-sensitive items into a steam sterilizer of any type; they will be destroyed.

3. Close the door tightly before activating either the automatic or the manual controls.
4. Unless it is an automatically controlled device, do not set a manually operated timer until the desired temperature registers on the thermometer and recording graphic chart. Thermometers, not pressure gauges, are the guides for sterilization.
5. Open the door only when the exhaust valve registers zero. Stand behind the door and open it slowly to avoid the steam that may escape around the door.
6. Wash the inside of the chamber according to the manufacturer's directions and with manufacturer-approved solution, rinse it with tap water, and dry it with a lint-free cloth every day. Remove and clean the filtering screen daily. Flush the discharge lines weekly with a hot solution of trisodium phosphate: 1 ounce (30 ml) to 1 quart (1000 ml) of hot water. Follow the flush with a rinse of 1 quart (1000 ml) of tap water.
7. Wipe the gasket daily with a lint-free cloth, and check for signs of wear and defects.
8. Provide routine preventive maintenance, including the evaluation of steam and air purity. The amount of solid, liquid, or vapor contamination in the steam is minimal. An ineffective air filter may contaminate a load when air is drawn into the chamber at the end of the cycle. A defective steam trap or clogged exhaust line can cause malfunction. Make sure the thermometer is correctly calibrated.

Preparing Items for Steam Sterilization

For effective steam sterilization, organic material and debris are first removed. Items are thoroughly rinsed and dried after cleaning and before sterilization.

Surgical Instruments   Special attention is given to cleaning surgical instruments before sterilization. Most instruments are made of metal, but many are difficult to clean. Instruments with removable parts should be disassembled, box locks should be opened, and heavy instruments should be placed on the bottom levels of the sterilizer, with lighter instruments on top.

Powered Equipment   Powered equipment should be placed in the cases provided by the manufacturer after appropriate decontamination and lubrication.

Basin Sets   If they are nested (placed one inside another), basins and solid utensils are separated by porous material, such as toweling. This permits the permeation of steam via wicking around all surfaces and the condensation of steam from the inside during sterilization. Sponges and drapes are not packaged in basins because steam could be deflected from penetrating through fabrics.

Drape Packs   Freshly laundered woven fabric drapes and gowns are fanfolded or rolled loosely to provide the least possible resistance to the penetration of steam through each layer of material. Packs must not exceed a maximum size of

12 × 12 × 20 inches (30 × 30 × 50 cm) and must not weigh more than 12 pounds (5.5 kg). Drapes are loosely crisscrossed so they do not form a dense, impermeable mass. Pack density should not exceed 7.2 lb/cu ft (see Box 17-2 for the calculation of density). The inner aspect of the outside wrapper becomes the sterile table drape when the pack is opened.

Rubber Goods and Thermoplastics   A rubber sheet or any other impervious material should not be folded for sterilization because steam can neither penetrate it nor displace air from the folds. It should be covered with a piece of fabric of the same size, loosely rolled, and then wrapped. For example, a layer of roller gauze is rolled between layers of an Esmarch bandage.

The mechanical cleaning of tubing, including catheters and drains, is a factor in reducing the microbial count inside lumen. A residual of distilled water should be left in the lumen of any tubing that is to be steam sterilized by gravity displacement. The residual becomes steam as the temperature rises, which helps to displace air in the lumen and to increase the temperature within it. (This is not necessary in a prevacuum sterilizer.) The tubing should be coiled without kinks.

Detachable rubber or plastic parts should be removed from instruments and syringes for cleaning and sterilizing. Rubber surfaces should not touch metal, glassware, or each other during sterilization; this prevents melting or sticking and permits steam to reach all surfaces. Rubber bands should not be used around solid items because steam cannot penetrate through or under rubber.

Wood Products   During sterilization, lignocellulose resin (lignin) is driven out of wood by heat. This resin may condense onto other items in the sterilizer and cause reactions if it gets into the tissues of a patient. Therefore wooden items are individually wrapped and separated from other items in the sterilizer.

Repeated sterilization dries wood so that during sterilization it adsorbs moisture from the saturated steam. As the water content of the saturated steam decreases, the steam

Box 17-2   Calculation of Density of Drape Pack

$$\frac{\text{Size of pack (in inches)}}{1728 \text{ (in/sq ft)}} = \text{Cubic feet of pack}$$

$$\frac{\text{Weight of pack (in lb)}}{\text{Cubic feet of pack}} = \text{Density factor (lb/cu ft)}$$

Example:

$$\frac{12" \times 12" \times 20"}{1728} = 1.666 \text{ cu ft}$$

$$\frac{12 \text{ lb}}{1.666 \text{ cu ft}} = 7.2 \text{ lb/cu ft (maximum density)}$$

becomes superheated and loses some of its sterilizing power. Because of this problem, the use of wood products that require steam sterilization should be minimized, and their repeated sterilization is avoided.

All Items Whether washed by hand, in a washer-sterilizer or washer-decontaminator, or in an ultrasonic cleaner, all items with detachable or separable parts are disassembled for cleaning, packaging, and sterilizing. Except for perhaps the lumen of tubing, all items are cleaned and dried before steam sterilization. Manuals (which often contain photographs) or index file cards are available in the room in which supplies are packaged; these materials provide ready reference during preparation and for wrapping single items, packs, or trays. Instructions are strictly followed to ensure safety in sterilizing items.

Loading the Sterilizer

All packages are positioned in the chamber to allow free circulation and steam penetration and to prevent the entrapment of air or water. A gravity displacement sterilizer is loaded so that steam can displace air downward and out through the discharge line. Wire mesh or perforated metal shelves separate layers of packages. Shelves may be contained within the chamber on sliding racks or on a transfer carriage. The shelves are loaded and rolled into the sterilizer. Floor loaders are easier to manage than off-floor carriage racks. Steam sterilizers should be loaded as follows:

1. Flat packages of textiles are placed on the shelf on edge so flat surfaces are vertical as shown in Figure 17-4. Instrument trays and closed container systems with perforated bottoms may be laid flat.
2. Large packs are placed 2 to 4 inches apart in one layer only on a shelf. Small packages may be placed on the shelf above with 1 or 2 inches between them. If small packages are placed one on top of another, they should be crisscrossed.
3. Packages must not touch the chamber walls, floor, or ceiling.
4. Rubber goods are placed on edge, loosely arranged and in one layer to a shelf; this allows free steam circulation and penetration. No other articles should be with the rubber goods.
5. Basins and solid containers are placed on their sides to allow air to flow out of them. They should be placed so that, if they contained water, all of it would flow out. If being sterilized in a combined load with fabrics, basins and containers should be placed on the lowest shelf.
6. Solutions are sterilized alone. At the completion of the sterilization cycle, the steam should be turned off and the temperature allowed to drop to 212° F (100° C) before the exhaust is opened; the selector should be set to slow exhaust. This prevents the solutions from boiling over. Allow the pressure gauge to reach zero before opening the door so caps will not pop off.

Figure 17-4 Proper loading of gravity displacement steam sterilizer; packs should be placed on edge, and the rack should not be overloaded. Steam must completely surround and penetrate every package in all sterilizers.

Timing the Load

The timing of a sterilization cycle begins when the desired temperature is reached throughout the chamber. If the sterilizer does not have an automatic timing device with a buzzer that sounds at the end of the cycle, a manual timer can be set after the proper temperature has been reached to time the load and to alert personnel when the cycle is completed.

Materials that need different lengths of exposure to ensure sterilization in a gravity displacement sterilizer should not be combined in the same load if the maximum time needed will be destructive to some items. Items may be sterilized either wrapped or unwrapped, and either alone or in combination with other items. The time of exposure varies according to these factors and the temperature of the steam. The minimum time standards, which are calculated after effective steam penetration of porous materials and the rate of heat transfer through wrapping materials, are listed in Table 17-2.

Most sterilizers are equipped with a graphic recorder and automatic electromechanical or microcomputer time-temperature controls. Some sterilizers print out a computer record to document each load. The time and temperature for each load are recorded for a 24-hour period. The record of each load should be checked before unloading to be certain that the desired temperature was achieved. Also, the temperature being recorded should be checked daily against the thermometer to see that the recording arm is working properly.

Drying the Load

After the sterilizer door is opened, the load of wrapped packages is left untouched to dry for 15 to 60 minutes. The time required for drying depends on the type of sterilizer and the type of supplies in a load. Large packages require a longer time than small ones. The packages are then unloaded onto a table or cart containing wire mesh shelves padded with absorbent material. Warm packages laid on a solid, cold surface become damp from steam condensation and thus contaminated by strike-through (capillary action).

TABLE 17-2	Minimum Exposure Time Standards for Steam Sterilization After Effective Steam Penetration and Heat Transfer		

	Gravity Displacement		Prevacuum
Materials	**250° F (121° C)**	**270° F (132° C)**	**270° F (132° C)**
Basin sets, wrapped	20 minutes	Not applicable	4 minutes
Basins, glassware, and utensils, unwrapped	15 minutes	Not recommended	3 minutes
Instruments, with or without other items, wrapped as set in double-thickness wrappers	30 minutes	Not applicable	4 minutes
Instruments, unwrapped but with other items, including towel in bottom of tray or cover over them	20 minutes	10 minutes	4 minutes
Instruments, completely unwrapped	15 minutes	3 minutes	3 minutes
Drape packs, 12 × 12 × 20 inches (30 × 30 × 50 cm) maximum size, 12 pounds (5.5 kg) maximum weight	30 minutes*	Not applicable	4 minutes
Fabrics, single items wrapped	30 minutes*	Not applicable	4 minutes
Rubber and thermoplastics, including small items and gloves but excluding tubing, wrapped	20 minutes*	Not applicable	4 minutes
Tubing, wrapped	30 minutes	Not applicable	4 minutes
Tubing, unwrapped	20 minutes	Not applicable	4 minutes
Sponges and dressings, wrapped	30 minutes	Not applicable	4 minutes
Solutions, flasked	(Slow exhaust)	Not applicable	Automatic selector determines correct temperature and exposure period for solutions
75-ml flask	20 minutes		
250-ml flask	25 minutes		
500-ml flask	30 minutes		
1000-ml flask	35 minutes		
1500-ml flask	45 minutes		
2000-ml flask	45 minutes		

*Fabrics and rubber deteriorate more rapidly with repeated sterilization for prolonged periods in gravity displacement sterilizer.

Packages are observed for water droplets on the exterior or interior and for absorbed moisture in the package. Packs wrapped in moisture-permeable materials that have water droplets on the outside or inside are unsafe for use because the moisture can be a pathway for microbial migration into the package via capillary action. A package should be considered contaminated if it is wet when opened for use. Packages should be completely dry after cooling at a room temperature of 68° to 75° F (20° to 24° C) for a minimum of 1 hour.

Biologic Testing of the Steam Sterilizer

Biologic test packs for steam sterilizers vary according to the type of sterilizer being tested. Each steam sterilizer is tested at least weekly for routine monitoring and as needed for a challenge test. Many hospitals test sterilizers daily. Because of the variations in sterilizers, the appropriate test is used for each type of sterilizer.

Gravity Displacement Sterilizer With a gravity displacement sterilizer, the test pack is placed on edge in the lower front of the load. This is the coldest area and therefore represents the greatest challenge in sterilization. The

chamber is fully loaded. The contents of the test pack may be any of the following:

- The equivalent of three woven fabric gowns, 12 towels, 30 gauze sponges (4 × 4 inches), five laparotomy tapes (12 × 12 inches), and one woven fabric drape sheet. Two biologic indicators are placed in the center of the pack, with a chemical indicator placed one towel above or below them. The pack is double wrapped. It should have a size of approximately 12 × 2 × 12 × 20 inches (30 × 30 × 50 cm) and should weigh 10 to 12 pounds.
- The equivalent of 16 freshly laundered reusable huck towels or absorbent towels in good condition, each approximately 16 × 26 inches (40 × 66 cm), folded 9 × 9 inches (23 × 23 cm), and stacked with a biologic indicator in the center. The pack is taped to provide a density of 12 lb/cu ft, and it should weigh 3 pounds.
- An equivalent commercial test pack.

Prevacuum Sterilizer With a prevacuum sterilizer, the contents of the test pack with biologic indicators can be the same as for a gravity displacement sterilizer. In addition, a Bowie-Dick test is conducted daily, usually on the first run of the day, to check for air entrapment in the prevacuum sterilizer. A biologic indicator may be put into this test pack. The test pack is placed horizontally on the bottom shelf at the front, near the door, and over the drain of an empty prevacuum chamber. The test pack consists of the following:

- Between 24 and 44 absorbent towels folded in a stack no smaller than 9 × 12 × 11 inches (23 × 30 × 28 cm)
- One Bowie-Dick test sheet placed in the center of the stack
- One double-thickness wrapper

Flash/High-Speed Pressure Sterilizer   For this type of sterilizer, the biologic indicator can be put in the bottom of a tray of unwrapped instruments. It should be positioned in the lower front of the chamber.

Dry Heat Sterilization

Dry heat in the form of hot air is used primarily to sterilize anhydrous oils, petroleum products, and talc, which steam and ethylene oxide gas cannot penetrate. The destruction of microbial life by dry heat is a physical oxidation or slow burning process that involves coagulating the protein in cells. Higher temperatures are required in the absence of moisture because the microorganisms are destroyed through a very slow process of heat absorption by conduction.

Advantages of Dry Heat Sterilization

1. Hot air penetrates certain substances that cannot be sterilized by steam sterilization or another method.
2. Dry heat is a protective method of sterilizing some delicate, sharp, or cutting-edge instruments. Steam may erode or corrode cutting edges.

Disadvantages of Dry Heat Sterilization

1. A long exposure period is required because hot air penetrates slowly and possibly unevenly.
2. The time and temperature required will vary for different substances.
3. Overexposure may ruin some substances.

Types of Dry Heat Sterilizers

Mechanical Convection Oven   The most efficient and reliable dry heat sterilizer is an electrically heated, mechanical convection hot air oven. A blower forces hot air in motion around items in the load to hasten the heating of substances and to ensure a uniform temperature in all areas of the oven.

Early models operated at 320° to 340° F (160° to 171° C) for a period of 1 to 2 hours. Faster portable tabletop models are available; these run at 375° to 400° F (190.5° to 204° C), with total cycle times of 6 minutes for unwrapped items and 12 minutes for wrapped ones. Optional cooling chambers are also available.

Gravity Convection Oven   A conventional gravity displacement steam sterilizer chamber can be used for dry heat sterilization. Heat is provided by steam in the jacket only; this heat may not be evenly distributed throughout the chamber. The hot air rises initially and by gravity displaces cooler air at the bottom of the chamber. The maximum temperature that can be obtained is 250° F (121° C)—or 270° F (132° C) in a high-pressure gravity displacement sterilizer. To ensure adequate heat conduction through all items, the exposure period is a minimum of 6 hours and preferably overnight.

Preparing Items for Dry Heat Sterilization

Oils   The amount of oil—including mineral oil and lubricating oil for electrically powered or air-powered instruments—put into a container should not exceed 1 ounce (30 ml). The depth of the oil is preferably not more than ¼ inch (6.35 mm). The greater the depth, the longer the exposure period.

Talc   A maximum of 5 g to 1 ounce of talc may be spread out in a glass container so the depth of the layer does not exceed ¼ inch (6.25 mm). The lid is secured, with the cap screwed tightly on the bottle or jar, and a dry heat process chemical indicator is affixed to the bottle. The sterilizing cycle for a gravity convection oven (steam sterilizer with steam in the jacket only) should be a minimum of 9 hours at 250° F (121° C) or 6 hours at 270° F (132° C).

An average quantity of 2 to 3 g of talc is usually needed as an intrapleural sclerosing agent. This smaller quantity may be evenly distributed inside a sealed glassine envelope or peel pouch, which is then inserted into a second envelope or pouch. The talc should not accumulate into a mass exceeding ¼ inch (6.25 mm); the package should lie flat in the sterilizer. Prepackaged sterile talc is commercially available.

Packaging Materials for Dry Heat Sterilization

Glass   Petri dishes, ointment jars, flasks, small bottles, or test tubes can be used for dry heat sterilization. Caps or lids are affixed or screwed tightly onto containers.

Stainless Steel Boats or Trays   Covers must fit tightly. They can be held in place with indicator tape.

Aluminum Foil   Foil conducts heat rapidly.

Woven Fabric and Peel Pouches   These materials can be used for wrapping instruments if the temperature in the chamber will not exceed 400° F (204° C). Powders and talc can be put in double glassine envelopes.

Loading the Sterilizer

When loading a dry heat sterilizer, it is necessary to allow space between the items and along the chamber walls so the hot air can circulate freely. The chamber is never loaded to full capacity.

Timing the Load

The time of exposure in a dry heat sterilizer varies depending on the characteristics of individual items, the layer depth in containers, and the temperature in the sterilizer. The timing of exposure begins when the thermometer registers the desired temperature. Items are exposed for the following minimum periods, assuming the amount in each container is kept to a minimum and the sterilizer is loaded according to the manufacturer's recommendations:

- Six minutes unwrapped at 400° F (204° C)
- Twelve minutes wrapped at 375° F (190.5° C)
- One hour at 340° F (171° C), wrapped or unwrapped
- Two hours at 320° F (160° C), wrapped or unwrapped
- Three hours at 285° F (140° C), wrapped or unwrapped
- Six hours at 250° F (121° C), wrapped or unwrapped

Biologic Testing of the Dry Heat Sterilizer

Biologic indicators with spores of *B. subtilis* are used to monitor the dry heat process. Commercially prepared spore strips in glassine envelopes should be used. Each load should be tested and the items quarantined until negative results are confirmed.

CHEMICAL STERILIZATION

The only chemicals used for sterilization are those that are registered as a sterilant by the EPA. They may be approved for use in either a gaseous, plasma, or liquid state.

Ethylene Oxide Gas Sterilization

Ethylene oxide gas is used to sterilize items that are sensitive to heat or moisture. Ethylene oxide (EO or EtO) is a chemical alkylating agent that kills microorganisms (including spores) by interfering with the normal metabolism of protein and reproductive processes, resulting in cell death. Used in the gaseous state, EO must have direct contact with microorganisms on or in the items to be sterilized. EO is highly flammable and explosive in air and therefore must be used in an explosion-proof sterilizing chamber in a controlled environment. When handled properly, EO is reliable and safe for sterilization, but the toxic emissions and residues of EO present health hazards to personnel and patients. Therefore the environment in which EO is used is constantly monitored for unsafe exposure levels.

EO gas sterilization is dependent on four parameters, each of which may be varied. Consequently, EO sterilization is a complex, multiparameter process. Each variable affects the other dependent parameters:

1. *Concentration of EO gas.* Liquefied EO is supplied in high-pressure metal cylinders or disposable cartridges. In the sterilization process, air is withdrawn from the chamber and the EO enters as gas under pressure. The only means for controlling EO concentration is to operate the sterilizer according to the manufacturer's instructions. The operating pressure of the cycle influences the rate of gas diffusion through the items to be sterilized. The absorbency of the items and packaging materials influence the concentration of the gas. EO gas may be diluted or used in pure form:

   a. *CFC-12, also referred to as 12/88.* This is a mixture of 12% ethylene oxide in 88% chlorofluorocarbon (CFC) by weight. Most EO gas sterilizers currently in use utilize this mixture.

   b. *HCFC-124 (trade name: Oxyfume 2000 Sterilant Gas).* Because CFCs cause destruction of the stratospheric ozone shield that protects the earth, 24 nations (including the United States) have signed the Montreal Protocol agreeing to reduce the production of CFCs. By the year 2000, no CFCs will be produced in the United States. HCFC-124 can be used in sterilizers that formerly used CFC. Conversion to this replacement gas requires minor changes in the sterilizing pressure and time, and more gas is used than with CFC. Manufacturers of EO gas sterilizers are researching alternative ozone shield–compatible flame retardants that can be used with no or only a minimal change in procedures and equipment.

   c. *100% EO.* Unit-dose cartridges of 67 g or 134 g pure EO are used in small, self-contained sterilizers. Because pure EO is highly flammable, only a small number of cartridges are kept in inventory.

   d. *EO/CO$_2$, referred to as 10/90.* This is a mixture of 10% ethylene oxide in 90% carbon dioxide. Because of the great pressure differential between EO and carbon dioxide, maintaining a uniform mix is difficult. A higher pressure cycle must be used, and therefore not all devices can be sterilized safely in this mixture.

2. *Temperature.* Temperature influences the destruction of microorganisms and affects the permeability of EO through cell walls and packaging materials. Higher density items and loads require a longer heat-up time. As temperature is increased, exposure time can be decreased. Gas sterilizers operate at temperatures ranging from 85° to 145° F (29° to 63° C). The uppermost limit for many heat-sensitive plastic materials is 140° F (60° C). The temperature in the chamber is raised by the injection of saturated steam.

3. *Humidity.* Moisture is essential in achieving sterility with EO gas. Desiccated or highly dried bacterial spores are resistant to EO gas; they must be hydrated. The moisture content of the immediately surrounding atmosphere and the water content within organisms are important to the action of EO gas. Therefore to hydrate the items during preparation, the relative humidity of the room in which the items are packaged and held for sterilization should be at least 50% and must not be less than 30%. The ability of the item and packaging material to absorb moisture affects the humidification

and diffusion of gas during the sterilization process. A humidity level of 30% to 80% is maintained throughout the cycle; excessive moisture will inhibit sterilization. Saturated steam provides the necessary humidity.

4. *Time.* The time required for the complete destruction of microorganisms is primarily related to the concentration and temperature of the gas. The cleanliness of items, type of materials, arrangement of load, and rate of penetration also influence exposure time. Drawing an initial vacuum at the start of the cycle aids in penetration of the gas.

Advantages of Ethylene Oxide Gas Sterilization

1. EO gas is an effective substitute agent to use with most items that cannot be sterilized by heat, such as plastics with low melting points.
2. EO gas provides an effective method of sterilization for items that steam and moisture may erode; it is noncorrosive and does not damage items.
3. EO gas completely permeates all porous materials; it does not penetrate metal, glass, and petroleum-based lubricants. Whether or not it penetrates oils, liquids, or powder depends on the amount in the containers. If the material is spread thin, the gas will penetrate; it will not go through bulk. EO gas sterilization is not recommended for oils, liquids, and powder (including talc).

    Solutions in glass ampules can be sterilized in EO because the gas does not penetrate glass. But a glass vial with a rubber stopper must not be put in the sterilizer because the gas will penetrate the rubber and may react with the drugs in solution and cause a potentially harmful chemical reaction.
4. Automatic controls preclude human error by establishing proper levels of pressure, temperature, humidity, and gas concentration. The sterilizer is operated according to the manufacturer's instructions.
5. EO gas leaves no film on items.
6. EO gas sterilization is used extensively in the preparation of commercially available, packaged, presterilized items, because packaging materials that prolong storage life can be used.

Disadvantages of Ethylene Oxide Gas Sterilization

1. EO gas sterilization is a complicated process that is carefully monitored.
    a. An item that can be safely steam sterilized should never be gas sterilized.
    b. Biologic tests, chemical indicators, sterilizer operation, and maintenance records should be reviewed to verify the adequacy of every cycle.
    c. Implants should not be used until the results of biologic testing are known—a minimum of 48 hours.

    d. Items are completely aerated before use to eliminate harmful residues.
2. EO sterilization takes longer than steam sterilization; it is a long, slow process.
3. EO gas requires special, expensive equipment. Gas is somewhat expensive per cycle.
4. Items that absorb EO gas during sterilization, such as rubber, polyethylene, or silicone, require an aeration period (see Table 17-3). Air admitted to the sterilizer at the end of the cycle only partially aerates the load.
5. Toxic by-products can be formed in the presence of moisture droplets during the exposure of some plastics, particularly polyvinyl chloride.
6. Repeated sterilization can increase the concentration of the total EO residues in porous items. These increased levels can be hazardous unless the gas can be dissipated.
7. EO is a vesicant when in contact with skin and mucous membranes.
    a. Liquid EO may cause serious burns if not removed immediately by thorough washing.
    b. Gloves made of neoprene, polyvinyl fluoride, nitryl or butyl rubber, or other material known to be impermeable to EO penetration should be worn for handling sterilized packages before aeration. If thick cotton gloves are worn, they should be placed in the aerator between uses.
    c. Personnel who wear contact lenses, especially soft lenses, should wear protective goggles when working around EO sterilizers to avoid eye irritation.
8. Inhaled EO gas can be irritating to mucous membranes. It is a colorless gas, but its presence is easily detectable by odor. Overexposure causes nasal and throat irritation. Prolonged exposure may result in nausea, vomiting, dizziness, difficulty breathing, and peripheral paralysis.
    a. Immediately following the completion of each cycle, the sterilizer door should be opened approximately 2 inches and the area cleared of all personnel for 15 minutes before unloading.
    b. Loading carts should be pulled, not pushed, from the sterilizer to the aerator. Air currents flowing over the load may accumulate a residual gas that could be inhaled.
9. Long-term exposure to EO is known to be a potential occupational carcinogen, causing leukemia. It is also a mutagen, causing spontaneous abortion, genetic defects, chromosomal damage, and neurologic dysfunction.
    a. The standards of the Occupational Safety and Health Administration (OSHA) limit an employee's exposure to ethylene oxide to 1 part per million (ppm) of air averaged over an 8-hour period to an active level of 0.5 ppm, and to a short-term limit of 5 ppm averaged over a 15-minute period. The short-term limit addresses exposure to bursts of gas, such as when opening a sterilizer. Breathing zone sampling is performed daily throughout an 8-hour shift on at least one employee for each job classification of exposed personnel. Passive dosimeter badges are the most popular

monitoring devices for personnel. Chromographs and other types of detectors are used for continuous gas analysis of the environment.

b. EO gas is vented from the sterilizer to the outside atmosphere to avoid personnel exposure. Audible and visual alarm systems should be installed to indicate a failure in the ventilation system. Most sterilizers have an exhaust hood over the sterilizer door.

c. The sterilizer door has locking and sealing mechanisms. The integrity of the seals are checked regularly. Automatic controls must function properly so the door cannot be opened until the gas is evacuated from the chamber.

Types of Ethylene Oxide Gas Sterilizers

The capacity of EO chambers varies from approximately 2 cu ft (57.5 L) in a tabletop size of 12 × 12 × 24 inches (30 × 30 × 60 cm) to very large floor loading units that are 28 × 67 × 78 inches (72 × 170 × 198 cm). These chambers automatically control gas concentration, temperature, humidity, and time. Most models have vacuum pumps to evacuate air from the chamber and steam ejectors to humidify and increase temperature. Microcomputer controls and digital printouts of cycle parameters provide evidence of proper operation. A purge cycle follows the timed gas exposure cycle to vent the chamber of airborne residual gas. Some chambers are a combination sterilizer/aerator, which eliminates the need for personnel to handle the load immediately after sterilization; the load is removed only after aeration.

Preparing Items for Ethylene Oxide Gas Sterilization

All Items All items to be sterilized with EO gas are thoroughly cleaned and dried. Detachable parts are disassembled, and syringes are separated. Impermeable items such as caps, plugs, and stylets are removed. All items must be completely dry.

Lumens Any tubing or other item with a lumen should be blown out with air to force it dry before packaging because water combines with EO gas to form ethylene glycol, a harmful acid.

Lensed Instruments Endoscopes with cemented optical lenses require special cement for EO gas sterilization.

Lubricated Instruments All traces of lubricant, especially petroleum-based lubricants, should be removed before sterilization. EO cannot permeate the film of the lubricant.

Camera As a permanent record or teaching aid, photographs are sometimes taken at the surgical site with a sterile, specially constructed camera. Some cameras and film can be sterilized with EO gas. The film is loaded before packaging for sterilization.

Packaging Materials for Ethylene Oxide Gas Sterilization

The type and thickness of the wrapper, the size and shape of the package, and the porosity of the contents used influence the time it takes for the EO gas to penetrate. Items wrapped for EO gas sterilization should be tagged for gas to prevent them from being inadvertently steam sterilized and damaged. Materials used for wrapping items are permeable to EO gas and water vapor and allow effective aeration. The materials discussed in the following sections are acceptable.

Woven Fabric Reusable double-thickness woven fabrics are used as they are for steam, with the same advantages and disadvantages.

Nonwoven Fabric Tyvek spunbonded olefin and other high-density polyethylene fabrics are highly permeable to EO and moisture. These single-use disposable wrappers offer the same advantages as the nonwoven fabrics described for use in steam, but not all of them can be used interchangeably; the cellulose/nylon/rayon combination should be used only for steam sterilization. Packages should be sequentially single wrapped or double wrapped or the material used according to the manufacturer's recommendations.

Peel Packs and Pouches Double wrapping may not allow adequate penetration of the gas and moisture. Peel pouches with either coated or uncoated paper on one side and coated Mylar on the other are generally acceptable for most gas sterilizers, and they allow visualization of contents. The manufacturer's instructions should be checked.

Materials not to be used for EO sterilization because of inadequate permeability include nylon, polyvinyl chloride film, saran, polyester, polyvinyl alcohol, cellophane, and aluminum foil. Combinations of materials that make a package insufficiently permeable for adequate humidification, gas penetration, and aeration are avoided.

Loading the Sterilizer

All packages are positioned in the chamber to allow free circulation and penetration of gas. Overloading creates conditions that can slow the penetration of EO gas, moisture, and heat. Air space should be provided between the chamber ceiling and the uppermost packages in the load, and packages should not touch the chamber walls and floor. Packages should not be stacked tightly; space is allowed between them. If paper/plastic pouches are used, the packages are placed on edge, with the plastic side of one facing the paper side of another.

Timing the Load

The timing of the EO cycle varies depending on the size of the chamber, the contents of the load, gas concentration, temperature, and humidity. For example, a cool cycle at 99° F (37° C) may require more than 5 hours, whereas the same load at 131° F (55° C) may take less than 3 hours. The instructions provided by the manufacturer of the sterilizer should be followed closely.

Aerating Items Following Ethylene Oxide Gas Sterilization

EO gas exerts toxic effects on living tissue. Therefore, following EO gas sterilization, adequate aeration is absolutely essential for all absorbent materials that will come in contact with skin or tissues, either directly or indirectly. Residual products after sterilization can include the following:

1. *Ethylene oxide.* Porous materials, such as plastic, silicone, rubber, wood, and leather, absorb a certain amount of gas that must be removed. The thicker the walls of items, the longer the aeration time required. Residual EO gas in plastic tubing or in parts of a heart-lung pump oxygenator causes hemolysis of blood. Rubber gloves or shoes worn immediately after exposure can cause irritation or burns on skin. The following are acceptable limits for residual EO:
   a. 25 ppm for blood dialysis units, blood oxygenators, heart-lung machines, and all implants
   b. 250 ppm for all topical medical devices
2. *Ethylene glycol.* Ethylene glycol is formed by a reaction of EO gas with water or moisture; this reaction leaves a clear or brownish oily film on exposed surfaces. This substance causes hemolysis of the red blood cells. It also can cause irritation to the mucous membranes if left on plastic or rubber endotracheal tubes or airways. The following are acceptable limits of ethylene glycol:
   a. 250 ppm for blood dialysis units, blood oxygenators, heart-lung machines, and all implants
   b. 1000 ppm for all topical medical devices
3. *Ethylene chlorohydrin.* This by-product is formed when a chloride ion is present to combine with EO, such as in polyvinyl chloride plastic. Rubber, soft nylon, and polyethylene items that have been in contact with saline solution or blood can retain enough chloride ions to cause this reaction in the presence of moisture. To avoid this hazard, disposable products should be discarded after use. The following are acceptable limits of ethylene chlorohydrin:
   a. 25 ppm for blood dialysis units, blood oxygenators, heart-lung machines, and all implants
   b. 250 ppm for all topical medical devices

Residuals are expressed as the weight of EO gas remaining in the item divided by the weight of the item. For example, 25 ppm in a device weighing 2500 g (approximately 5½ pounds) equals 0.01 mg of EO. Residues cannot be removed by rinsing items in water or liquids.

To purge residual gas, air is admitted into the chamber at the end of the sterilization cycle. In sterilizers with a pulse-purge cycle, the air is admitted and immediately removed as many as six times in 30 minutes. Additional aeration is required for all wrapped and porous items. Aeration to diffuse any residual products may be accomplished with ambient (room) air or preferably with an aerator chamber designed for this purpose.

Manufacturers of products suitable for EO sterilization should provide written instructions for the sterilizing cycle and for aerating. The available recommendations are followed. Polyvinyl chloride is one of the most difficult materials to aerate. If the composition of an item is not known, the minimum time for polyvinyl chloride should be followed (Table 17-3). Aeration time depends on the following:

- Composition, density, porosity, weight, and configuration of the item

TABLE 17-3	Minimum Aeration Times Following Ethylene Oxide Sterilization at Different Temperatures		
	Ambient Room Air	**Mechanical Aerator**	
Materials	**65°-72° F (18°-22° C)**	**122° F (50° C)**	**140° F (60° C)**
Metal and glass			
Unwrapped	May be used immediately		
Wrapped	2 hours	2 hours	2 hours
Rubber for external use—not sealed in plastic	24 hours	8 hours	5 hours
Polyethylene and polypropylene for external use—not sealed in plastic	48 hours	12 hours	8 hours
Plastics except polyvinyl chloride items—not sealed in plastic	96 hours (4 days)	12 hours	8 hours
Polyvinyl chloride	168 hours (7 days)	12 hours	8 hours
Plastic and rubber items—those sealed in plastic and/or those that will come in contact with body tissues	168 hours (7 days)	12 hours	8 hours
Internal pacemaker	504 hours (21 days)	32 hours	24 hours

- Packaging material
- Sterilizing conditions, such as the size of the load, the nature of the items in it, and variable required factors
- Aeration conditions, such as ambient vs. mechanical airflow and temperature
- Acceptable limits of residual products for the intended use of the item, such as external application or internal implantation

Aeration at an elevated temperature enhances the dissipation rate of absorbed gas, which results in faster removal. The entire load on the sterilizer carriage can be transferred into an aerator. A blower system draws air in from the outside to the heater in the upper part of the chamber to maintain a minimum rate of four air exchanges per minute. The aerator is vented to the outside atmosphere. Items cannot be safely used until they have been completely aerated.

All materials remain in the aerator for 8 hours at 140° F (60° C) to 12 hours at 120° F (50° C) or longer, depending on temperature and the instructions of the manufacturer of the aerator or item. In a combination sterilizer/aerator, aeration time varies according to temperature and airflow (e.g., 12 hours at 130° F [55° C] or 32 hours at 100° F [38° C]).

If an aerator is not available, packages may be moved on a cart or in a basket from the sterilizer into a well-ventilated clean storage area that has at least 10 air exchanges per hour. The cart should be pulled, not pushed, to this area to avoid being downwind of the EO gas adhering to the wrappers. Aeration time is prominently noted on the cart or basket. At a room temperature controlled between 65° and 72° F (18° and 22° C), a minimum aeration time of 168 hours (7 days) is required for polyvinyl chloride and plastic and rubber items sealed in plastic packages and for porous items that (1) will come in direct contact with blood; (2) will be implanted, inserted, or applied to body tissues; or (3) will be used for assisted respiration. Unwrapped, nonporous metal and glass may be handled immediately. Wrapped metal should be aerated for at least 2 hours. Intravenous or irrigation fluids in plastic containers must not be stored in a room where gas-sterilized items are aerating, because the residual diffusing gas could be absorbed through the plastic.

Biologic Testing of the Ethylene Oxide Gas Sterilizer

Biologic indicators carrying spores of *B. subtilis* are used to monitor EO gas sterilizers. Each sterilizer is tested in each load. Every load containing implantable devices should be tested. An implant should not be used until the test results are negative. The manufacturer's recommendations should be followed for the use of biologic test packs for EO gas sterilizers.

Formaldehyde Gas Sterilization

Formaldehyde kills microorganisms by coagulating the protein in cells. Used as a fumigant in gaseous form, formalde-hyde sterilization is more complex and less efficacious than other methods of sterilization. It should be used only if steam under pressure will damage the item to be sterilized and if EO gas and glutaraldehyde are not available. The use of formaldehyde for sterilization has been almost abandoned in the United States, Canada, and Australia. The method dates back to 1820, and it is still used in Europe and Asia.

Formaldehyde sterilization depends on gas concentration, temperature, humidity, and time. Formalin solution is heated in the Chemiclave sterilizer to produce fumes. The temperature is raised to at least 122° F (50° C) and may be raised as high as 176° F (80° C) by introducing saturated steam. The steam also humidifies the load. Humidity is close to 100% for gas penetration. A filtering system removes the residual condensate and formaldehyde and the odor of residual aeration vapors. The type of items, the size of the load, and the exchange of air and gas influence the time of the cycle. A cycle with a gas concentration of 40 to 80 mg/L (0.23% formaldehyde) at 131° F (55° C) will take 2 to 12 hours. Time may be decreased as temperature is increased.

Advantages of Formaldehyde Gas Sterilization

1. Formaldehyde can be used for heat-sensitive items.
2. It is nonexplosive and nonflammable.
3. It is noncorrosive.

Disadvantages of Formaldehyde Gas Sterilization

1. Formaldehyde is toxic. It is a potent allergen and is mutagenic and carcinogenic. An 8-hour exposure of 1 ppm in air is the accepted limit in several countries.
2. Formaldehyde has an unpleasant odor, and its fumes are irritating to the eyes and mucous membranes.
3. The residue of a gray or white film needs to be removed to prevent tissue irritation. Porous items are aerated.
4. Microorganisms must be hydrated for sterilization to be effective.

Considerations for Formaldehyde Gas Sterilization

1. Before sterilization, all items are thoroughly cleansed of organic material. The lumens of endoscopes and woven catheters should be blown out with air to force-dry them.
2. Paper, plastic, and a combination of paper and plastic pouches and tubes may be used as they are for EO gas sterilization.
3. Loading the sterilizer, timing the cycle, and aerating items should be carried out according to instructions provided by the manufacturer of the sterilizer.
4. Either *B. stearothermophilus* or *B. subtilis* biologic indicators can be used to monitor the process.

Hydrogen Peroxide Plasma/Vapor Sterilization

Hydrogen peroxide can be activated to create a reactive plasma or vapor. Plasma is a state of matter distinguishable from a solid, liquid, or gas. It can be produced through the action of either a strong electrical or magnetic field, somewhat like a neon light. The cloud of plasma created consists of ions, electrons, and neutral atomic particles that produce a visible glow. Free radicals of the hydrogen peroxide in the cloud interact with cell membranes, enzymes, or nucleic acids to disrupt the life functions of microorganisms. The plasma and vapor phases of hydrogen peroxide are highly sporicidal, even at a low concentration and temperature. The sterilizer chambers are simple in design, but the process of the sterilization cycle differs with the method used to convert hydrogen peroxide into plasma or vapor.

Advantages of Hydrogen Peroxide Sterilization

1. The process is dry and nontoxic.
2. The by-products of oxygen and water vapor are safely evacuated into the room atmosphere.
3. Aeration is not necessary.
4. A low temperature allows the safe sterilization of some heat-sensitive items, including endoscopes and fiberoptic devices.
5. Plasma has significantly less effect on metal than steam sterilization; corrosion does not occur on moisture-sensitive microsurgical and powered instruments.
6. The sterilizer is simple in design and connects to standard electrical outlets.

Disadvantages of Hydrogen Peroxide Sterilization

1. Metal trays block radiofrequency waves.
2. Hydrogen peroxide is not compatible with cellulose (i.e., woven textiles with cotton fibers and paper products).
3. Nylon becomes brittle after repeated exposure to hydrogen peroxide sterilization.

Low Temperature Gas Plasma Sterilizers

Sterrad by Advanced Sterilization Systems

This sterilizer connects to a standard electrical outlet. The supplies are placed in the chamber, and a strong vacuum is created. A solution of water and 58% hydrogen peroxide is vaporized by radiofrequency energy to create a pink, glowing reactive plasma. The reactive particles in the plasma are maintained at 104° F (40° C) and sterilize the heat- and moisture-sensitive load in approximately 1 hour. No aeration is necessary because the by-product is primarily oxygen and water.

Vapor Phase Sterilizer   A vacuum is created in the chamber for delivery of a cold vapor of hydrogen peroxide at 39° to 46° F (4° to 8° C). A vacuum exhausts vapor at the end of the cycle.

Considerations for Hydrogen Peroxide Sterilization

1. All items are thoroughly clean, free of organic debris, and dry.
2. Items are wrapped in nonwoven polypropylene. Tyvek peel pouches may be used.
3. The timing of the cycle varies with the process, capacity of the chamber, and contents of the load. The manufacturer's instructions are followed.
4. Biologic indicators with spores of *B. stearothermophilus* are used to monitor the hydrogen peroxide process.

Ozone Gas Sterilization

Ozone sterilizes by oxidation, a process that destroys organic and inorganic matter. It penetrates the membrane of cells, causing them to explode. Ozone is an unstable gas but can be generated easily from oxygen and water.

Advantages of Ozone Gas Sterilization

1. The sterilizer generates its own agent using hospital oxygen, water, and the electrical supply. It is simple and inexpensive to operate.
2. Ozone gas sterilization provides an alternative to EO gas sterilization of many heat- and moisture-sensitive items.
3. Ozone gas sterilization does not affect titanium, chromium, silicone, neoprene, and Teflon.
4. Aeration is not necessary; ozone leaves no residue and converts to oxygen in a short time.

Disadvantages of Ozone Gas Sterilization

1. Ozone can be corrosive. It will oxidize steel, iron, brass, copper, and aluminum.
2. It destroys natural rubber, such as latex, natural fibers, and some plastics.

Types of Ozone Sterilizers

A generator converts oxygen from a source within the hospital to ozone. A 6% to 12% concentration of ozone continuously flows through the sterilization chamber. The penetration of ozone may be controlled by a vacuum in the chamber or enhanced by adding humidity. When the exposure time is complete, the ozone is converted back into oxygen and is safe for release into room air. The cycle time may be up to 60 minutes depending on the size of the chamber or load.

Considerations for Ozone Sterilization

Preparing items, packaging, loading the sterilizer, and timing the cycle are done according to the instructions provided by the manufacturer of the sterilizer. *B. stearothermophilus* biologic indicators can be used to monitor the process.

Chemical Sterilants in Solution

Liquid chemical agents registered as sterilants by the EPA provide an alternative method for sterilizing minimally invasive, heat-sensitive items if a gas or plasma sterilizer is not available or if the aeration period makes EO gas sterilization impractical. Items are categorized as critical, semicritical, and noncritical according to the risk of infection to the patient. Items that enter tissue or the vascular system are considered critical and should be sterile. Items are sterilized with a liquid sterilant by immersing them in solution for the required time specified by the manufacturer to be sporicidal (i.e., to kill spores). All chemical solutions have advantages and disadvantages, and each sterilant has specific assets and limitations. Additional information is available at **www.fda. gov/cdrh/ode/germlab.html.**

Advantages of Chemical Sterilants

1. The solution has a low surface tension; it penetrates into crevices and is readily rinsed from items.
2. It is noncorrosive, nonstaining, and safe for instruments that can be immersed in a chemical solution.
3. It does not damage lenses or cement on lensed endoscopes.
4. It is not absorbed by rubber or plastic.
5. It has low volatility and is stable for the time specified by the manufacturer.

Disadvantages of Chemical Sterilants

1. Prolonged exposure to a chemical sterilant may be necessary for sterilization.
2. Some chemical sterilants have hazardous effects associated with exposure.
3. Even though the chemical has low toxicity and irritation, items must be thoroughly rinsed in sterile distilled water before use.
4. Failure to adequately rinse an endoscope can cause a chemically induced colitis.
5. Sterile transfer is difficult because items are wet.
6. Chemically sterilized items cannot be held in long-term sterile storage.
7. The solution can become diluted during use if an item is wet when placed in it.

Types of Chemical Sterilants

In addition to EPA registration, chemical sterilants are approved by the Food and Drug Administration (FDA) as a method of sterilization for critical items that are heat sensitive and can be immersed. The manufacturer is responsible for providing processing instructions on the container label, and the user is obligated to follow the instructions.

Acetic Acid   Acetic acid mixed with a solution of salts (Bionox) kills microorganisms by a process of oxidation to denature proteins. The process takes 20 minutes at room temperature 77° F (25° C). The solution is supplied in unit doses for each cycle.

Formaldehyde   A 37% aqueous solution (formalin) or 8% formaldehyde in 70% isopropyl alcohol kills microorganisms by coagulating protein in the cells. The solution is effective at room temperature. Formaldehyde has a pungent odor and is irritating to the eyes and nasal passages. Its vapors can be toxic.

Glutaraldehyde   According to the FDA, a 2.4%, 2.5%, or 3.4% aqueous solution of activated, buffered alkaline glutaraldehyde kills microorganisms by the denaturation of protein in cells. The solution is activated by adding a powdered buffer to the liquid. Alkaline glutaraldehyde solution changes pH and gradually loses its effectiveness after the date of activation. The expiration date specified by the manufacturer is marked on the container when activated (e.g., 14 or 28 days for aqueous Cidex activated dialdehyde solution). The solution is reusable until this date, after which it is discarded according to EPA requirements. In most locales, it may be discarded into the sanitary sewer, where it is bioxidized by sewer microorganisms into glutaric acid and then into carbon dioxide and water.

Most manufacturers claim that glutaraldehyde is a sterilant at 10 hours and a high-level disinfectant at 25 to 30 minutes, although the long-life varieties require 90 minutes to attain the same level of disinfection. These solutions are effective at room temperature 77° F (25° C).

Glutaraldehyde vaporizes rapidly. The fumes may have a mild odor and can be irritating to the eyes, nose, and throat. Although it is not classified as a teratogen, carcinogen, or mutagen, OSHA has established an exposure limit of 0.2 ppm in room air averaged over 8 hours. A glutaraldehyde exposure monitor should be worn by personnel who are at risk. Nitrile or butyl rubber or polyethylene gloves are worn to prevent skin sensitivity and contact dermatitis. Double gloving with latex provides protection. Neoprene and polyvinyl chloride gloves are not protective.

The concentration of glutaraldehyde in solution should be monitored. A test strip or kit of reagents is used for testing the concentration before and after each use. If the solution has become diluted below 1.5%, it is ineffective and should be discarded.

Peracetic Acid   A proprietary (Steris) chemical formulation of 35% peracetic acid, hydrogen peroxide, and water inactivates critical microbial cell systems. Peracetic acid is an acetic acid plus an extra oxygen atom that reacts with most cellular components to cause cell death. The mechanism may vary with each type of cell (e.g., vegetative bacterial spores, mycobacterium). The sterilant is supplied in unit doses for each cycle and is diluted during the sterilization process to 0.2% peracetic acid solution. During the 20- to 30-minute sterilization process, the solution is heated to 122° to 131° F (50° to 56° C) as it passes through the self-contained processing chamber. All items and internal components of the Steris unit are submerged in the heated sterilant.

On completion of the sterilizing cycle, the sterilant is discharged into the sanitary drain. The used chemical is not considered a hazardous material by the EPA. The instruments are automatically rinsed in tap water that is filtered through two external prefilters and a 0.22 μm internal microfiltration system. The smallest known bacterium, *Pseudomonas diminuta,* is unable to pass through the pores in this filter system. (This is the same method used by pharmaceutical manufacturers to make sterile injectable medications.)

The Steris unit uses a standard tap water supply, a sanitary drain, and a 110-volt electrical connection. This tabletop unit has a printout to document each cycle. Periodic maintenance includes filter changes based on the chemical components of the external water supply. Biologic monitoring according to the manufacturer's recommendation is performed daily with a commercially prepared spore strip containing *B. subtilis* or *B. stearothermophilus.*

Containers for Chemical Sterilization

With chemical sterilization, items are completely immersed in solution and in lumens filled with solution. The container is deep enough for total immersion. Trays or buckets with perforated liners and lids are convenient for solutions used at room temperature. A sterile container is preferable to facilitate the removal of items without contamination. The inside of the container and its lid should be kept sterile throughout the duration of use of the solution. Containers should also be kept covered to prevent evaporation and to minimize vaporization of the solution. Formaldehyde and glutaraldehyde solutions are used in a well-ventilated room.

Preparing Items for Sterilization by Chemical Immersion

Items should be clean and free of organic debris and blood. Glutaraldehyde will attack some organic materials. It remains highly active in the presence of protein matter in serum, mucus, and soap films. The human hepatitis virus cannot be isolated, so the removal of blood is critical. Items should be washed thoroughly in a nonfilming solution and rinsed; the items are thoroughly dried before submersion so the solution will not become diluted.

Timing the Immersion Cycle

The time required for sterilization varies with the sporicidal activity of the chemical agent:

- Acetic acid: 20 minutes at 77° F (25° C)
- Formalin, formaldehyde, and other glutaraldehydes: 12 hours at 77° F (25° C)
- Cidex solution: 10 hours at 77° F (25° C)
- Peracetic acid: 12 minutes at 131° F (55° C)

A load control record of the items sterilized in solution is kept as for other methods of sterilization (see the sample record in Box 18-2).

Rinsing Following Immersion

All items are thoroughly rinsed in sterile distilled water before use, except in the Steris unit. Sterile gloves are worn to transfer items from the solution to the container for rinsing. Items should then be dried with a sterile towel before being transferred to or placed on a sterile field.

RADIATION STERILIZATION

Microwave Sterilization

The nonionizing radiation of microwaves produces hyperthermic conditions that disrupt life processes. This heating action affects water molecules and interferes with cell membranes. Microwave sterilization uses low-pressure steam with the nonionizing radiation to produce the localized heat that kills microorganisms. The temperature is lower than conventional steam, and the cycle is faster—as short as 30 seconds. Metal instruments can be sterilized if placed under a partial vacuum in a glass container. Small tabletop units may be useful for rapid sterilization of a single instrument or a small number of instruments. Current models have a small chamber size—1 to 3 cubic feet.

Gamma Ray Sterilization

Some commercially available products are sterilized by irradiation. Ionizing radiation produces ions by knocking electrons out of atoms. These electrons are knocked out so violently that they strike an adjacent atom and either attach themselves to it or dislodge an electron from the second atom. The ionic energy that results becomes converted to thermal and chemical energy. This energy kills microorganisms by disrupting the DNA molecule, thus preventing cellular division and the propagation of biologic life.

The principal sources of ionizing radiation are beta particles and gamma rays. Beta particles are free electrons and are transmitted through a high-voltage electron beam from a linear accelerator. These high-energy free electrons penetrate into matter before being stopped by collisions with other atoms. Thus their usefulness in sterilizing an object is limited by the density and thickness of the object and by the energy of the electrons. They produce their effect by ionizing the atoms they hit, producing secondary electrons that, in turn, produce lethal effects on microorganisms.

Cobalt-60 is a radioactive isotope capable of disintegrating to produce gamma rays and is the most commonly used source for irradiation sterilization. Gamma rays are electromagnetic waves and have the capability of penetrating to a much greater distance than beta rays before losing their energy from collisions. Because they travel at the speed of light, they must pass through a thickness of several feet before making sufficient collisions to lose all of their energy.

Irradiation sterilization with beta or gamma rays is limited to industrial use. Depending on the strength of the source, the product is exposed to radiation for 10 to 20 hours.

Ionizing radiation penetrates most materials to sterilize reliably. However, the physical properties of some materials are altered by exposure to ionizing radiation, thus limiting its use. Irradiation can be used to sterilize heat- and moisture-sensitive items, because the rays have a very low temperature effect on materials and because the process is dry. Because gamma rays can penetrate large bulky objects, cartons ready for shipment can be sterilized in the cobalt 60 irradiator; this is cost-effective for the manufacturer.

Ionizing radiation is the most effective sterilization method. No residual radiation is generated. The process may be monitored with biologic indicators using *Bacillus pumilus*. However, products can be released for use on the basis of dosimetry (measurements of radiation dose) without the quarantine periods required for biologic testing.

CONTROL MEASURES

With the exception of items sterilized in a high-speed pressure flash steam sterilizer or by immersion in a chemical solution, all items are wrapped before sterilization. The integrity of the packaging material is maintained before use and during storage. Packages are labeled so the contents are known (unless they are visible through the packaging material). The label also includes the conditions of sterilization. A chemical indicator on each package verifies exposure to a sterilization process.

Load Control Number

Whether sterilized on or off site, a load control number should be imprinted on or be part of the label on every package of sterile items. This number designates the sterilization equipment used, the cycle, and the sterilization date. For sterilizers with microcomputer processor printouts, a label gun correlates the same control number for every package put in the load. Load control numbers are used to facilitate the identification and retrieval of supplies, if necessary, in the event of a sterilization failure. A load control number should also be assigned to items immersed in a chemical sterilant.

The sterilization date can be recorded as a Julian date (day 1 through 365) or as a Georgian date (month, day, year). An undated package is not considered sterile. The package may be stamped with the date of sterilization as it is removed from the sterilizer. The date also may be written or affixed on the package when it is wrapped. Monthly, color-coded, machine-labeling systems may be used. Peel-off bar code labels also help to control inventory and patient charges for items.

Wet Packs

All sterilizing methods in which humidity, usually steam, is a parameter of the process potentially present the hazard of producing wet packages. Microorganisms migrate easily through moisture when a pathway is provided from outside to inside a package. Water droplets may be visible on the outside or in-side, or absorbed moisture may be seen or felt. Unless the wrapper is completely impermeable to water, a pack should be considered unsterile and unacceptable for use if it is wet. A stain on a wrapper may indicate that moisture was present and has dried. The cause of the wet pack is investigated and promptly corrected. Reprocessing is necessary for a wet package or a load with one or more wet or suspect packages.

Causes/Conditions of Wet Packs

Excessive moisture may be related to the steam itself, to the load, or to the sterilizer.

Wet Steam   If the steam is abnormally wet, water droplets may form on the outside or inside of packages, and absorbent materials will become soaked with moisture. At the boiling point, water becomes steam. Saturated steam contains as much water in the vapor state as physically possible (98%) and minimal liquid water (2% water droplets). In a steam sterilizer, pressure increases the temperature to raise the boiling point to 250° F (121° C) or above at a pressure of 15 pounds or more above atmospheric pressure at sea level. The temperature of steam does not increase above the boiling point at normal atmospheric pressure in other types of sterilizers. If steam loses water vapor, it can achieve a higher temperature at the same pressure, thus becoming superheated. In steam sterilization, superheating decreases the effectiveness of steam to kill microorganisms.

The dryness (purity) of steam depends on the amount of water in the vapor state in proportion to the amount of solid, liquid, or vapor contamination. This contamination can come from particles in the boiler, steam lines, or sterilizer; from chemical additives in the water; or from moisture in the load. When steam contacts cold surfaces, a lowering of its temperature reverts steam to water, producing condensation on surfaces and raising the temperature of the remaining vapor, which causes superheating of the steam. Dry, dehydrated textiles and other porous materials will absorb water from steam, which changes the proportion of the water content of steam and causes superheating. The water content of steam should not fall below 97% during the sterilization cycle. Below this level, items in the load can become supersaturated with water, and subsequent drying will be inadequate.

Characteristics of the Load   Many factors affect the penetration of the sterilant through the load. The following characteristics are reiterated for emphasis:

1. Items are cleaned before they are packaged. Nonporous items must be dry. Porous materials, such as woven fabrics, are hydrated (i.e., humidified) but not wet.
2. Basins are separated by absorbent material and positioned so the water condensate will drain out.
3. Heat penetrates different materials at different rates. For even heating of the load, it is preferable not to mix materials. For example, a load may contain only instrument sets and metals or only packs of fabrics.

4. The density of a pack must allow the circulation of air, moisture, and sterilant within the pack. Porous items should not be wrapped tightly.
5. The permeability of packaging materials varies. A water droplet on an impermeable wrapper may not be a problem, but it can be absorbed by an adjacent package with a permeable wrapper.
6. Because condensation diffuses at different rates, the drying and cooling cycle depends on the materials in the load. Packages should not be handled until this cycle is complete.

Sterilizer Malfunctions   Clogged drains, steam traps and air filters, inoperable control valves, worn gaskets, and a dirty chamber can cause the sterilizer to malfunction. Routine cleaning and preventive maintenance techniques are imperative.

Reprocessing Wet Packs

Wet packs are disassembled and the items properly dried and repackaged before resterilization. Reusable woven fabrics should be sent to the laundry and are relaundered before use. Damp or wet fabrics will cause superheating during steam sterilization.

Shelf Life

Sterility is event related; it is not time related unless the package contains unstable components such as drugs or chemicals. Storage conditions are established to maintain the integrity of the package. An item is considered sterile on the basis of the following events:

- Handling of the package during transport and storage (i.e., the prevention of contamination and physical damage)
- Integrity, type, and configuration of packaging material
- Conditions of storage

Specific written policies should address the handling and storage of all stored sterile supplies. Expiration dates should be placed on a tray that contains medications or other unstable supplies. Most commercially sterilized products are considered sterile indefinitely or as long as the integrity of the package is maintained. An expiration date put on the label by the manufacturer indicates the maximum time the manufacturer can guarantee product stability and sterility on the basis of test data approved by the FDA.

Integrity of Packaging Material and Handling

The method of sterilization establishes the type of packaging material that may be used. Shelf life is affected by the permeability and density of the material, the type of closure used, and the method by which the package is handled. The following are considerations regarding the integrity of packaging materials:

1. An item is no longer considered sterile after an accidental puncture, tear, or rupture of the package. Paper may become brittle and crack.
2. Squeezing or crushing a package may force air out and draw unsterile air in, thus contaminating the contents. Packages wrapped in woven fabrics should be handled carefully and not packed tightly together for storage.
3. The accidental wetting of a package contaminates the contents. It is necessary to avoid the following:
   a. Handling the package with moist or wet hands.
   b. Handling the package with soiled gloves.
   c. Placing the package on a wet surface.
4. The density of nonwoven fabrics and plastic materials protects the integrity of the package.
5. Heat- or self-sealed pouches protect the contents from dust.
6. Commercially packaged, sterilized items are usually considered sterile until the package is opened or damaged or the stability of the product becomes outdated.

Dust Cover

A sealed, airtight plastic bag protects a sterile package from dust, dirt, lint, moisture, and vermin during storage. After sterilization and immediately following aerating or cooling to room temperature, infrequently used items may be sealed in plastic 2 to 3 mil thick. A dust cover will protect the integrity of the package.

Storage Conditions

The maintenance of sterility is related to the event and is not based on time. How sterile packages are handled and stored is as important as how long they can remain sterile. The following guidelines are helpful in maintaining the sterility of a package during storage:

1. Storage areas are clean and free of dust, lint, dirt, and vermin. Routine cleaning procedures are followed for all areas in the perioperative environment.
2. All sterile items should be stored under conditions that protect them from the extremes of temperature and humidity. Prolonged storage in a warm environment at high humidity can cause moisture to condense inside packages and thus destroy the microbial barrier of some packaging materials. Ventilating and air-conditioning systems with filtered air should maintain a temperature below 80° F (26° C) and a relative humidity between 30% and 60%. Ten air exchanges per hour are recommended.
3. Packages should be allowed to cool to room temperature before being put into storage to avoid condensation inside the package.

4. Peel pouches should be stored on their sides to minimize the pressure from items stacked on top of them.

5. For open shelving, the highest shelf should be at least 18 inches (46 cm) below the ceiling and 8 to 10 inches (20 to 25 cm) above the floor. Closed cupboards are preferred.

6. Sterile storage areas should have controlled traffic patterns.

Rotation of Supplies

When the standard number of packages kept sterile are adjusted according to daily needs, packages seldom need to be held for prolonged storage periods. In the interest of economy and good management, a stock supply of day-to-day items should be regulated to have enough for the busiest day, with used items replenished daily. Many items are seldom used, yet several are kept sterile at all times. These supplies should be sterilized, or commercially sterilized items ordered, only in quantities sufficient to ensure prompt use and rapid turnover.

Sterile supplies should be checked daily for the integrity of the packages. Some items deteriorate with repeated sterilization or prolonged storage (e.g., latex items). Any sterile packages that become contaminated are reprocessed and resterilized. Older supplies should always be used first to minimize storage. The acronym *FIFO* (first in/first out) is helpful to remember for the rotation of supplies, particularly sterile supplies.

Bibliography

Amsco technique manual, Erie, Penn, 1991, American Sterilizer.

Association for the Advancement of Medical Instrumentation: *AAMI standards and recommended practices for sterilization,* vol 1, *Sterilization,* Arlington, Va, 1992, American National Standards Institute.

Association for the Advancement of Medical Instrumentation: *Chemical sterilants and sterilization methods: a guide to selection and use (TIR7-008-HM),* Arlington, Va, 1990, American National Standards Institute.

Association for the Advancement of Medical Instrumentation: *Good hospital practice: flash sterilization steam sterilization of patient care items for immediate use,* Arlington, Va, 1992, American National Standards Institute.

Association of Operating Room Nurses: *AORN standards, recommended practices, and guidelines,* Denver, 1998, Association of Operating Room Nurses.

Belkin NL: Testing the efficacy of the sterilizer: what does it really prove? *Infect Control Today* 2(8):32, 34, 36, 1998.

Block SS: *Disinfection, sterilization, and preservation,* ed 4, Malvern, Penn, 1991, Lea & Febiger.

Fogg D: Clinical Issues: industry job descriptions, RN name tags, sterilization of wood, shoe covers, laminar airflow systems, *AORN J* 63(5):943-946, 1996.

Jacobs PT: The development of a new low temperature sterilization system, *Infect Control Today* 2(8):38, 40, 42, 43, 1998.

Muscarella LF: Are all sterilization processes alike? *AORN J* 67(5):966, 968-970, 973-976, 1998.

Patterson P: Controversy prompts revision of AAMI's flash sterilization standard, *OR Manager* 10(8):1, 12, 16, 1994.

Reichert M, Young J: *Sterilization technology for the health care facility,* Gaithersburg, Md, 1993, Aspen.

Schroeter K: Implementation of an event-related sterility plan, *AORN J* 60(4):595-602, 1994.

Steelman VM: Infection control, *AORN J* 59(2):476-482, 1994.

Sterilizing talcum powder used in surgery, *OR Manager* 8(7):18-19, 1992.

Chapter 18

Disinfection

 Chapter Objectives

After studying this chapter, the learner will be able to:

- Compare and contrast the three levels of disinfection.
- List several attributes of a hospital-grade disinfectant.
- Identify three safety issues associated with the use of chemical disinfectants.

Terminal decontamination, disinfection, and sterilization are the procedures carried out for the destruction of pathogens on items at the end of use for patient care during a surgical procedure. Methods and procedures for disinfection vary according to the intended use of the disinfected item. Personal protective attire should be worn while using chemical disinfecting agents. Terms associated with disinfection are defined in Box 18-1.

WHEN IS DISINFECTION APPROPRIATE?

Surfaces of items that will penetrate or separate tissue or invade the intravascular system must be sterile to prevent the introduction of potentially harmful microorganisms into the patient's body. Theoretically, all items used in the sterile field should be sterilized. Some specialized instruments and equipment cannot be sterilized between each patient use or will not withstand a sterilization process. Disinfection may be the only alternative. Items that cannot be sterilized by conventional methods discussed in Chapter 17 are disinfected to eliminate as many microorganisms as possible. Disinfection differs from sterilization by its lack of sporicidal power. Disinfection can be accomplished with chemical and physical agents. The application of disinfecting agents depends on the level of risk of infection or environmental contamination.

CLASSIFICATION OF PATIENT CARE ITEMS

Earle H. Spaulding developed a classification system in 1968 to determine the appropriate processing method to attain the desired level of disinfection required for patient care items. This system was adopted and later modified by the Centers for Disease Control and Prevention (CDC).

Critical items must be sterile because they enter sterile tissue, break the mucosal barrier, or come into contact with the vascular system. Examples include surgical instruments, endoscopic accessories that cut tissue, catheters, implants, and needles.

Semicritical items come into contact with nonintact skin and mucous membranes and require high-level disinfection, although they may also be sterilized. Examples include respiratory therapy equipment, anesthesia equipment, bronchoscopes, colonoscopes, gastroscopes, sigmoidoscopes, and cystoscopes.

Noncritical items are used in contact only with intact skin. Intermediate or low-level disinfection is adequate. Examples include blood pressure cuffs, furniture, linens, bedpans, and eating utensils.

Box 18-1
Terms Associated with Disinfection

bactericide   Kills gram-negative and gram-positive bacteria unless specifically stated to the contrary (adj.: *bactericidal*). Action may be specific to a species of bacteria (e.g., pseudomonacide kills *Pseudomonas aeruginosa;* tuberculocide kills *Mycobacterium tuberculosis*).
    fungicide   Kills fungi.
    sporicide   Kills spores.
    virucide   Kills viruses.
bacteriostatic   Inhibits growth of bacteria.
decontamination   Process by which chemical or physical agents are used to clean inanimate, noncritical surfaces. A specific contact time is not specified. A low-level disinfectant is commonly used for this purpose. If a known organism, such as hepatitis B virus (HBV), *M. tuberculosis,* or human immunodeficiency virus (HIV), is present on the surface, an intermediate-level disinfectant should be used.

disinfection   Chemical or physical process of destroying most forms of pathogenic microorganisms except bacterial spores; used for inanimate objects, but not on tissue. The degree of disinfection depends primarily on the strength of the agent, the nature of the contamination, and the purpose for the process.
    high-level disinfection   Process that destroys all microorganisms except high numbers of bacterial spores.
    intermediate-level disinfection   Process that inactivates vegetative bacteria, including *M. tuberculosis* and most fungi and viruses, but does not kill bacterial spores.
    low-level disinfection   Process that kills most bacteria, some viruses, and some fungi, but does not destroy resistant microorganisms, such as *M. tuberculosis* or bacterial spores.
sanitizer   Chemical used on inanimate surfaces to reduce the number of bacteria to a safe level.

LEVELS OF DISINFECTION

Disinfection is the process of destroying or inhibiting growth of pathogenic microorganisms on inanimate objects. It reduces the risk of microbial contamination, but it does not provide the same level of assurance as sterilization. Disinfection levels are classified by the effectiveness of the process (i.e., the ability of the agent to kill microorganisms) as follows:

- *High-level disinfection.* All bacteria, viruses, and fungi are killed. The process may kill spores if contact time is sufficient and other conditions are met. A high-level disinfectant should be used if a semicritical item is disinfected rather than sterilized for use in contact with nonintact skin or mucous membranes. Some chemicals used in high-level disinfection can produce sterilization if they are allow to remain in contact with the surface of the item for the time specified by the manufacturer. For example, exposure of a clean item to 2% glutaraldehyde for 20 minutes at 68° F (20° C) produces high-level disinfection. The item is then rinsed with sterile distilled water. High-level disinfection is not effective against Creutzfeldt-Jakob Disease (CJD). The agent that causes CJD is not a living microorganism like a bacteria or virus. It is a protein, referred to as a prion, that is extremely difficult to inactivate. This is discussed in detail in Chapter 14.
- *Intermediate-level disinfection.* Most bacteria, viruses, and fungi on noncritical items are killed. The process does not attack spores. It does inactivate *Mycobacterium tuberculosis*.
- *Low-level disinfection.* Kills most vegetative bacteria, fungi, and the least resistant viruses on noncritical items, including human immunodeficiency virus (HIV).

Box 18-2
Record for Sterilization or High-Level Disinfection with Chemical Solutions

Date: _____
Solution: Type/agent _____
         Strength _____
         Activation date _____
         Expiration date _____
         Temperature _____
         Immersion: Time in _____
                      Time out _____
Load: Control number _____
      Location _____
      Contents _____
                 _____
                 _____
                 _____

Sterilization is always preferable for critical items. High-level disinfection should not be confused with chemical sterilization. A record of the agent and time of exposure should be maintained for semicritical items that have undergone high-level disinfection (see sample in Box 18-2). The level of disinfection that can be achieved depends on the type and concentration of the agent, contact time, and bioburden. Items that are disinfected are patient safe for their intended uses to minimize risks of infection for the patient. An all-purpose disinfectant does not exist. The best housekeeping agents are not the best disinfectants and vice versa.

PRECLEANING BEFORE DISINFECTION

The Association for Professionals in Infection Control and Epidemiology (APIC) (**www.apic.org**) has established that organic debris and microbial bioburden should be removed before processing by high-level disinfection or sterilization. The biologic soil should be substantially reduced by decontamination so that items are safe to handle. Thorough cleaning is required before items are prepared for disinfection. Precleaning before high-level disinfection may include point-of-use cleaning, presoaking, manual cleaning, ultrasonic cleaning, and/or the use of a washer/decontaminator or washer/sterilizer.

Enzymatic presoaking solutions can be used to cleanse bioburden from instruments and equipment before they are disinfected. Items that are presoaked should be completely rinsed and dried before the disinfection process. Point-of-use cleansing removes gross debris and soil and prevents material from caking and becoming hardened in joints and crevices.

A washer/decontaminator does not reach the same temperature as a washer/sterilizer. It cleans at a maximum temperature of 140° to 180° F (60° to 82° C), rendering the instrument safe to handle without gloves at the end of the cycle. Prewashing by hand is not necessary. The instrument is also milked at the end of the cycle. Some models incorporate ultrasonic capabilities for select loads. The sets can be assembled and prepared for routine sterilization when the process is complete.

A washer/sterilizer requires instruments to be prewashed by hand in germicidal solution at 110° F (44° C) before being placed in the machine. All bioburden must be removed for the washer/sterilizer cycle to be effective. The temperature of the washer/sterilizer ranges from 250° to 280° F (121° to 138° C) and would cause coagulation and crusting of protein. The instruments should be thoroughly rinsed. At the end of the cycle, the instruments may be safely handled without gloves. The sets can be assembled and prepared for routine sterilization.

METHODS OF DISINFECTION

Methods of disinfection include manual wiping with a chemical-impregnated cloth or sponge, soaking by total immersion, or processing by flush-through machinery. The method employed depends on the desired resultant level of disinfection.

Chemical Disinfectants

Chemical agents, including sterilants, are registered with the Pesticide Regulation Division of the Environmental Protection Agency (EPA) to be sold in interstate commerce. An EPA registration number is granted only when requirements of laboratory test data, toxicity data, product formula, and label copy are approved. The product label should indicate sev-

Box 18-3 Information to Look for on a Disinfectant Label

Information About Active Ingredient
Trade and generic name
Concentration or strength
EPA registration number

Warnings
Toxicity alert
Cautionary statement
Treatment for untoward exposure
Poison control listing
Hot line number

Instructions for Use
Dilution information
Personal protective requirements
Intended use
Surfaces safe for use
Method of application
Duration of necessary contact

Intended Action
Antimicrobial activity
Residual action (if any)

Aftercare
Of equipment
Of treated surface
Of cleaning supplies
Disposal or storage of unused product

eral salient points important to the selection of the appropriate agent for the desired task. Sample labeling information is listed in Box 18-3.

To be labeled for hospital use, a chemical disinfectant should be proven effective against *Staphylococcus aureus* (gram-positive), *Salmonella choleraesuis* (gram-negative), and *Pseudomonas aeruginosa* (gram-negative); these are the most resistant gram-positive and gram-negative organisms. The agent can be classified as a hospital disinfectant without being pseudomonacidal, but the label is required to say whether or not it is effective against *Pseudomonas* organisms.

The EPA defines a disinfectant as an agent that kills growing or vegetative forms of bacteria. The terms *germicide* and *bactericide* may be used synonymously with the term *disinfectant* according to this definition. However, *Mycobacterium tuberculosis* has a waxy envelope that makes it comparatively resistant to aqueous germicides. Effective agents against *M. tuberculosis* should be labeled tuberculocidal. Agents also are labeled if they kill fungi (fungicide), viruses (virucide), and/or spores (sporicide). Agents effective enough to be labeled tuberculocidal will kill HIV. Those that meet the EPA testing requirements may be labeled specifically as HIV virucides. Hepatitis B virus (HBV) cannot be adapted to laboratory testing, but it is known to survive exposure to many disinfectants.

The safest products for use in the perioperative environment include all categories of biocidal action (Table 18-1). With the exception of the few cold sterilants previously discussed, most chemicals in solution are not sporicides. Analysis of the label statements helps determine whether a product is appropriate for a specific purpose in the operating room (OR). Factors to be considered in the selection of an agent include the following:

1. Microorganisms differ markedly in their resistance to chemicals. Factors influencing the microbial response include the active ingredient of the chemical, pH, hardness of the water, exposure time, and extent of precleaning before processing.
2. Disinfectants differ widely in the level of biocidal action they produce and mechanisms involved. All are protoplasmic poisons that either coagulate or denature cell protein, oxidize or bind enzymes, or alter cell membranes. In-use culture testing must determine the number of viable microorganisms after an agent is used for the intended purpose.
3. The nature of the microbial contamination influences the results of chemical disinfection. Bacteria, spores, fungi, and viruses are present in air and on surfaces throughout the environment. However, organic soil, such as blood, plasma, pus, feces, and tissue, absorbs germicidal molecules and inactivates some chemicals. Therefore good physical cleaning before disinfection helps reduce the number of microorganisms present and enhances biocidal action.
4. Requirements of the chemical agent vary.
   a. Housekeeping products should be detergent-disinfectants that meet the following requirements for both cleaning and disinfection:
      (1) They must be effective against a broad spectrum of microorganisms, including *P. aeruginosa* and *M. tuberculosis,* preferably in the presence of organic soil.
      (2) They must be compatible with tap water for dilution.
      (3) They must be low foaming and prevent waterborne deposits.
      (4) They must rinse easily and not leave a residual film that could affect electrical conductivity.
      (5) They should be nontoxic and nonirritating to patients and personnel.
      (6) They should be virtually odorless.
   b. Instrument and equipment disinfectants should be registered by the EPA and should kill as many species of microorganisms as possible to decontam-

TABLE 18-1   Activity of Disinfectants In Addition to Being Bactericidal, Pseudomonacidal, and Fungicidal*

Disinfectant	Activity Level	HIV	HBV†	Tuberculocide	Housekeeping	Hazards
Chemicals*						
Alcohol, 70%-95%						
Ethyl	Intermediate	Yes	Yes	15 minutes	Yes	Flammable
Isopropyl	Intermediate	Yes	No	15 minutes	Yes	Flammable
Chloride compounds	Low	Yes	Yes	N/A	Yes	
Formaldehyde						
37% aqueous	High‡	Yes	Yes	15 minutes	No	Toxic fumes
8% in alcohol	High‡	Yes	Yes	10 minutes	No	Toxic fumes
Glutaraldehyde, 2%	High§	Yes	Yes	45-90 minutes§	No	Irritating fumes
Iodophors						
450 ppm	Intermediate	Yes	Yes	20 minutes	Yes	
100 ppm	Low	No	No	N/A	Yes	
Mercurial compounds	None	No	No	N/A	No	Bacteriostatic only
Phenolic compounds	Low	Yes	No	20 minutes	Yes	Skin irritant
Quaternary ammonium	Low	Yes	No	N/A	No	
Physical						
Boiling water	Low	Yes	No	N/A	No	
Ultraviolet irradiation	Low	Yes	No	N/A	Air and water	Skin and eye irritant

N/A, No activity.
*Manufacturer's instructions for use and dilution must be followed.
†Probability cannot be tested.
‡Sporicidal in 12 hours.
§Formulation varies. Immersion time is 45-90 minutes for tuberculocide and 10-12 hours for sporicide.

Virucide spans HIV and HBV† columns. Immersion Time spans Tuberculocide column.

inate items effectively for handling by personnel or for preparing semicritical items for patient use, such as stethoscopes and monitors.

5. The kill time is correlated with the concentration of the agent and the number of microorganisms present. Most chemicals are used in aqueous solution. Water brings the chemical and microorganisms together. Without this water reaction, the process stops. Increasing the concentration of the chemical may shorten exposure time but not necessarily.
    a. All tap water has *Pseudomonas* bacteria in it. The pH, calcium, and magnesium in hard tap water can inactivate disinfectants. Therefore distilled water may be recommended for use in dilution.
    b. The temperature of hot water may make chemical agents unstable.
    c. Disinfectants should be premixed in required concentrations and stored in properly labeled containers to ensure that personnel use the product in the correct concentration.
    d. Instruments are completely submerged for the maximum time recommended by the manufacturer of the product used.
    e. All instruments should be clean and dry when put into solution. Drippy, wet items will dilute the solution and change the concentration of a chemical agent.
6. The composition of items to be disinfected varies. Nonporous items, such as metal instruments, are more easily disinfected than porous materials.
7. The method of application influences the effectiveness of the chemical agent.
    a. Direct application of a liquid disinfectant, either by mechanical action for housekeeping purposes or by immersion for instrument disinfection, is the most effective method of applying chemicals to the surface of inanimate objects.
    b. Aerosol spray from a pressurized container is an effective method of spot disinfection on smooth surfaces and into crevices not otherwise accessible.
    c. Fogging is the process of filling the air in a room with an aerosolized disinfectant solution in an attempt to control microbial contamination. Action on airborne contaminants is temporary because the agent dispersed through the air settles on surfaces or is exhausted through the ventilating system. This method is potentially toxic to personnel and patients. Unless all surfaces are completely covered by a layer of the disinfectant solution for the minimum exposure period, disinfection is incomplete. Fogging is impractical and too ineffective to be an acceptable method of disinfection in OR suites.
8. Disinfection should be done immediately before and after use or contamination. All patients are considered to be potential carriers of HIV and hepatitis. Therefore adequate bactericidal and virucidal disinfection is needed before and after every invasive procedure.

9. The shelf life and safe storage after reconstitution are other factors to be considered.

Disinfectants are labeled with the chemical properties and appropriate warnings of precautions. The labels must be read, and directions for dilution and/or use followed. Material Safety Data Sheets (MSDS), supplied by the manufacturer as required by the Occupational Safety and Health Administration (OSHA) for hazardous chemicals, must be available to users. Isopropyl alcohol, sodium hypochlorite, formaldehyde, glutaraldehyde, and phenol are considered hazardous chemicals. Some other chemicals can cause contact dermatitis. Gloves should be worn when handling chemical agents.

Alcohol

Ethyl or isopropyl alcohol, 70% to 95%, kills microorganisms by coagulation of cell proteins.

Effectiveness

1. It may be used as a housekeeping disinfectant for damp dusting furniture and lights or wiping electrical cords, without leaving a residue on treated surfaces. It is nonstaining.
2. It can disinfect semicritical instruments. To prevent corrosion of metal, 0.2% sodium nitrite is added.
3. It is bactericidal, pseudomonacidal, and fungicidal in a minimum of 10 minutes' exposure by total immersion. It is not sporicidal.
4. It is tuberculocidal and virucidal for most viruses (except hydrophilic viruses), including HIV, in a minimum of 15 minutes' exposure; isopropyl 70% to 95% ethyl alcohol is effective against HBV.

Precautions

1. The pattern of effectiveness of 95% isopropyl alcohol on HBV is irregular, because it evaporates rapidly and does not have prolonged moist contact with the microorganism. It should not be used for cleaning up blood or body fluid spills, because it is inactivated in the presence of biologic matter.
2. It is volatile; it will act only as long as it is in solution. Alcohol becomes ineffective as soon as it evaporates, and it loses its biocidal activity below a concentration of 50%; it should be discarded at frequent intervals.
3. It is inactive in the presence of organic soil. It does not penetrate skin oil that lodges on instruments through handling.
4. It will blanch asphalt floor tiles.
5. It cannot be used on lensed instruments with cement mountings because it dissolves cement.
6. With long exposure, it will harden and swell plastic tubing and items, including polyethylene.
7. It is flammable, so it is stored in a cool, well-ventilated area.
8. It is a skin irritant.

Chlorine Compounds

Inorganic chlorine is valuable for the disinfection of water. Chlorine compounds kill microorganisms by the oxidation of enzymes. Sodium hypochlorite (household bleach), 1:10 dilution of 5.25%, is a low-level disinfectant. Concentration may range up to 1:100, or 500 parts per million (ppm). Sodium dichloroisocyanurate (Presept disinfectant tablet) has a lowered pH, which enhances its biocidal action. Chloride compounds are limited to housekeeping disinfection.

Effectiveness

1. Chlorine compounds are housekeeping disinfectants for spot cleaning of blood and body fluid spills and for cleaning of floors and furniture.
2. They are bactericidal, fungicidal, and tuberculocidal and have a virucidal effect on HIV, HBV, and other viruses.

Precautions

1. Sodium hypochlorite is unstable and dissipates rapidly in the presence of organic soil. A dilution is prepared daily.
2. The odor may be objectionable. It can be a respiratory irritant.
3. Chlorine is corrosive to metal; it cannot be used for instrument disinfection and decontamination.
4. Chlorine compounds are potentially carcinogenic if combined with formaldehyde.

Formaldehyde

Formaldehyde kills microorganisms by coagulation of protein in cells. The solution may be 37% formaldehyde in water (Formalin) or 8% formaldehyde in 70% isopropyl alcohol. Formaldehyde is not used for housekeeping purposes.

Effectiveness

1. It is a high-level instrument disinfectant. To prevent corrosion of metal, 0.2% sodium nitrite is added.
2. It is bactericidal, pseudomonacidal, and fungicidal in a minimum of 5 minutes' exposure.
3. It is tuberculocidal and virucidal in a minimum of 10 minutes in alcohol solution and in a minimum of 15 minutes in aqueous solution.
4. It is sporicidal in a minimum of 12 hours.

Precautions

1. Fumes are irritating to the eyes and mucous membranes.
2. Fumes are potentially carcinogenic.
3. It is toxic to tissues, so instruments are thoroughly rinsed with sterile distilled water before use.
4. Since rubber and porous materials may absorb formaldehyde, they should not be disinfected in this agent.

Glutaraldehyde

An aqueous solution of glutaraldehyde kills microorganisms by denaturation of protein. It is most commonly used in an activated 2% solution that can be reused for the specified period of activation. Both alkaline and acid solutions are available for high-level disinfection of critical and semicritical items. A 1:16 dilution is not considered a high-level disinfectant; a 2% solution is. Glutaraldehyde is not used for housekeeping purposes.

Effectiveness

1. It is a noncorrosive high-level disinfectant for endoscopes and lensed instruments.
2. It is a safe high-level disinfectant for most plastic and rubber items, such as those used for administering anesthesia or respiratory therapy.
3. It is bactericidal, pseudomonacidal, fungicidal, and virucidal, including against HIV and HBV, in a minimum of 10 minutes' exposure at a temperature between 68° and 86° F (20° and 30° C).
4. It is tuberculocidal. Variations in formulations of products available affect the exposure time and temperature of the solution, especially after reuse. A 2% solution at 77° or 86° F (25° or 30° C) may be 100% tuberculocidal in 45 to 90 minutes, depending on the formulation. Label instructions of the manufacturer should be followed.
5. Most of the products labeled as cold sterilants are sporicidal in a minimum of 10 hours' exposure at room temperature.
6. Some products can be reused in closed containers or in an automatic machine for a period of activation specified by the manufacturer.
7. It remains active in the presence of organic matter; it does not coagulate protein material.

Precautions

1. Thorough and careful cleaning in a mild detergent is essential to remove organic debris and reduce microbial contamination. Detergent is rinsed off, and the item is dried before immersion.
2. Items are completely immersed and lumens are filled with solution for no longer than 24 hours.
3. Items are thoroughly rinsed before use.
4. Glutaraldehyde may be retained by woven polyester catheters and be an irritant to mucous membranes.
5. Odor and fumes may be irritating to the eyes, throat, and nasal passages. The solution should be kept covered and used in a well-ventilated area.
6. Its shelf life is limited after activation.

Iodophors

A complex of free iodine with detergent kills microorganisms through a process of oxidation of essential enzymes. An iodophor is an effective low- to intermediate-level disinfectant. The iodine-detergent complex enhances the biocidal activity of free iodine and renders it nontoxic, nonirritating, and nonstaining when used as directed. The concentration varies among the products available. The manufacturer's instructions for use should be followed.

Effectiveness

1. Iodophors are used as housekeeping disinfectants for surfaces such as floors, furniture, and walls. Iodine is effective as long as it is wet. An aqueous solution is more effective for cleaning than an alcohol solution because it dries more slowly.
2. An iodophor may be used as a semicritical instrument disinfectant. To prevent corrosion of metal, 0.2% sodium nitrite is added.
3. Iodophors are bactericidal, pseudomonacidal, and fungicidal in a minimum of 10 minutes' exposure in a concentration of 450 ppm of iodine or a minimum of 20 minutes' exposure in a concentration of 100 ppm of iodine.
4. They are tuberculocidal and virucidal, including against HIV and HBV, in a minimum of 20 minutes' exposure with a minimum concentration of 450 ppm of iodine. They are not sporicidal.

Precautions

1. Some iodophors are unstable in the presence of hard water or heat and are inactivated by organic soil.
2. Iodine stains fabrics and tissue; however, this is reduced or is temporary when iodine is used as an iodophor.

Mercurial Compounds

Mercurial compounds bind enzymes of bacteria but inhibit growth rather than kill the organisms. Therefore these agents are bacteriostatic, not germicidal. They have little if any value in hospital disinfection.

Phenolic Compounds

Derivatives of pure phenol kill microorganisms mainly by coagulation of protein. Depending on the phenol coefficient and species of organisms, phenolic compounds may cause rapid lysis of cells, leakage of cell constituents without lysis, or death by denaturing enzymes. Pure phenol, obtained from coal tar, is an extremely caustic agent and dangerous to tissue. Derivatives are used as low-level disinfectants, usually with a minimum of a 2% phenolic compound in an aqueous or detergent solution. Phenolic compounds are used primarily for housekeeping purposes.

Effectiveness

1. Phenolic compounds may be used as housekeeping disinfectants for cleaning surfaces such as floors, furniture, and walls. Phenolics retain a safe level of activity in the presence of heavy organic soil.
2. They are the disinfectants of choice when dealing with fecal contamination. They have good stability and remain active after mild heating and prolonged drying. Subsequent application of moisture to dry surfaces can redissolve the chemical so that it becomes bactericidal again.
3. They are tuberculocidal.

Precautions

1. Tissue irritation precludes use for semicritical instruments that will come in contact with skin and mucous membranes (e.g., anesthesia equipment).
2. Personnel should wear gloves when cleaning with these products to avoid skin irritation.
3. Rubber and plastics may absorb phenol derivatives.
4. The product may have an unpleasant odor.
5. Pure phenol is inactivated by the application of alcohol.

Quaternary Ammonium Compounds

"Quats," as these compounds are often called, cause gradual alteration of cell membranes to produce leakage of protoplasm of some microorganisms, primarily vegetative bacteria. These compounds possess detergent properties and are used to sanitize noncritical surfaces. Benzalkonium chloride, one of the most widely used of these compounds, should be used in a concentration of 1:750.

Effectiveness

1. They are rarely used as housekeeping disinfectants for surfaces such as floors, furniture, and walls.
2. For low-level, noncritical instrument disinfection, 0.2% sodium nitrite is added to the solution to prevent corrosion of metal.
3. They are bactericidal, pseudomonacidal, fungicidal, and lipid virucidal in a minimum of 10 minutes' exposure. They are nonirritating to skin.
4. There is no buildup on surfaces. They are not inactivated by hard water.

Precautions

1. Their biocidal effect can be reversed by adding a neutralizer, such as soap.
2. They are not effective against tuberculosis or hydrophilic viruses, such as poliovirus.
3. The active agent can be selectively absorbed by fabrics, thus reducing the strength perhaps to an ineffectively low level. Gauze or a towel must not be put in the basin used for immersing instruments.
4. Compounds are inactivated in the presence of organic soil.

Mercurial compounds and quaternary ammonium compounds are not recommended for hospital use because the hazards outweigh their effectiveness in the hospital environment. Other agents discussed are more efficacious.

Hydrogen Peroxide
Effectiveness

1. It is rapidly bactericidal, virucidal, fungicidal, and tuberculocidal.
2. It is useful for disinfection of noncritical items.

Precautions

1. It is inactivated by blood.

Physical Disinfectants
Boiling Water

Boiling water cannot be depended on to kill spores. Heat-resistant bacterial spores will withstand water boiling at 212° F (100° C) for many hours of continuous exposure. Inactivation of some viruses, such as those associated with hepatitis, is uncertain.

If no other method of sterilization or disinfection is available, boiling water can be rendered more effective by adding sodium carbonate to make a 2% solution, which reduces the hydrogen-ion concentration. At sea level the recommended boiling time for disinfection is 15 minutes. Rubber goods and glassware must not be boiled in sodium carbonate, since it is destructive to both. If sodium carbonate is not used, the minimum boiling period is 30 minutes. At high altitudes the boiling time is increased to compensate for the lower temperature of boiling water.

Boiling water is a nontoxic, high-level disinfection process, sometimes referred to as pasteurization, that can be used for items such as metal utensils and breathing circuits. For sanitization, the reduction or destruction of microbial contaminants to a relatively safe level for handling, the temperature of hot water ranges from 140° to 203° F (60° to 95° C).

Pasteurization is a method of hot water disinfection. Although not a sterilization process, exposure to hot water (160° to 180° F [60° to 70° C]) for 30 minutes kills microorganisms without killing spores. Respiratory breathing circuits can be processed this way.

Ultraviolet Irradiation

Ultraviolet (UV) rays at wavelengths of 240 to 480 nm photochemically transform nucleic acid bases to denature DNA and proteins. Generated by low-pressure mercury vapor bulbs, UV lights produce nonionizing radiant energy in sufficient wavelengths and intensity for low-level disinfection. The rays can kill select vegetative bacteria, fungi, and lipoprotein viruses on contact in air or water. The practical usefulness of UV irradiation is very limited, however, because the rays must make direct contact with the organisms and may actually support life for some varieties. Microorganisms are in a constant state of motion in the air currents of the ventilating system and in water. Moving across the ray of UV light, pathogens may be exposed for too short a time for effective contact with the radiant energy. The average UV lamp produces 45 microwatts per cubic centimeter. Many microorganisms require application of UV lights at 2000 to 100,000 microwatts per cubic centimeter to be effective.

UV lights have been installed in a few ORs to decrease airborne microorganisms to low levels. UV rays can cause skin burns, similar to sunburn, and conjunctivitis of the eyes. Therefore when working under exposure to UV rays, protective skin coverings and goggles or a visor over the eyes is worn. These lights may be turned on only when the room is unoccupied to reduce airborne and surface contamination.

UV irradiation is used in conjunction with activated carbon 5 micron filters for water purification. UV irradiation kills bacteria but does not remove impurities. The filtration process is followed by exposing water flowing at a constant rate and temperature to a 5-watt UV lamp. This produces purified water, not sterile water. UV irradiation is not sporicidal, and HBV can survive exposure to it.

Bibliography

Bays R: Changes and choices in cleaning and disinfecting, *Infect Control Today* 2(4):12, 16, 18, 1998.
Goncarovos V: The EPA registration number on disinfectant labels, *Infect Control Today* 2(4):33-34, 1998.
Hilgren J: The exposure time dilemma: how long to use disinfectants on environmental surfaces, *Infect Control Today* 2(3):12, 16-18, 1998.
Notarianni GL: Controlling glutaraldehyde exposure, part 2, *Infect Control Steril Tech* (4):16, 20, 24-25, 1995.
Otero RB: Cleaning formula efficacy, *Infect Control Today* 1(2):18-22, 1997.
Prince DL et al: Selecting cleaner-disinfectants, *Infect Control Today* 2(2):27-30, 32, 35-36, 1998.
Rutala WA, Weber DJ: Uses of inorganic hypochlorite (bleach) in healthcare facilities, *Clin Micro Rev* 10(4):597-610, 1997.
Schule RW: Pasteurization: is it only for milk? *Infect Control Today* 2(9):28, 32, 34, 36-38, 1998.
Springthorpe S: Disinfectants, *Infect Control Today* 2(11):40, 42, 1998.

Section
VI

Surgical Instrumentation and Equipment

Chapter 19

Surgical Instrumentation

Chapter Objectives

After studying this chapter, the learner will be able to:

- Identify the use and function of each type of surgical instrument.
- Demonstrate the appropriate methods for passing each type of instrument.
- Understand the rationale and methods of decontamination of instrumentation.
- Demonstrate the assembly and passing of sharps.

Surgical instrumentation is critical to the surgical procedure. The performance of the OR team is enhanced when team members know each instrument by name, know how each is safely handled, and know how each is used. Preparing the instrument for appropriate processing will prolong its use in patient care and decrease the costs for repair and replacement. Terms associated with surgical instrumentation are defined in Box 19-1.

HISTORICAL BACKGROUND

Perhaps as early as 10,000 BC, prehistoric man fashioned tools to cut human flesh for the purpose of either inflicting wounds or repairing them. Early writings describe cutting tools. The Incas of Peru used razor-sharp flint and sharpened animal teeth. The Code of Hammurabi (circa 1900 BC) describes a bronze lancet. The Egyptian Ebers papyrus mentions blades made of flint, reed, and bronze used around 1900 to 1200 BC. Hippocrates (460-377 BC) advocated heating the tips of rounded and pointed blades.

During the pre-Christian era in India, Shusruta made grasping tools designed for extracting objects such as arrowheads. Many of these tools were in the form of animal or bird heads, such as a toothed forceps that resembled a crocodile or

a smooth forceps that was shaped like the beak of a heron. He described more than 100 instruments, including scalpels, lancets, saws, bone cutters, trocars, and needles.

In the first century AD, Celsus described the use in Rome of scalpel handles with blunt dissecting ends, knives, saws, forceps, and clamps with locking handles, probes, and hooks for retraction. These crude and often heavy instruments were the armamentarium of medicine through the Dark and Middle Ages. Ambroise Paré (1510-1590) was the first to grasp blood vessels with a pinching instrument (the predecessor of the hemostat used today).

In the United States, amputations were the surgical trademark of the Civil War (1861-1865). In some instances these amputations were performed on kitchen tables with crude heavy knives and instruments, and table forks were even used as retractors.

Through the eighteenth and nineteenth centuries, surgical tools were made by skilled silversmiths, coppersmiths, and woodworkers. Some instruments had beautifully carved ivory, bone, or wood handles, and the surgeon kept them in velvet-lined cases. When sterilization became accepted around the turn of the twentieth century, instruments made entirely of metals such as carbon steel, silver, and brass replaced those with ornate but dirt-filled handles. The velvet

Box 19-1

Terms Associated with Surgical Instrumentation

atraumatic Without injury.

dilation Enlarging an opening in a progressive manner.

dissection Process of separating tissues through anatomic planes by using sharp or blunt instrumentation.

grasping Holding in a traumatic or atraumatic manner.

retraction Stabilizing a tissue layer in a safe position for exposure of a part. A retractor can be manual or self-retaining.

sharp Instrument with a cutting edge or pointed tip(s) that is used to cut or dissect tissue. These items include blades, scissors, needles, and other dissection devices.

traumatic Causing injury by penetration or crushing.

trocar A device used for penetration of tissue layers. It is commonly used for percutaneous endoscopy. It is used as a temporary pathway for gases, other instrumentation, or the removal of an organ or substance.

cases gave way to sterilizer trays. The development of stainless steel in the 1900s enhanced the art and craft of precision surgical instruments. Craftsmen—primarily in Germany, Sweden, France, England, Pakistan, and the United States—continue to provide the surgical instruments needed to extend the capabilities of the surgeons' hands.

Hippocrates wrote that the size, weight, and delicacy of an instrument ought to be well suited for its purpose. Consequently, instrument modifications vary from the strength needed for bone work, to the length needed to reach the depths of body cavities, to the delicacy needed to handle structures even under the microscope. All instruments are designed to provide a necessary tool to perform a basic surgical maneuver. The variations are numerous.

FABRICATION OF METAL INSTRUMENTS

Although some surgical instruments are made of titanium, cobalt-based alloy (Vitallium), or other metals, the vast majority are made of stainless steel. The alloys used must have specific properties to make them resistant to corrosion when exposed to blood and body fluids, cleaning solutions, sterilization, and the atmosphere. The manufacturer chooses the alloy for its durability, functional capacity, and ease of fabrication for the intended purpose.

Stainless Steel

Stainless steel is an alloy of iron, chromium, and carbon. It may also contain nickel, manganese, silicon, molybdenum, sulfur, and other elements to prevent corrosion or to add tensile strength. The formulation of the steel plus the heat treatment and finishing processes determine the qualities of the instrument. Chromium in the steel makes it resistant to corrosion. Carbon is necessary to give steel its hardness, but it also reduces the corrosion-resistant effects of chromium. Iron

alloys in the 400 series (low in chromium and high in carbon) are most commonly used for the fabrication of surgical instruments.

Steel is milled into blanks that are forged, spun, drawn, die cast, molded, or machined into component shapes and sizes. These components are assembled by hand, then heat hardened (tempered) and buffed. X-ray and/or fluoroscopy techniques are used to detect any defects that may occur as a result of the forging or machining operations. The stress and tension must be in balance, that is, the instrument must have the flexibility to withstand the stresses of normal use. The temper of the steel determines this balance.

The instrument is then subjected to processes that protect its surfaces and minimize corrosion. Oxidation of the surface chromium by a process called passivation forms a hard chromium oxide layer. Nitric acid both removes carbon particles and promotes the formation of this surface coating. Polishing creates a smooth surface for the continuous layer of chromium oxide. Passivation continues to form this layer when the instrument is exposed to the atmosphere and oxidizing agents in cleaning solutions. The term *stainless* is a misnomer. Steel does not tarnish, rust, or corrode easily; but some staining and spotting will occur with normal use.

Stainless steel instruments are fabricated with one of three types of finishes before passivation:

1. A mirror finish is shiny and reflects light. This highly polished finish tends to resist surface corrosion, but the glare can be a distraction for the surgeon or an obstruction to visibility.
2. An anodized finish, sometimes referred to as a satin finish, is dull and glareproof. Protective coatings of chromium and nickel are deposited electrolytically and reduce glare. This type of finish is somewhat more susceptible to surface corrosion than a highly polished surface, but the corrosion is usually easily removed.
3. An ebony finish is black, which eliminates glare. The surface is darkened by a process of chemical oxidation. Instruments with an ebony finish are used in laser surgery to prevent beam reflection. In other surgical procedures, instruments with an ebony finish may offer the surgeon better color contrast because they do not reflect the color of tissues.

Titanium

In comparison to stainless steel, the metallurgic properties of titanium are excellent for the manufacture of microsurgical instruments. Titanium is nonmagnetic and inert. Titanium alloy is harder, stronger, lighter in weight, and more resistant to corrosion than stainless steel. A blue anodized finish of titanium oxide reduces glare.

Vitallium

Vitallium is the trade name for an alloy of cobalt, chromium, and molybdenum. This inert alloy has the strength and corrosion-resistant properties suitable for some orthopaedic devices and maxillofacial implants. Instruments made of Vitallium must be used when these devices are implanted. In an electrolytic environment such as body tissues, metals of different potentials can cause corrosion if they come into contact with each other. Therefore an implant of a cobalt-based alloy is not compatible with instruments that are iron-based alloys (stainless steel) and vice versa.

Other Metals

Although most instruments are made of steel alloys, other metals are used. Some instruments are fabricated from brass, silver, or aluminum. Tungsten carbide is an exceptionally hard metal used for laminating some cutting blades or as inserts on the functional tips or jaws of some instruments.

Plated Instruments

A shiny finish can be put on a basic forging or tooling of an iron alloy. Chromium, nickel, cadmium, silver, and copper are used for coating or flash plating. When deposited directly on the steel, any of these metals is prone to rupturing, chipping, and spontaneous peeling. It is difficult to keep plated instruments from corroding, and rust can form beneath the plating. Plated instruments are used infrequently today.

CLASSIFICATION OF INSTRUMENTS

Various basic maneuvers are common to all surgical procedures. The surgeon dissects, resects, or alters tissues and/or organs to restore or repair bodily functions or body parts. Bleeding must be controlled during the process. Surgical instruments are designed to provide the tools the surgeon needs for each maneuver. Whether they are small or large, short or long, straight or curved, sharp or blunt, all instruments can be classified by their function. Because the nomenclature is not standardized, the names of specific instruments must be learned in the clinical practice setting. All instruments should be used only for their intended purpose, and they should not be abused.

Cutting and Dissecting

Cutting instruments have sharp edges. They are used to dissect, incise, separate, or excise tissues. These instruments should be kept separate from other instruments, and the sharp edges should be protected during cleaning, sterilizing, and storing. To prevent injury to the handler and damage to the sharp edges, proper precautions are necessary to take during the handling or disposing of all sharps, blades, or scalpels.

Scalpels

The type of scalpel most commonly used has a reusable handle with a disposable blade. Most handles are made of brass; the blades may be made of carbon steel. The blade is at-

Figure 19-1 Scalpel/knife blades: No./sizes 10, 11, 12, 15, 20 (actual size).

tached to the handle by slipping the slit in the blade into the grooves on the handle. An instrument, never the fingers, is used to attach and detach the blade; this instrument, usually a needleholder, should not touch the cutting edge. Blades vary by size and shape (Figure 19-1); handles vary by width and length:

1. A No. 10 blade is used most often. This blade has a rounded cutting edge along one side and fits on No. 3, 7, and 9 handles. No. 20, 21, and 22 blades are the same shape but are larger; they fit on No. 4 handles.
2. A No. 11 blade has a straight edge that comes to a sharp point. It fits on No. 3, 7, and 9 handles.
3. A No. 12 blade is shaped like a hook, with the cutting edge on the inside curvature. It fits on No. 3, 7, and 9 handles.
4. A No. 15 blade has a smaller and shorter curved cutting edge than a No. 10 blade. This blade also fits on No. 3, 7, and 9 handles. A No. 15C blade has the same shape but is smaller for tiny incisions, such as those for some pediatric procedures.
5. A No. 23 blade has a curved cutting edge that comes to more of a point than No. 20, 21, and 22 blades. The No. 23 blade fits on a No. 4 handle.

An assortment of blades with angulations and configurations for specific uses, such as a Beaver blade, are also used. These blades insert into a special universal handle that secures by turning a screw-in collar. Disposable scalpels also are available.

Knives

Knives come in various sizes and configurations. They usually have a blade at one end, like a kitchen paring knife, and the blade may have one or two cutting edges. The knives are designed for very specific purposes (e.g., a cataract knife). Other types of knives have detachable and replaceable blades (e.g., an adenotome, a dermatome). A knife blade may be incorporated into a multifunctional instrument, such as a GIA (gastrointestinal anastomosis) stapler that cuts and staples tissue.

Scissors

The blades of scissors may be straight, angled, or curved, as well as either pointed or blunt at the tips (Figure 19-2). The handles may be long or short. Some scissors are used only to cut or dissect tissues; others are used to cut other materials. To maintain sharpness of the cutting edges and proper alignment of the blades, scissors should be used only for their intended purpose:

1. Tissue/dissecting scissors must have sharp blades. The type and location of tissue to be cut determines which scissors the surgeon will use. Blades needed to cut tough tissues are heavier than those needed to cut fine, delicate structures. Curved or angled blades are needed to reach under or around structures. Handles to reach deep into body cavities are longer than those needed for superficial tissues.

2. Suture scissors have blunt points to prevent structures close to the suture from being cut. The scrub person may use scissors to cut sutures during preparation if needed.

3. Wire scissors have short, heavy blades. Wire scissors are used instead of suture scissors to cut stainless steel sutures. Heavy wire cutters are used to cut bone fixation wires.

4. Dressing/bandage scissors are used to cut drains and dressings and to open items such as plastic packets.

Bone Cutters and Debulking Tools

Many types of instruments have cutting edges suitable for cutting into or through bone and cartilage. These instruments include chisels, osteotomes, gouges, rasps, and files (Figure 19-3). Some have moving parts, such as rongeurs and rib cutters. Others, such as drills, saws, and reamers, are powered by air or electricity. The purpose of these instruments is to decrease the bulk of firm tissue.

Other Sharp Dissectors

Sharp dissection to cut tissue apart or to separate tissue layers may be accomplished with other types of sharp instruments:

- *Biopsy forceps and punches.* A small piece of tissue may be removed for pathologic examination with a biopsy forceps or punch. These instruments may be used through an endoscope.

Figure 19-2 Scissors. **A,** Tissue scissors. Blades may be straight or curved and either pointed/blunt, pointed/pointed, or blunt/blunt. **B,** Suture scissors. **C,** Wire cutters and scissors. **D,** Dressing/bandage scissors.

- *Curettes.* Tissue or bone is removed by scraping with the sharp edge of the loop, ring, or scoop on the end of a curette (Figure 19-4).
- *Snares.* A loop of wire may be put around a pedicle to dissect tissue such as a tonsil. The wire cuts the pedicle as it retracts into the instrument. The wire is replaced after use.

Blunt Dissectors

Friable tissues or tissue planes can be separated by blunt dissection. The scalpel handle, the blunt sides of tissue scissors blades, and dissecting sponges may be used for this purpose (Figure 19-5).

Grasping and Holding

Tissues should be grasped and held in position so the surgeon can perform the desired maneuver, such as dissecting or suturing, without injuring the surrounding tissues.

Tissue Forceps

Forceps are used to pick up or hold soft tissues and vessels (Figure 19-6). Forceps used to grasp and hold soft tissues and organs are too numerous to allow further elaboration. The configuration of each is designed to securely grasp but prevent injury to tissues.

Figure 19-4   Tissue curettes.

Figure 19-3   **A,** Osteotomes. **B,** Rasps.

Figure 19-5   Blunt dissectors, periosteal elevators.

Smooth Forceps Also referred to as thumb forceps or pick ups, smooth forceps resemble tweezers. They are tapered and have serrations (grooves) at the tip. They may be straight or bayonet (angled), short or long, and delicate or heavy. Smooth forceps will not injure delicate structures (see Figure 19-6, *A*).

Toothed Forceps Toothed forceps differ from smooth forceps at the tip. Rather than being serrated, they have a single tooth on one side that fits between two teeth on the opposing side or a row of multiple teeth at the tip. Heavy types are sometimes referred to as rat-toothed forceps. Toothed forceps provide a firm hold on tough tissues, including skin. Finer versions have delicate teeth for holding more delicate tissue (see Figure 19-6, *B*).

Allis Forceps An Allis forceps has a scissors action. Each jaw curves slightly inward, and there is a row of teeth at the end. The teeth hold tissue gently but securely (see Figure 19-6, *C*).

Babcock Forceps The end of each jaw of a Babcock forceps is rounded to fit around a structure or to grasp tissue without injury. This rounded section is circumferentially fenestrated (see Figure 19-6, *D*).

Stone Forceps

Either curved or straight forceps are used to grasp calculi such as kidney stones or gallstones. These forceps have blunt loops or cups at the end of the jaws.

Tenaculums

The curved or angled points on the ends of the jaws of tenaculums penetrate tissue to grasp firmly, such as when a uterine tenaculum is used to manipulate the uterus. Tenaculums may have a single tooth or multiple teeth, such as a Jacob tenaculum (Figure 19-7). Some uterine tenaculums have a built-in uterine cannula or probe elevator tip. The cannula, or probe, can be used during laparoscopy to raise the uterus into the visual field. The cannula is inserted into the cervical os as the tenaculum is clamped on the lip of the cervix. Dye can be instilled through the cannula into the uterine cavity.

Bone Holders

Grasping forceps, vice-grip pliers, and other types of heavy holding forceps stabilize bone.

Clamping and Occluding

Instruments that clamp and occlude are used to apply pressure.

Hemostatic Forceps

Most clamps used for occluding blood vessels have two opposing serrated jaws that are stabilized by a box lock and

Figure 19-6 Tissue forceps. **A,** Smooth thumb forceps may be straight, bayonet, or short and delicate. **B,** Toothed forceps tips. **C,** Allis forceps. **D,** Babcock forceps.

Figure 19-7 **A,** Single-tooth uterine tenaculum. **B,** Jacob multi-tooth tenaculum.

controlled by ringed handles. When the box locks are closed, the handles remain locked on ratchets (Figure 19-8).

Hemostats　Hemostats are the most commonly used surgical instruments and are used primarily to clamp blood vessels. Hemostats have either straight or curved slender jaws that taper to a fine point. The serrations go across the jaws.

Crushing Clamps　Many variations of hemostatic forceps are used to crush tissues or clamp blood vessels. The jaws may be straight, curved, or angled, and the serrations may be horizontal, diagonal, or longitudinal. The tip may be pointed or rounded or have a tooth (Figure 19-9). The length of the jaws and handles vary. Many forceps are named for the surgeon who designed the style, such as the Kocher or Ochsner forceps.

Some are designed to be used on specific organs, such as Péan intestinal forceps or kidney forceps. The features of the instrument will determine its use. Fine points are needed for small vessels and structures. Longer and sturdier jaws are needed for larger vessels, dense structures, and thick tissue. Longer handles are needed to reach structures deep in body cavities.

Noncrushing Vascular Clamps

Noncrushing clamps are used to occlude peripheral or major blood vessels temporarily, which minimizes tissue trauma. The jaws of these types of clamps have opposing rows of finely serrated teeth. The jaws may be straight, curved, angled, or S-shaped (Figure 19-10).

Exposing and Retracting

Soft tissues, muscles, and other structures should be pulled aside for exposure of the surgical site.

Handheld Retractors

Most retractors have a blade on a handle (Figure 19-11). The blades vary in width and length to correspond to the size and depth of the incision. The curved or angled blade may be solid or pronged like a rake. These blades are usually dull, but some are sharp. Some retractors have blades at both ends rather than a handle on one end. Handheld retractors are usually used in pairs, and they are held by the first or second assistant.

Malleable Retractors　With a malleable retractor, a flat length of low-carbon stainless steel, silver, or silver-plated copper may be bent to the desired angle and depth for retraction.

Hooks　Single, double, or multiple very fine hooks with sharp points are used to retract delicate structures. Hooks are commonly used to retract skin edges during a wide-flap dis-

Figure 19-8　Hemostatic forceps.

Figure 19-10　Noncrushing vascular clamp.

Figure 19-9　Crushing clamps. Jaws may be straight or curved. Tips may be pointed, rounded, or have a tooth *(inset)*. Serrations may be horizontal or longitudinal. Jaws and handles may be long or short.

Figure 19-11   Handheld retractors. **A,** Solid blade. **B,** Pronged/rake. **C,** Double-ended.

Figure 19-12   Self-retaining retractors.

section such as a face lift or mastectomy. Some styles of hooks have ball tips, which cause less trauma to tissues.

Self-Retaining Retractors

Holding devices with two or more blades can be inserted to spread the edges of an incision and hold them apart (Figure 19-12). For example, a rib spreader holds the chest open during a thoracic or cardiac procedure. A self-retaining retractor may have shallow or deep blades. Some retractors have ratchets or spring locks to keep the device open; others have wing nuts to secure the blades. Some retractors have interchangeable blades of different sizes. Some self-retaining retractors can be attached to the operating bed for stability.

Suturing or Stapling

Suture materials, surgical needles, and surgical staples are discussed in detail in Chapter 30. Only the instruments required for suture placement are mentioned here.

Needleholders

A needleholder is used to grasp and hold curved surgical needles. Most needleholders resemble hemostatic forceps; the basic difference is the jaws (Figure 19-13). A needleholder has short, sturdy jaws for grasping a needle without damaging it or the suture material. The jaws are usually straight, but they may be curved or angled; the inside surfaces of the jaws also may differ. In addition, the handles may be long to facilitate needle placement in surgical sites such as the pelvis

Figure 19-13 Needleholders. **A,** Crosshatched serrations on jaws. **B,** Smooth jaws.

Figure 19-14 Tungsten carbide insert in jaws of needleholder, with diamond-cut teeth, is designed to eliminate needle twisting and turning.

or chest. For example, the fine jaws of the needleholders used for ophthalmic surgery and microsurgery may be either diamond-cut or crosshatched, and the configuration of the handles is different; the jaws are squeezed together by a spring action. The size of the needleholder should match the size of the needle (i.e., heavy jaws for large needles and slim jaws for small needles). A needleholder should not be placed on a magnetic pad because it may become magnetized.

Tungsten Carbide Jaws Tungsten carbide is a hard metal. Jaws with an insert of solid tungsten carbide with diamond-cut precision teeth are designed specifically to eliminate the twisting and turning of the needle in the needleholder (Figure 19-14). These diamond-jaw needleholders can be identified by the gold plating on the handles.

Crosshatched Serrations The serrations on the inside surface of the jaws are crosshatched rather than grooved,

as in a hemostat. Crosshatching provides a smoother surface and prevents damage to the needle.

Smooth Jaws Some surgeons prefer needleholders that have jaws without serrations. These needleholders are used with small needles, such as those used for plastic surgery.

Staplers

Whether reusable or disposable, all surgical staplers are bulky, heavy instruments. Reusable staplers have many moving parts and are disassembled for cleaning and assembled at the sterile field before use. Sterile, single-use, disposable staplers that are completely assembled eliminate the many problems associated with reusable instruments. The staples are usually made from titanium, stainless steel, or absorbable material.

Clip Appliers Individual staples can be placed with a preloaded or single clip applier. These clips are used to mark tissue and to occlude vessels or small lumens of tubes. Powered or manual styles are available. Endoscopic clip appliers have been used for many years with laparoscopic tubal occlusion for reproductive sterilization.

Terminal End Staplers Terminal end staplers are designed for closing the end of a hollow organ (e.g., bowel or stomach) with a double staggered line of staples. The stapler is L-shaped and is positioned across the end of the hollow organ to be closed or the tissue to be amputated. A pin is positioned in the stapler head to contain the tissue neatly, and the instrument is closed and fired. A scalpel is used to trim the tissue extruding from the end of the closed instrument. The stapler is opened, and the staple line is inspected for integrity. Some types of terminal end staplers have articulating ends for placement across hard-to-reach areas, such as the vaginal cuff during a hysterectomy (Figure 19-15, *A*).

Internal Anastomosis Staplers Internal anastomosis staplers are designed to connect hollow organ segments to fashion a larger pouch or reservoir. Two tube-shaped organs are aligned side by side, and one fork of the two-forked stapler is positioned in each opening. The instrument is fired, and the tubes are stapled along the adjoining lengths. A trigger is pulled and a knife blade traverses between the two sets of double staple lines, creating a longitudinal opening on the inside of the anastomosed organ segments. Intestinal pouches can be fashioned in this manner. Some styles of side-to-side staplers do not have a self-contained knife. Endoscopic styles are available (Figure 19-15, *B*).

End-to-End Circular Staplers End-to-end circular staplers are designed to staple two hollow, tubelike organs end to end to create a continuous circuit. These staplers are commonly used for bowel anastomosis after resection. The instrument can be inserted via the rectum or inserted through a small incision in the wall of one limb of the tubes to be anastomosed. The ends of the tubes are positioned over

the distal and proximal tips of the stapler and are secured with circumferential purse-string sutures. The end of the stapler is closed, with the tissue of the tied ends completely enveloped in the closure. The instrument is fired, a double row of staples is placed, and a circular knife automatically trims the excess rim from the joined tubes. The instrument is opened and the trimmed rims (donuts) are examined for circular integrity. These trimmed rims should be carefully separated and identified as proximal and distal tissue for the pathologist; the margins may be examined for the presence or absence of cancer cells. End-to-end staplers may be curved or straight (Figure 19-15, *C*).

Viewing

Surgeons can examine the interior of body cavities, hollow organs, or structures with viewing instruments and can perform many procedures through them.

Speculums

The hinged, blunt blades of a speculum enlarge and hold open a canal (e.g., vagina, rectum) or a cavity (e.g., nose). An ear speculum is like a funnel.

Endoscopes

The round or oval sheath of an endoscope is inserted into a body orifice or through a small skin incision. Each type of endoscope is designed for viewing in a specific anatomic location. Many accessory instruments are used through endoscopes. Endoscopic procedures are discussed in each surgical specialty chapter of this text.

Hollow Endoscopes In a hollow endoscope, the rigid hollow sheath permits viewing in a forward direction through the endoscope. The sheath is made of brass, stainless steel, or plastic. A light carrier supplied by a fiberoptic cable provides illumination.

Lensed Endoscopes Lensed endoscopes have either rigid or flexible sheaths, and they have an eyepiece with a telescopic lens system for viewing in several directions. Lighting is provided through fiberoptic cable and an electric lamplight source. Used in combination with video-assisted technology, computerization permits recording action videos and still digital photography. Many endoscopes have working channels for performing specialized procedures. Lensed instruments are complex and require careful handling to avoid damage.

Suctioning and Aspirating

Blood, body fluids, tissue, and irrigating solution may be removed by mechanical suction or manual aspiration. Reusable suction tips and aspiration devices have lumens that are difficult to terminally clean and sterilize. Many of these items are available in disposable models.

Figure 19-15 Internal staplers. **A,** Terminal end stapler. **B,** Internal anastomosis stapler. **C,** End-to-end stapler.

Suction

Suction involves the application of pressure (less than atmospheric pressure) to withdraw blood or fluids, usually for visibility at the surgical site. An appropriate style tip is attached to sterile tubing; many tips are disposable. The style of the suction tip depends on where it is to be used and the surgeon's preference (Figure 19-16).

Poole Abdominal Tip   The Poole abdominal tip is a straight hollow tube with a perforated outer filter shield. It is used during abdominal laparotomy or within any cavity in which copious amounts of fluid or pus are encountered. The outer filter shield prevents the adjacent tissues from being pulled into the suction apparatus. This outer shield is completely removable.

Frazier Tip   The Frazier tip is a right-angle tube with a small diameter. It is used when encountering little or no fluid except capillary bleeding and irrigating fluid, such as in brain, spinal, plastic, or orthopaedic procedures. The Frazier tip keeps the field dry without the need for sponging. One model has a connection for an electrosurgical unit, and the tip can be used for fulguration. A fibdroptic cable can be attached to another model.

Yankauer Tip   The Yankauer tip is a hollow tube that has an angle for use in the mouth or throat. Large quantities of blood and fluid can be suctioned quickly with a Yankauer tip, which is useful for visualization during ruptured aneurysms.

Aspirating Tube   An aspirating tube is a long, straight tube that is used through an endoscope.

Autotransfusion   A double-lumen suction tip is used to remove blood for autotransfusion.

Aspiration

Blood, body fluid, or tissue may be aspirated manually to obtain a specimen for laboratory examination or to obtain bone marrow for transplantation. Suction is often performed with a needle and syringe.

Trocar   A trocar may be needed to cut through tissues for access to fluid or a body cavity. A trocar has sharp cutting edges at the end of a hollow tube. A cannula with a blunt end fits inside the trocar to keep fluid or gas from escaping until the cannula is removed. Endoscopic instruments may be manipulated through special trocars that have valves for insufflation, irrigation, and aspiration.

Cannula   A cannula with a blunt end and perforations around the tip may be used to aspirate fluid without cutting into tissue. Cannulas also are used to open blocked vessels or ducts for drainage or to shunt blood flow from the surgical site.

Dilating and Probing

A dilator is used to enlarge orifices and ducts, such as dilation of the uterine cervix. A probe is used to explore a structure or to locate an obstruction. Probes are used to explore the depth of a wound or to trace the path of a fistula. Tunneling devices can be used to make a passage for a vascular graft or shunt.

Measuring

Rulers, depth gauges, and trial sizers are used to measure parts of the patient's body. Some of these devices are used to determine the precise size needed for an implant, such as a joint or breast prosthesis.

Figure 19-16   Tips of suction tubes. **A,** Poole abdominal tip. **B,** Frazier tip. **C,** Yankauer tip.

Accessory Instruments

Many accessories are used in addition to the basic instruments previously discussed. For example, a mallet may be needed to drive a cutting instrument into bone. Screwdrivers are used to affix screws into bone. Each surgical specialty has its own accessories, many of which are described in the specialty chapters.

Of the thousands of instruments available, surgeons choose those that are most suitable to meet their particular needs. Differences in the size, curvature, or angulation of jaws or blades; in the length of handles; and in the weight and shape of the instruments can simplify, improve, and even shorten surgical time, which ultimately benefits the patient. Instruments should be maintained to provide the specific function each has been designed to do.

HANDLING INSTRUMENTS

Surgical instruments are expensive and represent a major investment. Surgical procedures have become more complicated and intricate and, as a result, instruments have become more complex, more precise in design, and more delicate in structure. Abuse, misuse, inadequate cleaning or processing, or rough handling can damage and reduce the life expectancy of even the most durable instrument, and the cost of repair or replacement becomes unnecessarily high. Instruments do deteriorate from normal use, but with proper care an instrument should have a life of 10 years or more.

Setting Up the Instrument Table

Standardized basic sets of sterile instruments are selected for each specific surgical procedure. A set is a group of instruments that may include all appropriate classifications of instruments or the instruments needed for a specific part of the procedure (e.g., a gallbladder set). The surgeon may prefer some specific instruments that are wrapped separately or added to the instrument set.

Instruments are usually prepared, wrapped, and sterilized several hours before the surgical procedure so they are dry and cool for safe handling. Instruments are sometimes steam sterilized immediately before use, but this method is not recommended as a routine practice. The instruments may be kept in an enclosed rigid container, or they may be sterilized in an unwrapped tray.

Exposed sterile instruments are never transported through corridors. The sterilizer may be located in the substerile room or in the OR. The scrub person or circulator may lift the tray from the sterilizer, depending on the physical location of the sterilizer in relation to the OR. The scrub person should not go beyond the confines of the OR, but this is the practice in some suites in which the sterilizer is immediately adjacent to the door of the substerile room. In lifting a tray from the sterilizer, the scrub person takes care not to brush the sleeves or the front of his or her sterile gown against the sterilizer. The circulator must not reach over the sterile instruments when lifting the tray or over the sterile table when placing it. The exterior of the sterilizing container is not considered sterile if handled by the nonsterile circulator.

When removed from the sterilizer, the instruments are hot. Condensate must not contaminate the sterile table cover. The tray can be set on the large basin in the ring stand if handled by the sterile scrub person.

The scrub person counts all instruments, sponges, and sharps with the circulator before setting up the Mayo stand and instrument table. Key points in handling instruments before the surgical procedure include the following:

1. Handle loose instruments separately to prevent interlocking or crushing.
   a. Instruments are never piled one on top of another on an instrument table; they are laid side by side. Close the box locks on the instrument to avoid entanglement.
   b. Microsurgical, ophthalmic, and other delicate instruments are vulnerable to damage through rough handling. Tip protectors are removed during setup.
   c. Metal-to-metal contact should be avoided or minimized. Scalpel blades should not be set in a metal basin. The edges can become dull, and small chips of metal can become dislodged and inadvertently transferred to the patient during irrigation.
2. Inspect instruments such as scissors and forceps for alignment, imperfections, cleanliness, and working conditions. Set aside or remove any defective instrument. Be sure to label it for repair and replace it in the set before it processing.
   a. Scalpel blades should be properly set in handles using a heavy instrument, not fingers.
   b. Teeth and serrations should align exactly.
   c. Tips should be straight and in alignment.
   d. Scissors should be snug and sharp in action.
   e. Cannulae should be clear and without obstruction. Stylets should be removed.
3. Sort instruments neatly by classifications.
4. Keep ring-handled instruments together with the curvatures and angles pointed in the same direction.
   a. Hang ring handles over a rolled towel or over the edge of the instrument tray or container.
   b. Remove instrument stringers or holders if used to keep box locks open during processing.
   c. Close box locks on the first ratchet.
5. Leave retractors and other heavy instruments in a tray or container or lay them out on a flat surface of the table.
6. Protect sharp blades, edges, and tips. They should not touch anything. Take care not to perforate the sterile table cover.
   a. Sets of instruments, such as osteotomes or microsurgical instruments, may be in sterilization racks so that the blades and tips are suspended. These instruments can remain in racks during the initial table setup and until they are needed during the surgical procedure.

b. Tip-protecting covers or instrument-protecting plastic sleeves should be removed and discarded before the instruments are used on the patient. Most covers and sleeves are not radiopaque and could become a retained foreign body.

c. If they are not in a rack, handles should be supported on a rolled towel or gauze sponge. This keeps the blades and tips of microinstruments suspended in midair for easy visualization.

Handling Instruments During the Surgical Procedure

Efficient instrument handling throughout the surgical procedure is the hallmark of an efficient scrub person. Key points in handling instruments during the surgical procedure include the following:

1. Know the name and appropriate use of each instrument. Using fine instruments for heavy tissue causes damage to the instrument.
2. Handle instruments individually. Tangled instruments are hard to separate in an emergency.
   a. If several instruments of the same type will be needed in rapid succession (e.g., hemostats to clamp subcutaneous vessels), three or four may be picked up at one time, but they are passed individually to the surgeon and/or assistant.
   b. Instruments with sharp edges and fine tips are more susceptible to damage than are standard instruments. The edges are easily dulled, and the tips are easily bent or broken. Extreme caution is necessary to prevent catching the tips of microinstruments on any object that could bend them.
3. Hand the surgeon or assistant the correct instrument for each particular task. Remember the following principle: Use for intended purpose only.
   a. Avoid placing fingers in the instrument rings as the instrument is passed. The instrument may inadvertently drop or snag on drapes, causing an untoward injury to the patient or a team member. The instrument may fall to the floor, thus becoming damaged and contaminated.
   b. Many surgeons use hand signals to indicate the type of instrument needed. An understanding of what is taking place at the surgical site makes these signals meaningful.
   c. Select instruments appropriate to the location of the surgical site; short instruments are used for superficial work, and long ones are used for work deep in a body cavity. Experience will facilitate instrument selection according to the surgeon's preference and need.
   d. Many instruments are used in pairs or in sequence. When the surgeon clamps and/or cuts tissue, he or she will usually request suture. After using suture, the surgeon or assistant will need scissors to cut or a hemostat to hold the end of the strand as a tag.

   e. Hand instruments around the incisional area, not directly over it, to prevent possible injury.
   f. A knowledge of anatomy is useful for determining which instrument is needed.
4. Pass instruments decisively and firmly. When the surgeon extends his or her hand, the instrument should be slapped or placed firmly into his or her palm in the proper position for use. In general, when passing a curved instrument, the curve of the instrument aligns with the direction of the curve of the surgeon's hand. The following points should be remembered when passing an instrument to the surgeon:
   a. If the surgeon is on the opposite side of the operating bed, pass across right hand to right hand (or with the left hand to a left-handed surgeon).
   b. If the surgeon or assistant is on the same side of the operating bed and to the right, pass with your left hand; if the surgeon or assistant is to your left, pass with your right hand.
   c. Hemostatic forceps are held near the box lock by the scrub person and passed by rotating the wrist clockwise to place the handle directly into the surgeon's waiting hand (Figure 19-17).
   d. Clip appliers are held between the fingers by the hinged joint during loading and passing. Placing fingers in the rings may cause the clip to be discharged unintentionally. The loaded applier is passed so the rings automatically pass over the surgeon's finger in a position of function for rapid use.
   e. Sharp and delicate instruments may be placed on a flat surface for the surgeon to pick up. This technique avoids potential contact with items such as cutting blades, sharp points, and needles in hand-to-hand transfer. Always protect the hands when manipulating sharp instruments. Some surgeons prefer to have all instruments placed on a magnetic pad or other flat surface to avoid hand-to-hand transfers (i.e., a free-hand technique).
5. Watch the sterile field for loose instruments. After use, remove them promptly to the Mayo stand or instrument table. The weight of instruments can injure the patient or cause postoperative discomfort. Keeping instruments off the field also decreases the possibility of their falling to the floor.
6. With a moist sponge, wipe blood and organic debris from instruments promptly after each use.
   a. Demineralized, sterile distilled water should be used to wipe instruments. Saline, blood, and other solutions can damage surfaces, causing corrosion and, ultimately, pitting.
   b. Blood and debris that are allowed to dry on surfaces, in box locks, and in crevices increase the bioburden that could be carried into the surgical site.
   c. A nonfibrous sponge should be used to wipe off microsurgical, ophthalmic, and other delicate tips.

Figure 19-17   Passing an instrument. Tip is visible; hand is free. Handle is placed directly into waiting hand. Avoid placing fingers in the rings as the instrument is passed.

This type of sponge prevents the snagging and breaking of delicate tips, and the potential for lint is decreased. Commercial microsurgical instrument wipes are available.

7. Flush the suction tip and tubing with sterile distilled water periodically to keep the lumens patent. Use only a few milliliters of solution if using irrigating fluids from the surgical field. Keep a tally of the amount used to clear the suction line, and deduct this amount from the total used to irrigate the surgical site. Accurate accounting of the solutions used for patient irrigation is necessary when determining the amount of blood lost during the surgical procedure.

8. Remove debris from electrosurgical tips to ensure electrical contact. Disposable abrasive tip cleaners are helpful for maintaining the conductivity and effectiveness of the surface of the tip. Avoid using a scalpel blade to clean electrosurgical tips because the debris may become airborne and contaminate the surgical field.

9. Place used instruments that will not be needed again (except sharp, cutting, delicate, or powered instruments) into a tray or basin during or at the end of the surgical procedure.
   a. Blood and gross debris are removed before actual cleaning.
   b. Carelessly dropping, tossing, or throwing instruments into a basin causes damage.
   c. Instruments that have been wiped can be immersed in a basin of sterile demineralized distilled water, not saline solution. The sodium chloride in saline solution and in blood is corrosive and can damage instrument surfaces. Bloody instruments should not soak in a basin of solution for a prolonged period.
   d. Heavy instruments such as retractors should not be placed on top of tissue and hemostatic forceps and other clamps. Place them in a separate tray.

   e. Reusable sharps should be kept separate from other instruments of the same or similar size to prevent injury to instrument processing personnel.
   f. Keep instruments accessible for final counts.

Dismantling the Instrument Table

Whether used or unused, all instruments on the instrument table are considered contaminated and must be promptly and properly decontaminated/cleaned, inspected, terminally sterilized, and prepared for subsequent use. Wearing gloves, a gown, a mask, and protective eyewear, the scrub person prepares instruments for the cleaning process. Instruments are cleaned in a designated instrument processing area, not in the OR. Key points in handling instruments when dismantling the instrument table include the following:

1. Check drapes, towels, and table covers to be sure that instruments do not go to the laundry or into the trash. A final quick count is a safeguard.
2. Collect instruments from the Mayo stand and any other small tables, and collect those that may have been dropped or passed off the sterile field.
3. Separate delicate, small instruments and those with sharp or semisharp edges for special handling.
4. Disassemble all instruments with removable parts to expose all surfaces for cleaning.
5. Open all hinged instruments to expose box locks and serrations.
6. Separate instruments of dissimilar metals. Instruments of each type of metal should be cleaned separately to prevent electrolytic deposition of other metals.
7. Flush cold, distilled water through hollow instruments or channels, such as suction tips or endoscopes, to prevent organic debris from drying.
8. Rinse off blood and debris with demineralized distilled water or an enzymatic detergent solution.

9. Follow the procedures for preparing each instrument for decontamination or terminal sterilization. Procedures vary depending on the type of instrument and its components and on the equipment available and its location.

CLEANING INSTRUMENTS

Decontamination is performed in a designated area, not in the OR, immediately after completion of the surgical procedure. Decontamination includes mechanical cleaning and a physical or chemical biocidal process to make instruments safe for handling. The decontamination process includes prerinsing, washing, rinsing, and sterilizing. Instruments may be prerinsed or presoaked and then cleaned manually or mechanically.

Prerinsing/Presoaking

The purpose of prerinsing or presoaking is to prevent blood and debris from drying on instruments or to soften and remove dried blood and debris. The circulator can prepare a basin of solution for the scrub person. For a short immersion period, instruments may be presoaked in the following:

- A dual proteolytic enzymatic detergent. Proteolytic enzymes dissolve blood and debris, and the detergent removes dissolved particulate from the surfaces of instruments, including otherwise inaccessible areas such as lumens.
- An enzymatic agent diluted per manufacturer's instructions.
- Water with a low-sudsing, near-neutral detergent. The detergent should be compatible with the local water supply.
- Plain, clean, demineralized distilled water.
- A noncorrosive detergent-disinfectant. Sodium hypochlorite (bleach) is corrosive. Instruments should not be soaked in any chlorine compound. Soaking in an iodophor should not exceed 1 hour. A phenolic or quaternary ammonium product with corrosion inhibitors is most suitable.

Instruments can be transported to the decontamination area in the soak basin or washer-sterilizer tray. The basin or tray should be enclosed in a plastic bag to keep the instruments moist and to contain contamination. Prerinsing or presoaking instruments in the OR can make further processing more efficient.

Manual Cleaning

If a washer-sterilizer is not available, instruments must be washed by hand. Even if a washer-sterilizer or decontaminator is available, some precleaning of instruments is necessary to remove gross debris. Delicate and sharp instruments should be handled separately. Microsurgical and ophthalmic instruments should be cleaned and dried by hand; they are never put in a washer-sterilizer. Because moisture is conducive to corrosion, these instruments should not remain wet for long periods of time. Some complex instruments require disassembly and precleaning before being put in a washer-sterilizer. Other instruments require special care. For example, the outside surfaces of powered instruments must be cleaned, but these instruments cannot be immersed in liquid.

Instruments may be prerinsed in the OR by the scrub person. They should not be cleaned in scrub sinks or utility sinks in the substerile room. The instruments may be covered and taken to a decontamination area in the OR suite or returned to sterile processing on the case cart. Personnel in these areas wear personal protective equipment such as gloves, waterproof aprons, and face shields to prevent accidental spray from contaminated solutions.

The purpose of manual cleaning is to remove residual blood and debris before terminal sterilization or high-level disinfection. The following steps should be observed when cleaning instruments manually:

1. Obtain clean, warm water to which a noncorrosive, low-sudsing, free-rinsing detergent has been added.
   a. Detergent should be compatible with the local water supply. The mineral content of water varies from one area to another; a water softener may be used in the system routinely to minimize mineral deposits. Regardless of the water content, the detergent should be anionic or nonionic and have a pH as close to neutral as possible. An alkaline detergent (pH over 8.5) will stain instruments; an acidic detergent (pH below 6) will corrode or pit them.
   b. Proteolytic enzymatic detergents dissolve blood and protein and remove dissolved debris from crevices. These detergents are effective in a wide range of water qualities.
   c. Liquid detergents are preferable because they disperse more completely than solids. Dilute the concentration before contact with instruments to avoid corrosion and staining. Do not pour liquid or put solid detergents directly on instruments.
2. Wash instruments carefully to guard against splashing and creating aerosols.
   a. Use a soft brush to clean serrations and box locks. A soft-bristled toothbrush may be used to clean ophthalmic, microsurgical, and other delicate instruments. Keep instruments submerged while brushing to minimize aerosolizing microorganisms.
   b. Use a soft cloth to wipe surfaces. A nonfibrous cellulose sponge will prevent damage to delicate tips.
   c. Remove bone, tissue, and other debris from cutting instruments.
   d. Never scrub surfaces with abrasive agents such as steel wool, wire brushes, scouring pads, or powders. These agents will scratch and may remove the protective finish on metal, thus increasing the likelihood of corrosion. The finish on stainless steel instruments protects the base metal from oxidation.

3. Rinse instruments thoroughly in hot distilled or deionized water. Inadequate rinsing can leave a surface residue that can stain instruments.
4. Load instruments into the appropriate trays for terminal sterilization or into containers for high-level disinfection.
   a. Put instruments back into sterilization racks or replace the protective guards as appropriate.
   b. Arrange instruments that can be steam sterilized in sterilizer trays for the washer-sterilizer or washer-decontaminator. The unwrapped tray is terminally steam sterilized.
   c. Unless an automatic cleaning, disinfecting, and sterilizing machine is available, immerse lensed instruments that are heat-sensitive in a high-level disinfectant after manual cleaning.
   d. Follow the manufacturer's instructions for the proper cleaning and sterilizing of powered instruments, which are discussed later in this chapter.

Washer-Sterilizer/Washer-Decontaminator

Mechanical cleaning and automated decontamination can be accomplished in a washer-sterilizer or washer-decontaminator. Gross debris is removed before instruments are put in these machines. A single cycle in a washer-sterilizer or decontaminator does not prepare instruments for immediate use.

A washer-decontaminator cleans with a spray-force action. It is similar to the washer-sterilizer in that the cycle includes a cold water prerinse to dissolve blood and protein, a detergent wash, a rinse and, finally, steam and heat. It does not sterilize but renders the instruments safe to handle without gloves. Unlike the washer-sterilizer, detergent solution in the washer-decontaminator enters under pressure through fixed or rotating arms for the wash cycle. Deionized or softened water is used for the rinse cycle to remove detergent residues. The final cycle includes drying with heated air. These automated thermal units are capable of consistent cleaning and disinfection.

Instruments should be arranged in perforated trays for processing in the washer-sterilizer or washer-decontaminator. The following steps should be observed when arranging the instruments:

1. Place heavy instruments in a separate tray or in the bottom of a tray, with smaller, lightweight instruments on top.
2. Turn instruments with concave surfaces, such as curettes and rongeurs, with the bowl side down; this facilitates drainage of the concave surface. Be certain that bone and tissue are removed from these surfaces.
3. Open the box locks and pivots of hinged instruments to expose maximum surface area.
4. Disassemble instruments that can be disassembled without tools (e.g., stapling devices).

5. Position sharp or pointed instruments carefully on top of other instruments to prevent contacts that could damage the cutting edges or surfaces of other instruments. An alternative is to either place sharp instruments in a separate tray or sterilize them after manual cleaning. Fine, delicate instruments should never be put in a washer-sterilizer or washer-decontaminator, because the mechanical agitation will damage them.
6. Always arrange instruments neatly. They should not be randomly piled on top of one another.

If the washer-sterilizer or washer-decontaminator is not located in an immediately adjacent room, the scrub person encloses trays in a covered cart for transport to the decontamination area.

An indexed washer-decontaminator has several chambers. The instrument tray automatically passes from chamber to chamber. It is indexed for the prerinse, ultrasonic cleaning, wash, rinse and lubrication, and drying cycles. The multiple chambers of the indexed washer-decontaminator can process several trays simultaneously.

Ultrasonic Cleaning

Surgical instruments vary in configuration from plane surfaces, which respond to most types of cleaning, to complicated devices that contain box locks, serrations, blind holes, and interstices that are difficult to clean. Using high-frequency sound waves, ultrasonic energy thoroughly cleans by a process of cavitation. These sound waves generate tiny bubbles in the solution of the ultrasonic cleaner. These bubbles are small enough to get into the serrations, box locks, and crevices of instruments that are impossible to clean by other methods. The bubbles expand until they become unstable and collapse in on themselves. This implosion generates minute vacuum areas that dislodge, dissolve, or disperse soil.

For ultrasonic cleaning, instruments should be completely immersed in the cleaning solution. The tank should be filled to a level of 1 inch (2.5 cm) above the top of the instrument tray. Suitable detergent, as specified by the manufacturer, is added. The temperature of the water should be between 100° and 140° F (37.7° and 60° C) to enhance the effectiveness of the detergent, but it should not coagulate with the protein on instruments. Instrument trays should be designed for maximum transmission of sonic energy. An important relationship exists between wire gauge, opening size, and sonic frequency. A large mesh of small wire size transmits more energy than heavy wire with narrow spacing.

The solution is degassed by turning on the ultrasonic energy. Gas, which is present in most tap water, impedes the transmission of sonic energy. An electrical generator supplies electrical energy to a transducer. The transducer converts the electrical energy into mechanical energy in the form of vibrating sound waves that are not audible to the human ear because they are of such high frequency. The presence of excess gas prevents the cleaning process from being fully effective because the cavitation bubbles fill with gas and the energy released during implosion is reduced. Tap water should be degassed for 5 minutes or longer each time it is changed. The solution should be changed or filtered at least once per shift, or whenever the detergent solution is visibly soiled. The inside of the tank should be cleaned between fillings.

An ultrasonic cleaner is not a sterilizer. Instruments must be cleaned and terminally sterilized before immersion in the ultrasonic cleaner. Most surgical instruments, including ophthalmic instruments, microinstruments, glassware, rubber goods, and thermoplastics, can be definitively cleaned by this method to remove the tiniest particles of debris from crevices. The manufacturer's instructions must be carefully followed. In general, these instructions include the following:

1. Arrange instruments as for sterilization, with heavy instruments at the bottom of the tray and lightweight instruments on top.
2. Open the box locks and pivots of hinged instruments. Leave the parts disassembled as appropriate.
3. Protect cutting edges from other instruments. Fine, delicate microsurgical and ophthalmic instruments may be damaged by vibrations or contact with each other. Some small units may be suitable for delicate instruments.
4. Separate dissimilar metals. Do not mix stainless steel instruments with other metals, because electrolysis with resultant etching may occur.
5. Do not clean plated instruments in an ultrasonic cleaner. Cavitation will accelerate the rupture and flaking of plating.
6. Rinse instruments thoroughly in hot demineralized water after the cleaning cycle to remove surface debris and detergent residue.
7. Dry instruments promptly and completely before reassembling or storing. Instruments will corrode if they are stored with trapped moisture.

Lubricating

All instruments with moving parts should be lubricated after cleaning. This is particularly important following ultrasonic cleaning because the sonic energy removes all lubricant. Instruments are immersed in an antimicrobial, water-soluble lubricant that is steam penetrable. The antimicrobial properties help prevent microbial growth in the lubricant bath, which can be reused for up to 7 days. A water-soluble lubricant deposits a thin film deep in box locks, hinges, and crevices but does not interfere with sterilization. Some lubricants also contain a rust inhibitor to prevent electrolytic mineral deposits. Mineral oil, silicones, and machine oils are never used to lubricate instruments because they leave a residue that interferes with steam or ethylene oxide sterilization. Oiling any surgical instrument constitutes a break in technique.

The lubricant should be used according to manufacturer's instructions for dilution, effectiveness, and exposure. To use most lubricants, instruments are completely immersed for 30 to 45 seconds; they are dipped and then allowed to drain dry. The solution is not rinsed or wiped off; excess solution can be shaken off. The thin film will evaporate during steam sterilization.

INSPECTING AND TESTING

Each instrument must be critically inspected after each cleaning. Instruments with movable parts should be inspected and tested following lubrication. Each instrument should be completely clean to ensure effective sterilization, and each should be inspected for proper function. The following key points should be observed when inspecting an instrument after cleaning:

1. Check hinged instruments for stiffness. Box locks and joints should work smoothly. Stiff joints are usually caused by inadequate cleaning. Lubrication eases stiffness temporarily. If box locks are frozen, leave the instruments in a water-soluble lubricant bath overnight, and then gently work the jaws back and forth. Reinspect the instrument for cleanliness.
2. Test forceps for alignment. A forceps that is out of alignment can break during use. Close the jaws of the forceps slightly; if they overlap, they are out of alignment. The teeth of forceps with serrated jaws should mesh perfectly. Hold the shanks in each hand with the forceps open, and try to wiggle them. If the box lock has considerable play or is very loose, the forceps will not hold tissue securely. If a surgeon continues to use it, jaw misalignment will occur and impair the effectiveness of the forceps.
3. Check the ratchet teeth. Ratchet teeth are subject to friction and metal-to-metal wear by the constant strain of closing and opening. Ratchets should close easily and hold firmly. To check this, clamp the forceps on the first tooth only. Hold the instrument at the box lock and tap the ratchet teeth lightly against a solid object. If the forceps springs open, it is faulty and should be repaired. A forceps that springs open when clamped on a blood vessel or duct is hazardous to the patient and is an annoyance to the surgeon. The ratchets must hold.
4. Check the tension between the shanks. When the jaws touch, a clearance of $\frac{1}{16}$ to $\frac{1}{8}$ of an inch (1.5 to 3 mm) should be visible between the ratchet teeth of each shank. This clearance provides adequate tension at the jaws when closed.
5. Test needleholders for needle security. Clamp an appropriately sized needle in the jaws of the needleholder and lock it on the second ratchet tooth. If the needle can be turned easily by hand, the needleholder needs repair.
6. Test scissors for correctly ground and properly set blades. The blades should cut on the tips and glide over each other smoothly. Use tissue/operating scis-

sors to cut through four layers of gauze at the tip of the blades (or through two layers if the scissors are less than 4 inches [10 cm] in length). The scissors should cut with a fine, smooth feel and a minimum of pressure.

7. Inspect the edges of sharp and semisharp instruments such as chisels, osteotomes, rongeurs, and adenotomes for sharpness, chips or dents, and alignment.

8. Test the penetration of cataract knives, keratomes, and other fine cutting instruments on a small kidskin drum. Slide the blade by gravity through the kidskin, with the handle resting on the palm of your hand. The blade should penetrate the drum as though it were passing through butter; it should not stick or tear.

9. Inspect microsurgical instruments under a magnifying glass or microscope to check alignment and to detect burrs on tips and nicks on cutting edges. The exact alignment of teeth on fine-toothed forceps is an absolute necessity. Microscopic teeth are very easily bent. Be certain that these instruments are thoroughly dry. A chamois is useful for drying to prevent snagging delicate tips.

10. Check pins and screws to be sure they are secure and intact. They can become loose or fall out during ultrasonic cleaning as a result of vibration.

11. Check plated instruments for chips, sharp edges, and worn spots. Chipped plating may harbor debris. Sharp edges will damage tissue or tear gloves. Worn spots will corrode.

12. Flatten or straighten malleable instruments such as retractors and probes.

13. Demagnetize instruments by passing them back through a magnetic field. Although this is a rare occurrence, instruments can become magnetized.

Unclean instruments should be returned to the cleaning area for ultrasonic cleaning. Instruments in poor working condition should be removed from the processing area. A place is usually designated in the OR suite or in the central service department for the collection of instruments for repair. A defective instrument must not be allowed to remain in circulation.

New instruments may be marked for identification of ownership before they are put in circulation. They can be imprinted with an electro-etching device. A vibrating or impact-type marking tool breaks the finish on the instrument and can cause hairline cracks. Electro-etching should be done on the shank rather than on the box lock to prevent it from fracturing. Some manufacturers will imprint identification when their instruments are purchased.

Some facilities affix colored tapes to instruments to differentiate them by sets or specialty. These tapes must withstand cleaning and sterilizing without peeling. They must be replaced if they loosen. The presence of marking tape allows debris to accumulate in the folds.

Instruments must be thoroughly dry if they will be stored for a period of time before packaging and sterilization.

Trapped moisture in hinges, box locks, serrations, and crevices will cause corrosion and rust. Stains or spots can appear on surfaces.

PACKAGING INSTRUMENTS FOR USE

To be effective, the sterilizing agent must come in direct contact with all surfaces of every instrument. Therefore instruments must be packaged (individually or in sets) in such a way to allow adequate exposure to the sterilant, to prevent air from being trapped and moisture from being retained during the sterilization process, and to ensure sterile transfer to the sterile field.

The majority of surgical instruments are made of stainless steel and can be sterilized by steam under pressure. Sterilization by steam and the methods of sterilization for heat- and moisture-sensitive items are discussed in Chapter 17. Instruments should be steam sterilized when possible. Disinfection of instrumentation is discussed in Chapter 18.

Effective steam sterilization involves the direct contact of all surfaces with steam and the revaporization of water condensate to produce a dry, sterile instrument. Retained moisture can cause corrosion that inhibits future sterilization of an instrument. A dry, sterile instrument set depends on the distribution of weight, the density of instruments, and their design.

Instrument Packaging

For sterilizing and transporting, instruments are put in a container or tray or are wrapped in a small set or individually. Instruments may be sterilized unwrapped in a high-speed pressure sterilizer immediately before use, may be prepared in advance as for a case cart, or may be retained in storage until needed. These variables determine the type of containment required to maintain sterility.

Rigid Containers

Metal or plastic containers provide the outermost enclosure for a set of instruments. The instruments are contained in a removable wire mesh tray or basket that can be lifted out of the rigid container. Air is evacuated from and steam enters into the container through filtered perforations or vents. For sterilization of porous load cycles in a pulsing prevacuum sterilizer, the bottom of the container may be solid, with perforations in the top or side vents along the top. For sterilization in a gravity displacement sterilizer, the container must have perforations in the top and bottom to allow air removal, steam penetration, and drying of contents.

Filter(s) on the inside cover the perforations. Disposable filters are changed after each use. The filter may have a chemical sterilization indicator in it. A textile or nonwoven liner may be necessary to absorb condensate from the instruments; this is not recommended for containers with valves. Containers may have sealing gaskets, locking devices, identification tags, and other accessories. Rigid containers ensure sterility if instruments are properly cleaned and loaded, if the correct container is used in each type of sterilizer, and if other sterilizing conditions are met. Sterility will be maintained during transport and storage.

Rigid containers usually have a locking mechanism on the lid latches to ensure integrity of the seal. The locking mechanism is secured with a tamperproof tag that is applied before the sterilization process. During sterilization, the tag shrinks to create a tight band around the latch. Many varieties of tamperproof tags have chemical sterilization indicators embedded on the surface. The tag also serves as a breakaway lock. An intact tag is reasonable proof that the container has not been opened.

To open a rigid container, the tamperproof tag is detached by pulling the latch to the open position, lifting the lid straight up, and then tilting it back toward self. The scrub person lifts the inner tray out by the handles on the ends of the tray. If an inner wrapper is packaged between the tray and the container, the scrub person opens the wrapper to cover the container and the table. Clips may be provided to hold this drape in place at the corners of the container.

Rigid containers designed specifically for high-pressure flash sterilization are available. These containers provide enclosed protection during transport and transfer to the sterile field. They must be used according to the manufacturer's instructions (e.g., whether to keep the lid open or closed during sterilization).

Wrapped Trays

To allow steam penetration around instruments and to prevent air from being trapped in the tray, trays cannot be solid. Therefore instruments are placed in open trays with mesh or perforated bottoms. Absorbent towels or foam may be placed in the bottom of the tray and over instruments to absorb condensate and to protect instruments from snagging in the perforations. Trays are sequentially double wrapped in woven or nonwoven wrappers. They must be allowed to cool and dry at the end of the sterilizing cycle before they are handled.

Prepackaged Instruments

A single instrument or a small set of instruments may be sequentially double wrapped in a woven or nonwoven wrapper. A single instrument may also be put in a peel-open pouch. Because a hinged instrument must be open during sterilization, the wrapping must ensure sterile transfer without contamination or damage to the instrument. A double peel pouch usually contains disassembled parts in the inner pouch for delivery to the sterile field. Instruments should never be tossed onto a sterile table. The circulator presents them to the scrub person using aseptic technique.

Some presterilized disposable instruments, such as staplers, are contained in sealed trays. The circulator peels back the cover for presentation to the scrub person.

The manufacturer may supply a fitted case or rack for a set of instruments or implants, such as orthopaedic devices. These cases or racks help to protect the instruments and keep them separated for sterilization and use. These cases or racks must be wrapped before sterilization; they are not rigid containers.

Assembly of Instrument Sets

The weight of instruments and density of metal mass is distributed in the tray to allow steam penetration for sterilizing and revaporization for drying. A large tray distributes instruments so they make minimum contact with one another. The size, design, and density of instruments are more important than their weight. The conditions necessary for steam sterilization are difficult to achieve in exceedingly heavy sets. Trays should not be overloaded. To assemble instrument sets for sterilization, the following steps should be performed:

1. Make sure the instruments are thoroughly dry.
2. Unless contraindicated, place an absorbent towel or foam in the bottom of the tray to absorb condensate, as for a rigid container with vacuum valves.
3. Count instruments as they are placed in the tray, and record the number of each type. A preprinted form is often used for this purpose. This form may accompany the tray to the OR for the circulator to verify the count, or it may remain in the processing area to verify that all instruments have been returned.
4. Arrange the instruments in a definite pattern to protect them from damage and to facilitate their removal for counting and use. Follow the instrument book or other listing of instruments to be included.
5. Place heavy instruments, such as retractors, in the bottom of the tray.
6. Open the hinges and box locks on all hinged instruments.
7. Place ring-handled instruments on stringers or holders designed for this purpose. The curved jaws of hemostatic forceps and clamps should point in the same direction. Instruments should be grouped together by style and classification (e.g., six straight hemostats, six curved hemostats). Do not band instruments together with rubber bands. Steam cannot penetrate through or under the bands to make contact with instrument surfaces.
8. Place sharp and delicate instruments on top of other instruments. They can be separated with an absorbent material or left in a sterilizing rack with the blades and tips suspended. The blades of scissors, other cutting edges, and delicate tips should not touch other instruments. If the instrument has a protective guard, leave it on. Tip-protecting covers or instrument-protecting plastic sleeves should be made of material that is steam permeable and does not melt or deform with heat.
9. Place concave or cupped instruments with the cupped surfaces down so that water condensate does not collect in them during sterilization and drying.
10. Disassemble all detachable parts. Some parts, such as screws and springs, can be put in a pouch that is left open.

11. Separate dissimilar metals. For example, brass knife handles and malleable retractors should be separated from stainless steel instruments. Preferably, put each metal in a separate tray, or separate metals with absorbent material.

12. Place instruments with a lumen, such as a suction tip, in as near a horizontal position as possible. These instruments should be tilted as little as possible to prevent the pooling of water condensate.

13. Distribute weight as evenly as possible in the tray. Some trays have dividers, clips, and pins that attach to the bottom, which helps to prevent instruments from shifting and keeps them in alignment.

14. Wrap the tray or place it in a rigid container. Check woven textile wrappers for holes or abrasion. Sequentially double wrap in a woven or nonwoven material.

15. Place a chemical sterilization indicator on the outside wrapper or container. An indicator may also be placed inside the tray.

16. Label the sets appropriately with their intended use (e.g., basic set), the date sterilized, and the control number.

REPAIRING OR RESTORING VS. REPLACING INSTRUMENTS

Instruments in poor working condition inhibit the surgeon and create a serious hazard for the patient. Instruments should be repaired at the first sign of damage or malfunction. If an instrument breaks during a procedure, all pieces should be accounted for.

Repair

Even with normal usage, the blades of scissors and the edges of other cutting instruments become dull over time, just as kitchen knives do at home. Cutting instruments must be sharp. For this reason, many blades are disposed of after a single patient use. Osteotomes, chisels, gouges, and meniscotomes can be sharpened by OR personnel with handheld hones or a honing machine designed for this purpose. Most manufacturers provide a service for sharpening and repairing instruments. Scissors, curettes, rongeurs, and reamers should be returned to the manufacturer for sharpening. Small, reusable drill bits and saw blades usually are discarded when dull. Disposable styles are preferred.

The misalignment of hinged instruments is a common problem that occurs primarily as a result of misuse. The instrument must be repaired if the teeth or serrations do not mesh perfectly or if the jaws overlap.

Stiff joints or frozen box locks are the result of inadequate cleaning or corrosion caused by trapped moisture or a corrosive. The instrument should be repaired before the box lock cracks and the instrument must be replaced.

After repeated use, instruments eventually wear, misalign, and stiffen. Parts such as inserts, screws, or springs may need to be replaced. The life of many instruments can be extended by preventive maintenance or prompt repair.

Restoration

Instruments may become spotted, stained, corroded, pitted, or rusted. Some surface discoloration will appear with normal usage, but the unusual or severe buildup of deposits may impair function or sterilization. The color of a stain may help identify a problem that needs to be corrected:

- *Light or dark water spots:* from mineral content in tap water or condensate in sterilizer caused by inadequate drying
- *Rust-colored film:* from iron content or softening agents in steam pipes
- *Bluish gray stain:* from some chemical sterilizing or disinfecting solutions
- *Brownish stain:* from polyphosphate cleaning compounds that are incompatible with local water supply, leaving a chromic oxide film on instruments
- *Purplish-black stain:* from detergents that contain ammonia or from amines in steam lines
- *Rust deposits:* from inadequate cleaning or drying, agents not thoroughly rinsed off, electrolytic deposits from exposed metal under chipped chrome plating onto stainless steel, or residues in textile wrappers

Blood, saline solution, or detergents that contain chloride can cause pitting if they are not rinsed off promptly and thoroughly. Detergents with high or low pH can destroy the protective chromium oxide layer on stainless steel.

If an instrument has been damaged, the surface can be repolished and passivated by the manufacturer to restore the finish. A plated instrument can be replated; this should be done as soon as the plating is chipped or begins to peel.

Replacement

Broken instruments must be replaced if they are beyond repair or restoration. With normal use, good-quality surgical instruments have an expected life of at least 10 years. Using these precise tools for only their intended purpose cannot be overemphasized. Misuse and abuse are the most common causes of instrument breakage. Replacing instruments that have been needlessly damaged is an unnecessary expense for the OR.

POWERED SURGICAL INSTRUMENTS

Most surgical instruments have movable parts that are manipulated by the surgeon. Some instruments are pneumatically powered by compressed air or nitrogen or are electrically powered by a battery or alternating current. Powered surgical instruments are complex assemblies of gears, rotating shafts, and seals. They require special handling during preparation and use and special considerations for cleaning and sterilizing.

Powered instruments are used primarily for precision drilling, cutting, shaping, and beveling bone. They also may be used for skin grafts and to abrade skin. Powered instruments increase speed and decrease the fatigue caused by manually driven drills, saws, and reamers. The instrument may have rotary, reciprocating, or oscillating action. Rotary movement is used to drill holes or to insert screws, wires, or pins. Reciprocating movement (a cutting action from front to back), and oscillating movement (a cutting action from side to side) are used to cut or remove bone or skin. Some instruments have a combination of movements and can be changed from one to another by adjusting controls.

Depending on the function desired, the surgeon chooses a drill, burr, blade, reamer, or abrader of appropriate size. These accessories attach securely into the handpiece. Small drill bits, burrs, cutting blades, and abraders may be disposable.

The heat generated by powered instruments can damage bone cells. Blood loss from bone is reduced by the tiny particles that these high-speed instruments pack into the cut surfaces. The speed of these instruments may disperse a fine mist of blood and bone cells. For this reason, the Occupational Safety and Health Administration (OSHA), the Centers for Disease Control and Prevention (CDC), and the American Academy of Orthopaedic Surgeons recommend wearing at least protective eyewear; a face shield or spacesuit-type headgear should be considered if splatter is anticipated.

Unless the instrument is carefully controlled, tissue can be unintentionally caught in a rapidly spinning drill or oscillating saw, or the instrument may cut more than desired. When a powered instrument is being used, particularly one with a rotating movement, all team members must be very careful to keep their hands away from the blade. Most powered instruments have a safety mechanism on the handpiece. Some are operated by foot pedals.

Power Sources

The type of power used by an instrument determines the accessories that are needed to operate the instrument.

Air-Powered Instruments

Air-powered instruments are small, lightweight, free of vibration, and easy to handle for pinpoint accuracy at high speeds. Compared with electrical instruments, they cause minimal heating of bone because they operate at a faster and higher speed.

In operating air-powered instruments, medical-grade compressed air or pure (99.97%) dry nitrogen is either piped into the OR or supplied from a cylinder tank on a stable carrier. The pressure must be set and monitored by the operating pressure gauges of the regulator. The correct pounds per square inch (psi), as determined by the manufacturer, is set after the instrument is assembled and turned on. The operating pressure is usually within a range of 70 to 160 psi, and storage pressure in the cylinder is at least 500 psi. Excessive pressure can damage the instrument and the hose that connects it to the regulator. A broken air hose under pressure can whip out of control and injure personnel or the patient.

Electrically Powered Instruments

Electrically powered instruments such as saws, drills, dermatomes, and nerve stimulators are potential explosion hazards in the OR. Most of the motors are designed to be explosion proof. All must have sparkproof connections.

Because of the heat generated when using electrical instruments, the surgeon usually has the assistant use a bulb syringe to drip saline solution on the area to cool the bone and wash away particles. Care must be taken so the syringe does not touch the blade, especially if it is glass. Plastic syringes are less hazardous.

Battery Power Some battery-operated instruments are cordless and have rechargeable batteries in the handpiece. Others have cords that attach to a battery charger, which is plugged into an electrical outlet. The batteries are charged and sterilized for use on the sterile table.

Alternating Current Power switches should be off before cords are plugged into electrical outlets. The power supply cord should be connected to the outlet before anesthetic gases are administered and should not be disconnected during anesthesia administration. The anesthesia provider should be alerted that electrical equipment will be used. The scrub person may be able to disconnect the instrument from its power source when it is not in use so a team member cannot inadvertently activate it. Many of these instruments are activated by foot pedals. The circulator can move the foot pedal away from the surgeon until it is needed.

Sonic Energy Some instruments are activated by sonic energy to move cutting edges in a linear direction. This is a power assist without the rotary motion and high speed of other electrically powered instruments.

Handling Powered Instruments

Before any new or repaired powered instrument is put into use, the biomedical technician should verify that the instrument is functioning according to the manufacturer's specifications. Powered instruments are not without some inherent dangers. Key points in handling powered instruments include the following:

1. Set the instrument and attachments alone on a small sterile table when they are not in use. This provides added protection from inadvertent activation.
2. Handle and store the air hose or electrical power cord with care. A broken air hose can whip out of control. A broken electrical cord can short-circuit the instrument. Always inspect the hose or cord for cracks or breaks.
3. To prevent inadvertent activation, assemble the appropriate handpiece, attachments (e.g., blades, drills, and reamers), and power source with the safety mechanism in position. Always be certain that attachments are completely seated and locked in the handpiece.
4. Test whether the instrument is in working condition before the surgeon is ready to use it and before it is applied to the patient. To prevent inadvertent activation, the safety mechanism must be set in position until ready to use and when changing attachments.

Cleaning and Sterilizing Powered Instruments

Powered instruments should always be operated, cleaned, and sterilized according to the manufacturer's directions for use and care. Each instrument has different cleaning, lubricating, packaging, and sterilizing requirements because of its various component parts. The bioburden is determined by the size, design, complexity, and condition of the instrument; the degree of contamination during use; and subsequent decontaminating and cleaning procedures. Microorganisms can become entrapped around the seals on rotating shafts. For instruments with a specific biologic challenge, manufacturers test in the area most difficult to sterilize and recommend sterilization cycles accordingly. The following general guidelines apply to the care of all powered instruments:

1. Clean and decontaminate the instrument immediately after use to maintain optimal function.
   a. During the surgical procedure, the scrub person should wipe off any organic debris between uses.
   b. The accessories are disassembled for cleaning.
   c. The air hose should remain attached to the handpiece during cleaning. The air hose or electrical cord should be wiped with detergent, damp cloth, and dry towel.
   d. The motor is not immersed in liquid. The power mechanism cannot be cleaned in a basin of solution or put in a washer-sterilizer, a washer-decontaminator, or an ultrasonic cleaner. The surface of the instrument is wiped with a mild detergent, and caution is used to prevent solution from entering the internal mechanism. The detergent is wiped off with a damp cloth, and the mechanism is dried with a lint-free towel.
2. Lubricate the instrument as recommended by the manufacturer.
   a. Some air-powered instruments can be lubricated with a sterile lubricant after sterilization and just before use.
   b. Some manufacturers supply lubricant, usually a silicone oil.
   c. Some instruments must be run after lubrication to disperse the lubricant through the mechanism.
3. Wrap the instrument for sterilization.
   a. Some manufacturers supply sterilizing cases. These cases can be wrapped in woven or nonwoven material.
   b. The instrument must be disassembled.

c. The sharp edges of accessories must be protected.
   d. Hoses or cords should be loosely coiled.
4. Sterilize the instrument in steam unless contraindicated by the manufacturer.
   a. A prevacuum sterilizer removes entrapped air and allows steam to access the internal mechanism; this type of sterilizer is therefore preferred to a gravity displacement sterilizer.
   b. Exposure time depends on the type of sterilizer, the design and complexity of the instrument, and packaging. In a gravity displacement sterilizer at 250° F (121° C), exposure time may be as long as 1 hour.
   c. Sterilization of an unwrapped instrument in a gravity displacement sterilizer at 270° F (132° C) must provide exposure that is long enough to sterilize the internal mechanism—usually at least 15 minutes.
   d. Ethylene oxide gas sterilization should be used only if the instrument cannot withstand the heat or moisture of steam sterilization. The instrument must be free of all traces of lubricant. The manufacturer should specify the aeration time.

Bibliography

Abbot P: The best of both worlds: "reposables," *Todays Surg Nurs* 19(2):35-38, 1997.

Association for the Advancement of Medical Instrumentation: *AAMI standards for the sterilization of patient care items for immediate use,* Arlington, Va, 1996, The Association.

Association of Operating Room Nurses: *AORN standards, recommended practices, and guidelines,* Denver, 1998, The Association.

Berguer R: Surgical technology and the ergonomics of laparoscopic instruments, *Surg Endosc* 12(5):458-462, 1998.

Chan-Myers H et al: Natural bioburden levels detected on rigid lumened medical devices before and after cleaning, *Am J Infect Control* 25(6):471-476, 1997.

DesCoteaux JG et al: A prospective comparison of the costs of reusable and limited reuse laparoscopic instruments, *Can J Surg* 41(2):136-141, 1998.

Dujovny M, Agner C: The use of high power drills for laminectomy in spinal stenosis: technical report, *Neurol Res* 19(2):219-221, 1997.

Finkelstein LE, Mendelson MH, Schneider NJ: Infection control: how to safely clean surgical instruments, *Am J Nurs* 97(6):59, 1997.

Hales M: Instrument decontamination methods that prolong instrument life, *Infect Control Today* 2(9):12, 16-18, 1998.

O'Neale M et al: Reusable instrumentation: patient and liability issues, *Point of View* 33(2):10-16, 1996.

Pezzella AT: Practical innovations: hand signals in surgery, *AORN J* 63(4):769-771, 1996.

Rutala WA et al: Levels of contamination on surgical instruments, *Am J Infect Control* 26(2):143-145, 1998.

Springthorpe S, Sattar S: Measuring instrument cleanliness, *Infect Control Today* 2(9):20, 22, 24, 26, 1998.

Tighe SMB: *Instrumentation for the operating room: a photographic manual,* ed 5, St Louis, 1999, Mosby.

Weber LA: The surgical tray, *Dermatol Clin* 16(1):17-24, 1998.

Chapter 20

Specialized Surgical Equipment

 Chapter Objectives

After studying this chapter, the learner will be able to:

- Distinguish between monopolar and bipolar electrosurgical units and applications.
- List the basic elements of electrosurgical safety.
- Identify three basic types of lasers.
- Describe the tissue effects of the different types of laser light in vivo.
- Discuss the application of minimally invasive endoscopic technique.
- Identify potential safety hazards associated with high technology in patient care.

Advances in technology have made possible the complex surgical techniques of the present. Technology may be defined as the branch of knowledge that deals with the creation and use of technical means for scientific purposes. In the context of surgery, technology refers to a system that uses both devices and people to perform specific tasks. Continuing research will further enhance technology in the future. New devices are usually adjuncts to or extensions of devices or techniques already in use. To enhance their use in patient care, perioperative team members constantly need to learn about new equipment and its applications.

Surgical residency and first assistant programs include education and training in electrosurgery, laser surgery, endoscopy, and microsurgery. Therefore on completion of postgraduate education, surgeons today are skilled in the use of these advanced technologies. Continuing surgical educational courses, including laboratory study, are available so that practicing surgeons can learn to use the newest technology. Before handling new equipment, patient care personnel on the perioperative team should be knowledgeable about its care and use. Some surgical procedures use more than one of these technologies (e.g., laser surgery through an attachment

to the operating microscope directed through an endoscope). Preparing and handling these expensive pieces of equipment are major responsibilities of perioperative nurses and surgical technologists. In addition, all operating room (OR) personnel should be aware of and safeguard against hazards associated with equipment. The perioperative environment should be safe for patients and personnel.

ELECTROSURGERY

Terms associated with electrosurgery are defined in Box 20-1.

Historical Background

The ancient practice of pouring boiling oil into a wound or searing it with hot irons to stop bleeding and infection was extreme. Patients usually were crippled if they survived. Surgeons continued to use these techniques, however, long after Ambroise Paré discredited their use in the sixteenth century. They recognized that application of heat accelerates the natural chemical reaction of blood to hasten clotting. This eventually led to the development of electrocautery (direct contact

313

Box 20-1 **Terms Associated with Electrosurgery**

active electrode Apparatus used to deliver electric current to the surgical site.
current Flow of electrical energy.
blended current Current that divides tissue and controls some bleeding.
coagulating current Current that passes intense heat through the active electrode used to sear vessels and control bleeding.
cutting current Current that arcs between tissue and the active electrode to divide tissue without coagulation.
electrosurgical unit (ESU) Generator, foot pedal, cords, active electrode, and inactive dispersive electrode designed to safely deliver electric current through tissue.
bipolar unit Current is delivered to the surgical site and returned to the generator by forceps. One side of the forceps is active; the other side is inactive. The current passes only between the tips of the forceps.
monopolar unit Current flows from the generator to the active electrode, through the patient to the inactive dispersive electrode, and returns to the generator.
generator Machine that produces electric current by generating high-frequency radio waves.
ground Conducting connection between the generator, the patient, and the earth.
inactive dispersive electrode Apparatus used to direct current from the patient back to the generator; also referred to as inactive electrode, return electrode, patient plate, or grounding pad.

of an electrically heated wire with tissue). Still in use, pencil-size, battery-operated units provide hemostasis by using a self-contained battery to heat a cauterizing wire. These are primarily used in plastic surgery. Electrosurgery, by contrast, delivers high-frequency oscillating electric currents through tissue between two electrodes to coagulate or cut tissue.

In 1906 Lee DeForest, the physicist commonly known as the father of radio, discovered by accident that a high-frequency electric current could sever tissue with only slight traces of generated heat. In conjunction with his vacuum tube generator, he patented an electrode that cut tissue with an electrical arc created at the point of a dull blade. Referred to as cold cautery, the device was used unsuccessfully by pioneers like Boston neurosurgeon Harvey Cushing (1869-1939).

Working with Cushing, W.T. Bovie, also a physicist, developed the first spark-gap tube generator in the 1920s. This became the universal basis of electrosurgical units (ESUs), often referred to as "Bovies" until the 1970s, when solid-state units became available. These solid-state units use transistors, diodes, and rectifiers to generate current. The spark-gap generator continues to be used in urology.

Principles of Electrosurgery

Electric current can be used to cut or coagulate most tissues. The initial incision is made by a scalpel to prevent charring

and scarring of skin. Electrosurgery can then be used on fat, fascia, muscle, internal organs, and vessels. High-frequency alternating or oscillating electric currents move at more than 20,000 cycles per second (10,000 for radiofrequency). ESUs operate at frequencies between 100,000 and 10,000,000 Hz. This current can be passed through tissue without causing stimulation of muscles or nerves. The heat produced is a direct result of resistance to its passage through tissue. The density of electric current flowing through a point of contact in tissue elevates temperature sufficiently to cause destruction of cells by dissolution of their molecular structure. The amount of heat produced by any amount of resistance is proportional to the current squared. For example, doubling the current increases the heat produced fourfold. Conversely, the amount of heat produced by any amount of current is directly proportional to resistance; doubling the resistance doubles the heat produced. Therefore current should be concentrated in a small area of high resistance to produce the high temperature required for electrosurgery, which is approximately 2000° F (1093° C).

Electrosurgical Unit

To complete the electrical circuit to coagulate or cut tissue, current flows from a generator (electrosurgical power unit) to an active electrode, through tissue, and back to the generator via an inactive dispersive electrode. Electrosurgery is used to a greater or lesser extent in all surgical specialties. Several different units are available. Some have selective uses; others are adaptable to many types of surgical procedures. Personnel should be familiar with the manufacturer's detailed manual of operating instructions for each type used.

Generator

The machine that produces high-frequency or radio waves is the generator or power component of the ESU. Some generators are grounded. This means that the machine acts as a ground to earth. Current returns to the machine, but if the circuit is broken, the current will find an alternate route back to earth, such as through metal in contact with a body. A balanced-output generator is referenced to earth. An isolated generator offers the advantage of a non–ground-seeking circuit. The flow of current is isolated and restricted to active and dispersive electrodes, and the current returns directly back to the generator. With an isolated generator, if the circuit is broken, current will not flow.

Solid-state generators are transistorized and use diodes (semiconductors) and rectifiers (devices that change AC to DC) to produce current. They usually operate at a lower output than spark-gap generators and have safety features such as return monitors to prevent burns and electrocution. Both solid-state and spark-gap generators provide two separate circuits within the housing of the machine. Controls on the outside of the housing allow selection of desired characteristic of current. The current may be identical in frequency, power (voltage), and amount (amperage) but vary in quality. Quality depends on the difference in damping (the pattern of waveforms by which oscillations diminish after surges of power). This difference determines tissue reaction to the current.

Coagulating Current

A damped waveform has a continuous pattern of surges of current that rapidly diminishes to short periods, or gaps, in which no current is delivered. This is produced by the spark-gap circuit. Damped current coagulates tissue. As it approaches the active electrode, the density of current increases to produce an intense heat, which sears the ends of small or moderate-size vessels to control bleeding on contact. Attempts to coagulate large vessels can result in an extensive burn and necrosis. Excess charring interferes with wound healing and may provide a medium for infection.

Cutting Current

An undamped waveform, which is produced by a vacuum tube oscillator, does not diminish but retains a constant output of high-frequency current. Undamped current cuts tissue. This continuous current forms an arc between tissues and an active electrode that is intense enough to divide fibrous tissue as it moves along lines of deep incision before sufficient heat builds up to coagulate adjacent tissues.

Blended Current

Undamped current can be blended with damped current to add a coagulating effect to the cutting current. At the same time that it cuts through or across tissue, cutting current accomplishes some coagulation of cells on the surface of the incision and prevents capillary bleeding. Some solid-state generators have a setting for blend or hemostasis for this function. This blend can also be achieved by a slightly damped waveform from a spark-gap generator.

Controls

The type and amount of current are regulated by controls on the generator. Most units provide up to 400 watts of power. It is seldom necessary to use full-power settings. A safe general rule for the circulator is to start with the lowest setting of current that accomplishes the desired degree of coagulation or cutting and then increase the current at the surgeon's request. The surgeon selects the type of current to be used with either a foot pedal or hand control switch. The circulator verbally confirms and documents the power settings before the generator is activated. The generator should be designed to minimize unintentional activation.

In solid-state units the power output is isolated to prevent overheating and is equipped with a warning buzzer and/or light to warn of too high a setting or a break in the circuit. Flow of current to and from the generator should be balanced. A return electrode monitoring system measures and compares current flowing from the active electrode with current returning from the inactive dispersive electrode. The generator deactivates if continuity in the electrical circuit is disrupted or inadequate in some units. Safety features should be tested before each patient use, and the generator should be periodically inspected by the biomedical engineering department.

The generator may be mounted on a portable stand. It should be moved carefully to avoid tipping. The machine should be cleaned before and after use. Unintentional activation or failure may occur if liquid or debris enters the generator. The facility may be held responsible for a defect causing patient injury. The generator should have an identification number. This should be recorded in the patient's record to verify the equipment used. This identification number also provides a means of maintaining records of routine inspections and maintenance. Operational instructions should be on or attached to every unit. Personnel using this equipment should be trained and knowledgeable in its use.

Active Electrode

The sterile active electrode directs flow of current to the surgical site. The style of the electrode tip (i.e., blade, loop, ball, or needle) will be determined by the type of surgical procedure and current to be used. The electrode tip may be fixed into or detachable from a pencil-shaped handle, or it may be incorporated into a tissue forceps or suction tube. It is attached to a conductor cord, which is connected to the generator. The scrub person hands the end of the conductor cord off of the sterile field to the circulator, who attaches it to the generator. The cord should be long and flexible enough to reach between the sterile field and the generator without stress. It should be free of kinks and bends that could deviate current flow. When the unit is not in actual use, although connected, the electrode tip should be kept clean, dry, and visible. It may be kept in an insulated holster/container attached to the drape over the patient to avoid the possibility of a fire being started by someone on the team inadvertently stepping on the foot switch or activating the hand control.

The surgeon places the active electrode tip on the tissue and then activates the foot switch or hand control to transfer electric current from the generator to the tissue. Some hand switches are color coded to identify coagulating and cutting functions. Some generators produce a buzzing sound that varies in pitch, depending on which current is being used. Charred or coagulated tissue should be removed from the tip because charred tissue absorbs heat and decreases the effectiveness of current. This can be done by scraping the tip on a disposable tip cleaner. Some specialized bipolar tips are wiped with hydrogen peroxide. Using a scalpel blade should be avoided because the debris may become airborne, creating a biologic hazard.

Rather than placing the tip directly on tissue, bleeding vessels may be clamped with hemostats or smooth-tipped tissue forceps. As little extraneous tissue as possible should be clamped to minimize damage to adjacent tissue. Vessels are coagulated when any part of the metal instrument is touched with the active electrode; this is frequently referred to as "buzzing." The electrode should be in contact with the instrument before activation to avoid arcing. The person holding it should have a firm grip on as large an area of instrument as possible and avoid touching the patient. The active current should not be applied for more than 3 seconds. Inadvertent patient injury can occur if the metal instrument is in contact with retractors or other instrumentation placed in the surgical field. Low-voltage cutting current should be used. Current can burn through surgical gloves if these precautions are not taken.

The electrode and cord may be disposable. Reusable electrodes should be inspected for damage before reprocessing and before use at the sterile field.

Inactive Dispersive Electrode

Electric current will flow to ground or a neutral potential. Therefore a proper channel should be provided to disperse current and heat generated in tissue. The inactive electrode disperses high-frequency current released through the active electrode and provides low current density return from tissues back to the generator. Resistance from the patient to the generator and from the generator to the wall electrical outlet should be less than 1 ohm. ESUs have either monopolar or bipolar mechanisms or both to direct the flow of electric current.

Bipolar Units   With bipolar units the dispersive electrode is incorporated into forceps used by the surgeon. One side of the forceps is the active electrode through which current passes to tissues. The other side is inactive. Output voltage is relatively low. Current flows only between the tips of the forceps, returning directly to the generator. Current does not disperse itself throughout the patient, as it does in monopolar units. This provides extremely precise control of the coagulated area. A grounding pad or plate is not needed because current does not flow through the patient.

Monopolar Units   With monopolar units current flows from the generator to the active electrode, through the patient to an inactive dispersive electrode, and back to the generator. Power is greater than through bipolar forceps. Because current supplied by the generator is dispersed from the active electrode, it seeks completion of the electrical circuit to ground or a neutral potential through the patient's body. An inactive dispersive electrode should be used to ground the patient. This is in the form of a patient grounding pad or plate placed in direct contact with skin. The contact area must exceed 100 mm² or have a diameter greater than 1.2 cm. Disposable styles are flexible to mold to any body surface. They must maintain uniform body contact. Some are prelubricated. If a metal plate is placed under the patient, a conductive electrode gel should be spread evenly over the entire plate to thoroughly wet the skin and thus reduce its electrical resistance to a minimum. Prelubricated pads should be checked for dry spots before placement.

Current flows from the active electrode through the body to the inactive dispersive electrode. It then returns to the generator via a conductor cord (Figure 20-1). This cord should be long and flexible enough to reach without stress on attachments to the electrode or generator. Attachments should be secure. The plug or adapter at the end of the cord fastens into the receptacle on the generator. This may be labeled and/or color coded to help ensure correct attachment of the dispersive electrode. Unless it is disposable, the cord should be checked before use for wire breakage or fraying by grasping the connecting plug and pulling firmly on the cord. If it stretches, wires inside are broken and should be repaired. Reusable cords should be inspected by the biomedical engineering department periodically for electrical integrity.

Figure 20-1   Path of electric current from ESU.

Figure 20-2   Placement of ESU dispersive electrode.

The dispersive electrode is properly placed and connected to the generator to avoid an electrical burn to the patient (Figure 20-2). The following safeguards are taken:

1. The dispersive electrode should be as close as possible to the site where the active electrode will be used to minimize current through the body. The patient should be in the desired position before the dispersive electrode is applied to prevent its becoming dislodged or buckled during patient positioning. Do not remove or reposition the disposable dispersive electrode because the integrity of the adhesive will be altered. A new electrode is used each time. The dispersive electrode should not be cut to fit.

2. The dispersive electrode must cover as large an area of the patient's skin as possible in an area free of hair or scar tissue, both of which tend to act as insulation. An area may need to be shaved. The surface area affects heat buildup and dissipation. Avoid areas where bony prominences might result in pressure points, which in turn can cause current concentration. Place the pad or plate on a clean, dry skin surface over or under as large a muscle mass area as possible. The gel conduction material on the pad is cold and sticky to the touch; a patient who is awake should be forewarned of its application.

3. The dispersive electrode should not be placed on skin over a metal implant, such as a hip prosthesis, because current could be diverted to the implant.

4. The dispersive electrode should be clean, free from bent edges, and adhere uniformly to skin. Some conductive lubricants will dry out and leave a high-resistance film that will prevent proper contact with skin. The integrity

of the package of a disposable dispersive electrode should be inspected before use. Do not use the electrode if the package is damaged or has been previously opened.

5. The metal connection between the pad or plate and the conductor cord must not touch the patient. Special care should be taken to ensure that the cord does not become dislodged. Do not put a safety belt over the electrode or cord, for example. The safest connectors are threaded or locked and also are insulated. The connector should not create a pressure point on the patient's skin.

6. The connection between the dispersive electrode and generator should be secure and made with compatible attachments. If the return circuit is faulty, the ground circuit may be completed through inadvertent contact with the metal operating bed or its attachments. If the grounded area is small, current passing through an exposed area of skin contact will be relatively intense. For example, one such contact point could be the thigh touching a leg stirrup while the patient is in the lithotomy position.

7. A dispersive electrode is not used with bipolar generators.

The circulator should record on the patient's chart the location of the inactive dispersive electrode, the condition of the patient's skin before and after electrosurgery, the generator identification number, and the settings used. Some institutions also require documentation of the dispersive electrode lot number.

Safety Factors

Electrical burn through the patient's skin is the greatest hazard of electrosurgery. These burns are usually deeper than flame burns, causing widespread tissue necrosis and deep thrombosis to the extent that debridement may be required. Isolated circuits for ESUs and return-electrode monitoring systems, if used, virtually eliminate these burns. Perioperative personnel should be aware of hazards and safeguard against injury to the patient. In addition to the precautions noted for preparing the ESU and for positioning the dispersive electrode used with monopolar units, other precautions should be taken as follows:

1. Electrosurgery should not be used in the mouth, trachea, around the head, or in the pleural cavity when high concentrations of oxygen or nitrous oxide are used. Flammable anesthetics are not used. Safety regulations for use with all inhalation anesthetic agents are followed.

2. Electrocardiogram electrodes should be placed as far away from the surgical site as possible. Burns can occur at the site of electrocardiogram electrodes and other low impedance points from invasive monitor probes if current diverts to alternate grounds.

3. Rings and other jewelry should be removed. Metallic jewelry, including that used in body piercing, presents

a potential risk of burn for the patient from diverted currents from the monopolar unit with either an isolated or ground-referenced output.

4. Flammable agents such as alcohol should not be used in skin preparation. If they are used, the skin surface should be completely dry before draping. Fumes and vapors may collect in drapes and ignite when the electrosurgical or cautery unit is used. The use of aqueous antiseptic solutions is preferred.

5. If another piece of electrical equipment is used in direct contact with the patient at the same time as the ESU, connect it to a different source of current if possible. The cutting current of the ESU may not work if another piece of electrical equipment is on the same circuit. The ESU may interfere with the operation of some equipment, such as older models of cardiac monitors. The isolated power system of solid-state generators may prevent these problems.

6. Monopolar electrosurgery may disrupt operation of an implanted cardiac pacemaker. New models of cardiac pacemakers are unaffected by monopolar ESU generators. Check with the pacemaker manufacturer regarding compatibility. The bipolar ESU may be used. The patient is continuously monitored. A defibrillator should be on standby in the OR.

7. Connection of a bipolar active electrode to a monopolar receptacle may activate current, causing a short circuit. Plugs on cords should be differentiated to prevent misconnections of active and inactive electrodes.

8. Secure the active electrode handle in an insulated holster/container when not in use. Do not immerse an active electrode in liquid.

9. To prevent fire, only moist sponges should be permitted on the sterile field while the ESU is in use. This includes using moist sponges during the use of battery-operated pencil cautery.

10. Investigate a repeated request for more current. The dispersive electrode or connecting cord may be at fault. Shock to those touching the patient may result. The patient may be burned.

11. For safety of the patient and personnel, follow instructions for use and care; these appear on the machine or in the manual provided by the manufacturer that accompanies each ESU. Grasp and pull only the plugs, not cords, when disconnecting attachments from the generator or the power source. Position the power cord away from the team to avoid tripping team members. Avoid rolling equipment over the power cord.

12. Any malfunctioning ESU should be taken out of service until cleared for use by the biomedical engineering department.

13. The patient and personnel should be protected from inhaling plume (smoke) generated during electrosurgery. A suction evacuator device should be placed as close to the source of plume as possible to maximize evacuation of smoke and enhance visibility at the surgical site.

Electrosurgery causes more patient injuries than any other electrical device used in the OR. Most incidents are caused by personnel error.

LASER SURGERY

The term *laser* is an acronym for *Light Amplification by Stimulated Emission of Radiation*. Terms associated with laser surgery are defined in Box 20-2.

Historical Background

Einstein's theory, purported in 1917, explaining the difference between spontaneous and stimulated emission of light, eventually led to the development of the laser. This development began in 1940 in the Soviet Union. Lasers depend on the capacity of atoms to become excited when struck by a quantum of electromagnetic energy known as a photon. Photons are the basic units of radiation that constitute light. When struck by a photon, the electrons of the atom move to a high energy level. On spontaneous return to a lower energy level toward normal ground state, these electrons emit another photon that will strike another atom also in the transitional pumped-up energy state. This reaction produces a second photon of the same frequency. This sets up a chain reaction of stimulated emission of photons at high energy levels. Production of this reaction in a sustained state, known as population inversion, was technically difficult. The introduction of practical lasers into scientific technology finally occurred almost simultaneously in the United States and Russia around 1960.

The laser as a surgical instrument was developed in the United States. The first surgical laser, the ruby laser, was used in ophthalmology for retinal hemorrhages. As scientists discovered that other materials could be electrically stimulated to produce lasers in a variety of wavelengths, the CO_2 and argon gas surgical lasers were developed in the mid-1960s. The argon laser replaced the ruby laser for use in ophthalmology. Not until after Jako adapted the CO_2 laser to the operating microscope in 1972 did lasers truly become viable adjuncts to the surgical arena.

Physical Properties of Lasers

The laser focuses light on atoms to stimulate them to a high point of excitation. The resulting radiation is then amplified and metamorphosed into the wavelengths of laser light. This light beam is monochromatic (one color) because all of the electromagnetic waves are the same length and collimated, or parallel to each other. The light is totally concentrated and easily focused. Unlike conventional light waves, which spread and dissipate electromagnetic radiation by many different wavelengths, the coherence of the laser beam is sustained over space and time with wavelengths in the same frequency and energy phase.

Lasers may emit their energy in brief, repeating emissions that have a duration of only an extremely small fraction of a second. These are pulsed laser systems. Or, they are capable of

Box 20-2 **Terms Associated with Laser Surgery**

emissions Surgical lasers emit nonionizing radiation, heat, and debris.

direct laser energy Nonionizing radiation is selectively absorbed by tissues with resultant destruction at the focal point.

indirect or reflective energy Radiation can become scattered if the beam strikes a reflective surface or is unintentionally activated. Direct or indirect exposure to laser energy can burn skin and injure eyes. It can also ignite flammable materials and combustible gases.

laser plume Carbonized cell fragments, toxic hydrocarbons, viruses, and noxious fumes can be dispersed from tissues exposed to the laser beam. Vaporization converts solid tissue to smoke and gas. This plume (smoke) is evacuated to maintain visibility and also to minimize the hazard of inhalation by personnel.

laser Acronym for *Light Amplification by Stimulated Emission of Radiation*. Light, concentrated and focused, stimulates atoms to emit radiant energy when activated.

laser beam Light beams, either pulsed or continuous, go through a medium to produce lasing effect. The beam has three distinct characteristics as follows:

coherent Light beams are sustained over space and time because electromagnetic waves are in same frequency and energy phase with each other.

collimated Light beams are parallel.

monochromatic Light beam is one color because waves are all the same length in the electromagnetic spectrum.

power All lasers have a combination of duration, intensity, and output of radiation when wavelengths are activated.

source Power to energize the light beam may be electrical, radiofrequency, or optical.

wavelength Electromagnetic waves transfer energy progressively from point to point through a medium. The wavelength is the distance traveled along the electromagnetic spectrum. Radiation penetration differs at different wavelengths. Each laser has a different wavelength and color, depending on the medium the light beam passes through.

medium Gases, synthetic crystals, glass rods, liquid dyes, free electrons, and semiconductors are used to produce the lasing effect.

producing continuous light beams; these are continuous-wave lasers. All lasers have a combination of duration, level, and output wavelengths of radiation emitted when activated. Power density, the irradiance, is the amount of power per unit surface area during a single pulse or exposure. This is expressed as watts per centimeter squared. Regardless of beam characteristics, components of a laser system are the same (Figure 20-3). These components include the following:

- A medium to produce a lasing effect of the stimulated emission. Gases, solid rods or crystals, liquid dyes, and free electrons are used. Each produces a different wavelength, color, and effect.

Figure 20-3 Basic laser components.

- A power source to create population inversion by pumping energy into the lasing medium. This may be electrical or radiofrequency power or an optical power source such as a xenon flash lamp or another laser.
- An amplification mechanism to change random directional movement of stimulated emissions to a parallel direction. This occurs within an optical resonator or laser cavity, which is a tube with mirrors at each end. As photons traveling the length of the resonator reflect back through the medium, they stimulate more atoms to release photons, thus amplifying the lasing effect. The power density of the beam determines the laser's capacity to cut, coagulate, or vaporize tissue.
- Wave guides to aim and control the direction of the laser beam. The optical resonator has a small opening in one end that permits transmission of a small beam of laser light. The smaller the beam, the higher its power density will be. Fiberoptic wave guides or a series of rhodium reflecting mirrors then direct the beam to tissue. The wave mode may be continuous, pulsed, or a Q-switched single pulse of high energy.
- Backstops to stop the laser beam from penetrating beyond the expected impact site and affecting nontargeted tissue. Quartz or titanium rods will stop the beam.

Types of Lasers

Lasers use argon, carbon dioxide, holmium, krypton, neodymium, phosphate, ruby, or xenon as their active media. When delivered to tissues, laser light can be absorbed, reflected, transmitted, or scattered, depending on the characteristics of the laser and the type of tissue. Only absorbed light produces thermal effects in tissue. Thermal penetration varies according to the ratio of absorption vs. scattering. Energy absorbed at the surface will destroy superficial cells; further penetration extends cell destruction in surrounding tissues. The wavelength of the laser light, power density, rate of delivery of energy, and exposure time will vary the effects on tissue. Energy density is based on the laser's wattage, beam or spot size, and time of exposure. The spot size depends on the laser fiber size and distance of the tip from tissue; it increases and becomes defocused as fiber is moved farther from tissue. Variables in tissue reaction are listed in Box 20-3.

Laser beams cut, vaporize, or coagulate tissue. Coagulative effect causes collagen bonding and welding of tissue surfaces. Each laser has selective uses. Laser light colors vary from the visible, near-ultraviolet range to the invisible, far-infrared range of the electromagnetic spectrum (Figure 20-4). Wavelengths also vary, providing different radiation penetration depths. Lasers are commonly used in conjunction with the operating microscope and/or an endoscope. The surgeon selects the appropriate laser for the tissue to be incised, excised, or coagulated.

Argon Laser

Argon ion gas emits a blue-green light beam in the visible electromagnetic spectrum at wavelengths of 450 and 530 nm, or 0.5 µm. This wavelength passes through water and clear fluid, such as cerebrospinal fluid, with minimal absorption. It is intensely absorbed by the brown-red pigment of hemoglobin in blood or melanin in pigmented tissue and converted into heat. Thermal radiation penetrates to a depth of 1 or 2 mm in most tissue.

The argon laser operates from electrical power. A water-cooling system is often required to dissipate heat generated in the argon medium.

The argon laser beam usually is transmitted through a flexible quartz fiberoptic wave guide that is 200 to 600 mm in diameter. This can be directed to a handpiece or through an endoscope or operating microscope. Most argon laser machines deliver a nonfocused beam that vaporizes tissue poorly and scatters more radiation than other types of lasers. Irradiance may vary from less than 1 watt to 20 watts, depending on the model.

Argon lasers coagulate bleeding points or lesions involving many small superficial vessels, such as a port-wine stain. They are used primarily to destroy specific cutaneous lesions while sparing adjacent tissue and minimizing scarring. Argon lasers may be used to treat vascular lesions and remove plaque and to coagulate superficial vessels in mucosa, such as in the gastrointestinal tract. They are also used in ophthalmology, otolaryngology, gynecology, urology, neurosurgery, and dermatology.

Carbon Dioxide Laser

Using a mixture of carbon dioxide, nitrogen, and helium molecular gases, the CO_2 laser emits an invisible beam from the mid- to far-infrared range of the electromagnetic spectrum at wavelengths of 9600 and 10,600 nm, or 10.6 µm. This wavelength is intensely absorbed by water. It raises water temper-

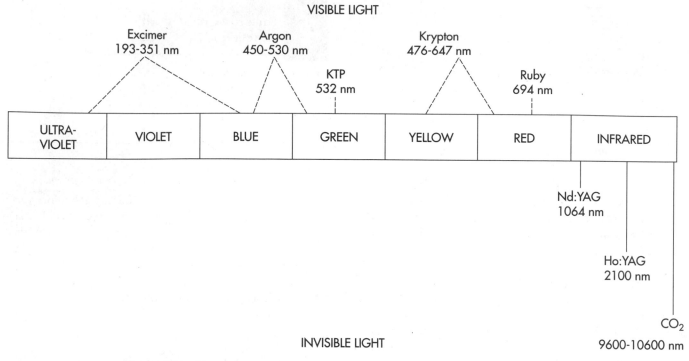

Figure 20-4 Electromagnetic spectrum of laser light beams at wavelengths in nanometers.

ature in cells to the flash boiling point, thus vaporizing tissue. Vaporization is the conversion of solid tissue to smoke and gas. This plume should be evacuated or suctioned through a filter device from the site of lasing. The intense heat of the CO_2 laser also coagulates vessels as it cuts through them. It penetrates the surface to a depth of 0.1 to 0.2 mm per application to tissue, with minimal thermal effect to surrounding tissue.

The CO_2 laser operates from electrical power. The machine has a self-contained cooling system. The CO_2 laser beam should be delivered in a direct line of vision. It can be directed through a rigid endoscope, but it cannot be transmitted through a fiberoptic wave guide because its longer wavelength prevents conduction through crystal fibers. It is transmitted through an operating microscope or an articulating arm with a series of mirrors. This arm allows precise focus and direction of the beam to a pencil-like handpiece. CO_2 lasers have a helium-neon laser coaxial target beam that superimposes the invisible carbon dioxide beam to provide a visible red aiming light. The wave generated may be continuous or pulsed. Irradiance can vary from less than 1 watt to up to 300 watts. A portable handheld laser tube with a hollow needle to deliver the carbon dioxide beam is available for use in vascular surgery and microsurgery.

The vaporization and hemostatic action of the CO_2 laser is of value to the surgeon in treating soft tissue and vascular lesions. Large or small masses of tissue can be removed rapidly and efficiently. The CO_2 laser cannot be used in a fluid environment. The peritoneal cavity is insufflated with gas before the beam is directed through an endoscope. This laser is used primarily in otolaryngology, gynecology, plastic surgery, dermatology, neurosurgery, orthopaedics, and cardiovascular and general surgery.

Excimer Laser

When organic molecular bonds are broken up by a photochemical reaction, cool laser energy is emitted. Short wavelengths in the ultraviolet to visible blue-green spectrum are produced by gas used in the excimer laser combining with a halide medium. Argon fluoride produces a wavelength of 193 nm; krypton fluoride, 248 nm; xenon chloride, 308 nm; and xenon fluoride, 351 nm. These gases are extremely toxic. The beams they produce offer precision in cutting and coagulating without thermal damage to adjacent tissue. Excimer lasers have been developed for use in ophthalmology, peripheral and coronary angioplasty, orthopaedics (to cut bone), and neurosurgery.

Free Electron Laser

Free electrons, which are not bound to a specific atom, pass from a particle accelerator through a series of magnets to create a light beam. The beam can be tuned anywhere within the electromagnetic spectrum from ultraviolet to infrared. The free electron laser (FEL) produces light waves as a series of rapid superpulses of high energy and short duration, with minimal thermal damage. These light waves can fragment calculi. The FEL can also be used for precise cutting of tissues.

Holmium:YAG Laser

A crystal that contains holmium, thulium, and chromium elements increases the wavelength of YAG laser energy to 2100 nm, or 2.10 μm. This invisible beam in the mid-infrared range of the electromagnetic spectrum is absorbed by tissues containing water. Combined with high-energy pulsed delivery, it penetrates less deeply into tissue than the neodymium (Nd):YAG laser for more precise cutting and less generalized heating of tissue. It may be used percutaneously through a laser fiber threaded through a hollow needle or be delivered through a fine fiberoptic fiber. It may be used in a fluid medium. It acts on water in cells without char or extensive tissue damage. Approved for use in all joints except the spine, the holmium (Ho):YAG laser is useful in orthopaedics to cut, shape, and sculpt cartilage and bone and to ablate soft tissues.

Krypton Laser

The krypton ion gas laser emits a red-yellow light beam in the visible electromagnetic spectrum at wavelengths of 476.2 to 647.1 nm, or 0.6 μm. It is intensely absorbed by pigment in blood and retinal epithelium. The krypton laser resembles the argon laser in construction and use. It operates from electrical power and is water cooled. Used in ophthalmology, it is more versatile than the argon laser in selective photocoagulation of the retina.

Neodymium:YAG Laser

Neodymium, yttrium, aluminum, and garnet (Nd:YAG) constitute the solid-state crystal medium from which the light beam of this laser emanates. This invisible beam in the near-infrared range of the electromagnetic spectrum has a wavelength of 1064 nm, or 1.06 mm. It is poorly absorbed by hemoglobin and water but is intensely absorbed by tissue protein. The wavelength penetrates to a depth of 3 to 7 mm to denature protein by thermal coagulation and shrinkage of tissue beneath the surface.

The Nd:YAG laser operates from electric current through the optical power source of xenon flash lamps. It must have an air, carbon dioxide, or water cooling system.

The Nd:YAG laser beam can be transmitted through a flexible quartz fiber, 200 to 600 mm in diameter, which passes through a rigid endoscope. It can also be transmitted through a fiberoptic wave guide to a handpiece or a flexible endoscope or be focused through an operating microscope. An aiming light of blue xenon or red neon-helium may be used in conjunction with the Nd:YAG beam. Sapphire or ceramic tips allow direct contact with tissue for cutting and vaporizing without diffuse coagulation, using less than 25 watts of power. These tips are available on handheld scalpels or to fit on the ends of fibers for endoscopic use. Many of these tips are reusable; some are for single use only.

The Nd:YAG laser has the most powerful coagulating action of all of the surgical lasers. Its continuous or pulsed wave penetrates deeper into tissues than other lasers (i.e., up to 2 cm) and will coagulate large vessels (up to 4 mm). It is used to coagulate and vaporize large volumes of tissue. This versatile laser has applications in rhinolaryngology, urology, gynecology, neurosurgery, orthopaedics, and thoracic and general surgery.

For ophthalmology the Nd:YAG laser uses a Q-switching mode to store energy in a resonator during pumping action,

followed by release of a single, short pulse of high energy. This does not burn tissue but disrupts it with minute shock waves.

Potassium Titanyl Phosphate Laser

The solid-state potassium titanyl phosphate (KTP) crystal emits a visible green light at a wavelength of 532 mm, or 0.5 μm. This laser produces less power than CO_2 or Nd:YAG lasers but can be focused to a smaller diameter for precision work, such as in the middle ear. KTP absorbs most effectively into red or black tissue for coagulation. The beam can be directed by a handpiece at or in contact with tissue or through a rigid or flexible fiberoptic fiber or micromanipulator. The beam cuts, vaporizes, or coagulates tissue with minimal lateral thermal damage and plume. Cooling gases are not necessary, but the system should be water cooled. Instruments are available that provide both KTP and Nd:YAG wavelengths selected by a button on the control panel or that pass the Nd:YAG beam through the KTP crystal. Many accessories are available for specific applications in all surgical specialties. The KTP laser has good cutting properties.

Ruby Laser

The ruby solid-state crystal laser emits a visible red light at a wavelength of 694 nm, or 0.6 μm. A synthetically machined crystal rod is placed in a resonator cavity with a xenon flash lamp that when activated creates the optical pumping to produce the ruby laser beam. Blood vessels and transparent substances do not absorb this beam. A pulsed system, the ruby laser is capable of generating large fields of energy on impact. This shock wave effect can injure internal tissues and bone. Irradiance is 1 watt. Originally used in ophthalmology, the ruby laser currently is used primarily to eradicate port-wine stain lesions of the skin.

Tunable Dye Laser

Fluorescent liquid dyes or vapors can produce lasing energy. When exposed to intense laser light, usually an argon beam, dye absorbs light and fluoresces over a broad spectrum from ultraviolet to the far-infrared range. The laser may be delivered interstitially, endoscopically, externally, or retrobulbarly. A tunable prism can adjust the laser wavelength from 400 to 1000 nm, in either continuous or pulsed mode, for the specific dye in use.

The argon tunable dye laser system emits a blue-green beam at a wavelength of 430 to 530 nm from an argon laser that pumps a rhodamine B dye laser to produce a red laser beam at a wavelength of approximately 630 nm for selective destruction of malignant tumor cells. A dye laser tuned to 577 nm can be used on vascular lesions. Other wavelengths, such as through copper vapor, may be used to treat skin lesions or superficial tumors, such as of the bladder wall. The site can be repeatedly treated as long as cells remain photosensitive. This tunable dye laser is used most commonly for photodynamic therapy.

Photodynamic Therapy For photodynamic therapy the patient is injected 24 to 48 hours before laser therapy with a photosensitive drug that is absorbed by normal and malignant tissue. Normal tissue gradually releases the drug, but abnormal tissue retains it. The abnormal photosensitive tissue is destroyed when exposed to the laser beam. Normal adjacent tissue appears sunburned but is not permanently damaged. All dyes used with tunable dye lasers are potentially toxic and are handled with caution.

Safety Factors

All surgical lasers present hazards to patients and to the OR team. This equipment should be used in accordance with established regulations, standards and recommended practices, manufacturer's recommendations, and institutional policies. Laser safety is based on knowledge of the specific laser to be used, its instrumentation, its mode of operation, its power densities, its action in tissues, and its risks.

Regulatory Agencies

Lasers are classified as medical devices and are subject to regulation. The Code of Federal Regulations' Performance Standards for Light Emitting Products* provides specifications for manufacturers of medical laser systems.

National Center for Devices and Radiological Health   The National Center for Devices and Radiological Health (NCDRH) is the regulatory section of the Food and Drug Administration (FDA) in the Department of Health and Human Services (DHHS). More than 250 types of lasers are regulated by the FDA. Those intended for medical and surgical use come under the jurisdiction of medical device regulations. They are categorized as class III, subdivision class 4, because lasers are potentially hazardous (Box 20-4). Manufacturers must verify that their products meet all safety requirements of the federal standard. They must receive approval from the NCDRH to market or test a laser for a particular clinical application or use, and they must comply with labeling requirements.

American National Standards Institute   The American National Standards Institute (ANSI) is a voluntary organization of experts who determine industry consensus standards in technical fields. The standard developed specifically for laser safety in health care facilities is intended for all users.† Existing federal legislation and state laser safety regulations are based on the ANSI standard. Simply stated, this standard implies that every health care facility that uses

---

*Performance standards for light emitting products, part 1040, Code of Federal Regulations, *Fed Register,* 1982; Laser products: amendments to performance standard, final rule, *Fed Register* 50(161), 1985; Regulations for the administration and enforcement of the Radiation Control for Health and Safety Act of April 1988, part 1040, sections 1040.10 and 1040.11, HHS Pub FDA 88-8035.
†American National Standards Institute: *American national standard for the safe use of lasers in health care facilities,* ANSI Z136.3, New York, 1988, The Institute.

| Box 20-4 | **Medical Device Regulations** |

FDA Classification of Medical Devices
Medical devices were classified in 1976 by the FDA according to their safety factors.

Class I
Subject to general controls.

Class II
Devices for which general controls are not enough.

Class III
Implants and life support devices.

Classification of Lasers
Lasers are classified according to potential hazard of exposure.

Class 1
Enclosed system, considered safe based on current medical knowledge. No light emission escapes the enclosure.

Class 2
Limited to visible light (400-780 nm). Output power is 1 mW or less. Momentary viewing (0.25-second maximum permissible exposure) is not considered hazardous. Staring into the beam is not recommended. Protective eyewear of the correct optical density should be worn.

Class 3A
Emitted laser light viewed directly through collecting optics would cause permanent eye damage. Output power is 0.5 mW or less. Protective eyewear of the correct optical density should be worn.

Class 3B
Continuous laser light with 0.5-watt or less output can cause permanent eye damage. Exposure to the beam should be avoided. Protective eyewear of the correct optical density should be worn.

Class 4
Laser light produced is hazardous to skin and eyes. Strict control measures are enforced. Protective eyewear of the correct optical density should be worn.

---

surgical lasers must establish and maintain an adequate program for control of laser hazards. This program shall include provisions for the following:

- *Laser safety officer.* This person should have authority to suspend, restrict, or terminate operation of a laser system if hazard controls are inadequate. A laser safety committee, often a subcommittee of the OR committee, may appoint this surveillance officer.
- *Education of users.* A safety training program must ensure that all users, including surgeons, perioperative nurses, surgical technologists, and biomedical engineers

and technicians, are knowledgeable of correct operation, potential hazards, and control measures.

- *Protective measures.* Protective measures are for patients, personnel, and the environment.
- *Management of accidents.* Management includes reporting accidents and developing plans of action to prevent a future occurrence.

Occupational Safety and Health Administration
The Occupational Safety and Health Administration (OSHA) is concerned primarily with the safety of health care workers. The agency can enforce ANSI standards.

State and Local Agencies
State regulations and local ordinances vary. Knowledge of and compliance with any requirements should be established.

Policies and Procedures

Specific policies and procedures related to use of lasers should be written by the laser safety committee before a laser program is instituted. These policies and procedures will need to be revised or updated when new equipment is installed. Applicable policies include, but are not limited to, the following:

1. *Credentialing and clinical practice privileges of medical staff.* Physicians authorized to use a laser should be required to complete a postgraduate laser course in their specialties. Hands-on experience and a preceptorship with a qualified user also should be required. The physician must have training for each type and wavelength of laser. A list of approved physicians should be available to the perioperative staff. Scheduling privileges should be denied to those surgeons who are not appropriately credentialed.
2. *Initial and ongoing educational laser use and safety programs for perioperative personnel.* Perioperative personnel should have thorough knowledge and understanding of laser equipment, laser physics, tissue reactions, applications, and safety precautions.
3. *Continuous quality improvement.* A program of continuous quality improvement includes appropriate care, use, and maintenance of equipment and prevention of laser-related accidents.
4. *Documentation.* The surgeon, procedure, type of laser used, length of use, and wattage should be recorded in the patient's medical record. This information, plus the patient's name, should also be recorded in the OR log.

Patient Safety

The surgeon must explain laser surgery and its potential complications to the patient before obtaining written consent. Some lasers are considered investigational devices by the FDA. The patient must sign a specific consent form permitting experimental use and data collection. With all lasers, appropriate precautions (including protection of the patient's eyes, skin, and tissue surrounding the target area

from thermal burns) are taken to ensure patient safety as follows:

1. The eyes and eyelids should be adequately protected from the specific laser beam in use.
   a. Patients who are awake must wear the same type of safety glasses or goggles as those worn by the laser team (see discussion of eye protection under Personnel Safety).
   b. The eyes can be taped shut on patients who are under general anesthesia.
   c. Eye pads moistened with saline solution should be taped securely in place for procedures around the head and neck, except for ophthalmic procedures and those using the Nd:YAG laser. Nonflammable material, such as aluminum foil with the reflective side down, can be taped over the eyes for Nd:YAG laser procedures. Moistened eye pads will not stop this laser beam.
   d. Protective shields should be used on the eyes during ophthalmic procedures. Corneal eye shields can be applied directly onto anesthetized eyes to protect corneal tissue.
2. Antiseptics used for skin preparation should be nonflammable.
   a. Aqueous solutions are safest, but they can retain laser heat if they are allowed to pool on or around skin. The skin should be thoroughly dry before the laser is activated.
   b. Alcohol and tinctures are flammable and volatile when wet. Vapors must not accumulate under drapes because they can ignite.
3. The immediate area around the incision and/or tissue surrounding the target site should be protected from thermal injury. Flammable materials are avoided or safeguarded to prevent fire.
   a. Flame- or fire-resistant drapes should be used. Metallic foil and polypropylene laser-retardant and ignition-resistant drapes are available. Polypropylene and plastic incise drapes can melt if a laser beam strikes them. Woven and nonwoven fabrics can be ignited.
   b. Woven textile or cellulose-based absorbent nonwoven towels saturated with sterile normal saline solution or water should be placed over fabric drapes around the incision before the laser is used.
   c. The laser handpiece should be laid on a moistened surface. The laser tip is extremely hot and may shatter if placed in contact with a cold surface.
   d. Moistened sponges, towels, or compressed patties should be placed around target tissue except when the Nd:YAG laser is used. Sponges and other material should be removed from tissue near the target site of the Nd:YAG laser because wetting will not stop this beam and they could be ignited.
   e. The rectum should be packed with a moistened sponge to prevent methane gas, which is potentially

explosive, from escaping from the intestinal tract during use of a laser in the perineal area. Placement of the sponge in the anal orifice and removal of the rectal packing should be recorded.

4. Anesthetic agents should be noncombustible. Non-flammable anesthetics and oxygen mixed with non-flammable agents are administered in a closed system.

   a. Oxygen and nitrous oxide concentrations around the head should be as low as possible during use of a laser in the aerodigestive tract (i.e., oral, laryngeal, bronchial, or esophageal procedures).

   b. Flexible metallic or insulated silicone endotracheal tubes are preferred for aerodigestive tract procedures. Laser-approved varieties are commercially available. If used, red rubber tubes are wrapped with reflective aluminum or copper tape to prevent ignition. Polyvinyl chloride endotracheal tubes should never be used, because they ignite easily. The endotracheal tube cuff should be inflated with saline solution, which may be tinted with methylene blue to facilitate detection of a leak.

5. The teeth should be covered during oropharyngeal procedures to protect against reflective radiation.

6. Patients who are awake may wear a protective high-filtration mask during CO_2 laser ablation, such as of condylomas (venereal warts), to prevent inhaling airborne material into the lungs. An intubated patient is not considered at risk for respiratory contamination.

7. Postoperative instructions should include care of a healing thermal skin wound.

Personnel Safety

Exposure to nonionizing laser radiation can be hazardous for personnel. Precautions are taken to avoid eye and skin exposure to direct or scattered radiation and inhalation of plume.

Eye Protection The eye is the organ that is most susceptible to laser injury. Different laser wavelengths affect eyes differently: argon and Nd:YAG lasers will be absorbed by retina, and the CO_2 laser will be absorbed by cornea. Therefore safety glasses or goggles of the correct optical density are worn at all times while the laser is in use. Optical density is the ability of the lens to absorb a specific wavelength (Table 20-1). The color of the lens is not the protective feature of the eyewear. Each type of wavelength requires protective eyewear of a specific optical density as recommended by the manufacturer of the laser. The following considerations apply to eye protection:

1. Protective eyewear is available outside the room near posted signs designating the specific type of laser in use. Only persons with appropriate eye protection are admitted in the room while the laser is in use.

   a. All protective eyewear (i.e., safety glasses or goggles) must shield the wearer's eyes from the top, bottom, and sides of the visual field.

TABLE 20-1	Optical Density Necessary for Protective Eyewear	
Optical Density	**Transmission of Light (% of Wavelength)***
0	1
1	0.1
2	0.01
3	0.001
4	0.0001
5	0.00001
6	0.000001

*Light transmission is measured with a spectrophotometer to calculate the optical density needed for protective eyewear.

   b. Goggles will fit over eyeglasses, or prescription lenses of the correct optical density can be obtained. Contact lenses do not provide eye protection.

   c. Scratches on the lens or breaks in the frame can negate eye protection.

2. Lens covers with filter caps are available for optical eyepieces of endoscopes and operating microscopes. Their use does not eliminate the need for the entire team to wear eye protection.

Skin Protection Skin sensitivities can develop from overexposure to ultraviolet radiation. Skin also can be burned from exposure to direct or reflected laser energy. These hazards are minimized if personnel are alert to precautions for environmental safety (see Environmental Safety). Other personnel safety precautions reduce risks and include the following:

1. Metallic jewelry should not be worn. It could absorb heat or reflect the beam.

2. Fire-resistant gowns may be worn.

Laser Plume Toxic substances, including carcinogens and viruses, may become airborne from vaporization of tissues, especially from CO_2 and Nd:YAG lasers. The smoke produced, referred to as laser plume, contains water, carbonized particles, mutated DNA, and intact cells. It may have a distinct odor. Laser plume should not be inhaled. One gram of plume is equivalent to smoking six cigarettes. Smoke evacuation from the site of lasing and high-filtration masks prevent personnel from inhaling plume. Removal of plume also enhances visibility at the target site for the surgeon. Plume can bend or refract the beam, thus inadvertently causing injury to adjacent tissues. The following precautions should be taken:

1. A mechanical smoke evacuator or suction with a high-efficiency filter should be turned on before or at the same time as the laser and should be run during activation and for 20 to 30 seconds after the laser is deactivated. The tip should be placed as close as possible, at

least within 2 inches (5 cm), to the lasing site of tissue vaporization.
  a. Several types of mechanical smoke evacuators are available. Many systems have charcoal filters.
  b. Charcoal filters in most evacuators are changed regularly. Gloves and a mask are worn when handling contaminated filters.
2. Masks should be tight fitting and should filter particles as small as 0.1 μm.

Environmental Safety

Only properly trained persons are authorized to participate in laser surgery. Others should be made aware of its hazards. The following considerations apply to environmental safety:

1. Warning sign(s), "Laser Surgery in Progress," should be posted on the outside of all OR doors when the laser is in use. The design, symbols, and wording on the warning sign should be specific for the type of laser in use.
2. Walls and ceilings should have nonreflective surfaces. Glass, as in windows, cabinet doors, and/or the x-ray viewing box, should be covered with nonreflective material to stop beams when lasers other than CO_2 lasers are used. CO_2 laser beams are absorbed by glass.
3. Warning labels on the machine, affixed by the manufacturer, must indicate points of danger to avoid personnel exposure to laser radiation.
4. The machine should be prepared, checked, and tested before the patient is brought into the room. A preoperative checklist is helpful. Any malfunction should be reported immediately, and the equipment should not be used until it is in proper working order.
5. When not in use, the machine should be kept on the "standby" setting with the beam terminated in a beam stop of highly absorbent, nonreflecting, fire-resistant material to avoid accidental activation. It should be turned off and locked with a key when left unattended. Only authorized personnel should have access to the key.
6. The foot switch should be operated by the surgeon who delivers the laser energy to the tissue. The foot pedal can be covered when not in use so that the surgeon will not inadvertently activate the laser. Foot pedals for other equipment should be moved away while the laser is in use. The laser pedal can then be removed after use.
7. Nonreflective instruments should be used in or near the beam. These instruments may be of a dull blue titanium alloy or an ebonized or anodized stainless steel. These finishes defocus and disperse the laser beam. Reflective instruments can cause burns or start fires.
8. Fire is a potential hazard that cannot be underestimated. Personnel should be aware of fire safeguards and adhere to precautions for their own and the patient's safety.
  a. A basin of sterile water or normal saline solution should be readily available at the sterile field.
  b. A halon fire extinguisher should be available.
  c. Oxygen concentration in the room should be as low as possible. Oxygen leaking from the side of a patient's face mask can be ignited by the laser beam. The anesthesia provider should be knowledgeable about flash points and fire retardation when the laser is in use.
  d. Liquids should never be placed on the machine. A spill could act as a conductor and short-circuit the mechanism.
9. Electrical codes and standards should be enforced to avoid electrical hazards. An isolation transformer is recommended for a high-power laser power source to avoid dangerous overload of the existing OR power system. Electrical circuitry must provide adequate amperage for power requirements. Preferably, the laser has its own dedicated circuit.
10. The manufacturer's instructions for operation, care, handling, and sterilization of the laser system should be followed. Proper care of lasers and accessory equipment is essential to patient, personnel, and environmental safety.

Laser Team

A laser team should be designated to carry out the duties that are different from those of the traditional OR team. This team may include the following personnel:

1. *Clinical laser nurse.* The responsibilities of the clinical laser nurse are different from those of the circulator. Duties include the following:
  a. Preparing and teaching the patient preoperatively, intraoperatively, and postoperatively.
  b. Bringing laser equipment to the OR and checking it. The chassis and the floor around it should be inspected for water leak. Using sterile technique, the clinical laser nurse and scrub person calibrate the laser as appropriate.
  c. Covering windows, posting signs, and distributing appropriate protective eyewear.
  d. Covering the patient's eyes.
  e. Positioning the laser foot pedal for the surgeon's convenience and removing it after use.
  f. Operating the key switch and monitoring activation of the laser. The wattage and exposure time are set according to the surgeon's orders. These should be repeated before and after adjusting controls.
  g. Cleaning and checking laser fibers after use and preparing them for sterilization.
  h. Completing the laser log.
  i. Collaborating with the laser safety officer and biomedical engineer and/or technician to ensure safe use of laser equipment.

2. *Biomedical technician.* The biomedical technician provides preventive maintenance and handles minor problems with the laser system. A log of laser use and maintenance is maintained.
3. *Camera operator.* Endoscopic procedures performed under video control may require an additional sterile team member to operate the camera attached to the endoscope while the surgeon controls the laser fiber.

Advantages of Laser Surgery

Surgical lasers emit nonionizing radiation. This radiation is selectively absorbed by different tissues with resultant penetration and destruction at the focal point but with differential thermal protection of surrounding tissues. Lasers offer the surgeon and the patient many advantages over other surgical techniques, including the following:

1. Precise control for accurate incision, excision, or ablation of tissue. The laser beam is precisely focused for localized tissue destruction. The depth of radiation penetration is precisely regulated by the duration of focus, power density, and type of tissue.
2. Access to areas inaccessible to other surgical instruments through minimally invasive techniques. The beam can be directed through endoscopes or deflected off of rhodium reflector mirrors.
3. An unobstructed view of the surgical site. The laser beam comes in contact with tissue to be cut, coagulated, or vaporized. It can be directed through the operating microscope.
4. Minimal handling of and trauma to tissues. Traction on target tissue is unnecessary.
5. A dry, bloodless surgical field. The laser beam simultaneously cuts and coagulates blood vessels, thus providing hemostasis in vascular areas.
6. Minimal thermal effect on surrounding tissue. Essentially no permanent thermal necrosis of tissue occurs beyond 100 mm from the edge of the area incised. This minimizes postoperative pain.
7. Reduced risk of contamination or infection. The laser beam vaporizes microorganisms, thus essentially sterilizing the contact area.
8. Prompt healing with minimal postoperative edema, sloughing of tissue, pain, and scarring.
9. Reduced operating time. Because procedures can be done more quickly, both anesthesia time and operating time are shorter. Many procedures can be done without general anesthesia. Many are done in ambulatory care facilities.

Disadvantages of Laser Surgery

1. The costs to start and maintain a program are high. Equipment, instrumentation, supplies, and staff education are expensive initial investments. Most aspects need frequent updates and maintenance.
2. Decisions should be made about the use of disposable vs. reusable supplies and the impact on patient care.

Most reusable supplies are fragile and should be replaced on a regular basis.
3. Liability may increase as the number of users increase. Specific credentialing and continuing education require planning and are time-consuming.

ENDOSCOPY, MINIMALLY INVASIVE, AND MINIMAL ACCESS PROCEDURES

The term *endoscopy* is a combined form of two Greek words: *endon* (ενδον), meaning *inside,* and *skopein* (σκοπην), meaning *to examine.* In medicine, endoscopy is a visual examination of the interior of a body cavity, hollow organ, or structure with an endoscope, an instrument designed for direct visual inspection. Terms associated with endoscopy, minimally invasive, and minimal access procedures are defined in Box 20-5.

AORN, the Association of periOperative Registered Nurses, has developed recommended practices for endoscopic minimally invasive surgery.

Historical Background

Although physicians sought to visualize the interior of body organs, development of endoscopy was slow. It was not until the early nineteenth century that attempts were made to examine the inside of the bladder. Instruments were inadequate because light was from a candle or lamp. Finally, Austrian urologist Max Nitze (1848-1906) developed an instrument in 1877 that is the basis of modern endoscopy. Dr. Chevalier Jackson of Philadelphia further enhanced endoscopy by developing a laryngoscope and bronchoscope. Only after the incandescent lamp was invented and an optical system was devised could an efficient instrument be made. Improvements started in about 1878, and the precise instruments of today have evolved since that time, making possible the conservative treatment of many conditions. Endoscopic inspection of the abdominal cavity, introduced in 1902, has become a common procedure since the advent of fiberoptic illumination.

An endoscope may be inserted into the body through a natural orifice (i.e., the mouth, anus, cervix, or urethra). Other

---

Box 20-5 **Terms Associated with Endoscopy, Minimally Invasive, and Minimal Access Procedures**

endoscopy Examination of a body part or cavity with an optical system in a tubular structure.
insufflation Act of filling with gas. Laparoscopy is performed with carbon dioxide.
trocar Surgical instrument that consists of a sheath with a sharp stylet used to puncture multiple layers of tissue. The sheath remains in place as the sharp stylet is removed. Additional instrumentation is passed through the sheath.

endoscopes are inserted through a small skin incision and/or trocar puncture, such as through a joint space or the abdominal wall. The endoscope is named for the anatomic area it is designed to visualize; for example, a laryngoscope is used for laryngoscopy. From head to foot, nearly every area of the body can be visualized with an endoscope.

All endoscopic procedures are considered minimally invasive except for ophthalmoscopy, because the scope is placed into a body orifice or cavity. Many require one or more small skin incisions for insertion of the scope and accessories. Endoscopy is used for many diagnostic and surgical procedures.

Design of Endoscopes

Although the sizes and shapes vary according to specific uses, all endoscopes have similar working elements.

Viewing Telescope

The surgeon views anatomic structures through a telescopic lens. The diameter of the scope varies from the 1.7-mm needle fetoscope to the 5 mm or less of the arthroscope to the 22 mm of an anoscope. The length varies but is appropriate to reach the desired structure. Endoscopes may be rigid or flexible.

Rigid Scopes A rigid scope is a narrow hollow tube that permits viewing in a forward direction only, such as a sigmoidoscope, or a tube with a telescopic lens system that permits viewing in a variety of directions, such as a cystoscope (Figure 20-5). Most rigid scopes are metal. Disposable plastic anoscopes and otoscopes are available. Rigid bron-

choscopes have additional side ports for administration of oxygen or anesthetics.

Flexible Scopes Flexible scopes have a dial adjuster that contours the lensed tip into and around anatomic curvatures to permit visualization of all surfaces of the wall of a hollow structure, such as the gastrointestinal tract. The user can look directly into the eyepiece, or an attachment can be placed over the eyepiece to project the image on a video screen. Flexible endoscopes have working channels that permit the use of biopsy forceps and laser fibers. A separate suction channel is on the opposite side. Two trumpet valves located near the eyepiece control suction and insufflation with air to expand the organ for viewing. The covering of flexible endoscopes is made of silicone-plastic material and is usually latex free (Figure 20-6).

Endoscopic Machinery

Lighting, insufflation, surgical accessories, and power sources are commonly stored and transported via an endoscopy cart or mounted on a ceiling boom (Figure 20-7).

Figure 20-6 Flexible endoscope.

Figure 20-7 Ceiling-mounted endoscopic machinery.

Figure 20-5 Basic rigid endoscopes. **A,** Standard rigid endoscope. **B,** Single-puncture laparoscope with working channel.

Light Source

Illumination within the body cavity is essential for visual acuity. The light source may be through a fiberoptic bundle or from an incandescent lightbulb. The light carrier may be an integral part of the viewing sheath, as in flexible scopes and rigid telescopes, or it may be a separate light carrier accessory to a hollow rigid scope.

Fiberoptic Lighting   With fiberoptic lighting, an intense cool light illuminates body cavities, including those that cannot be seen with other light sources. Light is conducted through a bundle of thousands of coated glass fibers encased in a plastic sheath attached to a light source generator. Each fiber is drawn from optical glass into a strand 10 to 70 mm in diameter that is coated to minimize loss of light by reflection. Light entering one end of the fiber is transmitted by refraction through its entire length. The light produced through the bundle of fibers is nonglaring and evenly distributed on the area to be visualized. Although it is of high intensity, the light is cool. A minimum rise of temperature in the tissues exposed to it may occur. Although the light inside the patient is cool, the cable should not be allowed to lie on the drapes, since it is a potential source of ignition.

Bulbs   Bulbs screw into the fitting either at the end of a removable light carrier or at the end of a built-in lens system. Electric current is conducted through a single-filament wire to illuminate the tiny incandescent lightbulb. Very few instruments use this lighting system.

Power Source

Electric current is transmitted to the light source connected to a fiberoptic bundle or a lightbulb. The electric current is entirely external to the patient with fiberoptic lighting. Current flows through a power cord attached to the endoscope inserted into the patient and through the instrument to the lightbulb at the distal end of the light carrier or sheath. The power source may or may not be connected to the electrical system in the room.

Projection Lamp   A quartz-halogen or mercury-arc lightbulb provides an intense light source, similar to a film projector, for transmission of light through a fiberoptic bundle to the distal end of the scope. Usually a portable, compact, self-contained unit, the light has an intensity that may be regulated from 400 footcandles to as much as 5200 footcandles, and up to 5500 Kelvin daylight in some illuminators. The bulb should be positioned securely in its socket so that output focuses on the center of the fiberoptic bundle. If the bulb is not properly positioned, light output will not be of maximum value.

Fiberoptic Cable   A fiberoptic cable transmits light from the projection lamp to the endoscope. Both ends of the cable must have the correct fittings to attach to the lamp and to the scope or removable light carrier. The diameter of the cable varies from 2.0 to 5.5 mm to be compatible with the aperture for the light source. Cable lengths also vary from 6 feet (180 cm) to 9 feet (275 cm), so the projection lamp can be positioned at a distance from a sterile field. Before use, the fiberoptic cable should be checked for damage. One end of the cable is held toward a low-power light, such as the overhead operating light. With a magnifying glass, the opposite end is examined. Broken fibers in the cable will appear as dark spots. The cable should be replaced if more than 20% of the area appears dark.

Battery Box   One or more sets of dry-cell batteries may be used as the power source for lightbulbs. The batteries may be recharged in some units, but eventually they should be replaced. A battery provides a good source of current, is safe, and can be used in conjunction with other electrical equipment.

Rheostat   A rheostat is a resistor for regulating flow of current from the electrical system. Rapidly introduced high voltage may burn out the delicate filament in a lightbulb. A rheostat reduces electrical potential and allows gradual increase of current to the desired brightness of the light. Safety precautions are observed when using this power source to prevent shock to the patient and operator. Rheostats that cannot be grounded should not be used. They also cannot be used when the cutting current of the ESU is in use. Cutting current will not work if another piece of equipment is on the same circuit.

Accessories

Accessories such as suction tubes, snares, biopsy forceps, grasping forceps, sutures, and sponge carriers are used in conjunction with endoscopes. These accessories can be passed through channels in the endoscope to remove fluid or tissue, coagulate or ligate bleeding vessels, inject fluid or gas to distend cavities, and so on. Some rigid scopes have an obturator, a blunt-tipped rod placed through the lumen, to permit smooth insertion of the instrument, such as into the anus. The accessories needed will be determined by the type of endoscope and purpose of the procedure.

Carbon Dioxide Insufflator   The peritoneal cavity is filled with carbon dioxide gas, creating a gas lake called a pneumoperitoneum, before a laparoscope is inserted through the abdominal wall. The pneumoperitoneum expands the abdomen and allows for visualization of organs and structures within the peritoneal cavity. The carbon dioxide insufflator is a specially designed machine that delivers a metered flow up to 9.9 L/min of carbon dioxide through a disposable tubing with an in-line hydrophobic filter. The filter should be single use and compatible with the insufflator. The filter acts to prevent contaminants and condensation from entering the abdominal cavity.

The carbon dioxide gas cylinder should be kept above the level of the patient's abdomen. If the cylinder is placed below the level of the patient, the pressure gradient on the patient's side increases, causing a backflow of biologic contaminants into the insufflator. As a result, the internal aspect of the insufflation machine can become biologically contaminated. This can be the source of cross-contamination between patients.

A small incision (1 to 1 mm) is made into the abdominal wall at the infraumbilical margin. A special spring-loaded Verres needle measuring 120 to 150 cm is inserted through the tiny incision at the thinnest portion of the abdominal wall. Carbon dioxide is delivered into the peritoneal cavity through the filtered tubing at a rate measured by pressure predetermined by the surgeon. The initial low flow is started at 6 to 7 mm Hg to establish a safe flow. It is maintained at a higher level between 12 to 18 mm Hg. Once the pneumoperitoneum is established, a 10- or 12-mm trocar is inserted and the insufflation tubing is attached to a port on the side of the trocar sleeve. Additional 5- to 12-mm trocars are inserted through the abdominal wall under direct video visualization at strategic points to create working portals for graspers, cutters, dissectors, staplers, and suturing devices for tissue manipulation.

Occasionally a surgeon will omit using a Verres needle for initial insufflation and create the gas lake (pneumoperitoneum) through a blunt Hasson trocar inserted into the abdomen through a small open incision. This procedure may be used for the patient who has many adhesions or has had multiple previous surgeries.

The circulator monitors the intraabdominal pressure and the amount of carbon dioxide delivered and may be asked to change the flow rate periodically throughout the procedure. Most insufflators are automatic and will maintain the pneumoperitoneum at a preset pressure. The insufflator readout should be visible to the anesthesia provider. The pressure should not be allowed to exceed 20 mm Hg. Pressures exceeding 20 mm Hg seriously compromise the hemodynamic status of the patient. Problems with kinked tubing can give a falsely high pressure reading. High pressures are immediately reported to the surgeon.

At the conclusion of the procedure, the carbon dioxide should be evacuated through the filtered suction port on the trocar and not expelled directly into the room air. The expelled carbon dioxide gas contains blood and body fluids that cause airborne contamination. Personal protective equipment, such as masks and eyewear, should be worn by all personnel in the room.

Some surgeons prefer to use a gasless method for displacing and expanding the abdomen during laparoscopy. A device referred to as a planar lift can be used to elevate the abdominal wall for minimal access procedures. Shorter instrumentation can be used because the internal organs are in closer proximity to the surface.

Electrosurgical Electrodes An active electrode connected to a monopolar ESU may be used through an endoscope, such as a laparoscope for general or gynecologic surgery or a resectoscope for urologic surgery. A variety of electrodes, both disposable and reusable, are available. They must have adequate insulation and be inspected before use for any defect. Electrical energy transfers by capacitance from the activated electrode through intact insulation into other nearby conductive materials. Unless a safe path is provided for current to return to ground, the current induced by capacitance might cause a burn on internal tissue. Direct coupling occurs when the activated electrode touches other metal instruments, particularly the laparoscope. An all-metal trocar/cannula system allows accidental contact to dissipate through the abdominal wall. The surgeon should avoid activating the electrode unless it is in contact with the tissue. A shielding and monitoring system is commercially available for monopolar endoscopic electrosurgical electrodes. Bipolar instruments, including dissectors, scissors, and graspers, eliminate the potential hazard of stray currents with monopolar electrodes.

Plane Expander A balloon device can be inserted between tissue layers and expanded with saline to separate and bluntly open the preperitoneal plane of dissection. After blunt dissection and expansion, the balloon is deflated and withdrawn. The space is then insufflated. This is useful for laparoscopic hernia repair procedures. Saphenous vein harvests and spinal surgery can be performed using this method (Figure 20-8).

Laser A laser beam can be focused through some endoscopes. Argon, Ho:YAG, and Nd:YAG lasers will pass light through a fiber. The CO_2 laser can be directed through a rigid endoscope or the interior mirror system of a multiarticulated arm of the operating microscope. The beam is then focused through the endoscope, which is usually held in a self-retaining device. A distal smoke evacuation suction device clears plume to maintain visibility through the scope and at the site of lasing. The endoscopes are specifically designed for adaptation to the articulated arm of the CO_2 laser (e.g., the CO_2 laser laparoscope and CO_2 laser bronchoscope).

Ultrasonic Transducer A high-frequency ultrasound transducer at the end of a fiberoptic endoscope provides visualization of the heart, liver, pancreas, spleen, and kidneys.

Operating Microscope The optical system of some endoscopes can be attached to a specially designed operating microscope such as the colpomicroscope. The illumination of the endoscope and binocular magnification of the microscope permit study of abnormal tissues and/or therapeutic procedures in areas otherwise inaccessible without an open surgical procedure.

Cameras Lensed scopes may be equipped with a still or motion picture camera so that organs or lesions can be photographed during a procedure. Video cameras with recorder/player/printer equipment can be adapted for use with some endoscopes. A high-powered light source may be needed with the camera for photographic applications and video documentation. An endoscopic video camera electron-

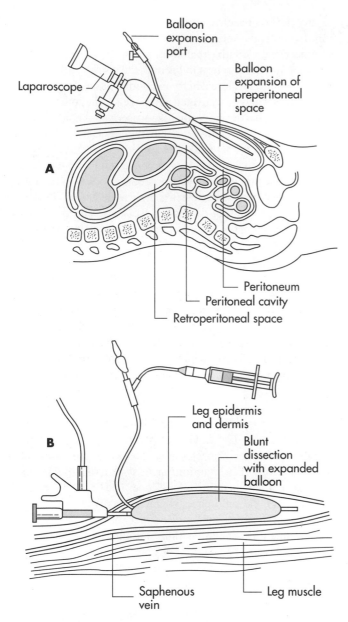

Figure 20-8 Balloon expansion of surgical planes. **A,** Preperitoneal expansion. **B,** Saphenous vein harvest using balloon dissection technique.

ically transmits images to a closed-circuit television screen. By viewing high-resolution monitor(s), the endoscopist can manipulate instruments for diagnostic examination or to perform a therapeutic procedure. Video documentation can be obtained by taping the examination or procedure. Microcomputer imaging systems with a printer reproduce these images into photographs. Fluoroscopy may be preferred to video images for certain procedures such as radioactive implantation.

Hazards of Endoscopy

Endoscopy is not without its hazards. Minimally invasive surgery requires appropriate credentialing. Surgeons who

wish to perform laparoscopy and other endoscopic techniques should be credentialed through the medical staff department. Personnel who are responsible for scheduling endoscopic procedures should confirm the surgeon's practice privileges. Serious complications of endoscopy include the following:

1. *Perforation.* Perforation of a major organ or vessel is a constant cause for concern when sharp trocars and rigid scopes are used. Flexible fiberoptic endoscopes have decreased this danger, but it remains a potential complication. Patient positioning from supine to the Trendelenburg position shifts the intraabdominal anatomy, causing elevation of the major vessels of the lower abdominal cavity. Care is taken to prevent inadvertent injury to these structures while holding cameras or other devices situated in intraabdominal trocar sleeves during repositioning of the operating bed.

   The sharp obturator should be examined briefly after it is withdrawn from the trocar sleeve. The presence of gross blood, stool, bile, or other unidentified substance may indicate perforation of an intraabdominal organ.

2. *Bleeding.* Bleeding can occur from a biopsy site, pedicle of a polyp, or other area where tissue has been cut. Endoscopic sutures or clips can become dislodged. Care is taken to observe for pooling of blood in the body cavity that may indicate venous oozing or other vessel disruption.

3. *Hypothermia.* Carbon dioxide gas is colder than body temperature. The patient may experience moderate to severe hypothermia if other warming measures, such as forced air warming or heating blankets, are not used. Hypothermia can alter the effects of propofol and increase the incidence of hypothermic coagulopathy.

Electrical systems used with endoscopy must conform with the standards and be subjected to the routine maintenance procedures prescribed by the National Fire Protection Association code for electrical safety. Two major electrical hazards associated with endoscopy are as follows:

1. *Improperly grounded electrical equipment.* If the surgeon will be using a monopolar ESU, place the inactive dispersive electrode with adequate skin contact to allow conduction of electric current. Only solid-state generators, and preferably bipolar active electrodes, should be used in order to avoid variances in voltage.

2. *Unsuspected current leaks.* Corrosion or accumulation of organic material can inhibit flow of current across the screw fitting between the light carrier and the bulb. Current can leak through the instrument to the patient. Ideally, endoscopes should not contain electrically conductive elements or metals that can corrode. Corrosion can be caused by repeated exposure to body fluids, hard water, or chemical agents.

Microorganisms, such as *Mycobacterium tuberculosis,* can be transmitted from one patient to another via a bronchoscope. *Streptococcus pneumoniae, Pseudomonas aeruginosa, Clostridium* organisms, and blood-borne pathogens also present potential hazards of cross-contamination. Personnel are exposed to potentially infectious body fluids and blood from aerosols, splashes, and contact with contaminated instrumentation. Gloves, masks, protective eyewear, gowns, and/or aprons are worn during endoscopic procedures and cleaning of equipment. Personnel should use standard precautions during endoscopic procedures and when handling and processing contaminated endoscopes and accessories.

Types of Endoscopic Procedures

Not all endoscopic procedures are performed as sterile procedures; some are surgically aseptic (high-level disinfection). An endoscope is introduced into the gastrointestinal tract through the mouth or anus. It touches only mucous membranes. The gastrointestinal tract normally harbors resident and transient microorganisms. Although the procedure is not considered sterile, patients and personnel are protected from cross-contamination. Endoscopes and their accessories are thoroughly cleaned and terminally sterilized or undergo high-level disinfection after use. Sterility is not maintained between and during patient uses. Instruments should be stored according to the manufacturer's recommendations. Many endoscopic procedures are performed in an endoscopy unit rather than in the OR.

Endoscopy is performed as a sterile procedure if body tissue will be incised or excised, or if a normally sterile organ or body cavity is entered, such as the bladder or uterus. Ideally, the endoscope and all accessories should be sterile regardless of the point of entry. It may not be feasible to sterilize some heat-sensitive parts, such as a lensed telescope, between patient uses when several procedures are scheduled in succession. Control of scheduling endoscopic procedures and adequate instrumentation will help to provide sterile endoscopes for every patient. In reality, high-level disinfection may be necessary between uses. Written policies and procedures must specify accepted practices for patient care and infection control. AORN has developed recommended practices for the use and care of endoscopes to be used as a guide in establishing processing procedures. Only sterile endoscopes and accessories should be used on patients with suppressed immune systems, such as from chemotherapy or steroid therapy or HIV-related diseases.

Often described as minimally invasive surgery, endoscopic minimal access surgery does not require the incisions of traditional open procedures, such as for removal of the gallbladder or appendix. The procedure is performed with instruments introduced through ports established through small, 5- to 10-mm, incisions. Routine practices should be established to reduce the risk of potential patient injuries and complications. These practices include, but are not limited to, the following:

- Training for and demonstrating competence in the use and care of endoscopic equipment by surgeons and perioperative personnel.
- Providing complete sets of properly prepared functional instruments.
- Monitoring the patient for changes in physiologic status. For example, development of hypercapnia and/or hypothermia can be caused by carbon dioxide insufflation.

All patients should be prepped and draped for conversion to an open procedure when warranted because of recognized or potential complications. Instrumentation and supplies for an open procedure should be precounted and readily available. The patient should be informed preoperatively of this possibility.

Care of Endoscopes

Endoscopes are delicate and expensive instruments. Rough handling, jarring, or bending of parts should be avoided. They should never be piled on top of each other or mixed with other instruments.

All parts of endoscopes and accessories are thoroughly disassembled, mechanically cleaned, and terminally sterilized or subjected to high-level disinfection after use. The primary causes of infection, such as herpes, hepatitis, or condylomas transmitted endoscopically, are inadequate cleaning and disinfection or sterilization of endoscopic equipment.

Cleaning

All parts of the endoscope should be cleaned as soon as possible after use while organic debris is still moist. Mucus, blood, feces, and protein-type residue can become trapped in the channels of the scope. This material is difficult to remove if it becomes dry and may render the scope useless.

Endoscopes should be washed in warm, never hot, water and a neutral, nonresidue liquid-detergent solution. A pipe cleaner or small brush may be used to clean inside the lumens of all channels. The stopcocks on some scopes should be thoroughly cleaned, too, because dirty ones will stick. Stopcocks are opened for cleaning; they should never be forced but can be loosen with a drop of solvent or lubricant. All removable parts are disassembled.

Particular attention should be paid to cleanliness of lenses, or viewing will be obstructed. Debris can be carefully removed from around the lens with a fine toothpick. Special lens paper is used on the lens itself. Lensed instruments should not be cleaned with any substance that contains alcohol, since it may dissolve cement around the lens.

The endoscope is rinsed thoroughly and dried well. If scopes are to be sterilized in ethylene oxide gas, they must be thoroughly dry. Gas combines with water on items that are damp to form ethylene glycol. Alcohol on cotton can be used on a wire stylet or a pipe cleaner to dry insertion tubes. Air can be forced through channels to dry inside them. Because organisms will multiply in a moist environment, all parts should be dry during the interval before further processing or storage.

An endoscope processor is available to clean long, flexible fiberoptic scopes, such as a colonoscope. It has two modes of operation to process the scope and its channels: a wash-and-dry cycle and a cycle of wash, disinfectant soak with activated glutaraldehyde solution, rinse, and dry. This equipment is an automated washer/disinfector.

Accessories are scrupulously cleaned. All debris is removed to ensure adequate steam sterilization. Disposable single-use biopsy forceps and cytology brushes are recommended because the configurations of these accessories are particularly difficult to clean. Some trocars, scissors, and forceps have disposable or replaceable points or tips on reusable shafts or handles. These combination instruments facilitate cleaning and also ensure a sharp cutting edge with each use.

Scopes and accessories should be inspected for damage after cleaning. Preferably, all endoscopic equipment should be terminally sterilized; otherwise it should be disinfected after thorough mechanical cleaning.

Sterilization

After cleaning and drying, each endoscope with all of its parts disassembled is placed in a well-padded perforated tray of convenient size. Some endoscopes, such as an arthroscope, are supplied in a perforated case lined with foam cut to fit each disassembled part. The tray or fitted case is wrapped for sterilization. Instruments should be packaged immediately and sent to be sterilized by steam or ethylene oxide gas as recommended by the manufacturer.

Some parts of endoscopes can be safely steam sterilized and therefore should be. Hollow, rigid metal sheaths, such as a sigmoidoscope, can be terminally steam sterilized after use but then may be stored to keep clean rather than sterile for a surgically clean procedure. Some fiberoptic cables also can be steam sterilized. Reusable biopsy forceps should be steam sterilized.

Parts with lenses and some fiberoptic carriers, such as a colonoscope, cannot be steam sterilized. High temperature and moisture will soften the cement holding lenses or fiberoptic fibers in place. The flexible shafts of some accessory instruments may erode when steam sterilized. These parts should be sterilized in ethylene oxide gas, hydrogen peroxide plasma, or formaldehyde gas, or soaked in a chemical sterilant solution if ethylene oxide or hydrogen peroxide is not available.

The manufacturer may recommend that the pressure not exceed 5 pounds during ethylene oxide sterilization of a fiberoptic lighting system. The manufacturer's instructions for handling, using, cleaning, and sterilizing these items should be followed. Aeration is necessary following ethylene oxide sterilization. Ethylene oxide is a vesicant if it comes in contact with skin. It also can cause eye irritation.

If endoscopes and accessories are immersed in activated glutaraldehyde, acetic acid, or formaldehyde solution, a plastic tray should be used without a towel in the bottom. Prolonged use of a stainless steel tray may create an electrolytic action between the metals and can cause metallic deposits on instruments. Scopes and all accessories should be well rinsed in sterile distilled water before they are used in order to prevent tissue irritation from solution.

Peracetic acid, another chemical sterilant in solution, is commercially available for sterilizing endoscopes for immediate patient use. The Steris system has specialized tray assemblies for endoscope processing. These assemblies are not intended for long-term storage of sterilized instruments. More information can be found in Chapter 17.

High-Level Disinfection

When immediate reuse of an endoscope that cannot be steam sterilized is necessary, the endoscope should be washed in nonresidue liquid-detergent solution, rinsed, dried, and immersed in activated glutaraldehyde, acetic acid, or peracetic acid solution with the parts disassembled. All channels should be filled with solution. Solution may become diluted if endoscopes are not dried before immersion.

A timer should be set for a minimum of 20 minutes to kill vegetative bacteria, fungi, and hepatitis B virus and human immunodeficiency virus (HIV). Time should be extended to 45 minutes for tuberculocidal activity of glutaraldehyde. The manufacturer's instructions should be consulted for specific information about chemical sterilization products.

Even though high-level disinfection is not sterilization, sterile gloves are worn to remove scopes from solution. A lensed instrument is never handled with forceps. Forceps could crush a telescope and ruin the optical system. Also, if an instrument is wet, the danger of dropping it is increased. All parts are rinsed thoroughly in sterile distilled water before use. More information is available at **www.cdc.gov.** Disinfection is discussed in Chapter 18.

Storage

If they are not immediately wrapped for sterilization and storage, endoscopes should be terminally sterilized or at least undergo high-level disinfection before being returned to their respective storage cabinets. Clean, dry, unwrapped instruments should be stored on a soft material such as plastic sheeting or foam. Towels hold a residue of laundry detergent that can cause tarnish on metal. Flexible endoscopes with detachable parts should be stored disassembled, in a vertical position with the distal end pointed downward. Accessories also may be hung.

The scope should be subjected to high-level disinfection or peracetic acid sterilization before use in patient care.

Considerations for Patient Safety

Endoscopy through a natural body orifice is usually performed on a patient who is not under general anesthesia. The following considerations should be included in the plan of care:

1. The patient should be monitored for signs and symptoms of reaction to drugs. Endoscopy is frequently performed with the use of sedatives and a topical or local anesthetic agent or with no anesthetic at all. The patient is awake during these procedures. Drugs such as midazolam (Versed) and diazepam (Valium), and narcotics such as meperidine hydrochloride (Demerol)

may be administered intravenously as an adjunct to other preoperative sedation to produce relaxation and cooperation during the procedure and amnesia afterward. Respiratory depression and transient hypotension can occur. Antagonistic drugs should be available to reverse narcotic depression. Emergency resuscitation equipment should also be available.

2. A topical agent is frequently applied to nasal or oral and pharyngeal mucosa before introduction of an endoscope into the tracheobronchial tree or gastrointestinal tract. A topical agent may be instilled into the urethra before introduction of a cystoscope.

3. The teeth, gums, and lips are protected if the endoscope is introduced through the mouth. Dentures are removed. A mouthpiece is inserted.

4. Hydrogen and methane gases are normally present in the colon. These gases are flushed out with carbon dioxide before laser surgery or electrosurgery through the colonoscope to avoid the possibility of explosion within the colon.

5. Power sources and lights should be tested before each use and after cleaning. They should be kept in working order.

6. The heat generated from the projection lamp of a fiberoptic illuminator is dissipated. It should not be enclosed in drapes because the heat could set them on fire. If the unit contains a fan for heat regulation, the direction of airflow should be away from the patient and the sterile field to minimize airborne contamination.

7. Endoscopes should be smooth, with no nicks on the surface. A scratch on the sheath could cause injury to tissue or the mucous membrane lining of an orifice. Metal endoscopes with metal-lifting forceps that can scratch the sheaths should not be handled. They should be handled only with the hands, usually gloved.

8. Extreme care should be taken to observe patients after endoscopic procedures for effects of respiratory or circulatory distress caused by trauma or medication. Many endoscopic procedures are performed on ambulatory outpatients. They must not leave the facility until vital signs are stable and side effects have passed. Follow-up phone calls are suggested within 24 to 48 hours to monitor patient progress.

Duties of the Assistant

Often only a circulator assists the surgeon with a minimally invasive procedure. The assistant's duties are as follows:

1. Set up the supplies and equipment as much as possible before the patient and surgeon arrive. Consult the procedure book. Remember that sterility must be maintained for a sterile procedure.

2. Explain the steps of the procedure to the patient as appropriate. It is important that the patient know the reasons for any discomfort that may be experienced so that symptoms of discomfort will be recognized as normal.

3. Explain the position and need for it before positioning the patient. The position the patient must assume during the procedure is often uncomfortable.

4. Drape the patient properly to prevent unnecessary exposure.

5. Adjust room lighting. The surgeon may want the room in semidarkness. A dimmer on the room light is helpful, but if one is unavailable, the x-ray view boxes may be illuminated to provide indirect lighting.

6. Divert the patient's attention as much as possible during the procedure. The patient may complain of pain more than is justified as a way of expressing displeasure at the invasion of the endoscope or the position required during the procedure. The circulator should stay with the patient to offer reassurance and emotional support. Suggest that slow, deep breaths may help relaxation and lessen the discomfort. Soft music may help the patient relax. The surgeon may allow the patient to watch the procedure through a viewing attachment on the endoscope or on a video monitor.

7. Evaluate the patient's level of discomfort and inform the surgeon of unusual reactions. The circulator also monitors the patient's respiratory status, blood pressure, and pulse. Pulse oximeter and automated blood pressure devices may be used routinely. Vital signs should be documented before the procedure begins, every 15 minutes during the procedure, and again at the conclusion. Additional vital signs should be recorded when medication is given or tissue samples are excised.

8. Know how to assemble the different scopes and their accessories and how to operate them. When passing the suction tube or biopsy forceps, place the tip directly at the lumen of the scope so that the surgeon can grasp the shaft and insert it without moving his or her eyes from the scope.

9. Take care not to drop endoscopic instruments; they are delicate and expensive. Fiberoptic bundles are glass; do not kink or bend them.

MICROSURGERY

The simplest magnifying instrument consists of a single lens with relatively high magnification (e.g., a magnifying glass or a jeweler's lens). Surgeons requiring lesser magnification than that provided by the microscope use an operating loupe. This simple lens magnifies approximately two times. It attaches to a headband or to the surgeon's spectacles. Loupe surgery terminates where microsurgery begins. From loupe surgery and refinements of the binocular microscope, microsurgery has evolved. Terms associated with microsurgery are defined in Box 20-6.

Historical Background

Use of the microscope has been an essential modality in scientific investigation for centuries. Pioneers such as Dutch

Box 20-6 Terms Associated with Microsurgery

beam splitter   Attachment to the microscope that splits light; one part is reflected laterally, and the other part is relayed upward to the binocular tube; can be 50%/50% or 30%/70%. The greater portion may be directed to a camera or video system.

binocular   Using two eyes to see in stereoscopic vision.

coaxial illumination   The light path follows the same direction as the visual image.

contraves stand   Series of weights used to balance some microscopes.

depth of field   Distance of focus.

diopter   Power of the lens to assist vision by refractive correction of reflected light.

focal length   Distance between the lens and the object in focus.

microscope   Instrument that uses a series of lenses to magnify very small objects.

monocular   Using one eye for vision. Depth of field is absent; the image is two-dimensional.

objective   Power of the lens that determines the focal distance of vision.

ocular   Eyepiece lens that multiplies the basic magnification of the microscope.

pupillary distance   Measurement between the pupils of the eyes; used to position the binocular eyepieces.

stereopsis   Vision with two eyes that enables objects to appear three-dimensional.

working distance   Physical space between the objective lens of the microscope and the surgical field.

zoom   To change the range of focus in continuous magnification; the change can be closer or more distant.

---

microscopist Anton van Leeuwenhoek (1632-1723), who in 1680 developed the compound microscope, which magnified objects 270 times, contributed to the adoption of the germ theory. Objects as small as protozoa and bacteria could be seen only through a light microscope, just as viruses can be seen only through the more recently developed electron microscope. Optician Joseph Jackson Lister (1786-1869), father of the English surgeon who introduced antiseptic surgery, perfected the achromatic lens to eliminate color aberrations in the compound microscope. Ernest Abbe (1840-1905) did further work in the nineteenth century to improve refraction through immersion of the lens in oil and concentration of illumination (1886). A basic system for binocular eyepieces was devised in 1902.

A microscope was first used for clinical surgery in 1921 when Nylen operated on patients with chronic otitis in Sweden. He used a monocular microscope. Subsequently, as binocular magnification, adequate illumination, and stable support were added, otolaryngology became the first surgical specialty to routinely use a microscope.

Ophthalmologists were the first to use the stereoscopic biomicroscope, commonly referred to as a slit lamp, in clinical examination to magnify objects in three dimensions. The principles applied to the biomicroscope led to the development of an operating microscope in 1953. Ophthalmologists quickly expanded applications and indications for ocular microsurgery. Most other specialties were slow to implement its use.

The first of the current operating microscopes was developed in 1960 by the Zeiss Instrument Company in collaboration with Julius Jacobson, a vascular surgeon in New York. Jacobson developed microsurgical instruments, introduced microvascular techniques, and began using the term *microsurgery*. Thus began the development of clinical applications of microsurgery in every surgical specialty.

Technique of Microsurgery

Performance of surgical procedures while directly viewing the surgical field under magnification affords surgeons greater visual acuity of small structures. The microscope provides a more limited, although more readily visible, surgical field. All things look considerably different under magnification. Tissues not otherwise visible can be manipulated. Use of microsurgical instrumentation and techniques is not simply a matter of adapting formerly learned conventional methods for use under the microscope. The techniques themselves for handling instruments, sutures, and tissues are different and infinitely more complex, precise, and time-consuming because of the meticulous skill involved. Coordination must be adapted to working with minute materials in a field of altered perception and position. Proficiency and facility in using the operating microscope entail laboratory practice in movements and manipulation of instruments and suture materials under various magnifications.

Divergence from tactile-manual to vision-oriented techniques requires that the surgeon and assistants pay maximum attention to detail. The most common maneuvers for placing and manipulating instruments, making an incision with scissors, and tying sutures involve a combination of several basic movements:

- *Compression-decompression:* to close scissors and forceps
- *Rotation:* to insert a needle, to cut, to extract, to engage or disengage
- *Push-pull, direct, or linear:* to incise with a razor knife

The surgeon also must be able to maintain a steady, stationary position during remote activation of equipment such as a laser beam. It is advisable that surgeons and assistants do no manual labor for at least a day before operating. Drinking coffee the morning of surgery may decrease steadiness in some individuals. Very little tremor is tolerable in microsurgery.

Advantages of Microsurgery

Microsurgery provides unique advantages in the restoration of wholeness and function of the body, such as restitution of hearing, vision, tactile sensation, circulation, and/or motion.

It is used in many surgical specialties to improve precision of already-established surgical procedures and to permit successful performance of procedures previously not possible. For example, blood vessels less than 3 mm in exterior diameter can be sutured. Nerves can be anastomosed. Replantation of amputated parts and some reconstructive surgery are possible only under magnification. In general, microsurgery allows the following:

- Dissection and repair of fine structures through better visualization
- Adaptation of surgical procedures to individual patient requirements (variation in anatomic landmarks is more distinct with magnification)
- Diminution of surgical trauma and complications because of safer dissection
- Superior focal lighting of the surgical field, particularly in deep areas

Operating Microscope

Compound microscopes use two or more lens systems or several lenses grouped in one unit. The operating microscope is a compound binocular instrument. Interchangeable objective lenses combined with interchangeable eyepieces allow a wide range of magnification and working distances adjustable to the surgeon's needs. The operating microscope uses light waves for illumination. These waves are bent as they pass through the microscope, causing the image seen by the viewer's eye to be magnified.

The users must understand the parts and their functions. Basically, all operating microscopes incorporate the same essential components: an optical lens system and controls for magnification and focus, an illumination system, a mounting system for stability, an electrical system, and accessories.

Optical Lens System

The ability to enlarge an image is known as magnifying power. This is the ratio of the size of the image produced on the viewer's retina by magnification to the size of the retinal image when the object is viewed without optical aid. To create a distinct image, adjacent images must be separated. An indistinct image remains unclear no matter how many times it is magnified. The ability to discern detail is known as resolving power.

Components The heart of the optical system is the body, which contains the objective lens (lens closest to the object). The head or binocular oculars (eyepieces) through which the surgeon looks are physically and optically attached to the body. The optical combination of the objective lens and the oculars determines the magnification of the microscope (Figure 20-9).

Objective lenses are available in various focal lengths ranging from 100 to 400 mm, with intervening increases by 25-mm increments. The 400-mm lens provides the greatest magnification. The designation of the objective lens enumer-

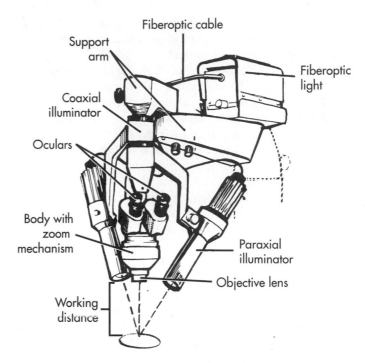

Figure 20-9 Microscope body in detail.

ates the working distance (the distance from the lens to the surgical field). Distances vary from 6 to 10 inches (15 to 25 cm). For example, a 200-mm lens will be in focus at a working distance of 200 mm, or approximately 8 inches (20 cm).

The oculars serve as magnifying glasses used to examine the real image formed by the objective. Most objectives are achromatic so that the true color of tissues can be viewed in sharp detail. The binocular arrangement provides stereoscopic viewing. Stereopsis is basically achieved through binocular viewing, wherein each eye has a slightly different positional view of the object under examination. The observer's brain then combines the two dissimilar images taken from points of view a little distance apart, thus producing a perception of a single three-dimensional image. If the user is wearing corrective lenses, the eyepieces are set to zero. If the user needs corrective lenses but is not wearing them, he or she should preset the eyepieces to a position of visual comfort and acuity before draping the microscope. Detachable rubber eyecups for the eyepieces are commercially available for the user's comfort.

Magnification The ability of the microscope to magnify depends on the design and quality of the parts in addition to the resolving power. The total magnification is computed by multiplying the enlarging power of the objective lens by that of the lenses of the oculars. The depth of the field, which is the vertical dimension within which objects are seen in clear focus, decreases with increases in magnification of power. Likewise, the width of the field of view narrows as the power of magnification increases. For example, at 20× magnification, the field of view narrows to ½ inch (10 mm, or less than 1.25 cm). Vertical viewing of the surgical field is extremely important, particularly in higher magnification ranges. It allows the surgeon more effective use of the increasingly limited depth of field.

In more complex microscopes a third set of lenses is interposed between the oculars and the objective lens to provide additional magnification in variable degrees as desired by the surgeon. A continuously variable system of magnification for increasing or decreasing images is possible with a zoom lens. A faster, easier-to-handle zoom lens is preferred by most surgeons to a simpler turret magnifier that manually changes magnification by fixed increments. The zoom lens is usually operated by a foot control that permits the surgeon to change magnification without removing the hands from the surgical field. The popular range of magnification in the zoom microscope is from $3.5\times$ to $20\times$ magnification. At $3.5\times$ magnification, the depth of the field is about $\frac{1}{10}$ inch (2.5 mm); at $20\times$ magnification, the depth is about $\frac{1}{25}$ inch (1 mm). Some microscopes magnify to 40 times.

Focus Focusing is accomplished manually or by a foot-controlled motor that raises and lowers the body of the microscope to the desired distance from the object to be viewed. Some microscopes divide the focus into gross and fine. The focus of the ocular lens usually is set at zero; the surgeon adjusts the focus as desired.

Illumination System

Illumination of the operating microscope uses light waves. The shorter the wavelength, the greater the resolving power. The intensity of illumination can be varied by controls mounted on the support arm of the body. The operating microscope has two basic sources of illumination: paraxial and coaxial.

Paraxial Illuminators One or more light tubes (paraxial illuminators) contain tungsten or halogen bulbs and focusing lenses. The illuminators are attached to the mounting of the body of the microscope in a position to illuminate the field of view. Light is focused to coincide with the working distance of the microscope.

One of the paraxial illuminators may be equipped with a diaphragm containing a variable-width slit aperture. This device permits a narrow beam of light to be brought into focus on the objective field. This slit image assists the surgeon in defining depth perception (i.e., in ascertaining the relative distance of objects within the field—which are closer, which are farther).

Coaxial Illuminators With fiberoptic coaxial illuminators, light is transmitted through the optical system of the microscope body. This type of illumination is called coaxial because it illuminates the same area in the same focus as the viewing, or objective, field of the microscope. The fiberoptic system provides intense, though cool, light that protects the patient's tissues and the optics of the microscope from excessive heat. The light intensity ranges from 600 to 2250 footcandles without creating shadows. Reflected glare may be a problem. Frequent wound irrigation with a cool solution is necessary to avoid tissue damage from radiant energy during long procedures.

If a fiberoptic system is not used for coaxial illumination, a heat-absorbing filter must be interposed in the illumination system. Direct heat from a high-intensity source can damage and even burn tissues. Tungsten and halogen bulbs are used in some housings.

Another type of optical prism assembly provides a larger area of coaxial illumination with a brighter light than that obtained with fiberoptic light bundles. Known as liquid light, it uses ionic, inorganic saline solution with quartz glass inserts inside a flexible aluminum spiral tube insulated with a polyvinyl chloride coating. Light is conducted throughout the cross section of the liquid, unlike the light provided by a fiberoptic bundle.

Mounting Systems

The stability of the microscope is of paramount importance. The body, the optical portion, is mounted on a vertical column that may be supported by the floor, ceiling, or wall, or by attachment to the operating bed. The body of the microscope is attached to the column by a hinged arm and a central pivot. The mounting permits positioning as desired. It may be adjusted horizontally or vertically, rotated on its axis, and tilted at different angles. The microscope can be aimed in any direction. The objective is aimed at the principal surgical site.

Floor and ceiling mounting systems are the most popular and versatile. All microscopes must have a locking mechanism to immobilize the microscope body over the surgical field.

Floor Mount The base of the vertical support, which rests on the floor, has retractable casters for ease in moving the entire instrument. When the base is lowered to working position, it is locked into position (Figure 20-10).

The base should be properly positioned in relation to the operating bed before the anesthetic is administered or the patient is prepped. To maintain balance and control, one should gently push (not pull) the microscope when moving it. Jarring or banging the scope should be avoided, since the lenses may dislocate and obscure vision. The brake should be released or casters activated before the microscope is moved. The arms should be folded close to the column with all of the attachments locked into place. Cords should be out of the way. Observation tubes should not be used as handles. Force should never be used in moving the microscope or in applying attachments; one should look for the problem instead. A floor-based microscope with column support is placed to the left of a right-handed surgeon. The base should not interfere with foot controls or power cables. It should be clear of any table attachments.

Some microscopes use a contraves stand. This is a counterbalanced weight system used to position the operating microscope in a suspended position over the surgical field. The weights are set and locked according to the type of attachments on the body of the microscope. The balance is set before activating the power switch.

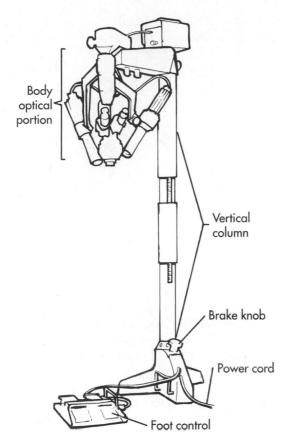

Figure 20-10 Floor-mounted operating microscope.

Figure 20-11 Ceiling track–mounted microscope.

As a safety factor, the base must not be moved when the microscope is positioned over the patient, because it is top-heavy. Gross adjustments, such as height in relation to the surgical field and focus, are made with the microscope swung away from the patient. The operating bed height, chair, and armrest heights are adjusted at the same time that gross adjustments are made. Fine focusing and adjustments arc done after the microscope is in position for the surgical procedure. The assistant's microscope is adjusted to the same focus as that of the surgeon. During prepping and draping, the microscope is rotated out of position, then brought over the surgical field for the procedure.

Ceiling Mount A ceiling mount, either a fixed or track-mounted model, provides freer floor space. The fixed unit is suspended from a telescoping column attached directly to the ceiling. Vertical support of a track-mounted unit is suspended from a ceiling rail. It can be moved out of the way when not in use (Figure 20-11). The microscope is positioned and focused after the patient is anesthetized. A ceiling-mounted instrument is operated by a control panel on a wall (on-off switch) and by foot controls for focusing, magnifying, raising, and lowering.

A ceiling mount is generally very stable, but it is only as stable as the supporting ceiling. Mechanical devices adjacent to the OR, such as air-conditioning units, may cause vibration. The microscope should be vibration free. A ceiling

mount permits the same flexibility of positioning as a floor mount.

The vertical support has a memory stop mechanism that can be preset for a preselected operating bed height. This setting should be checked and adjusted for each operating bed position change. The mechanism is a safety factor to prevent accidental lowering of the microscope at high speed too close to the patient. High-speed lowering should be done away from the patient until the memory stop is reached. As with the floor-mounted instrument, gross adjustments are never made over the patient. Fine adjustment and focusing are done after the microscope is over the surgical field.

Wall Mount The microscope is bracketed by a flexible arm to a stable wall. The swing-arm extension permits proper positioning.

Operating Bed Mount Smaller microscopes may be mounted on the framework of the operating bed. This system has many disadvantages and thus is not popular.

Electrical System

The same precautions are observed with the operating microscope as with any electrical equipment in the OR. Switches and wall interlocks should be explosion proof. Circuits are protected from overload by breaker relays and fuses. All light controls should be in the off position when the power plug is inserted or removed from the wall outlet to avoid short-circuiting or sparking. A red pilot light illuminates on the control panel when the electrical power is on.

Accessories

A number of accessories are available to enhance the versatility of microsurgery. The value of a good microscope is negated without proper ancillary equipment.

Assistant's Binoculars A separate optical body with a nonmotorized, hand-controlled zoom lens can be attached to the main microscope body for use by the assistant (Figure 20-12). This mechanism can be focused in the same

Figure 20-12   Surgeon's microscope on right with assistant's binoculars attached on left.

Figure 20-13   Microscope accessories.

plane as the surgeon's oculars. Its field of view may not coincide exactly with that of the surgeon. This can be rectified by using a beam splitter, which takes the image from one of the surgeon's oculars and transmits it through an observer tube, thereby providing the assistant with an identical image of the surgeon's view (see Figure 20-12). This is particularly important in critical areas where a difference of 1 or 2 mm is crucial.

Assistant's binocular co-observer tubes can be placed on the body so that the assistant can work and observe from the same side of the operating bed as, at a right angle to, or directly opposite, the surgeon. Binocular tubes, either tiltable, straight, or inclined, can be attached on the right or left side of the body. A dual viewing bridge, the quadroscope, is attached when the surgeon and assistant sit opposite each other. They have exactly the same view of the field with this accessory. Binoculars should be appropriately placed on the microscope body before the surgical procedure begins.

Broadfield Viewing Lens   A low-power magnifying glass is used for grasping needles or for getting an overall view of the field adjacent to the objective. This lens attaches to the front of the body of the surgeon's ocular (see Figure 20-12).

Couplings   Couplings allow versatility in positioning the microscope for specific applications. An automated mechanism, the X-Y attachment, provides precision in controlling small movements of the microscope in the field of view. A coupling piece lets surgeons change the angle for side-to-side or front-to-back viewing. A universal tilt coupling can be integrated into the X-Y coupling.

Cameras   Still photographic, motion picture, videotape, and television cameras may be attached to the beam splitter, permitting filming of the surgical procedure (Figure 20-13). The camera unit should be in the upright position when connected to the operating microscope. It may require the use of a stronger illumination source. One should check to be sure film is in the camera by trying to rewind the film

cartridge holder. The patient's and surgeon's names, the date, and the time are documented on the film or video cartridge to prevent mixing recorded images between patients. The use of recording equipment may require special patient consent in some institutions. The recorded procedure is useful in assisting, teaching, and research.

Laser Microadaptor   Laser beams can be directed through the operating microscope. The microscope and laser head couplings should be perfectly aligned in the grooves and protrusions on the metal adapters. A screw and locking pin secure the coupling. In the operating position the laser head is at approximately a 60-degree angle to the microscope. It will not fire in a horizontal or upside-down position. The microadaptor must have a compatible lens with a focal length of 200, 300, or 400 mm so that the surgeon can properly adjust the focal point of the laser beam. A CO_2 laser with electronic components that delivers milliwatt energy may be used to vaporize tissues or weld tissues together. Other types of lasers are directed through fiberoptics. To protect the surgeon's eyes, filter caps over optics should be appropriate for the wavelength of the laser being used. The entire team and patient must wear eye protection of the appropriate optical density when the laser is in use.

Remote Foot Controls   Simple microscopes are manually operated. It is more convenient for the surgeon to use motorized foot controls for functions such as focus, zoom, and tilt. Foot controls may be activated by switches of the push-button type, heel-to-toe, or side-to-side motion. The number of switches corresponds to the number of motor-controlled functions. There may be additional foot switches for the camera or for other non–microscope-associated equipment, such as cryosurgical, bipolar electrosurgical, or laser units. Switches may be separated by a vertical bar to prevent inadvertent contact. The bar also serves as a footrest for the surgeon. Because the surgeon and assistant usually are seated during microsurgical procedures, the height of the operating bed must permit them adequate knee room to operate foot controls.

Microscope Drape The entire working mechanism and support arm of the microscope are encased in a sterile drape. Draping the entire microscope permits it to be brought into the sterile field so that the surgeon can position the body and adjust the optics. Disposable drapes that are heat resistant, lint free, nonreflective, transparent, and quiet are available to fit the configuration of all microscopes and attachments. The scrub person slides the drape over the body, with hands protected as for draping a Mayo stand. The circulator helps guide the drape toward the vertical column and secures it. The scrub person secures the drape to the oculars. Sterile lens covers or rubber bands may be supplied with the drape for this purpose.

If it is not heat resistant, a plastic drape may cause heat buildup beneath it that can damage the microscope. A heat guard may be applied over the light source, or heat may be evacuated through an opening in the top of the drape.

Care of the Microscope

Persons responsible for the microscope should consult the manufacturer's manual. Any malfunction should be reported to the OR manager or appropriate person who can arrange for repair service. A checklist to verify care and functioning of various parts before the surgical procedure is helpful. All persons who assist with microsurgery must know how to set up, position, and otherwise care for the microscope as follows:

1. The microscope should be damp dusted before use.
   a. External surfaces, except the lenses, are wiped with a clean cloth saturated with detergent-disinfectant solution.
   b. Casters or wheels should be clean to reduce contamination and prevent interference with mobility.
2. Lenses should be cleaned according to the manufacturer's recommendations only, to avoid scratching or damage to antireflective lens coating. Most manufacturers recommend sterile distilled water and lens paper. They must not be soaked in any solution.
3. The circulator should prepare the microscope.
   a. When changing oculars, care is taken to avoid dropping and fingerprinting lenses. Avoid stripping the threads of screw mounts by seating the optics and turning in a counterclockwise direction until the threads align. Proceed by turning in a clockwise motion until secure. Take care not to overtighten. Right turns tighten; left turns loosen.
   b. Both hands should be used for attaching observation tubes, which are heavy.
   c. Extra lamp bulbs and fuses should be on hand. The circulator must know where they are stored and how to change them. It is advisable to check bulbs periodically to avoid the necessity of replacing them during a procedure. New bulbs should be inserted if a long procedure is anticipated. Bulbs should be changed with the power off.

   d. Check electrical connections for proper fit or wire fraying. Take special care of power cables to prevent accidental breakage from heavy equipment rolling over them.
   e. Check that all knobs are secured after the microscope is in operating position.
   f. Place foot controls in a convenient position so that the surgeon does not have to search for them.
4. The microscope and accessories should be properly stored. Store away from traffic but close to areas where used.
   a. Openings into the microscope body for attachment of accessory devices, such as the observer tube, should be closed with covers provided by the manufacturer when not in use to prevent accumulation of dust.
   b. Lenses and viewing tubes should be protected.
   c. The microscope and attachments should be enclosed in an antistatic plastic cover when not in use to keep them free from dust.
   d. Power cords should be neatly coiled for storage.

Microinstrumentation

Improved results of surgical intervention using microsurgical techniques are due in no small measure to the miniaturized precision instrumentation developed in association with the performance of these delicate procedures. The instruments are extremely fine, delicate, and miniature enough to handle in the very small working area. Manipulation becomes more difficult with increased size or bulk and weight. As with techniques, instruments are constantly being improved. Microsurgeons work with manufacturers to develop appropriate instruments, suture materials, and needles. Many surgeons purchase the instruments of their choice. Whether owned by the surgeon or the facility, microinstruments require exacting care to maintain desired function.

Instruments are designed to conform to hand movements under the microscope. They must permit secure grasp, ease of holding and manipulation, and fulfillment of their intended purpose. They are shaped to not obscure the limited field of view. Although these factors are important criteria for any instrument, they are especially vital for microinstruments. Everyone assisting in or setting up for microsurgical procedures must know the identification and functions of these unique instruments. Design is coincident to function.

Material and Surface

Microinstruments are made of stainless steel or titanium. Titanium alloy is considerably stronger yet lighter in weight than stainless steel. Some microinstruments are malleable for desired angling. Some are disposable. All are extremely vulnerable to abuse.

Finishes of at least the portions of instruments exposed to light in the surgical field are deliberately dulled during manufacture to reduce glare, which is both annoying and tiring to the surgeon. Titanium microinstruments have a dull blue finish.

Shape and Tips

Microinstruments are shorter than standard instruments and are often angulated for convenience of approach and avoidance of obstruction of the surgical field.

Instrument tips have minimal separation, which is compatible with their function. Finger pressure and movement necessary to close wide tips are undesirable because they may induce tremor.

Handles

Handles are designed for a secure and comfortable grasp, with a diameter comparable to that of a pen or pencil. Minimal diameter between fingers facilitates feel and accuracy of manipulation. Double-handled instruments (scissors, needleholders) have a slightly larger diameter than single-handled ones (razor knife). The shape of the handle is also important for manipulation. For example, instruments that are rotated between fingers when in use, such as forceps, must be turned easily. Their handles therefore are rounded or have six sides like a pencil (Figure 20-14). Those that are not rotated have finger grips or are flattened. Ring-handled instruments are not practical in microsurgery.

Many instruments, particularly scissors and some needleholders, have spring handles that return tips to the open posi-

tion between cutting or grasping functions (Figure 20-15). The distance from hinge to tip will vary according to function. Proper spring tension can be easily ruined by mishandling.

Handles should be long enough for comfort in the working position but must not extend beyond the working distance to contact the unsterile objective of the microscope. The maximum length of most microinstruments is about 4 inches (100 mm). Gripping surfaces should be functionally located to prevent fingers from slipping during manipulation. These surfaces serve as a guide to accurate finger positioning. The gripping area may have a six-sided, round, knurled, or flat and serrated surface.

Primary Uses

Appropriate instrumentation is used for specific types of procedures. Although all surgical instruments are structured for a definitive use, the function of microinstruments is even more restricted. Tissue can be severely injured by use of an improper or imperfect instrument. Instruments, too, can be damaged by use on inappropriate tissue. Primary usage includes cutting (knives, scissors, and saws), exposure (spatulas and retractors), gross and fine fixation (forceps and clamps), and suture and needle manipulation (needleholders). Instruments must not be used for manipulations other than the intended purpose.

Knives   Edges of razor, diamond, and dissecting knives have different degrees of sharpness and thickness of blades that are appropriate to the cutting function of each (i.e., to make penetrating or slicing incisions). A clean cut is desired to minimize trauma and tissue destruction.

Scissors   Like knives, scissors are designed to make a specific type of incision related both to the plane and to thickness. Incisions are vertical, horizontal, or of a special config-

1mm
straight

1mm
ring tips

Figure 20-14   Microsurgical forceps.

A

B

Figure 20-15   Microsurgical instruments with spring handles. **A,** Scissors. **B,** Needleholder.

uration, such as curved or two-planed. Use is governed by hinging and blade relationship. Scissors are hinged to cut vertically or obliquely. Cutting is usually done by the distal part of blades for better control. Some scissors come in pairs with right and left curves. Often a part number inscribed by the manufacturer on the handle will be an even number for a right-handed instrument and an odd number for a left-handed one. Blades may be sharp or blunt, long or short, and straight or angulated. Available with straight or curved blades, microsurgical scissors have a spring-type handle (Figure 20-15, *A*).

Powered Instruments Microsurgical air-powered drills and saws vary in sizes and shapes. They have a fingertip control; some have an optional foot control.

Spatulas and Retractors Spatulas and retractors are used to draw tissue back for better exposure or protection. Nerve hooks and elevators also are used for these purposes.

Forceps Straight and curved forceps may be toothed or smooth. They have light spring action and minimal tip separation. Teeth of some tissue forceps may be as small as $\frac{1}{250}$ inch (0.1 mm) in diameter. Therefore many tips are barely visible to the unaided eye. Toothed forceps are used for grasping tissue but never for grasping needles or sutures. Smooth forceps are used for tying delicate ligatures and sutures. For stability of grasp and avoidance of injury to the suture strand, the tips of the forceps should be absolutely parallel and have perfect apposition of grasping surfaces. Suture should be grasped firmly but without trauma, often from a slippery surface. Other smooth forceps are used on friable tissues. Bipolar forceps are used for electrocoagulation.

Clamps Mosquito hemostats and various clamps are used for vascular occlusion and for approximation of edges of tissues such as nerves and vessels. Crushing of vessels should be avoided.

Microsutures and Needles

Microsurgical closure is unique in that the smallest sizes of sutures and needles manufactured are used. Microsuture sizes range from 8-0 (45 μm) to 11-0 (14 μm) in diameter. Because of the minute size, proportionately small needles are swaged to suture. They range from 30 to 130 μm in diameter.

Suture materials include synthetic absorbable and nonabsorbable polymers. A strand is finer than a human hair. Packets provide ready access to the needle. When in use, the needle should always be kept in view in the surgical field because the strand may easily be lost from view and difficult to pick up. The surgeon should inspect the strand for damage while passing it through tissue to be sure holding power in situ is not threatened. It is safest and easiest for the scrub person to keep these sutures in packets until the surgeon is ready to use them.

Stainless steel microsurgical needles are measured in microns for wire diameter and millimeters for length. To achieve deep placement in tissue, the needle is short and

sharply curved. Less curvature is required for more superficial suturing. Straight needles may be preferred for some tissues.

To arm a needle in the needleholder, some surgeons want the scrub person to hold the open suture packet under the accessory broad-field viewing lens so that they may grasp the needle themselves from the foam that secures the needle. The scrub person then gently removes the packet from the strand. The surgeon grasps the needle lightly but firmly in the needleholder and takes it into the surgical field. Any readjustment of the position of the needle is done by the surgeon using the microscope.

Closure of an incision with the least trauma to produce minimal fibrosis and scarring is enhanced by placing sutures close together to yield a firm, even apposition line and anatomically secure wound. Integrity of the sutures compensates for minimal scar tissue in supporting the wound. Use of the zoom microscope facilitates tying and cutting sutures.

Needleholders Microsurgical needleholders are used only for suturing, not ligating, because the very fine suture materials would break if they were tied with a needleholder. They should be used to hold only minute microsurgical needles so as not to alter alignment. Handles are round to permit easy rotation between fingers. Some have spring handles. Although a lock on a needleholder may cause tips to jerk when engaged or released, some have a holding catch for use in deep wounds to prevent loss of small needles. Needleholders held closed by finger pressure, rather than a catch, firmly hold a needle shaft yet permit easy adjustment of the needle position. The tips can be curved or straight.

Sponges

Suitably small, nonfibrous sponges or lint-free patties of material such as compressed cellulose are used to accommodate the surgical field. Lint is visible under the microscope and could obstruct the view.

General Considerations in Microsurgery

Patient

The patient is prepared as for a standard surgical procedure. He or she should be positioned comfortably and safely with the operating bed locked in position. The surgical site is immobilized if possible.

Anesthesia

If general anesthesia is to be administered, the anesthesia provider should be informed in advance of the surgeon's intention to use the microscope. This is especially pertinent in procedures in which patient movements under light anesthesia could result in disaster. In addition, the anesthesia provider's position in relation to the patient should be considered to allow room for the microscope. The anesthesia provider should be aware that microsurgical procedures will take somewhat longer.

With local anesthesia the patient should be instructed to lie quietly and to tell the anesthesia provider or circulator of a desire to move. Many patients sleep during the procedure. A startle reflex on awakening or unexpected movement is especially hazardous in microsurgery, wherein the surgeon's mobility and field of view are limited. If the patient jerks or turns, he or she literally may move out of the surgeon's hands and often out of view of the microsurgical field. Therefore the patient should be closely monitored.

Stability of the Surgical Field

A vital factor for successful microsurgery is stability of the surgical field, microscope, and surgeon's hands. The complete microsurgical unit consists of the operating bed with the patient, the microscope, and the surgeon's chair. These should be functionally positioned in relation to each other so that major adjustments need not be made during the surgical procedure. The surgeon and circulator should check that all components are properly placed before the incision is made.

Armrests and Chair It is important that the surgeon's hands be adequately supported, because a shift of even ⅕ inch (1 mm) can alter the precision of motion, particularly at high magnifications. Support of the surgeon's arm should be continuous from shoulder to hand to give stability and to minimize tremor, especially in fine finger movements. A detachable, sterile, padded wrist support such as the Chan wrist rest may be affixed to the operating bed.

A chair with hydraulic foot controls for raising or lowering provides the necessary forearm support by means of attached armrests. These armrests are individually draped. Mayo stand covers are convenient. Armrests can be moved independently to a variety of levels and positions. They are secured in the desired position. The surgeon should be in a comfortable position to work.

Duties of the Scrub Person

Although a stabilized situation is crucial, a second fundamental necessity is for the surgeon to keep his or her eyes on the field of view through the microscope at all times. Looking away from the field requires readjustment of vision to the field. Cooperation and coordination by the scrub person in carrying out the following duties will prevent the surgeon's distraction from the surgical site:

1. Set up the Mayo stand and instrument table without touching the tips of instruments. Leave protective covers on them until they are needed for use. Holders are available to keep instrument tips in the air and to keep them separated. Microinstruments are handled individually. They are more susceptible to damage than standard instruments. Edges are easily dulled, and fine tips are easily bent or broken. Extreme caution is necessary not to catch tips on any object that could bend them.
2. Place instruments on the Mayo stand in anticipated order of use. Place the Mayo stand and instrument table

conveniently to the surgeon's hand so that he or she does not have to look around the microscope.
3. Pass instruments by placing them in the surgeon's hand in position for use and guide the hand toward the surgical field so that the surgeon may keep his or her eyes on the field.
4. Keep debris (i.e., blood, mucus, or suture ends) from the tips of instruments by wiping them gently on a nonfibrous sponge or lint-free gauze. Replace them in their original position on the Mayo stand, not touching each other.
5. Assist efficiently but never put hands in the surgical field unless requested to do so.
6. Understand the need for slow dissection at times. Do not let attention stray; observe the video monitor if one is available.

The increased time needed for use of the operating microscope can be minimized by adequate preparation and efficient assistance. Each team member should thoroughly understand the microscope and every aspect of microsurgical techniques.

Team members can be kept up to date by in-service explanation of new instruments and demonstration of the microscope. It is extremely helpful and contributory to understanding for the surgeon to show perioperative team members anatomic structures and instruments through the microscope. A comparison of microinstruments with standard instruments under the microscope is always a revelation. A television monitor is advantageous in providing the scrub person and anesthesia provider continuous observation of the surgical procedure. All members should be completely familiar with instrumentation. Not only are instruments then properly cared for, but even more important, surgical time is reduced.

ULTRASONOSURGERY

Ultrasonosurgery, also referred to as cytoreductive debulking surgery, is useful in removing or reducing tumors in highly vascular, delicate tissue such as the brain, liver, kidney, and spleen. The original prototypes of ultrasonic equipment were developed in 1967 to fragment and aspirate cataracts. An ultrasonic aspirator, such as the Cavitron, simultaneously fragments, irrigates, and aspirates tissue. During the fragmentation process, sterile fluid passes through the handpiece to emulsify target tissue. The emulsified tissue is aspirated and collected in a closed-container system.

A transducer in the handpiece converts electrical energy into mechanical motion. Ultrahigh-frequency sound waves produce vibrations at the tip. These vibrations are of the same physical nature as sound but with frequencies above the range of human hearing. Ultrasound has a frequency greater than 30,000 Hz. The vibrating tip of the ultrasonic aspirator fragments tissues at the cellular level. When the tip contacts tissue, vapor pockets within high-water-content cells cause cell walls to separate and collapse. The ultrasonic aspirator is used to disrupt tissues, or tracts, particularly in the central nervous system. It is also used to emulsify tumors with minimal mechanical trauma to surrounding nerves and blood vessels. A device that combines electrosurgery with ultrasonic dissection also allows coagulation during resection and aspiration of a tumor mass.

An ultrasonic probe can be inserted through an endoscope to fragment renal or ureteral calculi (i.e., kidney stones). A suction channel is incorporated into the probe to aspirate fragments as stone is pulverized by ultrasonic energy.

INTEGRATED TECHNOLOGIES

As implied in the previous discussion, several technologies may be used for minimally invasive surgical procedures. Video laseroscopy allows the surgeon to remove organs and tumors and to ablate or repair tissues without making a major incision. An endoscope is introduced into a body cavity through a small incision. The viewing area from the telescopic lens of the scope is magnified from a video camera to a video screen. While viewing the screen, the surgeon can direct a laser beam through the endoscope to the target tissue.

Other instrumentation may be introduced through adjacent small incisions for dissection, ligation, and suturing. These instruments can be manipulated while the surgeon looks through the endoscope or at a monitor. Manipulations may be observed with use of fluoroscopy or a video camera. Ultrasonic and thermal probes, electrosurgical electrodes, and laser beams can be directed through endoscopes. Laser beams can also be directed through the operating microscope.

Computers

Lasers and microscopes may be controlled by computerized systems. Computers can automatically scan tissues to select target tissue for the laser beam. Operating microscopes may contain voice-activated minicomputers that manipulate controls for fine adjustments, thus eliminating foot and hand switches.

ROBOTICS AND TELEMEDICINE

A computerized, robotic surgical assistant may be one of the team members. Computer Motion Corporation has developed a surgical robot, referred to by the mnemonic *AESOP* (Automated Endoscopic System for Optimal Positioning), that holds and moves a laparoscope into optimal position for the surgeon. Hand and foot directors move the computerized machine up to the surgical field. An articulated arm attaches to the side rail of the operating bed, and the positioning of the scope is controlled by voice commands. A computer connected to the robot is equipped with voice-activated software. Each surgeon has his or her own memory card that is inserted into the computer preoperatively. The computer responds only to the voice of the surgeon. Clear, concise directions are spoken into a headset worn under the surgeon's face mask. The articulated arm is draped with a sterile sleeve and moves into precise positions as verbally directed by the surgeon. More information about robotics in the OR is available at **www.computermotion.com.**

Other robotic systems include a central base platform wherein the surgeon verbally controls other computer-generated information during the surgical procedure. HERMES is a system by which all equipment in the OR is voice controlled by the surgeon. The surgeon can address the system and request the computed tomography (CT) scan to appear on the computer monitor. Real-time verbal and video documentation is recorded for the permanent record. The operative report is generated by electronic media, and a hard copy is printed simultaneously.

The ultimate surgical robotics example include the use of ZEUS, which is a totally hands-free system wherein the surgeon sits at a console to verbally command multiple robotic arms while observing their actions on a video screen. The system is voice activated and may be controlled by a surgeon who is many miles away.

Research is being done to develop virtual reality training for surgeons and operators of complex technologic equipment. Virtual reality is the computer science of simulating real-life motion, time, and space. Computer-generated images mimic real-life situations. The surgeon-in-training practices a procedure without touching a real patient. The surgeon dons a specialized headset/visor and sensor gloves and selects the training scenario to be practiced. The computer displays a video graphic of human anatomy in the headset/visor. The sensor gloves signal motion, direction, and pressure to a computer and in turn create a sensation of touch for the surgeon. The entire activity looks, feels, and responds as if the surgeon were performing surgery on an actual patient. This investigative technology can allow for "practice surgery" while evaluating the skill and dexterity of the surgeon.

The possibilities for integrating advanced technologies to simplify surgery and make it less painful and safer for patients seem endless as surgeons develop and refine innovative techniques. The challenges for all members of the OR team are to learn about technologic advances and to monitor the quality of patient care in their application. Engineering performance (i.e., clinical application of biotechnology) is measured by reliability, safety, maintenance, and effectiveness of equipment. Clinical performance is measured by the skills of users to achieve desired results—a successful outcome for the patient.

Bibliography

Ball KA: *Lasers: the perioperative challenge,* ed 2, St Louis, 1995, Mosby.

Ball KA: *Endoscopic surgery,* St Louis, 1997, Mosby.

Chin AK et al: Gasless laparoscopy using a planar lift device, *J Am Coll Surg* 178(4):401-403, 1994.

Conner R: Clinical issues: sterilizing endoscopes; spore testing; clinical attire; identifying operative limbs; combining OR/ICU lounges, *AORN J* 68(2):288-290, 1998.

Dunlap KD, Wanzer L: Is the robotic arm a cost-effective surgical tool? *AORN J* 68(2):265-266, 268-272, 1998.

Eckberg E: The future of robotics can be ours, *AORN J* 67(5):1018, 1020-1023, 1998.

Harrel GJ, Kopps DR: Minimizing patient risk during laparoscopic electro-surgery, *AORN J* 67(6):1194, 1196, 1199-1202, 1204-1205, 1998.

Hutchinson BA et al: Electrosurgical surgery, *AORN J* 68(5):830, 832-837, 1998.

Martin MA, Reichelderfer M: APIC guideline for infection prevention and control in flexible endoscopy, *Am J Infect Control* 22(2):19-38, 1994.

Mathias JM: Minimally invasive surgery: innovative devices expanding lap-aroscopy; telepresence lets surgeons operate from remote site, *OR Manager* 10(6):9-11, 1994.

Mathias JM: Robotic assistant for laparoscopic surgery, *OR Manager* 10(1):1, 9-10, 1994.

Mathias JM: The future of surgery: ahead . . . robots, digital surgeons, and virtual reality, *OR Manager* 11(1):1, 6-7, 9, 1995.

Steuer K: Pneumoperitoneum: physiology and nursing interventions, *AORN J* 68(3):412, 414-425, 1998.

Tsoi EK et al: Laparoscopic surgery without pneumoperitoneum, *Surg Endosc* 8(5):382-383, 1994.

Tucker RD, Voyles CR: Laparoscopic electrosurgical complications and their prevention, *AORN J* 62(1):51, 53, 55, 58-59, 61, 63-66, 68, 70-71, 1995.

Vanderhooft SL et al: Flashlamp-pumped pulsed dye laser treatment of vas-cular birthmarks, *AORN J* 67(6):1214-1220, 1222-1223, 1998.

Section
VII

Preoperative Patient Care

Chapter 21

Preoperative Preparation of the Patient

 Chapter Objectives

After studying this chapter, the learner will be able to:

- Discuss the importance of preoperative preparation.
- Describe the content of preoperative patient teaching.
- List several preoperative assessment factors relevant to all presurgical patients.
- Identify the key elements in a successful presurgical interview.

Regardless of the physical setting in which an invasive or surgical procedure will be performed, each patient should be adequately assessed and prepared so that the impact and potential risks of the surgical intervention are minimized. This involves both physical and emotional preparation. Perioperative caregivers should establish a baseline for the patient's preoperative condition so that changes that occur during the perioperative/perianesthesia care period can be easily recognized. Terms associated with preoperative patient care are defined in Box 21-1.

HISTORICAL BACKGROUND

For centuries before the proliferation of operating rooms (ORs) in hospitals, surgical procedures were performed on battlefields, in barber chairs, and on kitchen tables. Hospitals focused on the care of the poor, crippled, chronically ill, and insane until the eighteenth and nineteenth centuries. Even then, and on into the early twentieth century, many surgeons operated in their offices and in the homes of their patients.

Nurses were dispatched to the homes to prepare a suitable room and to prepare the patient for the surgeon.

From the late nineteenth century, the achievements in surgery as a medical discipline can be attributed to an increase in the understanding of physiology, the introduction of safe anesthetics and methods of blood transfusion, the development of antimicrobials, and the management of the patient before, during, and after invasive procedures. As surgeons moved into the OR arenas of hospitals, nurses became responsible for physically preparing patients for surgical procedures. In the early 1900s, patients were admitted 4 or 5 days before the procedure; by the late 1930s, this time was reduced to 24 hours or less.

From around 1920, nursing leaders advocated the importance of both the physiologic and the psychologic preparation of surgical patients. The individual needs of patients were recognized but were not emphasized in nursing education until the 1940s. During the 1950s, patient teaching became a limited part of preoperative preparation as surgeons recognized the value of early ambulation. It was not until the 1960s and 1970s that nursing research studies validated a link between preoperative preparation and postoperative recovery. The risk of postoperative physiologic complications can be reduced by teaching deep breathing, coughing, and leg exercises and by preparing the patient for early ambulation. Attention to the patient's preoperative psychosocial and spiritual needs also has important consequences for the management of postoperative pain and the promotion of desired outcomes. Studies showed that patients who received structured preoperative teaching had a smoother postoperative recovery. During these decades OR nurses were encouraged to visit patients preoperatively and prepare them psychologically for the surgical experience by helping to alleviate their fears and anxieties and by teaching appropriate postoperative behaviors. This visit could take place at the bedside the day before the scheduled procedure.

In 1983, amendments to the Social Security Act established a prospective hospital reimbursement system for Medicare patients. This system is based on diagnosis-related groups (DRGs), which have changed the time and place of the preoperative preparation of most surgical patients who require postoperative hospital support services. It has also stimulated the development of ambulatory surgery (i.e., minimally invasive procedures). The number of surgical procedures performed in ambulatory care facilities and on patients admitted to the hospital the same day of surgery increases annually.

HOSPITALIZED PATIENT

Although most patients undergoing a surgical procedure are admitted the day of surgery, some are admitted to the hospital one or more days before the scheduled procedure. The acuity of illness or the patient's general health status, as well as the surgical procedure to be performed, will influence whether the patient should be admitted to the hospital preoperatively or can arrive on the day of the procedure. Radiologic, endoscopic, or other diagnostic studies may be performed to confirm the medical diagnosis. Systemic disease or chronic illness, such as diabetes or heart disease, should be under control to the extent possible preoperatively.

Most patients who will remain in the hospital postoperatively are admitted the day of the surgical procedure. Often referred to as "AM admissions, TCI (to come in), or TBA (to be admitted)," these patients may be prepared for the procedure in a same-day admission unit before transferring to the OR suite. (Some facilities have a preoperative check-in area within the OR suite.) From the OR, some patients may go to the postanesthesia care unit (PACU) to recover from anesthesia before being transferred to a patient care unit; others are transferred directly from the OR to the intensive care unit (ICU). The magnitude of the surgical procedure and the patient's postoperative needs for complex care will determine when the patient can be discharged safely to home.

PREOPERATIVE PREPARATION OF ALL PATIENTS

Specific activities such as the preoperative history and physical are completed and documented before the patient arrives in the OR. This process can be performed before admission to the hospital or ambulatory care facility; other activities are performed when the patient arrives. The preoperative physical preparation is designed to help all patients overcome the stresses of anesthesia, pain, fluid and blood loss, immobilization, and tissue trauma. Preparation often begins before the patient's hospital admission with the institution of nutritional or drug therapy. An attempt is made to bring all patients to their best possible physical status before surgery. Appropriate consultations, such as a cardiac workup, are sought when necessary.

Preadmission Procedures

Some of the preoperative preparations can be performed in the surgeon's office. Patients are then referred to the preoperative testing center of the hospital or ambulatory care facility. Tests and records should be completed and available before the patient is admitted the day of the surgical procedure. Preadmission tests (PATs) are scheduled according to the guidelines of each facility. Some tests are acceptable only for a 30-day period or are repeated before admission. The preoperative preparations include the following:

1. *Medical history and physical examination.* These are performed and documented by a physician.
2. *Laboratory tests.* Testing should be based on specific clinical indicators or risk factors that could affect surgical management or anesthesia. Tests include age, sex, preexisting disease, magnitude of surgical procedure, and type of anesthesia. Ideally, these tests should be completed 24 hours before admission so the results are available for review. Some facilities perform laboratory studies the morning of the procedure.
   a. Hemoglobin, hematocrit, blood urea nitrogen (BUN), and blood glucose may be routinely tested for persons 60 years of age or older.

b. Hematocrit is usually ordered for women of all ages before the administration of a general anesthetic.

c. Complete blood count, SMA-6, SMA-12, SMA-18, or SMA-20 multichemistry profile may be indicated. (SMA stands for *sequential multichannel autoanalyzer.*) Differential, platelet count, activated partial thromboplastin time, and prothrombin time also may be ordered.

d. Urinalysis may be indicated by the type of surgical procedure, medical history, and/or physical examination.

3. *Blood type and crossmatch.* If a transfusion is anticipated, the patient's blood is typed and crossmatched. Many patients prefer to have their own blood drawn and stored for autotransfusion. Patients should be advised that blood banks charge an additional fee to store and preserve blood for personal use. Even if the patient is to have an autotransfusion, his or her blood should still be typed and crossmatched in the event that additional transfusions are needed. If the patient refuses to accept blood transfusions, the appropriate documentation of refusal should be completed according to the policies and procedures of the facility.

4. *Chest x-ray study.* A preoperative chest x-ray study is not routinely required for all patients. It may be required by facility policy or medically indicated as an adjunct to the clinical evaluation of patients with cardiac or pulmonary disease and for smokers, persons age 60 and older, and cancer patients.

5. *Electrocardiogram.* If the patient has known or suspected cardiac disease, an electrocardiogram (ECG) is mandatory. Depending on the policy of the facility, an ECG may be routine for patients 40 years of age or older.

6. *Diagnostic procedures.* Special diagnostic procedures are performed when specifically indicated (e.g., Doppler studies for vascular surgery).

7. *Written instructions.* The patient should receive written preoperative instructions to follow before admission for the surgical procedure. These instructions should be reviewed with the patient in the surgeon's office or in the preoperative testing center (Figure 21-1).

a. To prevent regurgitation or emesis and aspiration of gastric contents, the patient should not ingest solid foods before the surgical procedure. These instructions are usually stated as "NPO after midnight." (NPO is the Latin abbreviation for *nil per os,* or nothing by mouth.) Solid foods empty from the stomach after changing to a liquid state, which may take up to 12 hours. Clear fluids may be unrestricted until 2 to 3 hours before the surgical procedure but only at the discretion of the surgeon or anesthesia provider in selected patients. NPO time usually is reduced for infants, small children, patients with diabetes, and older adults prone to dehydration.

b. The physician may want the patient to take any essential oral medications that he or she normally takes. These can be taken as prescribed with a minimal fluid intake (a few sips of water) up to 1 hour before the surgical procedure.

c. The skin should be cleansed to prepare the surgical site. Many surgeons want patients to clean the surgical area with an antimicrobial soap preoperatively. Patients who will undergo a surgical procedure on the face, ear, or neck are advised to shampoo their hair before admission, because this may not be permitted for a few weeks after the procedure. Male patients may be requested to have their hair cut short and to shave on the day of the surgical procedure.

d. Nail polish and acrylic nails should be removed to permit observation of and access to the nail bed during the surgical procedure. The nail bed is a vascular area, and the color of the nail bed is one indicator of peripheral oxygenation and circulation. The oxisensor of a pulse oximeter may be attached to the nail bed to monitor oxygen saturation and pulse rate. A finger cuff may be used for continuous blood pressure monitoring. Nail polish or acrylic nails inhibit contact between these devices and the vascular bed. The patient should be advised to uncover at least one fingernail if the anesthesia provider will use these devices for monitoring.

e. Jewelry and valuables should be left at home to ensure safekeeping. If electrosurgery will be used, patients should be informed that all metal jewelry, including wedding bands and religious artifacts, should be removed to prevent possible burns.

f. Patients should be given other special instructions about what is expected, such as when to arrive. A responsible adult should be available to take the patient home if the procedure, medication, or anesthetic medication renders the patient incapable of driving. Family members or significant others should know where to wait and where the patient will be taken after the surgical procedure.

8. *Informed consent.* The physician should obtain informed consent from the patient or legal designee. After explaining the surgical procedure and its risks, benefits, and alternatives, the surgeon should document the process and have the patient sign the consent form. This document becomes part of the permanent record and accompanies the patient to the OR. Policy and state laws dictate the parameters for ascertaining an informed consent.

9. *Nurse interview.* A perioperative/perianesthesia nurse should meet with the patient to make a preoperative assessment. Ideally, an appointment with the perioperative nurse is arranged when the patient comes to the facility for preoperative tests. Through physiologic and psychosocial assessments, the nurse collects

GETBETTER HOSPITAL

PREOPERATIVE INSTRUCTIONS

Your doctor has scheduled your surgery to be performed at Getbetter Hospital on _____ (date) _____ at _____
AM/PM. Please arrive at _____ AM/PM.

If you develop a cold, flu, or illness before surgery or cannot keep your surgery appointment, please call your surgeon.

DIETARY RESTRICTIONS

- Avoid alcoholic beverages and cigarette smoking for at least 24 hours before surgery.
- Finish dinner the evening before surgery no later than 8 PM.
- Nothing to eat or drink after midnight the night before surgery.
  (This includes candy, gum, mints, lifesavers, ice chips, water.)
- Eating or drinking may result in the delay or cancellation of surgery.
- Medications to be taken the day of surgery _____ with sip (1 ounce) of water.
- Medications *not* to be taken the day of surgery _____ .

FOR YOUR SAFETY AND COMFORT

- No makeup—it may cause eye irritation or corneal abrasions while under anesthesia.
- Remove nail polish and artificial nails from at least one finger on each hand—oxygen is measured by placing a sensor on your finger tip.
- Do not bring valuables or jewelry—jewelry must be removed before surgery.
- Dress simply in loose-fitting clothes (sweatsuits are ideal).

UPON YOUR ARRIVAL

- Report to Main Lobby Admissions Desk.

AFTER YOUR SURGERY

- No driving, operating of heavy machinery, heavy physical activity, or decision making for 24 hours after receiving an anesthetic.
- If you are returning home on the same day as your surgery, please make arrangements for a responsible adult to accompany you. Your operation cannot be performed if a responsible adult is not with you.
- Call your surgeon for postoperative appointments.

If you have any questions, please do not hesitate to call the <u>Preadmission Testing Unit</u> at xxx-xxx-xxxx or <u>The Department of Anesthesia</u> at xxx-xxx-xxxx.

Patient signature: _____

RN signature: _____

Figure 21-1 Sample written preoperative instructions for the patient.

data for the nursing diagnoses, expected outcomes, and plan of care. From the assessment data and nursing diagnoses, the nurse establishes expected outcomes with the patient. The nurse develops the plan of care, which becomes a part of the patient's record. The nurse reviews the written preoperative instructions and consent form with the patient to assess the patient's knowledge and understanding. The nurse also provides emotional support and teaches the patient in preparation for postoperative recovery. Before or after the interview, the patient may view a videotape to reinforce information.

10. *Anesthesia assessment.* An anesthesia history and physical assessment are performed before a general or regional anesthetic is administered. The history may be obtained by the surgeon, or the patient may

be asked to complete a questionnaire for the anesthesia provider in the surgeon's office or in the preoperative testing center. An interview by an anesthesia provider or nurse anesthetist may be conducted before admission if the patient has a complex medical history, is high risk, or has a high degree of anxiety. All patients should understand the risks of and alternatives to the type of anesthesia to be administered. After discussion with the anesthesia provider, the patient should sign an anesthesia consent form.

A preoperative phone call by a perioperative nurse to the patient several days in advance of the scheduled surgical procedure may prevent cancellation because of inadequate preoperative testing. Testing requirements are reviewed with the patient, and arrangements for additional tests can be made as needed. The importance of preoperative preparations is reiterated, especially NPO status and the availability of a responsible adult for transportation home after the surgical procedure (if having ambulatory surgery).

Evening Before an Elective Surgical Procedure

In addition to the preadmission procedures previously described, the surgeon may write additional specific orders for other appropriate preoperative preparations. All preadmission assessment and testing procedures may be performed after the patient is admitted to a surgical unit before the surgical procedure. Some patients may require the following:

1. Bowel preparation. "Enemas till clear" may be ordered when it is advantageous to have the bowel and rectum empty (e.g., gastrointestinal procedures such as bowel resection or endoscopy, and surgical procedures in the pelvic, perineal, or perianal areas). An intestinal lavage with an oral solution that induces diarrhea may be ordered to clear the intestine of feces. Solutions such as Golytely or Colyte will normally clear the bowel in 4 to 6 hours. Because potassium is lost during diarrhea, serum potassium levels should be checked before the surgical procedure. Geriatric, underweight, and malnourished patients are prone to other electrolyte disturbances from intestinal lavage.
2. Bedtime sedation for sleep.

Preoperative Visit by the Perioperative/ Perianesthesia Nurse

The patient should be assessed preoperatively. Every effort should be made through supportive measures to minimize the potential hazards of adverse psychosocial distress. Ideally, this assessment takes place before the day of the surgical procedure; its purpose is to alleviate anxiety and fears. Factual information and clarification of misunderstandings will be helpful in this regard, as will the opportunity for the patient to express his or her feelings.

The broadened scope of perioperative nursing encompasses the phases of preoperative and postoperative care that contribute to the continuity of patient care. Preoperative visits to patients are made by registered nurse first assistants or perioperative/perianesthesia nurses skilled in interviewing and assessment. These interviews afford nurses an opportunity to learn about the patients, establish rapport, and develop a plan of care before the patients are brought to the perioperative environment.

Pros of Preoperative Visits

The advantages of preoperative visits with patients include the following:

1. An experienced perioperative/perianesthesia nurse is well qualified to discuss a patient's OR experience. The nurse can orient and prepare the patient and family for the procedure and for the postoperative period.
2. The perioperative/perianesthesia nurse can review critical data before the procedure and assess the patient before planning care.
3. Visits improve and individualize intraoperative care and efficiency and prevent needless delays in the OR.
4. Visits foster a meaningful nurse-patient relationship. Some patients are reluctant to reveal their feelings and needs to someone in a short-term relationship.
5. Visits make intraoperative observations more meaningful by establishing a baseline for the measurement of patient outcomes.
6. Visits contribute to patient cooperation and involvement by facilitating communication. Mutual goals and expected outcomes are more easily developed.
7. Visits enhance the positive self-image of the perioperative nurse and contribute to job satisfaction, which in turn reduces job turnover and is thus a benefit to the hospital. Because of increased patient contact, visits make perioperative and perianesthesia nursing more attractive to those who enjoy patient proximity and teaching.

Cons of Preoperative Visits

The disadvantages associated with preoperative visits include the following:

1. Cost-containment measures may not provide adequate staffing or allow time to visit patients.
2. The admission of patients on the day of the surgical procedure or late the day before the procedure makes the timing of visits difficult.
3. Visits may produce friction among different team factions if the program is not well planned and executed.
4. Repetitious interviewing may lead to a stereotyped manner and a lack of enthusiasm and spontaneity on the part of nurse interviewers.
5. If the nurse's interviewing skills are not practiced, patients may feel their privacy is being invaded.

6. Barriers to visits may arise from the nurse's inability to:
   a. Verbalize and communicate effectively.
   b. Handle or accept a patient's illness.
   c. Handle emotionally stressed persons.
   d. Understand cultural, ethnic, and value system differences.
   e. Function efficiently outside of his or her customary environment.
   f. Recognize how personal beliefs and biases can influence objectivity.

Interviewing Skills

Interviewing is a form of verbal interaction and is a valuable tool for obtaining information. The interview can be directive and structured with predetermined questions in a specific, predetermined order that limits responses. An example of a directive question is, "Have you had a surgical procedure before?" A nondirective interview gives the patient more of an opportunity to respond in an open manner. An example of a nondirective question is, "Tell me about your previous surgical experience." The choice of technique depends on the information desired.

A structured interview is valuable in learning about an individual's health history. The unstructured interview gives a portrait of the patient's emotional reactions, concerns, and personality. An effective preoperative interview usually includes questions about both facts and feelings. The informal observation of nonverbal behavior is an essential component of the interview. The setting should be conducive to communication, and all questions should be relevant. The interviewer should be able to handle the situation with spontaneity, judgment, and tact. The interview should be meaningful to both the patient and the nurse.

Structured Preoperative Visits

1. Review the patient's chart and records. Focus on medical and nursing diagnoses and the surgical procedure to be performed. Collect any information relevant to planning care in the OR. If the patient is admitted to the hospital, discuss the assessment data and the plan of care with the unit nurses before visiting the patient. Nursing data include the following pertinent information; these baseline parameters are essential for accurate intraoperative and postoperative assessment:
   a. Biographic information: name, age, sex, family status, ethnic background, educational level, patterns of living, previous hospitalization and surgical procedures, religion.
   b. Physical findings: vital signs; height; weight; skin integrity; allergies; the presence of pain, drainage, or bleeding; state of consciousness and orientation; sensory or physical deficits; and assistive aids or prosthetics.
   c. Special therapy: tracheostomy, inhalation therapy, hyperalimentation.
   d. Emotional status: understanding, expectations, specific problems concerning comfort, safety, language barrier, and other concerns.

2. Choose an optimal time and place without interruptions.
   a. Patients who will be admitted on the day of the surgical procedure may be interviewed in the preoperative testing center several days before the surgical procedure. If this is not feasible, a telephone call to the patient may provide an alternative means of contact.
   b. Patients who have been admitted to the hospital may be visited on a patient care unit the day before the surgical procedure. The best time to visit a patient is early evening—after dinner and before visiting hours.
   c. Allow adequate time for the interview, usually 10 to 20 minutes unless the patient has complex problems or special needs that require more time. Give the patient time to think and respond and to ask questions.
   d. If the patient is in acute physical or psychologic distress, offer support and consider rescheduling the visit. The visit may need to be canceled or conducted through a family member or significant other. An emergency surgical patient may be assessed in the preoperative holding area.
   e. Do not conduct the interview on the morning of the procedure! Patients are not psychologically receptive to preoperative teaching at this time. Premedicated patients may be susceptible to suggestions such as, "You will have minimal discomfort after the surgical procedure."

3. Greet the patient by introducing yourself and explaining the purpose of the visit. Tell the patient that the visit is a routine part of care so the patient does not feel singled out because of his or her medical diagnosis. Unless specifically requested to use a first name, demonstrate respect at all times by addressing the patient by his or her last name. Terms like "honey," "dear," or "sweetheart" are unacceptable. Children are usually addressed by their given first name unless the family uses a nickname.
   a. Put the patient at ease. Sit close so the patient can easily see and hear you.
   b. Secure the patient's attention and cooperation. Establish eye contact.
   c. Speak first with the patient alone (unless the patient is a small child, an individual who needs an interpreter, or an individual who is mentally impaired). This affords the patient privacy so he or she may feel free to talk. Then, if the patient is willing, the family may be invited to participate and ask questions. The family should be present during the preoperative teaching to learn how to assist the patient postoperatively.
   d. Allow the patient to maintain self-respect and dignity.
   e. Instill confidence in the patient by having a neat appearance and a positive attitude. Establish rapport by demonstrating warmth and genuine interest. Avoid displaying an authoritative manner.

f. Use language at the patient's level of development, understanding, and education.

4. Obtain information by asking about the patient's understanding of the surgical procedure.

a. Assess the patient's level of information and understanding and check its accuracy to determine whether further instruction or clarification is needed. Ask questions such as, "What has your surgeon told you about the surgical procedure?" Correct any misconceptions about the surgical procedure as appropriate within the scope of nursing.

b. Permit the patient to talk openly. The objective is to gather data that will generate the plan of care to be implemented by the perioperative team.

c. Direct questions should be used with caution and are not suitable for collecting all objective data. Construct open-ended questions to elicit information more detailed than one-word answers.

d. Listen attentively. To preserve self-esteem, the patient may tell you what he or she thinks you want to hear. A patient's statement that ends in a question may be either a request for more information or an expression of a feeling or attitude.

5. Orient the patient to the environment of the OR suite and interpret policies and routines.

a. Tell the patient the scheduled time of the surgical procedure, the approximate length of the procedure, and the probable length of stay in the PACU. Explain the procedures that will be performed in the preoperative holding area before the surgery, if this is the routine.

b. Ask the patient if family members or friends will be at the facility during the surgical procedure. They should be informed how early to be there to see the patient before sedation is given. Tell the patient and family where the waiting room is located.

c. Tell the patient that the family will be updated on the progress of the surgical procedure and informed when he or she arrives in the PACU, if this is hospital policy. Communicating the progress of the procedure, especially if it is prolonged, provides emotional support and decreases the family's anxiety.

6. Review the preoperative preparations that the patient will experience.

a. Familiarize the patient with who and what will be seen in the perioperative environment. Many perioperative nurses wear OR attire and laboratory coats with name tags when they visit patients, which familiarizes patients with the way they will see personnel the next day. Attire should be changed if the nurse reenters the OR suite after the visit.

b. Use discretion regarding how much the patient should know and wants to know. Use words that do not evoke an anxiety-inducing state of mind. Do not use words with unpleasant associations, such as knife, needle, or nausea.

c. Postoperative recovery begins with preoperative teaching, but keep the explanations short and simple. Excessive detail can increase patient anxiety, which reduces the attention span.

d. Give practical information about what the patient should expect, such as withholding fluids, drowsiness, and/or dry mouth caused by preoperative medications; transportation to the OR and the holding area; and where he or she will be taken after the surgical procedure. Instruct the patient not to hesitate to ask for assistance at any time. Explain any other relevant special precautions.

e. Give the basic reasons for procedures and regulations; this reduces patient anxiety. With children and older adults, the nurse may have to repeat information as a reinforcement.

f. Explain only the procedures of which the patient will be aware.

g. If patient will be going to the ICU after the procedure, tell the family what they will see there, such as monitors and machines.

7. Tell the patient that an anesthesia provider will visit to discuss specific questions relative to anesthesia, if this is routine.

8. Answer the patient's questions about the surgical procedure in general terms. Refer specific questions to the surgeon.

a. Be honest and responsible in communications about a proposed diagnostic or surgical procedure. Complement, but do not overlap, the surgeon's area of responsibility. Do not be unrealistic, falsify the truth, or give false reassurances to the patient or family.

b. Be extremely cautious about spelling out specific details of the treatment, procedure, and postoperative care unless you have been thoroughly briefed by the surgeon in charge. Surgeons individualize and tailor their plan of care to their own techniques and to the patient's needs, and certain forms of therapy may be controversial. Continual interdisciplinary communication is essential.

c. If unable or unprepared to answer a legitimate question, tell the patient that the concern will be answered by the appropriate personnel. For example, say, "I don't know, but I'll get that information for you." Then be certain to follow up with an answer.

9. Encourage the patient and family to discuss their feelings or anxieties regarding the surgical procedure and anticipated results.

a. Motivate and assist the patient and family to gain perspective, objectivity, awareness, and insight. A skilled professional nurse will know how to discourage wishful thinking for miraculous cures while communicating an understanding of their fears and wishes for an uncomplicated, fast recovery.

b. Observe emotional reactions.

c. As an interviewer, be objective about personal feelings. Listen to what the patient is asking without feeling threatened. Do not superimpose personal feelings onto what the patient is actually expressing. Empathy is appropriate in this environment.

d. Acknowledge the impact of the procedure on the patient's sexuality, if appropriate. Allow the patient to express personal feelings without evoking shame or guilt. Include the family or significant other as the patient desires.

e. Try to help the patient solve his or her own problems when possible. Ask open-ended questions that help explore a subject or feelings, but do not probe to elicit specific responses. Do not destroy the patient's coping mechanism; encourage an appropriate one. The visit is not a structured psychiatric counseling session.

f. Listen to the anxieties of the patient, family, or significant other in a realistic time frame, and get others to follow through as necessary. Do not attempt too full an agenda, but sort out what is legitimate. You cannot solve all problems in 20 minutes. For example, say, "I'll share this information with someone who can help you with this problem." Use a colleague's expertise to assist you or to make a proper referral.

g. Comfort the patient, and convey a sense of security and trust. Use touch as appropriate. Touch has a positive effect on physiologic parameters, such as respiration and circulation, and it can lower heart rate and blood pressure. Its calming effect can improve perceptual and cognitive abilities. It establishes rapport, provides reassurance, and conveys warmth, empathy, encouragement, and support. Touch should be comfortable. A perceptive nurse can tell when a patient resents being touched; respect the patient's feelings. Patients with decreased visual acuity appreciate the assurance that touch can give, but always speak first to avoid startling the patient.

h. Reassure the patient that he or she will not be alone but will be constantly attended by competent perioperative team members. Try to increase the patient's trust and confidence in the team as a whole.

i. Allow time to deal with the patient's questions or concerns. Ask the patient, "Do you have any other concerns?" Never bring a patient's feelings into the open and then cut off the conversation. Do not interrupt, interrogate, or belittle an expressed fear or seemingly irrelevant topic. All questions are significant to the patient. Answer the questions honestly and try to resolve concerns.

10. Identify any special needs of the patient that will alter the plan for intraoperative care. The preoperative visit is the time for a total assessment to guard against a traumatic experience for the patient.

a. Observe any physical characteristics of the patient that might affect positioning or require special setups.

The plan of care will include considerations for extra tall, obese, or left-handed patients. For example, an intravenous (IV) infusion should be started in the right arm of a left-handed person to minimize the limitation of manual dexterity.

b. Observe the patient for physical limitations such as pain on moving, an amputated extremity, paralysis, or sensory loss. This information enables the circulator to anticipate how much cooperation to expect from the patient and how much additional help may be needed. A pad of paper and pencil may be needed to communicate with a patient who is unable to speak or hear. In certain instances, an interpreter may be needed.

c. Ask the patient whether he or she wears any type of prosthetic device. Explain, per accepted hospital policy, that the device should be removed before the surgical procedure either at the bedside or in the OR. Explain that jewelry should be removed.

d. Determine how a preexisting medical condition should be managed in the OR. For example, it is important that the circulator know about the presence of an implanted pacemaker. Monopolar electrosurgery could cause certain models to malfunction and would therefore be contraindicated.

e. Know the patient's special requests.

11. Offer the patient reassurance when possible, and maintain an attitude of hope. Avoid using phrases such as, "Everything will be all right," or "You are okay." Reinforce the concept that the team will provide good care.

a. Help both yourself and the patient turn negative feelings into positive, useful responses.

b. Offer realistic hope, but do not minimize the seriousness of the surgical procedure.

12. Use audiovisual materials to supplement the interview, if available and appropriate.

a. Written instructions with photographs or drawings are useful for explaining procedures and equipment. These can be presented in a booklet or pamphlet that the patient can keep and share with family members or significant others.

b. Videotapes, slide/tape programs, or films help to reinforce the preoperative teaching.

Preoperative Teaching

Teaching is a function of nursing practice and embraces perception, thought, feeling, and performance. During the preoperative visit, the perioperative nurse supplements the instructions of the other perioperative team members and gives information unique to the patient's specific surgical procedure. The perioperative nurse teaches patients how to participate in their own postoperative recovery. Patients must have a readiness to learn. Preoperative teaching should take place at three levels:

1. *Information.* Explanations of procedures, patient care activities, and physical feelings that the patient may

encounter during the perioperative experience help the patient identify what is happening and what to expect. Such explanations also enhance patient satisfaction with care.

2. *Psychosocial support.* Interactions enhance coping mechanisms to deal with anxiety and fears and provide emotional comfort.

3. *Skill training.* Guided practice of specific tasks to be performed by the patient in the postoperative period can decrease anxiety, hasten recovery, and help to prevent complications.

Effective Teaching Patient teaching involves emotional energy on the part of the nurse. It can produce behavioral changes in patients as they become better prepared, both physically and emotionally, for the surgical procedure. They also learn how to use the health care system. Learning self-help has a positive effect. Discharge planning begins during preoperative teaching. The patient knows what to expect and where to go for help after discharge if needed, such as a support group.

Patient teaching may be conducted in an informal, individual manner or in a formal, group instructional setting. In conjunction with other team members, the nurse-instructor should first formulate attainable learning objectives with the patient's input. The development of learning objectives is based on the assessed level of the patient's emotional receptivity and mental capacity. The nurse also assesses, by observation and elicited response, factors such as the patient's developmental level, sight, hearing, and acceptance of his or her problem. Before beginning an explanation, the nurse should verify what the patient already knows, needs to know, and wants to know. An understanding relationship with the patient facilitates the teaching-learning experience.

The nurse must assist family members to cope with the situation to the extent of their ability. The success or failure of treatment often depends on what happens after the patient leaves the hospital. The family's knowledge and understanding of the patient's needs, their coping skills, and their willingness to help are important factors in recovery. Teaching should be presented at the family members' level of particular resources and knowledge base. Other points to consider include the following:

1. Arrange the environment so that a teaching-learning exchange may take place; a quiet, undisturbed environment and proper timing are important.

2. Language is the fundamental tool for education. Use understandable terms. Do not equate intelligence level with educational level. The nurse is accountable for what is taught.

3. Set priorities and teach what is significant and appropriate to the patient's particular needs.
   a. Break down instructions into manageable steps; for example, instruct the patient to deep breathe and then cough while he or she splints the site of the surgical incision with a pillow.

   b. Put content into a logical sequence of activities to facilitate learning. For example, to avoid the possibility of an inappropriate dosage, instruct the patient to write down the time he or she takes the medication when at home.

   c. Give the reasons for and the benefits of specific activities. For example, the movement of legs and toes and ambulation postoperatively, unless contraindicated, aids circulation and prevents venous stasis.

   d. Adapt the teaching method and timing to the specific situation. The patient may reject teaching not relevant to the immediate present. For example, a patient about to have a heart valve replacement procedure may listen to instructions but may actually be concentrating on the fact that his or her heart is going to be cut open.

   e. Do not overburden the patient with a multitude of facts.

4. Recognize the patient's need to know. This recognition, not pressure, should be the motivating factor in learning.

5. To evaluate understanding, ask the patient to repeat in his or her own words what has been explained during the instructional session and to demonstrate deep breathing and leg exercises.

6. Written information is helpful in reviewing verbal instruction. Go over the material with the patient, and test his or her comprehension by asking questions. A patient who is experiencing pain or anxiety or who is under the influence of medication may not fully understand verbal communication.

7. As the resource person, be consistent, concise, and organized. Repeat instructions to help the patient retain them.

Patients who receive preoperative instructions from and interact with the perioperative nurse may experience less apprehension, better tolerate the surgical procedure, and seem more secure and comfortable postoperatively. Patients usually remember what has been taught. They react more positively to their perioperative experience than patients who have not been given the benefit of this interaction.

At the end of the preoperative assessment and teaching session, the perioperative nurse should not depart from the patient abruptly but should briefly summarize the events that have taken place. The patient should be left with the understanding that a postoperative visit may be made after the procedure, if this is the policy.

Preoperative Visit by the Anesthesia Provider

The anesthesia provider is knowledgeable in the pathophysiology of disease as it pertains to anesthetic agents. Participation in the patient's preoperative preparation can reduce intraoperative complications. If the patient has been admitted, the anesthesia provider usually assesses a patient scheduled for anesthesia the evening before the surgical procedure. Otherwise the patient may be seen before admission in the preoperative testing center, in the same-day procedures unit, or in the preoperative holding area. All patients should be evaluated before the anesthetic is administered.

Judgment and skill are important in the selection of agents and in the administration of anesthesia, but firsthand knowledge of the patient is extremely valuable. The anesthesia provider visits the patient to seek information and to establish rapport, inspire confidence and trust, and alleviate fear. Preparation for anesthesia begins with this visit.

Before meeting the patient, the anesthesia provider reviews the patient's past and present medical records. If recent laboratory or other test reports are not in the chart, all decisions and the surgical procedure are delayed until all essential information is available. Special attention is given to past surgical procedures and any disease or complicating processes, especially those involving vital organs.

After introducing himself or herself to the patient, the anesthesia provider does the following:

1. Obtains a history pertinent to the administration of anesthetic agents by questioning the patient about past anesthetic experiences, allergies, adverse reactions to drugs, and habitual drug usage. Tranquilizers, cortisone, reserpine, alcohol, and recreational drugs, for example, influence the course of anesthesia. Smoking habits, genetic and metabolic problems, and reactions to previous blood transfusions also influence the choice of anesthetic.
2. Evaluates the patient's physical, mental, and emotional status to determine the most appropriate type and amount of anesthetic agent(s).
   a. Examines the patient as necessary to obtain the information desired, with particular interest in the heart and lungs.
   b. Palpates the needle insertion site and observes for skin infection if a regional block anesthesia is contemplated.
   c. Assesses the patient's mental state and cognitive ability subjectively and observes for signs of anxiety.
3. Investigates the patient's cardiac reserve and observes for signs of dyspnea or claudication during a short exercise tolerance test, if indicated.
4. Asks about teeth. If indicated, explains that dental work may be damaged inadvertently during airway insertion.
5. Evaluates the patient's physique for possible technical difficulties in the administration of the anesthetic.
   a. A short, stout neck may cause respiratory problems or difficult intubation. A stiff neck or unstable cervical spine such as from rheumatoid arthritis can make intubation difficult or dangerous, especially in a geriatric patient. Fiberoptic laryngoscope and/or awake intubation may be necessary.

   b. Active athletic persons and obese persons require more anesthetic than inactive persons.
   c. The patient's accurate weight should be known, because the dosage of many medications is calculated from body weight. Most dosages are calculated in milligrams per kilogram.
6. Explains his or her preference of anesthetic, pending the surgeon's approval, and informs the patient what to expect concerning anesthesia. The patient's wishes are taken into consideration, if expressed.
7. Tells the patient or asks about restricted or prohibited oral intake before anesthesia and gives the reasons for these restrictions. IV therapy is explained.
8. Discusses preoperative sedation in relation to the time the surgical procedure is scheduled to begin.
9. Reassures the patient that constant observation will be maintained during the surgical procedure and in the immediate postoperative period. The methods of monitoring vital functions are also explained.
10. Explains the risks of anesthesia without causing the patient undue stress.
11. Answers the patient's questions and allays his or her fears related to anesthesia.

Following this visit with the patient, the anesthesia provider does the following:

1. Estimates the effect of the necessary positioning during the surgical procedure on the patient's physiologic processes.
2. Records preliminary data on the anesthesia chart.
3. Writes preanesthesia orders, including times for medication administration.
4. Writes a summary of the visit and the proposed anesthetic management of the patient on the physicians' progress note. This summary has medicolegal value if a problem subsequently develops, and it is also necessary for regulatory accreditation, such as for the state or the Joint Commission on Accreditation of Healthcare Organizations (JCAHO).
5. Assigns the patient a physical status classification for the purpose of anesthesia, as per the taxonomy adopted by the American Society of Anesthesiologists (ASA):
   a. Class I theoretically includes relatively healthy patients with localized pathologic processes. An emergency surgical procedure, designated E, signifies additional risk. For example, a hernia that becomes incarcerated changes the patient's status to Class I-E.
   b. Class II includes patients with mild systemic disease (e.g., diabetes mellitus controlled by oral hypoglycemic agents or diet).
   c. Class III includes patients with severe systemic disease that limits activity but is not totally incapacitating (e.g., chronic obstructive pulmonary disease or severe hypertension).

d. Class IV includes patients with an incapacitating disease that is a constant threat to life (e.g., cardiovascular and renal diseases).

e. Class V includes moribund patients who are not expected to survive 24 hours with or without the surgical procedure. They are operated on in an attempt to save their life; the surgical procedure is a resuscitative measure, as in a massive pulmonary embolus. The patient may or may not survive the surgical procedure.

f. Class VI includes patients who have been declared brain dead but whose organs will be removed for donor purposes. Mechanical ventilation and life support systems are maintained until the organs are procured.

6. Consults with the surgeon and other physicians (e.g, a cardiologist) about a patient who has been assigned a Class III, IV, or V status. Consideration is given to the critical nature of the surgical procedure in relation to the risks of anesthesia.

a. In elective situations the surgical procedure is postponed until anesthesia will be less hazardous (e.g., following acute respiratory infection or cardiac decompensation).

b. In emergency situations, ideal practices may be altered or disregarded to meet the exigencies of the situation. For example, if a patient is hemorrhaging, there is no time to wait to restore a low red blood count. A multiple trauma victim with a full stomach may need a nasogastric tube inserted and suction applied, an endotracheal intubation while awake, or spinal anesthesia as applicable, and he or she may undergo a surgical procedure despite food ingestion.

In addition to the preoperative assessment of the patient and the administration and maintenance of the intraoperative anesthetic, the anesthesia provider may see the patient postoperatively. He or she has a responsibility to inform the patient of any unfavorable reaction to a medication or agent so that the patient is forewarned and can report these reactions to other physicians and anesthesia providers.

Before Leaving for the Operating Room

Before the patient goes to the OR suite, his or her physical and emotional status and vital signs should be assessed and recorded by the nurse on the surgical unit or in the same-day admission unit. Any untoward symptoms or extreme apprehension are reported to the surgeon because they could affect the patient's intraoperative course. The following preparations are made:

1. The patient puts on a clean hospital gown.
2. Jewelry is removed for safekeeping. If a wedding ring cannot be removed, it is taped loosely or tied securely

to prevent loss. The patient may be permitted to keep a religious symbol, but the patient must understand this may be removed before anesthesia is induced.

3. Unless otherwise ordered, dentures and removable bridges are removed before the administration of general anesthesia to safeguard them and to prevent them from obstructing respiration. Dentures may be permitted during local anesthesia, especially if the patient can breathe more easily with them in place. Some anesthesia providers prefer that securely fitting dentures be left in place to facilitate airway insertion. Dentures are necessary to retain facial contours for some plastic surgery procedures.

4. All removable prostheses (e.g., eye, extremity, contact lenses, hearing aids, and eyeglasses) are removed for safekeeping. In some instances the patient may be permitted to wear eyeglasses or a hearing aid to the OR. The circulator safeguards them and sends them to the PACU with the patient. Contact lenses are removed before the administration of a general anesthetic because they may become dry and cause corneal abrasions.

The patient's personal property is safeguarded to prevent loss or damage. Jewelry and valuables can be given to the family or sent to the hospital safe. The clothing of ambulatory surgery patients can be stored in a locker. The clothing of TCI patients can be sent to the room or unit where the patient will be admitted postoperatively.

5. Long hair may be braided. Wigs should be removed. Hairpins are removed to prevent scalp injury.

6. Antiembolic stockings or elastic bandages may be ordered for the lower extremities to prevent embolic phenomena. The stockings are applied before abdominal or pelvic procedures; for patients who have varicosities, are prone to thrombus formation, or have a history of emboli; and for some geriatric patients. They also are often applied for long procedures.

7. The patient voids to prevent overdistention of the bladder or incontinence during unconsciousness. This is especially important for abdominal or pelvic procedures in which a large bladder may be traumatized or may interfere with adequate exposure of the abdominal contents. The time of voiding is recorded. When indicated, an indwelling Foley catheter is usually inserted in the OR after the patient has been anesthetized.

8. If ordered, an antibiotic is given preoperatively to establish and reach a therapeutic blood level of antibiotic prophylaxis intraoperatively. This may be a one-time dose or may be continued into the postoperative period. If cultures or specimens are obtained during the surgical procedure, a notation should be made on the pathology specimen sheet to indicate antibiotic use.

9. Preanesthesia medications are given as ordered. Their purpose is to eliminate apprehension by making the patient calm, drowsy, and comfortable. Patients who

receive a preanesthesia medication should be cautioned to remain in bed and not to smoke. Many of the drugs cause drowsiness, vertigo, or postural hypotension. Therefore the side rails on the bed should be raised and the call bell placed within the patient's reach.

10. The patient, bed, and chart are accurately identified, and identifications are fastened securely in place. Allergies should be prominently noted on the chart and patient's wristband.

A preoperative checklist helps ensure that the patient has been properly prepared. If preparation is inadequate, the surgical procedure may be canceled. All essential records, including the plan of care, must accompany the patient.

Emotional Preparation

By fulfilling spiritual and psychosocial needs, the caregiver helps to provide the preoperative patient with as much peace of mind as possible. Understandably, the patient's tension level rises as the time for the surgical procedure approaches. The better prepared the patient is emotionally, the smoother his or her postoperative course will be.

If the patient has not seen his or her cleric or the hospital chaplain and makes such a request, the nurse should make every effort to contact that person for the patient.

Family members or significant others should be permitted to stay with the patient until he or she goes to the OR suite. Some hospitals permit parents to accompany infants and children into the OR suite. After leaving the patient, the family should be directed to the waiting area.

TRANSPORTATION TO THE OPERATING ROOM SUITE

Patients may be taken to the OR suite approximately 45 minutes before the scheduled time of the procedure. For safety, they are transported via a transport stretcher. The stretcher should be pushed from the head end so the patient's feet go first. Rapid movements through corridors and around corners may cause dizziness and nausea, especially if the patient has been medicated. The attendant at the head end can observe for vomiting or respiratory distress. The patient may be more comfortable if the head end of the stretcher is raised.

Ideally, certain elevators are designated "for OR use only," which ensures privacy and minimizes microbial contamination. The patient should be comfortable, warm, and safe during transport. Side rails are raised, and restraint straps are applied. The patient should be instructed to keep his or her arms, hands, and fingers inside the side rails during transport to avoid injury when going through doorways. IV solution bags hung on poles during transportation are attached securely and placed at the foot of the bed away from the patient's head; this minimizes the danger of injury to the patient if the container should fall. Gentle handling is indicated to prevent dislodging IV needles or indwelling catheters. A

unit nurse or nursing assistant should stay with the patient until relieved by a perioperative nurse or anesthesia provider, to whom the patient's chart is given. If the patient has a language barrier or is profoundly deaf, an interpreter may accompany him or her to the OR and stay until the induction of anesthesia.

ADMISSION TO THE OPERATING ROOM SUITE
Presurgical Holding Area

Outside personnel bring the patient through the outer corridor to the holding area. OR personnel may transfer the patient to an OR stretcher, where he or she remains until taken to the OR. After the procedure, this stretcher is used to transport the patient first to the PACU and then to the patient care unit. The stretcher is then brought back to a stretcher-cleaning room, where the entire stretcher (including the wheels) is decontaminated before being brought into the OR suite. This procedure is ideal from the standpoint of contamination control.

Some conditions justify bringing patients to the OR suite in their beds. Such conditions include patients in traction, patients on Stryker frames, or cardiac patients who must not be moved until transferred to the operating bed. A patient on a Stryker or similar frame may undergo surgery while on the frame. The surgeon chooses the course that best benefits the individual patient. After the surgical procedure, the bed or frame can be decontaminated in the exchange area and made up with clean linen before being brought into the OR.

Beds, stretchers, and frames are stabilized by personnel and by locking the wheels when a patient moves from one to the other. Mattresses also should be stabilized. Adequate personnel or a mechanical assist device should be available to ensure patient safety during transfer. The patient's head, arms, and legs are protected. The patient should be instructed and assisted to prevent a fall or injury. Once transferred to a stretcher, the patient is under constant surveillance with the restraining straps and side rails securely in place.

Some hospitals have individual rooms for anesthesia induction. The patient waits in this room and is administered an anesthetic before being taken into the OR.

Admission to the Presurgical Holding Area

The holding area nurse greets the patient by name and introduces himself or herself. The nurse stands next to the midsection of the stretcher so the patient can comfortably see him or her. The holding area nurse does the following:

1. Verifies patient identification.
2. Verifies the surgical procedure, site, and surgeon.
3. Reviews the patient's chart for completeness.
   a. Medical history and physical examination.
   b. Laboratory reports.
   c. Consent forms.

4. Measures the vital signs and blood pressure.
5. Verifies allergies and medication history.
6. Checks skin tone and integrity.
7. Verifies physical limitations.
8. Notes the patient's mental state.
9. Puts a cap on the patient to protect his or her hair (in case vomiting occurs), for purposes of asepsis, and to help prevent hypothermia. Patients who are bald are required to wear a head covering to prevent heat loss and dander shed.
10. Puts a clean gown and warm blanket on the patient.

The holding area nurse records pertinent findings in the perioperative patient care record. If a perioperative nursing assessment has not been performed, the holding area nurse must assess the patient's needs, formulate the nursing diagnoses and expected outcomes, and prepare an individualized plan of care. If the patient has been sedated, communication may be difficult.

Preanesthesia Preparations

The anesthesia provider or surgeon may wish to talk with the patient before sedation is given. The patient should be informed about procedures before they are initiated. The following procedures may need to be completed before the induction of anesthesia. Some or all of these procedures can be performed in the preoperative holding area if there are adequate facilities for patient privacy:

1. Removal of body hair, if ordered.
2. Insertion of IV infusion.
3. Insertion of invasive hemodynamic monitoring lines, as appropriate.
4. Insertion of a Foley catheter, if ordered.
5. Administration of the preanesthesia medication and other drugs such as antibiotics, as ordered. The preanesthesia medication can precipitate respiratory depression and hypotension, and the perioperative nurse should be alert and take prompt action if necessary. The holding area should be equipped for cardiopulmonary resuscitation.

The anesthesia provider may perform regional blocks in the holding area. All procedures performed in the holding area are documented on the patient's chart.

Despite the activities around them, patients may feel more alone in a holding area than in any other location. Time passes slowly, and anxiety can increase. An anxious patient looks to the nurse for comfort, reassurance, and attention. A compassionate expression in the eyes and voice and a reassuring touch of the hand can convey concern and understanding to the patient.

If the patient is drowsy, unnecessary conversation should be avoided. The nurse should answer questions and see to the patient's comfort. The patient should be kept warm, or the blanket should be turned down if he or she is too warm. An extra pillow should be placed under the patient's head or under an arthritic knee. Dry lips should be moistened, if appropriate. Any delay or unusual circumstances should be explained.

A quiet, restful atmosphere enables the patient to gain full advantage of the premedication. Some holding areas and ORs have piped-in recorded music, which diverts attention from the many other sounds in the environment. Music with a slow, easy rhythm and a low volume is most conducive to relaxation. Familiar music is more pleasing and relaxing because the patient can associate it with pleasant experiences. Some facilities provide earphones or headsets so patients can listen to the music of their choice. Earphones also muffle extraneous noises and conversations. Ideally, the patient should have a choice in selecting the music or in having no music at all; this is the advantage of individual headsets over piped-in systems.

Transfer to the Operating Room

When everything is ready, the circulator comes to the holding area for the patient. It is advantageous if this person is the perioperative nurse who made the preoperative visit, because the patient will appreciate seeing a familiar face. Before transporting the patient into the OR, the circulator has several important duties to fulfill:

1. Greet and check the identity of the patient, stretcher or bed, and chart.
   a. The circulator should introduce himself or herself if he or she has not previously met the patient. The patient should be addressed as Mr., Mrs., or Miss, not by the first name.
   b. When the patient arrives at the hospital, an identifying wristband is put on in the admitting office. The unit nurse checks the band before the patient leaves for the OR. The circulator compares the information on the wristband, including the identification number, with the information on the chart and with the information on the surgical schedule: name, anticipated surgical procedure, time, and surgeon.
   c. Identification on the stretcher or bed ensures the patient's return to the same stretcher or bed following surgery, if this is the procedure. If the patient is an infant or child, the identification tag on the crib should be out of his or her reach.
   d. Verification of the surgical procedure, site, and surgeon with the patient provides reassurance that this is the correct patient. If the patient is heavily sedated, the surgeon may be asked to identify the patient.
2. Check the side rails, restraining straps, IV infusions, and indwelling catheters.
3. Observe the patient for any reaction to the medication.
4. Observe the patient's anxiety level.
5. Check the history and physical, laboratory tests, x-ray reports, and consent form in the patient's chart.

6. Review the plan of care.
   a. Pay particular attention to allergies and any previous unfavorable reactions to anesthesia or blood transfusions.
   b. Become familiar with this patient's unique and individual needs.

The patient is taken into the OR after the surgeon sees him or her and the anesthesia provider is ready to receive the patient. The main preparations for the procedure should be complete so the circulator can devote undivided attention to the patient.

Before the Induction of Anesthesia

The anesthesia provider also has immediate preanesthesia duties, such as the following:

1. Checking and assembling equipment before the patient enters the room. Airways, endotracheal tubes, laryngoscopes, suction catheters, labeled prefilled medication syringes, and other items are arranged on a cart or table.
2. Reviewing the preoperative physical examination, history, and laboratory reports in the chart.
3. Making certain that the patient is comfortable and secure on the operating bed.
4. Checking for denture removal or any loose teeth. The latter may be secured with thread and taped to the patient's cheek to prevent possible aspiration.
5. Checking to be certain that contact lenses have been removed.
6. Asking patient when he or she last took anything by mouth.
7. Checking the patient's pulse, respiration, and blood pressure to obtain a baseline for the subsequent assessment of vital signs while patient is anesthetized.
8. Listening to the heart and lungs, then connecting ECG monitor leads and attaching the pulse oximeter and other monitoring devices.
9. Starting the IV infusion. This may be done in the holding area or in an induction room. Some patients arrive with an infusion line in place.
10. Preparing for and explaining the induction procedure to patient. If properly premedicated, the patient should be able to respond to simple instructions.

Circulator's Role During Induction

The patient's welfare and individual needs take priority over all other activities before and during the induction of anesthesia. The patient is the most important person in the OR. If the circulator gives more attention to the equipment than to the patient, the patient may feel abandoned. In addition, the equipment is not the best indicator of patient condition. At this time of stress, the patient wants the physical presence of a trusted, competent, and compassionate person.

The patient expects the circulator to be cognizant of his or her problems and conditions and willing to help relieve them. The patient will perceive the circulator's attitude as one of either acceptance or rejection. Consequently, the behavior of the circulator affects the patient in either a positive or a negative way. Positive actions include spending time with and staying close to the patient (distance may be interpreted as disapproval), paying attention to the patient's needs and discomfort, looking directly at the patient when he or she speaks, touching the patient with kindness, and appearing poised, confident, and professional. Negative actions include frowning, ignoring the patient, and failing to respond to the patient's feelings or needs. The way in which something is said and done is as important as what is said and done.

Human beings react through their senses. The positive effect of touch is a helpful nonverbal communication in establishing nurse-patient rapport within a short time. Touch communicates caring. A gentle touch can bridge a language barrier by establishing human contact. Holding a patient's hand warmly or laying a hand on an arm during the induction of anesthesia or a painful procedure can do much to alleviate anxiety and elicit trust.

A smile has been called the universal language. Even though the circulator is wearing a mask, his or her eyes can convey a smile or hope. Likewise, they can reveal anger or hostility. Physiognomy, the ancient Chinese art of discovering qualities of the mind and temperament from the expression of facial features, still has relevance. Facial expressions, eye contact, and body movements have either a positive or a negative effect on the patient. Warmth and caring can be conveyed by a pleasant manner and by the expression of the eyes.

Although routine procedures for care and teaching have been established, each patient deserves personalized care in the face of a disruptive life experience. The circulator should not become insensitive to patients because of depersonalized procedures and routines or his or her own prejudices. The patient must not be treated as inanimate or anonymous or categorized by the disease or surgical procedure. The patient is a living, feeling person, not "Dr. Brown's hysterectomy," "the cardiac in Room 4," "the arthritic I need help to move." Jargon such as this is depersonalizing, demoralizing, offensive, and totally unacceptable. The goal of perioperative patient care is to combine efficiency with caring.

The protection of modesty, dignity, and privacy is essential regardless of whether the patient is conscious or unconscious. Unnecessary exposure should be avoided. The gown and cotton blanket both protect modesty and keep the patient warm. The OR door should be kept closed for privacy; this is also important in terms of aseptic technique. Surgical procedures may be viewed only by authorized persons who have a definite function. All privileged information is kept confidential.

Patients are unnerved by stimuli such as strange odors and disturbing sights. A used but uncleaned operating room, with its soiled linen, instruments, equipment, unconscious patients, and bright lights, can be frightening. Patients feel isolation amidst the hustle and bustle of activity, and a lack of team preparedness increases the patient's stress level. The patient may feel embarrassment from body exposure, and loud noises such as voices, inappropriate conversation, staff disagreements, clattering instruments, and sterilizer noises contribute to the aura of fear perceived by the patient.

Anxiety and preoperative sedation tend to alter the patient's ability to interpret events objectively. The patient may relate everything heard to himself or herself, even though he or she may not actually be the subject of the conversation, and he or she may misinterpret or react unfavorably. Hearing is the last sense lost when becoming unconscious. It is not known at precisely what moment a person can no longer hear and interpret what is said, but it is known that patients remain aware of their environment much longer than their seemingly unconscious state would indicate.

A lack of consideration can destroy the patient's confidence in the team. An overheard thoughtless comment can create a lasting traumatic memory and fear. Negative recall can induce anxiety in similar future experiences. Therefore team members should think before speaking and should not converse near the patient while excluding him or her from the conversation. Sedation does not imply exclusion. The patient may be aware of conversation, even if he or she appears to be asleep! Out of the patient's hearing, conversation should pertain only to the work at hand. The OR is not the place for social discourse.

Time is of the essence to keep anesthesia and procedure time to a minimum, and it is a protective factor to provide as little disturbance to physiologic homeostasis as possible. However, efficiency and safety must not be sacrificed for speed. Safety is the prime concern. The OR suite imposes a high degree of vulnerability on patients and on the entire staff. Patients lack the power to defend and protect themselves during a surgical intervention; therefore the circulators are their advocates and protectors. They provide supportive care and safeguard patients from emotional or physical harm by maintaining constant vigilance. Circulators can minimize the potential hazards in the following manner:

1. Never leave a sedated patient unguarded. In addition to causing mental anguish from a feeling of abandonment, an unattended patient may fall or be injured by equipment.
2. Correctly identify patients, surgical sites, or medications. An incorrect surgical procedure on a patient or an error in medication is usually the result of inadequate identification.
3. Create, maintain, and control an optimally therapeutic environment in the OR. This involves control of the physical environment, such as temperature, humidity,

and personnel. Traffic flow in and out of the room should be kept to a minimum. The more movement and talking, the greater the microbial count in the room. Once the patient is in the OR, it should be kept quiet so the effects of sedation are not counteracted. A tranquil, relaxed atmosphere is conducive to team concentration and orderly functioning so all can go well. The standards of ethical conduct should be strictly enforced.

The impact inherent in any type of surgical intervention can be reconciled when the patient has hope and confidence in the caregivers. Nurses are the central figures in patient care and can do much to relieve fear and provide security. Preoperative preparations can influence the outcome of the surgical procedure.

Bibliography

American Society of PeriAnesthesia Nurses: *Standards of perianesthesia nursing practice,* Thorofare, New Jersey, 1998, The Society.

Badger JM: Calming the anxious patient, *AORN J* 94(5):46-50, 1994.

Brumfield VC et al: Preoperative patient teaching in ambulatory surgery settings, *AORN J* 64(6):941, 943-946, 948, 1996.

Cassidy J, Marley RA: Ambulatory surgery: preoperative assessment of the ambulatory patient, *J Perianesth Nurs* 11(5):334-343, 1996.

Conner R: Clinical issues: sterilizing endoscopes: spore testing, clinical attire, identifying operative limbs, combining OR/ICU lounges, *AORN J* 68(2):288-290, 1998.

Fortner PA: Preoperative patient preparation: psychological and educational aspects, *Semin Perioper Nurs* 7 (1):3-9, 1998.

Grossman D: Enhancing your cultural competence, *Am J Nurs* 94(7):58-62, 1994.

Kiernan M: Minor surgery in general practice: avoiding the pitfalls, *Commun Nurs* 3(10):50-51, 1997.

Lancaster KA: Patient teaching in ambulatory surgery, *Nurs Clin North Am* 32(2):417-427, 1997.

Mathias JM: NPO requirement challenged: clear liquids may be OK, *OR Manager* 10(1):1, 6, 1994.

Mitchell M: Patient's perceptions of preoperative preparation for day surgery, *J Adv Nurs* 26(2):356-363, 1997.

Morrisey J: Obtaining a "reasonably accurate" health history, *Plast Surg Nurs* 14(1):27-30, 1994.

Null SL: Preadmission testing, *AORN J* 59(5):1051-1060, 1994.

Oetker-Black SL, Taunton RL: Evaluation of a self-efficacy scale for preoperative patients, *AORN J* 60(1):43-49, 1994.

Pandit UA, Pandit SK: Ambulatory surgery: fasting before and after ambulatory surgery, *J Perianesth Nurs* 12(3):181-187, 1997.

Salzbach R: Presurgical testing improves patient care, *AORN J* 61(1):210-218, 1995.

Schwanitz LD: Battery of routine preoperative tests no longer recommended, *OR Manager* 10(9):14-19, 1994.

Seley JJ: Patient teaching: 10 strategies for successful patient teaching, *Am J Nurs* 94(11):63-65, 1994.

Voepel-Lewis T, Malviya S: Evaluation of a case management model for preanesthesia screening, *J Perianesth Nurs* 12(6):396-401, 1997.

Zalewski DE: Fine tuning preadmission surgical services, *Nurs Manage* 28(9):49, 51, 1997.

Chapter 22

Diagnostic Procedures

Chapter Objectives

After studying this chapter, the learner will be able to:

• List several invasive diagnostic tests.
• List several noninvasive diagnostic tests.
• List several interventional procedures that incorporate diagnostics.
• Describe several aspects of patient care associated with diagnostic testing.

Diagnosis of a pathologic disease, anomaly, or traumatic injury is established before a surgical procedure is undertaken. Many modalities and techniques help surgeons to assess each individual patient problem, guide them through the surgical procedure, and help them to verify the results of surgical intervention. The term *diagnosis* refers to the art or the act of determining the nature of a patient's disease. Diagnostic procedures can be classified as follows:

• *Noninvasive.* Noninvasive techniques use equipment placed on or near the patient's skin but outside body tissues.
• *Invasive.* Invasive techniques use equipment placed into a body cavity or vessel and/or substances injected into body structures.
• *Interventional.* Interventional techniques involve invasive diagnostics and procedures performed in a specialty department, such as in radiology.

Perioperative nurses and surgical technologists should be familiar with the modalities and equipment necessary to assist with diagnostic procedures in the operating room (OR) and specialty departments. Terms associated with diagnostic testing are defined in Box 22-1.

HISTORICAL BACKGROUND

Early diagnostic testing was surrounded by myths and legends. Most diseases were not detected until they became symptomatic or caused death. Primitive practitioners diagnosed illness as punishment from evil spirits and effected treatment by determining which taboo had been breached. One method of diagnosis included rubbing a small animal over the surface of the body and then dissecting it to observe the configuration of its internal organs.

Hippocrates used a format of history taking and physical examination that consisted of placing an ear on the patient's chest to hear heart and breath sounds. Other tests included smelling and tasting body fluids. Palpation was used for ascertaining body temperature and sampling the pulse. His philosophy was to study the patient, not the disease.

The discovery of the microscope and other tools of diagnosis improved patient outcomes by revealing previously unknown causes of disease and illness. In the sixteenth century Ambroise Paré performed routine autopsies after death to determine the cause of illness. He learned much about anatomy and physiology from studying the dead.

In 1895 German physics professor Wilhelm Conrad Roentgen discovered x-rays. An electromagnetic wave with

Box 22-1 Terms Associated with Diagnostic Testing

biopsy Procedure for obtaining a representative tissue sample for gross and/or microscopic examination. The specimen can be obtained surgically or by other means.

contrast media Use of a substance in the creation of density on a radiographic imaging device; radiopaque dye injected or instilled to outline an organ or a structure. A radiolucent substance, such as air, can help define a hollow space, such as a ventricle of the brain.

interventional radiology Invasive procedures performed under radiologic control. Examples include balloon angioplasty, coronary artery stent placement, and inferior vena cava filter placement.

nuclear medicine study Diagnostic test performed using radioactive substances to image a body part or system.

pathologic examination A series of tests and examinations conducted by a pathologist to determine the cause of changes in the structure or function of a body part or tissue.

percutaneous Directed through the skin and tissues of the external body surface. Diagnostics, treatments, or tissue removal can be performed by direct percutaneous routes.

plethysmography Procedure to determine variations in blood flow between parts.

scintigraphy Recording of the emissions of radiologic substances as they are collected or secreted by tissues and/or organs in body.

smear A sample of tissue cells or fluid aspirated or scraped from a mucous membrane or a potentially pathologic site. The material is stained and studied for cellular components to make a diagnosis.

stereotaxis Computerized localization of a lesion.

tomography Computerized method of imaging a structure in layers.

---

a short wavelength was emitted from a small screen that was placed near a cathode ray tube. He was able to see the bones in his hand. He termed the mysterious ray "X"-ray because "X" always represented an unknown quotient in science. He published his results and did not seek to patent his discovery. Boston was the first city in the United States to boast an x-ray machine for the diagnosis of physical disease. The use of the x-ray was extended to multiple body systems, including active physiology (e.g., the study of blood and urine flow during angiography and voiding cystometrics).

In 1927 Egas Moniz, a Portuguese physician, was the first to perform cerebral angiography. In 1929 in Germany, Werner Forssmann catheterized the right atrium by passing a ureteral catheter into it through a vein in the right arm. He was not successful in his attempt to inject a radiopaque substance through the catheter to visualize the pulmonary vessels. In 1931 Moniz was able to visualize the right chambers of the heart and pulmonary vessels using Forssmann's technique. Poor visualization and unfavorable reactions of patients to the contrast media discouraged pioneers in this procedure. By 1937 Robb and Steinberg had worked out the precursors to the cardiopulmonary visualization techniques as they are used today.

PATIENT CARE CONSIDERATIONS FOR DIAGNOSTIC PROCEDURES

1. Patients should be assessed for their physical condition and any metal implants, pacemakers, infusion pumps, sensitivities, or allergies.
2. Clear instructions should be given verbally and in writing before the test is performed.
3. Preprocedural preparations should be confirmed before the patient begins testing.
4. Explanations of procedures should be given to patients to allay fears and to ensure their understanding of the value of the procedure in making a diagnosis. Before the procedure begins, an explanation should be given of the equipment being used and of the necessity to remain quiet while films are being taken.
5. Sterile and aseptic techniques of invasive procedures are strictly observed.
6. Some surgical procedures are performed with the patient positioned on a fluoroscopic table equipped with an image intensifier for radiographic visualization of anatomic structures as the surgical procedure progresses. Positioning aids should be used as compatible with the machinery.
7. The x-ray tube or C-arm that will extend over the surgical site should be free from dust. It should be damp dusted with a disinfectant solution before the patient arrives and the surgical procedure begins. It may be covered with a sterile drape or sleeve before it is moved over the sterile field.
8. Time, distance, and shielding are the key factors in minimizing radiation exposure. Personnel should stand at least 6 feet (2 m) away from the x-ray beam and/or wear lead aprons or sternal and gonadal shields. Patients should be protected with gonadal shields if possible.
9. A stock of routine supplies should be kept on a portable cart if procedures are done in the radiology department or other interventional area. In general, the following items should be readily available:
   a. Sterile tray for the specific procedure
   b. Skin preparation tray and solutions
   c. Intravenous (IV) administration sets and solutions
   d. Local anesthetic agents, needles, and syringes
   e. Radiopaque contrast material
   f. Sterile gowns, gloves, drapes, and dressings
10. The following emergency equipment should be readily available:
    a. Cardiac resuscitation equipment, including a defibrillator and emergency medications
    b. Oxygen supply, ambu bag, and tubing
11. Patients should be carefully observed and monitored during all procedures for any change in condition. If a procedure is done with the patient under local anesthesia, a qualified registered nurse should monitor the patient's vital signs. A stand-by anesthesia provider should be available to check the patient's physiologic status as needed.

PATHOLOGIC EXAMINATION

Clinical pathology is the use of laboratory methods to establish a clinical diagnosis of a disease by examining tissue and organs. Surgical pathology is the study of alterations in body tissues removed by surgical intervention.

Biopsy

The removal of tissue or fluid for diagnosis is referred to as a biopsy. Biopsy specimens can be obtained by many methods. The pathologist determines and/or confirms the diagnosis by histologic and cytologic analysis (the study of cells).

Smear

Cells and small pieces of tissue are suspended in liquid and smeared on glass microscope slides. The specimen is "fixed" by being sprayed with fixative or immersed in liquid. The fixed slide is then stained and examined under a microscope by the pathologist or specially trained technician. This technique is useful for the examination of fine-needle aspirate or scrapings. Smears can be examined within minutes after they have been obtained from the patient. Instant diagnosis is possible in many cases.

Aspiration Biopsy

Fluid is aspirated through a 22- to 25-gauge needle placed in a lesion, such as a cyst or abscess, or in a joint or body cavity. Fine-needle aspiration biopsies are most commonly done to obtain cells from solid lesions in the breast, thyroid, neck, lymph nodes, or soft tissues. The needle is manipulated in the mass while suction is placed on the syringe. Several hundred cells are drawn into the syringe. The cells can be chemically fixed and then examined under the microscope. Aspiration biopsies can be performed under computed tomography (CT) or ultrasonic guidance with minimal local anesthesia.

Bone Marrow Biopsy

A trocar puncture needle or aspiration needle is placed into bone, through a small skin incision or percutaneous puncture. The sternum and iliac crest are common sites for bone marrow aspiration. Patients with abnormal blood counts or unusual blood morphology can benefit from cytologic studies of bone marrow.

Local anesthesia to the level of the periosteum is necessary. In obese patients a spinal-length needle may be needed to reach this depth. After satisfactory anesthesia, a larger-bore needle is introduced into the marrow space, and aspiration is performed. The aspiration may feel painful to the patient because the bone is not numb. A core sample of bone may be obtained at this time for pathologic examination.

Percutaneous Needle Biopsy

Tissue is obtained from an internal organ or solid mass by means of a hollow needle inserted through the body wall. Percutaneous puncture into a lesion may be guided by fluoroscopy under image intensification, by ultrasound, or by CT scanning. Special needles are used; some types are disposable.

Punch Biopsy

An instrument with a 3- to 4-mm circular, sharp, hollow tip is used to sample skin lesions in a cookie-cutter manner. The plug of tissue is sent for pathologic study. The circular wound is usually closed with 4-0 suture and heals without incident. Dermatologists or plastic surgeons use this method for skin biopsy.

Brush Biopsy

Stiff brushes of nylon or steel are passed through an endoscope to the interior of the respiratory tree or urinary tract. Tissue samples are collected as the brush rubs against the target organ. Smears are made on glass slides; the tip of the brush is then cut off and placed in formalin for a minimum of 1 hour for fixation. The slides and fixed tissue are subjected to histologic studies for diagnosis.

Excisional Biopsy

A mass or entire structure is cut from the body. The advent of fine-needle aspiration has decreased the need for full excisional biopsy with the exception of a friable organ or a breast mass. In diagnosing lymphoma, an entire lymph node is necessary for adequate diagnosis. Some excisional biopsies can be performed endoscopically.

Incisional Biopsy

A portion of a mass is removed. Soft tissue masses incised for diagnosis include muscle, fat, or other connective tissue.

Frozen Section Special preparation and examination of tissue can determine whether it is malignant and whether regional nodes are involved. When the surgeon removes a piece of tissue and wants an immediate diagnosis, it is placed in a basin or specimen container without any added preservative, such as formalin or normal saline solution. Formalin or normal saline solution will alter the freezing process used in the specialized pathologic study. The circulator should alert the pathologist that his or her services will be needed. In some facilities the pathologist comes to the OR suite to do a frozen section, which takes only a few minutes. When the tissue examination is complete, the pathologist will report the results directly to the surgeon in the OR. The patient's level of consciousness should be considered during report of pathologic results, especially if the patient is awake. The use of speakerphones should be avoided for patient confidentiality. If a malignant lesion is present and the individual situation calls for it, the surgeon proceeds with a radical resection of the affected organ or body area. In some situations additional tissue is needed for diagnosis.

Permanent Section The specimen is placed in fixative, commonly formalin, for several hours to cause the cells to become firm. The fixed specimen is placed in a machine that removes all of the water from the tissues, replacing it with paraffin. When this process is complete, the specimen is embedded into a block of wax. It is placed in a microtome and is sliced tissue-paper thin and floated in a bath of water. The slices are placed on glass slides, where the paraffin is

TABLE 22-1	Pathologic Specimens			
Specimen Type	**Test**	**Preparation**	**Example**	
Fluid	Bacteriology	Anaerobic or aerobic on culture swab in sterile tube	Exudate	
	Virology	Fresh, in sterile container	Cerebrospinal fluid	
	Cytology	Fresh or added solution of pathologist's choice in sterile container	Cell washings, urine	
	Genetic studies	Fresh, in sterile container	Amniotic fluid	
	Cell count	Fresh, in sterile container	Semen for infertility study	
Tissue	Permanent section	Fresh or added solution of pathologist's choice in sterile container	Diseased organ	
	Frozen section	Fresh, in sterile container	Margin of malignant lesion	
	Biopsy	Fresh or solution of pathologist's choice in sterile container	Suspicious lesion	
	Hormonal assay	Fresh, in sterile container	Breast tissue	
	Donor tissue	Fresh or added solution of pathologist's choice	Cadaver skin	
	Calculi	Dry, in sterile container	Gallstone	
	Ova	Fresh or added solution of surgeon's choice	Human egg for preservation	
	Muscle	Fresh, extended in special clamp in sterile container	Test for malignant hyperthermia	
Nonbiologic specimen	Foreign body	Fresh, in sterile container	Glass fragments	
	Projectile from crime scene	Dry, in nonmetallic container	Bullet	
	Clothing of crime or accident victim	Dry, in porous paper	Underclothes of rape victim	
	Explanted prosthesis	Dry, in sterile container	Orthopaedic screws or plates	

dissolved with solvent and the water is restored to the tissue on the slide. The slices readily accept dyes and stains used for diagnosis. Permanent section is the best diagnostic biopsy tool.

Surgical Specimens

All tissue removed during the surgical procedure is sent to the pathology laboratory for verification of the diagnosis.

Tissue specimens may be stored in a refrigerator in the laboratory or in some other location within the OR suite until they are taken to the pathology department at the end of each day's schedule of surgical procedures or at intervals during the day. Correct solutions for storage and correct labeling of specimens are critical for accurate diagnosis. Table 22-1 lists types of pathologic specimens.

RADIOLOGIC EXAMINATION

An x-ray is a high-energy electromagnetic wave capable of penetrating various thicknesses of solid substances and affecting photographic plates. X-rays are generated on a vacuum tube when high-velocity electrons from a heated filament strike a metal target (anode), causing it to emit x-rays. The photograph obtained by the use of x-rays may be referred to as an x-ray film, roentgenogram, radiograph, or other "-gram" name associated either with the specific technique used to obtain the photograph or with the anatomic structures identified (e.g., mammogram). X-rays are also used for diagnostic imaging with fluoroscopy, CT, and digital radiography. Computerized radiologic images may be stored on diskettes.

Types of Radiologic Equipment and Accessories

Many hospitals have one or more rooms within the OR suite that are equipped for diagnostic as well as intraoperative radiologic procedures. In some facilities OR personnel are cross-trained to assist with diagnostic and interventional procedures in the radiology department.

Contrast Media

Agents composed of nonmetallic compounds or heavy metallic salts that do not permit passage of radiant energy are radiopaque. When exposed to x-rays, the lumina of body structures filled with these agents appear as dense areas. Radiopaque contrast media frequently used for the procedures to be described are listed in Box 22-2. Some of these agents are fluorescent dyes. Most contain iodine. A history of sensitivity to substances that contain iodine, such as shellfish, or other allergies must be obtained before these agents are injected. A test dose of 1 or 2 ml may be given before the dose required for x-ray study. The patient should be observed

---

Box 22-2	**Radiopaque Contrast Media**

Barium sulfate for gastrointestinal studies
Diatrizoate meglumine, injectable:
    Cardiografin for angiography and aortography
    Hypaque Meglumine, 30%, for urography and CT
    Hypaque Meglumine, 60%, for urography, cerebral and
       peripheral angiography, aortography, venography, cholan-
       giography, hysterosalpingography, and splenoportography
Diatrizoate sodium, injectable:
    Hypaque Sodium, 25%, for urography and CT
    Hypaque Sodium, 50%, same uses as for Hypaque Meglu-
       mine, 60%
Diatrizoic acid, injectable, used as meglumine and sodium
   salts:
    Hypaque-M, 75%, for angiocardiography, angiography, aor-
       tography, and urography
    Renografin for cerebral angiography, peripheral arteriogra-
       phy and venography, cholangiography, splenoportogra-
       phy, arthrography, discography, urography, and CT
    Renovist for aortography, angiocardiography, peripheral
       arteriography and venography, venocavography, and
       urography
Ethiodized oil (Ethiodol) for splenoportography and CT
Iodipamide meglumine, injectable:
    Cholografin Meglumine for cholangiography and
       cholecystography
    Renovue for IV excretory urography
    Sinografin for hysterosalpinography
Iohexol (Omnipaque) for myelography
Iophendylate (Pantopaque) for myelography
Ioversol (Optiray) for arteriography and CT
Metrizamide (Amipaque) for myelography and CT
Propyliodone (Dionosil) for bronchography
Sodium iothalamate (Angio-Conray) for arteriography

for allergic reaction throughout the procedure. Signs of reaction may include the following:

- Red rash over face and chest
- Extreme agitation
- Sudden elevation of body temperature
- Complaints of muscle, joint, and back pain
- Respiratory distress
- Tachycardia
- Hypotension
- Blood-tinged urine
- Convulsions
- Loss of consciousness
- Cardiac arrest

Radiolucent Gases Filtered room air, oxygen, nitrogen, carbon dioxide, or a combination of gases may be injected into body spaces or structures that normally contain fluid other than blood. Gases are radiolucent (i.e., transparent to x-rays). Thus gas-filled spaces appear less dense on x-ray film than do surrounding tissues.

Radiologic Table

The tabletop the patient lies on is made of Bakelite, acrylic, or some other material capable of being penetrated by x-rays (radiolucent). Some operating beds have a tunnel top the length of the table that permits insertion of the x-ray cassette at any area. For fluoroscopy with image intensification, the entire top must be radiolucent because the image intensifier is positioned underneath the table. If the entire operating bed is not radiolucent, the foot section can be lowered and a radiolucent extension attached that will accommodate the C-arm.

Cassette

The lightproof holder for x-ray film is referred to as a cassette. The patient is positioned between the x-ray tube and the cassette. Holders for cassettes may be built into or attached to the operating bed. Intraoperative x-rays may require the use of a sterile disposable cassette cover. If a sterile cover is unavailable, a sterile Mayo stand cover may be substituted.

Processing Equipment

Conventional x-ray equipment projects a black-and-white image on x-ray film that is developed by a chemical process. Some OR suites have a darkroom where x-ray film is developed after exposure so that the surgeon can see results of the study without excessive delay. An automatic processor in which film can be developed within 90 seconds to 3 minutes may be available.

Fixed X-Ray Equipment

A fixed overhead x-ray tube with housing may be mounted on a ceiling track for unrestricted movement of the x-ray beam into the desired position over the patient. When not in use, it can be moved against a wall and retracted toward the ceiling. Some units are fixed to specially designed tables, such as the urologic table for cystoscopic examinations. The controls are in an adjacent room or behind a lead shield and are activated by the radiologist or radiology technician.

Portable X-Ray Machine

An x-ray tube mounted on a portable electric- or battery-powered generator of a nonexplosive design may be moved from one room to another in the OR suite and postanesthesia care unit (PACU). A portable x-ray machine offers the advantages of flexibility in scheduling procedures and availability for when and where it is needed.

Portable x-ray machines can be a source for cross-contamination. All portable equipment should be thoroughly disinfected before being brought into the OR/PACU and again after use. It should be stored within the perioperative environment between uses. Portable x-ray machines are used for intraoperative angiography, cholangiography, orthopaedic localization, and urologic contrast procedures. In the PACU the portable x-ray machine is used for stat chest and kidney-ureter-bladder (KUB) films. X-ray films can be used to check the location of implants and delayed passage of contrast media through an organ system.

Fluoroscope

Similar to an x-ray generator, a fluoroscope has an additional screen, composed of fluorescent crystals, which lies in contact with a photocathode. When an x-ray beam passes through this screen, it fluoresces. Fluorescent light sets electrons free from an adjacent photocathode to produce an electron image. Rather than this image of body structures being photographed on x-ray film, it is reproduced as an optical image on a luminescent screen. The image can be projected on a television monitor or retained on film or videotape by using a video camera. Known as fluoroscopy, examination under a fluoroscope allows visualization of both form and movement of internal body structures. Fluoroscopy is used frequently for both preoperative and intraoperative procedures.

It is an invasive technique because a fluorescent substance must be injected or a radiopaque device inserted. When exposure time is prolonged to perform a procedure with visual fluoroscopic control (e.g., cardiac catheterization), fluoroscopy exposes the patient and personnel to radiation at higher levels than do conventional x-rays. Personnel must wear lead aprons during fluoroscopy even though a lead shield is part of the installation. Patients should be protected with gonadal and thyroid shields.

Image Intensifier

The image intensifier is used with the fluoroscope. It amplifies the image onto a monitor screen. The surgeon activates the image intensifier with a foot pedal. Clarity of the image is an aid in diagnosis, particularly of vascular, urologic, neurologic, and bone disorders. The surgeon can observe the progression of an injected fluorescent substance as it moves through internal structures or the placement of a device, such as a catheter, into the body. When connected to other closed-circuit television facilities, the image can be transmitted to other rooms for teaching purposes. In addition, the image can be filmed for a permanent record and for teaching. The monitoring screen may be mounted on the ceiling above the operating bed to save space in the OR, or it may be portable.

Mobile C-Arm Image Intensifier Designed primarily for orthopaedic procedures, foreign body and calculi localization, and catheter placement, mobile image intensifiers offer the same advantages and disadvantages as do portable x-ray machines. The C-arm, so named because of its shape (Figure 22-1), keeps the image intensifier and x-ray tube in alignment; the intensifier is directly under the tube. It can be moved from an anterior to a lateral position. Utility of the mobile C-arm image intensifier is enhanced when the system is capable of making electronic radiographs for permanent records. An additional formatting device is required for this function.

Computerized Digital Subtraction Processor

Following IV injection of a radiopaque contrast medium, the computerized digital subtraction x-ray imaging system visually records perfusion within the cardiovascular system (e.g.,

Figure 22-1 C-arm keeps image intensifier and x-ray tube in alignment to amplify fluoroscopic optical image.

extracranial and intracranial vessels). Initially, before contrast medium is injected, fluoroscopic body images are converted to digital data for storage in a memory unit in the processor. Termed the mask image, these digitized data are integrated into single or multiple video frames. The video signal is logarithmically amplified and digitized. The mask image is electronically subtracted from subsequent images with the contrast medium. This process removes unwanted background, thus providing optimal visualization of vessels with contrast density that cannot be achieved by other image intensifiers. The resultant images (digital radiographs) are displayed on a video screen and can be recorded on diskette or videotape.

Radiologic Procedures
Chest X-Ray Films

Most surgeons consider a chest x-ray film as an extension of the patient's history and physical examination if it is clinically necessary. An x-ray study of the chest may be part of the admission procedure for elective surgical patients to rule out unsuspected pulmonary disease that could be communicable or would contraindicate the use of inhalation anesthetics. This procedure may be routine for patients over 40 years of age. It is always a part of the diagnostic workup in patients with suspected or symptomatic pulmonary abnormalities if they will be undergoing general anesthesia.

X-Ray Studies for Trauma

In addition to being an aid in determining the extent of traumatic injury, x-ray films and scans may be entered as legal evidence in a court of law to establish injuries sustained by the patient or to justify medical care given. Conventional noninvasive x-ray films will show the following:

- Fractures of bones
- Presence and location of some types of foreign bodies (e.g., bullets)
- Air or blood in the pleural cavity
- Gas or fluid in the abdominal cavity
- Outline of abdominal and chest organs and any deviation from normal size or location

Mammography

A technique for projecting an x-ray image of soft tissue of the breast, mammography is the most effective screening method for early diagnosis of small, nonpalpable breast tumors. Mammography may be performed in conjunction with ultrasonography if the woman has fibrocystic breasts and difficult to palpate masses less than ¼ inch (0.5 cm) in diameter. Three views of each breast are exposed to conventional x-rays. The procedure may be somewhat painful for the woman because compression is needed for radiologic imaging. Tumors appear on the mammogram as opaque spiculated areas or, occasionally, as areas of calcification. A small BB-like radiolucent bead with crosshairs is placed over a suspicious area by the radiologist. This area is x-rayed an additional time. Fine-needle aspiration may be performed under ultrasonic guidance to gather cells for cytologic study.

Patient Teaching Women 35 to 40 years of age should have a baseline screening mammogram. Between the ages of 40 and 50 years, they should have additional screening films yearly or every other year as recommended by their physician. After the age of 50 years every woman should have a yearly mammogram.

Mammography is not contraindicated in women with breast implants. The technician performing the radiograph should be informed of previous breast surgeries, hormone replacement therapy, and augmentation mammoplasty. Special breast-imaging techniques are employed to displace an implant or to x-ray extremely dense breast tissue.

Men with suspicious breast lesions or pronounced gynecomastia should have mammographic screening to rule out cancerous tissue.

Every patient should be taught breast self-examination and practice it every month as a baseline diagnostic test. Early diagnosis is the best chance for a cure. Figure 22-2 depicts the average sizes of masses discovered in patients who do and do not practice breast self-examination.

Stereotactic Core Breast Tissue Biopsy A needle biopsy device may be used in conjunction with mammography to obtain a tissue specimen from a lesion seen on the mammogram. The patient is positioned prone on a special

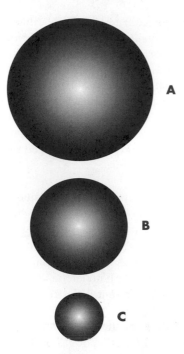

Figure 22-2 Average-size lumps found by breast self-examination (BSE). **A,** Woman not practicing BSE. **B,** Woman practicing occasional BSE. **C,** Woman practicing monthly BSE. (From Fortunato NM, McCullough SM: *Plastic and reconstructive surgery,* St Louis, 1998, Mosby.)

table with her breasts placed through a biopsy porthole. Imaging equipment is used to stereotactically isolate breast lesions that may not be palpable. Percutaneous needle biopsies are performed with the patient under local anesthesia.

Computed Tomography

In CT, special complex and expensive equipment uses an x-ray beam in conjunction with a computer. Because the x ray beam moves back and forth across the body to project cross sectional images, the technique is referred to as computed tomography (CT), computed axial tomography (CAT), or simply scanning. It produces a highly contrasted, detailed study of normal and pathologic anatomy. The x-ray tube and photomultiplier detectors rotate slowly around the patient's head, chest, or body for 180 degrees in a linear fashion along the vertical axis. The computer processes the data and constructs a three-dimensional or two-dimensional picture on a black-and-white monitor or in colors that correspond to the density of tissue. Structures are identified by differences in density. This picture is photographed for a permanent record. The computer also prints out on a magnetic disk the numerical density values related to the radiation-absorption coefficients of substances in the area scanned. The radiologist uses this printout to determine whether a substance is fluid, blood, normal tissue, bone, air, or a pathologic lesion. The exact size and location of lesions in the brain, mediastinum, and abdominal organs are identified.

CT becomes an invasive procedure when a radiopaque contrast medium is injected IV to enhance visualization of the vascular and renal systems. Oral diluted barium contrast can be used to examine the gastrointestinal tract. Tissue biopsy can be performed under CT guidance. Needle aspiration can be performed under direct CT visualization.

CT exposes the patient to ionizing radiation and a potential allergic reaction to contrast medium, if used. To ensure proper use of this complex equipment, as well as to protect the patient from excessive or unnecessary radiation, the procedure is done under the supervision of a qualified radiologist.

Ventriculography

Ventriculography is the radiographic study of the ventricles following injection of gas directly into the lateral ventricles of the brain. It may be used to evaluate a patient with signs of increased intracranial pressure as a result of blockage of cerebrospinal fluid circulation. Ventricular needles or catheters are inserted into one or both lateral ventricles through holes made in the skull. The ventricular needle has a blunt, tapered point that prevents injury to the brain as it is inserted into the ventricle. Openings on the side near the point permit removal of spinal fluid and injection of gas. If the patient is an infant whose suture lines in the skull are not yet closed, needles are inserted through these.

The entire ventriculographic procedure may be done in the OR. Otherwise, the holes are drilled and the ventricular needles or an intraventricular catheter is inserted, and the patient is then transferred to the radiology department or special procedures room within the OR suite. If a lesion is identified, the diagnostic procedure may be followed immediately by a surgical procedure because of the possibility of a further increase in intracranial pressure. If the patient is returned to the unit following the procedure, sterile ventricular needles should accompany the patient. If intracranial pressure becomes too great after gas injection, a needle can be inserted to remove the gas.

Arthrography

Arthrography is the study of a joint following the injection of gas or contrast media into it. Conventional x-ray films show only the bony structure of a joint. Through injection of a dye or gas, injury to cartilage and ligaments may be visualized. A double-contrast study uses both gas and contrast, which is particularly useful in knee arthrograms.

Angiography/Arteriography

Angiography is a comprehensive term for studies of the circulatory system following injection of a radiopaque substance to permit visualization of a specific blood vessel system. These procedures are useful in the differential diagnosis of arteriovenous malformations, aneurysms, tumors, vascular accidents, or other circulatory abnormalities caused either by traumatic injury or by an acquired structural disease.

Intraoperative studies often are essential to assess the results of vascular reconstruction. Angiography is one method of assessment to confirm the position and patency of an arterial or venous graft or the quality of a restored vessel lumen. Intraoperative angiography frequently is indicated for

these assessments in the peripheral vessels of extremities. After insertion of a bypass graft or endarterectomy, patency of the graft or vessel is checked by pulsations and also by arteriography.

Angiography is also used at the time of the surgical procedure to identify vascularity or the exact location of some types of lesions in the extremities, brain, and thoracic and abdominal cavities. After injection of radiopaque contrast medium, radiologic studies are made. Techniques and equipment to be used will vary according to the specific procedure, but all types of angiography have the following features in common:

1. Access to the vessel to be injected with a radiopaque contrast medium may be made by a percutaneous puncture or a cutdown. An IV drip is maintained when the latter approach is used.
   a. Cannulated needles with or without a radiopaque plastic catheter, similar to those used for IV infusions, may be used for a percutaneous puncture. To prevent backflow of blood, cannulated needles have an obturator that remains in place until the contrast medium is injected. Long catheters have a guidewire to assist threading through the vessel.
   b. A Seldinger (18-gauge) needle has a sharply beveled inner cannula and a blunt outer cannula. The blunt end of the outer cannula prevents trauma to the vessel. After insertion, the inner cannula is replaced with a guidewire and the outer cannula is removed. A 20-cm vessel dilator (which is approximately 8 inches) is threaded over the guidewire to create a track for a radiopaque catheter. After it is removed, the catheter is positioned and the guidewire is withdrawn. This method is generally preferred for angiography because blood vessels other than the one punctured can be injected with contrast medium.
   c. A Cournand needle has a curved flanged guard that contours to the body. It is particularly useful in carotid arteriography to hold the needle in position in the neck during injection.
   d. A Robb cannula is blunt, with a large lumen and a stopcock at the hub. It is inserted via a cutdown and is used with a Robb syringe that has a large opening in the tip for fast injection.
   e. A Sheldon needle has an occluded point with an opening at 90 degrees to the lumen. When the vertebral artery is entered, a right-angle injection is made into the lumen of the artery.
2. The amounts of radiopaque contrast substances injected into blood vessels are computed for infants and children according to weight. In adults the amount is measured so that it can be repeated safely for more exposures if necessary. Radiopaque agents dissipate very rapidly in the bloodstream.
3. Radiopaque contrast material should be warmed to body temperature to prevent precipitation and to reduce viscosity.

4. If awake, the patient should be told to expect a warm feeling and possibly a burning sensation when the contrast medium is injected. Procedures may be done with the patient under local anesthesia.

5. Sterile plastic tubing, 30 inches (76 cm) long with a syringe on one end and an adapter on the other, is connected to the needle or catheter in the vessel to prevent jarring from the pressure of injection and to keep the hands of the operator out of the x-ray beam.

6. An automatic injector may be used instead of injecting contrast medium by hand. This device correlates injection and x-ray exposure. When an automatic injector is used, special high-pressure nylon tubing is used that does not pull apart with pressure. When this tubing is used, a stopcock is placed on the end for closing it off at the syringe connection because nylon tubing cannot be clamped.

7. Automatic seriogram equipment takes rapid multiple exposures while the contrast medium is in sufficient concentration to visualize the vessels. It can be set at ½- to 2-second intervals to take multiple pictures in succession.

8. Digital subtraction angiography converts the x-ray beam into a video screen image. A small amount of contrast medium is injected IV. Vessel catheterization is unnecessary, and less contrast medium is used. This procedure may be done on an ambulatory basis.

Bronchography

Study of the tracheobronchial tree is performed by instillation of a contrast medium to aid in the diagnosis of bronchiectasis, cancer, tuberculosis, and lung abscess or to detect a foreign body. The location of a lesion can be determined and the surgical procedure planned accordingly. The procedure should be explained in detail to the patient because cooperation is necessary to accomplish the desired result. This radiologic study may be done in conjunction with bronchoscopy. In most patients, bronchoscopy is performed alone without the use of bronchographic contrast media.

Cholangiography

In addition to preoperative diagnostic x-ray studies, some surgeons routinely request radiologic studies in conjunction with cholecystectomy or cholelithotomy to identify gallstones in the biliary tract. Other surgeons selectively include cholangiography at the time of the surgical procedure in patients in whom they suspect stones might be present or retained in the bile ducts. Conventional x-ray equipment or an image intensifier may be used for these intraoperative studies.

The basic difference between preoperative and intraoperative cholangiography is the site of administration of the radiopaque contrast medium. For preoperative invasive cholangiography, the contrast medium injected IV through percutaneous venipuncture is excreted by the liver into the bile ducts. During open surgical procedures the medium is injected directly into bile ducts.

Gastrointestinal X-Ray Studies

Studies are performed to identify lesions in the mucosa of the gastrointestinal tract, such as an ulcer, stricture, or tumor. Inflammatory lesions and partial or complete obstructions may also be identified. Barium sulfate is either swallowed by the patient or instilled by enema to outline the lumina of segments of the tract to be studied. These studies are done in the radiology department, but surgeons often refer to films during the surgical procedure. Care is taken not to use natural latex rubber enema tubing for this procedure if the patient is sensitive to latex. Latex sensitivity is discussed in Chapter 13.

Myelography

Lesions in the spinal canal are studies by myelography. It is helpful to localize a filling defect, spinal cord tumor, or herniated nucleus pulposus. Most surgeons do not rely entirely on this method of diagnosis; the patient's symptoms and signs are important in making a final diagnosis. Arachnoiditis is a potential complication of intrathecal injection of iophendylate (Pantopaque). Therefore a water-based contrast medium such as metrizamide (Amipaque) may be preferred.

Urography

Urography is a comprehensive term for radiologic studies of the urinary tract. Most procedures are performed in the radiology department, but some are done in conjunction with cystoscopic examinations. Urographic studies are described as follows:

1. Cystography is the study of the bladder following instillation of a contrast medium. It is valuable in detecting ureterovesical reflux, a malfunction of the sphincter valves.

2. Cystourethrography is the study of the bladder and urethra to determine whether there is an obstruction or abnormality in contour or position. X-ray films may be taken as contrast medium is injected into the bladder or when the patient voids the material.

3. Intravenous pyelography (IVP) is the study of structures of the urinary tract and kidney function. Contrast medium is introduced into the circulatory system by rapid IV injection or slow IV infusion drip. It is excreted through the kidneys. X-ray films are taken at carefully timed intervals. If the medium is poorly excreted through the kidneys, the last film may be taken as late as 24 hours after injection. Tomograms also may be taken while the contrast material is still in the urinary tract. These procedures are done in the radiology department rather than in the cystoscopy room.

4. Retrograde pyelography is the study of the shape and position of the kidneys and ureters. Contrast medium is injected through catheters placed in each ureter. This procedure is used to visualize the renal pelves and calyces.

5. Voiding cystourethrography is the study of contour and patency of the urethra. Contrast medium may be instilled into the bladder. X-ray films are taken as the

patient voids. The medium must flow well but be viscous enough to distend the urethra and provide good detail on the x-ray film. If the patient is anesthetized, a very viscous contrast medium is injected into the urethra and films are taken. Because the urethra is quite short, the latter technique is of little value in female patients.

Incidental X-Ray Films

An unanticipated need for an x-ray film occurs when a sponge, needle, or instrument is unaccounted for at the time the final count is taken during wound closure. An x-ray film will confirm whether the item is still in the patient. Unless the patient's condition demands immediate wound closure, a film may be taken before closure is completed.

Interventional Radiology

The radiologist may work in collaboration with the surgeon to insert catheters for infusion of pharmacologic and cytotoxic drugs, dilation, or embolization of vessels or organs. Cardiac catheterization, angioplasty, and stent placement are performed in an interventional radiology department. Biopsies may be performed percutaneously under radiologic C-arm control. Foreign bodies and thrombi may be extracted.

MAGNETIC RESONANCE IMAGING

Magnetic resonance imaging (MRI) was introduced in hospitals in the United States in 1981. Unlike CT scanning, MRI does not use radiation. The patient lies flat inside a large electromagnet. In this static magnetic field the patient is exposed to bursts of alternating radiofrequency energy waves. The magnetic nuclei of hydrogen atoms in the water of body cells are stimulated from their state of equilibrium. As nuclei return to their original state, they emit radiofrequency signals. These signals are converted by a digital computer into two-dimensional color images displayed on a monitor and recorded on film. Cross-sectional views of the head and all body soft tissue planes can be obtained. A computer software system has been developed that produces three-dimensional images.

MRI is based on the magnetic properties of hydrogen in the body rather than on the radiodensity of calcium, which is the basis of radiology. MRI looks at both the body's structure and function. It defines soft tissues in relationship to bony and neurovascular structures. It distinguishes between fat, muscle, compact bone and bone marrow, brain and spinal cord, fluid-filled cavities, ligaments and tendons, and blood vessels. The major applications of MRI are detection of tumors, inflammatory diseases, infections, and abscesses, and evaluation of functions of the cardiovascular and central nervous systems and other organs.

MRI paramagnetic IV contrast media, such as gadopentetate, are sometimes used to localize tumors in the central nervous system. These media do not contain iodine, and allergic reactions are rare. All metals can cause artifacts that distort

Figure 22-3   Conventional closed MRI.

Figure 22-4   Open MRI.

MRI scans, some more so than others. Titanium ligating clips, for example, create less distortion than do ferromagnetic (iron) or stainless steel clips. Iron-containing pigments used in tattoos and permanent eyeliner can alter the image produced. The magnetic field can cause ferromagnetic components of implants, such as pacemakers and cochlear implants, to malfunction. The magnetic field will also disable metallic devices in the area, such as cardiac monitors, infusion pumps, and wristwatches.

Some patients feel a sense of claustrophobia in a conventional MRI machine (Figure 22-3). The procedure lasts from 30 to 90 minutes, and the patient must remain still. As the magnets switch on and off, a banging noise echoes through the chamber. Ear plugs and cassette players help reduce the sound. Newer open MRI technology has decreased the feeling of being closed in and has decreased the noise level caused by the scanning (Figure 22-4).

NUCLEAR MEDICINE STUDIES

Radionuclides

Radioactive isotopes used in medicine are referred to as radionuclides. A nuclide is a stable nucleus of a chemical element, such as iodine, plus its orbiting electrons. A nuclide bombarded with radioactive particles becomes unstable and emits radiant energy; it becomes a radionuclide. Radionuclides that emit electromagnetic energy are used for diagnostic studies to trace the function and structure of most organs of the body. They may be given by the oral, intracavitary, or IV route, including slow IV infusion. These agents may be used to visualize specific areas rather than radiopaque contrast media in some of the procedures previously described. They are particularly useful in studies of the bone marrow, liver, spleen, biliary tract, thyroid, brain, urinary tract, and peripheral vascular system. Because they provide better quantification of arrival times for vascular perfusion above and below lesions, radionuclides may be a more accurate index of the functional significance of a lesion than are other radiopaque contrast media.

Total-Body Scanning

Total-body scanning does not refer to CT but to a radiologic scanning procedure following IV injection of a radionuclide material. Uptake of the radionuclide within the tissues depends on blood flow. Therefore the imaging procedure may be delayed for several hours after the dose is given, not because it takes long for the material to localize in a tumor or inflammatory lesion, where the uptake is high, but because differentiation is achieved after washout from normal structures. Scanning may include the whole body or only areas of specific interest. Total-body scanning includes identification of structures in the skeletal and vascular systems for diagnosis of a pathologic process such as metastatic bone tumors or thrombotic vascular disease. The scanner can be angled for many views of the same structure.

Scintigraphy

Distribution of gamma radioactivity, such as from gallium-67 citrate, may be determined by an external scintillation detector. This is referred to as scintigraphy; the record produced is a scintigram or scintiscan. A sterile probe may be used intraoperatively to count gamma emissions from cancer cells. A radionuclide, such as iodine-125, and specific antibodies for antigen-producing tumors are injected approximately 3 weeks before the surgical procedure. The computerized display unit emits an auditory signal when the probe detects radioactivity in tissue.

Lymphoscintigraphy

Spread of cancer from the primary tumor starts with cells entering an adjacent lymph node. This node is referred to as the sentinel lymph node. Some patients have multiple sentinel nodes in some areas of the body. The degree of tumor progression is measured, and the prognostics of the disease can be predicted by evaluating the findings in the sentinel node(s). It is possible to detect spread to other nodes in the area. If the sentinel node is disease free, then it can be assumed that the cancer has not spread to other nodes in the area.

Lymphoscintigraphy uses technetium-99m sulfur colloid, which is an isotope that emits gamma rays as it spontaneously degrades. The isotope is injected around the primary tumor and taken up by the lymphatics. A high-resolution gamma camera follows the isotope's path. Images are captured on digital media until the sentinel node is visualized. An excisional biopsy is performed in the OR.

Some surgeons prefer to use isosulfan blue dye, which is selectively picked up by lymphatic vessels, to visually observe the location of the sentinel node. The dye is injected 1 hour before the excisional biopsy. Care is taken not to transect the lymphatic vessels that carry the dye—other tissue could be stained, and the location of the node in question would be obscured. The excised specimen is sent to the laboratory for fixation or frozen section. Before permanent slides are made, the specimen is stored in the nuclear medicine department for 2 or 3 days until the isotope has degraded to normal. At this point, the permanent slide is sent to the pathology department for further diagnosis.

Positron Emission Tomography

Positron emission tomography (PET) is a form of nuclear imaging that combines elements of CT scanning and nuclear scanning to create a picture representing the brain or other organ structure. The radioisotopes used emit positrons that cause pairs of gamma rays to be discharged. The rays are detected by the scanner and are relayed to a computer that converts them into cross-sectional, three-dimensional color images. PET studies provide detailed measurements of biochemistry and physiologic activity. They are used to study blood flow and metabolic functions, primarily in the brain and heart. Higher metabolic activity appears red, lesser activity appears yellow, still lesser activity appears green, and the least activity appears blue.

A PET scan can be used with fludeoxyglucose-F18 to identify and localize lymph node activity. Metastasis can be detected, and/or the patient's response to therapy can be assessed.

This method is costly because the radioisotopes have a short half-life. The patient is placed on a table that slides into a tubelike opening. A similar form of scan is the single photon emission computed tomography (SPECT) scan, which is done with a rotating gamma camera and is commonly used in brain, liver, and cardiac imaging.

ULTRASONOGRAPHY

Ultrasonography uses vibrating high-frequency sound waves in the frequency of 20,000 to 10 billion cycles per second, beyond the hearing capability of human ears, to detect alterations in anatomic structures or hemodynamic properties within the body. The basic component of any diagnostic ultrasound system is its specialized transducer, which is a piezoelectric crystal. The transducer converts electrical impulses to ultrasonic waves at a frequency greater than 1 million cycles per second. These ultrasonic frequencies are transmitted into tissues through a transducer placed on the skin. A water-soluble gel is applied to the skin to maintain airtight contact between the skin and the transducer because ultrasonic waves do not travel well through air. A portion of the transmitted ultrasonic waves are reflected back as real-time images to a receiving crystal. The transducer, connected to a microprocessing computer, is held on the skin long enough to obtain a graphic recording of the reflected high-frequency sound waves. Uniform imaging of a wide range of body tissues is possible. Ultrasound is not effective in the presence of bone or gases in the gastrointestinal tract. Whether used as a preoperative or intraoperative diagnostic technique, ultrasonography is a rapid, painless, noninvasive procedure that distinguishes between fluid-filled and solid masses.

Ultrasonic frequencies are reflected when the beam reaches target anatomic structures of different densities and acoustic impedance. The reflected signal is picked up by the transducer/receiver as an echo. The intensity of the returning echo is determined not only by the angle formed between the ultrasound beam and the reflecting surface of the anatomic structure, but also by the acoustic properties of that surface. The resulting echo is described in terms of time and intensity and displayed on a computerized monitor for immediate interpretation of movements and dimensions of structures. The image can be recorded on videotape or printed to provide a permanent record known as an echogram or sonogram. Sonograms can be obtained on multiple planes. Ultrasonography is a useful adjunct in the diagnosis of the following:

- *Space-occupying lesions in the neonatal brain.* The echoencephalogram will show a shift of the brain caused by tumor.
- *Lesions in the breast, thyroid, and parathyroid glands and in abdominal or pelvic organs.* Ultrasound can distinguish between a cystic and a solid tumor mass in the kidney, pancreas, liver, ovary, and testis. It is the best imaging method in patients with gallbladder disease.
- *Emboli (air, blood, or fat).* Ultrasonography is particularly useful in the early diagnosis of pulmonary embolism. Fat embolus syndrome can develop following long bone fractures.
- *Fetal maturation.* Fetal head size is an aid in the determination of fetal maturation. This can be measured by ultrasound before an elective cesarean section (C-section) or to determine the need for a C-section if the head is too large for vaginal delivery. Ultrasonography is also used to determine the position of the fetus and placenta, to identify sex, and to detect fetal abnormalities.
- *Cardiac defects.* Structural defects, insufficient valvular movement, and blood flow volumes within the heart chambers and myocardium can be detected. This diagnostic technique is known as echocardiography. The echo probe is inserted into the esophagus to obtain a transesophageal echocardiogram (TEE) or placed over the chest for a two-dimensional effect. The esophageal method is useful during open heart surgery.

Doppler Studies

Blood flow velocity and pressure measurements are possible with ultrasound because moving blood cells produce a sufficient interface with surrounding vessels to independently re-

flect high-frequency sound waves. The Doppler ultrasonic velocity detector emits a beam of 5 to 10 MHz that is directed through the skin into the bloodstream. A portion of the transmitted ultrasound is reflected from moving particles in the blood. Known as the Doppler effect, the reflected sound wave changes in frequency because the source of the sound is in motion. This shift in frequency is proportional to the velocity of the blood flow. Originally introduced for use in detecting obstruction in arterial blood flow, the Doppler instrument is used extensively to locate and evaluate blood flow patterns in peripheral arterial and venous diseases or defects:

- *Arterial disease.* Detection of altered hemodynamics in arterial flow is significant in diagnosis of obstructive or occlusive arterial lesions. For example, the Doppler instrument will indicate regions in the neck where carotid artery blood flow to the brain is obstructed by atherosclerosis. A surgical procedure can be performed to remove or bypass the obstruction to prevent the patient from suffering a cerebrovascular accident (stroke). It also may help the surgeon determine the appropriate level of lower extremity amputation for ischemia caused by peripheral arterial occlusive disease. It is useful in diagnosis of aortoiliac aneurysms.
- *Venous disease.* Occlusion of superficial or deep veins and the presence of incompetent valves can be located and identified by sounds made by the flow of blood through the peripheral venous system. This qualitative information of abnormal venous hemodynamics in patients with varicose veins and thrombotic disease helps the surgeon plan surgical intervention.

Intraoperative Ultrasonography

A sterile ultrasound transducer probe or scan head may be placed on tissue to evaluate vascularity or density. A pathologic condition can be diagnosed or localized. The handheld transducer must make an acoustic coupling with tissue. Tissues are moistened with sterile normal saline solution, acoustic gel, or peritoneal fluid (if the transducer is placed in the abdomen). The flexible transducer cable is attached to the ultrasound machine, which has a visible display screen. Permanent recordings of images may be made on a videocassette incorporated into the machine. The sound waves may be either continuous or pulsed. A 7.5-MHz focused transducer is usually used. Ultrasonography is less time-consuming and requires less tissue manipulation than other intraoperative diagnostic procedures and does not expose the patient to radiation and contrast medium.

Hemodynamics

Ultrasound imaging is used to evaluate the adequacy or restoration of blood flow during vascular reconstruction procedures, such as of peripheral vessels in the lower extremities, hepatic and portal shunts, and carotid arteries. A TEE may be obtained during coronary revascularization by placing the transducer in the esophagus. Doppler instruments are frequently used to assess blood flow through reconstructive tissue flaps and grafts and microvascular anastomoses.

Air Embolus

The Doppler instrument can be used to monitor patients during open heart surgery or during procedures on the great vessels in the chest to detect the escape of air into the circulation. Air entering an artery to the brain (cerebral air embolism) may cause brain damage or death. If an air embolism is detected at the time it occurs, therapy can be initiated immediately.

Localization of Lesions

Ultrasound imaging is used for intraoperative localization of subcortical brain lesions, spinal cord lesions, pancreatic and hepatic tumors, pelvic masses, and lesions in other soft tissues to determine whether the lesion is resectable. The exact location of gallbladder and kidney stones can also be identified.

Percutaneous Puncture

The direction and depth of needle punctures to locate lesions in various abdominal organs, such as a pancreatic cyst, can be determined by following the ultrasound that is continuously visualized on the monitor. The echo from the tip of the needle is easily visible on the scope when the lesion is entered. These procedures are performed to aspirate cytologic specimens for diagnosis.

SENSORY EVOKED POTENTIAL

Sensory evoked potential (SEP), used to measure neural pathways, involves placement of multiple recording electrodes over peripheral nerves or the scalp and ears. The evoked potentials generated in response to stimulation are recorded. Components of the computerized system provide sensory stimulation; acquisition, amplification, and filtering of electrophysiologic signals; signal processing; and display, measurement, and storage of SEP waveforms. These noninvasive measurements may be taken preoperatively to assist in the diagnosis of a pathologic condition, such as acoustic neuroma. The techniques may also be used for intraoperative monitoring to assess the status of the central nervous system. Multimodality evoked potentials aid in assessment of patients with trauma. Three modalities are used:

1. Somatosensory evoked potential is objective evaluation of peripheral and central neural pathways. Pairs of surface or needle skin or scalp electrodes are placed in desired patterns over the appropriate peripheral nerves and areas of the spinal cord and cerebral cortex. These electrodes record somatosensory responses elicited on application of electrical stimuli, such as to the peroneal peripheral nerve at the knee or from over the spinal column or scalp. These impulses along neural pathways

are charted to determine if the nerve is functioning properly or if a lesion is impeding impulses to the brain. Testing time can range from 45 minutes to 4 hours, depending on the number of peripheral nerves stimulated and sites necessary to assess neural pathways.

2. Auditory brainstem evoked potential is a test of the eighth cranial nerve and the auditory pathway to the cerebral cortex. The patient, wearing headphones or earphones, responds to auditory clicks or tones. Multiple electrodes on the scalp and ears record responses. This study is used to assess the physiologic condition of the brainstem and the patient's hearing threshold.

3. Visual evoked potential is a test of responses to visual pattern-reversal stimulation of the optic nerve and its associated pathways to the cerebral cortex. The patient receives stimuli via a television monitor or special eye goggles. Multiple electrodes on the scalp and ears record the evoked potentials.

PLETHYSMOGRAPHY

In plethysmography, pressure-sensitive instruments placed on an organ or around an extremity record variations in volume and pressure of blood passing through tissues. Pen-recorded tracings reflect pulse wave impulses transmitted from moving currents within arteries and veins. These impulses may be measured, computed by electronic circuits, and displayed as digitized data. Plethysmography does not identify the exact anatomic location, extent, or characteristics of vascular disease. It will quantitatively measure the rate of blood flow or degree of vascular obstruction. Four techniques are used:

1. Oculoplethysmography is a technique for determining hemodynamically significant carotid artery stenosis or cerebrovascular obstruction. The instrument is placed on each eyeball to record pulse waves emanating from the cerebrovascular system.

2. Strain-gauge plethysmography is a technique to evaluate altered venous hemodynamics in deep venous thrombosis and varicose veins. Two pneumatic cuffs are placed on the leg snugly around the thigh and calf, or ankle and great toe. A mercury strain gauge attached to the plethysmograph is secured around the leg or foot between the two cuffs. Cuffs are inflated sequentially for distal arterial occlusion and proximal venous occlusion. Changes in blood flow volume are measured as the gauge detects changes in the circumference of the calf or foot caused by sequential inflation and deflation of the pneumatic cuffs.

3. Venous impedance plethysmography is a technique to measure venous reflux in the lower extremity. Impedance electrodes are attached to the calf under a pneumatic boot. As the boot is inflated, blood is forced proximally out of the veins. Tissues are compressed, causing a concomitant increase in impedance and decrease in calf volume.

Box 22-3   Endoscopic Procedures

angioscopy   Heart and major vessels
anoscopy   Lower rectum and anal canal
antroscopy   Maxillary sinus
arthroscopy   A joint, usually the knee
bronchoscopy   Tracheobronchial tree
cholangiopancreatoscopy   Biliary and pancreatic ducts
choledochoscopy   Common bile duct
colonoscopy   Colon from ileocecal valve to anus
colposcopy   Vagina and cervix
culdoscopy   Through the vaginal wall into the retrouterine space for visualization of female pelvic tissues, especially the ovaries
cystoscopy   Urinary bladder
esophagoscopy   Esophagus
fetoscopy   Through the abdominal wall and uterus for visualization of the fetus in utero
gastroscopy   Stomach
hysteroscopy   Uterus
laparoscopy   Through the abdominal wall for visualization of abdominal organs and female pelvic organs
laryngoscopy   Direct visualization of the larynx; indirect laryngoscopy is an examination with a laryngeal mirror
mediastinoscopy   Mediastinal spaces in the chest cavity
nasopharyngoscopy   Nasopharynx
nephroscopy   Renal pelvis
ophthalmoscopy   Direct and indirect examination of the eye
otoscopy   Auditory canal and tympanic membrane
peritoneoscopy   Within the peritoneal cavity for visualization of abdominal and pelvic organs
pleuroscopy   Pleural cavity
proctoscopy   Rectum and anal canal
sigmoidoscopy   Sigmoid colon and rectum
sinoscopy   Nasal sinuses
thoracoscopy   Pleural surfaces
ureteroscopy   Ureter
urethroscopy   Urethra
ventriculoscopy   Ventricles of the brain

---

4. Cutaneous pressure photoplethysmography is a technique to identify peripheral arterial occlusive disease. An infrared light source in a handheld photoplethysmograph probe is applied to the skin with increasing pressure until the pulse is occluded. Infrared light is absorbed by blood. The intensity of the reflected light changes as the volume of blood increases as pressure is released. The probe measures the ability of the vascular system to force arterial blood into skin tissue.

ENDOSCOPY

Direct visualization within body cavities and structures aids in determination of the appropriate course of therapy for many conditions. Specific endoscopic procedures are discussed in other chapters when they are pertinent to diagnostic and surgical procedures in the appropriate surgical specialties. Box 22-3 lists endoscopic procedures.

Diagnostic endoscopy is frequently performed in conjunction with radiologic studies or to obtain specimens for pathologic examination. A radiolucent or radiopaque contrast material may be injected through the endoscope or an accessory before radiologic studies. Fluid and secretions may be withdrawn for culture or chemical analysis. Biopsy specimens are frequently obtained. Direct visualization alone may confirm the presence or absence of a suspected lesion or abnormal condition. This may be enhanced by an ultrasonic transducer at the end of a flexible fiberoptic scope. Endoscopic diagnosis often provides the information necessary to proceed with an open procedure or to cancel an anticipated surgical procedure.

Intraoperative Endoscopy

Vascular endoscopy and visualization of other vessels, such as the biliary and hepatic ducts, following either removal or bypass of an obstruction confirm the patency of the vessel before completion of the surgical procedure. Colonoscopy may be performed intraoperatively to locate soft, nonpalpable tumor masses that will be removed transabdominally. Flexible fiberoptic scopes are used for these procedures. A rigid proctoscope or sigmoidoscope may be inserted transrectally to assess an anastomosis in colon surgery.

Therapeutic procedures are performed through endoscopes without subjecting the patient to an open surgical procedure. Removal of a foreign body, excision of a small tumor or polyp, application of a medication, aspiration of fluid, permanent hemostasis of bleeding, and ligation of a structure are examples of therapeutic procedures. Electrosurgery, cryosurgery, and laser procedures may be performed through an endoscope to destroy or remove tissue following confirmation of a diagnosis such as cholecystitis or appendicitis. These procedures are often referred to as minimal access or minimally invasive surgery.

Bibliography

Bennert KW, Abdul-Karim FW: Fine needle aspiration cytology vs. needle core biopsy for soft tissue tumors, *Acta Cytol* 38(3):381-384, 1994.
Brenner H: Measures of differential diagnostic value of diagnostic procedures, *J Clin Epidemiol* 49(12):1435-1439, 1996.
Gurney JW: Why chest radiography became routine, *Radiology* 195(1):245-246, 1995.
Hader DJ et al: Sentinel lymph node biopsy using lymphoscintigraphy, *AORN J* 68(4):572, 575-576, 579-580, 582, 585, 588, 1998.
Lightdale CJ: Indications, contraindications, and complications of endoscopic ultrasonography, *Gastrointest Endosc* 43(2 pt 2):S15-S19, 1996.
Maresca G et al: New prospects for ultrasound contrast agents, *Euro L Radiol* 27 (suppl 2):S171-S178, 1998.
McConachie NS et al: Computed tomography and magnetic resonance in the diagnosis of intraventricular cerebral masses, *Br J Radiol* 67(795):223-243, 1994.
Newman PG, Rozycki GS: The history of ultrasound, *Surg Clin North Am* 78(2):179-195, 1998.
Raptopoulos V: Abdominal trauma, *Radiol Clin North Am* 32(5):969-987, 1994.
Rogers LF: The mammography muddle, *AJR* 168(5):1151, 1997.
Whittingham TA: New and future developments in ultrasonic imaging, *Br J Radiol* 70(spec No):S119-S132, 1997.

Chapter 23

Surgical Oncology

 Chapter Objectives

After studying this chapter, the learner will be able to:

- Identify the clinical signs that may indicate a cancerous condition.
- List several factors that may predispose a patient to cancer.
- Discuss the role of chemotherapy.
- Discuss the role of radiation therapy.
- Describe several diagnostic surgical procedures.
- List several side effects of cancer treatment.

Oncology is the study of scientific control over neoplastic growth. It concerns the etiology, diagnosis, treatment, and rehabilitation of patients with known or potential neoplasms. A neoplasm is an atypical growth of abnormal cells or tissues that may be a benign or malignant tumor. Table 23-1 compares the characteristics and effects of benign and malignant tumors. Four characteristics distinguish malignant from benign tumors, with a malignant tumor having the following characteristics:

1. It is anaplastic. Cancer cells resemble normal cell forms but are morphologically and functionally differentiated from the normal tissue of origin. They vary in size, shape, and texture.
2. It infiltrates and destroys adjacent normal tissue.
3. It grows in a disorganized, uncontrolled, and irregular manner, usually increasing in size both rapidly and perceptibly within weeks or months.
4. It has the power to metastasize. Cancer cells migrate from the primary focus to another single focus or to multiple foci in distant tissues or organs via lymphatic or vascular channels.

Cancer is a potentially curable disease, but it is the second leading cause of disease-related death in the United States. Treatment and prognosis are based on the type of cancer and the extent of the disease. Each type differs in its symptoms, behavior, and response to treatment. Terms pertinent to surgical oncology are defined in Box 23-1.

HISTORICAL BACKGROUND

The first drug used for cancer chemotherapy was synthesized in 1854. This type of therapy did not attract much attention until after World War II, when published reports purported that tumor cells circulate in the venous blood of patients undergoing surgical procedures. The administration of chemotherapeutic agents during and shortly after a surgical procedure, in the hope of destroying cancer cells, seemed justified in select patients. Nitrogen mustard was first used in 1942. A cooperative clinical study involving 23 medical centers was begun in 1958 to evaluate the efficacy of triethylenephosphoramide following radical mastectomy. Since then, many researchers have investigated more than a quarter of a million compounds in search of systemic antineoplastic substances that can kill tumor cells without excessive toxicity or damage to normal cells.

Ancient Chinese and Arabic writings describe stimulation of the body's immune system to combat infectious diseases. Immunization against smallpox was practiced in Turkey long before Edward Jenner (1749-1823) developed a vaccine in England in the late eighteenth century. The concept developed by Jenner, Pasteur, Salk, Sabin, and others—using vaccinations and immunizations to treat or prevent infectious disease—forms the basis of modern immunotherapy.

POTENTIAL CAUSES OF CANCER

Cancer is a broad term that encompasses any malignant tissue change. The exact cause of cancer is unknown. Cancerous tumors can be caused by exposure to chemical toxins, ionizing radiation, chronic tissue irritation, cigarette smoke, ultraviolet rays, viral invasion, and genetic predisposition. Studies have shown that immunosuppression may contribute to the incidence of cancer by altering biochemical metabolism and cellular enzyme production. Other research has shown that dietary influences, such as nitrates, salt-cured or smoked foods, and high-fat diets, may contribute to cancer in certain individuals.

Both malignant and benign neoplasms consist of cells that divide and grow uncontrollably at varied rates. The stimulus for growth can be intrinsic (e.g., hormonal) or extrinsic (e.g., exposure to external elements). Neoplastic overgrowth or the invasion of surrounding tissue causes dysfunction and may eventually cause the death of the patient.

The early detection of cancer decreases the incidence of morbidity and mortality. A screening examination may identify

TABLE 23-1	Comparison of Benign and Malignant Tumors	
Benign		**Malignant**
Characteristics		
Expansive		Invasive
Localized		Spreads to distant sites
Encapsulated		No capsule
Slow growth		Rapid growth
Resembles parent tissue		Varied differentiation
Normal cell reproduction		Disorganized cell reproduction
Organized mitoses		Abnormal mitoses
Effect on Patient		
Pain uncommon		Severe pain common
Little nutritional effect unless mechanical obstruction is involved		Cachexia, nausea, and vomiting

---

Box 23-1 **Terms Used in Surgical Oncology**

anaplasia Change in cellular differentiation and orientation that causes a more primitive structural appearance and function. Anaplastic cell changes are characteristic of malignancy.

brachytherapy Placement of radioactive material inside of or close to a tumor. Radioactive elements are introduced through catheters inserted into the tumor.

cancer Broad term that describes any malignant tumor within a large class of diseases. More than 100 different forms of cancer are known, each with histologic variations. Cancerous tumors are divided into two broad groups:

   carcinoma Malignant tumor of epithelial origin that affects glandular organs, viscera, and skin.

   sarcoma Malignant tumor of mesenchymal origin affecting bones, muscles, and soft tissue.

chemotherapy Use of chemical or pharmacologic agents to treat diseases, such as cancer.

cytoreductive surgery Mechanical reduction in cell volume at the tumor site by sharp or blunt tissue dissection. Vessel- and nerve-sparing procedures include the use of an ultrasonic aspirator and/or hydrostatic pulsed lavage.

cytotoxin Chemical or pharmacologic agent that causes cell damage or death. Some cytotoxic agents alter cellular metabolism or physical characteristics, which makes the cell vulnerable to destruction by other means, such as a laser.

immunotherapy Use of agents that stimulate or activate the body's own host defense immune system to combat disease.

neoplasm Atypical new growth of abnormal cells or tissues, which may be malignant or benign.

-oma Suffix denoting a tumor or neoplasm.

oncogene Potentially cancer-inducing genetic material derived from viral or host DNA. Rapidly dividing cells may be transformed to a malignant state by viral invasion, radiation, chemical exposure, or other mutagenic agent.

oncologist Specialist in the study and treatment of neoplastic growths. A surgical oncologist has been trained to perform specialized surgical procedures.

radiation therapy Localized use of ionizing radiation to injure or destroy malignant cells.

tumor Any neoplasm in which cells are permanently altered but have the capability of growth and reproduction. A tumor consists of two elements: the tumor cells themselves and a supporting framework of connective tissue and vascular supply.

   benign tumor Aggregation of cells that closely resemble those of the parent tissue of origin. The tumor usually grows slowly by expansion, is localized, and is surrounded by a capsule of fibrous tissue.

   malignant tumor Progressively growing tumor that originates from a specialized organ such as the lung, breast, or brain, or a tumor localized to a specific body system such as bone, skin, lymph nodes, or blood vessels.

a neoplasm before clinical symptoms develop. Recommended cancer screening examinations are listed in Table 23-2.

Risk-Related Factors

Risk factors for cancer include the following:

1. Age, sex, or racial, genetic, or hereditary predisposition. Table 23-3 identifies neoplasms associated with familial cancer syndromes.
2. Exposure to carcinogens (cancer-producing agents) such as cigarette smoke, coal tar, ionizing radiation, ultraviolet rays, and chemicals. Table 23-4 lists examples of chemical carcinogens.
3. Predisposition from specific environmental conditions or acquired conditions or diseases. Table 23-5 gives examples of viral-mediated carcinogens.

Risk-Avoidance Behaviors

Patient education should include information about avoiding cancer-causing behaviors and how to minimize the risk for cancer. Behaviors to discuss include the following:

1. Avoiding smoking and exposure to smoke. The Department of Health and Human Services reports that exposure to cigarette smoke is responsible for 83% of all cases of lung cancer. Each year more than 100,000 children 12 years of age and younger begin smoking, which leads to habitual use. Secondhand smoke, referred to as passive smoking, has been implicated in the development of cancer in nonsmoking persons who are exposed to smoke on a regular basis.
2. Increasing dietary intake of fiber and low-fat foods. Antioxidants such as vitamins C and A may reduce an individual's risk for developing cancer. High-fat diets have been implicated in the development of breast, colon, and prostate cancers. According to reports of the American Cancer Society, 35% of cancer deaths are related to dietary causes and are possibly preventable. A desirable weight should be maintained, and obesity should be avoided. Excessive alcohol intake should also be avoided.
3. Minimizing sun exposure, especially between the hours of 10:00 AM and 3:30 PM. Sun exposure has been shown to be the major cause of skin cancer, especially melanoma. Severe sunburn in childhood may be linked to the development of skin cancer later in life. Certain medications, such as tranquilizers, antidiabetic agents, diuretics, antiinflammatories, and antibiotics, can predispose an individual to sunburn. Certain cosmetic products, such as tretinoin (Retin-A) and alphahydroxy acid are extremely reactive to sunlight and can increase the risk of sunburn within 30 minutes of exposure. Tanning booths can also be hazardous to the skin.

A waterproof sunscreen lotion with a sun protection factor (SPF) of at least 15 should be applied whenever

TABLE 23-2	Cancer-Screening Examinations	
Sex	**Age**	**Frequency of Examination**
Pelvic Examination by Palpation and Inspection		
Female	18–40 years	Every 1–3 years
	Over age 40	Every year
Pelvic Examination by Palpation and Inspection, Including Pap Smear		
Female	Start at age 18 or at age of onset of sexual activity if younger	Yearly; may be performed less frequently on advice of physician if patient has had three negative Pap smears in 3 consecutive years
Endometrial Tissue Sample		
Female	At menopause or sooner at recommendation of physician	Sample for baseline in high-risk patient
Breast Self-Examination		
Female and male	Start at age 18 and throughout life span	Female: monthly after menses or at same time each month after menopause Male: monthly
Clinical Breast Examination		
Female	Start at age 18 and throughout life span	Corresponds with pelvic examination sequence unless patient has a previous history of breast disease or is at high risk for breast disease
Mammography		
Female	Baseline at age 35, yearly after age 40	Frequency after base-line is individualized according to age, health, and risk-factor analysis by physician; mammography, when performed, should precede clinical breast examination so that data analysis will be complete

Continued

TABLE 23-2 Cancer-Screening Examinations—cont'd

Sex	Age	Frequency of Examination
Testicular Self-Examination by Palpation and Inspection		
Male	Start at age 16 and throughout life span	Monthly
Prostate		
Male	Over age 50; start at age 40 for men at high risk	Yearly, prostate-specific antigen (PSA) blood test
Digital Rectal Examination		
Male and female	Over age 40	Yearly; frequency may vary according to individual risk factors or the recommendation of physician
Stool Guaiac Examination		
Male and female	Over age 50	Yearly; age and frequency may vary according to symptoms and the recommendation of physician
Sigmoidoscopy or Colonoscopy		
Male and female	Over age 50	Every 3-5 years or according to the advice of physician; age and frequency may vary in the presence of risk factors or individual symptoms; colonoscopy may be advised according to risk factors
Generalized Physical with Health Counseling		
Includes palpation of thyroid, gonads, and lymphatics, as well as inspection of oral mucosa		
Male and female	Over age 20	Every 3 years
Male and female	Over age 40	Every year

TABLE 23-3 Familial Cancer Syndromes

Syndrome	Associated Neoplasm
Autosomal Dominant Gene	
Familial polyposis coli	Adenocarcinoma of colon, adenomatous polyps
Gardner's syndrome	Adenocarcinoma of colon, musculoaponeurotic tumors
Peutz-Jeghers syndrome	Adenocarcinoma of small intestine, colon, ovary
Neurofibromatosis	Neurofibroma, neurogenic sarcoma, pheochromocytoma
Multiple endocrine neoplasia (MEN type I), or Wermer's syndrome	Pituitary, pancreatic islet cells, parathyroid glands
Multiple endocrine neoplasia (MEN type IIA), or Sipple's syndrome	Thyroid, parathyroid glands, pheochromocytoma
Multiple endocrine neoplasia (MEN type IIB)	Thyroid, parathyroid, pheochromocytoma, mucosa ganglioneuromas
Autosomal Recessive Gene	
Xeroderma pigmentosum	Basal and squamous cell carcinoma of skin, malignant melanoma
Ataxia-telangiectasia	Acute leukemia, lymphoma, some gastric cancers

TABLE 23-4 Examples of Chemical Carcinogenesis

Chemical	Site of Neoplasm
Alkylating Agents	
Nitrogen mustard, cyclophosphamide, chlorambucil	Leukemia, urinary bladder
Vinyl chloride	Angiosarcoma of liver
Polycyclic Hydrocarbons	
Tar, soot, oils	Skin, lung
Aromatic Amines and Azo Dyes	
β-Naphthylamine, benzidine	Urinary bladder
Food Products	
Saccharin	Urinary bladder
Aflatoxin (mold on peanuts)	Liver
Betel nuts	Oral mucosa
Medication	
Androgenic metabolic steroids	Liver
Diethylstilbestrol	Vagina
Phenacetin	Renal pelvis
Inorganic Compounds	
Chromium	Lung
Nickel	Lung, nasal sinuses
Asbestos	Serosal membranes, lung
Arsenic	Skin

TABLE 23-5	Viral-Mediated Carcinogenesis
Viral Family	**Type of Neoplasm**
DNA-Associated	
Papilloma (condyloma)	Squamous papilloma and squamous cell carcinoma
Hepatitis B	Hepatocellular carcinoma
Herpesvirus	
Epstein-Barr	Burkitt's lymphoma, nasopharyngeal carcinoma
Cytomegalovirus	Kaposi's sarcoma
Herpes simplex type II	Uterine cervical carcinoma
RNA-Dependent	
Human T-cell lymphotrophic type I (retrovirus C)	T-cell leukemia, lymphoma

sun exposure is likely. Sun-blocking products of SPF 30 to 45 are preferred. The sun-blocking product should provide protection from both ultraviolet A and ultraviolet B (UVA, UVB) rays. (UVA rays can increase the damage caused by UVB rays.) Sunscreen should be applied at least ½ hour before going outdoors and reapplied every hour thereafter.

4. Having regular checkups, especially yearly checkups after 40 years of age. Knowing the warning signs of cancer may promote prompt diagnosis and treatment. Signs to consider in young children include frequent swelling (lymphadenopathy) or bruising, unexplained headaches or fevers, dramatic weight loss or gain, and localized pain.
5. Self-examining the skin, breast, and testes, which may reveal an early sign of cancer. These self-examinations should be performed on a monthly basis.

CLINICAL SIGNS AND SYMPTOMS

According to the American Cancer Society, the following are the clinical signs and symptoms of cancer:

- Palpable mass or abnormal thickening of tissue
- Abnormal bleeding or discharge
- Obvious change in a wart or mole
- Lesion that does not heal
- Steady decrease in weight, appetite, and energy
- Chronic cough
- Change in bowel or bladder habits

Extent of Disease
Carcinoma in Situ

With carcinoma in situ, normal cells are replaced by anaplastic cells, but the growth disturbance of epithelial surfaces shows no behavioral evidence of invasion and metastasis.

This cellular change is noted most often in stratified squamous and glandular epithelium. Carcinoma in situ is also referred to as intraepithelial or preinvasive cancer. Common sites include the following:

- Uterine cervix
- Uterine endometrium
- Vagina
- Anus
- Penis
- Lip
- Buccal mucosa
- Bronchi
- Esophagus
- Eye
- Breast

Localized Cancer
Localized cancer is contained within the organ of its origin.

Regional Cancer
With regional cancer, the invaded area extends from the periphery of the organ or tissue of origin to include tumor cells in adjacent organs or tissues (e.g., the regional lymph nodes).

Metastatic Cancer
In metastatic cancer the tumor extends, by way of lymphatic or vascular channels, to tissues or organs beyond the regional area.

Disseminated Cancer
In disseminated cancer, multiple foci of tumor cells are dispersed throughout the body.

Tumor Identification System

A standardized tumor identification system, which includes classification and staging, is essential for establishing treatment protocols and evaluating the end result of therapy. Hospitals maintain a tumor registry of patients to evaluate therapeutic approaches to specific types of tumors. Classification includes the anatomic and histologic description of a tumor, whereas staging refers to the extent of the tumor. There are three basic categories of the tumor identification system:

T Primary tumor
N Regional nodes
M Distant metastases

The TNM categories are identified by pretherapy clinical diagnosis, tissue biopsy, and/or histopathologic examination following surgical resection of the tumor. Numeric subscripts are used to describe the findings; for example, bronchogenic carcinoma $T_1 N_1 M_0$ means a primary tumor in the lung without positive regional nodes or distant metastases. If a positive lymph node is identified in the area, it is indicated in a subscript (e.g., $T_1 N_1 M_0$). If a metastatic site also is diagnosed, it too is indicated in the subscript (e.g., $T_1 N_1 M_1$). The subscripts correspond to the number of separate tumors at the identified primary site, positive lymph nodes, or metastatic sites (Box 23-2). Other staging systems are referred to in the literature as stages I, II, III, and IV. After treatment, the estimation of residual tumor volume is indicated by the letter *R.*

Monitoring Tumor Markers

Tumor markers are serum studies used to measure specific enzymes emitted by tumor cells. Elevated tumor markers in the patient's blood and tissues can help determine the patient's treatment and prognosis. Table 23-6 describes common blood tests for tumor markers and their implication in cancer prognostication.

Box 23-2	Tumor Identification Scale

Primary Tumor

TX   Primary tumor is discovered by the detection of malignant cells in secretions or cell washings but not directly visualized

T_0 No evidence of primary tumor

Tis   Tumor (carcinoma) in situ

T_1 Tumor is 2 cm or less at largest dimension

T_2 Tumor is larger than 2 cm at largest dimension

T_3 Tumor directly invades surrounding tissue

T_4 Tumor invades surrounding tissue and adjacent structures, such as blood vessels or bone

Regional Lymph Nodes

NX   Unable to assess nodes

N_0 No regional lymph node metastasis

N_1 Metastasis to ipsilateral nodes or direct extension to nodes

N_2 Metastasis to contralateral nodes

Distant Metastasis

MX   Distant metastasis cannot be assessed

M_0 No distant metastasis

M_1 Distant metastasis is confirmed

Posttreatment Residual Tumor

RX   Unable to assess residual tumor

R_0 No residual tumor

R_1 Microscopic residual tumor

R_2 Macroscopic residual tumor

TABLE 23-6 Common Serum Tumor Markers

Test	Value	Indication
Carcinoembryonic antigen (CEA)	0-2.5 ng/ml	Colorectal
Alpha-fetoprotein (AFP)	10 ng/ml	Testicular Liver
Human chorionic gonadotropin (HCG)	0-1.0 ng/ml	Choriocarcinoma Testicular
Prostate-specific antigen (PSA)	0-4.0 μg/L (>40 years)	Prostate

CURATIVE VS. PALLIATIVE THERAPY

Cancer is a systemic disease. Therapy is curative if the disease process can be totally eradicated, but the success of therapy depends largely on early diagnosis. Tumors are classified to determine the most effective therapy. When a cure is not possible, palliative therapy relieves symptoms and improves quality of life but does not cure the disease.

ADJUVANT THERAPY

Surgical resection, endocrine therapy, radiation therapy, chemotherapy, immunotherapy, hyperthermia, or combinations of these procedures are used in the treatment of cancer. The surgeon or oncologist determines the most appropriate therapy for each patient. When determining the most appropriate therapy, consideration is given to the following:

- Type, site, and extent of tumor and whether lymph nodes are involved
- Type of surrounding normal tissue
- Age and general condition of the patient, including nutritional status and whether or not other diseases are present
- Whether curative or palliative therapy is possible

Before beginning therapy, a patient with cancer undergoes an extensive pretreatment workup. Each form of cancer therapy has certain advantages and limitations. Several factors affect a patient's response to treatment: host factors, clinical stage of malignancy, and type of therapy. The patient is followed carefully to determine the effectiveness of treatment at routine intervals.

SURGICAL RESECTION

Surgical resection is the modality of choice to remove solid tumors. The resection of a malignant tumor is, however, localized therapy for what may be a systemic disease. Each patient is evaluated and treated individually, and the surgical procedure is planned appropriately for the identified stage of disease. Depending on localization, regionalization, and dissemination of the tumor, the surgeon selects either a radical curative surgical procedure or a salvage palliative surgical procedure. Surgical debulking, in which the tumor is partially removed, may be the procedure of choice for some types of surgically incurable malignant neoplasms. With surgical debulking, the intent is not to cure but to make subsequent therapy with irradiation, drugs, or other palliative measures more effective and thereby extend survival. In planning the surgical procedure, the surgeon considers the length of expected survival, the prognosis of surgical intervention, and the effect of concurrent diseases on the postoperative result.

Accessible primary tumors are often treated by excision. An extremely wide resection may be necessary to avoid recurrence of the tumor. The pathologist is able to make judgments about questionable margins by evaluating frozen sections while the surgical procedure is in progress. The pathologist's findings guide the surgeon during resection so that residual tumor is not left in the patient. The specimen is also tested after permanent section fixation in the pathology laboratory. Final results are available in 2 to 3 days.

Many surgical procedures are performed for ablation of tumors by primary resection. In addition, a lymphadenectomy may be performed as a prophylactic measure to inhibit the metastatic spread of tumor cells via lymphatic channels. Other modalities of therapy may be administered preoperatively, intraoperatively, and/or postoperatively to reduce or prevent a recurrence or metastasis. Other palliative surgical interventions are described in Box 23-3.

Perioperative Patient Care

Malignant tumor cells can be disseminated by manipulation of tissue. Because of their altered nutritional and physiologic status, patients with cancer also may be highly susceptible to the complications of postoperative infection. To minimize these risks, the following specific precautions are taken in the surgical management of patients with cancer:

1. The skin over the site of a soft tissue tumor should be handled gently during hair removal and antisepsis. Vigorous scrubbing could dislodge underlying tumor cells; this is avoided by the use of "no-touch" techniques. With vascular tumors, manipulation during positioning or skin preparation could cause vascular complications such as emboli or hemorrhage.
2. Gowns, gloves, drapes, and instruments may be changed following a biopsy (e.g., a breast biopsy) before incision for a radical resection (e.g., a mastectomy). The tumor is deliberately incised to obtain a biopsy for diagnosis.
3. Instruments placed in direct contact with tumor cells may be discarded immediately after use. Even when the tumor appears to be localized, most cancers have disseminated to some degree. Therefore some surgeons prefer to use each instrument once and then discard it.

Box 23-3 | Palliative Oncologic Surgical Procedures

Reduction of tumor to prevent obstruction
Reduction of tumor cells to aid effectiveness of chemotherapy
Treatment of oncologic emergencies such as hemorrhage or compression
Removal of enlarged organs such as the spleen
Repair of perforations in irradiated parts such as the rectum
Removal of a hormone-producing part such as a gonad or other gland
Removal of a diseased organ such as the uterus, prostate, or breast
Insertion of a nutritional support device such as a feeding gastrostomy or total parenteral alimentation line
Pain control such as nerve blocks or the severing of a neural pathway or receptor site

---

4. Some surgeons prefer to irrigate the surgical site with sterile water instead of sterile normal saline solution to cause the destruction of cancerous cells by crenation. This practice is common during mastectomy.
5. As a prophylactic measure, antibiotics are administered preoperatively, intraoperatively, and postoperatively to provide an adequate antibacterial level to prevent wound infection.
6. Time-honored precautions such as handling tissue gently, keeping blood loss to a minimum, and avoiding an unduly prolonged surgical procedure influence the outcome for the patient.

During a long surgical procedure, messages should be conveyed periodically to the patient's anxiously waiting family members or significant others to reassure them that their loved one is receiving care from a concerned perioperative team.

ENDOCRINE THERAPY

Tumors arising in organs that are usually under hormonal influence (e.g., breast, ovary, and uterus in female patients; prostate and testes in male patients) may be stimulated by hormones produced in the endocrine glands. Cellular metabolism is affected by the presence of specific hormone receptors in tumor cells: estrogen and/or progesterone in a female and androgens in a male. Certain breast, endometrial, and prostatic cancers depend on these hormones for growth and maintenance. Therefore the recurrence or spread of disease may be slowed by therapeutic hormonal manipulation. Endocrine manipulation does not cure, but it can control dissemination of the disease if the tumor progresses beyond the limits of effective surgical resection or radiation therapy.

Hormonal Receptor Site Studies

Identifying the hormonal dependence of the primary tumor through studies of the receptor site is a fairly reliable way of selecting patients who will benefit from preoperative or postoperative endocrine manipulation. Following a positive diagnosis of cancer, either by a frozen section biopsy or by pathologic permanent sections, the surgeon will probably request a receptor site evaluation of a primary breast, uterine, or prostatic tumor. The tissue specimen removed by surgical resection should be sent fresh or in saline. It should not be placed in formalin preservative solution, because doing so will alter the receptor cells enough to negate the hormonal study.

Endocrine Ablation

Since 1896, surgeons have described positive clinical responses in patients with metastatic breast cancer after treatment by endocrine ablation, the surgical removal of endocrine glands. If the surgeon plans to eliminate endocrine stimulation surgically in a patient with a known hormone-dependent tumor, all sources of the hormone should be ablated chemically, hormonally, or surgically.

Bilateral Adrenaloophorectomy

Both adrenal glands and/or ovaries may be resected to prevent the recurrence of endocrine-derived cancer. These may be removed as a one-stage surgical procedure (i.e., bilateral adrenaloophorectomy). If two separate surgical procedures are preferred, the bilateral oophorectomy precedes the bilateral adrenalectomy, except in menopausal women in whom only the latter surgical procedure may be indicated.

Bilateral Orchiectomy and Adrenalectomy

Following prostatectomy for advanced carcinoma of the prostate, both testes may be removed (i.e., bilateral orchiectomy) to eliminate androgens of testicular origin. Bilateral adrenalectomy may also be indicated.

Hormonal Therapy

Hormones administered orally or via injection can alter cell metabolism by changing the systemic hormonal environment of the body. To be effective, tumor cells must contain receptors. Hormones must bind to these receptors before they can exert an effect on cells.

Antiestrogen Therapy

Patients with medical contraindications to endocrine ablation may receive antiestrogen therapy. An estrogen antagonist deprives an estrogen-dependent tumor of the estrogen necessary for its growth. Nafoxidine hydrochloride and tamoxifen citrate (Nolvadex) are synthetic nonsteroidal drugs that inhibit the normal intake of estrogen at estrogen receptor sites; they are taken orally.

Corticosteroids

Prednisone, cortisone, hydrocortisone, or some other preparation of corticosteroids may be administered as an antiinflammatory agent along with the chemotherapeutic agents given to control disseminated disease.

PHOTODYNAMIC THERAPY

For photodynamic therapy (also referred to as photoradiation), an argon tunable dye laser is used to destroy malignant cells by photochemical reaction. A photosensitive drug, either hematoporphyrin derivative (HPD) from cow's blood (Photofrin) or purified dihematoporphyrin ether, is absorbed by malignant and reticular endothelial cells. The photosensitive drug is injected intravenously via venipuncture or Hickman catheter 24 to 48 hours before the photodynamic therapy and is taken up by cells to make them fluorescent and photosensitive. It remains longer in malignant cells than in normal cells before being excreted from the body. When exposed to light from an argon laser, the tunable rhodamine B dye laser produces a red beam of approximately 630 nm. Other dyes, such as dicyanomethylene, may produce different wavelengths. HPD in cells absorbs the laser light, which leads to a photochemical re-

action that causes tissue-oxygen molecules to release cytotoxic singlet oxygen and destroy tumor cells. Depending on tumor site, the laser can be delivered interstitially, endoscopically, externally, or retrobulbarly.

Photodynamic therapy may be used to debulk tumors of the eye, head and neck, breast, esophagus, gastrointestinal tract, bronchus, and bladder. The tunable dye laser may also be used to diagnose tumor cells. The operating room (OR) should be darkened or have shades to block outside daylight during the laser treatment. The patient is cautioned to avoid exposure to sunlight or other sources of ultraviolet light both after injection of the dye and postoperatively. Photosensitivity is the primary side effect of the dye and may last 4 to 6 weeks.

RADIATION THERAPY

Radiation is the emission of electromagnetic waves or atomic particles that result from the disintegration of nuclei of unstable or radioactive elements. The treatment of malignant disease with radiation may be referred to as radiation therapy, brachytherapy, or radiotherapy. Ionizing radiation is used for this type of therapy, which involves the use of high-voltage radiation and other radioactive elements to injure or destroy cells. Like surgical resection and photodynamic therapy, radiation therapy is localized therapy that is applicable for a limited number of specific tumors.

Ionizing Radiation

Ionization is the physical production of positive and negative ions capable of conducting electricity. Ionizing radiation is radiation with sufficient energy to disrupt the electronic balance of an atom. When disruption occurs in tissue cells or extracellular fluids, the effect can range from minor changes to profound disturbances. Radiation may come either from particles of the nuclei of disintegrating atoms or from electromagnetic waves that have no mass. Types of ionizing radiation include the following:

- *Alpha particles.* Alpha particles are relatively large particles that have a very slight penetrating power. They are stopped by a thin sheet of paper. They have dense ionization but can produce tremendous tissue destruction within a short distance.
- *Beta particles.* Beta particles are relatively small, are electrical, and travel with the speed of light. They have greater penetrating properties than do alpha particles. Their emissions cause tissue necrosis, and they produce ionization, which has destructive properties.
- *Gamma rays and x-rays.* Gamma rays and x-rays are electromagnetic radiations of short wavelength but high energy, and they are capable of completely penetrating the body. They affect tumor tissue more rapidly than normal tissue. These types of rays are stopped by a thick lead shield. Protons ranging in energy from 30 kilovolts (kV) to 35 million electron volts (eV) are available for

the treatment of various cancers. Gamma rays are emitted spontaneously from the nucleus of an atom of a radioactive element.

Effects of Radiation on Cells

Cancer cells multiply out of normal body control; they are in a state of active, uncontrolled mitosis (the nuclear division of the cytoplasm and nucleus). Radiation affects the metabolic activity of cells. Cells in an active state of mitosis are most susceptible. Over time, gamma rays and x-rays cause a cessation of cell growth and a regression of the tumor mass. Cells die and are replaced by fibrous tissue.

The sensitivity of a tumor to radiation varies. Some tumors can be destroyed by a small amount of radiation, whereas others require a large amount. The sensitivity of the tumor cells is determined by the sensitivity of the normal cells from which the tumor cells are derived. The effects of radiation therapy also depend to a large extent on tissue oxygenation. As a tumor grows, the periphery is well oxygenated, but the central portion becomes necrotic and poorly oxygenated. The number of cells killed by radiation therapy is directly related to the amount of tissue and oxygen within the tumor. Therefore the hypoxic effect is a factor in determining therapeutic dose of radiation.

Radiation therefore cannot be limited solely to the area being treated. The danger of injuring normal surrounding tissue is a limiting factor in the dosage and selection of the most appropriate type of radiation therapy. A factor in dosage is the ratio of tumor tissue to the surrounding normal tissue. The dosage is computed in rads (roentgen-absorbed doses). A rad is the unit used to measure the absorbed dose of radiation. One rad is the amount of radiation required to deposit 100 ergs of energy per gram of tissue. Radiophysics or instruments such as Geiger counters or scintillation probes are used to determine the dose of radiation delivered to a specific tissue site; the dose is measured by distance from the source and duration of exposure. Doses are measured in rads to determine whether the dosage is adequate for therapy but not so excessive that it would cause damage to normal tissues.

The penetration of radiation energy is calculated from the rate of decay or disintegration, known as half-life. Half-life is the time required for half of the radioactive element to disintegrate and to lose one half its activity through decay.

Sources of Radiation

Although the effects of the different types of radiation therapy are similar, their sources and applications do differ. Some sources are implanted into the body in direct contact with tumor tissue, whereas other sources use an external beam to pass the radiation through the body to the tumor.

Radium

Radium is a radioactive metal. Mme. Marie Curie (1867-1934), a research chemist, and her husband, Pierre (1859-1906), a physicist, discovered and named this metal in 1898. Several years earlier, Mme. Curie had been given the task of finding out why pitchblende would record its image on a photographic plate. She and her husband knew this material emitted more radiation than would be justified by the known minerals contained in it. It took 6 years of painstaking, difficult work for the Curies to isolate radium as a pure element and to learn of its radioactive properties. Their research eventually led to the use of radium in the treatment of malignant tumors.

Metallic radium is unstable in air. Radium chloride or bromide salts emit fluorescence and heat. One gram gives off 134 calories per hour. Alpha and beta particles and gamma rays are products of its disintegration. The half-life of radium is approximately 1620 years; half the remaining life is lost in another 1620 years, and so on. The final product is lead.

Radon

Radon is a dense radioactive gas liberated as the first by-product of the disintegration of radium. Mme. Curie discovered this gas and first named it *emanation*. Radon is collected by an intricate process in radiopaque glass or gold capillary tubing, and the seeds for implantation are then cut and sealed. The dosage is computed according to the hours of insertion into tissue. It is measured in millicurie-hours. The half-life of radon is 4 days; its total life is approximately 30 days.

Radionuclides

A radionuclide is an element that has been bombarded with radioactive particles in a nuclear reactor. A radionuclide shows radioactive disintegration and emits alpha and beta particles or gamma rays. Radionuclides that emit beta particles and gamma rays are used primarily for treating malignant tumors. Therapeutic radionuclides may also be referred to as radiopharmaceuticals. Historically they were known as radioactive isotopes, or radioisotopes, and these terms are still found in the literature. Cesium, cobalt, iodine, iridium, and yttrium are the most commonly used elements for therapy. Brachytherapy, an internal application with sealed sources of radionuclides, has almost totally supplanted the use of radium and radon. For example, the gamma rays of cesium-137 have greater penetrating power than do those of radium.

Radionuclides are controlled by the Atomic Energy Commission and are released only to individuals trained and licensed to use them. Available in liquid or solid forms, they may be ingested orally, infused intravenously, instilled into a body cavity, injected or implanted into a tumor, or applied to the skin externally. The ionizing radiation emitted has an action on tissue similar to that of radium, but radionuclides differ from radium in the following ways:

1. The half-life of radionuclides is short. Radionuclides disintegrate at varying rates depending on their type. Each element has a specific half-life that varies from a few hours (e.g., the 6 hours of technetium-99) to the 8 days of iodine-131 or the 5.3 years of cobalt-60.

2. Irradiation with radionuclides does not spread so much into adjoining tissue; therefore a stronger dose can be used in a malignant tumor. Radiation is not absorbed by bone and other normal body tissues.
3. Irradiation with radionuclides can be more easily shielded. The surgeon and other personnel get less radiation exposure in placing or removing radionuclides.

As with exposure to radium and radon, exposure to radionuclides is always potentially dangerous. Radiation may treat cancer, but it can also cause a malignant neoplasm.

Implantation of Radiation Sources

All radiation sources for implantation are prepared in the desired therapeutic dosages by the nuclear medicine department. Many types of sources are used to deliver maximum radiation to the primary tumor. No single type is ideal for every tumor or anatomic site.

Interstitial Needles

Interstitial needles are hollow sheaths and are usually made of platinum or Monel metal. Radium salts or radionuclides are encased in platinum or platinum-iridium short units or cells, which in turn are sealed in the metal sheath of the needle for implantation into tumor tissue. A needle may contain one or several short units or cells of the radiation source, depending on the length of needle to be used. Needles vary in length from 10 to 60 mm, with a diameter of 1 to 2 mm. The choice of length depends on dosage and on the area involved. Dosage is measured in milligram hours, which can be converted to rads.

The interstitial needles, which usually contain cesium-137, are implanted in tumors near the body surface or in tissue accessible enough to permit their use (e.g., the vagina, cervix, tongue, mouth, or neck). In certain patients, stereotactic techniques are used to implant needles for the irradiation of brain tumors.

In the OR, these needles are inserted at the periphery of and within the tumor. One end of the needle is pointed, and the other end has an eye for a heavy (size 2) suture. Needles are threaded to prevent loss while in use and to aid in removal. After the surgeon inserts the needles, the ends of the sutures are tied or taped together and are taped to the skin in an adjoining area or secured to buttons. Depending on the anatomic site, a template may be used to position and secure the needles. A template consists of two acrylic plates that are separated by rubber O-rings and held together with screws. The plates have holes for insertion of the interstitial needles. The template remains in place until the needles are removed. Depending on the planned dosage to the tumor bed, needles are usually left in place for 4 to 7 days.

Interstitial Seeds

Sealed radionuclide seeds may be implanted permanently or temporarily. Because they have a short half-life, gold seeds are permanently implanted, most commonly into the prostate, lungs, or pancreas. Seeds containing cesium-137, iridium-192, or iodine-125 implanted directly into tumor tissue are removed after the desired exposure. Seeds are useful in body cavities, in localized areas, and in tumors that are not resectable because of their location near major vessels or the spinal cord. Because they are small, the seeds can be placed to fit a curved area without requiring immobilization. However, they may move about if there is much motion.

Radionuclide seeds are 7 mm or less in length, are 0.75 mm in diameter, and have a wall 0.3 mm thick. The length of the seed depends on the desired dosage. Seeds can be inserted with or without an invasive surgical procedure. They may be strung on a strand of suture material or placed in a hollow plastic tube with sealed ends. With a needle attached, the strand or tube is woven or pulled through the tumor. Seeds in a plastic tube may be inserted through a hollow needle, such as a catheter through a trocar. Empty tubes may be inserted in the OR and afterloaded (i.e., the seeds are put into the tube at a later time and place). A microprocessor-controlled machine that pulls wire attached to radioactive material through the tube may be used for remote afterloading.

Intracavitary Capsules

A sealed capsule of radium, cesium-137, iodine-125, yttrium-192, or cobalt-60 may be placed into a body cavity or orifice. The capsule may be a single tube of radioactive pins fixed in a tandem loader or a group of individual capsules, each of which contains one radioactive pin. Usually used to treat tumors in the cervix or endometrium of the uterus, a capsule is inserted via the vagina for treatment of the uterine body.

In a patient with cervical cancer, an instrument such as an Ernst applicator is used. A metal or plastic tube with radioactive pins is inserted in the uterus. Metal pins are used in conjunction with heat. The tube is attached to two vaginal ovoids, each of which contains a radioactive pin, that are placed in the cul-de-sac around the cervix. This type of application delivers the desired dosage in a pear-shaped volume of tissue, which includes the cervix, corpus, and tissue around the cervix but spares the bladder and rectum from high doses of radiation.

A blunt intracavitary applicator is used to position the parts. The applicator is held securely and remains fixed to ensure proper dosage to the tumor without injuring the normal surrounding structures. For stabilization, the surgeon may suture the applicator to the cervix, and vaginal packing also is used. Two different methods of application are used for inserting the radiation source: afterloading techniques and preloading techniques.

Afterloading Techniques Afterloading techniques afford the greatest safety for OR personnel. In the OR, a cold, unloaded, hollow plastic or metal applicator, such as the Fletcher afterloader, is inserted into or adjacent to the tissues that will receive radiation. After x-ray verification of correct placement, the radiation source is loaded into the applicator at the patient's bedside.

Preloading Techniques Preloading techniques require insertion of the "hot" radiation capsule in the OR by the surgeon. OR personnel should not be permitted in the OR during this procedure. To deliver a uniform dose to the desired area, the surgeon inserts an adjustable device designed to hold the radiation source in proper position in the tissues (e.g., the Ernst applicator). The bladder and rectum are held away from the area with packs to avoid undesired irradiation. To calculate the necessary dosage, the surgeon uses x-ray films of the pelvis to check the position of the radiation source and to measure its distance from critical sites.

All preparations for insertion are made by nursing team members before they leave the room. (They wait in the substerile room during insertion.) Preparations include setting the sterile table with vaginal packing, antibiotic cream for packing, radiopaque solutions for x-ray studies, and a basin of sterile water; placing the x-ray cassette on the operating bed and notifying the radiology technician; obtaining the radiation source; positioning the patient; and putting a radiation sheet on the patient's chart and a card on the stretcher.

Intracavitary Colloidal Suspensions

Sterile radioactive colloidal suspensions of gold or phosphorus are used as palliative therapy to limit the growth of metastatic tumors in the pleural or peritoneal cavities. Radioactive colloidal gold-198 is most commonly used; it has a half-life of 2.7 days. It may also be instilled within the bladder. The effect of these suspensions is caused by the emission of beta particles, which penetrate tissue so slightly that radioactivity is limited to the immediate area in which the colloidal suspension is placed. A trocar and cannula are introduced into the pleural or peritoneal cavity, and the colloidal suspension is injected through the cannula from a lead-shielded syringe. After use, these instruments are stored in a remote area until the decay of radioactivity is complete.

External Beam Radiation Therapy

Ionizing radiations of gamma or x-rays generated from machines are used externally to alter tumor cells within the body. This type of radiation therapy is noninvasive.

A maximum dose of radiation is concentrated on the malignant tumor below the skin, with a minimum dose to surrounding tissue. The angle of approach is changed a number of times during treatment to spread the amount of radiation to normal tissue over as wide an area as possible. Both orthovoltage equipment (low-voltage equipment that produces 200 to 500 kV) and megavoltage equipment (e.g., cobalt-60 beams and linear accelerators or betatrons) are used for external beam radiation therapy.

With some cancers, external radiation may be the only therapeutic modality used. It is difficult to determine the dosage of radiation that will provide the optimal cure with an acceptable balance of complications. With the advent of stereotactic techniques and the use of megavoltage equipment, intense rays can deliver cancericidal doses without permanently injuring normal tissue and causing skin irritation.

Even so, for many tumors most oncologists recommend a combination of radiation therapy and surgical resection; radiation therapy may be administered preoperatively and/or postoperatively or intraoperatively. External radiation therapy may also be combined with internal sources, such as intracavitary radiation capsules, to build up the dosage to large tumor areas.

Intraoperative Radiation Therapy

During a surgical procedure, a single high dose of radiation may be delivered directly to an intraabdominal or intrapelvic tumor or tumor bed to provide an additional palliative or localized means of control. Normal organs or tissues can be shielded from exposure. Radiation may also be used following resection of the bulk of the tumor.

An orthovoltage unit may be installed in a lead-lined OR for performing intraoperative radiation therapy. The sterile Lucite cone is placed directly over the tumor site. All team members leave the room during treatment. In some hospitals the patient is transported from the OR to the radiation therapy department. Following exposure to a megavoltage electron beam, the wound may be closed in the treatment area, or the patient may be returned to the OR for further surgery and/or wound closure. The open wound is covered with a sterile drape during transport, and sterile technique is used for closure.

Stereotactic Radiosurgery

Gamma knife technology was developed in Sweden in the early 1950s by surgeon Lars Leksell and Borge Larson, Ph.D. They experimented with guiding devices and proton beams. Cobalt-60 was found to be most effective in the treatment of brain tumors and was selected as the energy source for the gamma knife. In 1975, the device was used to treat brain tumors in humans.

With stereotactic radiosurgery, fiberglass fixation pins are used to apply a bone ring (the Leksell head frame) to the patient's head preoperatively. Two small rods are placed in the ear canals to stabilize the head frame during fixation. Care is taken not to injure the ear canal or tympanic membrane during this process. A calibrated ring is affixed to the frame to form X, Y, and Z coordinates to localize the brain lesion. The frame and ring sit within a larger helmet that aims the radiation at the tumor.

The gamma knife delivers highly concentrated doses of gamma rays to inoperable or deep-seated vascular malformations or brain tumors 1 cm^3 to 10 cm^3 in size. The localized area is determined by precision stereotaxis. The neurosurgeon places the patient's head, with the Leksell head frame and localizing ring, into the collimator helmet so that the focusing channels direct 201 pinpointed cobalt-60 beams to the tumor. (The radiation sources are housed in a large spherical chamber that is housed within a special room.) The patient is placed on a sliding bed that accommodates and aligns with the helmet as it enters the spherical chamber. The gamma knife process lasts 3 to 4 hours. During the procedure, the patient is in video and voice communication with the perioperative team. All personnel leave the room during treatment because of the intensity of the radiation and its cumulative effects.

Safety Rules for Handling Radiation Sources

The cardinal factors of protection from radiation sources are distance, time, and shielding. For both personnel and patients, the following principles of radiation safety apply to handling all types of radioactive materials:

1. The intensity of radiation varies inversely with the square of the distance from it—double the distance equals one quarter the intensity. Personnel should stay as far from the source as is feasible.
2. Radiation sources (e.g., needles, seeds, capsules, and suspensions) are prepared by personnel in the nuclear medicine department. Personnel prepare these sources behind a lead screen, and their hands are protected by lead-lined gloves, if possible, or special forceps during handling.
3. Radiation sources are transported in a long-handled lead carrier so they are as close to the floor and as far away from the body of the transporter as possible. The lead carrier should be stored away from personnel and patient traffic areas while it is in the OR suite.
4. When radiation sources are delivered to the OR, each needle, seed, or capsule is counted by the surgeon with the radiation therapist. This number is recorded.
5. Glutaraldehyde solution is poured into the lead carrier to completely submerge the radiation sources. When ready to use, the lead carrier is transported into the OR. The needles, seeds, or capsules are removed from the lead container with sterile, long-handled instruments and are rinsed thoroughly with sterile water.
6. All radiation sources are handled with special, long, ring-handled forceps from behind a lead protection shield. Never touch radiation sources with bare hands or gloves. Radiation sources are never handled with a crushing forceps because the seal of hollow containers can be broken. A groove-tipped forceps that is designed for this purpose is used.
7. Radiation sources are handled as quickly as possible to limit the time that personnel are exposed to radiation.
8. All radiation sources are accounted for before and after use, and any loss is immediately reported to the OR nurse manager. Do not remove anything from the room. To locate a lost radiation source, call a radiation therapist or nuclear medicine department technician to bring a Geiger counter. A Geiger counter has a radiation-sensitive gauge with an indicator that moves and a sound that increases when near radioactive substances.
9. A radiation documentation sheet is completed and put in the patient's chart. The surgeon fills in the amount and exact time of insertion and the time the source is to be removed. Each nurse who cares for the patient on the unit signs this sheet just before going off duty, thereby passing responsibility for checking the patient

and radiation source to the nurse who relieves. To check needles, the sutures attached to each needle are counted.
10. The patient's bed and door to the room are conspicuously labeled with a radiation-in-use card or symbol (Figure 23-1).
11. The radiation source is removed by the surgeon at the exact time indicated so the patient will not be overexposed.
12. Radiation is neither seen nor felt. Therefore be careful to observe the rules. Monitor and minimize exposure.

Figure 23-1 Universal symbol for radiation. Symbol is dark purple on a solid yellow background.

Box 23-4	Physiologic Effects of Radiation Therapy
External Beam	**Internal Implants**
Gastroenteritis	Bleeding tendency
Nausea and vomiting	Increased infections
Diarrhea	Sexual dysfunction
Menstrual irregularities	
Miscarriage	**Intracavitary Implants**
Sexual dysfunction	Bleeding
Fatigue	Infection
Cystitis	Sexual dysfunction
Erythema	
Skin desquamation	**Intraoperative Radiation**
Decreased circulation	Anorexia
	Nausea and vomiting

Effects of Radiation Therapy on the Perioperative Patient

The patient may be undergoing several treatment modalities and may experience the specific tissue and systemic effects of each. The perioperative nurse should understand how radiation affects the patient and how it affects the attainment of desired outcomes. The plan of care should include consideration for the potential side effects of radiation therapy. Box 23-4 describes the patient's responses to the physiologic effects of radiation.

CHEMOTHERAPY

Either alone or in combination, a variety of chemotherapeutic agents are capable of providing measurable palliative remission or regression of primary and metastatic disease, with a decrease in the size of the tumor and no new metastases. In some instances a complete response, with the disappearance of all clinical evidence of the tumor, is achieved.

The trend is toward earlier and greater use of adjuvant chemotherapy. More than one agent may be administered to enhance the action of another cytotoxic or antigenic substance. Adjuvant therapy is designed to maximize the benefits of each agent in the combination while avoiding overlapping toxicities. The following factors are important in determining the ability of tumor cells to respond to chemotherapy:

- *Size and location of the tumor.* The smaller the tumor, the easier it will be to reach cells. The mechanism for the passage of drugs into the brain differs from that for other body organs.
- *Type of tumor.* For example, cells of solid tumors in the lung, stomach, colon, and breast may be more resistant than cells in the lymphatic system.
- *Combinations of adjuvant therapy.* In select patients, chemotherapy may be used as an adjunct to all other types of therapy. Precise scheduling of dosages is necessary to attain effective results.
- *Specific biochemical requirements of the tumor.* Agents are selected according to the appropriateness of their structure and function. More than one agent is usually given.
- *State of life cycle of the cancer cells.* Cancer cells and normal cells go through the same life-cycle phases. An understanding of this phenomenon is necessary for understanding chemotherapy.

Cell Life Cycle

Deoxyribonucleic acid (DNA) is a double molecule in the cell nucleus; it contains the genetic code. DNA is capable of reproducing itself and of producing ribonucleic acid (RNA), which in turn synthesizes protein. Protein is essential for cellular function, and therefore DNA is vital to cell viability. It regulates the growth, mitosis, differentiation, specialization, and death of cells. Cell division requires the assimilation of nutrients in the cell, their incorporation into DNA, the synthesis of new DNA, and the splitting of DNA to form two new cells. RNA is synthesized in the rest intervals between phases of DNA replication. The duration of the rest interval is related to the proliferative activity of the tissue cells. Malignant tumor cells may proliferate more rapidly than normal cells.

Action of Chemotherapeutic Agents

Antineoplastic cytotoxic agents are destructive to rapidly dividing cells. Each dose kills only a fraction of the tumor cells present. The action of these agents takes place within the cell, but each agent acts differently to interrupt the life cycle of the cell. Antineoplastic agents are classified according to their structure and function. Cytotoxic action may be one of the following, and only a few of the many agents in use are mentioned as examples of each classification:

1. *Cell-cycle specific.* An agent may affect the cell during one or more phases and have no adverse effect during other phases. Some cytotoxic agents interfere with DNA synthesis, others inhibit mitosis when the cell is most susceptible, and still others prolong the rest intervals.
   a. Antimetabolites affect cells as they enter the DNA synthesis phase, thus interfering with RNA synthesis. This causes death of the cell by inhibiting the DNA cycle. Antimetabolites include floxuridine (FUDR), 5-fluorouracil (5-FU), and methotrexate.
   b. Mitotic inhibitors prevent cell division in a subphase of mitosis. These agents may be plant alkaloids such as vinblastine sulfate (Velban), vincristine sulfate (Oncovin), and paclitaxel (Taxol), or enzymes such as L-asparaginase (Elspar).
2. *Cell-cycle nonspecific.* These agents affect the cell throughout the entire life cycle. They have a more prolonged action that is independent of the phases of the life cycle.
   a. Alkylating agents denature or inhibit DNA to interfere with mitosis and synthesis, thereby preventing rapid cell growth. Alkylating agents include cyclophosphamide (Cytoxan), melphalan (L-phenylalanine mustard [L-PAM]), mechlorethamine hydrochloride (Mustargen), chlorambucil (Leukeran), and cisplatin (Platinol).
   b. Antibiotics bind with DNA to block RNA production, thus disrupting cellular metabolism. The antibiotics used as antineoplastic agents include dactinomycin (Cosmegen), bleomycin sulfate (Blenoxane), doxorubicin hydrochloride (Adriamycin), and daunorubicin hydrochloride (Cerubidine).

Indications for Chemotherapy

Patients who are at risk for or who have systemic signs of advanced or disseminated disease (generally indicated by extranodal involvement) may be candidates for preoperative or postoperative chemotherapy.

Preoperative Chemotherapy

The objective of preoperative chemotherapy may be to shrink the tumor sufficiently to permit surgical resection. Adjuvant radiation therapy may be used in combination with chemotherapy to increase tumor regression and necrosis. Agents may also eliminate subclinical microscopic metastatic disease.

Postoperative Chemotherapy

Surgical resection followed by regional chemotherapy often can control local disease to keep a tumor in remission. Residual metastatic disease may be treated with systemic chemotherapy to cure the patient or to prolong life. Multiple doses may be given over a long period (several months to a year or more) to delay or eliminate recurrence of the tumor.

Administration of Agents

The method of chemotherapy administration depends on the extent of dissemination or localization of the tumor cells and on the agent or combination of agents selected. Agents can be instilled locally into a target site by continuous infusion, injected intramuscularly or intrathecally, infused by intravenous push or drip, or ingested orally. A patient with widely disseminated metastatic disease usually receives systemic chemotherapy via the intravenous, intramuscular, or oral route. Agents may be infused regionally for patients whose tumor cannot be removed because of its location (e.g., a primary or metastatic tumor in the liver). The patient may come to the OR for insertion of an indwelling catheter or implantable infusion pump of the brain.

Infusion Catheters

An indwelling infusion catheter may be placed percutaneously or directly into a vein, artery, or body cavity. Continuous or intermittent infusion of the chemotherapeutic agent can be maintained by means of a portable infusion pump attached to the catheter, or the catheter may be used on an intermittent basis.

Central Venous Catheter Under local anesthesia, a long-term Hickman, Quinton, Groshong, or other central venous catheter is inserted percutaneously through a particular blood vessel and into the right atrium of the heart. The catheter also may be used for hyperalimentation. Varieties include single-, double-, and triple-lumen styles and require heparinized saline flushes between uses. Groshong catheters do not require heparinization and are available in single-, double-, and triple-lumen styles. Therefore the Groshong catheter can be used for patients with bleeding tendencies without the same risk associated with added heparinization. Sterile normal saline for injection is used to flush the line between uses.

Short-term subclavian catheters in double- and triple-lumen styles can be used for the administration of chemotherapeutic agents and total parenteral nutrition (TPN). These types of catheters require heparin flushes between uses.

Hepatic Artery Catheter Hepatic artery catheterization may be performed to establish regional chemotherapy to treat primary or metastatic disease of the liver. With the use of a local anesthetic, the catheter may be inserted percutaneously into the left axillary artery and threaded into the common hepatic artery. This technique eliminates the need for a laparotomy to cannulate the hepatic arteries. However, some patients have variant anatomy that requires a dual-catheter delivery system. Vascular reconstruction, ligation, and/or occlusion of an artery may be necessary for local/

regional perfusion. Regardless of the method of catheterization, an infusion pump is attached to the catheter(s) to deliver the cytotoxic agent to the tumor.

Intraperitoneal Catheter Intraperitoneal chemotherapy permits the delivery of high concentrations of an agent to an ovarian or colorectal tumor without exposing normal tissues systemically. With the use of a local anesthetic, a Tenckhoff catheter is inserted into the peritoneal cavity. An incision in the anterior abdominal wall is usually located just lateral to the right or left of the rectus abdominis muscle at the level of the umbilicus. The anterior rectus sheath is incised to allow a Verres needle to penetrate the peritoneum. To prevent the catheter from kinking, air is injected before the catheter is placed in the peritoneal cavity. A subcutaneous tunnel is made between the initial incision and stab wound to secure the catheter. A Dacron cuff is embedded in the subcutaneous tissue to anchor the catheter in place. The agent exits the peritoneal cavity via the portal circulation.

Infusion Devices

Devices with reservoirs for the chemotherapeutic agent are implanted into body tissues.

Subcutaneous Infusion Port With the use of a local anesthetic, a venous access device is implanted subcutaneously for continuous or intermittent injections of cytotoxic agent(s), TPN, or blood products. Depending on the manufacturer, the device consists of a plastic or silicone rubber self-sealing port on a plastic or stainless steel reservoir. The catheter attached to the reservoir is inserted into a central vein, hepatic artery, peritoneal cavity, or epidural space. A tunnel is created from the point at which the catheter enters the vessel, cavity, or space to a subcutaneous pocket. The pocket is made wherever necessary to stabilize the port. The reservoir is sutured to the underlying fascia. A Huber needle with an angled tip is used to enter the port for heparinizing and infusing agents. Extension tubing may connect the needle to an infusion pump for continuous infusion. After use, the port is flushed with 10 ml sterile normal saline followed by 3 to 10 ml heparinized saline (100 U/ml). Thrombosis and infection are potential complications of long-term venous access devices and catheters.

Implantable Infusion Pump With the patient under local, regional, or general anesthesia, an infusion catheter is placed into an artery, vein, body space, spine, or ventricle for localized chemotherapy to a tumor in the liver, head, neck, or brain. The infusion pump device is implanted in a subcutaneous pocket created in the abdominal wall, beneath the clavicle, or under the scalp. The titanium, stainless steel, and silicone rubber device resembles a hockey puck and delivers the agent by means of a bellows device (Infusaid) or by radio signals (Medtronic). The inner reservoir is filled with the cytotoxic agent. When the reservoir is collapsed by pressure, the agent is infused into the catheter. The pump is warmed initially to activate the fluorocarbon propellant in the chamber around the reservoir. It is placed over a bony prominence for support when refilling. The drug is replenished periodically by percutaneous injection. A bolus can be administered through a side port on the pump. These implanted infusion devices also are used to control severe systemic conditions such as diabetes, thromboembolic disease, or pain from a malignancy. Insulin, heparin, or morphine is infused, respectively.

Safe Handling of Agents

Antineoplastic cytotoxic agents have carcinogenic and mutagenic properties, and most can cause local and/or allergic reactions. During handling, personnel should avoid inadvertent inhalation and ingestion of these agents or direct contact with the skin or eyes. Written precautions and procedures for handling, preparing, administering, and disposing of cytotoxic agents are followed. Basic guidelines include the following:

1. Protect yourself from skin and respiratory contact. Prepare agents under a vertical laminar flow hood. Whether or not a containment hood is available, wear thick gloves, a mask, eye protection, and a gown.
2. Wash hands after handling agents and all items that have been in contact with them, including those used for administration.
3. Place all cytotoxic waste in sealed, leakproof bags or containers. Incineration is recommended for all materials used in preparing and administering cytotoxic agents.
4. Spills should be reported promptly to appropriate personnel who are trained in safety procedures. Material Safety Data Sheets (MSDSs) should be available for information about the chemical spilled and the procedures for cleanup. Eyewash stations should be immediately accessible in the event of a splash.

Side Effects

Cytotoxic agents are destructive to rapidly dividing cancer cells, but they also affect rapidly dividing normal cells such as hematopoietic cells of the bone marrow, epithelial cells of the oral cavity and gastrointestinal tract, and hair follicles. Patients should be informed of the toxic side effects they can expect from the specific agents they are receiving. Side effects can include the following:

1. *Alopecia.* Hair loss can occur suddenly or gradually, usually 10 to 21 days after treatment. This can be devastating to the patient's self-image. It is most often caused by the alkylating and plant alkaloid agents and by some antibiotics. A patient with thinning hair should be discouraged from using hair dryers or curling irons because the scalp may be irritated and easily burned. Hair grows back after therapy is discontinued.
2. *Bone marrow suppression.* Suppression of bone marrow function begins 7 to 14 days after treatment starts and is the most hazardous toxic effect of the cytotoxic

agents. Bone marrow can be harvested before treatment and readministered to the patient after the treatments are complete. Patient teaching should include instructions on avoiding infection. Therapy may need to be discontinued to allow bone marrow to recover. Bone marrow suppression increases the patient's susceptibility to the following:

   a. *Leukopenia.* With leukopenia, the white blood cell count is lower than normal. Leukocytes protect the body against the invasion of microorganisms. Therefore patients with leukopenia are highly vulnerable to the spread of infection from one part of body to another or to acquiring a nosocomial infection from the environment.

   b. *Thrombocytopenia.* With thrombocytopenia, the number of platelets in the blood decreases below normal, with variable consequences. Spontaneous hemorrhage into the skin, sclera, joints, or brain may occur. Normal blood clotting time can be prolonged. The patient should be instructed to consult his or her physician if any sign of bleeding, such as bruising, menorrhagia, or tarry stools, should occur. The patient may require a platelet transfusion.

3. *Anemia.* The patient may experience a decrease in circulating red blood cells, which results in decreased hemoglobin and hematocrit. The causes of anemia include red blood cell loss, a defect in red blood cell manufacturing, or red blood cell destruction in excess of production.
4. *Gastrointestinal disturbances.* Anorexia, nausea, vomiting, and/or diarrhea are common complaints. An antiemetic may be administered routinely 30 minutes before meals for several days after therapy begins. Usually these symptoms subside within a few hours or days after each dose is administered. Laboratory results should be observed for a decrease in the levels of total protein and albumin. Weight should be monitored every other day; any weight loss should be reported to the physician.
5. *Neurotoxicity.* Symptoms of neurotoxicity to plant alkaloids may begin with constipation. Toxicity can progress to impaired sensation, ataxia, and an unsteady gait. The effects are cumulative during the course of therapy and may be reversible when therapy is discontinued.
6. *Stomatitis.* Ulcerative lesions in the mouth and oropharynx may appear 5 to 7 days after the start of therapy and last up to 10 days. These lesions are signs of toxicity from antimetabolite and antibiotic agents. They can be very painful and may lead to a secondary infection.
7. *Vein hyperpigmentation.* A dark discoloration of a vein may occur over the length of the arm during prolonged infusion of some agents. A vesicular rash around the injection site may develop from the use of some other agents. Although unsightly, these effects are not uncomfortable for the patient.

8. *Extravasation.* The chemotherapeutic vesicant (blistering) or sclerosing (scarring) agent can escape from the IV catheter into the surrounding tissue. Damage may extend into the muscles, nerves, and tendons and cause neurologic effects or loss of function. Significant damage may cause tissue loss that requires debridement and/or grafting. The antidotes used include sodium thiosulfate 10%, ascorbic acid, sodium bicarbonate, hyaluronidase, and pyridoxine. Alternating heat and cold may be used for relief of symptoms associated with extravasation.

9. *Respiratory insufficiency.* Alveolitis, interstitial fibrosis, and other symptoms of respiratory insufficiency may include dyspnea, cough, fine or coarse crackles, and fever. Respiratory infection can disseminate rapidly as a result of bone marrow suppression and/or an altered immune system.

10. *Nephrotoxicity.* Agents excreted exclusively in urine (e.g., methotrexate and cisplatin) may be toxic to renal function. Adequate hydration and measurement of intake and output before administration is necessary to ensure urinary creatinine clearance. Other agents may cause hematuria.

IMMUNOTHERAPY

Immunotherapeutic agents stimulate or activate the body's own host defense immune system to combat disease. This is the same immune system that normally wards off the microorganisms that cause infection. Cancer may become clinically apparent only when the immune system ceases to function properly. The immune response may be defective or become compromised as the disease progresses. Immunosuppression can stimulate tumor growth and prolong wound healing. If the patient can be helped to regain partial or complete immunocompetence, the immune system can be utilized against tumor cells.

Attempts to treat cancer by immunization date back to 1895. However, it was not until 1957 that tumor-specific antigens were conclusively demonstrated in animals. Although intensive research has been conducted since that time, the applications of immunotherapy as a therapeutic modality remain selective and adjunctive. Active nonspecific immunotherapy, thought to be promising in the 1960s, was used to stimulate the production of antibodies and lymphocytes by injecting vaccines of bacille Calmette-Guérin (BCG, a bovine tubercle bacillus), methanol-extracted residue of BCG (MER), and *Corynebacterium parvum* (a gram-positive anaerobic bacillus). Further research led to the development in the 1980s of monoclonal antibodies for identifying tumor-associated antigens and the selective use of active specific immunotherapy and biologic response modifiers.

Types of Agents

The objective of immunotherapy is to augment, direct, and restore the body's immune functions. When the immune system detects antigens, such as tumor cells, it evokes an immune response to destroy them. This may be a humoral response of antibodies that occurs in blood and tissue fluid outside the cells, or it may be a cell-mediated immunity that occurs within or on the surface of cells. A cell-mediated reaction binds an antigen with an antigen receptor on the surface of T lymphocytes. T lymphocytes differentiate into antigen-specific killer cells, suppressor cells, helper cells, memory cells, and lymphokine-producing killer cells. Tumor-specific cytotoxic T cells can be generated from the lymphocytes of a tumor-bearing host or from syngeneic lymphocytes.

Active Specific Immunotherapy

Active tumor-specific cytotoxic T lymphocytes (CTLs) are obtained from lymphocytes in a removed tumor mass, such as from the kidney or spleen, or by the resection of melanoma or metastatic lymph nodes. A vaccine is produced from these CTLs. The vaccine also can be produced from peripheral blood lymphocytes used to generate CTLs for specific adoptive cellular immunotherapy. The vaccine of the specific tumor antigen stimulates the immune response by making antibodies that attack live cancer cells. A series of small doses of these vaccines are administered intradermally.

Biologic Response Modifiers

Biologic therapy is defined as a treatment that is derived from biologic sources that produce a biologic response in the patient. Biologic agents that have the potential to alter the patient's own reaction to tumor cells (i.e., biologic response modifiers) may be used as single agents or in conjunction with other therapy. Lymphokines are soluble protein molecules produced by sensitized T-helper lymphocytes in contact with specific antigens. Lymphokines enhance the body's immune response.

Interleukins Interleukin-1 through interleukin-7 (IL-1 through IL-7) are cytokines found in the body in small amounts. They can be cloned and are named for their amino acid sequences, and they help stimulate and regulate cellular immunity. They stimulate T lymphocytes to multiply and become activated. Lymphocytes activated with interleukins, known as lymphokine-activated killer (LAK) cells, preferentially lyse malignant cells.

By a recombinant process of DNA fusion, an optimal immunomodulating dose of IL-2 (a glycoprotein discovered in 1976) with LAK cells is produced. By leukopheresis, the patient's lymphocytes are collected by a blood cell separator. The IL-2 is extracted and fused with cells of *Escherichia coli*, which produce large quantities of IL-2 when they reproduce. This IL-2 is incubated to generate LAK cells before being prepared for reinfusion into the patient. The LAK cells seem to be tumor specific when reinfused in combination with recombinant IL-2. Clinical application includes the use of IL-2 in combination with other biologic modalities, such as monoclonal antibodies, with great success.

Interferon Interferon, a glycoprotein first isolated in 1957, directly interacts with T lymphocytes to stimulate the production of killer cells. It also directly inhibits the growth and division of tumor cells and stimulates antigens. Interferon can be produced from human donor blood, tissue culture, or a recombinant DNA process. Therapy supplements the body's natural supply of interferon.

Monoclonal Antibodies Monoclonal antibodies (MOABs) can be produced by hybridoma to react with specific antigens. Tumor cells are fused with antibody-producing cells (B lymphocytes) from the spleen of an immunized mouse. The cells that survive, called hybridomas, are cloned for the production of MOABs. MOABs are used for radioimmunoimaging to locate both primary and metastatic tumors. They may be given therapeutically for immunoconjugate therapy to target tumor cells.

Active Nonspecific Immunotherapy

Levamisole is a putative immunostimulant given to stimulate host defense. It may be administered alone or with a chemotherapeutic agent such as 5-FU as adjuvant therapy for colorectal cancer.

Advantages of Immunotherapy

Immunotherapeutic agents have a relatively weak killing capacity but no limitation on the types of cells they can destroy. They are highly specific and can destroy small numbers of tumor cells, but they are not effective against large numbers. They can regress or eradicate a small tumor mass or eliminate cells resistant to chemotherapy. Combining immunotherapeutic agents may accomplish what neither can do alone, either with or without surgical resection—delay the recurrence of cancer and prolong survival. An immunotherapeutic agent has the following characteristics:

- Attacks only cancer cells
- Does not damage normal cells
- Can be continued for long periods with fewer hazardous side effects than chemotherapy

HYPERTHERMIA

Hyperthermia at temperatures of 105.8° to 113° F (41° to 45° C) has a regressive tumoricidal effect, with the necrosis proportional to the thermal dose. Thermal energy inhibits DNA synthesis. Increasing the temperature of tumor cells sensitizes them to the effects of radiation therapy or chemotherapy; therefore for some tumors hyperthermia is used as an adjunct to these therapeutic modalities. Because drug action is greater at higher temperatures, the perfusate is warmed before the regional infusion of cytotoxic agents. The extremity also is warmed externally during regional perfusion. Systemic total-body hyperthermia may be applied externally by placing the patient on a hyperthermia blanket or mattress. Systemic hyperthermia can also be produced with extracorporeal circulation via a shunt placed in the thigh.

For localized palliative management of some solid tumors, a surface or interstitial hyperthermia device applies microwave energy. The temperature is measured by probes in target and surrounding normal tissue and is controlled by the computer adjustment of power. When tissue absorbs microwave radiation, energy converts into heat that dissipates by blood perfusion. Solid tumors with less blood perfusion dissipate heat slowly and hence retain heat longer than normal surrounding tissue.

FUTURE OF ONCOLOGY

As described in this chapter, many therapeutic modalities are used to treat cancer, and researchers are constantly seeking other modalities to improve survival rates and quality of life for patients with neoplasms. The complex nature of cancer makes adjuvant therapy and research a multidisciplinary effort. Early diagnosis, while the disease is still localized, is crucial for the selection of appropriate curative therapy. In poor-risk patients with extensive tumors and advanced disease, only palliative therapy may be possible.

Oncologists study the cause (epidemiology) of cancer, as well as the diagnosis, treatment, and rehabilitation of cancer patients. Moreover, patients are demanding that their surgeons give attention to the reconstruction of body image and rehabilitation to a useful life. Therefore the management of patients with cancer must be accomplished through the efforts of a multidisciplinary team of oncologic surgeons in conjunction with pathologists, radiation oncologists, pharmacists, immunologists, medical oncologists, and others. In addition to physical care, nurses in all patient care settings provide psychologic support for cancer patients and their families.

Bibliography

Bertolone K: Pediatric oncology: past, present, and new modalities of treatment, *J Intraven Nurs* 20(3):136-140, 1997.

Bloom JR: Early detection of cancer, *Cancer* 74(suppl 4):1464-1473, 1994.

Calzone KA: Genetic predisposition testing: clinical implications for oncology nurses, *Oncol Nurs Forum* 24(4):712-718, 1997.

Davis DL: Prostate cancer treatment with radioactive seed implantation, *AORN J* 68(1):18, 21-23, 26-30, 33-34, 37-40, 1998.

Engleking C: New approaches: innovations in cancer prevention, diagnosis, treatment, and support, *Oncol Nurs Forum* 21(1):62-71, 1994.

Larson SM et al: Overview of clinical radioimmunodetection of human tumors, *Cancer* 73(suppl 3):832-835, 1994.

Nag S et al: Comprehensive surgical radiation oncology, *AORN J* 60(1):27-37, 1994.

Page MS, Rabbitt JE: Issues in metastatic disease, *Crit Care Nurs Clin North Am* 7(1):143-149, 1995.

Pasacreta JV, Pickett M: Psychosocial aspects of palliative care, *Semin Oncol Nurs* 14(2):110-120, 1998.

Rieger PT: Emerging strategies in the management of cancer, *Oncol Nurs Forum* 24(4):728-737, 1997.

Rospond RM, Mills W: Hepatic artery chemoembolization therapy for hepatic tumors, *AORN J* 61(3):573-576, 1995.

Strohl RA: Radiation therapy in tumors of the central nervous system, *Semin Oncol Nurs* 14(1):26-33, 1998.

Wells NL, Balducci L: Geriatric oncology: medical and psychosocial perspectives, *Cancer Pract* 5(2):87-91, 1997.

White SK et al: Hyperthermic intraoperative intraperitoneal chemotherapy safety considerations, *AORN J* 63(4):716-718, 720-724, 1996.

Section

VIII

Anesthesia Concepts and Considerations

Chapter 24

General Anesthesia: Techniques and Agents

 Chapter Objectives

After studying this chapter, the learner will be able to:

- Identify three methods of general anesthesia.
- Describe the physiologic effects of general anesthesia.
- Discuss the purpose for cricoid pressure.
- List key points in providing safety for the anesthetized patient.

Anesthesiology is the branch of medicine that is concerned with the administration of medication or anesthetic agents to relieve pain and support physiologic functions during a surgical procedure. It is a specialty that requires knowledge of biochemistry, clinical pharmacology, cardiology, and respiratory physiology. The American Board of Anesthesiology has defined anesthesiology as the practice of medicine dealing with the management of procedures for rendering a patient insensible to pain during surgical procedures, and with the support of life functions under the stress of anesthetic and surgical manipulations.

Perioperative nurses and surgical technologists should be aware of the effects of general anesthesia on the patient. During several aspects of the administration and maintenance of the anesthetic process, the perioperative caregivers should be readily available to assist the anesthesia provider as needed. Continuing education is advised for the entire team. Internet Web sites included with links to educational information, such as Anesthesiology Village at **www.hp.com/go/anesthesia**,

are excellent resources. Common terms associated with the administration of anesthesia are found in Box 24-1.

HISTORICAL BACKGROUND

During the time of Nero (37 to 68 AD), Greek and Roman surgeons gave their patients a mixture of wine and vinegar. Called a "potion of the condemned," the mixture was used to relieve anguish such as that suffered during crucifixion. These surgeons also experimented with a form of local anesthesia by placing a carbonate stone directly over the surgical site and pouring vinegar over it; they noted a numbing sensation, resulting from the formation of carbon dioxide. Sleep-producing inhalants were first used by the Egyptians and Arabs, who concocted many potions from plants such as poppy and hemlock. Sponges saturated in these solutions were held to the patient's nostrils. Death often resulted from them and from root juices used as reviving agents because dosage was unregulated and drug action unknown. The Egyptians and Assyrians

Box 24-1

Terms Associated with Anesthesiology

amnesia   Loss of memory; an indifference to pain.

analgesic   Drug that relieves pain by altering perception of painful stimuli without producing loss of consciousness; acts on specific receptors in the nervous system.

anesthesia   Loss of feeling or sensation, especially loss of the sensation of pain with loss of protective reflexes.

anesthetic   Drug that produces local or general loss of sensibility.

anoxia   Absence of oxygen.

anticholinergic   Antagonist to action of parasympathetic and other cholinergic nerve fibers.

apnea   Suspension or cessation of breathing.

depolarization   Neutralization of polarity; reduction of differentials of ion distribution across polarized semipermeable membranes, as in nerve or muscle cells in the conduction of impulses; to make electrically negative.

dysrhythmia   Defective rhythm, as of heart rate or brain waves; may be used interchangeably with arrhythmia.

emergence   Return of sensation and reflexes; to regain consciousness following general anesthesia.

endotracheal   Within the trachea. An endotracheal tube may be placed in the trachea to maintain a patent airway during loss of consciousness.

   extubation   Removal of an endotracheal tube.

   intubation   Insertion of an endotracheal tube.

fasciculation   Incoordinate skeletal muscle contraction in which groups of muscle fibers innervated by the same neuron contract together.

general anesthesia   Reversible state of unconsciousness produced by anesthetic agents in which motor, sensory, mental, and reflex functions are lost.

hypercapnia   Excessive amount of carbon dioxide in the blood; may also be termed hypercarbia.

hypnotic   Drug or verbal suggestion that induces sleep.

hypothermia   State in which body temperature is lower than the physiologic normal (i.e., below 95° F [35° C]).

hypoxia, hypoxemia   Oxygen deficiency; state in which an inadequate amount of oxygen is available to or utilized by tissue; inadequate tissue oxygenation.

induction   Period from the beginning of administration of an anesthetic until the patient loses consciousness and is stabilized in the desired plane of anesthesia.

laryngospasm   Involuntary spasmodic reflex action that partially or completely closes the vocal cords of the larynx.

narcosis   State of arrested consciousness, sensation, motor activity, and reflex action produced by drugs.

narcotic   Drug derived from opium or opium-like compounds, with potent analgesic effects associated with significant alteration of mood and behavior.

Paco$_2$ Arterial carbon dioxide tension (partial pressure of carbon dioxide in arterial blood). Normal: 35 to 45 torr.

pain threshold   Individual's tolerance for pain. It may be influenced by factors such as anxiety.

Pao$_2$ Arterial oxygen tension (partial pressure of oxygen in the arterial blood); degree of oxygen transported in the circulating blood. Normal: 80 to 100 torr.

pH   Expression for hydrogen ion concentration or acidity. In blood, alkalemia: values above 7.45; acidemia: values below 7.35; normal: 7.4.

tachycardia   Excessive rapidity of heart action, heartbeat. Pulse rate is higher than 100 beats per minute.

tachypnea   Abnormally rapid rate of breathing.

---

produced unconsciousness by pressing on the carotid vessels in the neck, causing cerebral anoxia.

Army surgeons have always contributed to medical advancement. Ambroise Paré (1510-1590) dulled the pain of his soldiers in the sixteenth century by compressing blood vessels and nerves near the surgical area. At this time also, half-frozen soldiers were found to have a higher pain threshold. Refrigeration anesthesia was revived in 1941 for use in amputations during World War II.

Joseph Priestley (1733-1804), an English chemist, experimented with oxygen and nitrous oxide, setting the stage for modern anesthesia. This combination and ether were first used at parties for entertainment. Traveling chemists administered these agents to induce incoherence and giddy laughter, hence the term *laughing gas*. The anesthetic properties were realized when injuries sustained during inhalation of these agents were not felt.

Crawford Williamson Long (1850-1878), a physician in Georgia, administered the first ether anesthetic in 1842 for the painless removal of a tumor of the neck, but he did not publish the results of this and subsequent cases until 1849. In 1846, however, two Boston dentists, William T.G. Mor-

ton and Horace Wells, used nitrous oxide for tooth extraction. In October of that year, Morton first demonstrated ether for surgical anesthesia before an astounded group of clinicians; a new era in surgery was born. Oliver Wendell Holmes (1804-1894), an American physician, as well as professor of anatomy and literature, devised the term *anesthesia* from the Greek words meaning *negative sensation.*

Sir James Simpson (1811-1870), a Scottish obstetrician, instituted the use of chloroform anesthesia in 1847. In the late nineteenth and twentieth centuries surgical procedures within the abdomen, thorax, and cranium evolved with administration of ether and chloroform for anesthesia as demonstrated by John Snow (1813-1858), an English physician and epidemiologist. He administered chloroform to Queen Victoria during childbirth. Development of the surgical specialties was concurrent with the refinement of anesthesia methods and instrumentation.

Purification of drugs such as morphine, the invention of the hollow needle in the 1850s, and the development of gas machines hastened the finding of new anesthetic techniques and agents. Endotracheal anesthesia, first used by open tracheotomy, was developed by German physician Friedrich

Trendelenburg (1844-1924). The development of the laryngoscope by American laryngologist Chevalier Jackson (1865-1949) greatly aided intubation.

Methods for monitoring and supporting the patient's condition during anesthesia were developed by American surgeons George Crile (1864-1943) and Harvey Cushing (1869-1939). Studies on surgical shock and blood pressure emphasized the importance of keeping accurate records of the patient's condition during the surgical procedure. In 1896 Cushing brought to the United States from Italy one of the first sphygmomanometers invented and founded the basis for opioid administration during anociassociative (unconscious/unaware) anesthesia.

The use of muscle-paralyzing agents, such as curare in 1942 in Montreal, required the use of endotracheal intubation for safe administration. Education and qualifications of anesthesia providers included the complexities of respiratory physiology. Postanesthesia care units (PACUs) were developed to monitor the patient who had received general anesthesia. Special techniques such as hypothermia and extracorporeal circulation opened new vistas. Complex procedures lasting 6 to 24 hours are not uncommon using these techniques.

Salient features of modern anesthesia include assessment of patients preoperatively; selection of appropriate agents and techniques; management of induction, maintenance, and emergence processes; and continuous monitoring of vital functions during anesthesia. The American Society of Anesthesiologists (ASA), founded in 1905 and incorporated in 1936, and the American Association of Nurse Anesthetists (AANA), founded in 1931, have established guidelines and standards for safely administering and monitoring anesthesia care. ASA also developed the taxonomy for classifying patients by physical status from class I, the lowest risk, to class VI, the highest risk. Historically, specialists in anesthesia have been advocates of patient safety and risk management.

With the proliferation of pain clinics, anesthesia providers are essential members of multidisciplinary teams concerned with management of acute and chronic pain. Because of their familiarity with anesthetic drugs, nerve pathways, and nerve block techniques, anesthesia providers are well qualified to assess and treat pain.

PAIN

Pain is a perceptual phenomenon, a disturbed sensation causing suffering or distress. Physical pain is often what induces the patient to seek medical assistance. Realization of pain commences with stimulation of the nerve endings of pain fibers, which in turn produces a nerve impulse that travels to the brain. The impulse is processed and registered as an unpleasant sensation. The quality, intensity, location, duration, and memories of pain influence perception and emotional response to it..

Pain may be phasic, of short duration (e.g., from a needle stick), acute (e.g., postoperative from tissue trauma), or chronic (e.g., from disease). Any patient with trauma/tissue damage from a surgical procedure, ischemia from localized

tissue pressure, or an infarct from a localized area of ischemic tissue necrosis will experience pain. Understanding the anatomy and physiology of pain is necessary in order to assess and measure it and to attempt to relieve it. Discovery of the body's endogenous endorphins that bind to opiate receptors in the brain and spinal cord opened new horizons in understanding pain control. Pain is beyond the domain of a single specialty, but in the perioperative environment every effort is made to relieve the patient's awareness of pain.

The anesthesia provider uses many drugs and agents to safely produce analgesia and amnesia. Some surgeons use a preemptive approach to postoperative pain management in general anesthesia patients by injecting the incision line before incising with local anesthesia. The rationale for this involves prevention of the brain from recognizing neurologic signals from the incision of the skin. Other surgeons inject local anesthesia into the incision before closing to block the pain impulse from incised skin and tissue.

Pain is undoubtedly not purely organic or strictly functional; most pain also carries a psychogenic factor. An individual's tolerance for pain, his or her pain threshold, may be a reaction to stress, anxiety, fear, and/or external stimuli. Cultural traditions can influence expectations of pain and appropriate actions to deal with it.

PREANESTHESIA PREMEDICATION

Preanesthesia medication may be given to allay preoperative anxiety, produce some analgesia and amnesia, and dull awareness of the perioperative environment. Elevating the pH of gastric secretions and reducing the risk of nausea and vomiting also are desirable effects. An ideal preoperative medication has a quick onset, short duration of action, and minimal side effects. Some drugs decrease secretions in the respiratory tract, diminish vagal nerve effects on the heart, counteract undesirable side effects of the anesthetic, and raise the pain threshold. Preoperative medication constitutes to a greater or lesser extent a part of the overall anesthetic technique. Certain drugs may prolong the effect of the anesthetic and increase a respiratory-depressant effect.

The administration of an anesthetic actually begins with the giving of preanesthetic drugs as needed. A discerning choice can lead to smooth, effective anesthetic management and an uncomplicated postanesthetic course.

Choice of Drugs

Selection of drugs is made by the anesthesia provider based on an assessment of the patient's physical and emotional status, age, weight, medical and medication history, laboratory tests, and x-ray and electrocardiographic (ECG) findings; the demands of the surgical procedure; and the patient's concerns. If the patient is scheduled for local anesthesia, the surgeon may order minor preoperative sedatives if the patient is extremely apprehensive. In choosing premedication, the anesthesia provider tries to disturb respiration and circulation as little as possible. Since more than one pharmacologic response is desired, a combination of drugs is used. Most anesthesia providers prefer to have the patient arrive in the OR awake, free of apprehension, and fully cooperative. Drowsiness and lack of fear are not synonymous; for some patients relief from anxiety is attained only by dulling the consciousness.

Special Considerations

The patient's metabolic rate varies with age, body build, and general health. Heavy smokers, alcoholics, and patients who have problems involving hyperthyroidism, emotional instability, toxicity, or high fever have high metabolic rates and require more medication, oxygen, and anesthetic. A lower metabolic rate (e.g., as a result of a debilitating disease or hypothyroidism) requires a smaller dosage.

Patients with a history of substance abuse (e.g., alcohol, barbiturates, narcotics, or amphetamines) present special problems concerning premedication, anesthesia, and venipuncture. These patients may have contracted human immunodeficiency virus (HIV) infection or hepatitis. Heroin and cocaine abusers may be given an opiate for premedication. They must be closely observed for withdrawal symptoms, especially during and after prolonged procedures.

Drugs taken simultaneously or in close sequence may act independently, may interact to reduce or increase intended effects, or may produce an undesired reaction. The anesthesia provider queries the patient about allergies, previous drug intolerance or incidence of adverse reactions, and any family history of reactions, and carefully notes any medications the patient is currently taking. Minimal, if any, premedication is given to ambulatory surgery patients. A sedative and antiemetic may be given just before surgery. Drugs associated with prolonged physiologic effects are avoided if possible.

Time Given

Time is calculated to maximize the effect of premedication. Peak effect is desired at the time of induction. Premedication is usually given at least 45 minutes before induction; some drugs require 60 to 90 minutes to reach peak effect.

Drugs Used

Drugs may be given orally (PO) or intramuscularly (IM), often in combination to cause drowsiness, amnesia, analgesia, and narcosis and to control vagal reflexes. Their efficacy depends on the rate and extent of absorption, distribution in tissues, site of injection, degree of protein binding, and rapidity of detoxification and excretion. Drugs used for premedication include sedatives and tranquilizers, narcotics, anticholinergics, and antiemetics. The dosages indicated in this chapter are average for adult patients.

Sedatives and Tranquilizers

Sedation reduces the effect of anxiety. Amnesia helps to provide comfort. Sedatives and tranquilizers produce a calm, hypnotic state. Many drugs are available. Each has its advantages and side effects.

Benzodiazepines   Benzodiazepines produce excellent amnesia and mild sedation sufficient to reduce anxiety and fear. They cause an inhibitory effect on interneuronal transmission to sites in the central nervous system (CNS) associated with anxiety and fear. They are metabolized by the liver. Side effects are associated with overdosage. Adverse reactions are rare. Examples include the following:

- Diazepam (Valium); 5 to 10 mg PO is the usual dose for a 70-kg adult. It is metabolized by the liver.
- Lorazepam (Ativan); 2 to 4 mg PO is given for better amnesic effect than that achieved through the IM route. It has good antiemetic action and acts more quickly than diazepam.
- Midazolam (Versed); 0.05 to 0.1 mg/kg (2 to 3 mg) is given IM. It is short acting, metabolizing in 4 to 6 hours. Midazolam may cause respiratory depression and delayed metabolism. Dosage is highly individualized.

Barbiturates   Because barbiturates have a prolonged duration of action, they are seldom used for premedication on the day of the surgical procedure. They may be given orally for sleep the night before to help allay anxiety. Secobarbital (Seconal), pentobarbital (Nembutal), and phenobarbital have a hypnotic and sedative effect.

Narcotics

Narcotics produce analgesia by acting on opiate receptors in the CNS. They effectively raise the pain threshold and lower the metabolic rate, thus moderately decreasing the amount of anesthetic needed during the surgical procedure. They also decrease alveolar ventilation and depress respiration. They should not be given to patients with asthma or those with cardiopulmonary disease. Narcotics may cause circulatory depression and hypotension. They stimulate and constrict smooth muscles, sometimes causing nausea, vomiting, and urinary retention. Examples include the following:

- Morphine sulfate, a natural opiate (usually not given for premedication because of its prolonged duration of action, unless the patient is in pain); when used, the typical dosage is 0.1 to 0.15 mg/kg given 1 hour preoperatively. It is metabolized by the liver and excreted by the kidneys.
- Meperidine hydrochloride (Demerol), a synthetic opioid; 50 to 100 mg is given IM or subcutaneously (SQ) 30 to 90 minutes preoperatively for premedication. It is metabolized by the liver and is short acting with fewer side effects than morphine.
- Fentanyl (Sublimaze), a synthetic opioid; dosage for a 70-kg adult is 50 to 100 μg intravenously (IV) immediately before induction of general anesthesia. It is short acting with good analgesia and sedation. Fentanyl is metabolized by the liver and excreted by the kidneys.

Anticholinergics

Anticholinergics interfere with stimulation of the vagus nerve. They are useful in the prevention and treatment of reflex slowing of the heart, which may occur intraoperatively with stimulation of the carotid sinus, intrathoracic manipulation, or traction on the viscera or extraocular muscles. They are given preoperatively to prevent vagal-mediated hypotension, cardiac dysrhythmias, and bradycardia. They increase the heart rate. Anticholinergics are also bronchodilators and parasympathetic depressants. Because they inhibit mucus secretions, they may be given to decrease oral and respiratory secretions, causing the patient to complain of dry mouth. Examples include the following:

- Atropine sulfate may be given preoperatively for peripheral effects. The patient will experience dry mouth and blurred vision. The preoperative dose of 0.3 to 0.6 mg IM does not provide significant vagal blocking action but will decrease secretions. Supplemental doses may be given during the surgical procedure to reduce gastric acidity.
- Glycopyrrolate (Robinul) has an atropine-like effect with a longer duration of action. Dosage of 0.2 to 0.3 mg IM reduces volume and acidity of gastric secretions, thus elevating their pH. Because it does not cross the blood-brain barrier, it has less autonomic effect and causes less tachycardia than atropine.
- Scopolamine decreases secretions and provides some amnesia. Typical dosage is 0.3 to 0.6 mg IM or IV, 2 mg PO, or a transdermal patch. In combination with a narcotic, it may produce an altered state of consciousness, but it can also produce excitement, rage, and hallucinations.

Antiemetics

Some sedatives also have antiemetic effects to minimize nausea and vomiting. They may potentiate effects of narcotics. Usually they are used in combination with other drugs. Examples include the following:

- Promethazine hydrochloride (Phenergan), 0.7 mg/kg IM or 0.3 to 0.7 mg/kg IV. Sedation and side effects are secondary to interactions with other drugs on the CNS.
- Chlorpromazine hydrochloride (Thorazine), 25 to 50 mg IM or IV, or 10 to 25 mg PO.
- Prochlorperazine (Compazine), 5 to 10 mg PO, 5 to 10 mg IM, 2.5 to 10 mg IV.
- Hydroxyzine hydrochloride (Vistaril), 25 to 100 mg PO or IM, often with a narcotic. Hydroxyzine causes drowsiness. This antiemetic also has antihistaminic and anticholinergic actions that cause dry mouth.
- Droperidol (Inapsine), 0.005 to 0.175 mg/kg IV or 0.25 to 7.5 mg IM. Droperidol has good sedative and antiemetic action. It may cause hypotension and tachycardia.

TYPES OF ANESTHESIA

Anesthesia may be produced in a number of ways:

- *General anesthesia.* Pain is controlled by general insensibility. Basic elements include loss of consciousness, analgesia, interference with undesirable reflexes, and muscle relaxation.
- *Balanced anesthesia.* The properties of general anesthesia (i.e., hypnosis, analgesia, and muscle relaxation) are produced, in varying degrees, by a combination of agents. Each agent has a specific purpose. This often is referred to as neuroleptanesthesia.
- *Local or regional block anesthesia.* Pain is controlled without loss of consciousness. The sensory nerves in one area or region of the body are anesthetized. This is sometimes called conduction anesthesia. Acupuncture is sometimes used.
- *Spinal or epidural anesthesia.* Sensation of pain is blocked at a level below the diaphragm without loss of consciousness. The agent is injected in the spinal canal.

CHOICE OF ANESTHESIA

Selection of anesthesia is made by the anesthesia provider in consultation with the surgeon and the patient. The primary consideration with any anesthetic is that it should be associated with low morbidity and mortality. Choosing the safest agent and technique is a decision predicated on thorough knowledge, sound judgment, and evaluation of each individual situation. The anesthesia provider uses the lowest concentration of anesthetic agents compatible with patient analgesia, relaxation, and facilitation of the surgical procedure. An ideal anesthetic agent or technique suitable for all patients does not exist, but the one selected should include the following characteristics:

- Provide maximum safety for the patient
- Provide optimal operating conditions for the surgeon
- Provide patient comfort
- Have a low index of toxicity
- Provide potent, predictable analgesia extending into the postoperative period
- Produce adequate muscle relaxation
- Provide amnesia
- Have a rapid onset and easy reversibility
- Produce minimum side effects

The patient's ability to tolerate stress and adverse effects of anesthesia and the surgical procedure depend on respiration; circulation; and function of the liver, kidneys, endocrine system, and CNS. The following factors are important:

- Age and size/weight of the patient
- Physical, mental, and emotional status of the patient
- Presence of complicating systemic disease or concurrent drug therapy
- Presence of infection at the site of the surgical procedure
- Previous anesthesia experience
- Anticipated procedure
- Position required for the procedure
- Type and expected length of the procedure
- Local or systemic toxicity of the agent
- Expertise of the anesthesia provider
- Preference of the surgeon and patient

ANESTHETIC STATE

Both the central and the autonomic nervous systems play essential roles in clinical anesthesia. The CNS exerts powerful control throughout the body. The effect of anesthetic drugs is one of progressive depression of the CNS, beginning with the higher centers of the cerebral cortex and ending with the vital centers in the medulla. The cerebral cortex is not inactive during deep anesthesia. Afferent impulses continue to flow into the cortex along primary pathways and to excite cells in appropriate sensory areas. Also, the cerebral cortex is integrated with the reticular system. The brain represents approximately 2% of body weight but receives about 15% of cardiac output. Various factors cause alterations in cerebral blood flow and are of considerable importance in anesthesia. These factors are oxygen, carbon dioxide, temperature, arterial blood pressure, drugs, the age of the patient, anesthetic techniques, and neurogenic factors.

The autonomic nervous system is equally important because of its role in the physiology of the cardiovascular system, the anesthesia provider's ability to block certain autonomic pathways with local analgesic agents, specific blocking effects of certain drugs, and the sympathomimetic and parasympathomimetic effects of many anesthetic agents.

The anesthetic state involves control of motor, sensory, mental, and reflex functions. The anesthesia provider constantly assesses the patient's response to stimuli to evaluate specific anesthetic requirements. Specific drugs are used to achieve the desired results: amnesia, analgesia, and muscle relaxation.

KNOWLEDGE OF ANESTHETICS

Anesthesia involves the administration of potentially lethal drugs and gases. Interactions of these with human physiology can be profound. Using discerning observation, astute deduction, and meticulous attention to the minutiae, the anesthesia provider provides skilled induction, careful maintenance of anesthesia, and prophylaxis to avoid postoperative complications. Being responsible for vital functions of the patient, the anesthesia provider must know physical and chemical properties of all gases and liquids used in anesthesia. These properties determine how agents are supplied, their stability, systems used for their administration, and their uptake and distribution in the body. Important factors are diffusion, solubility in body fluids, and relationships of pressure, volume, and temperature. The synthesized general anesthetic agents are nonflammable, in contrast to the older agents.

Perioperative and PACU nurses need to be cognizant of the pharmacologic characteristics of the most commonly used anesthetics. Anesthesia and surgical trauma produce multiple systemic effects, which are continually monitored.

GENERAL ANESTHESIA

Anesthesia is produced as the CNS is affected. Association pathways are broken in the cerebral cortex to produce more or less complete lack of sensory perception and motor discharge. Unconsciousness is produced when blood circulating to the brain contains an adequate amount of the anesthetic agent. General anesthesia results in an unconscious, immobile, quiet patient who does not recall the surgical procedure.

Most anesthetic agents are potentially lethal. The anesthesia provider must constantly observe the body's reflex responses to stimuli and other guides to determine the degree of CNS, respiratory, and circulatory depression during induction and the surgical procedure. No one clinical sign can be used as a reliable indication of anesthesia depth. Continuous watching and appraisal of all clinical signs, in addition to other available objective measurements, are necessary. In this way the anesthesia provider judges the level of anesthesia, referred to as light, moderate, or deep, and provides the patient with optimal care (Table 24-1).

TABLE 24-1	**Depth of General Anesthesia**		
From	**To**	**Patient's Responses**	**Patient Care Considerations**
Induction of general anesthesia and beginning of inhalant and/or IV drug	Begins to lose consciousness; will have recall. Bispectral state 100	Drowsy, dizzy, amnesic	Close OR doors. Keep room quiet. Stand by to assist. Initiate cricoid pressure if requested.
Loss of consciousness: excitement phase	Relaxation, light hypnosis; low probability of recall. Bispectral state 70 to 50	May be excited with irregular breathing and movements of extremities; susceptible to external stimuli (e.g., noise, touch)	Restrain patient. Remain at patient's side, quietly, but ready to assist anesthesia provider as needed.
Surgical anesthesia stage of relaxation	Loss of reflexes: depression of vital functions. Bispectral state 40: maintenance range	Regular respiration; contracted pupils; reflexes disappear; muscles relax; auditory sensation lost	Position patient and prepare skin only when anesthesia provider indicates this stage is reached and under control.
Danger stage: vital functions too depressed	Respiratory failure; possible cardiac arrest. Bispectral state 0	Not breathing; little or no pulse or heartbeat	Prepare for cardiopulmonary resuscitation.

The three methods of administering general anesthesia are inhalation, IV injection, and rectal instillation. The latter method is obsolete, except occasionally in pediatrics, because absorption in the colon is unpredictable. Control of each method varies.

Induction of General Anesthesia

Induction involves putting the patient safely to sleep (i.e., into a state of unconsciousness). A patent airway and adequate ventilation must be ensured. If one is not already running, an IV infusion is started. The anesthesia provider should wear gloves for venipuncture. A nasogastric tube may be inserted to evacuate stomach contents.

Preoxygenation

The anesthesia provider may have the patient breathe pure (100%) oxygen by face mask for a few minutes. This provides a margin of safety in the event of airway obstruction or apnea during induction, with resultant hypoxia.

Loss of Consciousness

Unconsciousness is induced by IV administration of a drug or by inhalation of an agent mixed with oxygen. Because the technique is rapid and simple, an IV drug usually is preferred by anesthesia providers and often is requested by patients.

Barbiturates Ultrashort-acting barbiturates given IV in small dosages offer a rapid, pleasant induction within 30 seconds. They provide marked sedation and amnesia. Because excessive secretions in the respiratory passage predispose the patient to coughing or laryngospasm, he or she should be asked to clear air passages as necessary before injection of the drug. Also, minor laryngeal or pharyngeal stimulation of the head and neck, such as during airway insertion, can precipitate coughing and laryngospasm. The most commonly used barbiturates are thiopental sodium (Pentothal Sodium), methohexital sodium (Brevital), and sodium thiamylal (Surital).

Benzodiazepines Benzodiazepines are not as predictable and are slower acting than barbiturates, but they cause less hypotension, bradycardia, and respiratory depression. Their sedative effects facilitate awake intubation. The most commonly used IV benzodiazepines are diazepam (Valium) and midazolam (Versed).

Etomidate (Amidate) An ultrashort-acting IV hypnotic agent can be given for induction of general anesthesia or, in smaller amounts, for maintenance with nitrous oxide for short procedures. Like thiopental, etomidate has no analgesic activity. Its main advantage is the relative absence of cardiopulmonary effects. This drug has little or no effect on cardiac output, peripheral or pulmonary circulation, or myocardial metabolism. Pain on injection and myoclonic muscle movements can occur. But when etomidate is administered in combination with a narcotic, skeletal muscle contractions are reduced. Laryngospasm, coughing, and hiccups can occur during induction.

Etomidate is useful for patients who are sensitive to other induction agents because it does not seem to cause histamine release. Its use is contraindicated in children under 10 years of age and in obstetric procedures, including cesarean section.

Intubation

A patent airway must be established to provide adequate oxygenation and to control breathing of the unconscious patient. The patient's tongue and secretions can obstruct respiration in the absence of protective reflexes. An oropharyngeal airway, laryngeal mask, or endotracheal tube may be inserted.

Intubation is insertion of an endotracheal tube between vocal cords, usually with an oral tube by direct laryngoscopy. A nasal tube may be inserted by blind intubation or with a lightwand to aid in positioning the tube in the posterior oropharynx. Tubes may be made of metal, plastic, silicone, or rubber. Most styles for adult sizes have a built-in cuff that is inflated with a measured amount of air, water, or saline after insertion to completely occlude the trachea. The anesthesia provider is informed if a laser will be used in the mouth or throat so that a laser-resistant endotracheal tube can be inserted. The endotracheal tube must be securely fixed in place to prevent irritation of the trachea and to maintain ventilation. The anesthesia provider should wear a mask and protective eyewear to prevent secretions from splashing in the eyes during intubation. An oropharyngeal suction tip and tubing should be kept close at hand.

Neuromuscular blocking agents are given before intubation to relax the jaw and larynx. Pediatric patients and patients susceptible to malignant hyperthermia may experience jaw tightness, which is referred to as masseter muscle rigidity (MMR) or trismus. Intubation during induction and extubation during emergence from anesthesia are precarious times for the patient. The patient may cough, jerk, or experience laryngospasm from tracheal stimulation. Hypoxia commonly precedes dysrhythmia. Cardiac dysrhythmias may occur. Hypoxia is a potential complication.

Aspiration is also a hazard, particularly in a patient with a full stomach or with increased intraabdominal or intracranial pressure. Any patient who arrives in the operating room (OR) unconscious or who is a victim of trauma should be treated as though he or she has a full stomach. Pregnant patients and obese patients should also be considered in this category because of increased intraabdominal pressure in the supine position and possible decreased gastric motility.

Cricoid Pressure The circulator may be asked to apply pressure to the cricoid cartilage to occlude the esophagus and immobilize the trachea. Referred to as Sellick's maneuver, this action prevents regurgitation and aspiration of stomach contents. The cricoid cartilage forms a complete ring around the inferior wall of the larynx below the thyroid cartilage prominence. Exerting pressure with one or two fingers to compress the cricoid cartilage against the body of the sixth cervical vertebra obstructs the esophagus (Figure 24-1). Compression must begin with the patient awake before

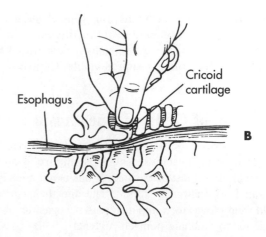

Figure 24-1   Cricoid pressure. **A,** Index finger displaces cricoid cartilage posteriorly, thus obstructing esophagus. **B,** Two-finger technique obstructs esophagus between body of sixth cervical vertebra and cricoid cartilage.

induction drugs are injected. It must continue until the endotracheal tube cuff is inflated and the anesthesia provider states that it is safe to release pressure.

Awake Intubation   Based on preoperative physical assessment, the anesthesia provider may determine that intubation must be performed before the induction of general anesthesia. Acromegaly, an anterior larynx, an enlarged tongue, a limited oral cavity, jaw fixation, a short neck, or limited cervical range of motion are the most common indications for awake intubation. These conditions may inhibit visualization of the vocal cords by direct laryngoscopy and thus increase the potential risk of airway obstruction in the absence of protective reflexes, such as following the induction of anesthesia. Most awake intubation is performed with a fiberoptic laryngoscope for direct visualization of vocal cords after the administration of IV sedation and application of a topical spray anesthetic to the posterior pharynx. The anesthesia provider may inject a local anesthetic around the laryngeal nerve to suppress the patient's gag and cough reflex. Usually two anesthesia providers work together during awake intubation. After the patient is sedated and the topical anesthetic agent is applied, one anesthesia provider inserts the endotracheal or nasotracheal tube as the second anesthesia provider gives a rapid-acting barbiturate to induce general anesthesia.

Key Points During Induction

Induction of general anesthesia is a crucial period requiring maximum attention from the OR team. The following key points are critical to the patient's welfare:

1. The perioperative nurse should remain at the patient's side during induction to provide physical protection and emotional support, assist the anesthesia provider as needed, and closely observe the monitors.
2. Although induction is quiet and uneventful for most patients, untoward occurrences are possible. Excitement, coughing, breath holding, retching, vomiting, ir-

regular respiratory patterns, or laryngospasm can lead to hypoxia. Secretions in air passages, from irritation by the anesthetic, can cause obstruction and dysrhythmias. Induction is gentle and not so rapid as to cause physiologic insult. To prevent these events, avoidance of stimulation of the patient is necessary. (Avoid venting steam from the sterilizer in the adjacent substerile room, clattering instruments, or opening paper wrappers. Do not move or begin prepping the patient until the anesthesia provider says it is safe to do so.)
3. Precautions to be taken during induction include continuous ECG monitoring, use of a precordial chest stethoscope, and having resuscitative equipment, including a defibrillator, readily available.
4. Induction is individualized. For example, an obese or pregnant patient may be induced with the head raised slightly to avoid pressure of the abdominal viscera against the diaphragm. The patient is placed flat, however, if the blood pressure begins to drop.
5. Small children need gentle handling. The perioperative nurse can help the anesthesia provider in making the induction period less frightening by staying close to the child. Sometimes a drop of artificial flavoring (e.g., orange, peppermint) put inside the face mask facilitates the child's acceptance of it. Parents are often allowed in for induction according to the institution's policy. After induction, the parent is escorted back to the waiting area.
6. The speed of induction depends on the potency of the agent, administration technique, partial pressure administered, and the rate at which the anesthetic is taken up by blood and tissues.

Maintenance of General Anesthesia

The anesthesia provider attempts to maintain the lightest level of anesthesia in the brain compatible with operating conditions. The following are five objectives of general anesthesia:

1. *Oxygenation.* Tissues, especially the brain, must be continuously perfused with oxygenated blood. The color of the blood, amount and kind of bleeding, and pulse oximetry are indicators of the adequacy of oxygenation. Controls on the anesthesia machine and monitors of vital functions keep the anesthesia provider aware of the patient's condition.

2. *Unconsciousness.* The patient remains asleep and unaware of the environment during the surgical procedure.

3. *Analgesia.* The patient must be free of pain during the surgical procedure.

4. *Muscle relaxation.* Muscle relaxation must be constantly assessed to provide necessary amounts of drugs that cause skeletal muscles to relax. Less tissue manipulation is required when muscles are relaxed.

5. *Control of autonomic reflexes.* Anesthetic agents affect cardiovascular and respiratory systems. Tissue manipulations and systemic reactions to them may be altered by drugs that control the autonomic nervous system.

Anesthesia Machine

General anesthesia is maintained by inhalation of gases and IV injection of drugs. An anesthesia machine is always used to deliver oxygen-anesthetic mixtures to the patient through a breathing system.

The anesthesia machine includes sources of oxygen and gases with flowmeters for measuring and controlling their delivery; devices to volatilize and deliver liquid anesthetics; a gas-driven mechanical ventilator; devices for monitoring the ECG, blood pressure, inspired oxygen, and end-tidal carbon dioxide; and alarm systems to signal apnea or disconnection of the breathing circuit. Breathing tubes of corrugated rubber or plastic carry gases from the machine to the face mask and breathing system. The reservoir (breathing) bag compensates for variations in respiratory demand and permits assisted or controlled ventilation by manual or mechanical compression of the bag. Sterile disposable sets containing tubing, a mask, a Y-connector, and a reservoir bag are commercially available in conductive and nonconductive materials.

Machine design includes fail-safe alarm systems to prevent delivery of a hypoxic gas mixture and to reduce the possibility of human error or mechanical failure. Reference to a daily machine performance checklist by the anesthesia provider before induction should be routine as recommended by the Food and Drug Administration (FDA) in 1986. Studies have shown that many complications associated with the administration of anesthesia could have been avoided if the equipment had been checked before use.

All anesthesia machines have the following features (Figure 24-2):

1. Sources of oxygen and compressed gases. These may come from piped-in systems, but mounted oxygen tanks are necessary in the event of failure of systems.

2. Means for measuring (flowmeters) and controlling (reservoir bag) delivery of gases.

3. Means to volatilize liquid (vaporizer) and deliver (breathing tubes) anesthetic vapor or gas.

Figure 24-2 Anesthesia machine for maintenance of general anesthesia. *1,* Anesthetic and respiratory gas monitor; *2,* physiologic monitor (channels include ECG, blood pressure, temperature, heart rate, and pulse oximeter); *3,* flow-through vaporizers; *4,* face mask; *5,* reservoir "breathing" bag; *6,* carbon dioxide absorber canister; *7,* patient breathing circuit; *8,* ventilator; *9,* flowmeters for gases; *10,* sphygmomanometer for manual blood pressure.

4. Device for disposal of carbon dioxide (carbon dioxide absorption canister).

5. Safety devices:
   a. Oxygen analyzers
   b. Oxygen pressure interlock system or equivalent to automatically shut off the flow of gases in the absence of oxygen pressure
   c. End-tidal carbon dioxide monitors
   d. Pressure and disconnect alarms to notify the anesthesia provider if the flow of oxygen and gases becomes disproportional
   e. Pin-index safety system to release excess gases
   f. Gas scavenger system to collect exhaled gases

Waste Gases The elimination of waste gas, vented through an exhaust valve into a waste gas scavenger system, controls pollution of the room air. Nitrous oxide and halogenated agents can escape into room air if they are not directed through the scavenger system. Substantial amounts may be an occupational health hazard to OR team members. Valves on the machine and tubing connections should be checked daily and must be secure for the system to work properly. Room air should be monitored. This may be done by an infrared spectrophotometer, for example, to monitor the escape of gases from the patient's exhalations and from the anesthetic delivery system. Passive dosimeters may be used to monitor air in team members' personal breathing spaces.

Trachea

Figure 24-3 Laryngeal mask.

Inhalation Systems

The method for administration of inhalation anesthetics through the anesthesia machine can be classified as semiclosed, closed, semiopen, or open:

- *Semiclosed system.* The most widely used system, a semiclosed system permits exhaled gases to pass into the atmosphere so that they will not mix with fresh gases and be rebreathed. A chemical absorber for carbon dioxide is placed in the breathing circuit. This reduces carbon dioxide accumulation in blood. Induction is slower but with less loss of heat and water vapor than with open methods.
- *Closed system.* A closed system allows complete rebreathing of expired gases. Exhaled carbon dioxide is absorbed by soda lime or a mixture of barium and calcium hydroxide (Baralyme) in the absorber on the machine. The body's metabolic demand for oxygen is met by adding oxygen to the inspired mixture of gases or vapors. This system provides maximal conservation of heat and moisture. It reduces the amount and therefore the cost of agents and reduces environmental contamination.
- *Semiopen system.* With the semiopen system some exhaled gas can pass into surrounding air but some returns to the inspiratory part of the circuit for rebreathing. The degree of rebreathing is determined by the volume of flow of fresh gas. Expired carbon dioxide is not chemically absorbed.
- *Open system.* In an open system, valves direct expired gases into the lower portion of the canister, where it is removed by vacuum. The patient inhales only the anesthetic mixture delivered by the anesthesia machine. The composition of the inspired mixture can be accurately determined. However, anesthetic gases are not confined to the breathing system. High flows of gases are necessary because resistance to breathing varies. Water vapor and heat are lost. Inspired gases should be humidified for respiratory mucosa to function properly, especially for children and during long surgical procedures.

Administration Techniques

Inhalation gases and vapors can be delivered from an anesthesia machine via a face mask, laryngeal mask, or endotracheal tube. Respirations must be assisted or controlled.

Mask Inhalation Anesthetic gas or vapor of a volatile liquid is inhaled through a face mask attached to the anesthesia machine by breathing tubes. The mask must fit the face tightly to minimize escape of gases into room air. Significant leakage occurs around an ill-fitting mask, particularly in the area above the nose. Several sizes should be available.

Laryngeal Mask An airway can be maintained by inserting a laryngeal mask into the larynx. This flexible tube has an inflatable silicone ring and cuff. When the cuff is inflated, the mask fills the space around and behind the larynx to form a seal between the tube and the trachea. Reusable and disposable styles are commercially available (Figure 24-3).

Endotracheal Administration Anesthetic vapor or gas is inhaled directly into the trachea through a nasal or oral tube inserted between the vocal cords by direct laryngoscopy. The tube is securely fixed in place to minimize tissue trauma. The patient is given oxygen before and after suctioning of a tracheal tube.

Advantages of endotracheal administration are the following:

1. It ensures a patent airway and control of respiration. Secretions are easily removed from the trachea by suctioning. Positive pressure can be given immediately by

pressing the reservoir bag on the machine without danger of dilating the stomach.

2. It protects the lungs from aspiration of blood, vomitus of gastric contents, or foreign material.
3. It preserves the airway regardless of the patient's position during the surgical procedure.
4. It interferes minimally with the surgical field during head and neck procedures.
5. It helps minimize the escape of vapors or gases into the room atmosphere.

Intubation and extubation can cause tracheal stimulation. The patient may cough, jerk, or develop spasms of the larynx (laryngospasm). Other potential complications of endotracheal administration include the following:

- *Trauma to the teeth, pharynx, vocal cords, or trachea.* Postoperatively the patient may experience sore throat, hoarseness, laryngitis, and/or tracheitis. Laryngeal edema is more common in children than in adults. Ulceration of the tracheal mucosa or vocal cords may cause granuloma.
- *Cardiac dysrhythmias.* Cardiac dysrhythmias may occur in light anesthesia or be caused by suctioning through the endotracheal tube.
- *Hypoxia and hypoxemia.* Hypoxia is a common complication during intubation and extubation. Endotracheal tube suctioning can cause hypoxemia.
- *Accidental esophageal or endobronchial intubation.* The latter results in ventilation of only one lung.
- *Aspiration of gastrointestinal contents.* This is a hazard in a patient with a full stomach or a patient who has increased intraabdominal or intracranial pressure. It can also occur in a patient with intestinal obstruction who is extubated before protective reflexes return.
- *Tracheal collapse.* This may follow extubation.

Controlled Respiration Respirations may be assisted or controlled. Assistance, to improve ventilation, may easily be given by manual pressure on the reservoir (breathing) bag of the anesthesia machine. Assisted respiration implies that the patient's own respiratory effort initiates the cycle. Controlled respiration may be defined as the completely controlled rate and volume of respirations. The latter is best accomplished by means of a mechanical device that automatically and rhythmically inflates the lungs with intermittent positive pressure, requiring no effort by the patient. Gas moves in and out of the lungs. The combination of a volume preset ventilator with an assist mechanism maintains the integrity of the respiratory center. Controlled respiration is initiated after the anesthesia provider has produced apnea by hyperventilation or administration of respiratory depressant drugs or a neuromuscular blocker.

Controlled ventilation is used in all types of surgical procedures, especially in lengthy ones. The anesthesia provider's artificial control of respiration or the patient's respiratory efforts influence the minute-to-minute level of anesthesia. Advantages of controlled respiration are the following:

1. It provides for optimal ventilation.
2. It puts the diaphragm at rest for thoracic procedures.
3. It provides access to deep regions of the thorax and upper abdomen.
4. It permits deliberate production of apnea to facilitate surgical manipulation below the diaphragm, ligation of deep vessels, or the taking of x-ray films.

The patient is taken off the respirator gradually near the end of the surgical procedure, and spontaneous respiration resumes. Assisted ventilation may be continued postoperatively after lengthy procedures until reflexes and spontaneous respirations return.

Inhalation Anesthetic Agents

Inhalation is the most controllable method of administration because uptake and elimination of anesthetic agents are accomplished mainly by pulmonary ventilation. The lungs act as avenues of entrance and escape, although the agents are metabolized in the body in varying degrees. The anesthetic vapor of a volatile liquid or an anesthetic gas is inhaled and carried into the bloodstream by passing across the alveolar membrane into the general circulation and on to the tissues. Ventilation and pulmonary circulation are two critical factors involved in the process. Each can be affected by components of the anesthetic experience, such as a change in body position, preanesthetic medication, alteration in body temperature, or respiratory gas tensions.

In inhalation anesthesia the aim is to establish balance between the content of the anesthetic vapor or gas inhaled and that of body tissues. The blood and lungs function as the transport system. Anesthesia is produced by the development of an anesthetizing concentration of anesthetic in the brain. The depth of anesthesia is related to concentration and biotransformation (see Table 24-1).

Pulmonary blood-gas exchange is important to tissue perfusion. Defective gas exchange can cause hypoxemia and respiratory failure. It also interferes with delivery of the anesthetic. Potent inhalation agents, such as myocardial depressants, affect oxygenation. Most of them induce a dose-related hypoventilation. The deeper the anesthesia, the more depressed ventilation becomes. Surgical stimulation partially corrects depression, but respiration must be controlled to keep oxygen and carbon dioxide exchange constant to prevent hypoventilation and cardiac depression.

Although the respiratory system is employed for distribution of the anesthetic, it also must carry on its normal function of ventilation (i.e., meeting tissue demands for adequate oxygenation and elimination of carbon dioxide and helping to maintain normal acid-base balance). The amount of anesthetic vapor inspired is influenced by the volume and rate of respirations. Gas or vapor concentration and the rate of delivery are also significant. Pulmonary circulation is the vehicle for oxygen and anesthetic transport to the general circulation. The large absorptive surface of the lungs and their extensive microcirculation provide a large gas-exchanging surface. In optimal gas exchange, all alveoli share inspired gas and cardiac output equally (ventilation-perfusion match).

Because respiratory and anesthetic gases interact with pulmonary circulation, alveolar anesthetic concentrations are rapidly reflected in circulating blood.

Alveolar concentration results from a balance between two forces: ventilation that delivers the anesthetic to the alveoli and uptake that removes the anesthetic from the alveoli. Certain factors influence uptake of the anesthetic and thus induction and recovery. Uptake has the following two phases:

1. *Transfer of anesthetic from alveoli to blood.* The rate of transfer is determined by the solubility of the agent in the blood, the rate of pulmonary blood flow (related to cardiac output), and the partial pressure of the anesthetic in arterial and mixed venous blood.
2. *Transfer of anesthetic from blood to tissues.* Factors influencing uptake by individual tissues are similar to those for uptake by blood. They are the solubility of the gas in tissues, the tissue volume relative to the blood flow (flow rate), and the partial pressure of the anesthetic in arterial blood and tissues. Tissues differ; thus uptake of the anesthetic differs. Highly perfused tissues (heart) equilibrate more rapidly with arterial tension than poorly perfused tissue (fat), which has a slow rise to equilibrium and retains anesthetic longer.

Elimination of the anesthetic is affected by the same factors that affected uptake. As an anesthetic is eliminated, its partial pressure in arterial blood drops first, followed by that in tissues.

The most important factors influencing safe administration of any anesthetic are the knowledge and skill of the anesthesia provider. A perfect agent has not been found, and no agent is entirely safe. Commonly used agents are listed in Table 24-2. Advantages and disadvantages are relative.

Synthesis of potent, nonflammable, halogenated, volatile liquids has replaced cyclopropane and ether, which are highly flammable agents. All inhalation agents are administered with oxygen. Volatile liquids are vaporized for inhalation by oxygen, which acts as a carrier, flowing over or bubbling through liquid in the vaporizer on the anesthesia machine. The oxygen picks up 0.25% to 5% concentration of the halogenated agent. Known sensitivity to halogenated agents or a history significant for the risk of malignant hyperthermia are contraindications for their use.

Nitrous Oxide
Usually used as an adjunct to an IV drug, nitrous oxide gas can be inhaled for a comfortable, rapid induction. It has a pleasant, fruitlike odor and is administered by face mask. Relaxation is poor. Excitement and laryngospasm may occur. It is the only gas in use for anesthesia.

ADVANTAGES When used in combination with other forms of inhalants and IV drugs, excessive depth of anesthesia is avoided. Nitrous oxide is rapidly cleared from the circulation. The incidence of nausea and vomiting is minimal. The gas has a rapid uptake and elimination and few aftereffects except headache, vertigo, and drowsiness. It causes minimal physiologic change; adverse effects can be quickly reversed. It is an excellent analgesic for procedures not producing severe pain.

DISADVANTAGES Nitrous oxide can cause bowel distention and increased volume in other air pockets. The use of nitrous oxide can cause displacement of tympanoplasty grafts or increase intracranial pressure. It should not be used during laparoscopy. There is no muscle relaxation. There is possible excitement or laryngospasm. Hypoxia is a hazard. There is a depressant effect on myocardial contractility.

USE Because it lacks potency, nitrous oxide is rarely used alone but rather as an adjunct to barbiturates, narcotics, and other IV drugs. In combination, the concentration of potent drug is reduced, thereby lessening circulatory and respiratory depression. Because exposure can be an occupational hazard for personnel, measures are taken to minimize levels of nitrous oxide in room air.

Halothane (Fluothane)
A widely used halogenated hydrocarbon, halothane reduces myocardial oxygen consumption more than it depresses cardiac function.

ADVANTAGES Halothane is nonflammable, potent, versatile, chemically stable, and rapid, and it has a smooth induction. High potency makes possible the use of high concentrations of oxygen for adequate ventilation. The depth of anesthesia can be rapidly altered. There is little excitement. It permits early intubation because of minimal laryngeal irritation. Spontaneous ventricular dysrhythmias are rare if anoxia and respiratory acidosis are avoided. Halothane is useful for patients with bronchial asthma because it induces bronchodilation and is nonirritating to the respiratory tract.

DISADVANTAGES Halothane is potentially toxic to the liver. It is progressively depressant to respiration. It is especially depressant to the cardiovascular system, causing hypotension, bradycardia, and, in rare cases, cardiac arrest. It sensitizes the myocardial conduction system to catecholamines; epinephrine should be avoided. It may cause dysrhythmias in the presence of aminophylline. It raises intracranial pressure. There is limited relaxation of the abdominal muscles (necessitating muscle relaxants). Halothane has a profound effect on body temperature control; it may cause hypothermia. It exerts undesirable effects on rubber, some metals, and plastics. It is highly soluble in rubber and is retained in it during prolonged administration. Complete elimination of halothane takes some time.

USE Halothane is used in a wide spectrum of all types of surgical procedures for adults and children except routine obstetrics, where uterine relaxation is not desired. It is a profound uterine relaxant. Because its metabolites have a possible effect as a hepatotoxin, some anesthesia providers avoid repeated administration within an arbitrary time (e.g., a 3-month period) in adults. Recent jaundice and known or suspected liver disease (past or present) are usually contraindications to its use.

Enflurane (Ethrane)
A widely used, nonflammable, stable, halogenated ether, enflurane is similar in potency and versatility to halothane.

ADVANTAGES Enflurane has a rapid induction and recovery with minimal aftereffects. Pharyngeal and laryngeal reflexes are obtunded easily, salivation is not stimulated, and

TABLE 24-2	Most Commonly Used General Anesthetic Agents			
Generic Name	**Trade Name**	**Administration**	**Characteristics**	**Uses**
Inhalation Agents				
Nitrous oxide	—	Inhalation	Inorganic gas; slight potency; pleasant fruitlike odor; nonirritating; non-flammable but supports combustion; poor muscle relaxation	Rapid induction and recovery; short procedures when muscle relaxation unimportant; adjunct to potent agents
Halothane	Fluothane	Inhalation	Halogenated volatile liquid; potent; pleasant odor; nonirritating; cardio-vascular and respiratory depressant; incomplete muscle relaxation; po-tentially toxic to liver	Rapid induction; wide spectrum for maintenance; depth of anesthe-sia easily altered; rapid reversal
Enflurane	Ethrane	Inhalation	Halogenated ether; potent; some mus-cle relaxation; respiratory depressant	Rapid induction and recovery; wide spectrum for maintenance
Isoflurane	Forane	Inhalation	Halogenated methyl ether; potent; mus-cle relaxant; profound respiratory depressant; metabolized in liver	Rapid induction and recovery with minimal aftereffects; wide spec-trum for maintenance
Intravenous Agents				
Thiopental sodium	Pentothal sodium	Intravenous	Barbiturate; potent; short acting with cumulative effect; rapid uptake by circulatory system; no muscle relax-ation; respiratory depressant	Rapid induction and recovery; short procedures when muscle relaxation not needed; basal anesthetic
Methohexital sodiuim	Brevital	Intravenous	Barbiturate; potent; circulatory and respiratory depressant	Rapid induction; brief anesthesia
Propofol	Diprivan	Intravenous	Alkylphenol; potent short-acting sedative-hypnotic; cardiovascular depressant	Rapid induction and recovery; short procedures alone; prolonged anesthesia in combination with inhalation agents or opioids
Ketamine hydrochloride	Ketaject, Ketalar	Intravenous, intramuscular	Dissociative drug; profound amnesia and analgesia; may cause psycho-logic problems during emergence	Rapid induction; short procedures when muscle relaxation not needed; children and young adults
Fentanyl	Sublimaze	Intravenous	Opioid; potent narcotic; metabolizes slowly; respiratory depressant	High-dose narcotic anesthesia in combination with oxygen
Sufentanil citrate	Sufenta	Intravenous	Opioid; potent narcotic, respiratory depressant	Premedication; high-dose narcotic anesthesia in combination with oxygen
Fentanyl and droperidol	Innovar	Intravenous	Combination narcotic and tranquilizer; potent; long acting	Neuroleptanalgesia
Diazepam	Valium	Intravenous, intramuscular	Benzodiazepine; tranquilizer; produces amnesia, sedation, and muscle relaxation	Premedication; awake intubation; induction
Midazolam	Versed	Intravenous, intramuscular	Benzodiazepine; sedative; short-acting amnesic; central nervous system and respiratory depressant	Premedication; conscious sedation; induction in children

bronchomotor tone is not affected. The cardiac rate and rhythm remain relatively stable, although caution is advised when it is used with epinephrine. Muscle relaxation is produced, but small supplementary doses of muscle relaxants may be re-quired; nondepolarizing relaxants are potentiated by enflurane.

DISADVANTAGES Enflurane has a pungent odor. Respira-tion and blood pressure are progressively depressed with deepening anesthesia. Although biotransformation (metabo-lism) of enflurane is less than what occurs with other halo-genated agents, small amounts of fluoride ion are released. Severe renal disease is a contraindication to use. At deeper

levels an electroencephalographic (EEG) pattern resembling seizures may occur. The agent is absorbed by rubber.

USE Enflurane is used in a wide spectrum of procedures.

Isoflurane (Forane)

Of the potent halogenated agents, isoflurane comes closer to ideal than other inhalation agents. Isoflurane is a nonflammable, fluorinated, halo-genated methyl ether similar to halothane and enflurane yet different. It is a more potent muscle relaxant, but, unlike the others, it protects the heart against catecholamine-induced dysrhythmia. Heart rhythm is remarkably stable. The blood pressure drops with induction but returns to normal with intraoperative stimulation. A dose-related lowering of the blood pressure occurs, but cardiac output is unaltered, mainly as a result of increased heart rate. Isoflurane potentiates all commonly used muscle relaxants, the most profound effect occurring with the nondepolarizing type.

ADVANTAGES There is less cardiac depression; there is increased cardiac output with a wide margin of cardiovascular safety. Isoflurane does not sensitize the myocardium to the effects of epinephrine. There are no CNS excitatory effects. There is rapid induction and, especially, rapid recovery with minimal aftereffects (less postoperative nausea and confusion). Isoflurane is innocuous to organs; it has low organ toxicity because of its low blood solubility and minimal susceptibility to biodegradation and metabolism. It provides superb muscle relaxation. Pharyngeal and laryngeal reflexes are easily obtunded. Isoflurane depresses bronchoconstriction; it may be used in patients with asthma and patients with chronic obstructive pulmonary disease.

DISADVANTAGES Isoflurane is expensive. It is a profound respiratory depressant and reduces respiratory minute volume. Respirations must be closely monitored and supported. Assisted or controlled ventilation is used to prevent respiratory acidosis. In the absence of intraoperative stimulation, the blood pressure may drop as a result of peripheral vasodilation. Cerebral vascular resistance decreases, cerebral blood flow increases, and intracranial pressure rises but is reversible with hyperventilation. Secretions are weakly stimulated.

USE Isoflurane is used for induction and maintenance in a wide spectrum of procedures except routine obstetrics. Isoflurane produces uterine relaxation. Safety to the mother and fetus has not been established. Because the drug is metabolized in the liver, it may be given to patients with minimal renal disease.

Desflurane (Suprane)
A nonflammable, halogenated liquid with low solubility, desflurane has faster uptake by inhalation and elimination than halothane and isoflurane.

ADVANTAGES There is rapid emergence and recovery from anesthesia. Desflurane resists biotransformation (metabolism) and degradation; it produces few urinary metabolites. The dosage of nondepolarizing muscle relaxants to maintain neuromuscular blockade may be reduced.

DISADVANTAGES Desflurane has a pungent odor that may be irritating during induction. Increasing alveolar concentration may lower the blood pressure, which may be corrected by reducing the inspired concentration. Hemodynamic effects, including an elevated heart rate, preclude use of desflurane by itself in a patient with cardiovascular disease; it may be combined with IV opioids or benzodiazepines.

USE Desflurane is used in induction and maintenance of anesthesia in adults. It may be used for maintenance in infants and children, but it is not used for induction because of its potential for causing coughing and laryngospasm. Because it has a high vapor pressure, desflurane is delivered only through a vaporizer specifically designed for this agent. Desflurane vaporizers require electrical power to heat the liquid. It works well for ambulatory surgery patients.

Methoxyflurane (Penthrane)
A partially halogenated methyl ether, methoxyflurane is the most potent inhalation agent, but it is rarely used. Its high solubility makes induction slow and prolongs recovery. Its disadvantages outweigh its advantages.

ADVANTAGES It provides excellent muscle relaxation and good analgesia.

DISADVANTAGES It is a depressant to the cardiovascular and respiratory systems. Renal and hepatic toxicity are potential complications. Nausea and vomiting, headache, hypotension, and delirium may accompany recovery.

USE Use of methoxyflurane is limited to low concentration for short duration or for analgesia in combination with nitrous oxide.

Intravenous Anesthetic Agents

IV anesthesia became popular with the introduction in the 1930s of rapidly acting barbiturates. A drug that produces hypnosis, sedation, amnesia, and/or analgesia is injected directly into the circulation, usually via a peripheral vein in the arm. Diluted by blood in the heart and the lungs, the drug passes in high concentration to the brain, heart, liver, and kidneys, the organs of highest blood flow. Concentration in the brain is rapid. With recirculation, redistribution occurs in the body, decreasing cerebral concentration. Dissipation of effects depends on redistribution and biotransformation. Because removal of drug from the circulation is impossible, safety in use is related to metabolism. It is advisable for the anesthesia provider to give a small test dose at induction.

Oxygen is always given during IV anesthesia. A barbiturate, dissociative agent, or narcotic may be given (see Table 24-2). Each has advantages, disadvantages, and contraindications. They may be supplemented with other drugs.

Barbiturates
Thiobarbituric acid derivatives are commonly used, but they do not produce relief from pain, only marked sedation, amnesia, and hypnosis. Repeated administration has a cumulative, prolonged effect. Thiopental sodium (Pentothal Sodium), methohexital sodium (Brevital), and sodium thiamylal (Surital) must be supplemented with other drugs to produce analgesia and relaxation during the surgical procedure. They are excellent, rapid induction agents.

ADVANTAGES Barbiturates are nonirritating to the mucous membranes of the trachea or bronchi; they do not stimulate salivation. Recovery is rapid, but with possible excitement. Nausea and vomiting are rare.

DISADVANTAGES Administration of large doses can cause rapid, pronounced respiratory and circulatory depression; small, divided doses are well tolerated, with rapid uptake. Respiratory depression may be marked immediately following injection. Barbiturates can produce hypotension. The range of CNS depression is from mild sedation to coma or cardiac arrest.

USE Barbiturates are most commonly used for induction before administration of more potent agents, such as inhalants. They may be used as a basal anesthetic for short procedures not requiring relaxation. They are used for control of convulsions in patients with increased intracranial pressure; as an adjunct to spinal, nitrous oxide, and antimuscarinic drugs; and for hypnosis during regional anesthesia.

CONTRAINDICATIONS Caution is necessary for patients with bronchial asthma, acute or chronic respiratory infections, or porphyria. IV barbiturates are not appropriate for patients with small, superficial veins. Because solutions are highly alkaline, they are always administered via tubing of an IV infusion. Extravasation can cause thrombophlebitis, nerve injury, or tissue necrosis.

Intraarterial injection is avoided. Inadvertent intraarterial injection is evidenced by sudden excruciating pain that requires immediate treatment to prevent a chemical endarteritis with tissue destruction. Arterial spasm and ischemia must be counteracted to prevent gangrene of fingers. Treatment is with intraarterial injection of lidocaine (10 ml of 0.5% solution), which dilutes the barbiturate solution; local heparinization via the arterial needle to prevent arterial thrombosis; and stellate ganglion block or general anesthesia with halothane to promote vasodilation. For extravasation, 5 to 10 ml of 0.5% lidocaine injected into the involved area dilutes the barbiturate to prevent vasoconstriction.

Propofol (Diprivan)

A short-acting alkylphenol, propofol is a sedative-hypnotic that produces anesthesia. It is used for rapid induction and maintenance of anesthesia for short procedures. It can also be used in combination with inhalation agents or opioids for prolonged anesthesia. Propofol is supplied in a sterile milky, soybean oil–in–water emulsion. In low doses it produces sedation (i.e., drowsiness and decreased responsiveness). Continued IV administration leads to hypnosis and unconsciousness. Propofol is twice as potent as thiopental sodium.

ADVANTAGES Propofol is rapidly distributed, metabolized, and eliminated. Emergence is very rapid, with few postoperative side effects.

DISADVANTAGES Propofol produces dose-related cardiorespiratory depression. Cardiovascular depressant action will decrease the blood pressure. Its hypotensive effect is potentiated by narcotics. The solution supports rapid growth of microorganisms if the infusion pump or syringes become contaminated. Moderate to severe pain may be felt at the injection site in the small vein of the hand or forearm; the larger antecubital vein should be used, or the site injected with lidocaine.

USE Propofol is used for general anesthesia for ambulatory surgery patients and for maintenance of sedation during local and regional anesthesia. It is acceptable for patients who are allergic to barbiturates or who have porphyria.

CONTRAINDICATIONS Propofol is used with caution in geriatric, debilitated, and hypovolemic patients. It is not recommended for pediatrics, obstetrics, and some neurosurgical procedures.

Ketamine Hydrochloride (Ketalar, Ketaject)

General anesthesia may be produced by a phencyclidine derivative to produce a state referred to as dissociative anesthesia. The drug acts by selectively interrupting associative pathways of the brain before producing sensory blockage. This permits a surgical procedure on a patient who appears to be awake (i.e., eyes are open and may move) but who is anesthetized (i.e., unaware and amnesic). Ketamine may be given IV or IM to yield profound analgesia. It is swiftly metabolized. Individual response varies, depending on the dose, route of administration, and age. Because of a dose-response relationship, careful patient selection and dose selection are important. Ketamine is used alone or with nitrous oxide.

ADVANTAGES Ketamine has a rapid induction. Respirations are not depressed unless the drug is administered too rapidly or in too large a dose. A mild stimulant action on the cardiovascular system may elevate the blood pressure. The effects of ketamine are potentiated by narcotics and barbiturates.

DISADVANTAGES Psychologic manifestations (e.g., delirium, vivid imagery, hallucinations, and unpleasant dreams) may occur during emergence. These can be reduced by giving preanesthetic diazepam and by allowing the patient to lie quietly, undisturbed during recovery except for essential procedures. Reactions are more common in adults than in children. IV thiopental sodium or diazepam may be given to treat emergence delirium.

USE Ketamine is used mainly in children between the ages of 2 and 10 years and in young adults under 30, for short procedures not requiring skeletal muscle relaxation, for plastic and eye procedures when combined with local agents, for diagnostic procedures, as an induction agent before other general agents are used, and to supplement nitrous oxide when adequate respiratory exchange is maintained. For longer procedures repeated doses are given that may prolong recovery time. If relaxation is needed, muscle relaxants and controlled ventilation are indicated.

Low-dose ketamine (1 mg/kg) has been used as an induction agent for obstetric procedures because of rapid onset, intense analgesia and amnesia, and minimal fetal effects. With its cardiovascular-stimulating properties, it is useful in hypovolemic and hypotensive patients, allowing the use of high oxygen concentration, both in obstetric and trauma procedures.

CONTRAINDICATIONS Ketamine is contraindicated in procedures involving tracheobronchial stimulation because pharyngeal and laryngeal reflexes are usually active. If the drug is used alone, mechanical stimulation of the pharynx should be avoided. Other contraindications include hypertension, increased intracranial pressure, intraocular procedures, and previous cerebrovascular accident because this agent increases cerebrospinal fluid and intraocular pressure.

High-Dose Narcotics

Historically, natural opiates and synthetic opioids have been given to produce analgesia and sedation preoperatively and postoperatively. In addition, they are used intraoperatively as supplemental agents and/or in combination with oxygen for complete anesthesia for short procedures and in patients with little cardiovascular reserve. Cardiovascular depression must be avoided in these patients. Halogenated agents are contraindicated in patients with liver and renal disease and malignant hyperthermia risk.

The most popular narcotics for general anesthesia are the opioids fentanyl (Sublimaze), sufentanil citrate (Sufenta), alfentanil (Alfenta), and meperidine hydrochloride (Demerol), and the opiate morphine sulfate. Although they are analgesics, to reliably achieve anesthesia, markedly larger doses of narcotics are needed (e.g., 10 to 30 times as much morphine [3 to 8 or more mg/kg body weight]). High doses of fentanyl range from 50 to 100 μg/kg body weight. The drugs may be given in bolus doses or continuously via IV infusion. Surprisingly, side effects seem to occur less frequently as the potency of narcotics increases. They reduce adverse physiologic responses to the stress of the surgical procedure, such as increased work of the heart, potential dysrhythmia, sodium and water retention, and increased blood glucose levels. Narcotics produce a dose-related respiratory depression. The respiratory effects of narcotics are as follows:

- Reduction of responsiveness of the CNS respiratory centers to carbon dioxide (less stimulation)
- Impairment of respiratory reflexes and alteration of rhythmicity (prolonged inspiration, delayed expiration)
- Reduction in the respiratory rate before reduction in the tidal volume
- Production of bronchoconstriction (morphine, meperidine) or rigidity of the chest wall (fentanyl)
- Impairment of ciliary motion

Factors that influence narcotic respiratory actions include age, pain, sleep, urinary output, other drugs, intestinal reabsorption, and disease.

The neurophysical state obtained by use of large doses of narcotics is not the same as "the general anesthesia state" resulting from use of volatile inhalation agents such as halothane. Narcotics are more selective in action. Narcotics do not produce muscle relaxation. Conversely, they cause an increase in muscle tone. Neuromuscular blocking agents can block or treat this action or rigidity.

Following high-dose narcotic anesthesia, patients are awake and pain free, with adequate though not good ventilation. These patients need careful monitoring by a well-trained PACU staff because narcotization after large doses of narcotics can occur rapidly in an apparently awake and responsive patient. The patient can hypoventilate, become hypoxic, and stop breathing when intraoperative stimuli cease. The vital signs, pupils, and skin color must be monitored. Clinical signs of narcotic toxicity are pinpoint pupils, depressed respiration, and reduced consciousness. A narcotic antagonist (see Narcotic Agonists-Antagonists) is given to reverse narcotic-induced hypoventilation. The potential for delayed toxicity following IM injection of narcotics, as opposed to IV administration, exists because absorption from muscle mass may be irregular.

Adjunctive Drugs

Many drugs are used to supplement nitrous oxide, halogenated inhalation agents, and IV drugs to maintain amnesia and analgesia, control hypertension, attenuate the extent of postoperative respiratory depression, or maintain or control other effects of general anesthesia. These drugs must be carefully controlled to avoid adverse drug interactions. For example, morphine sulfate and nitrous oxide have a synergistic action with thiopental sodium (i.e., when they are given together, each potentiates the action of the other). Therefore they are given concomitantly with caution because of their combined respiratory depressant effect.

Some drugs are given preoperatively, during induction, and/or intraoperatively. Adjunctive drugs are used primarily for analgesia and amnesia or to counteract side effects of anesthesia. Some are particularly useful for ambulatory surgery patients because they are short acting.

Morphine Sulfate   An opiate narcotic, morphine produces analgesia for pain relief without loss of motor, sensory, or sympathetic functions. Amnesia is incomplete (i.e., sporadic episodes of awareness may occur). Cardiovascular stability is good, but a significant dose-related vasodilatory effect can increase intraoperative blood loss. Respiratory depression is the most serious side effect; pulmonary blood volume is decreased, and pulmonary artery blood pressure is increased. Morphine may be given by IM, IV, epidural, or intrathecal injection. The duration of action varies with the route of administration.

Fentanyl (Sublimaze)   An opioid narcotic, fentanyl produces analgesia. It is 70 times more potent than morphine. It has minimal cardiac effects and is not associated with venous dilation. Although it has a short duration of action, it becomes concentrated in well-perfused tissue, such as in the brain. It metabolizes slowly, with possible consequent respiratory depression and chest wall rigidity. It may be given in bolus, incrementally, or as a continuous IV infusion.

Sufentanil Citrate (Sufenta)   An opioid narcotic, sufentanil produces analgesia/anesthesia and effectively reduces anxiety. It is 5 times more potent than fentanyl and 625 times more potent than morphine. Sufentanil does not depress the myocardium or change vascular resistance. It is short acting because the onset of action is immediate, accumulation is limited, and elimination is rapid. It can cause respiratory depression and skeletal muscle rigidity. It is given IV or epidurally.

Alfentanil (Alfenta)   An opioid narcotic, alfentanil is a rapid and short-acting analgesic. Respiratory depression outlasts analgesia. It is given IV by bolus or continuous infusion.

Meperidine Hydrochloride (Demerol)   An opioid narcotic, meperidine produces analgesia. It causes myocardial depression and tachycardia as a result of peripheral vasodilation. It causes bronchoconstriction but has fewer undesirable side effects than morphine. Meperidine is 1000 times less potent than fentanyl and sufentanil. Commonly used for premedication and postoperative pain relief, meperidine is available in a liquid preparation that may be useful when an oral medication is preferred (e.g., in children). It is usually given IM or IV.

Hydromorphone Hydrochloride (Dilaudid)

An opioid narcotic analgesic, hydromorphone has a rapid onset and shorter duration than morphine but is 8 to 10 times more potent. It has less hypnotic quality and causes less nausea and vomiting. Hydromorphone suppresses coughing and may cause respiratory depression. It is not used in children.

Narcotic Agonists-Antagonists An agonist combines with receptors, such as the opiate receptors, to initiate drug actions. An antagonist neutralizes or impedes the action of another drug (i.e., reverses its effects). For example, narcotics produce a dose-related respiratory depression that can be reversed by opiate antagonists. These drugs are given IV, IM, or SQ.

NALOXONE HYDROCHLORIDE (NARCAN) A specific narcotic antagonist, naloxone reverses respiratory depression caused by narcotics. It has no respiratory or circulatory action of its own in the presence or absence of a narcotic or other agonist-antagonist. Complications can include hypertension and tachycardia if naloxone is combined with opioids.

NALBUPHINE HYDROCHLORIDE (NUBAIN) A narcotic agonist-antagonist, nalbuphine is a potent analgesic. It has limited respiratory and cardiovascular effects.

BUTORPHANOL TARTRATE (STADOL) A narcotic agonist-antagonist, butorphanol is an analgesic. It produces dose-related respiratory depression and some hemodynamic changes in the cardiovascular system.

PENTAZOCINE HYDROCHLORIDE (TALWIN) A weak narcotic antagonist, pentazocine is a potent analgesic and mild sedative. It does not completely reverse cardiovascular and respiratory depression induced by narcotics.

BUPRENORPHINE HYDROCHLORIDE (BUPRENEX) A narcotic antagonist, buprenorphine is an analgesic with a high affinity for opiate receptors. It has slight respiratory and circulatory depressant action.

Droperidol (Inapsine)

A tranquilizer, droperidol produces sedation. It may be used to prevent nausea and vomiting. It is a CNS depressant. It may be given IM or IV.

Diazepam (Valium)

A sedative, diazepam produces amnesia, sedation, and muscle relaxation. It can lower the body temperature when given preoperatively. When used for induction, it causes less hypotension and bradycardia than thiopental sodium but is slower acting. Its sedative effect facilitates awake intubation. It may extend CNS depression and somnolence during emergence, especially in geriatric patients. Diazepam may be given PO, IM, or IV.

Midazolam (Versed)

A sedative, midazolam is given IV or deep IM for its short-acting amnesic effect. It is a CNS and respiratory depressant. This depression can be significantly prolonged in geriatric patients, the obese, and patients with liver dysfunction. For pediatric surgery it may

be given orally or rectally preoperatively for a smooth induction of general anesthesia and a less eventful emergence postoperatively. Since its introduction in 1986, it has rapidly replaced diazepam as the drug of choice for IV conscious sedation.

Flumazenil (Romazicon) A benzodiazepine antagonist, flumazenil may be used for complete or partial reversal of the sedative effects of diazepam or midazolam after anesthesia. An initial dose is given IV, followed by additional doses IV every 30 to 60 seconds until consciousness is restored. The effect peaks 6 to 10 minutes after injection.

Muscle Relaxants

Skeletal muscle relaxant drugs, referred to as neuromuscular blockers, facilitate muscle relaxation for smoother endotracheal intubation and working conditions during the surgical procedure. Their use has eliminated the need for deep inhalation anesthesia to produce relaxation. Administered IV in small amounts at intervals, they interfere with the passage of impulses from motor nerves to skeletal muscles. They act primarily at autonomic receptor sites, the neuromuscular junction, and at prejunctional and postjunctional acetylcholine-binding sites, causing paralysis of variable duration. They also can affect transmission of impulses at preganglionic and postganglionic endings in the autonomic nervous system. Neuromuscular blockers paralyze all skeletal muscles, including the diaphragm and accessory muscles of respiration. Therefore the chief danger in their use is that they decrease pulmonary ventilation, causing respiratory depression. They also may cause circulatory disturbance. Special attention to anesthesia depth, ventilation, and electrolyte balance is required.

Neuromuscular blockers are classified as nondepolarizing and depolarizing. Although theoretically they are antagonistic, combinations are used. They may widen the scope of less potent anesthetics, such as nitrous oxide, or lessen the overall amount of anesthetic needed. Depolarizing and nondepolarizing drugs behave differently; depolarizers stimulate whereas nondepolarizers inhibit autonomic receptors. Duration of action should be balanced against duration of effect on ventilation.

Nondepolarizing Neuromuscular Blockers

Nondepolarizing neuromuscular blockers act on enzymes to prevent muscle contraction. They produce tetanic electrical impulses that gradually fade, but they do not cause muscular fasciculation on IV injection. Their effects are decreased by anticholinesterase drugs, acetylcholine, epinephrine, and depolarizing neuromuscular blockers. Action is potentiated by halogenated inhalation agents and some aminoglycoside antibiotics. Interactions with other drugs can result in delayed recovery. For example, antibiotics may act synergistically to produce prolonged paralysis, such as occurs when the peritoneal cavity is irrigated with an antibiotic solution or antibiotic is injected IV. Box 24-2 lists some antibiotics that can potentiate neuromuscular blockers. Synergism also occurs with local and inhalation anesthetic agents. They are useful for patients on mechanical ventilators. Nondepolarizing blockers may be referred to as competitive antagonists. A peripheral nerve stimulator is useful for assessing neuromuscular transmission as a guide to the dosage, degree and nature of the blockade, and evidence of muscle-response recovery during and after the use of nondepolarizing agents. The anesthesia provider can choose from several drugs.

SHORT-ACTING NEUROMUSCULAR BLOCKING AGENT: MIVACURIUM CHLORIDE (MIVACRON) Blockade lasts 15 to 20 minutes. It has minimal cardiovascular effect but can cause skin flushing.

INTERMEDIATE-ACTING NEUROMUSCULAR BLOCKING AGENTS

Atracurium Besylate (Tracrium) With a duration of action of about 30 minutes, atracurium metabolizes more quickly than the other blockers, which may be an advantage in patients with liver or renal disease. Repeated doses are not cumulative. Atracurium causes histamine release, vasodilation, and hypotension.

Cisatracurium (Nimbex) Cisatracurium can cause bradycardia, hypotension, and skin flushing.

Vecuronium Bromide (Norcuron) Similar to pancuronium, vecuronium has a shorter duration of action and is more potent. It does not noticeably increase the heart rate or blood pressure unless it is combined with opioids.

Rocuronium Bromide (Zemuron) With a rapid onset of action, rocuronium facilitates intubation. The duration of action is about 30 minutes, with minimal overall effect on cardiovascular stability. Tachycardia is possible.

LONG-ACTING NEUROMUSCULAR BLOCKING AGENTS

Tubocurarine Chloride (Curare) Obtained from plants, tubocurarine was used centuries ago by South American Indians for poison arrows. The poison caused death by suffocation from respiratory paralysis. The effects of tubocurarine on the neuromuscular junction were first described in 1856. Blocking transmission of nerve impulses to muscle fibers results in paralysis, predominantly of voluntary muscles. D-Tubocurarine releases histamine. Autonomic blockade can

cause vasodilation, hypotension, and histamine release. Tubocurarine is used as pretreatment if succinylcholine is used, to decrease the possibility of fasciculation.

Gallamine Triethiodide (Flaxedil) Similar in action and duration to D-tubocurarine, gallamine does not cause hypotension or bronchospasm. It may increase arterial pressure and cause tachycardia. It is contraindicated in iodide and sulfide allergy.

Metocurine Iodide (Metubine) Metocurine iodide produces less hypotension and releases less histamine than D-tubocurarine. It is contraindicated in patients with iodide allergy.

Pancuronium Bromide (Pavulon) Pancuronium is similar in action to D-tubocurarine but about five times more potent. It has a vagolytic action that may raise the blood pressure, pulse rate, and heart rate. It can cause dysrhythmia if used with digoxin.

Pipecuronium (Arduran) Pipecuronium can cause decreased arterial pressure with moderate histamine release.

Depolarizing Neuromuscular Blockers Depolarizing neuromuscular blockers have the opposite effect of the nondepolarizing drugs. They stimulate autonomic receptors. For example, they cause muscular fasciculation (i.e., involuntary muscle contractions). These contractions, the result of depolarization of nerve-muscle end plate, are seen following injection. They are followed by fatigue. Drugs may be given IM, but IV use is more common.

SUCCINYLCHOLINE CHLORIDE (ANECTINE, QUELICIN, SUCOSTRIN) An ultrashort-acting synthetic drug with an onset of action in seconds, succinylcholine produces paralysis for up to 20 minutes. It is used primarily for endotracheal intubation. A dilute solution may be used to provide continuing muscle relaxation. Repeated IV administration may effect changes in the heart rate and rhythm (i.e., bradycardia and ventricular dysrhythmia) until the drug is metabolized by enzymes. Muscle pain may occur after use unless fasciculation is prevented by a small preliminary dose of a nondepolarizing agent. Succinylcholine is contraindicated in patients with a known or suspected history of malignant hyperthermia. It can cause increased intracranial and intraocular pressures.

DECAMETHONIUM (SYNCURINE) A very potent synthetic with a rapid onset and short duration of action, decamethonium is not cumulative and has little effect on vital systems. It is used for deep relaxation of a short duration, such as for endoscopy, treatment of laryngeal spasm, abdominal closure, and endotracheal intubation. It is excreted through the kidneys. Prolonged blockade may result if decamethonium is given to a patient in renal failure.

• • •

The anesthesia provider must constantly verify the degree of paralysis present by noting the amount of relaxation of the abdominal wall or the limpness of extremities, or by using a nerve stimulator connected to the patient through needle electrodes. The use of neuromuscular blockers requires surgeon–anesthesia provider teamwork and communication. Use of these drugs always presents the hazard of overdosage, a danger alleviated by the anesthesia provider's familiarity with the surgeon's technique and the requirements of the particular surgical procedure; thus the anesthesia provider can regulate the dosage of anesthetic and relaxant necessary to produce the conditions required at the appropriate time. For example, a major use of neuromuscular blockers is in intraabdominal procedures. At different times during the surgical procedure, blockade may be more or less essential. Although tightness of tissues and inadequate exposure may be a result of factors other than relaxation, it is helpful to the anesthesia provider to be told before pertinent action, such as closure of the peritoneum, is taken. Inadequate muscle relaxation makes closure difficult. Controlled respiration during upper abdominal manipulation can prevent descent of the diaphragm into the surgical field.

Monitoring the Depth of Anesthesia

The anesthesia provider monitors the level of anesthesia, balancing doses of medications, throughout the surgical procedure. The FDA has approved a compact system for monitoring the effects of anesthesia on the brain. Known as Bispectral Index (BIS) anesthesia monitoring, the BIS monitor allows the anesthesia provider to accurately track the patient's level of consciousness by using an electrode applied to the patient's forehead that sends EEG-like signals to a small monitor. The readout is a single number ranging from 100 (wide awake) to 0 (absence of brain activity). The device can be used as a stand-alone unit or be integrated into other monitoring devices. The result of its use is decreased amounts of anesthetic administration and a faster postoperative return to alertness. More information is available on the Internet at **www.aspectms.com.**

Emergence from General Anesthesia

The anesthesia provider attempts to have the patient as nearly awake as possible at the end of a surgical procedure. Pharyngeal and laryngeal reflexes must be recovered to prevent aspiration and respiratory obstruction. The degree of residual neuromuscular blockade must be determined and treated if necessary for respiratory adequacy. The action of nondepolarizing muscle relaxants may be reversed with antagonists, such as long-acting neostigmine methylsulfate (Prostigmin) or pyridostigmine bromide (Regonol), or short-acting edrophonium (Tensilon, Enlon). These anticholinesterase drugs are accompanied or preceded by atropine sulfate to minimize side effects, such as excessive secretions and bradycardia.

Extubation is delayed until spontaneous respiration is ensured. The endotracheal tube is carefully removed when this maneuver is deemed safe. A patent airway and adequate manual or mechanical ventilation are maintained until full recovery. In the absence of a means of respiratory control, such as when a maxillofacial procedure endangers the airway, the endotracheal tube may be left in place.

Retching, vomiting, and restlessness may accompany emergence. Slight cyanosis, stertorous respiration, rigidity, and shivering are not uncommon as a result of a temporary disturbance of body temperature–regulating mechanisms, thus altering circulation to the skin and muscles. Administering oxygen and pain medication and applying warm blankets help relieve these aftereffects. The anesthesia provider should flush the patient's lungs with oxygen to minimize exhalation of gases in the PACU.

BALANCED ANESTHESIA

Balanced anesthesia has become a widely used technique to achieve physiologic homeostasis, analgesia, amnesia, and muscle relaxation. A combination of agents is used with many possible variations, depending on the condition of the patient and requirements of the procedure. The technique is especially useful for preventing CNS depression in older and poor-risk patients.

Induction

Induction can be accomplished with a thiobarbiturate derivative (thiopental sodium [Pentothal], methohexital [Brevital]), diazepam (Valium), midazolam (Versed), or other induction agent. Oxygen is administered in physiologic quantities. Neuromuscular blockers permit control of ventilation while providing muscle relaxation during intubation.

Maintenance

Different combinations of narcotics and neuroleptic drugs (tranquilizers) are administered IV whether they are used alone or in combination with inhalation agents. Neuroleptics reduce motor activity and anxiety; produce a detached, apathetic state; and potentiate hypnotic and analgesic narcotic effects. The dosage can be regulated to produce the desired state.

Neuroleptanalgesia

Neuroleptanalgesia refers to an intense analgesic and amnesic state resulting from the combination of a narcotic (potent analgesic) and a neuroleptic (psychotropic tranquilizer). The analgesia, amnesia, and sedation produced are not true anesthesia. Unconsciousness may or may not occur. The dosage can be controlled so that the patient can cooperate and respond to commands, if desirable (e.g., for some diagnostic procedures). A single drug or combination of drugs may be used.

Innovar Injection Innovar injection is a combination of fentanyl and droperidol. Fentanyl, a potent, short-acting opioid narcotic, may cause respiratory depression, hypotension, and bradycardia. Therefore some anesthesia providers prefer to individualize doses separately to allow more controlled injection of fentanyl (Sublimaze). An advantage of the combination is an apparent absence of toxic effects on the kidneys and liver and only slight cardiac depression. Droperidol, a potent long-acting tranquilizer, also exerts an antiemetic effect. Consciousness returns within minutes after injection, but psychotropic effects persist for 4 to 6 hours, causing drowsiness and indifference to discomfort. Respirations must be closely watched, and the patient is encouraged to breathe.

Neuroleptanesthesia

When the narcotic-neuroleptic drug combination is reinforced by an anesthetic, the resulting state is referred to as neuroleptanesthesia. Supplementation is necessary for extensive surgical procedures. Nitrous oxide or a halogenated inhalation agent and IV narcotics provide analgesia. Neuromuscular blockers permit optimal conditions for the surgeon. An opioid agonist-antagonist may be a useful supplement. For example, nalbuphine hydrochloride (Nubain) has limited potency and toxicity. It has cardiovascular stability and limited respiratory effects.

Emergence

Residual effects of narcotics or muscle relaxants may require reversal by antagonists during and/or at the conclusion of the surgical procedure. Other precautions are taken as for any patient emerging from general anesthesia.

CONTROLLED HOMEOSTASIS

Functions controlled by homeostatic mechanisms include body temperature, heartbeat, blood pressure, electrolyte balance, and respiration. These parameters may be altered by anesthetic and other pharmacologic agents and by physiologic stresses during surgical manipulations. In the hands of a skilled anesthesia provider, adjunctive methods of control may be used concurrently with the administration of general anesthesia, but only when the expected outcomes will outweigh the inherent risks.

Induced Hypothermia

Hypothermia is an artificial, deliberate lowering of body temperature below the normal limits (Box 24-3). It reduces the metabolic rate and oxygen needs of the tissues in conditions causing hypoxia or during a decrease or interruption of circulation. Bleeding is also decreased, and less anesthetic is needed. The patient can therefore better tolerate the surgical procedure. Hypothermia may be used as follows:

- For direct-vision intracardiac repair of complex congenital defects in infants and in other cardiac procedures. This is the most common usage.
- After cardiac resuscitation, to decrease oxygen requirements of vital tissues and limit further damage to the brain following anoxia.

Box 24-3	Hypothermia

Normal core temperature: 98.2° to 99.9° F (36.8° to 37.7° C)
Systemic hypothermia may be:
  Light: 98.6° to 89.6° F (37° to 32° C)
  Moderate: 89.6° to 78.8° F (32° to 26° C)
  Deep: 78.8° to 68° F (26° to 20° C)
  Profound: 68° F (20° C) or below
Sensorium fades at 91° to 93° F (33° to 34° C)

- In treatment of hyperpyrexia and some other nonsurgical conditions, such as hypertensive crisis.
- To increase tolerance in septic shock.
- In neurosurgery, to decrease cerebral blood flow, brain volume, and venous and intracranial pressures.
- To aid in transplantation of organs.

Attaining Hypothermia

To achieve hypothermia, heat must be lost more rapidly than it is produced. The following methods may be used:

1. *Surface-induced hypothermia.* External cooling of infants and small children weighing less than 20 pounds (10 kg) may be attained by immersion in iced water, packing the body in ice, or alcohol sponging. A hypothermia/hyperthermia machine with a cooling blanket or mattress is used for adults and larger children.
2. *Internal cooling.* A decreased or interruption of blood flow can be achieved by placing sterile iced saline slush packs around a specific internal organ or by irrigation of cold fluids within a body cavity, such as intraperitoneal lavage. The cold cardioplegia technique combines cold from saline slush with drugs injected into coronary arteries for myocardial protection during heart surgery. Drugs may also be used to lower metabolism and to increase resistance to shivering during cooling.
3. *Systemic hypothermia.* The bloodstream is cooled by diverting blood through heat-exchanging devices of extracorporeal circulation and returning it to the body by a continuous flowing circuit (e.g., core cooling by cardiopulmonary bypass or IV administration of cold fluids). Systemic hypothermia is used in adults and larger children to 78.8° F (26° C). Oxygen consumption and metabolism of different organs vary, making uniform hypothermia impossible. The temperature is not deliberately lowered below about 84.5° F (29° C) unless arrest of the heart is desired by means of deep hypothermia (below 78.8° F [26° C]). This is accompanied by perfusion of the rest of the body with the extracorporeal circulation method, permitting an open, motionless dry field while the blood flow is interrupted. A noncontracting heart requires very little oxygen.

The patient is progressively rewarmed at the close of the surgical procedure until the temperature is 95° F (35° C) or until consciousness returns. Sometimes a degree of hypothermia is maintained for a day or two postoperatively to allow the patient to adapt more readily. Oxygen therapy and intubation, if advised, are part of postoperative care.

Complications in the Use of Hypothermia

Hypothermia carries many inherent risks. Primarily it affects the myocardium, decreasing its resistance to ventricular fibrillation and predisposing the patient to cardiac arrest. This is more likely to happen with deep hypothermia or during manipulation of the heart itself. Other dangers are heart block, effects on the vascular system, atrial fibrillation, embolism, microcirculation stasis, undesired downward drift of temperature, tissue damage, metabolic acidosis, and numerous effects on other organs and systems.

Time is required for cooling and rewarming. Shivering and vasoconstriction, normal defenses of the body against cooling, can be problems during the use of hypothermia. This muscle activity greatly increases oxygen needs. Shivering can be overcome by the administration of a muscle relaxant drug or IV injection of chlorpromazine or an analgesic such as meperidine.

Rewarming can be accomplished by circulating warmed blood by means of extracorporeal circulation or by using a heating mattress with circulating fluid and warm blankets. If external heat is applied, care should be taken not to burn the patient. Rewarming carries potential problems such as reactive bleeding or circulatory collapse. If the patient is rewarmed too rapidly, vasodilation causes the blood pressure to drop. Organ ischemia can occur from severe shivering. These superficial and systemic events impair perfusion (oxygenation) of tissues. "Rewarming shock" may be prevented by slow warming, adequate oxygenation, and prevention of massive sudden vasodilation or vasoconstriction associated with shivering.

Induced Hypotension

Induced, deliberate hypotension is the controlled lowering of arterial blood pressure during anesthesia as an adjunct to the surgical procedure. Hypotensive anesthesia is used to shorten the operating time, reduce blood loss and the need for transfusion, and facilitate dissection and visibility, especially of tumor margins in radical procedures. Visible vessels are ligated, even in the absence of active bleeding.

Adequate oxygenation of blood and tissue perfusion in vital organs (heart, liver, kidneys, lungs) and in the cerebrum must be maintained to prevent damage. The degree and duration of hypotension must be carefully controlled so that the state can be rapidly terminated at any time.

Naturally, controlled hypotension is not indicated as a routine procedure. It is used only when the expected gain for a particular patient requiring a specific surgical procedure outweighs the risks. Hypotension may be specifically induced for the following:

- Surgical procedures in which excessive blood loss is anticipated to decrease gross hemorrhage or venous oozing, such as spinal surgery.
- Surgical procedures on the head, face, neck, and upper thorax, especially radical dissection, in which the position of the patient allows blood to pool in dependent areas and reduces venous return to the heart and cardiac output.
- Neurosurgical procedures when control of intracranial vessel hemorrhage may be difficult. It reduces leakage, makes an aneurysm less turgid and prone to rupture, decreases blood loss in the case of rupture, and facilitates placement of ligating clips.
- Surgical procedures in which blood transfusions should be avoided, such as when compatible blood is unavailable or transfusion is against the patient's religious belief.
- Surgical procedures on the spine or posterior torso. Blood loss is decreased in the prone position.
- Total hip replacement.

Precautions in the Use of Hypotension

Potential complications of hypotensive anesthesia include cerebral or coronary ischemia or thrombosis, reactionary hemorrhage, anuria in acute renal failure, delayed awakening, and dermal ischemic lesions. Primary contraindications are vascular compromise to any vital organ system or the brain. Precautions include the following:

- Careful selection of the patient
- Preoperative cardiac, renal, and hepatic evaluation of the patient to avoid circulatory insufficiency in vital organs
- Selection of an appropriate but not arbitrary level of blood pressure
- Administration and evaluation by expert anesthesia providers
- Use for only a short time and lowering of blood pressure only enough to obtain the desired result
- Maintenance of blood volume at an optimal level by continuous infusion
- Controlled ventilation with adequate oxygenation via an endotracheal tube because hypotension increases susceptibility to hypoxia
- Extensive monitoring: ECG; core temperature; esophageal stethoscopy; urinary output, central venous pressure and arterial catheters; electrophysiologic brain monitoring or EEG via Bispectral Index monitoring

Attaining Hypotension

Several techniques will produce hypotension. The blood pressure may be lowered chemically by direct arterial or venous dilators or by ganglionic blocking drugs. Perfusion pressure drops in proportion to a decrease in vascular flow resistance, but adequate tissue blood flow exists. Fine adjustment of the desired level of hypotension can be achieved by mechanical maneuvers—namely, alterations in body position or changes in airway pressure, control of the heart rate or blood volume, or addition of other vasoactive drugs in conjunction with hypotensive drugs. Properly used, these maneuvers can reduce the total dose of potentially toxic drugs needed for maintenance of hypotension.

Methods to produce hypotension include the following:

1. Deep general anesthesia with halothane or isoflurane, followed by a vasodilator, produces the desired minute-to-minute effect. With increased concentration, halogenated agents produce hypotension as a result of myocardial and peripheral vascular depression.
2. Sodium nitroprusside is a potent, fast-acting vasodilator that reduces virtually all resistance in vascular smooth muscle (resistance vessels). It also reduces preload and afterload of the heart and pulmonary vascular resistance. To achieve safe arterial pressure control, administration is via a calibrated drug pump. The acid-base status and blood cyanide level are determined frequently to guard against metabolic acidosis and sodium nitroprusside–induced cyanide and thiocyanate toxicity.
3. Nitroglycerin, primarily a venodilator, directly dilates capacitance vessels. It reduces preload and improves myocardial perfusion during diastole, a protection against potential ischemia. Nitroglycerin for IV infusion (Nitrostat), after dilution in 5% dextrose or physiologic saline, dilates both venous and arterial beds. Arterial pressures are reduced. Nitroglycerin migrates into plastic. To avoid its absorption into plastic parenteral solution containers, dilution and storage are done in glass parenteral solution bottles. A special non-absorbing infusion set prevents loss of nitroglycerin.
4. Trimethaphan camsylate (Arfonad) blocks sympathetic ganglia, which results in relaxation of resistance and capacitance vessels and reduces arterial pressure.
5. Fentanyl may be used as a basal anesthetic for hypotension. The blood pressure can be maintained at the desired level by the addition of a small amount of a volatile agent. Fentanyl lowers arterial pressure; volatile agents reduce cardiac output.
6. Other drugs such as verapamil, nifedipine, phentolamine, tetrodotoxin, or adenosine triphosphate may be used.

Safe lower limits of arterial pressure may vary. Average values are 50 mm Hg mean and 65 to 70 mm Hg systolic, with lower values for short periods only.

Normovolemic Hemodilution Anesthesia

Intraoperative normovolemic hemodilution has been used in cardiac surgery for several decades but more recently as an anesthetic technique in other types of major surgery when large blood loss is anticipated. It is especially useful in infants and children and in patients, such as Jehovah's Witnesses, who for religious reasons do not accept administration of blood products.

At the beginning of the surgical procedure, whole blood is withdrawn from the patient to a hematocrit of 14% to 15% and replaced with three times the volume of a balanced electrolyte solution to maintain intravascular volume. This di-

luted blood is transparent, giving the surgeon a clearer, almost bloodless field. This may decrease operating time. The patient is maintained under controlled hypotension with halothane anesthetic and a supplemental narcotic. The body temperature may be lowered to 89.6° F (32° C) or below for moderate hypothermia to help protect vital organs against hypoxia and hypotension.

After significant blood loss has ceased, the patient's own blood is reinfused. Diuresis is stimulated to remove electrolyte solution. Normovolemic hemodilution can make a difficult surgical procedure easier and in some patients makes an otherwise impossible resection possible.

CARE OF THE ANESTHETIZED PATIENT

Anesthetic agents and drugs vary in potency. Therefore they differ in the amount of analgesia, amnesia, or muscle relaxation produced. Each patient's ability to detoxify anesthetic agents and to tolerate physiologic stress differs. Impairment of pulmonary function accompanies general anesthesia to some degree. General anesthesia is usually more complicated than local or regional anesthesia.

Considerations

The anesthesia provider keeps the surgeon informed of significant physiologic changes detected by monitoring vital functions. The following should be considered:

1. A deficit in pulmonary and/or cardiac functions is detrimental to the patient's physiologic status. Abnormalities of pulmonary ventilation and diffusion influence the course of anesthesia and diminish tolerance to stress or the insults from the anesthetic and the procedure.
   a. Respiratory patterns vary from breath holding and apnea to deep breathing and tachypnea.
   b. Drug action affecting respiratory stimulation or depression is related to changes in oxygen tension (Pao_2) or arterial carbon dioxide tension ($Paco_2$).
   c. Hypoxia, anemia, and decreased cardiac output may produce inadequate tissue oxygenation. Subnormal cardiac reserve or oxygen-transporting ability, combined with anemia or hypoxia in an arteriosclerotic patient, for example, can be lethal.
2. Circulation is affected both centrally and peripherally. Individual agents are associated with characteristic hemodynamic patterns. Generally, the agents are circulatory depressants that reduce arterial pressure, myocardial contractility, and cardiac output.
3. The liver is affected by general agents (e.g., the rate of visceral blood flow). Alterations in liver function tests may follow anesthesia. Halogenated hydrocarbons have been associated with hepatotoxicity. The liver metabolizes many anesthetic agents and other medications.
4. Kidney function is affected by disturbances in systemic circulation, since kidneys normally receive 20% to 25% of the cardiac output. A reduced renal plasma flow and

glomerular filtration rate depress renal functions related to hemodynamics and to water and electrolyte excretion. Oliguria, with reduced sodium and potassium excretion, accompanies induction. Postoperative fluid retention may result from a reduction in urine volume from anesthesia, intraoperative trauma, and the use of narcotics. In the absence of renal disease, changes in renal function are usually transitory and reversible. Endocrine effects on renal function during anesthesia are important. Many drugs and agents are excreted by the kidneys.

5. Biotransformation of agents varies with metabolites excreted by the kidneys. Urinary secretion of IV agents may be slow and unpredictable. Studies indicate that nitrous oxide may be exhaled as long as 56 hours after anesthesia, and metabolites of halothane have been recovered from patients' urine as long as 20 days after anesthesia.
6. Agents may cause nausea, emesis, or systemic complications.

General anesthesia may be contraindicated for the following:

- Elective procedures on patients who are medically at high risk or severely debilitated.
- Elective procedures during the first 5 months of pregnancy. Some anesthesia providers avoid general anesthesia because of unknown teratogenic effects of inhalation anesthetics.
- Emergency surgical procedures on patients who have recently ingested food or fluids. Gastric suction and awake intubation are indicated if the surgical procedure cannot be delayed.

Intraoperative Awareness

Although seemingly anesthetized, the patient may be aware of conversations, noises, and even pain. Is it possible to imagine anything more terrifying than to feel intraoperative maneuvers but be unable to communicate this discomfort? Intraoperative awareness varies, depending on the type of procedure and depth of anesthesia. Newer monitoring techniques, such as Bispectral Index monitoring, have decreased the incidence of intraoperative awareness.

The common use of narcotics and muscle relaxants as adjuncts has consequently decreased the amount of anesthetic used to induce and maintain unconsciousness. This is particularly true in balanced anesthesia. As a result, studies have shown evidence of intraoperative awareness (i.e., recall), consciously or unconsciously, of events and sounds during a state of anesthesia. Even though the patient may not consciously recall or remember the experience, unconsciously it may affect behavior and attitudes postoperatively. Subconscious memory may cause anger, generalized irritability, anxiety, repetitive nightmares, preoccupation with death, or physiologic complications.

Patient awareness of pain is rare in the hands of skilled anesthesia providers. However, hearing is the last sensation

to surrender to anesthesia. Therefore perioperative caregivers should be constantly aware of the patient's vulnerability to auditory stimuli, including conversations and room noise. Even potent amnesic drugs may not totally block recall of stimuli, especially disturbing stimuli.

Safety Factors

Team members, especially the anesthesia provider and the circulator, must be constantly aware of potential trauma to the patient, since he or she is unable to produce a normal response to painful or injurious stimuli. Although safety factors are stressed throughout the text, important factors in the care of the anesthetized patient are reiterated here for emphasis:

1. The patient's position is changed slowly and gently to allow circulation to readjust (i.e., to compensate for physiologic changes caused by motion or position).
2. Proper positioning and padding are important to avoid pressure points, stretching of nerves, or interference with circulation to an extremity.
3. The patient's chest must be free for adequate respiratory excursion during the surgical procedure. The airway must be patent. Leaning on the patient during the procedure can cause permanent injury. Remember that the patient under the drapes is unable to complain!
4. The lungs must be adequately ventilated intraoperatively and postoperatively by either voluntary or mechanical means. Anesthetic agents are basically depressants that affect the vasomotor and respiratory centers, predisposing the patient to postoperative respiratory complications.
5. The anesthesia provider assists in transferring the patient to a stretcher or bed, safeguarding the head and neck, when it is safe to move the patient. The transfer is made carefully and gently to avoid strain on ligaments or muscles of the patient and the caregivers. The relaxed, unconscious patient is adequately supported.
6. The anesthesia provider gives the PACU nurse a verbal report, including specific problems in regard to this patient, and completes records before the transfer of responsibility. The perioperative nurse gives a report of preoperative and intraoperative care to the PACU nurse.

CARE OF ANESTHESIA EQUIPMENT

The anesthesia equipment is a potential vector in the spread of infection. The anesthesia provider may become the victim of an acquired infection from contact with a patient's body fluids or blood. Studies have found that nearly 20% of anesthesia providers have had hepatitis B infections.

Standard Precautions

The need for anesthesia staff to strictly adhere to standard precautions (formerly known as universal precautions) while caring for patients and equipment should be emphasized.

Gloves should be worn to prevent skin contact with patient's blood and body fluids, such as when starting the IV infusion, when intubating and/or extubating, or when suctioning the patient. Protective eyewear should be worn to prevent a splash in the eye. Hands should be washed and the mask should be changed between patient contacts. Needles must be handled carefully without recapping to avoid accidental needle sticks. All anesthesia equipment that has come in contact with mucous membranes, blood, or body fluids is cleaned, disinfected, or sterilized after use to render it safe for handling and for subsequent patient use. Disposable items are discarded in the appropriate receptacles.

Hazards of Equipment

Anesthesia techniques encompass the use of drugs for parenteral administration and gases and volatile liquids for inhalation administration by means of anesthesia machines. These machines and their component parts (reservoir bags, canisters, connecting pieces, ventilators) accumulate large numbers of microorganisms during use. Consequently, the parts that come in contact with the patient's skin or respiratory tract are sources of cross-contamination. Inhalation, exhalation, and the forcible expulsion of secretions create moist conditions favorable to the survival and growth of a multitude of organisms (streptococci, staphylococci, coliform bacteria, fungi, yeasts). Therefore the anesthesia circuit can become a veritable reservoir for microorganisms and a pathway for transmission of disease. When the apparatus is used on a patient with a known respiratory disease, such as tuberculosis, the risk increases.

All used accessories must be terminally cleaned and either undergo high-level disinfection or be sterilized before reuse, because clinical respiratory cross-infection has been traced to contaminated apparatus. Valves of the breathing circuit become contaminated from essentially healthy patients at an average rate of 35 organisms per minute. *Pseudomonas aeruginosa* has been cultured from carbon dioxide absorption devices. Many microorganisms accumulate in valves and air passages and in soda lime canisters. Although the alkalinity of soda lime inhibits many organisms, it is not a dependable germicide or effective mechanical filter, nor is it meant to be one. Respiratory therapy equipment, mechanical ventilators, resuscitators, and suction machines and bottles present the same problems. Resistant strains of organisms, as well as opportunists, have caused nosocomial infections. Patient-to-patient infection must be eliminated. The following are points to remember:

1. The patient's respiratory tract is a portal of entry for pathogenic organisms and a source of delivering pathogens into the environment.
2. The respiratory tract loses some of its inherent defense mechanisms during anesthesia.
3. Aseptic precautions are necessary to prevent needless exposure of air passages to foreign, potentially pathogenic, organisms from equipment and hands of anesthesia personnel.

4. Anesthesia machines and equipment, unless properly treated, increase the danger of airborne contamination and contact transmission of pathogenic microorganisms capable of causing postoperative wound infections and systemic infections.

In the presence of tuberculosis or a virulent respiratory infection, the anesthesia provider should wear a gown and strictly adhere to universal precautions. Some contacts require donning a mask with high-efficiency particulate air (HEPA) filters. The patient should wear a mask during transportation and until induction of anesthesia.

Disposable Equipment

Disposable equipment warrants use for reasons of safety, efficiency, and convenience. Presterilized, disposable airways, endotracheal tubes, tracheotomy tubes, breathing circuits, masks and canisters (with soda lime sealed in the plastic), and spinal trays reduce the hazard of cross-infection. They are especially recommended for the compromised host and the bacteriologically contaminated patient. Single-use components of the anesthesia system are discarded after use. Needles are disposed of in puncture-resistant containers.

Care of Reusable Equipment

All parts of patient-exposed, reusable equipment must be thoroughly cleaned after every use to prevent pulmonary complications. Thorough cleaning to remove organic debris and drying must precede any high-level disinfection or sterilization process. All items that can be sterilized should be sterilized. Manufacturers strive to make the machines that cannot be sterilized more amenable to adequate terminal cleaning and freedom from microorganisms. The following points should also be considered:

1. The anesthesia machine should be disinfected immediately whenever it is soiled by blood and secretions.
2. The surfaces of anesthesia machines, carts, or cabinets should be disinfected after each patient use. The specific work area used for airways, endotracheal tubes, and other items should also be cleaned. The top of a cart or tray should be draped with a disposable impervious material that is changed between patients. All equipment for maintenance of the airway should be set up on and returned to this drape. Disposable items should be discarded in suitable containers after use. Nondisposable equipment must be set aside after use for terminal cleaning and testing, thereby diminishing the risk of contaminating clean equipment needed for subsequent patients. A biohazard disposal container should be placed by the anesthesia machine.
3. Monitoring equipment, including ECG and other electrodes and blood pressure cuffs, should be cleaned with a detergent-disinfectant when contaminated and preferably after each use.

4. All equipment that comes in contact with mucous membranes of the patient and the inside of the breathing circuit must be terminally cleaned and sterilized, preferably, or undergo high-level disinfection.

   a. Endotracheal tubes, stylets, airways, laryngoscope blades, face masks, and suction equipment should be sterile for each patient. Suction catheters and tubing should be sterile, single-use disposable items.

   b. Disposable breathing circuits are preferred to reusable equipment because of the complexities of cleaning and maintaining cleanliness. The interior of reusable breathing circuits remains sterile if they stand unused in their normal position on the machine, but contamination rapidly occurs when the circuits are used on patients. The parts of the circuit nearest the patient are the most heavily contaminated. Therefore reusable corrugated hoses, breathing tubes, and reservoir bags are sterilized or undergo high-level disinfection between each patient use.

   c. Items located farther away, such as circle systems and ventilators, are cleaned and sterilized according to a regular schedule, at least once or twice a month.

5. For cleaning, an automated process is available for decontamination. Machines wash equipment in mild detergent and hot water, and rinse and dry it. Some machines incorporate a chemical disinfection cycle. If automatic equipment is not used, anesthesia and respiratory therapy equipment must be disconnected and manually cleaned before sterilization. Prompt immersion in a detergent-disinfectant solution prevents crusting of secretions. Tubing takes a long time to dry. Commercial dryers are available.

6. Sterilization methods:

   a. Steam is the preferred method for all heat-stable materials.

   b. Ethylene oxide is used for materials that are deteriorated by heat, such as rubber, plastics, mechanical ventilators, and electronic equipment. Thorough aeration, according to the manufacturer's recommendations, is necessary before use to remove all residual gas from the material sterilized. Otherwise, facial burns, laryngotracheal inflammation, and obstruction or bilateral vocal cord paralysis may be caused by use of the equipment.

   c. Buffered glutaraldehyde solution does not impair conductivity of antistatic rubber. Although its use is the least convenient method, it is preferred if ethyl-ene oxide is not available for heat-sensitive items. The manufacturer's recommendations should be followed for a 100% kill of *Mycobacterium tuberculosis* by immersion methods. When glutaraldehyde is used, the items must be thoroughly rinsed with sterile water because tap water contains microorganisms and pyrogens.

7. Sterile packaged equipment should be stored in a closed, clean, and dry area. Anesthesia and respiratory therapy equipment should be kept sterile until used.

8. Policies and procedures regarding processing of equipment should be written, available, and reviewed annually.

Checking Anesthesia Equipment

Inhalation systems are tested biologically at regular intervals and checked daily for proper functioning. Preventive maintenance is essential to avoid mechanical failures, which could be fatal. Goals for quality control are to ensure that equipment is available and that it performs reliably when needed.

Bibliography

Benumof JB, Saidman LJ: *Anesthesia and perioperative complications,* ed 2, St Louis, 1999, Mosby.

Davidson JK: *Clinical anesthesia procedures of the Massachusetts General Hospital/Department of Anesthesia and Harvard Medical School,* ed 4, Boston, 1993, Little, Brown.

Mathias JM: New anesthetics have fewer side effects, *OR Manager* 11(1):16-19, 1995.

New drugs: rocuronium (Zemuron): a safer fast muscle relaxant? *Am J Nurs* 95(3):56-57, 1995.

Ouellette SM, Simpson C: Monitoring for intraoperative awareness, *AORN J* 68(6):950, 952-953, 955-956, 959-961, 1998.

Patterson P: NIOSH alerts ORs to excessive nitrous oxide levels, *OR Manager* 10(7):1, 13, 1994.

Phillip BK: New approaches to anesthesia for day case surgery, *Acta Anaesthesiol Belg* 48(3):167-174, 1997.

Pittman SK et al: Video-assisted fiberoptic endotracheal intubation, *Anesth Analg* 78(1):197, 1994.

Proposed recommended practices for cleaning and processing anesthesia equipment, *AORN J* 60(3):487-489, 1994.

Rogers MC: *Current practice in anesthesiology,* ed 2, St Louis, 1992, Mosby.

Song D et al: Fast-track eligibility after ambulatory anesthesia: a comparison of desflurane, sevoflurane, and propofol, *Anesth Analg* 86(2):267-273, 1998.

Struys M et al: Clinical usefulness of the Bispectral Index for titrating propofol target effect–site concentration, *Anaesthesia* 53(1):4-12, 1998.

Tong D et al: Predictive factors in global and anesthesia satisfaction in ambulatory surgical patients, *Anesthesiology* 87(4):856-864, 1997.

Vilke GM et al: Intubation techniques in the helicopter, *J Emerg Med* 12(2):217-224, 1994.

Walker SM et al: A comparison of sevoflurane with halothane for paediatric day case surgery, *Anaesth Intensive Care* 25(6):643-649, 1997.

Chapter 25

Local and Regional Anesthesia

 Chapter Objectives

After studying this chapter, the learner will be able to:

- Differentiate between local and regional anesthesia.
- Compare the differences in expected and unexpected responses between local anesthesia and regional anesthesia.
- Describe how a patient should be monitored during the administration of local anesthesia and during the administration of regional anesthesia.

Local and regional anesthetic techniques are used to decrease intraoperative stimuli, thereby diminishing stress response to surgical trauma. Injected at or near the nerves of the surgical site, the anesthetic drug temporarily interrupts sensory nerve impulses during manipulation of sensitive tissues.

When a local anesthetic drug is used, the patient usually remains conscious. Local infiltration anesthesia is particularly advantageous for procedures performed in ambulatory surgery settings from which the patient is discharged to home soon after completion of the procedure. Oral, intramuscular (IM), or intravenous (IV) sedation may be given to relieve anxiety and to produce amnesia. IV sedation is commonly used and is referred to as intravenous conscious sedation (IVCS).

Anesthetic may be administered locally during general anesthesia for postoperative pain control. When injected before the incision is made, the patient's nervous system is preempted from sensory stimulation associated with the initial trauma of incision. Some surgeons elect to inject local anesthesia drugs before the skin is closed for additional delay of sensory stimulation associated with postoperative pain.

Regional blocks are useful for more extensive procedures. Regional anesthesia may be used, with or without IVCS,

when general anesthesia is contraindicated or undesired. Nerve blocks, intrathecal blocks, peridural blocks, and epidural blocks are examples of regional anesthesia techniques. These techniques block conduction of pain impulses from a specific area or region. The anesthetic drug is injected around a specific nerve or group of nerves to prevent pain of the surgical procedure.

Local anesthetics and regional blocks, with or without supplementary sedation, are administered as the anesthetic of choice for many diagnostic and therapeutic surgical procedures. Terms associated with local and regional anesthesia are defined in Box 25-1.

HISTORICAL BACKGROUND

Historically, the Incas used the coca leaf for local pain relief. Anthropologists have found evidence that liquid derivatives were used for trephination (creating holes in the skull). More formalized experimentation with cocaine began in 1860. European physicians found it had a numbing effect on the tongue and caused the pupils to dilate. Theories of the day held that cocaine had potential as a replacement for morphine. Sigmund Freud (1856-1939), an Austrian psychiatrist,

Box 25-1   Terms Associated with Local and Regional Anesthesia

conduction anesthesia   Loss of sensation in a region of the body produced by injecting an anesthetic drug along the course of a nerve or a group of nerves to inhibit conduction of impulses to and from the area supplied by that nerve or nerves (block anesthesia, nerve block anesthesia).

epidural anesthesia   Loss of sensation below the level of peridural injection of an anesthetic drug into the epidural space in the spinal canal for relief of pain in the lower extremities, abdomen, and pelvis without loss of consciousness.

intrathecal injection   Instillation of solution, such as an anesthetic drug, into the subarachnoid space for diffusion in spinal fluid, as for spinal anesthesia.

intravenous conscious sedation (IVCS)   Depressed level of consciousness produced by IV administration of pharmacologic agents. The patient retains the ability to continuously maintain a patent airway independently and to respond to physical or verbal stimulation. Sedation may relieve anxiety and produce amnesia.

local anesthesia   Loss of sensation along specific nerve pathways produced by blocking transmissions of impulses to receptor fibers. The anesthetic drug injected depresses sensory nerves and blocks conduction of pain impulses from their site of origin. The patient remains conscious, with or without IV sedation.

local infiltration   Injection of an anesthetic drug intracutaneously and subcutaneously into tissues to block peripheral nerve stimuli at their origin.

nerve block   Loss of sensation produced by injecting an anesthetic drug around a specific nerve or nerve plexus to interrupt sensory, motor, or sympathetic transmission of impulses.

regional anesthesia   Loss of sensation in a specific body part or region produced by blocking conductivity of sensory nerves supplying that area. The anesthetic drug is injected around a specific nerve or group of nerves to interrupt pain impulses. The patient remains conscious, with or without IV sedation. Regional anesthetic techniques include nerve, intrathecal, peridural, and epidural blocks.

sedative   Pharmacologic agent (drug) that suppresses nervous excitement, allays anxiety, and produces a calming effect. Benzodiazepines, barbiturates, and opioids (narcotics) are the most commonly used drugs for conscious sedation.

spinal anesthesia   Loss of sensation below the level of the diaphragm, produced by intrathecal injection of an anesthetic drug into the subarachnoid space without loss of consciousness.

topical anesthesia   Depression of sensation in superficial peripheral nerves by application of an anesthetic agent directly to the mucous membrane, skin, or cornea.

---

and an ophthalmology student performed experiments in the use of cocaine as a local anesthetic for the eye. Freud also experimented with cocaine as a substitute for chemically dependent patients. Unfortunately, the patients ultimately became addicted to cocaine.

James Corning (1855-1923), an American neurologist, experimented with cocaine as a local infiltrate in the spinal column. In 1885 he successfully induced spinal anesthesia and published a textbook on the subject of local anesthesia the following year. August Bier (1861-1949), a German surgeon, continued the experimentation and the use of regional anesthesia in Europe. His technique of regional anesthesia using double tourniquets was introduced in 1908.

Refinement of other drugs followed and was strongly enhanced by the isolation of epinephrine by John Abel (1857-1938), an American pharmacologist. Heinrich Braun (1847-1911), a German surgeon, used epinephrine mixed with cocaine for local anesthesia during nasal and urologic surgery. He found that the tissues bled less and a lower concentration of the drug could be safely used. Local agents procaine (1904) and lidocaine (1948) advanced the use of local anesthesia by many practitioners.

Modern refinements and the development of additional drugs for injection have increased the use of local and regional anesthesia for surgical procedures.

PREPARATION OF THE PATIENT

Preparation of the patient who will receive a local or regional anesthetic depends on the extent of the procedure to be performed and on the anticipated technique of administration. Although it is anticipated that the patient will remain conscious, it is sometimes desirable or necessary to supplement the local or regional anesthesia with IVCS. Careful preoperative assessment, history taking, and a clear explanation of what to expect are part of the preparatory process. More information can be found at **www.nursingnet.org.**

Preoperative assessment of the patient who is scheduled for a procedure provides baseline data and identifies risk factors. Data that should be documented include the following:

- Baseline vital signs, blood pressure, laboratory values, and results of electrocardiographic (ECG) monitoring and any other tests that were performed.
- Weight, height, and age. Dosage of some drugs is calculated on the basis of body weight in kilograms (milligrams per kilogram of body weight). Some drugs are contraindicated for age extremes (i.e., pediatric or geriatric patients).
- Current medical problem(s) and past history of medical events, including a history of substance abuse.

TABLE 25-1	Comparison of Toxicity and Allergy Caused by Local Anesthetic Drugs	

Toxic Reaction	Allergic Reaction*
Symptoms vary depending on the drug	Immediate localized reaction followed by generalized body reaction
Subjective	
Dizziness, somnolence, paresthesia, nausea, visual/speech problems	Sense of uneasiness, pruritus, agitation, paresthesia
Objective	
Decreased breathing rate and depth, muscle twitches, tremors, slurred speech, seizures, vomiting, unconsciousness, coma	Erythema, urticaria, wheals
Vasovagal	
Dysrhythmia, bradycardia, vasodilation, hypotension, myocardial depression, cardiac arrest	Coughing, sneezing, wheezing, bronchospasm, hypotension, hypovolemia, vasodilation, cardiovascular collapse, cardiac arrest
Treatment	
Supportive, airway management; need IV line; Trendelenburg position; muscular contractions are treated with diazepam (Valium)	Especially with amino ester type: airway management, IV fluids, epinephrine, diphenhydramine, and steroids as needed

*Not common with amino amide.

- Current medications or drug therapy, such as insulin for diabetes or hypertensive drugs.
- Allergy or hypersensitivity reactions to previous anesthetics or other drugs.
- Mental status, including emotional state and level of consciousness.
- Communication ability. A patient with hearing impairment or language barrier may be unable to understand verbal instructions during the procedure or to respond appropriately.

Preoperative orders regarding the time when the patient should cease taking anything by mouth vary with the circumstances; 6 to 8 hours before the surgical procedure is the usual minimum for adults. If possible, the adult patient is instructed to remain on NPO (nothing by mouth) status after midnight. Some patients are permitted a few sips of water to take oral medications, such as hypoglycemics or antihypertensives. Suggested criteria for preoperative oral intake for pediatric patients varies and is described in Chapter 8.

Many ambulatory surgical patients scheduled for same-day procedures have no premedication and are permitted to walk to the operating room (OR). Some facilities require the use of a stretcher or wheelchair for transport. The patient should be transported via a stretcher if sedated.

INTRAOPERATIVE PATIENT CARE

The patient must be able to respond cooperatively and to maintain respiration unassisted. The patient needs careful observation throughout the surgical procedure and for a period of time afterward for symptoms of delayed reaction or com-

plications. The care the patient will need depends on the type and length of the procedure, the amount of sedation given, and the type and amount of local anesthetic used. Psychologic support and reassurance are given before and during the surgical procedure. The patient should be told what to expect and what is expected of him or her. The patient should be monitored by qualified personnel and observed for adverse effects of the medication or the procedure.

LOCAL ANESTHESIA

The surgeon injects the anesthetic drug or applies it topically. The anesthesia provider is not in attendance for this method. Supplemental agents should be available for analgesia or anesthesia, if necessary, or for adverse reactions (Table 25-1). Resuscitative equipment, suction, and oxygen must be at hand before administration of any anesthetic. Qualified personnel should be immediately available to assist in the event of an emergency.

Administration of Local Anesthesia

In the absence of an anesthesia provider, a qualified registered nurse is responsible for monitoring the patient's physiology and safety during local anesthesia. This should be the only activity assigned to this nurse for the duration of the procedure. Circulating duties should not be performed simultaneously. The perioperative nurse who assumes the responsibility for patient monitoring should have the knowledge, skill, and ability to use and interpret data from monitoring equipment. The perioperative nurse also should be able to recognize symptoms of abnormal reactions to local anesthetic drugs and to provide interventions to prevent further complications.

The patient who is under local anesthesia requires observation of physiologic changes in pulse, blood pressure, oxygenation, and respiration. Baseline data obtained during preoperative assessment are compared with intraoperative and postoperative findings. The vital signs, including blood pressure, pulse, and respirations, are continuously monitored. Monitoring devices may include an electrocardiograph and pulse oximeter. Monitoring equipment is used to assess the patient's physiologic status in combination with direct observation. Data from monitoring and direct observation are documented at frequent intervals and with any significant event, such as the injection of medication or the removal of a specimen. The patient is monitored for reaction to drugs and for behavioral and physiologic changes. It is important for the perioperative nurse to be aware of the maximum dosages of local anesthetics in milligrams per kilogram of body weight. The total amount of anesthetic and supplementary drugs administered is also recorded in the patient's record. AORN, the Association of periOperative Registered Nurses, has established recommended practices for the care of patients receiving local anesthesia. Policies and procedures should be in place to delineate patient care, monitoring activities, and documentation during the use of local anesthetics.

Intravenous Conscious Sedation

During procedures performed with the patient under local anesthesia, mild sedation may be given by IV infusion. IVCS refers to a mild to moderate depressed level of consciousness that allows the patient to maintain a patent airway independently and to respond appropriately to verbal instructions or physical stimulation. A benzodiazepine, such as midazolam (Versed) or diazepam (Valium), is most commonly given either alone or in combination with a narcotic and atropine or scopolamine. Benzodiazepines provide amnesia with sedation, but they also may cause respiratory depression and fluctuations in blood pressure and heart rate and rhythm.

All team members need to understand the objectives and desired effects of IVCS. If the primary objective is to allay the patient's anxiety and fear, the therapeutic effects of the drugs given should produce relaxation and some degree of amnesia. Because consciousness is maintained, the patient has intact protective reflexes to respond to physical stimuli. The patient also can easily be aroused with verbal commands as necessary. In this state vital signs may fluctuate to a minimal extent. Documentation in the patient's record should reflect evidence of continuous assessment and identification of any untoward or significant reactions during administration of local anesthesia with IVCS.

The Perioperative Nurse's Role During Local Anesthesia and Intravenous Conscious Sedation

The patient under IVCS should be monitored continuously for cardiac status, blood pressure, pulse, respiration, and oxygen saturation. Monitoring devices may include, but are not limited to, an electrocardiograph and pulse oximeter. In the absence of an anesthesia provider, a qualified registered nurse should be assigned to monitor the patient's physiologic state. This registered nurse should not be assigned to simultaneously circulate and should be competent in the use and interpretation of monitoring devices. For patients with unstable physiology, an anesthesia provider should be in attendance to monitor the patient. Policies and procedures should be in place that address the registered nurse's competency in patient monitoring and the nurse's role during the use of IVCS.

Monitored Anesthesia Care

When an anesthesia provider's presence is necessary, the surgical procedure is scheduled as monitored anesthesia care (MAC), attended local, or anesthesia standby. Terminology may vary at different institutions. Patients with particular medical problems or age-extreme patients (pediatric or geriatric) may require supervision by anesthesia personnel. Patients receiving a local anesthetic because they are too ill to undergo general anesthesia should have an anesthesia provider in attendance. The type and length of procedure also may be factors that influence the surgeon's request for an anesthesia provider to be available to give and monitor IVCS. The anesthesia provider may initiate and maintain a regional nerve block, such as an axillary brachial plexus block for hand surgery. IVCS and regional blocks with MAC have gained popularity for ambulatory surgery.

Monitoring the Patient Receiving a Local Anesthetic

The extent of monitoring, determined in consultation with physicians in the department of surgery and anesthesiology where applicable, depends on the seriousness of the procedure, sedation required, and/or patient's condition. The perioperative nurse assigned to monitor the patient receiving a local anesthetic, with or without IVCS, continuously attends the patient. This nurse does not have other responsibilities during the surgical procedure. *AORN Standards, Recommended Practices, and Guidelines* provide guidance for the perioperative nurse in monitoring the patient receiving a local anesthetic and the patient receiving IVCS. The guidelines may be summarized briefly as follows:

1. The patient is monitored for reaction to drugs and for behavioral and physiologic changes. The perioperative nurse should recognize and report to the physician significant changes in the patient's status and be prepared to initiate appropriate interventions.
2. The nurse attending the patient should have basic knowledge of the function and use of monitoring equipment, ability to interpret information, and working knowledge of resuscitation equipment.
3. Accurate reflection of perioperative care should be documented on the patient's record.
4. Institutional policies and procedures in regard to patient care, including monitoring, should be written, re-

viewed annually, and readily available. This information should be included in orientation and in-service programs. It should include policies regarding permissible drug administration and emergency interventions by the nurse.

In addition to preoperative assessment and postoperative evaluation for a continuum of care, intraoperative activities include determining and documenting the patient's baseline physiologic status before administration of sedatives, analgesics, and anesthetic drugs and monitoring the patient throughout the procedure. Parameters include, but are not limited to, the following:

- Blood pressure
- Heart rate and rhythm
- Respiratory rate
- Oxygen saturation by pulse oximetry
- Body temperature
- Skin condition and color
- Mental status and level of consciousness

Vital signs are taken before injection of a drug and at 5- to 15-minute intervals after injection. Changes in the patient's condition are reported to the surgeon immediately. If an adverse reaction occurs, emergency measures should be instituted on request as per policy. These may include maintaining a patent airway, starting oxygen therapy when clinically indicated, and/or administering IV therapy.

Considerations in the Selection of Local Anesthetics

A local anesthetic depresses superficial peripheral nerves and blocks conduction of pain impulses from their site of origin. Regional nerve blocks interrupt conduction of pain impulses from a specific area or region. These techniques may be employed, with or without IVCS, when general anesthesia is contraindicated. As with any anesthetic agent, local anesthetics offer advantages in some circumstances but have disadvantages and are contraindicated in others.

Advantages

1. Use of local anesthetic agents can minimize the recovery period. The patient can ambulate, eat, void, and resume normal activity.
2. Local anesthesia uses minimal equipment and is economical.
3. Loss of consciousness does not occur unless anesthesia is supplemented with additional drugs.
4. Local anesthesia avoids the undesirable effects of general anesthesia.
5. Local anesthesia is suitable for patients who recently ingested food or fluids (e.g., before an emergency procedure).
6. Local anesthesia is useful for ambulatory patients having minor procedures.
7. Local anesthesia is ideal for procedures in which it is desirable to have the patient awake and cooperative.

Disadvantages

1. Local anesthesia is not practical for all types of procedures. For example, too much drug would be needed for some major surgical procedures; the duration of anesthesia is insufficient for others.
2. There are individual variations in response to local anesthetic drugs.
3. Rapid absorption of the drug into the bloodstream can cause severe, potentially fatal reactions.
4. Apprehension may be increased by the patient's ability to see and hear. Some patients prefer to be unconscious and unaware.

Contraindications

Local anesthesia is generally contraindicated in patients with the following:

- Allergic sensitivity to the local anesthetic drug.
- Local infection or malignancy at the site of injection, which may be carried to and spread in adjacent tissues by injection. A bacteriologically safe injection site should be selected.
- Septicemia. In a proximal nerve block a needle may open new lymph channels that drain through a region, thereby causing new foci and local abscess formation from the perforation of small vessels and escape of bacteria.
- Extreme nervousness, apprehension, excitability or inability to cooperate because of mental state or age.

SPINAL AND EPIDURAL ANESTHESIA

Intraspinal injection of an anesthetic drug is a technique of regional anesthesia performed by a person who has been properly trained and has acquired the necessary skill. Regional anesthesia is delivered to select areas, referred to as dermatomes, to affect motor and sensory nerves as desired (Figure 25-1). The patient's dermatome levels can be tested by touch and by asking the patient to move his or her extremities. Dermatome level T12 is near the iliac crest, T10 is near the umbilicus, and T6 is near the xiphoid.

Assessment of the patient's level of consciousness, pulse, respirations, and blood pressure is essential for early detection of hypotension associated with high spinal anesthesia. If regional anesthesia extends above the level of T4, a full sympathetic block may follow, causing cardiorespiratory arrest. Ventilatory support equipment and naloxone (Narcan) should be immediately available.

Spinal and Epidural Drugs

The choice of drug depends on factors such as the duration, intensity, and level of anesthesia desired; the anticipated surgical position of the patient; and the surgical procedure. Patient factors include the anesthetic history, physical condition, and preference of the patient and surgeon. The duration of action depends on physiologic and metabolic factors. The

Figure 25-1 Dermatomes of the body.

addition of a vasoconstrictor, usually epinephrine 1:200,000, prolongs the duration. Diffusion of the drug into the cerebrospinal fluid (CSF) is affected by solubility, molecular weight, and volume. Glucose may be added to make the drug heavier than CSF (hyperbaric). Anesthesia diminishes as the drug is absorbed into the systemic circulation. The most commonly used anesthetic drugs for spinal and epidural anesthesia are listed in Table 25-2.

Spinal Anesthesia

Spinal anesthesia, also referred to as an intrathecal block, causes desensitization of spinal ganglia and motor roots. The agent is injected into the CSF in the subarachnoid space of the meninges (the three-layered covering of the spinal cord) using a lumbar interspace in the vertebral column (Figure 25-2). The subarachnoid space is located between the pia mater (the innermost membranous layer covering the spinal cord) and the arachnoid (the thin vascular, weblike layer immediately beneath the dura mater, which is the outermost sheath covering the spinal cord). Spinal ganglia, motor nerve roots, and blood

vessels pass through the meninges. The drug diffuses into the CSF around ganglia and nerves before it is absorbed into the bloodstream. Absorption into nerve fibers is rapid.

Spinal anesthesia is often used for abdominal (mainly lower) or pelvic procedures requiring relaxation, inguinal or lower extremity procedures, surgical obstetrics (cesarean section without effect on the fetus), and urologic procedures. It is preferred for patients with alcoholism, substance abusers, or obese or muscular patients (who would need large doses of general anesthetic and muscle relaxant), and for emergency surgical procedures on patients who have eaten recently. It is also used in the presence of hepatic, renal, or metabolic disease because it causes minimal upset of body chemistry.

The level of anesthesia attained depends on various factors, such as the patient's position during and immediately after injection; CSF pressure; site and rate of injection; volume, dosage, and specific gravity (baricity) of the solution; inclusion of a vasoconstrictor, such as epinephrine; spinal curvature; interspace chosen; uterine contractions with labor; and coughing or straining, which can inadvertently raise the level. Spread of the anesthetic is controlled mainly by solu-

| TABLE 25-2 | Local and Regional Anesthetic Agents | | | | |

Generic Name	Trade Name(s)	Uses	Concentration	Duration of Effect (Hours)	Maximum Dosage
Amino Amides					
Bupivacaine hydrochloride	Marcaine Sensorcaine	Local infiltration* Regional block* Surgical epidural	0.25% to 0.50%	2 to 3	400 mg
Dibucaine hydrochloride	Nupercaine Percaine Cinchocaine	Local infiltration Peripheral nerves	0.05% to 0.1%	3 to 3½	30 mg
Etidocaine hydrochloride	Duranest	Peripheral nerves Epidural	0.5% to 1%	2 to 3	500 mg
Lidocaine hydrochloride	Xylocaine Lignocaine	Topical Infiltration* Peripheral nerves* Nerve block* Spinal Epidural	2% to 4% 0.5% 1% to 2%	½ to 2	200 mg 500 mg or 7 mg/kg body weight
Mepivacaine hydrochloride	Carbocaine	Infiltration Peripheral nerves Epidural	0.5% to 1% 1% to 2%	½ to 2	500 mg
Prilocaine hydrochloride	Citanest	Infiltration Peripheral nerves Regional block Epidural	1% to 2% 2% to 3%	½ to 2½	600 mg
Amino Esters					
Chloroprocaine hydrochloride	Nesacaine	Infiltration* Peripheral nerves* Nerve block* Epidural	0.5% 2% 2% 2% to 3%	¼ to ½	1000 mg
Cocaine hydrochloride		Topical	4% or 10%	½	200 mg or 4 mg/kg body weight
Procaine hydrochloride	Novocain	Infiltration Peripheral nerves Spinal	0.5% 1% to 2%	¼ to ½	1000 mg or 14 mg/kg body weight
Tetracaine hydrochloride	Cetacaine Pontocaine	Topical Spinal	2% 1%	2 to 4	20 mg

*Epinephrine may be used.

tion baricity and patient position. The period immediately following injection is decisive; the anesthetic is becoming "fixed" (i.e., absorbed by the tissues and unable to travel). Further control of the anesthetic level is attained by tilting the operating bed at that time. The direction of tilting depends on whether the drug is hyperbaric (specific gravity greater than that of spinal fluid) or hypobaric (lighter than spinal fluid). Isobaric anesthetics (same weight as spinal fluid) are made hyperbaric by the addition of 5% or 10% dextrose to the anesthetic before injection.

Immediately after injection, the anesthesia provider carefully tests the level of anesthesia by pinprick, touch, or nerve stimulation, tilting the bed as necessary to achieve the desired level for the surgical procedure. After anesthetic fixation and with the anesthesia provider's permission, the patient is placed in surgical position. The patient is asked to relax and let the team turn him or her. Straining or holding breath can precipitate hypotension or an inadvertent rise in the level of anesthesia. The incision is not made until it is certain that anesthesia is adequate. Supplementation of spinal anesthesia is necessary if anesthesia or muscular relaxation is insufficient or the patient is unduly apprehensive. Sometimes the patient is given IVCS but can still be roused.

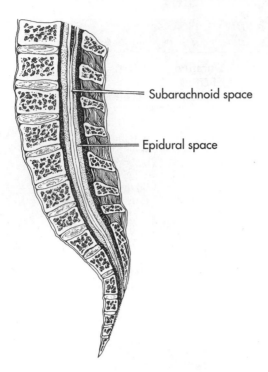

Figure 25-2   Agent is injected into subarachnoid space for spinal anesthesia or into epidural space for epidural anesthesia.

Figure 25-3   Lateral position for administration of spinal anesthetic.

Choice of Agent

The drug used depends on various factors such as the duration, intensity, and level of anesthesia desired, the anticipated surgical position of the patient, and the surgical procedure.

Duration of Agent

The desirable duration of anesthesia depends on physiologic [and meta]bolic factors. It is prolonged by the addition of a [vasoconstr]ictor. Anesthesia diminishes as the agent is ab[sorbed into] the systemic circulation.

Spinal Anesthesia Procedure

For injection, the patient is placed in the position desired by the anesthesia provider, depending on patient condition, solution baricity, and level of anesthesia to be produced:

1. *Lateral position.* The patient lies on the side with the back at the edge of the operating bed. The knees are flexed onto the abdomen, and the head is flexed to the chest. The hips and shoulders are vertical to the operating bed to prevent rotation of the spine (Figure 25-3).
2. *Sitting position.* The patient sits on the side of the operating bed with the feet resting on a stool. The spine is flexed, with the chin lowered to the sternum; the arms are crossed and supported on a pillow on an adjustable table or Mayo stand.

The circulator or an anesthesia assistant supports the patient in position, observes and reassures him or her, and assists the anesthesia provider as possible. Attention to asepsis is extremely important. The anesthesia provider dons sterile gloves before handling sterile items. Sterile disposable spinal trays eliminate the need for cleaning and sterilizing of nondisposable equipment. They also avoid the hazards of sterilizing ampules, but the dates on the drugs supplied by the manufacturer should be checked.

A spinal tray usually contains the following:

- Fenestrated drape.
- Ampules of local anesthetic, spinal anesthetic, vasoconstrictor drug, 10% dextrose.
- Gauze squares, forceps, and antiseptic solution. Some kits include disposable sponges on plastic applicator sticks.
- Needles: 25-gauge hypodermic needle for infiltration of local anesthetic into the skin; 22-gauge × 2-inch (5-cm) needle for IM injection; blunt 18-gauge needles for mixing drugs; 22- or 26-gauge × 3½-inch (9-cm) spinal needle with stylets for intrathecal injection.
- Syringes: 5-ml syringes for spinal anesthetic, 10-ml syringes for hypobaric solutions, 2-ml syringes for superficial anesthesia.

The lumbar puncture site is cleansed with an antiseptic solution and draped with a fenestrated drape. The blood pressure is checked before, during, and after spinal anesthesia, since hypotension is common.

Advantages

The patient is conscious if desired. The procedure can be performed with IVCS as necessary. Throat reflexes are maintained; breathing is quiet, without airway problems, because the respiratory system is not irritated. The bowel is contracted. Muscle relaxation and anesthesia are excellent if the procedure is properly executed.

Disadvantages

Spinal anesthesia produces a circulatory depressant effect: hypotension, and stasis of blood as a result of interference with venous return from motor paralysis and arteriolar dilation in the lower extremities. A change in body position may be followed by a sudden drop in blood pressure; after fixation of the anesthetic, a slight elevation of the feet and legs may increase venous return to the heart. The agent cannot be removed after injection. Nausea and emesis may accompany cerebral ischemia, traction on viscera, or premedication. There is possible sensitivity to the agent and danger of trauma or infection. The patient can hear.

Complications

Transient or permanent neurologic sequelae from cord trauma, irritation by the agent, lack of asepsis, and loss of spinal fluid with decreased intracranial pressure syndrome are potential complications. Examples include spinal headache; auditory and ocular disturbances, such as tinnitus and diplopia; arachnoiditis; meningitis; transverse myelitis; cauda equina syndrome (failure to regain use of the legs or control of urinary and bowel functions); temporary paresthesias, such as numbness and tingling; cranial nerve palsies; and urinary retention. Late complications include nerve root lesions, spinal cord lesions, and ruptured nucleus pulposus.

True spinal headache caused by a persistent CSF leak through the needle hole in the dura usually responds to supine bed rest, copious oral or IV fluids, and systemic analgesia. Refractory postspinal headache may be treated by an epidural blood patch: 5 to 10 ml of the patient's own blood is administered at the puncture site. This usually affords prompt relief.

If a high level of anesthesia is reached, extreme caution is essential to prevent respiratory paralysis ("total spinal"), an emergency situation requiring artificial ventilation until the level of anesthesia has receded. Respiratory arrest, although rare, is thought to be a result of medullary hypoperfusion caused by a sympathetic block. Apnea also can be produced by respiratory center ischemia resulting from precipitous hypotension.

The anesthesia machine, oxygen, and IV line must be in readiness before injection. Constant vigilance of respiration and circulation is critical. The blood pressure and heart rate are monitored and maintained at normal levels.

Epidural Anesthesia

The terms *epidural, peridural,* and *extradural* are used synonymously. The epidural space lies between the dura mater, the outermost sheath covering the spinal cord, and the walls of the vertebral column. It contains a network of blood vessels, lymphatics, fat, loose connective tissue, and spinal nerve roots. Injection is made into this space surrounding the dura mater (see Figure 25-2). The drug diffuses slowly through the dura mater into CSF. Anesthesia is prolonged while the drug is absorbed from CSF into the bloodstream. The spread of anesthetic and duration of action are influenced by the concentration and volume of solution injected (total drug mass) and the rate of injection. The anesthetic diffuses toward the head (cephalad) and toward the coccyx (caudad). In contrast to spinal anesthesia, patient position, baricity, and gravity have little influence on anesthetic distribution. The high incidence of systemic reactions is attributed to absorption of the agent from the highly vascular peridural area and the relatively large mass of anesthetic injected. Epinephrine 1:200,000 is usually added to retard absorption. Approaches used for epidural anesthesia and analgesia include thoracic, lumbar, and caudal approaches. Skin and ligaments are infiltrated with a local anesthetic agent before epidural catheter placement is performed.

The management and sequelae of epidural anesthesia are similar to those of spinal anesthesia. An epidural approach may be used for lower extremity, abdominal, urologic, anorectal, vaginal, or perineal procedures. It is used commonly for postoperative pain management and in obstetrics during labor and delivery or during and after cesarean section. The patient is attended constantly by a qualified registered nurse once the block is initiated for analgesia. Vital signs should be monitored at regular intervals, and any deviation of level of consciousness, pulse, respirations, or blood pressure should be reported immediately to the anesthesiologist. Use of an apnea monitor may be indicated. In an obstetric patient the fetal heart rate should be electronically monitored continuously because the patient is insensitive to uterine contractions.

Epidural narcotic analgesia may provide sustained postoperative relief or control of pain in patients with intractable or prolonged pain. This may be administered by a percutaneous indwelling epidural catheter, an implanted epidural catheter with infusion port or reservoir and pump, or an implantable infusion device. A patient may come to the OR for placement of an epidural catheter or pump device for ongoing pain management.

An epidural catheter for administration of a narcotic for prolonged postoperative pain relief, usually for 2 or 3 days, may be inserted before induction of general anesthesia for postoperative use. Morphine sulfate, fentanyl, sufentanil citrate, and buprenorphine hydrochloride are the drugs most commonly used for prolonged pain relief. Although probability of respiratory depression is less when the epidural route is used as compared with spinal narcotics, use of an apnea monitor is advisable. Side effects include nausea and vomiting, urinary retention, and pruritus. Epidural narcotics block pain at the level of opiate receptors in the dorsal horn of the spinal cord, not in the brain, so the patient is mentally alert and able to ambulate.

Thoracic and Lumbar Approaches

The thoracic and lumbar approaches are peridural blocks. Equipment is similar to that for a spinal block with the addition of a 19-gauge × 3½-inch (9-cm), thin-walled needle with a stylet with a rigid shaft and a short, beveled tip to minimize the danger of inadvertent dural puncture. Insertion of a catheter allows repeated injections for continuous intraoperative and postoperative epidural anesthesia, requiring additional needles, stopcocks, and a plastic catheter in the setup.

Caudal Approach

The caudal approach is an epidural sacral block. Epidural injection is through the caudal canal, desensitizing nerves emerging from the dural sac. The patient position for injection is prone with the hips flexed, sacrum horizontal, and heels turned outward to expose the injection site. The sacral area is prepared and draped, with care taken to protect the genitalia from irritating solution. The left lateral position is used in the pregnant patient. The spread of agents in epidural anesthesia is enhanced in pregnancy, atherosclerosis, and advanced age.

The tray includes the addition of a 20-gauge × 1½ inch (4-cm) spinal needle with a stylet. Commercial sets are available.

Advantages

Compared with spinal anesthesia, there is a decreased incidence of hypotension, headache, and potential for neurologic complications with epidural anesthesia, although a higher failure rate is reported.

Disadvantages

There is less controllable height of anesthesia; it is a more difficult technique; there is a greater area of potential infection from anaerobic organisms with the caudal approach; it is unpredictable; it is time-consuming (i.e., a longer time is required for complete anesthesia); a larger amount of agent is injected; continuous technique may slow the first stage of labor.

Complications

Intravascular injection, accidental dural puncture and total spinal anesthesia, blood vessel puncture and hematoma, profound hypotension, backache, and transient or permanent paralysis (paraplegia) are possible complications. The patient may suffer hypoxia, respiratory arrest, and/or cardiac arrest.

TECHNIQUES OF ADMINISTRATION OF LOCAL OR REGIONAL ANESTHESIA

Topical Application

The anesthetic is applied directly to a mucous membrane, to a serous surface, or into an open wound. A topical agent is often applied to the respiratory passages to eliminate laryngeal reflexes and cough, for insertion of airways before induction or during light general anesthesia, or for therapeutic and diagnostic procedures such as laryngoscopy or bronchoscopy. It is also used in the urethral meatus for cystoscopy. Mucous membranes readily absorb topical agents because of their vascularity. The onset of anesthesia occurs within minutes. The blood level of a topical agent may equal the same level obtained by IV injection. The duration of anesthesia is 20 to 30 minutes. If a spray or atomizer is used, it should contain a visible reservoir so that the quantity of drug administered is clearly observed because droplets vary in size, causing variations in dosages.

Preanesthetic anticholinergics are important before topical application within the respiratory tract. Saliva can dilute the topical anesthetic and prevent adequate duration of contact with mucous membranes. Also, a dry throat is necessary to prevent aspiration until the anesthetic effect has disappeared and throat reflexes have returned. Adverse reactions to topical anesthetic agents are uncommon when dosage is carefully controlled. Sudden cardiovascular collapse can occur, more commonly following topical anesthesia of the respiratory tract.

Topical local anesthetic ointment may be used on the skin surface before starting an IV line. The ointment should be applied and allowed to remain in contact with the skin for several minutes to an hour for optimal effect. A transparent cover dressing may be placed over the application point to prevent accidental smearing of the medication. Care is taken to prevent contact with the eyes and other mucus membranes.

Cryoanesthesia

Cryoanesthesia involves blocking local nerve conduction of painful impulses by means of marked surface cooling (i.e., freezing) of a localized area. It is used in such brief procedures as the removal of warts or noninvasive papular surface lesions. Cryotherapy units are commercially available.

Simple Local Infiltration

The agent is injected intracutaneously and subcutaneously into tissues at and around the incisional site to block peripheral sensory nerve stimuli at their origin. It is used to suture superficial lacerations or for excision of minor lesions.

Regional Injection

The agent is injected into or around a specific nerve or group of nerves to depress the entire sensory nervous system of a limited, localized area of the body. The injection is at a distance from the surgical site. A wider, deeper area is anesthetized than with simple infiltration. There are several types of regional blocks.

Nerve Block

A selected nerve is anesthetized at a given point. Nerve blocks are performed to interrupt sensory, motor, and/or sympathetic transmission. Blocks may be used preoperatively, intraoperatively, and postoperatively to prevent pain of the procedure; diagnostically to ascertain the cause of pain; or therapeutically to relieve chronic pain. Blocks are useful in various circulatory and neurosurgical syndromes, such as reflex sympathetic dystrophy (RSD). For prolonged pain relief (e.g., during a long procedure or to treat chronic pain associated with disease or trauma), a continuous infusion or incremental injections through a catheter may sustain regional anesthesia. Some examples of blocks are as follows:

1. Surgical blocks
   a. Paravertebral block of the cervical plexus for procedures in the area between the jaw and the clavicle
   b. Intercostal block for relatively superficial intraabdominal procedures, such as drain placement
   c. Brachial plexus or axillary block for arm procedures
   d. Median, radial, or ulnar nerve block for the elbow or wrist

e. Hand and digital block for fingers (an additive vasoconstrictor, such as epinephrine, is not added to the local agent because necrosis can result from inadequate circulation to the digit)

f. Blocks in other specific areas, such as a penile block for circumcision in adults

2. Diagnostic or therapeutic blocks

a. Sympathetic nerve ganglia block to produce desired vasodilation by paralysis of the sympathetic nerve supply to the constricting smooth muscle in the artery wall

b. Stellate ganglion block to increase circulation in peripheral vascular disease in the head, neck, arm, or hand

c. Paravertebral lumbar block to increase circulation in the lower extremities

d. Celiac block for relief of abdominal pain of the pancreatic origin

Bier Block

A Bier block is a regional IV injection of a local anesthetic to an extremity below the level of a double-cuffed tourniquet. An IV catheter is introduced into a vein in the arm or leg close to the intended surgical site. A double-cuffed (proximal and distal cuff) tourniquet is applied to the proximal portion of the extremity, and the extremity is elevated. Blood is drained from the extremity by wrapping it from distal to proximal with a rubber compression Esmarch's bandage as the limb remains elevated. The upper (proximal) cuff is inflated to stop blood flow after the extremity has been exsanguinated. Local anesthetic is injected into the IV catheter. When the anesthetic takes effect over the limb, the lower (distal) cuff of the tourniquet is inflated. When the lower cuff is fully inflated, the upper (proximal) cuff is released. The patient feels less discomfort related to the tourniquet because the lower cuff is over an anesthetized region.

On release of the tourniquet at the conclusion of the surgical procedure, entry of a bolus of the remaining drug into systemic circulation may cause cardiovascular or CNS symptoms of toxicity. A Bier block is used for upper extremity procedures and for those that last an hour or less.

Field Block

The surgical site is blocked off with a wall of anesthetic drug. A series of injections into proximal and surrounding tissues will provide a wide area of anesthesia, as in an abdominal wall block for herniorrhaphy.

Complications of Blocks

Each type of block carries unique complication potential. Examples of complications include the following:

- *Intercostal blocks:* pneumothorax, atelectasis, total spinal anesthesia, air embolism, transverse myelitis
- *Brachial plexus blocks:* pneumothorax, hemothorax, recurrent laryngeal nerve paralysis, phrenic paralysis, sub-

arachnoid injection, Horner's syndrome (axillary approach may be preferred to interscalene approach)
- *Stellate ganglion blocks:* pneumothorax
- *Celiac blocks:* large vessel perforation, pancreatic injury, total spinal anesthesia

ACTIONS OF LOCAL AND REGIONAL ANESTHETICS

Local and regional anesthetics interfere with the initiation and transmission of nerve impulses by interacting with the membranous sheath that covers nerve fibers. By physical and biochemical mechanisms, drugs retard and stop the propagation of nerve impulses, eventually blocking conduction.

Drug Pharmacodynamics

The duration of action depends not only on pharmacologic properties of drugs, but also on the volume and concentration of the solution and its systemic interactions. Drugs vary in potency, penetration, rapidity of hydrolysis or destruction, and toxicity.

Conduction Velocity

Nerve fibers vary in their susceptibility to drugs. The larger the fiber, the greater the concentration required. The least amount and lowest concentration to achieve the desired effect should be administered. Conduction of a peripheral stimulus is blocked at its origin by topical application or local infiltration of the drug. Transmission of stimuli along afferent nerves from the surgical site is blocked in regional anesthesia. Conductive pathways in and around the spinal cord are blocked for spinal and epidural anesthesia.

Blocking Quality

Drugs of high potency, minimal systemic activity, and prompt metabolism, and those that lack local irritation are most effective. Blocking qualities include the following:

- Latency time between administration and maximum effect
- Duration of action
- Regression time between beginning and end of pain perception

Sensory nerves are blocked initially. Motor nerves are also affected, with resultant paralysis of both voluntary and involuntary muscles. Some degree of vasodilation occurs with all local and regional use of anesthetic drugs except cocaine.

Absorption Rate and Additives

Local blood flow, vasodilation, and vascularity of tissues can markedly influence local anesthetic action and systemic absorption of drugs. Fibrous tissue and fat in some injection sites act as diffusion barriers and nonspecific binding sites. Supplemental drugs added to anesthetic drugs to facilitate or retard absorption include, but are not limited to, the following:

- *Hyaluronidase (Wydase).* A soluble protein derived from bovine testicular enzyme, hyaluronidase is sometimes added to a local anesthetic to facilitate its spread through subcutaneous tissues to all desired nerves. This action causes more rapid absorption of anesthetic and may reduce the intensity and duration of its effect. Rapid absorption may increase the possibility of a systemic reaction. Hyaluronidase should be refrigerated and used within 14 days of reconstitution.
- *Epinephrine (Adrenalin).* A catecholamine, epinephrine is a potent stimulant. When combined with an anesthetic drug, it causes vasoconstriction to slow circulatory uptake and absorption, thus prolonging anesthesia. It is used to counteract cardiovascular depressant effects of large doses of local anesthetic. It also decreases bleeding, which is a desired effect in many surgical procedures. A concentration of epinephrine that is 1:1000 (1000 mg/1000 ml = 1 mg/ml) to 1:200,000 (0.005 mg/ml) may be optimal for absorptive and hemostatic purposes. Epinephrine is premixed in commercially prepared solutions. If it is added to an anesthetic drug, it is best to do so with a calibrated syringe to avoid overdosage. Epinephrine can produce an acute adrenergic response: nervousness, pallor, diaphoresis, tremor, palpitation, tachycardia, and hypertension. The patient receiving epinephrine should be well oxygenated.

Toxicity

Allergic reactions to anesthetic drugs can occur but are rare. Toxic reactions occur when the concentration of drug in the blood affects the central nervous system (CNS). Slurred speech, numbness of the tongue, blurred vision, and tinnitus are symptoms of toxicity that can progress to drowsiness and confusion. The maximum recommended dosage for each drug should not be exceeded. Severe toxic reaction can quickly lead to cardiovascular collapse. In topical anesthesia extremely rapid systemic absorption from the mucous membranes explains the relatively high frequency of toxic reactions. In local or regional anesthesia, inadvertent intravascular injection and use of fairly large quantities in highly vascular areas will contribute to local anesthetic toxicity.

Pharmacologic Agent Overview

Many different local or regional anesthetic drugs are in use. All are direct myocardial depressants, but the CNS effects precede this depression. Detoxification occurs in the liver. They differ in structure and therefore in action. These drugs are hydrochloride salts of weak bases in solution. They are categorized by chemical structure as amino amides and amino esters (see Table 25-2).

Amino Amides

Amino amides are metabolized in the liver by enzymes and are excreted by the kidneys. Patients with hepatic disease may become toxic with normal dosages because of ineffective metabolism. The amides include the following:

- *Lidocaine hydrochloride (Xylocaine).* Probably the most widely used agent, this potent anesthetic slowly hydrolyzes in circulating plasma. It undergoes hepatic degradation. Dosage should be reduced if hepatic function or blood flow is impaired. Its major advantages are a rapid onset of anesthesia and lack of local irritant effect. Allergic reactions are rare. Used extensively for surgical procedures and dentistry, it has moderate potency and a moderate duration of action. For infiltration: 0.5%; for peripheral nerves: 1% to 2%; maximum dose: 500 mg (0.5 g) or 7 mg/kg body weight. It is a good topical anesthetic, although it is not as effective as cocaine. For topical use in the respiratory tract: 2% to 4%; maximum dose: 200 mg. It is commonly used topically before intubation.

  Clinical indications of lidocaine toxicity usually are related to the CNS. Excessive doses can produce myocardial and circulatory depression.
- *Mepivacaine hydrochloride (Carbocaine).* Similar to lidocaine hydrochloride, mepivacaine takes effect rapidly but produces a 20% longer duration of anesthesia. It has moderate potency and a moderate duration of action. It is commonly employed for infiltration and nerve block. It produces minimal tissue irritation and few adverse reactions. Epinephrine may not be added to it because of its duration of action. For infiltration: 0.5% to 1%; for peripheral nerves: 1% to 2%; maximum dose: 500 mg.
- *Bupivacaine hydrochloride (Marcaine, Sensorcaine).* Four times more potent than lidocaine, bupivacaine has high potency of long duration. The onset of anesthesia is slow, but the duration is two to three times longer than that of lidocaine or mepivacaine, with toxicity approximate to that of tetracaine. Cumulation occurs with repeated injection. The drug affords prolonged pain relief following caudal block for rectal procedures. It is contraindicated for obstetric paracervical block and epidural anesthesia and for a Bier block. For local infiltration or a regional block, with or without epinephrine: 0.25% to 0.50%; maximum dose: 175 mg per dose without epinephrine or 225 mg with epinephrine 1:200,000 to a total dose of 400 mg.
- *Prilocaine hydrochloride (Citanest).* With prilocaine the onset of anesthesia is slower than with lidocaine, but the duration of action is longer. It is particularly useful for patients with diabetes or cardiovascular disease. It is used without epinephrine. For infiltration and peripheral nerves: 1% or 2%; for regional blocks: 2% or 3%; maximum dose: 600 mg.
- *Etidocaine hydrochloride (Duranest).* The onset of anesthesia is slower than that of lidocaine, but the block is of greater potency and toxicity, with a longer duration of action. For peripheral nerves: 0.5%; maximum dose: 500 mg.

• *Dibucaine hydrochloride (Nupercaine, Percaine, Cinchocaine)*. Dibucaine is a very potent drug with a high rate of systemic toxicity. The onset is slow, and the duration of action is long. For infiltration and peripheral nerves: 0.05% to 0.1%, maximum dose: 30 mg.

Amino Esters

Amino esters are hydrolyzed in plasma by pseudocholinesterase enzymes produced by the liver. Para-aminobenzoic acid (PABA), a factor in the vitamin B complex, is a product of this metabolism. Some patients are allergic to PABA. The esters include the following:

• *Cocaine hydrochloride*. The first known local anesthetic, introduced in 1884, cocaine is a crystalline powder with a bitter taste in solution. It is the most toxic of the local drugs and, in contrast to all but lidocaine hydrochloride, is a vasoconstrictor and a CNS stimulant. Cocaine reduces bleeding and shrinks congested mucous membranes. It causes temporary paralysis of sensory nerve fibers, produces exhilaration, lessens hunger and fatigue, and stimulates pulse and respiratory rates. Administration is by topical application only, because of its high toxicity; the solution rapidly penetrates mucous membrane and spreads into highly vascular tissue. Absorption is self-limiting because of vasoconstrictive properties associated with the drug. Epinephrine should not be added. When applied to the throat, cocaine abolishes throat reflexes. The patient is awake and can cooperate, but its limited use and possible addiction are disadvantages.

Cocaine is used topically in 4% or 10% concentration for anesthesia of the upper respiratory tract (nose, pharynx, tracheobronchial tree). Concentrations of 10% are used less frequently and may not be available in all facilities. Untoward reactions may occur rapidly in response to even a very small amount of the drug. Maximum dose: 200 mg or 4 mg/kg body weight. Cocaine is metabolized by the liver and excreted by the kidneys. It should be used with caution in patients with impaired liver or kidney function.

• *Procaine hydrochloride (Novocain)*. Procaine is similar to cocaine but less toxic. Concentrations used: 0.5% for infiltration; 1% to 2% for peripheral nerves. It is injected subcutaneously, intramuscularly, or intrathecally. It has low potency, is of short duration, and is ineffective topically. Its advantages include minimal toxicity, easy sterilization, low cost, and lack of local irritation. Newer agents are used more frequently. Maximum dose: 1000 mg (1 g) or 14 mg/kg body weight.

• *Chloroprocaine hydrochloride (Nesacaine)*. Chloroprocaine is possibly the safest local anesthetic from the standpoint of systemic toxicity because of its fast metabolism. It has moderate potency of short duration. It is rapidly hydrolyzed in the plasma. Its action is fast, but it is not active topically. When used in obstetrics, it does not detectably alter neurobehavioral responses of newborn infants. For infiltration: 0.5%; for peripheral nerves: 2%; maximum dose: 1000 mg (1 g).

• *Tetracaine hydrochloride (Cetacaine)*. With tetracaine the onset of analgesia is slow, but the duration of its effect is longer than that of many other drugs. It has high potency of long duration. It is also more toxic systemically because of the slow rate of destruction in the body, but low total dosage tends to reduce the chances of reaction. It is not used for local tissue infiltration or nerve block. Tetracaine in 2% solution is used only for topical anesthesia on accessible mucous membranes such as the oropharynx. Maximum dose: 20 mg. Tetracaine hydrochloride is used primarily for spinal anesthesia.

COMPLICATIONS OF LOCAL AND REGIONAL ANESTHESIA

Minor or transient complications of local and regional anesthesia are common. Serious complications, although rare, are usually permanent. Complications may be caused by the mechanical effect of needles or pharmacologic effect of the drug administered. As with general anesthesia, the prevention of complications requires patient assessment and preparation, knowledge of anatomy and physiology, and attention to detail. Proper choice of drug, equipment, and constant monitoring are as necessary in local and regional anesthesia as in general anesthesia. Complications of local and regional anesthesia may be summarized briefly as local effects, systemic effects, and effects unrelated to the anesthetic drug.

Local Effects

Tissue trauma, hematoma, ischemia, drug sensitivity, and infection can be minimized by the use of proper drugs and equipment, sterile technique, avoidance of local anesthetics with vasoconstrictors in sites with smaller vascular structures (digits, penis), and avoidance of repetitive injection that promotes trauma, edema, tissue necrosis, and infection.

Systemic Effects

Systemic effects are primarily cardiovascular, neurologic, or respiratory (e.g., hypotension, seizure, or respiratory depression). Drug interactions also are systemic. Following high blood levels, toxicity that affects more than one system may occur. Blood levels depend on the amount of drug used, its physical characteristics, the presence or absence of vasoconstrictors, and the injection site. For example, because of vascularity of surrounding tissue, intercostal blocks produce higher anesthetic blood levels in a shorter time than axillary or epidural blocks. Absorption and the blood level of drugs are related to their uptake and rate of removal from the circulation. A linear relationship exists between the amount of drug administered via a given route and the resultant peak anesthetic blood level.

Predisposing Factors for Hypersensitivity

True hypersensitivity that produces an allergic response can occur, but it is less frequent than reactions from overdosage of pharmacologic agents. The following may predispose a patient to hypersensitivity:

- *Immunologic sensitization.* Allergies are thought to be more common with the amino esters than with the amide group of compounds. An allergic reaction to the preservative in some solutions, such as methylparaben, also is possible. Some local anesthetics release histamine, which is the basis of an allergic response. True allergy, mediated by antigen-antibody reaction, can cause anaphylaxis, urticaria (skin wheals), dermatitis, itching, laryngeal edema, and possibly cardiovascular collapse.
- *Overdosage.* An excessive amount of drug may enter the bloodstream if the injection exceeds maximum dose or is absorbed too rapidly. The IV route is the most dangerous route of injection because histamine is released into the systemic circulation. The injection site is also pertinent. Hazardous sites involve vascular areas of tracheobronchial mucosa, and tissues of the head, neck, and paravertebral region. The least hazardous areas are subcutaneous tissue of the extremities and trunk (abdominal wall and buttocks).

Precautions

Extraordinary precautions must be taken for a patient with a history of any allergies, hypersensitivities, or reactions to previous anesthetics or other drugs. Atopic individuals, those with a hereditary tendency or with multiple allergies, may be more prone to adverse reactions to anesthetics or other drugs. Prediction of allergic reactions is unreliable. If testing for sensitivity to specific drugs is done, it is executed cautiously under well-controlled conditions.

Precautions for preventing adverse drug reactions in all patients include the following:

1. Assessing the patient's preoperative physiologic and psychologic condition to determine potential problems and abnormal stress responses:
    a. Identify all medications the patient has recently received or is currently taking, including any history of substance abuse. If local anesthesia is planned, ask the patient if he or she has ever had local anesthesia at the dentist's office and if there were any adverse effects.
    b. Question the patient about known or suspected previous drug reactions. Any chemically related drug is not given.
    c. Help the patient cope with anxiety and fears by giving preoperative instructions and answering questions.

2. Handling drugs with care. Before administering or placing drugs on the sterile table:
    a. Read the label correctly. Check the expiration date.
    b. Discard the ampule or vial if the label is not completely legible or has been disturbed.
    c. Open, unlabeled, undated, multiple-use vials should be discarded and not used.
    d. Observe the solution for clarity and discard any suspicious ampule or vial.

3. Administering drugs selected by a physician in appropriate concentrations and dosages for anesthesia and IVCS:
    a. Give the minimum effective concentration and smallest volume needed. Adjust the precise amount to the weight of the patient in kilograms as appropriate.
    b. Limit the total amount of drug injected or applied to prescribed safe limits. Sterile single-dose ampules and prefilled syringes are recommended.
    c. Inject slowly to retard absorption and avoid overdosage. Use incremental titration of drug.
    d. Pull back on the syringe plunger frequently while injecting tissues to be sure the solution is not entering a blood vessel inadvertently. Intravascular injection of an anesthetic drug can release histamine into the systemic circulation, causing an anaphylactoid (nonimmunologic) reaction.
    e. Exercise caution with drugs that depress respiratory or cardiovascular functions, such as sedatives, when the upper dose limit of the anesthetic drug is used.
    f. Provide continuous IV access for administering drugs for IVCS or adverse reactions. An IV line should be established in case of adverse reaction or inadvertent intravascular injection or bolus of anesthetic. A heparin lock device or infusion of IV fluids may be used to maintain continuous access.
    g. Cease administration of the drug immediately at the sign of any sensitivity.
    h. Record the drug name, dosage, route, time, and effects of all drugs or pharmacologic agents used.

4. Continuous patient monitoring:
    a. Observe the patient, including facial expressions, and note responses to conversation and the patient's state of alertness.
    b. Assess the patient's physical signs and symptoms, such as skin color and temperature. Use assessment knowledge and skill and avoid total reliance on monitoring equipment.
    c. Monitor the patient's vital signs as appropriate (ECG, blood pressure, pulse, oxygen saturation, and respiration).
    d. Know resuscitation measures and be able to assist or initiate them as necessary, as per institutional policies and procedures. Basic cardiac lifesaver certification (BCLS) is required of all registered nurses who monitor patients. Advanced cardiac lifesaver certification (ACLS) is preferred.

Symptoms of Systemic Reactions

Symptoms of systemic reaction may be CNS stimulation or depression. Conversely, stimulation may be followed by depression and cardiovascular collapse (see Table 25-1). The cardiovascular system seems more resistant than the CNS to toxic effects of local anesthetics. The seizure threshold may differ enormously in individual patients, as may the relationship of the dose to symptoms of CNS effect. For example, lidocaine usually produces drowsiness before a convulsion, whereas bupivacaine may cause sudden seizure, disorientation, decreased hearing ability, paresthesias, muscle twitching, or agitation in a wide-awake patient without premonitory signs. Hypercapnia or hypoxemia from hypoventilation lowers the seizure threshold. Toxicity of local anesthetics is manifested primarily by CNS effects resulting from high blood levels. Symptoms of systemic reaction include, but are not limited to, the following:

- *Stimulation:* talkativeness, restlessness, incoherence, excitation, tachycardia, bounding pulse, flushed face, hyperpyrexia, tremors, hyperactive reflexes, muscular twitching, focal or grand mal convulsions
- *Depression:* drowsiness; disorientation; decreased hearing ability; stupor; syncope; rapid, thready pulse or bradycardia; apprehension; hypotension; pale or cyanotic moist skin; coma
- *Other signs:* nausea, vomiting, dizziness, blurred vision, sudden severe headache, precordial pain, extreme pulse rate or blood pressure change, angioneurotic edema (wheeze, laryngeal edema, bronchospasm), rashes, urticaria, severe local tissue reaction

Systemic reactions or undesired effects of IVCS used in combination with local anesthetics may include slurred speech, agitation, combativeness, unarousable sleep, hypotension, hypoventilation, airway obstruction, and apnea. Other symptoms may be related to specific drugs.

Benzodiazepines and sedatives used in IVCS may cause somnolence, confusion, diminished reflexes, depressed respiratory and cardiovascular function, and coma. Nystagmus (involuntary eye movements), which may be normal with large doses of diazepam (Valium), may be an abnormal reaction with other drugs. Opioids (narcotics) may cause nausea and vomiting, hypotension, and respiratory depression.

Treatment of Adverse Reactions

Treatment of an adverse reaction is aimed at preventing respiratory and cardiac arrest. Treatment must be prompt. ACLS protocol may need to be started.

Administration of the agent thought to produce the reaction is stopped immediately at the first indication of reaction. Therapy is generally supportive, the specifics dictated by clinical manifestations. Treatment consists of the following:

1. Maintaining oxygenation of vital organs and tissues with ventilation by manual or mechanical assistance to give 100% oxygen with positive pressure. Tracheal intubation may be indicated.
2. Reversing myocardial depression and peripheral vasodilation before cardiac arrest occurs. The patient is supine with the legs elevated. IV fluid therapy is begun, and a vasoconstrictor drug may be given IV or IM for hypotension or a weak pulse, which are signs of progressive circulatory depression. The choice of vasopressor is suggested by the symptoms, and the drug is used with caution. Drugs that may be used include the following:
   a. Epinephrine (IV) counteracts hypotension, bronchoconstriction, and laryngeal edema. It also stimulates beta- and alpha-adrenergic receptors and inhibits further release of mediators. It increases arteriolar constriction and force of the heartbeat. When appropriate, application of a tourniquet or subcutaneous injection of epinephrine in an area of drug injection may delay absorption of toxic drug.
   b. Ephedrine and other vasoconstrictors such as phenylephrine (Neo-Synephrine) or mephentermine (Wyamine) cause peripheral vasoconstriction, increased myocardial contraction, and bronchodilation.
   c. Antihistamines block histamine release but are not generally advocated.
   d. Steroids enhance the effect of epinephrine and inhibit further release of histamine. The effect is not immediate, and use is directed toward late manifestations of allergic response.
   e. Isoproterenol (Isuprel) is used predominantly in asthma and heart attacks; it is a bronchodilator.
   f. Antagonist drug may be given in situations in which the causative agent is identified.
3. Stopping muscle tremors or convulsions if they are present, since they constitute a hazard for further hypoxia, aspiration, or bodily injury. Diazepam in 5-mg doses or a short-acting barbiturate is given IV to inhibit cortical irritation.

For patients in whom the adverse response is caused by hypersensitivity, the previous measures are applicable. However, aminophylline may be administered to help alleviate bronchospasm, hydrocortisone (IV) to combat shock, and sodium or potassium iodide (IV) to reduce mucosal edema.

The perioperative nurse who is monitoring the patient must know resuscitation measures and be able to assist in or initiate them when necessary. An emergency cart with emergency resuscitative drugs and a defibrillator should be immediately available to the room where local or regional anesthesia with or without IVCS is administered. The following equipment should be in the room and ready for use:

- Oxygen and positive pressure breathing device (e.g., Ambu bag and mask)
- Oral and nasopharyngeal airways and endotracheal tubes in an assortment of sizes
- Cardiac and oxygen saturation monitoring equipment
- Suction

Unrelated Effects

A nerve deficit, such as pain or neuritis, that occurs in the postoperative period may be related to a preexisting condition such as multiple sclerosis. Alternatively, it may be from a cause unrelated to the anesthetic drug, such as faulty positioning; trauma from retractors; a tourniquet inflated for an inordinately long period, resulting in ischemia or pressure on peripheral nerves; or an improperly applied cast. Less common causes involve bleeding around the nerve or reaction to epinephrine.

ALTERNATIVES TO CONVENTIONAL ANESTHESIA

When local or regional anesthesia may be contraindicated but consciousness is desirable, acupuncture or hypnoanesthesia may offer alternative methods to control pain. An altered state of awareness of painful stimuli may be advantageous in selected patients.

Hypnosis

Hypnoanesthesia refers to hypnosis used as a method of anesthesia. Hypnosis produces a state of altered consciousness characterized by heightened suggestibility, selective wakefulness, reduced awareness, and restricted attentiveness. Although hypnosis has a long history of misuse, modern application by highly trained medical specialists is appropriate. Hypnoanesthesia, although seldom used, has been successfully employed in adult and pediatric patients. Motivation and concentration in the patient is an important factor. The method may be combined with the use of a small dose of a chemical anesthetic or muscle relaxant drug. Hypnosis should not be used indiscriminately in place of standard treatment.

Hypnosis may be used as a therapeutic aid in very selected patients in the following situations:

- When chemical agents are contraindicated (patient may be kept pain free, asleep or awake, without toxic side effects)
- As an adjunct to chemical anesthesia to decrease the amount of anesthesia needed
- When it is desirable to free the patient from certain neurophysical effects of an anesthetic
- When anxiety and fear of anesthesia are so great as to contribute to serious anesthetic risk
- When posthypnotic suggestion may be valuable in the postoperative period
- When it is desirable to raise the pain threshold
- When it is desirable to have the patient respond to questions or commands

Hypnoanesthesia is advantageous for burn dressings and debridement and for patients with severe respiratory or cardiovascular disease or multiple drug allergies. The anesthesia provider must establish rapport with the patient preoperatively so that the patient will listen to and obey hypnotic commands. Hypnosis is a time-consuming method and is unreliable as compared with chemical anesthesia.

Acupuncture

The ancient Chinese art of acupuncture has been practiced for more than 5000 years. Its acceptance by Western medical practitioners is fairly recent. Acupuncture is a technique of providing intense stimulation at meridian points, or planes of energy referred to as Ch'i. This stimulation prompts the brain to release endorphins and other chemicals that can relieve or block pain. Some meridians are associated with prevention of nausea and vomiting postoperatively. An example of Ch'i points in a meridian line for the lung is depicted in Figure 25-4.

Stimulation is effected by manually rotating or applying electric current to very-fine-gauge needles inserted into meridian points. When acupuncture is used for anesthesia, a minute electric current is used to speed and enhance analgesia or anesthesia in the desired body region. The meridian points generally correspond to the area where the somatic nerve supply is located. It is a time-consuming technique. It may be used immediately after premedication is given to reduce postoperative nausea and vomiting following short procedures with the patient under general anesthesia.

Acupuncture is gaining popularity in surgical and dental procedures and for postoperative or intractable pain. The patient remains conscious. Procedures are limited to use by physicians or appropriate personnel under their direct supervision in keeping with acceptable standards of medical practice.

Figure 25-4 Example of Ch'i points in meridian line used in acupuncture for treatment of the left lung.

Bibliography

Association of Operating Room Nurses: *AORN Standards, Recommended Practices, and Guidelines,* Denver, 1998, The Association.

Bouaziz H et al: The use of selective axillary nerve block for outpatient hand surgery, *Anesth Analg* 86(4):746-748, 1998.

Liguori GA et al: Transient neurologic symptoms after spinal anesthesia with mepivacaine and lidocaine, *Anesthesiology* 88(3):619-623, 1998.

Liu SS: Optimizing spinal anesthesia for ambulatory surgery, *Reg Anesth* 22(6):500-510, 1997.

Muller CM et al: Sedation and anaesthesia outside the OR, *Acta Anaesthesiol Scand* 111(suppl):196-198, 1997.

Pasero CL, Vanderveer BL: Pain control: epidural infusions: not just for labor anymore, *Am J Nurs* 94(12):51-52, 1994.

Phillip BK: New approaches to anesthesia for day case surgery, *Acta Anaesthesiol Belg* 48(3):167-174, 1997.

Roberge CW, McEwen M: The effects of local anesthetics on postoperative pain, *AORN J* 68(6):1003-1012, 1998.

Smith CJ: Preparing nurses to monitor patients receiving local anesthesia, *AORN J* 59(5):1033-1041, 1994.

Tarkkiila P et al: Home-readiness after spinal anaesthesia with small doses of hyperbaric 0.5% bupivacaine, *Anaesthesiology* 52(12:1157-1160, 1997.

Watson DS: *Conscious sedation/analgesia,* St Louis, 1998, Mosby.

Willins JS: Giving fentanyl for pain outside the OR, *Am J Nurs* 94(2):24-28, 1994.

Chapter 26

Physiologic Maintenance and Monitoring of the Perioperative Patient

 Chapter Objectives

After studying this chapter, the learner will be able to:

- Identify pertinent body systems that should be monitored during a surgical procedure.
- Discuss the differences between invasive and noninvasive means of patient monitoring.
- Discuss why personnel monitoring a patient should be knowledgeable about the monitoring devices used.
- Describe how monitoring parameters provide information about interrelated body systems.

The development of successful, controllable anesthesia has made modern surgery possible. Because anesthesia is an adjunct to most surgical procedures, familiarity with various anesthetic agents, their interaction with certain drugs, and their potential hazards is a necessity. The perioperative nurse responsible for patient monitoring may detect the onset of complications and help to avert an undesired outcome.

Working with anesthesia providers in the perioperative environment gives the learner an unparalleled opportunity to master immediate resuscitative measures and their effectiveness, as well as an understanding of the care of unconscious and critically ill patients. For example, the learner daily observes endotracheal intubation, ventilatory control, insertion of arterial and venous cannulas, fluid replacement, and sophisticated hemodynamic monitoring.

No surgical procedure is minor. Surgery and anesthesia impose on the patient certain inescapable risks, even under supposedly ideal circumstances. Overall, however, the anesthetic-related surgical mortality rate is relatively low. Preexisting patient factors, such as age and/or medical condition, and those related to the circumstances of the surgical procedure, such as type, duration, and elective vs. emergency procedure, are more significant in determining surgical mortality. The American Society of Anesthesiologists (ASA) has established standards for basic perioperative monitoring. Specialization in monitoring equipment and the use of computers to record monitoring data are facets of contemporary anesthesia practice. Terms associated with monitoring and maintaining the perioperative patient are defined in Box 26-1.

Box 26-1   Terms Associated with Monitoring and Maintaining the Perioperative Patient

hemodynamics   Study of blood circulation, blood pressure, peripheral vascular physiology, and cardiac function.

monitoring   Observing, evaluating, and reporting physiologic function.

pulse   Palpable sensation of blood passing through an artery.

respiration   Exchange of oxygen and carbon dioxide at the molecular level.

   expiration   Exit of waste gases from the body through the mouth and nose.

   external respiration   Exchange of gases between the lungs and blood at the alveolar level.

   internal respiration   Exchange of gases between the blood and cells at the capillary/tissue level.

   ventilation/inspiration   Bringing air into the lungs through the mouth and nose.

sinus rhythm   Electrical impulse in the heart that originates at the sinoatrial node of the right atria of the heart, passes through the atrioventricular node at the atrial-septal junction, and continues down the length of the Purkinje fibers in the ventricular septum, causing contraction of the ventricles.

HISTORICAL BACKGROUND

Iatrophysics was the study of the application of the principles of mechanics to human physiology. As early scientists and physicians learned more about anatomy and physiology, assessment of precise physiologic measurements improved patient care. The most significant discovery of the seventeenth century was cardiopulmonary circulation. English physiologist William Harvey (1578-1657) described the circulation of blood through the body in 1628. Spanish physician Michael Servetus (1511-1553) had paved the way by describing theories of pulmonary circulation through the lungs. Conceptually, these discoveries disproved theories developed by the Roman father of physiology, Claudius Galen (130-200 AD), that blood flowed between the heart chambers via pores. Earlier myths included the belief that blood actually originated in the heart and was pumped one drop at a time.

Expanding knowledge of circulation and its effects on the body led to the ability to monitor physiologic function. Italian physicist Galileo Galilei (1564-1642) experimented with temperature measurement in 1592. His theories were followed by those of Santorio Santorio (1561-1637), who developed a prototype of a thermometer. Dutch physician Herman Boerhaave (1668-1738) was the first to use a thermometer in clinical practice and taught that clinical discussions of patient condition improved the outcome of treatment. The glass thermometer as used in current practice was developed by Clifford Allbutt in 1870.

Monitoring techniques began to improve with the development of the sphygmomanometer for the measurement of blood pressure in 1896 by Italian physician Scipione

Riva-Ricci (1863-1943). The development of watches with second hands allowed physicians to count a patient's pulse and respirations.

Techniques for monitoring patients have improved significantly over the past decade. Automated monitoring devices have become more sensitive and accurate. Electrocardiographic (ECG) monitors, blood pressure machines, and pulse oximeters display the patient's hemodynamics electronically. Specialized probes measure core temperature, and skin patches measure surface temperature without the use of a glass thermometer. Appropriate monitoring techniques can assist the perioperative team in patient care.

MONITORING PHYSIOLOGIC FUNCTIONS

Preoperative patient assessment establishes a baseline and provides valuable information by which intraoperative and postoperative patient care is planned and evaluated. Establishing a preoperative baseline enables the caregiver to be alerted to changes in the patient's physiologic condition that may require prompt attention.

Surgical and anesthesia techniques have become increasingly complex, allowing many critically ill patients of all ages to undergo surgical procedures. The anesthesia provider carefully monitors the patient's condition through the entire perioperative process and keeps the surgeon informed of important changes.

Monitoring implies keeping track of vital functions. During extensive surgery with the patient under anesthesia, the body is subjected to physiologic stress. Bleeding, tissue trauma, potent drugs, large extravascular fluid shifts, multiple transfusions, and a surgical position that may inhibit breathing and circulation all contribute to altered physiology. These factors can induce significant cardiopulmonary dysfunction.

Evaluation of the patient's responses to these stressors includes observation, auscultation, and palpation. The assessment is enhanced by the use of electronic or mechanical devices that reveal physiologic trends and subtle changes and indicate responses to therapy. Most of this equipment is expensive and is incorporated into the anesthesia machine. Compact, precise devices with miniaturized circuitry, better visibility, and easier maintenance are incorporated into portable models that allow for continued monitoring after the patient leaves the operating room (OR).

Computers improve and expedite analysis of data. They are sophisticated data collection and management tools to assist in physiologic assessment, diagnosis, and therapy. Clinical computers vary from single-function devices to complex, multifunction, real-time systems that acquire, store, and display data; organize information; display trends; and perform calculations.

Personnel using electronic and computerized monitoring equipment must understand its use and function, be experienced in its interpretation, and be able to determine equipment malfunction easily. Instrumentation should augment, not replace, careful observation of the patient. Monitoring equipment can be inaccurate. Information from monitors should be compared with physical assessment data. Perioperative nurses involved with patient monitoring should remain current in the knowledge of physical assessment and the use of the equipment in use. Periodic competency testing should be performed. Written policies, procedures, and guidelines should be available for reference.

The spectrum of monitoring devices is broad. It ranges from noninvasive to invasive. Noninvasive monitors do not penetrate the body or a body orifice. Conversely, invasive monitors penetrate skin or mucosa, or they enter a body cavity. Some parameters can be measured by both noninvasive and invasive methods. Perioperative nursing responsibilities may include assisting with sophisticated hemodynamic monitoring to evaluate the interrelationship of blood pressure, blood flow, vascular volumes, physical properties of blood, heart rate, and ventricular function. Detection of early changes in hemodynamics allows prompt action to maintain cardiac function and adequate cardiac output. Monitoring facilitates rapid, accurate determination of decreased perfusion. It reflects immediate response to therapeutic measures and stress.

Invasive Hemodynamic Monitoring

Hemodynamics is the study of the movement of blood. Measurements of cardiac output and intracardiac pressures provide information related to functions of the heart and other major organ systems.

Invasive hemodynamic monitoring uses basic physiologic principles to detect and treat a wide variety of abnormalities. Its purpose is to avoid problems in high-risk patients and to accurately diagnose and treat patients with established life-threatening disorders. It involves direct intravascular measurements and assessments by means of indwelling catheters connected to transducers and monitors. Pressures and forces within arteries and veins are converted to electrical signals by the transducer, a device that transfers energy from one system to another. These electrical signals are then processed and amplified by the monitor into a continuous waveform displayed on an oscilloscope or monitoring screen that reproduces images received via the transducer; or the monitor may digitally display the values. These measurements yield specific information that is otherwise not usually attainable or as accurate. Although these measurements may be pertinent in guiding patient care, they present additional risks because obtaining them requires invasion of the great vessels or heart. The benefits of invasive monitoring must be balanced against the risks.

Various types of equipment, monitors, and catheters are in use. All persons caring for patients with invasive monitors must have knowledge of anatomy and physiology and understanding of the entire monitoring circuit. Every precaution must be taken to ensure patient safety. Strict adherence to policies and procedures, manufacturer's instructions for use, and sterile technique is absolutely essential to minimize complications and misinterpretation of data that could lead to errors in therapy.

Indwelling arterial, venous, and intracardiac catheters permit rapid, accurate assessment of physiologic alterations in high-risk patients. Intravascular access is justified because of the high yield of information with minimal discomfort to patients. But hemodynamic monitoring techniques must not be abused. Cardiac dysrhythmias, thrombosis, embolism, and infection are serious, sometimes fatal, complications of intravascular cannulation. Some facilities require the patient to sign an informed consent form before insertion of an invasive catheter.

Intravascular Cannulation

Intravascular catheters usually are inserted before induction of anesthesia by a physician; a certified registered nurse anesthetist (CRNA) may be permitted to insert some types. They may be inserted percutaneously or by cutdown, depending on the type of catheter, intended purpose(s), and location of the vessel to be cannulated. Intracardiac catheters may be placed under fluoroscopic control, or their position may be verified on a chest x-ray film after insertion. In addition to their use in hemodynamic monitoring, intravenous (IV) catheters can be used to administer blood, drugs, and nutrients. Catheters may be inserted via the vena cava into the right atrium or pulmonary artery through a subclavian, jugular, brachial, or femoral vein or via an antecubital vein.

Intraarterial catheters are inserted for direct pressure measurements and to obtain blood for arterial blood gas (ABG) analyses. Potential sites for cannulation include the radial, ulnar, axillary, brachial, femoral, and dorsalis pedis arteries. The radial artery is most commonly used if ulnar circulation to the hand is adequate. A Doppler ultrasonic device may be used to determine a dominant artery and to locate a weakly palpable one. When radial artery dominance exists, the ulnar, brachial, or other artery is used. As a precaution, adequacy of perfusion to the extremity below the catheter should be established before insertion, in case thrombosis or occlusion occurs. A radial artery distal to a brachial artery previously used for cardiac catheterization is avoided because of the possibility of distorted pressures or occlusion. Some physicians cannulate the femoral artery if the catheter is to remain in place for more than 24 hours. The incidence of thrombosis is lower when a large vessel is used. Thrombosis may result from irritation of the vessel wall or hypercoagulation or inadequate flushing of the catheter and line. The larger the catheter in relation to the artery lumen, the greater the incidence of thrombosis. Other complications of arterial cannulation include embolic phenomena, blood loss from a dislodged catheter or disconnected line, bruise or hematoma formation, arteriovenous fistula or aneurysm formation, systemic infection, and ischemic fingers from arterial spasm.

Catheters

Most catheters are radiopaque and have centimeter calibrations. They are flexible. They may be made of silicone, polyethylene, polyvinyl chloride, polytetrafluoroethylene (Teflon), or polyurethane. Those with soft, pliable tips are safer than stiff catheters. Shearing of a vessel with extravascular migration of the catheter has occurred from stiffness and sharpness of the catheter and movement of the patient. Soft catheters must be introduced over a guidewire or by flow-directed balloons. The catheter and related introducer, guidewire, and caps may be supplied as a prepackaged sterile kit.

Many catheters have a heparin coating to prevent clot formation. Polyurethane or other uncoated catheters are available for the patient who is allergic to heparin. The catheter is kept open with a slow, continuous infusion. Routine flushing of the catheter is necessary. Normal saline may be used if heparin is unnecessary or contraindicated. Continuous-flush devices with fast-flush valves release small amounts of solution. Limited pressure diminishes the possibility of ejecting a large clot. The catheter usually is fast flushed both hourly and after blood samples are withdrawn. Air bubbles in the line must be avoided. After flushing, the drip rate in the drip chamber is checked.

A catheter may have a single lumen or two or three lumens. The catheters to be discussed are used for hemodynamic monitoring of the following:

- ABGs and pressure via a single-lumen intraarterial catheter
- Central venous pressure via a central venous, Hickman, or Broviac catheter
- Pulmonary artery pressures via a pulmonary artery or Swan-Ganz catheter

Catheter Insertion   Catheter insertion is a sterile procedure. The necessary sterile supplies should be collected before the patient arrives. Although catheters are different, the technique for insertion is basically the same for all types. Insertion is a team effort. The circulator's responsibilities may vary but usually include the following:

1. Explain the procedure and reassure the patient. If the patient will be awake, sedation may be ordered.
2. Document the patient's vital signs and pulse distal to the selected insertion site. If the pulse weakens after cannulation, circulation may be inadequate in an extremity and the catheter may have to be removed.
3. Position the patient as appropriate.
   a. For radial artery cannulation, affix the forearm to an armboard with the hand supinated and wrist dorsiflexed to an angle of 50 to 60 degrees over a towel. Avoid extreme dorsiflexion; this can obliterate the pulse. Tape the thumb to the armboard to stabilize the artery at the wrist.
   b. For subclavian or jugular vein insertion, place the patient in a 25- to 30-degree head-down Trendelenburg position to reduce the potential for air embolism. Elevate the scapular area with padding or a rolled towel underneath the shoulders to allow the physician to identify anatomic landmarks and

locate the vein more easily. Turn the patient's head away from the insertion site.
4. Prepare the skin per routine procedure. Wearing sterile gloves, the physician then drapes the area. Warn the patient if his or her face will be covered.
5. Inform the patient, if awake, that he or she may have a burning sensation for a few seconds when the local anesthetic is injected before the area becomes numb. Explain that he or she may feel pressure, but not pain, during insertion. The skin and subcutaneous tissues are infiltrated with a local anesthetic because the skin is incised to facilitate entrance of the catheter. A cutdown to a vein may be necessary.
6. Assist the physician as appropriate. Be familiar with and follow the manufacturer's directions for the brand of catheter and monitoring equipment being used.
7. Make sure the connections between the catheter and infusion line are secure after the catheter has been inserted and properly placed. The catheter is sutured in place to prevent inadvertent advancement or removal and is taped to the skin. Lumens on the three-way stopcock and catheter may be capped to prevent fibrin deposits and retrograde contamination.
8. Connect the catheter line to the transducer or monitor and take baseline pressure readings.
9. Dress the puncture site. An antibacterial ointment may be put around the site. Tape must not apply pressure directly over the insertion site or catheter. A transparent dressing is preferable. The catheter beneath it must not be bent or curled.
10. Take the patient's vital signs. Using a sphygmomanometer with the blood pressure cuff on the opposite arm from the insertion site, check the blood pressure to compare with the monitor's pressure reading to verify the monitor's accuracy. The monitor will probably read higher systolic and lower diastolic pressures than the blood pressure cuff readings.
11. Document the procedure and initial readings. Include the insertion site; type and gauge of catheter; type of infusion solution and amount of heparin, if added; flow rate and pressure; pulse before and after insertion; tolerance of the procedure; color, sensation, and warmth of the area distal to the insertion site; time of insertion; and names of insertion team members.

Frequent checks of circuitry and calibrations are necessary to validate the recorded data. Conscientious attention to every detail is mandatory during catheter insertion and monitoring.

Drawing Blood Samples   When the arterial or venous catheters are in place, the perioperative nurse may be asked to collect blood samples for analysis or to take measurements, although this is not universal practice. These procedures require special training, skill, and knowledge of equipment and hazards involved. An on-line tutorial is available at **nursing.about.com/mbody.htm?COB=home&PID=2789&PM=68_910_T.**

Samples for ABG measurements are sometimes drawn from an indwelling catheter line kept open by a continuously running infusion. The tubing incorporates a plastic three-way stopcock, usually close to the catheter insertion site. One lumen of the stopcock goes to the infusion solution, one to the cannulated vessel, and one to outside air. The last-mentioned one is normally closed or covered with a sterile cap, or a sterile syringe is kept inserted in the lumen to prevent bacteria and air from entering. With a three-way stopcock, two of the three lumens are always open. More information can be found at **www-medlib.med.utah.edu/kw/ecg/ecg_outline.**

In drawing blood samples from an indwelling catheter, always use strict sterile technique. Blood may be drawn through a stopcock on a single-lumen catheter or from one lumen of a multilumen catheter. A sterile ABG monitoring kit with administration tubing and pressure transducers may be used for intraarterial pressure monitoring. The manufacturer's instructions should be followed for turning the stopcock to draw blood samples and to flush lines. Drawing blood from a multilumen catheter is simplified when an injection port can be used. The basic procedure is similar to the following, using a stopcock (always wipe the stopcock or end of the catheter with alcohol before entering the system):

1. Wear sterile gloves. A sterile heparinized syringe is used to prevent the blood samples from clotting. To heparinize, draw 1 ml of aqueous heparin 1:1000 into a 10-ml syringe. While rotating the barrel, pull the plunger back beyond the 7-ml calibration. With the syringe in an upright position, slowly eject the heparin and air bubbles while rotating the barrel.
2. Attach a sterile 5-ml syringe to the stopcock lumen going to outside air. Turn off (close) the infusion lumen. This automatically opens the line between the patient and the syringe. Aspirate to clear the line of fluid and close the lumen to the patient. Discard this diluted sample.
3. Quickly attach the sterile heparinized syringe to a lumen to outside air and open the lumen to the patient. This closes the lumen to the infusion, permitting aspiration of undiluted blood for analysis. Arterial pressure forces blood into the syringe. Withdraw 3 to 5 ml of blood. Hold the barrel, as well as the plunger, of the syringe to avoid their separation. Cap the syringe for placement in a properly labeled specimen bag.
4. Close the lumen to the patient and flush the line and stopcock by letting the infusion solution run through them to prevent clot formation inside the catheter wall or stopcock, which could result in arterial embolization.
5. Close and recap the lumen to outside air (being careful not to contaminate the cap), thereby restarting the infusion to the patient. Regulate the infusion rate with the clamp on the infusion tubing.
6. If air bubbles are in the syringe, remove them. Send the samples immediately to the laboratory. If more than 10 minutes elapses between blood drawing and analysis, the analysis cannot be considered accurate. In the event of delay, the syringe with blood should be immersed in ice immediately and refrigerated at near-freezing temperature. Iced specimen bags may be used.
7. Attach the appropriate laboratory slips that include information such as the patient's name and location, the time and date, and the use of oxygen or room air.

Physiologic Parameters Monitored

Noninvasive methods can be used to monitor some cardiopulmonary and neural functions and to determine body temperature and urinary output (Box 26-2). Both noninvasive and invasive techniques are used for monitoring hemodynamic parameters to show minute-to-minute changes in physiologic variables. Normal ranges of hemodynamic parameters are given in Table 26-1.

Electrocardiogram

Every heartbeat depends on the electrical process of polarization. Muscles in the heart wall are alternately stimulated and relaxed. An electrocardiogram (ECG/EKG) is a recording of electrical forces produced by the heart and translated as waveforms (Figure 26-1). It shows changes in rhythm, rate, or conduction, such as dysrhythmias; appearance of premature beats; and block of impulses. An ECG does not provide an index of cardiac output (CO). Cardiac monitoring has become standard procedure in the OR and postanesthesia care unit (PACU). Review of cardiac anatomy and physiology can be found on-line at **www.innerbody.com/indexbody.html.** An on-line tutorial for ECG review can be found at **www-medlib. med.utah.edu/kw/ecg/ecg_outline.**

Cardiac monitoring systems generally consist of a monitor screen; a cathode ray oscilloscope, on which the ECG is continuously visualized; and a printout system, which transcribes the rhythm strip to paper to permit comparison of tracings and provide a permanent record. The printout may be controlled or automatic. A heart rate meter may be set to print out a rhythm strip and sound an alarm if the rate goes above or below a preset figure. Lights and beepers may provide appropriate visual and audible signals of the heart rate. Monitor leads or electrodes are attached to the chest and/or extremities. These electrodes detect electrical impulses that the heart generates. Connecting lead wires and cables transmit them to the cardiac monitor. A complete cardiogram includes 12 different leads, but usually only two or three electrodes are used. Careful placement of leads is important to show waves and complexes on the ECG rhythm strip. Leads to the anterior, lateral, or inferior cardiac surfaces, where ischemia most often occurs, provide myocardial ischemia monitoring. Use of multiple leads allows better definition of dysrhythmia and ischemia, the main reason for cardiac monitoring in the OR. The choice of leads is made by the anesthesia provider or by the surgeon in unattended local anesthesia.

In placing disk electrodes, one must be sure that the underlying skin is clean and dry for adequate adherence. The sites are shaved, if necessary, because hair can interfere with adherence. The skin is abraded slightly with a gauze pad or rough material to facilitate conduction. The paper

Box 26-2 Noninvasive Methods of Monitoring Vital Functions

Cardiopulmonary Functions

blood pressure (BP) Measurement of pressure exerted against arterial vessel walls to force blood through circulation.

capnometry Measurement of end-tidal concentration of carbon dioxide by exposing expired air to infrared light.

cardiac index (CI) Measurement of cardiac output in relation to body surface with ultrasound.

chest x-ray study Determination of the position of intravascular catheters and endotracheal or chest tubes by radiology.

echocardiogram Assessment of intraventricular blood volume by observing two-dimensional color images of the beating heart produced by an ultrasonic probe placed in the esophagus.

electrocardiogram (ECG/EKG) Recording of electrical forces produced by the heart to evaluate changes in rhythm, rate, or conduction.

near-infrared reflectance Determination of the amount of oxygen in hemoglobin being delivered to the brain with a niroscope (NIRS).

pulse oximetry Determination of arterial hemoglobin oxygen saturation by measuring the optical density of light passing through tissues.

respiratory tidal volume (V_T) Measurement of the volume of air moved with each respiration with a respirometer.

stethoscopy Detection of cardiac rate and rhythm and pulmonary sounds by ausculation.

total blood volume (TBV) Measurement of plasma and red blood cell volumes with an electronic device.

Neural Functions

electroencephalogram (EEG) Recording of electrical activity in the brain.

evoked potentials Recording of electrical responses from the cerebral cortex after stimulation of a peripheral sensory organ.

Other Functions

temperature Measurement of core body temperature with a thermometer probe.

urinary output Measurement of urine to assess renal perfusion via an indwelling catheter attached to a calibrated collection device.

TABLE 26-1 Hemodynamic Monitoring Parameters

Parameter	Abbreviation	Normal Range for Adults
Arterial oxygen content	CaO_2	17-20 ml/dl blood
Blood pressure	BP	Systolic 90-130 mm Hg
		Diastolic 60-85 mm Hg
Cardiac index	CI	2.8-4.2 L/min/m²
Cardiac output	CO	4-8 L/min
Central venous pressure	CVP	2-8 mm Hg, 3-10 cm H_2O
Cerebral perfusion pressure	CPP	80-100 mm Hg
Coronary perfusion pressure	CPP	60-80 mm Hg
Ejection fraction	EF	60%-70%
Glomerular filtration rate	GFR	80-120 ml/min
Heart rate	HR	60-100 beats/min
Intracranial pressure	ICP	0-15 mm Hg
Left ventricular end-diastolic pressure	LVEDP	8-12 mm Hg
Mean arterial pressure	MAP	70-105 mm Hg
Mean pulmonary artery pressure	MPAP	9-19 mm Hg
Oxygen saturation in arterial blood	SaO_2	95%-97.5%
Oxygen saturation in mixed venous blood	SvO_2	75%
Partial pressure of carbon dioxide in arterial blood	$PaCO_2$	35-45 mm Hg (torr)
Partial pressure of oxygen in arterial blood	PaO_2	80-100 mm Hg (torr)
Partial pressure of oxygen in venous blood	PvO_2	40 mm Hg (torr)
Pulmonary artery pressure	PAP	Systolic 15-25 mm Hg
		Diastolic 8-15 mm Hg
Pulmonary capillary wedge pressure	PCWP	6-12 mm Hg
Right atrial pressure	RAP	3-6 mm Hg
Right ventricular pressure	RVP	Systolic 15-25 mm Hg
		Diastolic 0-5 mm Hg
Stroke volume	SV	60-130 ml/beat
Systemic vascular resistance	SVR	800-1600 dyne/sec/cm
Total blood volume	TBV	8.5%-9% of body weight in kg
Venous oxygen content	CvO_2	15 ml/dl blood

Figure 26-1 Electrocardiogram complex. *P wave* before each QRS complex represents atrial depolarization. *PR interval* of sinus rhythm occurs between each P wave and R wave. *PR segment* represents conduction of impulse through atrioventricular (AV) node, bundle of His, bundle branches, and Purkinje fibers. *QRS complex* following each P wave represents ventricular depolarization and occurs at regular intervals, but rate can vary. *T wave* represents ventricular repolarization.

backing is peeled off the disk. As much as possible, touching the adhesive is avoided. The conductive gel within the gauze pad at the center of the disk is checked. If it is not moist, another disk is used. The electrode is placed on the desired site, adhesive side down, and secure tightly by applying pressure. One begins at the center and moves outward to avoid expressing gel from beneath the electrode. Placing gel over a bony area is avoided, since bone will interfere with conduction.

One ECG tracing is taken before induction of anesthesia as a baseline. An ECG is especially valuable during induction and intubation, when dysrhythmias are prone to occur. Early detection and rapid identification of abnormal rhythms and irregularities of the heart's actions permit treatment to be more specific. Tracings may show changes related to the anesthetic itself or to oxygenation, coronary blood flow, hypercapnia (increased $PaCO_2$), or alterations in electrolyte balance or body temperature. The ECG tracing becomes a flat line when heart action ceases, but preceding tracings may define the type of cardiac arrest, which is of value in treatment. It is beyond the scope of this text to describe normal and abnormal cardiac rhythms interpreted by the ECG. However, perioperative nurses who monitor patients under local anesthesia should become familiar with them. Box 26-3 shows the characteristics of sinus rhythm, and Figure 26-2 shows an example of sinus rhythm in each of 12 leads.

Box 26-3	**Characteristics of Sinus Rhythm**

P wave is present before each QRS complex.
There is equal space between P wave and R wave (PR interval) in each complex.
QRS complex follows each P wave (ratio 1:1).
P wave and QRS complex occur at regular intervals (rate can vary).

ECG monitors should be insensitive to electrical interference. Occasionally, recording may be affected by a high-frequency electrosurgical unit. If a tracing problem occurs, lead contacts, the integrity of the leads, and the choice of monitoring axis are checked.

The ECG monitor may be connected to a computer for analysis and storage of data. From the ECG readings, a device within the computer may be able to measure the amount of blood being pumped by the heart. This gives a continuous assessment of pumping capacity and CO. Impedance cardiography also provides data based on the mechanical activity of the heart. This is also a noninvasive, computer-assisted measurement of CO, an alternative to the thermodilution technique.

Figure 26-2 Example of normal sinus rhythms as they appear in each of 12 leads. (From Kinney MR et al: *Andreoli's comprehensive cardiac care,* ed 8, St Louis, 1996, Mosby.)

Echocardiogram

Sound waves from a sonarlike device provide two-dimensional color images of the beating heart. An ultrasonic probe on the end of a small gastroscope is placed in the esophagus. Also referred to as transesophageal echocardiography, the echocardiogram can help the anesthesia provider immediately assess intraventricular blood volumes. This can be useful information for the surgeon during cardiac surgery.

Stethoscopy

Auscultation, the act of listening to the chest, detects both cardiac rate and rhythm and pulmonary sounds. A stethoscope is taped over the precordium, the region over the heart and stomach at the level of the diaphragm, or a pressure-sensitive detector may be placed within the patient's esophagus. With the trachea protected by a cuffed endotracheal tube to prevent aspiration, the stethoscope is inserted in the esophagus to the level of the heart. Esophageal stethoscopy is especially valuable during thoracic and abdominal procedures, when auscultatory monitoring is ineffective because of tissue manipulation or movements of the members of the operating team.

Arterial Blood Pressure

Blood pressure (BP) signifies the pressure exerted against vessel walls to force blood through the circulation. Evaluation of BP during anesthesia requires consideration of blood volume, CO, and the state of the sympathetic tone of the vessels. Tissue perfusion is dependent on these factors. Arterial BP is used to assess hemodynamic and respiratory status during every surgical procedure, with very few exceptions. BP measures contraction of the heart (systolic pressure) and relaxation of the heart between contractions (diastolic pressure). Blood is forced through the arteries between contractions. Pressure is higher during systole and lower during diastole. Many factors can cause BP to vary. It is measured in millimeters of mercury. Normal range is 90 to 130 mm Hg systolic and 60 to 85 mm Hg diastolic.

The arm used for measurements should be opposite the one cannulated for IV fluid therapy or invasive monitoring and should be protected from contact with team members standing beside the operating bed. BP readings can be obtained by indirect or direct methods, either intermittently or continuously.

Sphygmomanometer A pneumatic cuff is wrapped around the circumference of the upper arm. When the cuff is inflated, measurements are obtained on the sphygmomanometer as the cuff deflates. Through a stethoscope placed over an artery distal to the cuff, the systolic pressure is heard when blood begins to flow through the artery. The diastolic pressure is noted by a change in sound. This is an indirect, noninvasive method for intermittent monitoring of BP.

Doppler Ultrasonic Flowmeter With ultrasound, BP can be monitored automatically at preset intervals. The Doppler ultrasonic flowmeter monitor automatically inflates the cuff, takes a reading, and deflates the cuff. It can be programmed to sound an alarm if systolic pressure reaches a preset high or low level. The readings are more accurate than with sphygmomanometer pressure cuff monitoring because the ultrasonic transducer amplifies blood flow sounds. Automated, noninvasive BP monitors function well in a noisy environment. However, they do not provide continuous BP measurement or detect extremely low pressures. Frequent inflations of the cuff can bruise the skin, especially of geriatric patients.

Infrared Beams Noninvasive infrared beams (Finapres technique) may be used to indirectly monitor BP. A small cuff fits on a finger. The beams from the cuff shine through tissue. They continuously measure arterial pressure from one heartbeat to the next.

Direct Arterial Pressure From an invasive modality, beat-to-beat direct pressures are obtained through an artery, usually the radial or femoral, via an indwelling catheter inserted percutaneously. A very slow drip of slightly heparinized saline keeps the catheter open. The fluid-filled tubing from the catheter is connected to a mechanical electric transducer. The transducer is attached to an amplifier. A waveform of the amplified pulse, which represents force imposed on the transducer, is displayed. The monitor also converts waveforms into numerical measurements of systolic and diastolic rates. An alarm sounds if deviations are significant.

Mean Arterial Pressure Mean arterial pressure (MAP), calculated by most monitors and shown on digital display, portrays perfusion pressure of the body. This is significant in evaluating myocardial perfusion. Normal MAP is between 70 and 105 mm Hg. Direct intraarterial pressure monitoring is valuable in patients with major multiple trauma or burns, inaccessibility of an extremity, unstable vital signs, or inaudible BP. Other indications are complex, extensive procedures, such as a cardiopulmonary bypass with an open chest; major vascular surgery with large potential fluid shifts or blood loss; total hip replacement; and major neurosurgery with the patient in the sitting position. Also included are patients in shock or with preexisting cardiac or pulmonary disease who must undergo major surgery. Direct pressure monitoring is necessary in deliberate hypotensive anesthesia, as well as in treatment of hypotensive or hypertensive crisis with continuous infusion of vasopressor or hypertensive drugs.

Blood Gases and pH

Monitoring of tissue perfusion is indispensable in evaluating pulmonary gas exchange and acid-base balance. Measurements are considered in relation to other parameters, such as vital signs, venous pressure, and left atrial pressure. Oxygen and carbon dioxide in blood exert their own partial pressures (P). Measurements are expressed in millimeters of mercury or torr. They may be differentiated as arterial (Pa) or venous (Pv). The gas being measured is identified. The partial pressure of oxygen is expressed as Po_2, or specifically in arterial blood as Pao_2 and in venous blood as Pvo_2. Oxygen saturation (So_2) in arterial blood (Sao_2) is expressed in percentages. The partial pressure of carbon dioxide is specified as $Paco_2$ or $Pvco_2$. (See Table 26-1 for normal ranges.) Monitoring techniques can be either noninvasive or invasive.

Pulse Oximetry A pulse oximeter measures arterial oxyhemoglobin saturation (Sao_2). It provides a reading within seconds by measuring optical density of light passing through tissues. A sensor probe is clipped on each side of a pulsating vascular bed. Fingers, toes, earlobes, and the bridge of the nose are suitable sites. The patient's skin should be clean and dry. An area with fingernail polish should be avoided or the polish removed. Skin integrity under the sensor must be intact. The sensor must be maintained flush with the skin surface and positioned so that the light source and photodetector are in direct alignment. The sensor is attached to an oximeter, which is plugged into a power source. Some power sources are battery powered. The oximeter may have an earphone adapter and an alarm system. The alarm is usually set for audible alert within 10 seconds if the oxygen saturation falls below the preset range.

Wavelengths of red (660-nm) and infrared (940-nm) light pass through tissues from the light source side of the probe. Light is picked up by a receptor in the sensor on the opposite side of the tissue. The oximeter continuously calculates the amount of oxygen present in the blood by processing the ratio of red to infrared light absorbed. The presence of oxygen in hemoglobin influences this absorption (oxyhemoglobin).

The oximeter reading should remain above 95%. A reading below 90% probably signifies developing hypoxia. Some patients have significant respiratory disease and have prolonged trends of low readings. Oximeters give no information about the retention of carbon dioxide and are not indicators of respiratory failure caused by carbon dioxide retention. Falsely high readings may occur in cigarette smokers because carbon monoxide (carboxyhemoglobin) can prevent red blood cells from picking up oxygen. Carboxyhemoglobin closely resembles oxyhemoglobin and is perceived by the sensor to be oxygenated. These cells may absorb light from the oximeter, however, so the reading may be higher than the actual Sao_2. Other factors may influence reliability, such as shielding of the sensor, excessive ambient light, patient movement, or intravascular dyes. Oximeter readings should always be compared with patient assessment. More information about the use of pulse oximetry can be found on-line at **www.nicl.com/labnotes/pulseox.html.** Information about competency testing for the use of pulse oximetry can be found at the National Institutes of Health (NIH) Web site: **www.cc.nih.gov/nursing/pulsoxim.html.**

Niroscope Oxygen reserves in the brain can be assessed with a near-infrared reflectance scope (NIRS), a noninvasive technique. A specific form of infrared light passes through the skull. The portion of light reflected back to sensors outside the skull is measured to determine the amount of oxygen in the hemoglobin being delivered to the brain. The niroscope provides a continuous reading of the brain's oxygen reserves.

Capnometry Changes in exhaled carbon dioxide reflect changes in respiration, circulation, or metabolism. Capnometry measures end-tidal concentration of carbon dioxide. Normal concentration is 38 torr (5%). Carbon dioxide production is in direct relationship to cellular metabolism. Monitoring carbon dioxide can detect the onset of inadvertent hypothermia or malignant hyperthermia. Capnometry, a noninvasive technique, also can detect anesthesia equipment problems, inadvertent esophageal intubation, inadequate neuromuscular blockage, air embolus, or a ventilation-perfusion problem.

A mainstream or sidestream adapter is placed in the breathing circuit as close to the face mask as possible so that expired carbon dioxide will approximate alveolar concentration. The analyzer, attached to the adapter, exposes expired air to infrared light. The amount of light absorbed by carbon dioxide determines the end-tidal concentration. A sidestream analyzer can be used to monitor patients receiving local or regional anesthesia by placing the sampling end of the tubing in the patient's nostril or mouth.

A capnographic waveform printout provides data to evaluate respiratory rate and rhythm. Some gas monitors continuously measure carbon dioxide, oxygen, and nitrous oxide parameters of the patient's airway. Digital values are displayed on the monitor.

Optode An optode is an optical fiber inserted through an 18- or 20-gauge radial artery cannula. The tip contains chemicals that react to oxygen, carbon dioxide, and acidity of the blood. The optode is connected to a monitor that generates light through the fiber. The chemicals produce luminosities that vary in intensity for oxygen and carbon dioxide. These are measured. Readings are instantaneously and continuously shown on a digital display. Precautions must be taken to maintain sterile technique with this equipment as with other methods of percutaneous radial artery cannulation.

Direct Arterial Blood Analysis Blood samples may be drawn intermittently from arterial or venous indwelling catheters. ABG determinations of PaO_2, Pco_2, and

So_2 monitor adequacy of oxygenation and carbon dioxide elimination. This is especially important in patients requiring mechanical ventilation. The tidal volume, respiratory rate, and concentration of oxygen can be appropriately adjusted. ABG monitoring also permits laboratory analyses of pH, base excess, bicarbonate, and electrolytes to evaluate metabolic processes and acid-base status. Differentiation of respiratory or metabolic acidosis or alkalosis is a guide to appropriate treatment. Samples may be taken also for other analyses (e.g., glucose or coagulation factors). More information on drawing blood from arterial lines can be found at **critcare.lhsc.on.ca/icu/cctc/procprot/nursing/procedures/ bldwithd.htm.**

Hypoventilation, uneven ventilation in relation to blood flow, impairment of diffusion, and venous-to-arterial shunting lead to anoxemia unless oxygen in inspired air is increased. Hypoventilation of the whole lung or a major portion leads to retention of carbon dioxide and predisposes the patient to cardiac dysrhythmias. Disturbances of acid-base balance have many serious consequences in many organs. They must be corrected to achieve normal physiologic functioning.

Central Venous Pressure

Because it accurately measures right atrial BP, which in turn images right ventricular BP, central venous pressure (CVP) assesses function of the heart's right side. It measures the pressure under which blood returns to the right atrium. It reflects pressure in the major veins as blood returns to the heart. In other words, CVP represents the amount of venous return and filling pressure of the right ventricle. This information helps determine the patient's circulatory status.

CVP monitoring also aids in evaluating blood volume and the relationship between circulating blood volume and the pumping action of the heart (i.e., adequacy of volume presented to the heart for pumping). Therefore CVP monitoring is a useful guide in blood or fluid administration to avoid circulatory overload in patients having limited cardiopulmonary reserve. Too great or too rapid replacement can cause pulmonary edema. Generally, a low CVP indicates that additional fluid can be given safely. CVP monitoring may be used during shock or hypotension to judge the adequacy of blood replacement. However, CVP is not a measure of blood volume per se or of CO.

Indications for CVP monitoring include major surgical procedures in patients with preexisting cardiovascular disease, in surgical procedures in which large-volume shifts are anticipated (e.g., open heart surgery), in critically ill patients (e.g., massive trauma), in surgical procedures in which venous air emboli are a risk (e.g., craniotomy in sitting position), and in rapid administration of blood or fluid.

Although CVP monitoring provides valuable data for assessing the adequacy of vascular volume, it only indirectly reflects the function of the left side of the heart. There is no direct relationship between right and left ventricular filling pressures. Because of the distensibility (compliancy) of the pulmonary blood vessels, the lungs can accept a marked increase in blood flow before significant congestion appears.

Backup of blood caused by impaired function of the left ventricle and a subsequent increase in pulmonary vascular resistance (PVR) may occur before this increased pressure affects the right side of the heart, as exhibited by CVP values. Thus CVP does not correlate with left-sided heart performance in patients with left ventricular dysfunction or pulmonary congestion.

Central Venous Cannulation   CVP may be monitored with a single-lumen or multilumen radiopaque catheter. A double- or triple-lumen Hickman or Broviac catheter is used most commonly. The right atrial lumen of a Swan-Ganz pulmonary artery catheter also can be used to obtain CVP readings. The lumens are labeled and color coded on multilumen catheters.

The catheter is inserted, preferably percutaneously through a subclavian vein. A brachial, external or internal jugular, or femoral vein may be used or, by cutdown, the antecubital vein. If the patient is awake, he or she is asked to bear down (Valsalva maneuver) as the vein is punctured. This increases intrathoracic pressure and counteracts negative pressure from the vein, thus reducing the possibility of air embolism.

The catheter is threaded through the vein and advanced into the superior vena cava or right atrium. This may be done under fluoroscopy, or a chest x-ray may be taken to verify accurate placement of the catheter tip.

The catheter may be attached to a transducer and monitor. Pressure readings are expressed in millimeters of mercury. The catheter can be attached to a fluid-filled manometer that measures pressure in centimeters of water. To set up this line, the IV solution bag is connected to the tubing; the manometer is inserted into the line by attaching it to the stopcock between the IV tubing and the extension tubing; air is run out of the line, and the line is clamped; and the manometer is secured upright to an IV pole. The hub of the catheter lumen is connected to the stopcock. Connections to the three-way stopcock should be taped to prevent inadvertent disconnection and air leaks. Cyclic variations in intracaval venous pressure occur; pressure becomes negative during atrial filling and respiratory inspiration. Sucking of air into the system during negative venous pressure can result in air embolus.

Baseline measurement is taken as soon as the catheter is in place and attached to the monitor. This is also a presumptive check for proper placement of the cannula tip. Because expansion of the lungs increases intrathoracic pressure and deflation decreases it, fluid in the manometer should fluctuate with each breath. To obtain a CVP reading on the manometer, adjust the scale to zero level with the patient's right atrium. The lumen of the stopcock to the catheter is shut off, allowing the IV fluid to run into the manometer to the desired level. The infusion is shut off, and the catheter is opened. After obtaining the reading, the infusion lumen to the catheter is opened to keep the line open.

Electronic transducer systems provide continuous monitoring of venous pressure. Continuous monitoring supplies good measurement of the right side of the heart and portrays the trend of heart function that is more valuable than are isolated readings obtained with a manometer. CVP values may vary somewhat, but normal readings range from 2 to 8 mm Hg, or 3 to 10 cm H_2O.

Multilumen central venous catheters provide access for administration of drugs, blood, fluids, and hyperalimentation. Blood can be removed for blood gas analyses or autotransfusion. These catheters also provide access for removal of air embolism.

Pulmonary Artery Pressures

Because a pulmonary artery catheter measures function of both the right and left sides of the heart, it provides faster, more accurate indication of impending left ventricular failure than does CVP alone. Pressures of the left side of the heart are reflected in pulmonary artery and pulmonary capillary wedge pressures, measured by the pulmonary artery catheter. This is more sensitive to rapid changes in the cardiovascular system than CVP and more sensitive to the ability of the heart to accommodate fluid loads. Measurement of pulmonary pressures enables precise, rapid assessment of the left ventricle's ability to eject adequate CO. Continuous evaluation of left ventricular function is extremely important in patients whose left-sided heart dysfunction has a greater direct effect on CO, circulating volume, and respiratory function than impaired right-sided heart function. Data procured include PAP, pulmonary capillary wedge pressure (PCWP), right atrial pressure (RAP), and CO computation. These pressures reveal the hemodynamic status of cardiovascular and pulmonary functions. They also serve as guidelines for administration of fluids, diuretics, or cardiotonic drugs to obtain optimal CO.

Indications for pulmonary artery monitoring include preexisting cardiac or pulmonary disease in a patient undergoing a major vascular, intraabdominal, or neurosurgical procedure, and a potential risk of development of cardiopulmonary instability from the stress of the surgical procedure. Other conditions may include shock, burns with large fluid shifts, renal failure with low CO, or pulmonary embolism. Pulmonary artery catheters may be used in patients who require long-term monitoring. Some multipurpose catheters may be used with ventricular and atrial pacing wires in patients with heart block or severe bradycardia. These catheters may be used to measure CO in patients with intracardiac shunts or during titrated drug administration.

Contraindications to invasive pulmonary catheter monitoring are abnormal cardiac anatomy in the patient, as well as inadequate monitors or lack of personnel trained in their use.

Pulmonary Artery Cannulation   Various pulmonary artery catheters are available. The number of lumens vary from two to five, depending on the range of functions desired. These catheters are used with transducers for monitoring. The type of transducer varies according to the balloon flotation device in the catheter.

In setting up the monitoring system, the manufacturer's instructions must be followed explicitly. All equipment, including the oscilloscope, should be checked. The stopcocks and flush devices in the lines to the transducer head(s) need to be attached. Preassembled tubing systems and disposable transducer domes are commercially available. If the patient also will have a peripheral arterial line, two transducers and a triple stopcock manifold are needed. Simultaneous monitoring of PAP and RAP is thus possible. The transducer dome is backflushed. The monitor should be balanced and calibrated according to the manufacturer's directions. There must be no air bubbles remaining in the lines or system.

Before insertion, the physician inspects the catheter for defects and tests the balloon for leakage by inflating it, submerging it in sterile saline solution, and watching for air bubbles. The balloon must then be deflated. Moistening the catheter tip with saline solution or lidocaine reduces the possibility of venospasm at insertion.

Vital signs are taken before insertion of the catheter. An ECG should be monitored for dysrhythmias during insertion. With the introducer set, the catheter is inserted and advanced rapidly to prevent kinking or knotting. It is advanced through the vein into the inferior or superior vena cava and on into the right atrium. Continued manipulation irritates or damages vessel walls. Watching the increment markings on the side helps determine how far the catheter has advanced. It is possible to keep pushing the catheter while it is not going into the right place. It can coil up and knot in the ventricle.

When the catheter tip reaches the right atrium and a right atrial waveform appears on the oscilloscope screen or readout strip, the balloon is inflated slowly with air with a tuberculin syringe to enable it to float with the flow of blood. The balloon is never inflated without a visible oscilloscope trace. If the patient is awake, a voluntary cough confirms the position of the catheter in the thoracic cavity if the right atrial wave fluctuates. The amount of air is specified by the manufacturer (usually about 1.3 to 1.5 ml). Overinflation could rupture the balloon. Carbon dioxide is used for balloon inflation in patients with intracardiac shunts. If the balloon ruptures in arterial circulation, carbon dioxide is more soluble than ambient (room) air in blood. A feeling of resistance should accompany inflation. Absence of resistance is a sign of a ruptured balloon; inflation should be stopped immediately. Fluid is never used for inflation because it would prevent proper catheter flotation and complete deflation.

Passing through the tricuspid valve, the catheter enters the right ventricle. A typical right ventricular waveform should appear. If dysrhythmia develops or is persistent, a bolus of lidocaine may be injected. Then after the catheter floats through the pulmonary semilunar valve into the pulmonary artery, a pulmonary artery tracing should appear on the monitor. This waveform has a steep upstroke at the beginning from right ventricular ejection and opening of the pulmonic valve, followed by a dicrotic notch on the downstroke at the closing of the pulmonic valve. Pulmonary artery blood flow carries the balloon into one of the artery's smaller branches. When the vessel diameter becomes too narrow for it to pass, the balloon wedges in the vessel and occludes it. A PCWP

waveform should appear. After recording of this wedge pressure, the physician permits the balloon to deflate passively; air is not aspirated with the syringe. The catheter will then slip back into the main branch of the pulmonary artery. A PAP waveform should reappear on the monitor. Thus the physician depends on these sequential characteristic pressure waveforms to reveal the catheter tip's location at all times. The circulator records pressure at each location. The catheter remains in the pulmonary artery with the balloon deflated, continuously recording the PAP, except when a PCWP reading is desired. If a PAP waveform persists and a PCWP reading is unobtainable, or if resistance is not felt with an attempt to inflate the balloon, it may be that the balloon is ruptured. An x-ray film is taken to confirm the catheter position. In the case of rupture, the catheter may be left in place to record the PAP, provided that it has not slipped back to the right ventricle. The physician may also elect to remove it. The balloon is always inflated during catheter advancement and deflated during catheter withdrawal.

To prevent an air embolus after catheter insertion, the catheter must not be attached to the monitoring system until all air has been expelled. All lines and transducers should be checked for secure connections and patency. Each transducer's balancing port must be leveled with the patient's right atrium. Right atrial, pulmonary artery, and pulmonary capillary wedge pressures and waveforms, as well as the patient's response to the procedure, must be documented.

Swan-Ganz Thermodilution Catheter The No. 7 Swan-Ganz thermodilution catheter has four separate lumens or passages within its outside wall. It is versatile and widely used. It is 43¼ inches (110 cm) long, with 10-cm increments marked on the side to permit observation of how far the catheter has advanced during insertion. Like all pulmonary artery catheters, it is a balloon-tipped flotation catheter that is inserted into a major vein and advanced to the inferior or superior vena cava. When inflated, the thin latex balloon at the tip permits the catheter to float with the flow of blood through the right atrium, tricuspid valve, right ventricle, pulmonary semilunar valve, and pulmonary artery, and to wedge in a small pulmonary artery branch (arteriole) for recording the PCWP during occlusion of the vessel. When the balloon is not inflated, the catheter lies in the pulmonary artery to record the PAP. It is essential to achieve proper catheter placement to minimize the risk of vessel damage and complications, as well as to validate pressure readings.

The end of the catheter inserted in the patient is referred to as the distal end; the opposite one is the proximal end. The latter comprises the lumen ports or external openings. The pulmonary artery port is used for monitoring PAP and PCWP. A syringe is connected to the balloon port for the desired balloon inflation. The thermistor port is used for CO calculation. The right atrial port is used for measuring RAP. This port also can be used to administer fluids or can be connected to a flush system for maintenance of catheter patency. For CO measurement, normal saline or dextrose solution is injected into the cardiovascular system via the proximal lumen. The pulmonary artery and right atrial ports should be labeled.

The catheter has four separate lumens or passages. The pulmonary artery lumen, the largest and most distal, terminates in the opening at the catheter's tip. With proper catheter positioning, this opening lies in the pulmonary artery. In this position with the balloon deflated, pulmonary artery systolic, diastolic, and mean pressures are recorded on the monitor. These are indicative of pulmonary function. When the balloon is inflated and the catheter migrates to a pulmonary artery branch to wedge, the PCWP is recorded. PCWP is sometimes referred to as PAWP (pulmonary artery wedge pressure) or PAOP (pulmonary artery occlusion pressure). Occlusion of a pulmonary artery branch creates a no-flow system, thereby blocking blood flow from the right side of the heart to the lungs and permitting pressure equilibration in the pulmonary vascular bed distal to the catheter. Occlusion of an arteriole and low resistance of the pulmonary systems give a pressure measurement equal to the left atrial pressure (LAP), which in turn is equal to the LVEDP. To prevent pulmonary infarction, ischemia, or hemorrhage from prolonged wedging, the balloon is always deflated immediately after a reading is taken. The catheter will float back into the main pulmonary artery. The pulmonary artery lumen can provide blood samples for blood gas measurements and mixed venous blood, which is also of value in judging cardiac function.

The balloon lumen opening, permitting inflation and deflation, is about 1 cm from the catheter tip. When inflated, the balloon surrounds, but does not cover, the opening in this tip.

The thermistor lumen opening is about 4 cm from the catheter tip. This lumen contains temperature-sensitive wires that run its length and transmit the temperature of blood flowing over them from the thermistor to the computer used to determine CO by the thermodilution technique.

The proximal right atrial lumen opening is about 30 cm from the catheter's tip. This opening lies in the right atrium to monitor RAP when the catheter is in place.

Interpretation of Pressures

The range of normal pressure values may vary slightly from one authority to another. Characteristic waveforms appear on the oscilloscope or screen, depending on the location of the catheter tip during insertion and continuous monitoring. These waveforms must be watched carefully to ascertain that the catheter is in the desired position. The catheter enters the right atrium via the vena cava.

RIGHT ATRIAL PRESSURE Normal RAP is 3 to 6 mm Hg. RAP reflects right atrial filling diastolic pressure, equivalent to CVP and RVEDP—pressure at the end of filling just before contraction. A rise in RAP may indicate right or left ventricular failure, volume overload (hypovolemia), or air embolism. A fall in RAP may indicate vasodilation, hypovolemia, or peripheral blood pooling.

RIGHT VENTRICULAR PRESSURE Normal right ventricular pressure (RVP) is 15 to 25 mm Hg systolic, 0 to 5 mm Hg diastolic. A rise in RVP may indicate mitral insufficiency, congestive heart failure, hypoxemia, or left ventricular failure.

PULMONARY ARTERY PRESSURE Normal PAP is 15 to 25 mm Hg systolic, 8 to 15 mm Hg diastolic; the mean is 9 to 19 mm Hg. These pressures estimate venous pressure in the lungs, as well as mean filling pressure of the left atrium and left ventricle. They reflect right ventricular function unless the patient has pulmonary stenosis, because commonly the pulmonary artery systolic pressure approximates the right ventricular systolic pressure. Changes in pulmonary artery systolic and mean pressures indicate changes in PVR. Alterations in PVR occur in hypoxemia, respiratory insufficiency, pulmonary edema, pulmonary embolism, shock, or sepsis. Thus these pressures are indices of pulmonary function. A rise in PAP may indicate left ventricular failure; increased pulmonary arteriolar resistance, as in pulmonary hypertension and hypoxia; or fluid overload.

PULMONARY CAPILLARY WEDGE PRESSURE Normal pressure is 6 to 12 mm Hg. Pulmonary artery diastolic pressure and PCWP are prime determinants of function of the left side of the heart because they reflect left ventricular end-diastolic pressure (LVEDP) just before the left ventricle contracts, except in patients with mitral valve impairment.

Normally, when the mitral valve between the right atrium and right ventricle is open (ventricular diastole), flow of blood from the pulmonary artery to the pulmonary veins and left side of the heart is unimpeded. Then pressures throughout the pulmonary circulation and left side of the heart are comparable. Because PCWP usually approximates LAP, an indicator of left heart function, it is an important determinant of left ventricular preload. Intraoperative monitoring of PCWP usually can give early disclosure of left ventricular dysfunction. A rise in PCWP may indicate left ventricular failure, mitral insufficiency, pulmonary hypertension, fluid overload, or pulmonary congestion. A rise also may occur during anesthesia induction. A fall in PCWP may indicate a reduction in LVEDP and CO, or hypovolemia.

Complications of Pulmonary Artery Catheter Monitoring

Invasion of the great vessels and heart carries many inherent perils. Probably the most common one during insertion is cardiac dysrhythmia, especially premature contractions. Other problems include local or systemic infection (septicemia, endocarditis), thrombus formation, pulmonary embolism, pulmonary infarction, pneumothorax, hemothorax, major vessel or heart chamber perforation, kinking or knotting of the catheter, balloon rupture, postoperative bleeding, or erroneous diagnosis from misinterpretation of data.

Although rare, pulmonary artery perforation is very serious. Predisposing factors are pulmonary hypertension, anticoagulation, hyperthermia, or an overinflated balloon or catheter. Hemoptysis and sudden hypotension are symptoms of pulmonary artery rupture. Equipment for endobronchial intubation, chest tube insertion, and surgical intervention must be available.

Complications that are potentially life threatening increase markedly after 48 to 72 hours of indwelling catheterization. The physician must be notified of any change in patient status.

Catheter withdrawal is performed by and at the discretion of a physician. To prevent injury to the heart valves, the balloon is slightly inflated until the catheter is withdrawn to the right atrium. Then the balloon is completely deflated for withdrawal. Dysrhythmias may occur. Pressure is applied to the insertion site to prevent bleeding. The pulse and BP are checked before and after withdrawal. A postwithdrawal dressing is applied. The patient is monitored for at least 24 hours.

In addition to patient problems, monitoring problems may arise. Each requires a specific intervention. A major problem is a damped pressure or PAP waveform. This means decreased amplitude in pressure tracings or loss of sharpness in the image that suggests a defect in the circuit. Common causes are air in the system or blood in the transducer; loose connections; a kinked, overwedged, or malpositioned catheter; falling systolic pressure in the patient; or a clot in the monitor system. If the last-mentioned cause is suspected, one should gently try to aspirate blood. If no blood can be aspirated, the catheter should not be flushed. Flushing could dislodge a clot. The physician, who may withdraw the catheter, should be notified.

Another problem involves a sudden change in configuration of a pressure tracing. Potential causes include the following: the transducer is not at the right atrial level, the transducer is in need of calibration, the transducer connection to the catheter is not secure, the catheter is no longer in proper position, or there is a loss of pressure in the pressure bag. If a PCWP waveform persists after a reading, the balloon may not be completely deflated or the catheter tip may be caught in the wedge position, requiring immediate attention. Circulators must be familiar with the appropriate interventions in both patient problems and monitoring problems, in addition to being knowledgeable about the causes and preventive measures. Only in this way can patient safety be maximized in invasive monitoring.

Cardiac Output

CO is measured by the thermodilution technique to determine liters of blood pumped per minute by the left ventricle into the aorta. Normal resting value is 4 to 8 L/min. A known amount of fluid at a known temperature is injected into a lumen of an arterial catheter, and a temperature gradient at a point downstream is measured via a second lumen. Iced cold or room-temperature physiologic saline solution or 5% dextrose in water (10 ml) usually is used. Blood flow supplies the thermal dilution; for example, saline mixes with blood in the superior vena cava or right atrium, depending on the catheter location, reducing the temperature of blood in the heart. The cooled blood flows past a transistorized intravascular thermistor in the thermodilution catheter that detects changes in blood temperatures that are then used to compute CO. When the solution is injected via the proximal right atrial lumen of a pulmonary artery Swan-Ganz catheter, a digital display of CO is seen within 4 to 5 seconds.

CO reflects the mechanical activity of the heart and represents total blood flow to all tissues and vascular shunts. It depends on the heartbeat rate, the contractile strength of the heart muscle (myocardial contractility), the peripheral resistance of vessels, and venous return. Inotropic agents such as digitalis or epinephrine increase contractility and CO except in patients with loss of functioning ventricular muscle (e.g., after myocardial infarction or an aneurysm of the left ventricle). Agents such as beta-blockers decrease the work of the heart by reducing contractility and CO. Calculation of the left ventricular stroke work index reflects pumping ability. During systole the ventricle does not totally eject the blood received during diastole. The amount of blood ejected with each contraction is referred to as the stroke volume (SV). Normal resting SV is 60 to 130 ml per beat. Determinants of the SV are the LAP, afterload, contractile state of the myocardium, and LVEDP. The ejection fraction (EF), a commonly used indicator of ventricular function, is the percentage value of the SV. Normal EF is 60% to 70%. Major SV determinants of CO are preload, contractility, and afterload. Only in limited circumstances does adjustment of the heart rate therapeutically enhance CO.

Preload, the amount of blood in the ventricle at the end of diastole, may be referred to as left ventricular end-diastolic volume (LVEDV) or filling pressure (LVEDP). Assessment of changes in volume by measurement of changes in filling pressure helps to describe cardiac function. Starling's principle concerns the relationship between volume, stretch, and contractility. It relates myocardial fiber length to the force of the contraction. The greater the preload and stretch of myocardial fibers, the greater the subsequent contraction, thereby increasing the SV until at some point ventricular failure commences. Fiber overstretch weakens contractions. As the pumping ability decreases, the left ventricle is unable to empty completely. Residual blood, combined during diastole with incoming oxygenated blood from the pulmonary veins and left atrium, increases workload and elevates the left ventricular volume and pressure. As ventricular efficiency declines, CO falls. Unpumped blood in the left ventricle backs up into the left atrium and pulmonary circulation, increasing these pressures. Pulmonary edema and respiratory insufficiency result as fluid is impelled into the alveoli. The CVP catheter measures the right-sided heart preload; the pulmonary artery catheter measures left atrial and left ventricular end-diastolic pressures.

Cardiac function may be classified as normal, compromised, or failing. In normal hearts maximum ventricular performance seems to be achieved at 8 to 12 mm Hg filling pressure. In compromised hearts this pressure is higher.

A reduced CO results in decreased perfusion of the capillary circulation. During hemorrhage, when circulating blood volume is reduced, the resulting diminished venous return and preload lead to a lowered CO. Atrial fibrillation also can modify the filling of the ventricles. Venous dilation contributes to pooling of blood, with subsequent decreased venous return to the heart. Low CO states result from reduced preload, as in hypovolemia, venous dilation, or cardiac tamponade; reduced contractility (e.g., from anesthetic drugs, ischemia, infarction, or cardiac decompensation); dysrhythmias; or increased afterload, as in hypertension, pulmonary embolism, or an elevated or diminished heart rate. Body position can influence circulation, as can age, body surface area, oxygen consumption, body temperature, basal metabolic rate, and activity. Thus many factors can affect CO.

Afterload indicates the resistance the heart must overcome to eject blood into the systemic circulation. This impedance to flow is called systemic vascular resistance (SVR). Left ventricular pressure must exceed pressure in the aorta to open the aortic valve and force blood from the heart into the circulation. Afterload, not a direct measure, is deduced by calculating the SVR. An elevated afterload can produce increased left ventricular wall tension in an attempt to generate adequate intracavitary ventricular pressure to overcome resistance and permit systolic ejection. The subsequent increase in myocardial oxygen demand must be met, or ventricular function deteriorates. Diminution of afterload reduces wall tension, thereby improving ventricular contraction. Improving cardiac function involves cost in myocardial oxygen consumption. Augmenting CO by increasing the heart rate and contractility increases myocardial oxygen consumption. Improving CO by augmenting preload or by reducing afterload results in relatively little oxygen cost to the myocardium.

A comprehensive view of cardiac function can be obtained by measurements of filling pressure, CO, and calculation of peripheral resistance. Repeated measurements offer evaluation of treatment. More information about cardiac output can be found at **critcare.lhsc.on.ca/icu/cctc/procprot/nursing/procedures/cardout2.htm**.

Cardiac Index The cardiac index (CI) assesses the heart's ability to meet the body's need for oxygen and other nutrients. With noninvasive ultrasound, the CI measures CO in relation to body surface. A CI less than 2 L of blood per minute per square meter of body surface identifies high risk for untoward cardiovascular events during or following anesthesia. The BP may drop; irregular heartbeats may develop. If these adverse events are anticipated, they can be prevented or treated.

Total Blood Volume

Blood volume is useful in determining the total amount of blood replacement required. An accurate method of total blood volume (TBV) measurement involves measuring plasma and red blood cell volumes separately, then adding the results together. To measure red blood cell volume, cells are tagged with detectable, nontoxic, radioactive chromium, subsequently injected intravenously, and counted after an appropriate mixing time. Or radioactive iodinated human serum albumin, in standard-dose packages, can be injected, mixed, and counted. Counting may be done rapidly by an electronic device. This technique may be used in place of estimation of blood loss.

Respiratory Tidal Volume

The respiratory tidal volume (VT), the volume of air moved with each respiration, may be measured with a respirometer placed on the expiratory limb of the anesthesia machine or mechanical ventilator. Alarms may be incorporated to signal disconnection, failure to cycle, or excessive pressure.

Body Temperature

The body continuously produces heat through metabolic activities and loses heat through convection, evaporation, conduction, and radiation. When the rate of production is equal to the rate of loss, a heat balance of constant core body temperature is maintained. Core temperature is that of the interior of the body as opposed to the body surface temperature. Normal core temperature ranges from 98.2° to 99.9° F (36.8° to 37.7° C). Under anesthesia, the average adult loses 0.9° to 2.7° F (0.5° to 1.5° C); the greatest loss occurs during the first hour through convection from exposure to the environment, through evaporation via respiration, through conduction from contact with cool surfaces, and through radiation from tissues. Intraoperative hypothermia, or core temperature below 96° F (35° C), is a common complication of surgery under general anesthesia, especially in pediatric and geriatric patients. Some anesthetic agents inhibit heat production; halogenated agents cause vasodilation that contributes to surface cooling; muscle relaxants prevent shivering, which is a thermoregulatory protective reflex. Other factors can change core temperature. Hyperthermia (retention of heat) may be caused by premedication, drapes, a closed anesthesia breathing circuit, or fever from sepsis. Physical reactions are not seen in the anesthetized patient. Therefore the body temperature should be continuously monitored for metabolic changes.

Electronic telethermometers with dial or digital readouts measure body and surface temperatures with thermistor or thermocouple probes. A core temperature probe can be inserted into a body orifice (i.e., nasopharynx, esophagus, bladder, or rectum). An esophageal probe measures body temperature at the level of the right side of the heart and is responsive to changes in body heat. A rectal probe responds slowly to changes in body temperature. These probes are available in various sizes and have flexible tips; some are disposable. The sensor of a bladder probe is in the tip of a sterile Foley catheter. A sterile catheter probe may also be inserted into the pulmonary artery. A probe can be placed on the tympanic membrane via the external auditory canal of the ear. This measures temperature closest to the hypothalamus, which is the thermoregulatory center in the brain.

Skin surface probes have either small tips or disks that are attached to the skin, often on an extremity, with an adhesive-backed foam pad. Cutaneous liquid crystal thermography, with temperature-sensitive chemicals laminated within an adhesive plastic strip, may be used for surface monitoring. The strip is usually applied to the forehead; its chemicals visibly change color with a temperature variation. Proximity to major arteries, insulation from the external environment, and the location of an inflammatory process and the surgical site are considerations in the choice of the temperature monitoring site.

Urinary Output

Urinary output can be measured by an indwelling Foley catheter attached to a calibrated collection bag. The sterile disposable collection system must be below the level of the bladder to prevent distention and allow flow without reflux. Output is valuable in assessing effective blood volume and fluid administration, except when a diuretic is given. Volume, electrolytes, osmolarity, and pH are important.

A reduction in urinary volume may indicate reduced renal perfusion. Oliguria can result from stress of the surgical procedure, antidiuresis from the anesthetic agent, impending renal failure, or reduced volume of circulating blood. Urinary output above 30 to 60 ml/hr usually shows adequate intravascular volume and BP.

The collecting system should be able to accurately measure a half-hour output between 1 and 200 ml and provide observation of the urine. Hemoglobinuria can be a manifestation of transfusion of incompatible blood. An electronic monitoring system is available with digital display of data that can be fed into a computer. The system records output in milliliters for both the present and the immediately past hours. It also shows the number of minutes elapsed in the current hour. Early warning of possible cardiovascular or renal problems is facilitated by visual alert signals if urine flow falls below 15 ml/hr or ceases.

Chest X-Ray Study

A chest x-ray study is essential for checking the position of the pulmonary artery (Swan-Ganz) catheter, CVP line, endotracheal tube, and chest tube and for observing changes in the lung and heart during therapy.

Electroencephalogram

Electrical activity of the nervous system reflects neurologic function. Therefore electrophysiologic monitoring provides information about the functional integrity of the central nervous system during anesthesia and is especially valuable in patients undergoing high-risk neurosurgical, cardiac, vascular, or orthopaedic procedures. Electrodes placed on the scalp transmit the electrical signals, alpha rhythms, from brain activity. Alpha rhythms normally occur at a rate of 8 to 13 waves per second. On the electroencephalogram (EEG) these wave patterns vary among individuals in response to anesthetics, drugs, and pathologic and physiologic changes. They reveal the presence of organic brain damage, abnormal physiologic alterations, and actions of drugs.

Regional cerebral blood flow correlates well with EEG activity. Computer analysis offers visual recognition of cerebral hypoperfusion or ischemia. The EEG is used particularly in surgical procedures involving expected localized brain ischemia caused by intentional surgical occlusion. An EEG also is a means of determining cessation of circulation, an index of expected prognosis, and brain vitality.

Scalp electrodes (cups or disks of silver/silver chloride, gold, or tin) are fixed in place with paste or collodion. Or subdermal platinum electrodes can be used. Electrodes are placed over areas of cerebral cortex according to a system that uses measurements of head circumference, distance between the ears, and distance from the nasion (point where the sagittal plane intersects the frontonasal suture) to the inion (external protuberance of the occipital bone). The small neurophysiologic signals recorded are amplified for analysis and display. Multiple channels are necessary to detect regional vs. global alterations in function. As many as 8 to 32 channels may be recorded simultaneously. Paper records or strip-charting provides comparisons of EEG activity during crucial periods with the activity seen before anesthesia induction or surgical manipulation. Methods of EEG analysis that permit automated pattern recognition and alarm generation enhance monitoring in the OR or intensive care unit (ICU). Devices are available that process EEG signals to simplify and facilitate the complex EEG analysis.

Cerebral Function Monitor The cerebral function monitor provides trend recording of amplitude and amplitude variability for a single channel of the EEG and is mainly useful for detecting marked global alterations in EEG activity during cardiopulmonary bypass, induced hypotension, or metabolic coma. During carotid endarterectomy, paired monitors can detect EEG asymmetries. Although they simplify monitoring, they may be less sensitive to ischemia than the 16-channel strip-chart recording.

Compressed Spectral Array Compressed spectral array (CSA) programs may give a time-compressed mountain-and-valley representation of brain activity. The mountains move to the left with slower brain activity and to the right with faster activity. CSA helps determine if the brain is ischemic because of a lack of contralateral circulation during vascular surgery, such as carotid endarterectomy. This type of computerized EEG can be run on general-purpose minicomputers or microcomputers.

Neurometrics Monitor A neurometrics monitor is also a single-channel device for displaying processed EEG signals. From 4 to 32 minutes of EEG can be seen at one time, but trends are less easily seen.

Bispectral Index Monitoring Bispectral Index (BIS) monitoring is a noninvasive method of monitoring the anesthesia level through processed EEG parameters. An electrode patch is placed on the patient's forehead, and the brain signals are relayed to a monitor. Readings are displayed as a single number (100, wide awake, to 0, absence of brain electrical activity) and indicate the level of anesthesia. The results are reduced drug use, faster wake-up time, and decreased risk of patient awareness during the surgical procedure. This potentially translates into faster discharge for ambulatory surgery patients.

Evoked Potentials

Sensory information (sight, sound, smell, taste, and touch) evokes an electrical response when it reaches the brain. Evoked potentials are those electrical responses recorded from the cerebral cortex after stimulation of a peripheral sensory organ. A computer is programmed to average the brain's repetitive responses to the stimuli. The computer displays these as waves on a video screen or prints them on a plotter.

Auditory Evoked Potentials   A clicking sound is delivered in the ear to stimulate the auditory nerve. Brain waves are recorded by the evoked potential computer. The evoked potentials can be used to assess function of the auditory nerve (e.g., during removal of acoustic neuroma). Because the auditory nerve enters the brainstem, evoked responses provide an indirect assessment of brainstem activity.

Somatosensory Evoked Potentials   Intraoperative monitoring of somatosensory evoked potentials is used to continuously assess spinal cord function and to protect the cord from injury during orthopaedic or neurosurgical procedures on the spine or spinal cord. Because hypotension increases the insult of direct pressure on the cord and heightens damage to cord function, the spinal cord is monitored when induced hypotension is employed for spinal surgery. Impulses generated below the site of the surgical procedure travel over lateral afferent neural pathways and through the operative spinal area and are recorded by electrodes at brain level. Abnormal brain responses are marked by changes in the arrival time of electrical impulses or amplitude of the waves on a graph. Change in latency and amplitude of the recorded signal, which normally averages 30 to 50 evoked responses, alerts the team to the danger of spinal cord compression or ischemia. Corrective measures taken immediately can prevent serious sequelae. Evoked responses then return to normal.

Bibliography

Barrie PS: Advances in critical care monitoring, *Arch Surg* 132(7):734-739, 1997.

Bayne CG: Technology assessment: vital signs: are we measuring the right parameters? *Nurs Manage* 28(5):74-76, 1997.

Cowan T: Pulse oximeters, *Prof Nurs* 12(10):744-745, 747-748, 750, 1997.

Dennison RD: Making sense of hemodynamic monitoring, *Am J Nurs* 94(8):24-31, 1994.

Leiberman K: Beyond the basics: monitoring with a pulmonary artery (Swan Ganz) catheter, *J Emerg Nurs* 24(3):218-222, 1998.

Nash CA, Jensen PL: When your surgical patient has hypertension, *Am J Nurs* 94(12):38-44, 1994.

O'Neal PV: How to spot early signs of cardiogenic shock, *Am J Nurs* 94(5):36-40, 1994.

Pasero C, McCaffery M: Avoiding opioid-induced respiratory depression, *Am J Nurs* 94(4):24-30, 1994.

Pearlman RC, Schneider PL: Intraoperative neural monitoring, *AORN J* 59(4):841-849, 1994.

Smith EA, Kilpatrick ES: Intraoperative glucose measurements: the effect of hematocrit on glucose monitoring strips, *Anaesthesia* 49(2):129-132, 1994.

Stein E: *Rapid analysis of electrocardiograms: a self-study program,* ed 2, Malvern, Pa, 1992, Lea & Febiger.

Taylor L et al: Hemodynamic monitoring: theory and application, *J Perianesth Nurs* 12(6):453-455, 1997.

Taylor L et al: Time out: hemodynamic monitoring: troubleshooting, *J Perianesth Nurs* 13(1):74-77, 1998.

War JA et al: Pulse oximetry, *Respir Care Clin North Am* 1(1):77-105, 1995.

Wilson BA et al: *Nurse's drug guide,* Norwalk, Conn, 1994, Appleton & Lange.

Section

IX

Intraoperative Patient Care

Chapter 27

Coordinated Roles of the Scrub Person and the Circulator

 Chapter Objectives

After studying this chapter, the learner will be able to:

- Describe the activities of the scrub person.
- Describe the activities of the circulator.
- Discuss the preliminary care of the patient by the circulator.
- Differentiate between counting and being accountable for items used in patient care.

DIVISION OF DUTIES

The circulator and the scrub person should plan their duties so that, through coordination of their efforts, the sterile and unsterile parts of the surgical procedure move along simultaneously. From the time the scrub person starts the surgical scrub until the surgical procedure is completed and dressings are applied, an invisible line separates the duties of the scrub person and the circulator, which neither person may cross. In this chapter, the duties of the two positions are listed separately, but a spirit of mutual cooperation is essential to move the schedule of surgical procedures efficiently and to serve the best interests of the patient.

As a coordinated effort, the scrub person and the circulator should complete the preparation of the environment as described in Chapter 12—whether it is for the first case of the day or for a subsequent case performed during the course of the day. One suggested room arrangement is illustrated in Figure 27-1. Both caregivers should double check the needs for the case to prevent needing to run to the supply room dur-

ing the procedure. Box 27-1 contains a mental checklist for consideration before the scrub person scrubs to set up and before the patient arrives at the room.

Scrub Person Duties

When all supplies have been obtained and opened and the room is ready for the patient's arrival, the scrub person prepares for the surgeon's arrival. At all times, the integrity of the sterile field is closely monitored. The principles of asepsis and sterile technique as described in Chapters 17 and 18 are followed.

Preparation of the Sterile Field

Open the gown and gloves on a surface separate from the sterile field. Don protective eyewear with sideshields. Perform a complete scrub according to the facility procedure. Gown and glove using the closed gloving method. If double gloving, wear gloves one size larger as the first layer and the

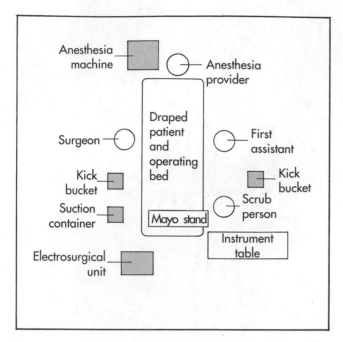

Figure 27-1 Arrangement of sterile field, team members, and unsterile equipment *(shaded).*

usual size gloves as the second pair. The larger size underneath provides an air pocket and helps to prevent a sensation of tightness around the hands. If hypoallergenic gloves are worn, these should be donned as the first pair, with generic gloves worn as the outside pair. Wipe the powder from gloves before handling drapes, instruments, and other sterile items.

Drape tables according to the standard departmental setup procedure. Select from the drape pack the appropriate drapes for covering unsterile surfaces to create a sterile field. The scrub person may drape and set a small table for preparation of the patient's skin, but more commonly the circulator opens and prepares a disposable or prepackaged prep tray. A second instrument table may be needed for extensive surgical procedures or special types of instrumentation (e.g., tables for preparation of an implant or organ for transplant).

When draping an unsterile table with a separate table drape, unfold it to cover the front edge of the table first; this minimizes the possibility of self-contamination from the unsterile edge of the table. Unfold the remainder of the table drape over the surface of the table and away from the front of the sterile gown. The edges are allowed to fall over the ends of the table and are no longer considered sterile. After the ends of the drape are unfolded over the sides of the table, be careful not to lift them to table level again while opening the crosswise folds. Avoid leaning over the table.

Place the remaining contents of the drape pack on a corner of the instrument table if they are not prepositioned in a convenient place on the table drape. Custom packs usually contain disposable supplies that are nested within each other and require minimal handling when setting up the field. Reusable woven fabric drapes may be arranged within the drape pack according to the size or direction of the folds.

Box 27-1 — Checklist to Consider When Preparing for a Surgical Procedure

All Surgical Procedures
Housekeeping: room cleaned
Furniture: present and arranged
Suction: connected and functional
Operating light and bed: prepositioned and functional

Specific to Scheduled Procedure
Correct operating bed in working order
Basic instrument and basin sets
Basic drape pack
Skin preparation setup
Sterile supplies

Specific to Surgical Specialty
Electrosurgical unit (ESU)
Laser
Microscope
Tourniquet
Endoscope
Drapes
Instruments
Sterile supplies
Fluoroscopy or x-ray
Specific implant

Specific to Surgeon
Gloves
Instruments
Sutures
Table medications and solutions
Personal preferences/preference card

Specific to Patient
Special considerations/plan of care
Age
Body build
Allergies
Physical limitations/impairments
Autotransfusion/blood transfusion
X-ray, CT, or MRI films

A standard number of each item is contained within a drape pack. The disposable or reusable drape pack usually contains, at a minimum, the following items:

- One Mayo stand cover
- Six to eight towels
- Two to four medium drape sheets (optional)
- One fenestrated sheet

Drape both the frame and the tray of the Mayo stand. The Mayo stand cover is like a long pillowcase. It is fanfolded with a wide cuff to protect gloved hands. With hands in the cuff, support the folds of the drape on the arms, in the bend of the elbows, to prevent it from falling below waist level (Figure 27-2). While sliding the cover on the Mayo stand, place

Figure 27-2 Starting to drape Mayo stand. Scrub person's hands are protected in cuff of drape. Folds of drape are supported on arms, in bend of elbows, to prevent their falling below waist level. Foot is placed on base of stand to stabilize it.

Figure 27-3 Completing draping of Mayo stand. Hands are protected in cuffs.

a foot on the base of the stand to stabilize it (Figure 27-3). Some sterile custom packs contain an impervious disposable Mayo tray as the bottom layer of the pack. At some facilities, a stainless steel tray is wrapped snugly and sterilized separately. The tray can be set into the draped Mayo stand.

If reusable basin sets are used, leave the large solution basin in the ring stand and take the remainder of the basins to the instrument table. The wrapper on the basin set serves as the cover for the ring stand with the large basin. The use of these basins as "splash basins" is discouraged, but some surgeons still prefer to use them to wash their hands at the start of the case. If basins are used for this purpose, the circulator should fill them with sterile normal saline. The preferred methods for removing powder or blood from gloves is either to use a sterile towel moistened with sterile saline or to pour sterile saline directly over the gloved hands. The basin should not be permitted to sit after being used to remove glove powder; it should be emptied into the dirty sink in the utility room.

Some facilities use the large solution basin to collect and rinse used instruments. Only demineralized sterile water should be used for this purpose. Disposable custom packs usually contain plastic basins that can remain on the sterile instrument table.

Separate basins are arranged close to the edge of the instrument table for holding sterile warm irrigation solution (usually Ringer's lactate or saline), for securing the specimen after it is procured, and for moistening sponges. All basins and containers should be clearly labeled to identify their contents. The practice of dipping sponges into the irrigation solution should be discouraged because this releases lint into the solution, which in turn can be introduced into the patient during irrigation. Lint can contribute to foreign body reactions in the tissues of the patient. An Asepto syringe can be used to moisten sponges with warm saline in their own basin.

The basin set also may contain solution cups for the skin preparation table and/or a basin specifically intended for trash (waste suture packaging) disposal. Attaching a trash bag to

the side of the table compromises the sterility of the field because the bag hangs lower than the sterile table surface. If these bags are used, the inside is not considered sterile because it is below the level of the sterile field.

Arrange on the Mayo stand the instruments and accessory items needed to create the primary incision. Arrange other instruments and items on the instrument table (Figure 27-4). Table 27-1 describes the "Eight *P*'s" of table and room organization, which can help the scrub person and circulator improve the efficiency of the setup procedure.

The instruments for each surgical procedure are selected and placed according to standard basic sets and the preferences of the surgeon. Instruments of suitable size, shape, strength, and function are needed for each step of the surgical procedure. The styles and numbers of instruments are dictated by the type of surgical procedure. A discussion of instrumentation is found in Chapter 19.

A few of each classification of instruments, plus sutures, surgical needles, and sponges, may be put on the Mayo stand initially. If a local anesthetic will be used, a syringe and injection needle are also needed. One possible setup of the Mayo stand is illustrated in Figure 27-5. As the surgical procedure progresses, additional instruments and supplies can be added or deleted as necessary. Long-handled forceps and clamps and deep retractors can be substituted for those used on superficial structures. The Mayo stand should be kept neat throughout the surgical procedure.

Count sponges, surgical needles, other sharps, and instruments with the circulator according to established institutional policy and procedure. After completing the count with the circulator, place on the Mayo stand a few appropriate-size sponges for the initial incision. Many different types of sponges are available. These sponges may be opened to their full length. Fix two or three sponges on sponge forceps (if these will be used), but leave the forceps on the instrument table. Put x-ray–detectable rings on tapes (large sponges), if used. These items and counting procedures are discussed later in this chapter.

Figure 27-4 Example of basic instrument table setup. Contents will vary according to the type of surgical procedure.

Figure 27-5 Example of setup for Mayo stand.

After completing the counts with the circulator, secure surgical needles and all other sharps, including knife blades. Surgical needles and sharps should never be loose on the Mayo stand. If eyed reusable needles are used, each needle must be inspected before threading for cleanliness, burrs, and integrity of the eye. Disposable needles are preferred.

Put blades on knife handles. To avoid injury, always use an instrument to attach the blade; never use the fingers.

Holding the cutting edge down and away from the eyes and other personnel in the room, grasp the widest and strongest part of the blade with a heavy clamp, and slip the blade into the groove on the knife handle. A click indicates the blade is in place. To prevent damage to the blade, the instrument should not touch the cutting edge of the blade (Figure 27-6). Blades being dispensed to the field should not be placed in a metal basin; this may dull the edge. They should be placed

TABLE 27-1	The "Eight P's" of Operating Room and Sterile Field Setup and Management*	
The Eight *P*'s to Consider When Preparing for a Surgical Procedure	**Environment Considerations for the Circulator**	**Sterile Field Considerations for the Scrub Person**
Proper Placement Items should be placed so they will not need to be moved during the procedure.	Suction canisters, tourniquet, and the ESU need to be stationary. The operating lights should be directed toward the field.	The Mayo stand and instrument table should not be moved during the procedure. Drapes may not be moved on the patient's skin.
Proper Function Items should be tested for safety and usefulness before they are needed to prevent delay in the case.	Test the ESU, tourniquet, laser, and other equipment before the patient enters the room.	Test the efficiency of instruments (scissors, needleholders, and clamps) as they are closed and positioned on the field. Replace as needed.
Place It Once Items should not be manipulated during the procedure. Energy and attention should not be diverted to resetting the field.	The operating bed should be in the right place for the procedure. The dispersive electrode should not be moved or displaced.	When setting up the field, each item (e.g., a basin) should be placed where it will be used during the procedure with minimal handling.
Point of Contact Items used within the field could cause harm or be rendered useless if they do not reach the intended point of contact.	The circulator should evaluate the delivery of items to the sterile field. Some items (e.g., staplers) should be handed; others can be transferred in other ways.	The scrub person should be aware of the passing of instruments and how they are securely placed in the waiting hand of the surgeon or first assistant.
Position of Function Items should positioned so they will be useable during the procedure.	The use of a C-arm, laser with articulating arm, or microscope should be preplanned so they may be positioned while the procedure is in progress.	When passing instruments, they should be placed in the surgeon's hand in a useable way. For example, the curve of the instrument should match the curve of the hand.
Point of Use Items should be as close to the area of use as possible.	Pour solutions directly into the basins, open and hand sponges or sutures directly to the scrub person as they are needed.	Basins should be placed close to the edge of the table so the circulator can pour without requiring the basin to be repositioned. The ESU pencil holder should be close to the field for safe containment of the tip.
Protected Parts Items and surfaces should be rendered safe for the patient and the team.	Cords, cables, and tubing should be secured and appropriately directed away from the field. Pad the operating bed and patient as appropriate. Use safety belts.	Apply jaw liners to instruments during setup. Hand instruments with care to avoid causing injury with the tip or sharp surface. Do not lay items on or rest them against the patient's body.
Perfect Picture Items within and around the field should not be at risk for causing harm or becoming damaged. The environment should not be cluttered.	The entire room should appear neat and tidy. The door should be closed, and the temperature and humidity should be appropriate. Forethought to having a clear path for the crash cart or emergency equipment is essential.	The sterile field should remain neat and orderly, with instruments and supplies within easy sight and reach. Consistent setup fosters a sense of comfort and confidence in the scrub role.

*The examples used for each "P" will vary according to the type of procedure and equipment, the position of the patient, and the surgeon's preference. The "Eight *P*'s" apply to both the scrub person and the circulator.

in clear vision of the scrub person, who places them on the knife handles.

Prepare sutures in the sequence in which the surgeon will use them. The surgeon may ligate (tie off) large blood vessels shortly after the incision is made, unless electrosurgery is preferred to seal vessels. Prepare ligatures (free-hand ties) first if they will be used. Remove suture material from the packet, unless the packet is designed for single-strand dispensing. Work over the instrument table and hold onto the ends of the suture material to prevent strands from dropping over the edge of the table and thus becoming contaminated.

Dispensing packets or strands of ligating material can be placed in a suture book (a fanfolded towel), with the ends extended far enough for rapid extraction. Place the largest size

Figure 27-6 Putting scalpel blade on knife handle. To avoid injury, always use an instrument; never use fingers. The blade is attached with a heavy instrument. Grasp blade at its widest, strongest part and slip it into groove on handle. The handle and blade are pointed down and away from eyes and other personnel.

in the bottom layer along the fold that is farthest away when placed on the Mayo stand. The next smaller size is placed in the next layer so that the ends are not overriding those below; if three sizes are prepared, the medium size can be placed midway between the other two. The smallest size will be along the closest fold. The suture book may be placed on the Mayo stand with the ends of the strands on the stand, not over the edges, and toward the sterile field. To prevent possible contamination, strands are pulled out toward the surgical field, never away from it.

A few packets of suture may be opened and prepared for suturing (sewing or stitching). Seldom is it necessary to prepare large amounts of suture material in advance. Suture materials, preparation, and handling are discussed in detail in Chapter 30.

If a local anesthetic is to be used, fill a syringe with the correct agent. Attach an appropriate-size needle and put it on the Mayo stand. This will be the first thing the surgeon will use after the patient is draped. State the type and percentage of the solution when handing the syringe to the surgeon. The solution label should be checked by a registered nurse when it is poured and verified when it is given. Sterile labels and marking pens are commercially available for labeling containers for medications, radiopaque dyes, and other solutions used in the sterile field. Labeling should include the name and strength of the solution. An appropriate label should be placed on syringes, basins, and medicine cups to prevent inadvertent use of the wrong solution in the wrong manner.

Syringes with needles are used for injection and aspiration, and syringes without needles are used for irrigation. Most hospitals use sterile disposable syringes and needles. Glass syringes and reusable needles in the same models and sizes are occasionally used. When using a sterile syringe, be very careful not to touch the plunger, even while wearing gloves. Contamination of the plunger contaminates the inner wall of the barrel and thus the solution that is drawn into it. Glove powder and other debris can act as a contaminant and cause a for-

eign body reaction. Care is taken to determine if the patient is at risk for latex sensitivity. Nonlatex injection and irrigation syringes are commercially available, and reusable sterile glass syringes are available at many facilities.

The following types of syringes are commonly used for injection or aspiration:

- *Luer-Lok tip.* This type of syringe has a tip that locks over the needle hub. It is used whenever pressure is exerted to inject or aspirate fluid. Sizes range from 2 to 100 ml.
- *Ring control.* This type of syringe has a Luer-Lok tip. The barrel has a thumbhold and one fingerhold, which gives the surgeon a secure grip when injecting with only one hand. Sizes range from 3 to 10 ml.
- *Luer slip tip.* This type of syringe has a plain, tapered tip that may not give a secure connection on a needle hub. It is necessary when using some catheter adapters or a rubber connection for aspiration. Sizes range from 1 to 100 ml.

The size of injection needles is designated by length and gauge. Gauge is the outside diameter of a needle, which gets smaller as the number gets larger (i.e., a 30-gauge needle is smaller than a 20-gauge needle). Although numerous sizes of needles are available, only a few representative sizes and their uses are mentioned here:

- ½ inch (12.7 mm) × 30 gauge, for intradermal local anesthetic
- ¾ inch (19 mm) × 24 or 25 gauge, the usual needle for any subcutaneous injection
- 1½ inches (3.8 cm) × 22 gauge, for subcutaneous or intramuscular injection
- 2 inches (5 cm) × 18 or 20 gauge, for aspiration
- 4 inches (10 cm) × 20 or 22 gauge, for deep injections into joints or for intracardiac injections

The following types of syringes are used for irrigation:

- *Bulb with tapered barrel.* With this type of syringe (commonly referred to by the trade name Asepto syringe), a plastic or rubber bulb is attached to the neck of the barrel. The barrel has a tapered or blunt end (like a turkey baster) and can be made of plastic or glass. It is used for one-hand control of irrigation during many types of surgical procedures. This type of syringe has a solution capacity of ¼ to 4 ounces (7.6 to 118 ml).
- *Tapered bulb without barrel.* This type of syringe contains a one-piece bulb that tapers to a blunt end. It is used to irrigate small structures, and it may be used for suctioning nasal and oral fluids from neonates during deliveries by cesarean section. This variety is usually disposable because it is not possible to clean the interior of the bulb after use.

To fill an irrigation syringe, depress the bulb, submerge the end in solution, and release the bulb. The bulb will reinflate, thus drawing solution into it. Warm, not hot, solution is usually used for irrigation; check the temperature before giving the syringe to the surgeon. Irrigating solution may be stored in a warmer maintained at a temperature that ranges from 99° to 122° F (37° to 50° C). For use, solution usually should not exceed body temperature.

After the Surgeon and Assistant(s) Scrub

Gown and glove the surgeon and assistant(s) as soon after they enter the room as possible, if this is routine procedure. This procedure should take precedence over other setup activities, but do not interrupt a sharps, instrument, or sponge count to do so; such interruptions lead to incorrect counts. The surgeon and assistant(s) may take their gowns and gloves from a separate table that has been set up for this purpose. They should never take towels, gowns, or gloves from the primary sterile field.

After the patient is positioned and prepped, assist in draping according to the type of procedure and the surgeon's preference. Many surgeons use towels secured with towel clips to square off the incision. To prevent reaching over the unsterile operating bed, go to the same side of the table as the surgeon to hand towels and towel clips. For hard-to-drape areas, skin towels may be held in place with sutures or staples rather than clips. Some surgeons use self-adhering plastic sheeting directly over the squared-off incision site; the adherent sheeting may be plain or impregnated with iodophor. To apply this adherent drape, stand on the opposite side of the operating bed to assist as the surgeon positions the adherent surface over the patient's prepped skin. The fenestrated drape sheet is placed over this. During the draping process, care is taken not to allow sterile gloves to touch unsterile surfaces. Drapes are cuffed over the hands as they are placed.

Once a perforating towel clip has been fastened through a drape, do not remove it, because the points are contaminated. If it is necessary to remove a perforating towel clip, discard it from the field and cover the punctured area with another sterile drape or towel. Nonperforating ball-tip towel clips are preferred for securing drapes. Because of the risk of contamination, drapes should not be moved once they have been positioned.

After draping is completed, bring the Mayo stand into position over the patient, making sure it does not rest on the patient. Position the instrument table at a right angle to the operating bed. Assist the surgeon in securing sterile light handles for adjustment of the operating light. The beam of light should pass the surgeon's right ear and center at the tip of the index finger of his or her right hand (or left hand for a left-handed surgeon).

Lay a towel or magnetic pad for instruments below the fenestration (opening) in the drape, and lay two dry sponges on the pad. Use a nonperforating clamp to attach suction tubing and electrosurgical unit (ESU) cords to drapes. Allow ample length to reach both the incision area and the equipment. Drop the ends off the side of the operating bed nearest the unit to which the circulator will attach them. It is helpful to have the cables and tubing directed over the same side of the field.

Figure 27-7 Passing the knife with the blade down and protected. The scrub person's hand is pronated.

The tip of an ESU pencil becomes hot and could burn the patient or a team member. Accidental activation can occur if pressure is exerted on the handpiece; this can cause ignition of the draping material or dry sponges. Therefore attach a container (holder/holster) to the drape with a nonperforating clip for containment of the ESU pencil. When not in use, the tip of the ESU pencil is cleaned and placed into the holder.

If the instrument towel on the sterile field becomes bloody, do not remove it but cover it with a fresh, sterile towel. Remember that drapes should not be repositioned once they have been placed. Take care not to lay the clean towel over a sponge or instrument.

During the Surgical Procedure

Pass the skin knife to the surgeon (Figure 27-7), and pass a hemostat to the assistant. When passing the knife, take care to direct the blade away from yourself and all other personnel. Hold the hand pronated, with thumb apposed against the tip of the index finger, and flex the wrist. Eye contact is recommended when passing the scalpel. Some surgeons do not want the knife handed to them but prefer to use a no-passing technique for sharps. When using the no-passing technique, lay the knife on an instrument towel, magnetic pad, or tray for the surgeon to pick up. The surgeon will replace the knife onto this surface or tray after the incision is made. The scrub person should not allow the knife to remain on the field after its use.

Because skin cannot be sterilized, the initial skin knife is considered contaminated whether or not the surgeon has cut through an adhering plastic skin drape. The skin incision exposes deep skin flora of the hair follicles and sebaceous gland ducts. If an existing scar is excised, it may be sent to the pathology department as a specimen for gross identification. Some surgeons discard this tissue. Determine the surgeon's preferences and the facility policies.

Hand up sterile towels or lap sponges if requested for covering skin at the edges of the incision. Throw soiled sponges

Figure 27-8   Passing an instrument. The scrub person holds the instrument by the hinge and avoids entangling fingers in the rings. Tip is visible, and handle is free. Handle is placed firmly and directly into waiting hand. A soft snap may be heard as the instrument contacts the waiting hand.

into the appropriate sponge receptacle for counting, and add clean sponges to the field. If sponges or tapes are added during the surgical procedure, count all of them with the circulator before use. Do not mix types of sponges and tapes on the table. Keep them separated for ease of identification and tracking.

If the surgeon uses a sterile towel as packing within the wound, this is relayed to the circulator and the number is tracked with all other counted items. The circulator is informed when the packing towel is removed, and it is accounted for at the conclusion of the procedure. The practice of using towels for packing is discouraged unless a mechanism is in place for accounting for their removal from the patient at the end of the procedure. Commercially precounted and packed disposable towels with radiopaque markers are available from several manufacturers. Most reusable towels are processed in-house and do not have x-ray detectable markers.

Watch the field and try to anticipate the needs of the surgeon and assistant. Keep one step ahead of them in passing instruments, sutures, and sponges and in handing up the specimen basin. Notify the circulator if additional supplies are needed or if the surgeon asks for something not on the table. Ask quietly for supplies to avoid distracting the surgeon. Consideration is given to the patient who has received a local or regional anesthetic and may be awake.

When bleeding is obvious, the surgeon needs a hemostatic forceps and/or the ESU pencil. If the bleeding is in a deep wound, the ESU pencil tip may need to be changed to a longer type. After making a deep stitch, the surgeon may want to tag the ends of the suture with a hemostat. Scissors are needed for cutting the suture. Some surgeons use hand signals to indicate the type of instrument needed. These signals eliminate the need for talking, but such signs should be clearly understood. An understanding of what is taking place at the surgical site makes these signals meaningful.

Pass instruments in a decisive and positive manner. When instruments are passed properly, surgeons know they have them; their eyes do not need to leave the surgical site. When the surgeon extends his or her hand, the instrument should be placed firmly into his or her palm in the proper position for use (Figure 27-8). Return instruments to the Mayo stand or instrument table promptly after use. Their weight or a sharp tip could injure the patient.

Keep instruments as clean as possible. Wipe blood and organic debris from them with a moist sponge. Remove debris from electrosurgical tips. To keep the suction tip and tubing patent, periodically flush the suction tip with a few milliliters of saline or sterile water. Keep track of the amount of solution used to clear the line, and inform the circulator. The volume of fluid in the suction canister may be confused with blood loss.

Place a ligature in the surgeon's hand. The surgeon keeps both eyes on the field and does not reach for a ligature except to hold out a hand to receive it. Draw a strand out of the suture book and toward the sterile field, grasp both ends, and place the strand securely in the surgeon's outstretched hand. The end of a ligature may be placed in a long curved forceps, such as Kelly forceps or a right-angled clamp, in a maneuver referred to as "a tie on a passer" (Figure 27-9). This method is used when the structure will be circumferentially tied off instead of being sutured, such as a vessel in the mesentery. When handing a tie on a passer, place the forceps in the surgeon's hand in the same manner used to pass any hemostatic forceps. Trail the end of the ligature until it is taken by the assistant during the tying procedure.

At all times during the surgical procedure, have ready a fine and a heavy suture on needles placed in needleholders. Load the needle into the needleholder in a left- or right-hand manner according to the hand dominance of the surgeon or the direction of the suturing motion (Figure 27-10). After handing a suture to the surgeon, hand the suture scissors to

Figure 27-9 Tie on a passer.

the assistant and immediately prepare another suture just like it. The surgeon will probably need a forceps for manipulation of tissue during the suturing process. Account for each needle in its entirety as the surgeon finishes with it, because a suture or needle can break. Check the integrity of the needle as it is returned in the needleholder. Tell the surgeon immediately if a needle is broken so that all pieces can be retrieved.

Repeat the size of a suture or ligature when handing it to the surgeon. Obviously, this repetition is not necessary if the surgeon is using a long series of interrupted sutures or many ligatures in rapid succession. Use good judgment. Be logical in selecting the instruments used for suturing. Give the surgeon long needleholders to work deep in a cavity; short ones may be used for surface work. Give the assistant a needleholder to pull the needle through tissue for the surgeon. Have scissors ready when the knot is tied. Hemostatic forceps are sometimes used to secure the ends of multiple interrupted sutures placed in rapid succession. Often the knot tying and cutting take place after all sutures are in position.

Remove the waste ends of suture material from the field, Mayo stand, and instrument table, and place them in the trash disposal container. Put used needles on a magnet, in a needle rack, or into the suture book (or other container for this purpose) until the needle count is complete. Follow established institutional policy and procedure for securing sharps during the surgical procedure.

Save and care for all tissue specimens according to policy and procedure. Some facilities require that all tissue removed from a patient, including exudates, be sent for pathologic examination. Therefore it is advisable to send all tissue to the laboratory even though it may appear to be of no value for examination or diagnostic purposes.

Specimens are put in a specimen basin or another container. Never put a large clamp on a small specimen; this may crush cells and make tissue identification difficult. Some specimens have borders or margins that the surgeon will mark with specific sutures as tags for the pathologist's identification of and attention to certain areas. Keep the specimen basin on the field until all tissue has been removed or all contaminated items have been placed in it. Specimens designated as right or left should be kept separate in clearly marked containers.

When handing a specimen from the field to the circulator, hand it in a basin or appropriate container; never place it on a sponge. Tell the circulator exactly what the specimen is, if there are any identifying notations for the pathologist, or if the specimen is to have special testing (e.g., frozen section). If there are any doubts about the specimen's identification, markers, or processing, ask the surgeon for clarification.

Before closure, the surgeon may request several liters of fresh, warm irrigation solution to rinse the abdomen (or smaller amounts to irrigate other surgical wounds). Some surgeons may pour the irrigation directly from the basin, and others may request an Asepto syringe. If a Poole suction is used to evacuate the solution, make sure the guard is slipped over the tip to protect the tissues. Keep track of the amount of irrigation used and report it to the circulator for the permanent record.

During Closure

Alert the circulator that closure is about to begin, and hand up the wound closure materials. In accordance with established procedures, count sponges, sharps, and instruments with the circulator as the surgeon begins closure of the wound. Verify that intraabdominal or other cavity packing materials and towels have been removed.

As time permits, clear unnecessary instrumentation from the Mayo stand, leaving a tissue forceps, suture scissors, and four hemostats. Place unneeded instruments and supplies on the instrument table. The instrumentation setup and the Mayo stand should remain sterile until the patient has left the room. Cardiac arrest, tracheal collapse, hemorrhage, or other emergencies can occur in the immediate postoperative-postanesthesia period. Even though sterile instrument sets are nearby, valuable time can be lost in opening sterile supplies, and every second counts in an emergency situation. Regardless of their previous use, sterile instruments on the Mayo stand can be used for an emergency intervention. These instruments can be lifesaving until other ones become available.

Have a clean, warm, saline-moistened sponge ready to wash blood from the area surrounding the incision as soon as skin closure is completed. Have the dressings ready. After the dressing is in place, assist the team in undraping the patient. Place the soiled drapes in the appropriate receptacle.

Circulator Duties

Before entering the OR at the beginning of the day, circulators should wash their hands and arms as required by institutional policy and procedure, but they do not don sterile gowns and gloves. The circulator is an unsterile team member. Persons

Figure 27-10 **A,** Loading a needleholder for right-handed suturing. **B,** Right-handed needle in needleholder. **C,** Hand signal for suture on a needle. **D,** Passing right-handed needle.

who wear sterile attire touch only sterile items; persons who are not sterile touch only unsterile items. The circulator should assist the sterile scrub person by providing and opening sterile supplies needed to prepare for arrival of the patient and the surgeon. The circulator should test all equipment before bringing the patient into the room.

After the Scrub Person Scrubs

Fasten the back of the scrub person's gown. Check with the scrub person to see if additional supplies or instruments are needed. If instruments have been autoclaved between cases,

clear a path to the sterilizer so the scrub person can access the sterilized items without becoming contaminated. Open the packages of sterile supplies (e.g., syringes, suction tubing, sutures, sponges, and gloves) as needed. Use an appropriate method of sterile transfer to the sterile field. Methods of transfer include, but are not limited to, the following:

1. Place the item on the edge of the sterile instrument table with the inside of the wrapper everted over your hand. Never reach over the sterile field and shake an item from its package.

Figure 27-11 Scrub person taking contents from suture packet opened and held by circulator. Scrub person avoids touching unsterile outer wrapper.

Figure 27-12 Flipping a packet of suture to the sterile field.

2. Expose the contents so the scrub person can remove the item from the wrapper or package by using a forceps or by grasping the item (Figure 27-11). The scrub person avoids touching the unsterile outside. Remember that the sterile boundary of a peel-open package is the inner edge.
3. Flip only small, rigid items (e.g., suture) with caution (Figure 27-12). Flipping an item from a package may result in the item missing the intended sterile surface and landing on the floor. Flipping creates air turbulence and thus is the least preferred method of sterile transfer. Larger items, such as staplers or implants, can become contaminated or damaged and therefore are never flipped.

Check the list of suture materials and sizes on the surgeon's preference card, but verify with the surgeon before opening packets. Avoid opening suture packets that will not be used. The surgical procedure might be canceled or the patient's condition may warrant something different, and then the sutures would be wasted. If the surgeon's need for sutures cannot be anticipated and further instructions have not been given, dispense a packet or two ahead of actual need during the surgical procedure. Once the surgical procedure is started, more suture can be added to the field; this method prevents waste.

Pour warmed solution (usually normal saline or Ringer's lactate) into the round basin on the instrument table for irrigation and moistening sponges. Pour sterile water into the instrument basin if one is used. For the skin preparation, pour a small amount of antiseptic agent into the solution cups on the prep table.

To establish a baseline of table contents for the record, count sponges, sharps, and instruments with the scrub person as required by institutional policy and procedure. Record this number immediately to begin the ongoing tally.

After the Patient Arrives

The circulator attends to the patient while the scrub person continues to prepare for the arrival of the surgeon. Although time is limited during the check-in process, the circulator should perform a brief assessment of the patient. Assessment data about the patient's health status that can be gathered without using equipment or taking an extraordinary amount of time are listed in Box 27-2.

Greet and identify the patient. Introduce yourself and identify your title and role. Offer the patient a blanket from the warming cabinet. Check the wristband for identification by name and number. Ask the patient to verbally identify himself or herself and (in his or her own words) describe an understanding of the surgical procedure. If the surgical site is designated left or right, validate the area by having the patient point to the spot. Double check this spot against the permanent record and the scheduled procedure. In some facilities this spot is actually marked with an ink marker. If the patient is a minor or is unable to respond for himself or herself, this process is performed in the presence of a parent or legal guardian. Check the plan of care and the patient's chart for pertinent information, including consent. Immediately report any discrepancies or questions to the surgeon.

Verify any allergies or environmental and/or chemical sensitivities the patient may have. These may be identified by an additional wristband and/or by a special notation on the patient's chart. Ask the patient to describe his or her reaction to the drug or substance.

Be sure the patient's hair is covered with a cap; this prevents dissemination of microorganisms and protects the hair from being soiled. Loosen the neck and back ties on the patient's gown, and untuck the blanket from the foot of the transport stretcher. Align the transport cart with the operating bed and lock the wheels. Ask the anesthesia provider to stand on the opposite side of the bed as the patient moves over. Assist the patient as needed, taking care that the patient's gown, blanket, intravenous (IV) infusion tubing, or catheter drainage tubing is not caught between the stretcher and the operating bed. Protect the patient's modesty, and use good body mechanics. Additional personnel should be summoned to help if the patient is unable to move himself or herself.

Box 27-2	**Brief Physical Assessment That Can Be Performed by the Circulator During the Check-In Period Before Entering the OR***

Review of Body Systems (Brief History)	**Head-to-Toe Assessment (Brief Physical)**
Is the patient a reliable historian, or is a family member translating or communicating on his or her behalf?	Is the patient here for a scheduled procedure, urgent or emergent care or, possibly, a redo from an earlier surgery? This may alter the needed supplies for the case.
Ask the patient if he or she is taking any medication on a regular basis (e.g., heart or blood pressure medications). This should include vitamins, hormones, or herbal preparations.	Is the patient a child or adult? Is a parent present?
	Observe the color of the patient's skin and body tissues.
Does the patient have any allergies? What are the patient's reactions when exposed to the offending substance? Is the reaction localized or systemic?	Listen to the sound of the patient's voice as he or she speaks. Is it raspy or breathless? Is the patient coughing?
Ask about the patient's last meal and oral intake. If this is an emergency, ask what the foods were in this meal. Red foods may falsely imply gastrointestinal bleeding if the patient vomits.	Touch the patient's skin as the dialogue progresses. Is it cool, hot, damp, dry, or in any other condition? This assessment can be performed as part of shaking hands. Does the patient have a weak or strong handshake or grasp? Is the patient shaky?
Ask if the patient has ever had any surgery before. This may reveal a condition that requires special positioning or other modification to the standard plan of care.	Is there eye contact, and do the eyes move appropriately? Is one or the other eyelid drooping? Is the patient crying?
Has the patient experienced any complications during previous surgeries?	Does the patient have enough physical coordination to point to the surgical site?
Ask if the patient if he or she wears contact lenses or prosthetic parts.	Does the patient appear to understand what is being said? Can the patient speak and respond appropriately?
Ask the patient if he or she has any trouble moving limbs.	
Is the patient extremely large or small? This may indicate the need for additional instruments or a weight-appropriate operating bed.	Does the patient have a Foley catheter or an ostomy? Is the patient continent?
Is the patient aware of the procedure being performed?	Are IV fluids running? Is the line infusing? Are additives in the container?
Are laboratory studies and blood work reports included with the chart? Are they current?	

*Most of these assessment activities can be performed simultaneously in just a few minutes and may lead to additional nursing diagnoses that require a modification of the plan of care.

After the patient has transferred to the operating bed, apply the safety belt over the thighs 3 to 4 inches above the patient's knees, and secure his or her arms. The safety belt should be placed over the blanket so it is visible, and it should not impair circulation to the extremities. Avoid placing additional blankets over the belt, because there is no way to be sure the belt is secure if it is not visible. Other considerations include the following:

1. The patient's legs should not be crossed. A small pillow may be placed under the patient's knees to decrease strain on the back.
2. Remove the patient's arm from the sleeve of the gown before securing it to the armboard. The angle of abduction of the arm on the armboard should not exceed 90 degrees—a right angle with the body. The brachial nerve plexus can be damaged by lengthy, severe abduction of the arm.

Help the anesthesia provider as needed. Apply and connect monitoring devices, and assist with IV infusion, induction, and intubation as necessary. Some facilities have anesthesia technicians to assist the anesthesia provider. Before the patient arrives, obtain the following equipment:

- Unsterile gloves for the person who will do a percutaneous venipuncture. Sterile gloves are required for a venous cutdown or for insertion of arterial monitoring lines.
- A tourniquet to help expose the vein for percutaneous insertion. An unsterile Penrose drain is sometimes used for this purpose.
- Sponges saturated with antiseptic solution for skin preparation. Thorough skin antisepsis is imperative.
- A sterile IV administration tubing set and angiocaths. A cutdown tray (may be needed).
- 1½-inch (3.8-cm) × 20- or 21-gauge angiocaths, which are usually used for IV fluids when blood transfusion is not anticipated; 1½ inch (3.8-cm) × 18-gauge or 2-inch (5-cm) × 20-gauge needles are used when blood transfusion is anticipated.
- Adhesive tape strips to firmly secure the needle or catheter and tubing to the patient's skin, which prevents motion that may traumatize the vein or cause microorganisms to enter into the skin wound. If the patient is sensitive to adhesives, paper tape may be used.
- A stopcock to regulate or stop the flow of solution through the tubing into the vein. Ports should remain covered until needed to prevent microbial migration into the system.
- IV crystalloid solutions, which include the following:
  Normal saline
  Dextrose, 5% or 10%, in water (D_5W)
  Dextrose in 0.25% saline
  Ringer's lactate solution
  Dextrose in Ringer's lactate solution

When prolonged postoperative fluid therapy or hyperalimentation is anticipated, an inert, nontoxic, radiopaque plastic single-, double-, or triple-lumen catheter is inserted through either a venipuncture through the skin (percutaneous insertion) of the neck or subclavian area or a cutdown through a skin incision to expose the vein. A venous cutdown is performed in other selected situations: for central venous pressure monitoring, for thrombosed superficial veins, or for superficially collapsed veins caused by shock or prolonged preoperative IV therapy. The cutdown site is a sterile procedure that creates an open wound. Sterile gloves, drapes, and a tray of sterile instruments and sutures are needed. Assorted sizes of IV catheters should be available so the anesthesia provider can choose the size best suited to the vein. A soft, pliant catheter takes the contour of the anatomy and is not easily dislodged by movement of the patient.

Gently squeeze the plastic bag to detect leaks, and check the glass for cracks. Check the solution for clarity or discoloration; a cloudy solution is contaminated. A registered nurse or physician must check the label on the container before it is administered. All solutions given are charted and monitored to see that they are running at the proper speed. Usually this is the responsibility of the anesthesia provider.

During the Induction of General Anesthesia

Remain at the patient's side during the induction of anesthesia. Assist the anesthesia provider during induction and intubation.

Maintain a quiet environment. Tactile or auditory stimulation may produce excitement in the patient during induction. Hearing is the last sense lost. A strong startle reaction to sound can provoke life-threatening cardiac dysrhythmias in any patient. Undue stimulation while the patient is under light anesthesia should be avoided. A quiet, undisturbed induction makes for a much safer and easier maintenance of and recovery from anesthesia.

After the Patient Is Anesthetized

Attach the anesthesia screen and other table attachments as needed. Reposition the patient only after the anesthesia provider says the patient is anesthetized to the extent that he or she will not be disturbed by being moved or touched. If the patient is to be placed in the prone position, be sure a transport cart remains outside of the door for the duration of the case in the event of an emergency. In the event of cardiac arrest, the patient will need to be rapidly turned to a supine position for treatment.

If an electrosurgical unit is to be used, place the inactive electrosurgical dispersive electrode pad or plate in contact with the patient's skin. Avoid scar tissue and hairy or bony areas. Expose the appropriate area for skin preparation and/or Foley catheter insertion. Turn the blanket downward and the gown upward neatly to make a smooth area around the surgical site. Other areas are exposed as necessary. Before prepping and draping begins, note the patient's position to be certain all measures for his or her safety have been observed. The circulator or first assistant then prepares the patient's skin with antiseptic solution.

Turn on the overhead spotlight over the site of the incision. Preoperative medication affects the protective pupillary reflex, and therefore bright light should not be focused on the patient before he or she is asleep or the eyes are covered. Dim light is restful and not irritating.

Cover or bag the prep tray immediately after use. Preparation sponges are not detectable on x-ray films. Because they are not included in the sponge count, they are not discarded in the kick bucket. A disposable tray may be bagged for disposal with trash at the completion of the surgical procedure.

After the Surgeon and Assistant(s) Scrub

Assist with gowning of the team. Reach inside the gown to the shoulder seam. If a closed gloving technique is used, pull the gown sleeves only so far that the hands remain covered by the knitted cuff. If an open technique is used, pull each sleeve over the hands so the gown cuffs are at the wrists. Fasten the waist tie first, followed by the neck closure. Securing the back of the gown in this order allows the upper body more freedom of motion for gloving.

After gloving, the surgeon and assistant(s) should wipe their gloves with a sterile damp towel to remove glove powder. If the surgeon rinses his or her gloves in a splash basin, the basin should be removed from the sterile field immediately after use; this prevents powder from being carried into the surgical wound if the gloves are rinsed of blood and debris during the surgical procedure.

Observe for any breaks in sterile technique during draping. Stand near the head end of the operating bed to assist the anesthesia provider in fastening the drape over the anesthesia screen or around an IV pole next to the armboard. The drainage bag of the Foley catheter should be placed in view of the anesthesia provider and the circulator.

Assist the scrub person in moving the Mayo stand and instrument table into position, being careful not to touch the drapes. Place steps or platforms for team members who need them, or place stools in position for a surgeon who prefers to operate while seated. If the surgeon is seated, the entire team should be seated to protect the level of the sterile field.

Position kick buckets on each side of the operating bed. Connect suction, the ESU cord, the dispersive electrode cable, or any other powered equipment to be used. If possible, these cords should be directed off the same side of the operating bed to avoid creating a stumbling hazard. Place foot pedals within easy reach of the surgeon's foot. Tell the surgeon which foot pedal is placed by which foot, and confirm and document the desired settings on all machines.

During the Surgical Procedure

Be alert to anticipate the needs of the sterile team, such as adjusting the operating light, removing perspiration from brows, and keeping the scrub person supplied with sponges, sutures, warm saline, and other necessary items. Ideally, the circulator watches the surgical procedure closely enough to see when routine supplies are needed and gives them to the scrub person without him or her having to ask for them. The circulator should know how to use and care for all supplies, instruments, and equipment and be able to get them quickly. This is particularly important in emergency situations, such as cardiac arrest.

Stay in the room. Inform the scrub person if you must leave to get something. Be available to answer questions, obtain supplies, and assist team members.

Keep discarded sponges carefully collected, separated by sizes, and counted. Sponge forceps or gloves are used to handle and count sponges. Soiled sponges should be placed away from traffic, cabinets, and doors but in full view of the scrub person and anesthesia provider. The preferred method is to gather them directly into containers, such as clear plastic bags that can be closed.

Assist the surgeon and the anesthesia provider in monitoring blood loss. Weigh sponges if requested to do so. Estimate the blood volume in the suction container by subtracting irrigation and body fluids from the total volume in the container. Determinations of total blood volume may be used for estimation of the surgical blood loss. Obtain blood products for transfusion from the refrigerator as necessary, or send a patient care assistant to the blood bank. If the patient's own blood will be recovered for intraoperative autotransfusion, obtain the necessary equipment.

Know the condition of the patient at all times. Inform the operating room (OR) manager of any marked changes, unanticipated procedure, or delays. In a busy department it may be necessary to rearrange the schedule. Communicate periodically with the patient's family or significant other(s) to inform them of the progress of the procedure as appropriate.

Prepare and label specimens for transportation to the laboratory. An error in labeling a tissue specimen or culture could cause an inaccurate diagnosis or improper therapy or necessitate another operation. Each container is labeled with the patient's name, identification number, and type of specimen. Accompanying the specimen is a requisition that specifies the laboratory test requested by the surgeon. The requisition includes the date, name of the surgeon, preoperative and postoperative diagnoses, surgical procedure, desired test, and tissue to be examined, including its source.

Containers for storing specimens may be plastic containers, waxed cardboard cartons, or glass jars with preservative solution. The closed, labeled container is placed into a plastic bag or additional container for transport to the laboratory. The handling of specimens should be kept to a minimum and only while wearing gloves and appropriate personal protective gear, such as eyewear. Use care to avoid contaminating the outside of a specimen container. If it is contaminated, wipe it with a tuberculocidal disinfectant. Always wash hands thoroughly after removing gloves that have been worn to handle specimens. If instruments are used for handling, be careful not to tear, crush, or damage tissue. The routine care for each type of tissue specimen may vary as follows:

1. Pathologic tissue specimens should not be allowed to dry out. Saline or a solution of aqueous formaldehyde (10% formalin) is most often used as the fixative until the specimen is processed further in the laboratory. Some pathology laboratories prefer moistening the specimen with sterile normal saline. Check for the preference of the laboratory that will be examining the specimen. Fresh tissue and frozen sections are not placed in preservative solution.

2. Cultures should be refrigerated or sent to the laboratory immediately. Cultures that are immediately placed into media can be stored in an incubator. Cultures are obtained under sterile conditions. The tips of swabs must not be contaminated by any other source. The circulator may hold the tube with gloved hands, but swabs are handled only by sterile team members. OR and laboratory personnel must be protected from contamination. If the tube is handed off the sterile field, the circulator (wearing gloves) can hold open a small plastic bag into which the scrub person drops the tube.

3. Cultures for suspected anaerobic pathogens require immediate attention. Exposure to room air may kill anaerobes in a few minutes. Most laboratories provide special transport devices or media for their survival. If such devices are not available, purulent material can be aspirated into a sterile disposable syringe through a disposable needle. This needle is removed and placed with counted sharps on the instrument table. Air is expelled away from the field, and the syringe is capped with the syringe tip supplied with the syringe; the syringe is then sent immediately to the laboratory. The syringe should not be sent to the laboratory with the needle attached, and the needle should not be recapped by hand because of the potential for a needle-stick injury.

4. Smears and fluids should be taken to the laboratory as soon as possible. These may be placed on glass slides or drawn into evacuation tubes.

5. Stones are placed in a dry container so they will not dissolve.

6. Foreign bodies should be disposed of or preserved according to policy, and a record is kept for legal purposes. A description of the object is recorded. A foreign body may be given to the police, surgeon, or patient, depending on legal implications, policy, or the surgeon's wishes.

7. Amputated extremities are wrapped in plastic before sending them to a refrigerator in the laboratory or morgue. Avoid placing the amputated limb in the patient's field of vision. Most patients needing amputation have spinal or epidural anesthesia for the procedure. The sight of the body part may cause emotional distress in the patient.

The patient may request that an amputated extremity be sent to a mortuary for preservation for burial with his or her body after death. This request must be noted on the requisition sent to the laboratory. Refer to institutional policy and procedure for the care of amputated limbs.

As required, complete the documentation in the patient's chart, permanent OR records, and requisitions for laboratory tests or chargeable items. Information to be included in the documentation of direct intraoperative care is identified in Box 27-3. Additional information about documentation in the perioperative environment is listed in Chapter 4.

During Closure

Count sponges, sharps, and instruments with the scrub person. Report counts as correct or incorrect to the surgeon. Complete the count records. Collect used sponges for disposal in the appropriately marked receptacles.

If another patient is scheduled to follow (TF), the following procedures should be observed:

1. Phone or ask the clerk-receptionist to call the unit where the next patient is waiting and request that preoperative medication be given if ordered; this should

---

Box 27-3	**Documentation by the Circulator of Direct Intraoperative Patient Care**

Initial assessment of the patient on arrival to the OR. The identity of the patient and verification of the procedure should be validated.

The significant times, such as arrival, start, completion, and room exit times.

Disposition of sensory aids or prosthetic devices accompanying the patient on arrival in the OR.

Position, supports, safety devices, and/or restraints used during the surgical procedure.

Placement of monitoring and ESU electrodes, tourniquets, and other special equipment and identification of units or machines used, as applicable. The settings and duration of use should be recorded.

The names and times of all personnel in the room for the procedure.

The type of anesthetic administered, and by whom.

The surgical site preparation, the antiseptic agent administered, and by whom.

Medications, solutions, and doses administered, and by whom.

A description of the actual surgical procedure performed.

Contact with the patient's family or significant other(s).

Type, size, and manufacturer's identifying information (lot numbers) of prosthetic implants, or the type, source, and location of tissue transplants or inserted radioactive materials.

Use of x-ray study or imaging.

Disposition of tissue specimens and cultures.

Correctness or incorrectness of surgical counts (if incorrect, the remedial measures to locate the lost item).

Placement of drains, catheters, dressings, and packing. Output is recorded if receptacle is emptied in the OR.

Wound classification.

Charges to patient for supplies, according to hospital routine.

Piece of equipment sent from OR with patient to unit (e.g., tracheotomy set that accompanies patient following thyroidectomy, wire scissors if patient has had teeth wired together). These items are to be returned.

Disposition of the patient after leaving the OR.

Any unusual event or complication.

---

be done at least 45 minutes before the scheduled time of the surgical procedure. This procedure usually is not necessary for the first scheduled patient of the day but is important for subsequent patients when the exact time of the surgical procedure is uncertain. For these patients the anesthesia provider usually orders medication "on call."

2. Send a nursing assistant for the patient or notify the unit to transport the patient. The patient should be in the OR suite 30 minutes before the anticipated time of incision. If a holding area is included in the OR suite, the patient may arrive earlier to receive the preoperative medication there.

Check the surgeon's preference card and procedure book. Collect supplies that will be needed, and get them organized to the extent possible. These supplies can be assembled in the substerile room or left in a cabinet. They cannot be put on furniture in the room until it is cleaned after completion of the current surgical procedure. Advance preparation for the following case may vary if a case cart system is used.

Prepare for room cleanup so that minimal time is expended between surgical procedures:

1. Remove x-ray films from the viewbox, place them in an envelope, and take them to the designated area to be returned to the x-ray department.

2. Obtain the washer-sterilizer tray, instrument tray, and other items necessary for the cleanup procedure.

Send for a postanesthesia care unit (PACU) stretcher or an intensive care unit (ICU) bed, or prepare the patient's stretcher or bed with a clean sheet, whatever is the institutional procedure. Obtain a transfer monitor and oxygen tank with tubing if needed. Also alert patient care assistants and housekeeping personnel that the surgical procedure is nearing completion so they can be ready to assist in room turnover as needed. This helps shorten the downtime between surgical procedures.

After the Surgical Procedure Is Complete

Assist with dressing the surgical wound and managing the surgical drainage systems. The scrub person should roll the drapes off the patient before the outer layer of dressing is applied. Secure the outer layer of the dressing with the appropriate type of tape. Open the neck and back closures of the surgeon's and assistants' gowns so they can remove them without contaminating themselves.

See that the patient is clean. Wash off body substances or plaster. Put on a clean, warm gown and blanket. Have a patient care assistant bring in a clean PACU stretcher or ICU bed. Check the patient's name on the stretcher or bed if the procedure is to return the patient to same one used for transport to the OR suite. Align the cart with the operating bed and lock the wheels. Remove the arm and leg safety belts and table appliances.

A lifting frame or patient roller is a great help in moving unconscious and obese patients. The Davis patient roller consists of a series of rollers that are mounted in a frame long enough to accommodate the trunk of an adult patient. The edge of the roller is placed under the lift sheet and the patient's side. With the patient's head and feet supported, the lift sheet is pulled and the patient is rolled onto the stretcher or bed. A minimum of four people is required to move the patient with this device: one to lift the head, one to lift the feet, one beside the stretcher or bed to pull, and one beside the patient to lift him or her from the operating bed. The action of all four people should be synchronized, and the count of three is called by the anesthesia provider. The following precautions should be taken in lifting or rolling an unconscious patient:

1. Protect the IV, drains, and urinary drainage bag. Secure IV solution bags on an IV pole. It is preferable to attach the IV pole near the foot end of the stretcher or bed, where there is less danger of injury to the patient if it should fall or break.
2. Use the lift sheet to support the arms at the sides so the arms do not dangle.
3. The anesthesia provider guards the head and neck from injury.
4. Lift or roll the patient gently and slowly to avoid circulatory depression.

After the patient is safely on the transport cart, remove the lift sheet by rolling the patient gently from side to side. Brush burns result if the fabric is pulled from under the patient. Place the patient in a comfortable position that is most conducive to the maintenance of respiration and circulation. The appropriate position may vary with the type of surgical procedure; usually the patient should:

- Be supine following a laparotomy, with the head of the stretcher elevated 15 degrees, especially if he or she is still intubated
- Be semiprone following a tonsillectomy, for drainage, if extubated
- Be lateral, on the affected side, following transthoracic surgical procedures, thus splinting the side, usually extubated
- Have the affected extremity supported on a pillow

Raise the side rails before the patient is transported out of the OR. Be sure the completed chart and proper records accompany the patient, and send other supplies as indicated. Help transport the patient to the PACU or patient care unit.

Patient Transfer from the Operating Room

During transport, the patient should be constantly observed by someone familiar with his or her condition. If the patient has had local anesthesia, the circulator and transporter may accompany the patient during the return to an ambulatory unit. The anesthesia provider and circulator should accompany an anesthetized patient during transport to the PACU, where they give a verbal report to the PACU nurse. This postoperative report is important for the continuity of care. A concise verbal report from the anesthesia provider and/or circulator includes the following:

- Name and age of the patient
- Type of surgical procedure and the name of the surgeon
- Type of anesthesia and the name of the anesthesia provider
- Vital signs (baseline, preoperative, and intraoperative), including current body temperature
- Types and locations of drains, packing, and dressings
- Preoperative level of consciousness and current status
- Medications given preoperatively and intraoperatively, as well as those regularly taken by prescription or self-medication
- Medical history, including previous surgical procedures
- Allergies and responses to allergens, substance sensitivity
- Positioning on the operating bed and devices attached to the skin
- Complications during the surgical procedure
- Intake and output, including IV fluids and blood
- Location of the waiting family or significant other(s)
- Special considerations:
  Sensory and/or physical impairments; eyewear, hearing aids, dentures, or other personal property brought to the OR is returned to the patient when the level of consciousness is appropriate
  Language barrier and level of understanding
  Use of tobacco, alcohol, and/or addictive drugs
  Orders such as "no code," "do not resuscitate," or "do not attempt resuscitation"

SPONGE, SHARP, AND INSTRUMENT COUNTS

The counting of sponges, needles and other sharps, and instruments has been mentioned throughout this chapter. These supplies are crucial to the surgical procedure and must be accounted for throughout every procedure. Items are counted before and after use. The types and numbers of sponges, needles and other sharps, and instruments vary for each surgical procedure.

Accountability is a professional responsibility. The surgeon and patient rely on the accuracy of this accountability by the team. There are several reasons why is it important for the scrub person and circulator to count and be accountable for all items used during the procedure. Counts are performed for patient and personnel safety, infection control, and inventory purposes. A needle, instrument, sponge, tape, or towel left in the wound after closure is a possible cause for a lawsuit following a surgical procedure. Containment and control is also important for infection control.

A retained foreign object made of woven textile is referred to as a *gossypiboma* or a *textiloma*. A foreign body unintentionally left in a patient can be the source of wound infection or disruption. The longer the object remains in the body, the more it incorporates ingrowth of tissue. An abscess can form, and fistulae may develop between organs. The foreign body reaction may be immediate or may be delayed for years. Diagnosis is sometimes difficult and costly, and removal of the object usually requires major surgery. The literature reports the removal of some retained sponges through laparoscopic surgery if they are discovered before adhesions develop.

A contaminated sponge or needle that is unaccounted for at the close of procedure could also inadvertently come in contact with the personnel who clean the room. Blood or body fluids are sources of pathogens such as human immunodeficiency virus (HIV) or hepatitis B virus (HBV). A surgical pattie that has become saturated with cerebrospinal fluid during a neurologic case may also be contaminated with Creutzfeldt-Jakob disease (CJD).

Inventory control is monitored by accounting for the instrument set in its entirety. Counting ensures that expensive instruments such as towel clips and scissors are not accidentally thrown away or discarded with the drapes. Injury to laundry and housekeeping/environmental services personnel by the contaminated sharp edges of surgical instruments, blades, and needles is a potential risk. Surgical instruments also can cause major damage to equipment in the laundry services.

Counting Procedures

A counting procedure is a method of accounting for items put on the sterile table for use during the surgical procedure. Sponges, sharps, and instruments should be counted and/or accounted for on all surgical procedures. This includes any materials introduced into the patient during the procedure, such as rectal or vaginal packs or sterile towels used to pack off viscera.

First Count

The person who assembles and wraps items for sterilization will count them in standardized multiple units. Some facilities enclose a copy of this tray inventory count sheet in the instrument set. In commercially prepackaged sterile items (e.g., sponges or disposable towels), this count is performed by the manufacturer.

Second Count

The scrub person and the circulator together count all items before the surgical procedure begins and during the surgical procedure as each additional package is opened and added to the sterile field. These initial counts provide the baseline for subsequent counts. Any item intentionally placed in the wound, such as packing towels, is recorded. A useful method for counting is as follows:

1. As the scrub person touches each item, he or she and the circulator number each item aloud until all items are counted.
2. The circulator immediately records the count for each type of item on the count record. Preprinted forms are helpful for this purpose.

3. Additional packages should be counted away from counted items already on the table in case it is necessary to repeat the count or to discard an item.
4. Counting should not be interrupted. The count should be repeated if there is uncertainty because of interruption, fumbling, or any other reason.
5. If either the scrub person or the circulator is permanently relieved by another person during the surgical procedure, the incoming person should verify all counts before the person being relieved leaves the room. Persons who perform the final counts are held accountable for the entire count.

Third Count

Counts are taken in three areas before the surgeon starts the closure of a body cavity or a deep or large incision:

1. *Field count.* Either the surgeon or the assistant assists the scrub person with the surgical field count. Additional items (e.g., vaginal or rectal packing, sterile towels used as intraabdominal packing) are accounted for at this time. This area should be counted first. Counting this area last could delay closure of the patient's wound and prolong anesthesia.
2. *Table count.* The scrub person and the circulator together count all items on the Mayo stand and instrument table. The surgeon and assistant may be closing the wound while this count is in process.
3. *Floor count.* The circulator counts sponges and any other items that have been recovered from the floor or passed off the sterile field to the kick buckets. These counts should be verified by the scrub person.

Fourth or Final Count

A fourth count is performed to verify any counts and/or if institutional policy and procedure stipulates additional counts before any part of a cavity or a cavity within a cavity is closed. A final count may be taken during subcuticular or skin closure. The circulator totals the field, table, and floor counts. If the final counts match the totals on the tally sheet, the circulator tells the surgeon the counts are correct. A count should be reported to the surgeon as correct only after a physical count by number actually has been completed.

The circulator documents on the patient's record what was counted, how many counts were performed and by whom, and if the counts were correct or incorrect. A registered nurse should participate to verify that all counts are correct, but the personnel actually performing the counts are responsible for the accuracy of the counts. The counting procedure, the outcome, and participating personnel should be documented according to institutional policy and procedure.

Omitted counts because of an extreme patient emergency should be recorded on the patient's record, and the event should be documented according to institutional policy and procedure. If a sponge or sponges are intentionally retained for packing or if an instrument remains with the patient, the number and type should be documented on the patient's record. Any time a count is omitted, refused by a surgeon, or aborted, the reason should be fully documented.

Records can be subpoenaed and admitted as evidence in court. The accountability for all items used during the surgical procedure is placed on the scrub person and the circulator, who jointly perform the counting procedures as defined by institutional policy and procedure.

Incorrect Count

If any count is incorrect, a specific policy and procedure should be defined by each institution and include, but not be limited to, the following:

1. The surgeon is informed immediately.
2. The entire count is repeated.
3. The circulator searches the trash receptacles, under the furniture, on the floor, in the laundry hamper, and throughout the room.
4. The scrub person searches the drapes and under items on the table and Mayo stand.
5. The surgeon searches the surgical field and wound.
6. The circulator should call the immediate supervisor to check the count and assist with the search.
7. After all search options have been exhausted, policy should stipulate that an x-ray film be taken before the patient leaves the OR. The surgeon may wish an x-ray film be taken at once, with a portable machine, to determine whether the item is in the wound. Alternately, the surgeon may prefer to complete the closure first because of the patient's condition or because there is reasonable assurance, based on wound exploration, that the item is not in the patient.
8. The circulator should write an incident report and document on the OR record all efforts and actions to locate the missing item, even if the item is located on the x-ray film. This report has legal significance for verification that an appropriate attempt was made to find the missing item. If the item is not found on the x-ray film, the report brings to the attention of personnel the need for more careful counting and the control of sponges, sharps, and instruments.

Sponges

Sponges are used for absorbing blood and fluids, protecting tissues, applying pressure or traction, and dissecting tissue. Many different types of sponges are available. Those placed on the sterile table and field should be detectable by x-ray study. A radiopaque thread or marker is incorporated into commercially manufactured sponges.

Types of Sponges

The following list is representative of the types of sponges used:

1. Gauze sponges (which are called "swabs" in some countries) are supplied sterile, precounted, and folded.

When opened out to a single ply during blunt dissection, fibers along the raw edges could become foreign bodies in the wound.
   a. 3 × 3 inch (7.6 × 7.6 cm) sponges may be used in small incisions. These are packaged in groups of ten.
   b. 4 × 4 inch (10 × 10 cm) sponges are the most common size of sponge and are usually used dry. They are usually opened to their full length for blotting superficial tissues. They may be folded into a 2 × 2 inch (5 × 5 cm) square and used on sponge forceps deep in body cavities. They are packaged in groups of ten.
   c. 4 × 8 inch (10 × 20 cm) sponges may be used for sponging or as a moist pack in a large exposed area. These are packaged in groups of ten.
2. Tapes, also called lap pads or packs, are used for walling off the viscera and keeping them moist and warm. Tapes are either square or oblong and may have a loop of twilled tape sewn on one corner; a metal or plastic radiopaque ring, approximately 1½ inches (3.8 cm) in diameter, can be fastened over this corner. If rings are used, they remain outside the edges of the incision while the tape is inside. A small radiopaque marker is sewn into one corner of the tape. Normal saline or Ringer's lactate are isotonic solutions and are thus commonly used to moisten tapes. Tapes are packaged in groups of five. Sizes include 4 × 18 inch, 12 × 12 inch, 18 × 18 inch, and 8 × 36 inch. Larger varieties are commercially available.
3. Dissecting sponges have a self-contained x-ray–detectable element incorporated into the weave.
   a. Peanut sponges are very small, ovoid gauze sponges used for blunt dissection or absorption of fluid in delicate procedures. They are clamped into the tip of a forceps during use. They are packaged in groups of five.
   b. Kitner dissectors are small cylindrical rolls of heavy cotton tape that are held in a forceps for use. They are packaged in groups of five.
   c. Tonsil sponges are ball-shaped, cotton-filled gauze sponges with an attached cotton thread. They are held in a forceps for use. They are packaged in groups of five.
4. Compressed absorbent patties (cottonoids) are squares or rectangles made of compressed rayon or cotton; they are very absorbent. They are moistened with Ringer's lactate or saline for use on delicate structures such as the nerves, brain, and spinal cord. They are pressed out flat after moistening and before handing them to the surgeon. The surgeon will pick up the pattie with a forceps (commonly bayonet forceps) and apply it to the area of intended use. Patties have a radiopaque thread attached so they can be located in the wound.
5. Towels are occasionally but not universally used for protecting the viscera. The scrub person and circulator are responsible for accounting for the tracking and retrieval of towels or anything placed in the patient.

The scrub person informs the circulator that a towel has been used for packing or protecting viscera, and the circulator documents the event. During the first closing count at the conclusion of the case, the circulator checks with the scrub person to verify that the towel has been removed before closure. Disposable varieties of sterile, precounted, packaged towels with x-ray detectable elements are commercially available. Towels can be white, blue, or green. Some have twill tags with rings like those on lap tapes.

Retained surgical towels have been the subject of several liability suits. Case law demonstrates that the hospital, on behalf of the scrub person and the circulator, has been successfully sued in these cases, while the surgeon has been exonerated (*Good Samaritan Hospital* vs. *Dr. Ramondelli; Court of Common Pleas,* Montgomery, Ohio, 1997). The premise for these findings is based on the fact that the scrub person and circulator are responsible for the counts and the fact that the surgeon relies on their accurate performance in this role.

Counting Sponges

Radiopaque, x-ray–detectable gauze sponges, tapes, towels, dissecting sponges, and cottonoid patties are counted in multiples of 5 or 10 per package. The types of sponges and number of different sizes should be kept to a minimum. To count them, the scrub person will do the following:

1. Hold the entire pack of sponges of whatever type, including tapes, in one hand. The thumb should be over the edges of the folded sponges.
2. Break the paper band. Breaking the band is good way to designate which stacks have been counted and which ones have not.
3. Shake the pack gently to separate the sponges and loosen the twill-tape tails on tapes.
4. Pick each sponge separately from the pack with the other hand and number it aloud while placing it in a pile on the sterile instrument table.

If a pack contains an incorrect number of sponges, the scrub person should hand the entire pack to the circulator. There should be no attempt to correct errors or to compensate for discrepancies. The pack should be isolated and not used.

Methods of Accounting for Sponges

Regardless of the types and numbers of sponges counted, various methods may be used to help ensure that one is not misplaced or left in the patient.

By the Scrub Person
1. Keep sponges, tapes, peanuts, and other such materials separated on the instrument table and far away from each other and from any draping material, especially towels.
2. Keep sponges far away from small items (e.g., needles and hemostatic clips) that might be dragged into the wound by a sponge or tape.

3. Do not give the surgeon or assistant a sponge to wipe the powder off his or her gloves. It may end up in the laundry hamper or trash. Use a sterile towel instead.
4. Do not cut sponges or tapes. It may be hard to account for the item in its entirety.
5. Do not remove the radiopaque thread or marker. Either the marker or the sponge could be lost.
6. Never mix sponges and tapes in a solution basin at the same time; this prevents the danger of dragging a small sponge unknowingly into the wound along with a tape.
7. Do not give the pathologist a specimen on a sponge to take from the room; instead, put the specimen in a basin or on a towel.
8. Discard all soiled sponges into the kick bucket, and leave no more than two clean sponges on the sterile field at a time. If the surgeon needs more, keep a mental count of the number of sponges or tapes on the field. Put up clean ones before removing soiled ones on an exchange basis.
9. Do not be wasteful of sponges. Besides the economy factor, the more sponges that are used, the more there are to count and the greater the chance for error.
10. Once the peritoneum is opened or the incision is made and extends deep into a body cavity (where a sponge could be lost), three alternative precautions can be taken:
    a. Remove all small gauze sponges from the field, and use only tapes. Rings, if used, hang over the edges of the wound.
    b. Use 4 × 4 sponges on sponge forceps only.
    c. Give sponges to the surgeon one at a time on an exchange basis.
11. With the circulator, count sponges and tapes added during the surgical procedure before moistening or using them. Break the paper band to signify they have been counted.
12. Do not add or remove sponges from the surgical field during a sponge count until the count is verified as complete and correct. Before beginning the final count, place one or two tapes or sponges on the field for use while the count is being taken.

By the Circulator
1. To prevent the possibility of confusion in the count, different types and sizes of gauze squares should be used on different trays (e.g., spinal, shave, or prep trays) and should be contained before the incision is made. Gauze sponges from these trays are non–x-ray detectable and should placed in a plastic bag and discarded in a separate trash receptacle.
2. Unfold each discarded sponge and gently shake the tapes to be sure no saturated sponges are tangled with them. To avoid the transmission of blood-borne pathogenic organisms, wear gloves and protective eyewear to separate sponges for counting, stacking, and bagging.

3. Count and bag sponges in the same total number in which they are supplied, such as groups of five or ten of like sponges. These numbers should be recorded on the sponge count record and counted and stacked as a counted unit.

   The kick bucket should be lined with a plastic bag. Sponges may be hung over the rim of the bucket until the count unit of five or ten is complete. To minimize airborne contamination, the collective unit is bagged and the next collection of five or ten is counted and bagged. The scrub person should verify the count with the circulator before the bagged unit is closed. The number of sponges in each unit and the number of units are recorded so that the circulator has a record of the number bagged when it is time for the final count. The bagged soiled units can be placed within sight of the anesthesia provider and scrub person.

4. Give additional sponges or tapes to the scrub person when it is convenient for him or her to count them. The scrub person counts them, and the circulator records the numbers immediately.

5. Give dressings to the scrub person after the final sponge count. Radiopaque sponges are not used for dressings because they could distort a postoperative x-ray study of the site.

6. Do not remove sponges from the room.

Sharps

Sharps include surgical needles, hypodermic needles, knife blades, electrosurgical needles and blades, and safety pins. Each item must be accounted for. Surgical needles are the most difficult to track and are used in the largest quantity. All surgical needles and other sharps are counted as they are added to the sterile table and/or separated from other instruments in the instrument tray.

Types of Sharps

Surgical needles are used for suturing. The type will determine the method of transfer to the sterile table:

1. Reusable eyed needles put in a needle rack or a suture book are uniformly counted into sets in multiples of two or three of each type and size the surgeon will need. These needles are usually packaged and sterilized separately from the instrument sets.

2. Disposable suturing needles are precounted, packaged, and sterilized by the manufacturer. The label will specify whether the sterile pack contains single or multiple needles.

Counting Sharps

Each sharp or packet containing sharps is separated for individual counting. Suture packets containing swaged needles can remain unopened. The count is taken according to the label on each packet. Some packets contain multiple needles. The scrub person must verify the count when the packet is opened.

Methods of Accounting for Sharps

If a needle has broken, both the scrub person and the circulator must make sure all pieces are recovered or accounted for. Sometimes the risk of retrieving a piece of a needle is more hazardous than letting it encapsulate in tissue. The surgeon makes this determination.

Many smaller gauge needles do not appear on x-ray film. Needles, knife blades, safety pins, and other small sharps should never be left loose on the Mayo stand because they could be dragged into the incision or knocked onto the floor.

By the Scrub Person

1. Leave needles swaged to suture material in their inner folder or dispenser packet until the surgeon is ready to use them. These folders or packets can be placed in a fold of the suture book or secured on the Mayo stand. Suture packets can remain sealed until the scrub person anticipates their use, thus minimizing the number of loose, unused needles on the sterile table.

2. Give needles to the surgeon on an exchange basis; that is, one is returned before another is passed. Account for each needle as the surgeon finishes with it.

3. Use needles and needleholders as a unit. The following is a good rule: No needle on the Mayo stand without a needleholder, and no needleholder without a needle.

4. Secure used needles and sharps until after the final count. Many methods for efficient handling are available:

   a. Sterile adhesive pads with or without magnets facilitate counting and safe disposal. Separate pads can be used for needles that may be used again and for those that will not be. When a large number of swaged needles will be used, the scrub person and circulator may determine the number of needles a pad will hold and work out a unit system. When this maximum number is reached and counted by the circulator and scrub person, the pad is closed. This method eliminates the hazard of handling loose needles on the Mayo stand or instrument table. Disposable plastic boxes of various sizes for the containment of sharps are commercially available.

   b. Used eyed needles can be returned to the needle rack or threaded into the top layer of the suture book. Reusable suture or injection needles are not encouraged because they become dulled with use and could harbor microorganisms if not properly cleaned.

By the Circulator

1. Open only the necessary number of packets of sutures with swaged needles. Overstocking the instrument table not only is wasteful but also complicates the needle count.

2. Counted sharps should not be taken from the OR during the surgical procedure. If a scalpel with a counted knife blade is given to a pathologist to open a specimen, the scalpel must remain in the room after gross

examination of the specimen; it is not be taken to the laboratory with the specimen.

3. A sharp is passed off the sterile field if it punctures, cuts, or tears the glove of a sterile team member. These sharps are retained and added to the table and field counts to reconcile the final sharp count.

4. A magnetic roller may be used to locate a surgical needle or blade that has dropped on the floor.

Instruments

Surgical tools and devices are designed to perform specific functions that include cutting or dissecting, grasping and holding, clamping and occluding, exposing, or suturing. For each basic maneuver, an instrument of suitable size, shape, strength, and function is needed. Variation in the style and number of instruments will be dictated by the type of surgical procedure and, to some extent, by the personal preferences of the surgeon.

Counting Instruments

Instrument counts are recommended for all surgical procedures. Specific written policies and procedures are followed without deviation. To count instruments, the scrub person should do the following:

1. Remove the top rack of instruments from the instrument tray or container and place it on a rolled towel or over the lip of a tray or container. Instruments are counted as they are assembled in standardized sets. Groups of even numbers of each of the basic clamps facilitate handling and counting.

2. Expose all instruments left in the tray for counting. Remove knife handles, towel clips, tissue forceps, and other small instruments from the tray and place them on the instrument table. Do not put instruments on the Mayo stand until they are counted; they can be put on the stand as they are being counted.

3. Account for all detachable and disassembled parts. These must be counted or accounted for during assembly.

4. Recover and retain all pieces of an instrument that breaks during use. A replacement instrument is added to the count sheet.

5. After the initial count is taken, count any instruments added to the table, with one exception. If the circulator decontaminates and sterilizes an instrument that has dropped to the floor or has been passed off the table, an adjustment in the count is unnecessary. Instruments that are recovered from the floor or passed off the table and not sterilized are retained by the circulator and added to the designated counts.

Simplifying Instrument Counts

Counting is easier if the number and types of instruments are reduced and if standardized sets are streamlined. Inform the OR manager if unused, unnecessary instruments are routinely included in basic sets. Keep the surgeon's preference cards up-to-date. Instruments peculiar to specific surgical procedures or surgeons can be wrapped separately and added to the basic set only when needed.

Standard count sheets for each basic instrument set will facilitate the counting process. The sheet accompanies the set. The person who prepares the set verifies the initial count as listed. The circulator can check the items as they are counted with the scrub person.

EFFICIENCY OF THE OPERATING ROOM TEAM

A discussion of the duties of the scrub person and the circulator would not be complete without consideration of efficiency, productivity, and work habits. The scrub person and circulator together coordinate their efforts to accomplish the tasks necessary to achieve a common goal in the OR: to provide for the safety and welfare of every patient. Therefore efficiency depends primarily on individual effort and the working relationship among team members.

Productivity

Productivity and efficiency go hand in hand. Productivity is directly related to what a person does and how he or she does it. Productivity is also the quantity and quality of work (output) in relation to the costs in terms of labor and time (input). Labor costs can amount to as much as 60% of the OR budget. To be productive, perioperative nurses and surgical technologists should develop their psychomotor skills, competencies, and mental capacities. This requires an accurate perception of the factors and conditions that affect the patient, surgeon, and other team members. The concept of situational awareness means staying in touch with the environment and thinking ahead in preparing for and participating in the surgical procedure. Productivity is enhanced by a person's ability to do the following:

1. Organize work efficiently and effectively. Efficiency is important to minimize the length of time during which a patient is anesthetized and the anxious family is waiting.

2. Work rapidly with precision and dexterity. Learn to follow directions quickly and accurately, and give attention to the smallest detail. Carelessness creates waste and unnecessary hazards for the patient and team.

3. Adapt to changes or unexpected situations quickly, calmly, and efficiently. A change in diagnosis during the surgical procedure may require an altogether different setup and a different surgical approach from the one anticipated. Emergencies will arise. Knowing what to do and why to do it in a particular way decreases the anxiety of rapid performance. Exercise good judgment, and learn to prioritize actions and function competently under pressure.

4. Anticipate the needs of the surgeon and the team, and keep one step ahead. The surgeon becomes distracted if handed the wrong instrument or is made to wait for supplies. Be alert and try to anticipate procedural needs logically.
5. Maintain physical and emotional stamina. Situational awareness can be compromised by fatigue, poor physical health, and emotional distress. Be sensitive to the health and well-being of other team members.

Time and Motion Economy

Time is money; do not waste it. Know the policies and procedures, and follow them efficiently. Learn to do things right the first time and continue to do them that way; time is wasted in correcting errors. Motions should be productive.

Time Is Costly

Time is an important element in the OR. If time is wasted between surgical procedures, the day's schedule is slowed down and later procedures are delayed. The surgeons' time is wasted, and they then tend to come late because they anticipate delays. The patients and families become anxious during these delays.

Workers with poor time management skills tend to become less efficient and drift into poor work habits. Common sense is a great ally. Take time to stop and think. Is there a quicker, easier, or more efficient way of doing the job? Most work habits can be improved. Analyze them in a methodic manner.

Recognition that a problem exists is the first step toward solving that problem. Gather the facts needed to support the desirability of adopting alternatives. Seek to develop more efficient and more economical work methods.

Associations

Each patient, surgeon, and surgical procedure is unique, but all have commonalities. A logical thought process will simplify the necessary OR preparations for the patient and the surgeon. Supplies and equipment must be ready before the procedure can begin. Developing a mental checklist can help you to make quick associations of the requirements for a specific procedure according to the surgical specialty, the surgeon, and the individualized needs of the patient (see Box 27-1).

Association is a great aid to memory and organization of work. With association, the mention of one article brings to mind the others used with it. For instance, the scrub person knows a suture calls for a tissue forceps to the surgeon, a needleholder to the assistant, and then scissors. Watch for and try to establish associations to increase efficiency. Think of the order in which instruments and supplies are going to be needed, and do first things first (e.g., prepare sutures for closing deep tissue layers before preparing sutures for the skin).

To be proficient, know the organization of work and the relative importance of the factors in accomplishing it. If, as the patient is being prepped, the surgeon requests stainless steel retention sutures for closure instead of the usual sutures, the circulator should realize there is plenty of time to get these sutures after the other duties have been completed. Before getting these closing sutures, the circulator must perform the duties necessary to start the surgical procedure—tie the gowns, supervise the draping, adjust the Mayo stand and instrument table, connect the ESU and suction, and so on. When getting these steel sutures, association tells the circulator to also get wire scissors and bumpers or bridges.

Motion Economy

Wasted motion is not only time-consuming but also adds to physical fatigue. Fatigue is the result of body movement. Ten principles of motion economy can reduce fatigue from physical activity and improve personal levels of efficiency:

1. *Motions should be productive.* Once the steps in a procedure are learned, work to increase speed and the psychomotor skill needed to perform them. Make each movement purposeful; avoid rushed or disorganized motions. Work quietly and quickly. Work as fast as possible without sacrificing accuracy and technique for speed.

   The corollary to this principle is *a place for everything and everything in its place.* Keep an orderly work area to avoid fumbling and rehandling items. Arrange the items properly and leave them there. This corollary is justification for standardization of procedures, such as setting up a standardized instrument table and stocking supplies in cabinets or on carts. If everything has a place and is in its place, supplies are easily obtained by instinct when needed. A neat and orderly work area is one of the first requirements for productive motions. Consider the work flow so that minimal motions can be made to accomplish productive work.

2. *Motions should be simple.* Body movements should be confined to the lowest classification with which it is possible to perform work properly. Movements of the upper extremity are classified into five levels:
   a. Class 1 involves the fingers. The knuckle provides the pivot for motion for such tasks as fingering through a card file, turning a set screw on an instrument, and using a pair of scissors.
   b. Class 2 involves both the hand and the fingers. The wrist is the pivot for motion for tasks such as passing instruments, counting sponges, and picking up or writing on an intraoperative record.
   c. Class 3 includes the forearm. The elbow is used as a pivot to open a peel-open package, unfold drapes, and unwrap small supplies. More effort and time are expended in the third and succeeding classifications because the movements of any one class involve the movements of all classes preceding it. It takes longer and requires more effort to turn the pages of a procedure book or a patient's chart than to thumb through a file of surgeon's preference cards.

d. Class 4 includes the upper arm. The shoulder pivot is used when opening a door, setting up the Mayo stand, and prepping a patient.

e. Class 5 adds the torso. The trunk bends or stretches to lift a patient, take supplies from a low shelf or drawer, hang an IV bag, or count the sponges in a kick bucket.

Upper extremity work should be arranged to reduce work to the lowest possible classification. Finger motion is the least fatiguing, and shoulder motion is the most fatiguing. The scrub person should be positioned at the operating bed so that elbow, wrist, and finger motions can be used. To prevent prolonged shoulder motion for both of them, he or she should be positioned opposite the surgeon so that both can work with their elbows at their sides.

It is quicker for the circulator to stretch to hang an IV bag than to take time to use finger action to loosen the set screw on an IV pole, lower it with shoulder movement, hang the bag with elbow action, and repeat the sequence in reverse. However, stretching is more fatiguing. Increasing fatigue causes slower motion as the day progresses. Maybe 30 seconds was saved with the first patient of the day, but what happens to the last patient of the day? Time is lost because energy wanes.

3. *Motions should be curved.* Motions should follow curved rather than straight paths whenever possible. A circular motion to clean the flat surfaces of furniture is less fatiguing than straight push-and-pull strokes.

4. *Motions should be symmetric.* Motions should be rhythmic and flow smoothly; when possible, both hands should be used symmetrically. Damp cloths in both hands, going in opposing circles, will get flat surfaces cleaned faster and easier.

5. *Work should be within grasp range.* To avoid changes in body position, all work materials should be arranged so they are within grasp range. Grasp range is within the radius from the pivot point of the elbow or shoulder, either horizontally or vertically. The minimum grasp range is within the radius of the arcs formed with only the forearms extended, using the elbows as pivot points on the horizontal plane (Figure 27-13).

The optimum grasp range is within the area where the left-hand and right-hand arcs overlap. This is the area in which two-handed work, such as putting a needle in a needleholder, can be performed most conveniently.

The maximum grasp range is within the arcs formed from the shoulder pivots. The overlapping of these arcs is the maximum extent at which two-handed work can be performed within reach without changing body position.

The Mayo stand should be placed over the operating bed at a height and in a position within the minimum and optimum grasp range of the scrub person. It must not rest on the patient, but it can be lowered to an inch or two above the patient. The in-

Figure 27-13   Grasp ranges. Minimum range is within radius of arcs formed with only forearms extended, using elbows as pivotal points. Optimum range is within area where arcs of hands overlap. Maximum range is within the arcs formed from shoulder pivots.

strument table should be positioned as close as possible to the horizontal plane within maximum grasp range. Instruments or supplies that require two-handed work should be placed on the Mayo stand and instrument table as close to the optimum grasp range as possible.

6. *Hands should be relieved of work.* Hands should be relieved of any work that can be performed more advantageously by other parts of the body. Many electrical instruments have foot pedals to facilitate operation.

7. *Work materials should be prepositioned.* Supplies can be arranged for convenient use and minimal handling. Drapes are packaged in order of use so they do not need to be handled by the scrub person, except to move the stack to a corner of the instrument table, until ready to use. Instruments can be arranged in containers so that all of them do not need to be removed until needed.

Economize time and effort by placing items on the instrument table and Mayo stand in the order in which they will be used, and put them in their proper places without rearranging them. Arrange instruments on the Mayo stand in position to hand to the surgeon or assistant. In passing an instrument, place it in the surgeon's hand in the position in which it will be used so that readjustments will not be necessary. Grasp the instrument with the thumb and the first two fingers, far enough away from the handle so the surgeon can grasp it. Hand a needle in a needleholder in the same way, supporting the suture so it does not drag; hand it with the needle pointing in the direction in which the surgeon will start to use it. Hand thumb forceps so the surgeon can grasp the handle; do the same with retractors.

8. *Gravity should be used.* Dispensers for scrub sponges and brushes operate on the principle that gravity should be used whenever possible. Cabinets for smaller packages in the sterile supply room can be vertical and divided into appropriate-size slots. These cabinets can be filled from the top and dispensed from the bottom of each slot. This method is convenient, saves space, and ensures that older items are used first. Shelves for large, heavy packs can be made of rollers and slanted slightly to facilitate handling. Gravity-feed and drop-delivery installations eliminate or reduce motions. The quickest way to dispose of an object is to drop it. Because this also may be the quickest way to break or contaminate the object, the application of this principle requires good judgment.

9. *Supplies should be combined.* Items should serve two or more purposes whenever possible. For example, sterilizer indicator tape serves a dual purpose: to hold the package closed and to show if it has been exposed to a sterilization process. And only inches, not a yard, of tape accomplish the job.

   Disposable kits and trays are purchased, or sets are made up of reusable items so that all the supplies and materials needed for a procedure are combined into a single unit. This eliminates opening many separate packages.

10. *The worker should be at ease.* Tiring body motions or awkward or strained body postures should be avoided. A pleasant, quiet environment is less fatiguing, has fewer psychologic and physiologic adverse effects on team members, and enhances greater efficiency.

Economical Use of Supplies and Equipment

As the cost of supplies increases, circulators and scrub persons should be conscious of ways in which to eliminate wasteful practices. For example, throw away disposable items only. Avoid throwing away reusable items.

The OR suite is one of the most expensive departments of a hospital. Adequate instruments and supplies are necessary for patient care, and cost is not always the primary consideration. Economy becomes a hazard when exercised beyond the point of safety. Nevertheless, supplies do not need to be used lavishly just because they are available. Remember the principles mentioned in the following sections.

"Just Enough Is Enough"

The varieties and numbers of instruments and supplies needed for each surgical procedure can be kept to a minimum. If the procedure book and surgeon's preference cards are kept up-to-date, articles no longer used can be eliminated. Items to "have available" are not opened unnecessarily. The following procedures should be observed:

1. Pour just enough antiseptic solution for skin preparation according to the manufacturer's recommenda-

tion; it takes only a small amount. Do not open a bottle unnecessarily for a small amount if you know the remainder will not be used.

2. Follow the procedures for draping to provide an adequate sterile field without wasting disposable draping material or opening reusable woven fabric drapes unnecessarily.

3. Do not open another packet of sutures for the last stitch unless absolutely necessary. A few leftover pieces are usually long enough to complete the closure.

4. Suction tubing, syringes, hypodermic needles, drains, catheters, extra drapes, and other such materials are kept sterile. Supplies should be opened only as needed, not routinely "just in case" they may be needed.

5. Do not soak too much plaster or fiberglass casting material when helping with cast applications. Keep just ahead of the surgeon. Ask if more is needed before soaking an extra roll.

6. Turn off lights when they are not needed.

7. Separate trash into contaminated and noncontaminated waste. Contaminated waste is processed at a cost per pound.

Use Supplies and Equipment for Intended Use

1. Use operating bed appliances according to the manufacturer's instructions for positioning and stabilizing patients.

2. Use unsterile gloves for unsterile procedures in which the use of gloves is for hand protection. Open sterile gloves for sterile procedures only.

3. Do not use hemostats to clamp drapes or tubing; doing so ruins both the hemostat and the tubing. Use a stopcock or a special tubing clamp for tubes, and use a nonpiercing towel clip to secure drapes.

4. Give the assistant a needleholder for pulling needles through tissue for the surgeon. A hemostat can be ruined by using it for this purpose, and the needle can be damaged.

5. Use wire scissors for cutting wire, tissue scissors for cutting tissue, dressing scissors for cutting drains and dressings, and suture scissors for cutting sutures.

Avoid Damage

Handle all supplies and equipment carefully to avoid damage and breakage:

1. Slip off the patient's gown sleeve before the preoperative IV transfusion is started. This prevents having to cut off a wet, soiled gown at the completion of the surgical procedure.

2. Rotate sterile and older supplies to prevent items from deteriorating or the integrity of packaging from being compromised.

3. Take special care to preserve the edges of sharp instruments.

4. Follow established procedures for the proper sterilization and care of instruments, electrical equipment,

and other materials. If uncertain how to sterilize or care for any equipment, find out; do not ruin items by guessing. Items for ethylene oxide gas sterilization should be plainly tagged "for gas" to help prevent the possibility of inadvertent steam sterilization.

5. Remove all tape from packages wrapped in reusable woven fabrics. Tape will clog the washers in the laundry. Do not handle adhesive with rubber gloves; it sticks to the gloves and tears them.

6. Check drapes to be certain that instruments are not discarded in disposable drapes or sent to the laundry. At end of the surgical procedure, the scrub person should look for instruments, needles, and equipment before discarding drapes. This is part of the inventory control reason for counting instruments.

7. If an instrument or piece of equipment is defective, immediately remove it from use. Tag the device with a description of the problem, and report the malfunction promptly for corrective action. In addition, report a surgeon's complaints about the function or quality of an instrument or equipment.

8. Adhere to the routine preventive maintenance schedule for equipment.

Bibliography

Abbott CA: Intraoperative nursing activities performed by surgical technologists, *AORN J* 60(3):382-393, 1994.

Allen GJ: Reducing waste and costs in the operating room, *Surg Technol* 26(12):15-17, 25, 1994.

Association of Operating Room Nurses: *AORN standards, recommended practices, and guidelines,* Denver, 1998, The Association.

Cekirge S et al: Percutaneous retrieval of a surgical laparotomy sponge from the peritoneal cavity, *Cardiovasc Intervent Radiol* 18(1):59-61, 1995.

Ibrahim IM: Retained surgical sponge, *Surg Endosc* 9(6):709-710, 1995.

Kaiser CW et al: The retained surgical sponge, *Ann Surg* 224(1):79-84, 1996

Meeker MH, Rothrock JC: *Alexander's care of the patient in surgery,* ed 11, St Louis, 1999, Mosby.

Moyle H et al: Gossypiboma of the abdomen, *Arch Surg* 131(5):566-568, 1996.

Pezzella AT: Hand signals in surgery, *AORN J* 63(4):769-771, 1996.

Phippen ML, Applegeet C: Clinical issues: unlicensed assistive personnel in the perioperative setting, *AORN J* 60(3):455-458, 1994.

Ponder KS: The RN circulator, *AORN J* 60(3):459-462, 1994.

Sahin-Akyar G et al: Pseudotumor due to surgical sponge: gossypiboma, *Australas Radiol* 41(3):288-291, 1997.

Smith CD: Clinical issues: instrument use; contaminated glove removal; used sponge display; foot pedal operation; instrument disassembly for processing, *AORN J* 59(3):687-690, 1994.

Chapter 28

Positioning the Patient

 Chapter Objectives

After studying this chapter, the learner will be able to:

- Identify the safety hazards associated with moving a patient from one surface to another.
- List the anatomic considerations for positioning.
- Describe the effects of positioning on the patient's body systems.

HISTORICAL BACKGROUND

The historical methods of patient positioning were not standardized for safety or comfort. Surgical procedures were commonly performed with the patient in a seated position and with persons in the room holding him or her down. This method of restraint was common because anesthetics were not always available. Lithographs depict patients lying on unpadded tables, such as those used for meals. Some drawings illustrate dogs at the surgeons' feet.

PRELIMINARY CONSIDERATIONS

Proper positioning for a surgical procedure is a facet of patient care that is as important to patient outcome as adequate preoperative preparation and safe anesthesia. Proper positioning requires a knowledge of anatomy and the application of physiologic principles, as well as familiarity with the necessary equipment. Safety is a prime consideration. Terms associated with patient positioning are defined in Box 28-1.

Patient position is determined by the procedure to be performed, with consideration given to the surgeon's choice of surgical approach and the technique of anesthetic administration. Factors such as age, height, weight, cardiopul-

monary status, and preexisting disease (e.g., arthritis) also influence positioning and should be incorporated into the plan of care. Preoperatively, the patient should be assessed for alterations in skin integrity, for joint mobility, and for the presence of joint or vascular prostheses. The expected outcome is that the patient will not be harmed by positioning for the surgical procedure.

Responsibility for Patient Positioning

The choice of position for a surgical procedure is made by the surgeon in consultation with the anesthesia provider. Adjustments are made as necessary for the administration of anesthetic and for maintenance of the patient's physiology. The circulator or first assistant may be responsible for placing the patient in a surgical position, with guidance from the anesthesia provider and the surgeon. In essence, patient positioning is a shared responsibility among all team members. The anesthesia provider has the final word on positioning when the patient's physiologic status and monitoring is in question.

In cases of complex positioning or positioning patients who are obese, the plan of care includes the need for additional help in lifting and/or positioning. Special devices or

Box 28-1 Terms Associated with Patient Positioning

body habitus   Generalized physiologic configuration of the patient's size, weight, and shape.
caudad   Toward the foot of the patient.
cephalad   Toward the head of the patient.
dorsa   Back of a part.
lateral   Toward the side of the patient.
prone   Face down.
supine   Face up.

positioning aids may be necessary. Consideration should be given to the weight tolerance of the mechanism and balance of the operating bed. The manufacturer's recommendations should be consulted for guidance in selecting the appropriate bed.

Timing of Patient Positioning and Anesthetic Administration

After transfer from the stretcher to the operating bed, the patient is usually supine (face up on his or her back). The patient may either be anesthetized in this position and then positioned for the surgical procedure or first positioned and then anesthetized. If the patient is having a procedure performed while in a prone position and under general anesthesia, he or she is anesthetized and intubated on the transport stretcher. A minimum of four people is required to place the patient safely in the prone position on the operating bed.

Several factors influence the time at which the patient is positioned: the site of the surgical procedure, the age and size of the patient, the technique of anesthetic administration and, if the patient is conscious, pain on moving. The patient is not positioned or moved until the anesthesia provider indicates it is safe to do so.

Preparations for Positioning

Before the patient is brought into the operating room (OR), the circulator should do the following:

1. Review the proposed position by referring to the procedure book and the surgeon's preference card.
2. Ask for assistance if unsure how to position the patient.
3. Consult the surgeon as soon as he or she arrives if not sure which position is to be used.
4. Check the working parts of the operating bed before bringing the patient into the room.
5. Assemble all attachments and protective pads anticipated for the surgical procedure.
6. Test positioning devices for patient safety. Check for cleanliness.
7. Review the plan of care for unique needs of the patient.

Safety Measures

Safety measures, including the following, are observed while transferring, moving, and positioning patients:

1. The patient is properly identified before being transferred to the operating bed, and the surgical site is affirmed.
2. The patient is assessed for mobility status.
3. The operating bed and transport vehicle are securely locked in position, with the mattress stabilized during transfer to and from the operating bed.
4. Two persons should assist an awake patient with the transfer by positioning themselves on each side of the patient's transfer path. The person on the side of the transport stretcher assists the patient in moving toward the operating bed. The person on the opposite side prevents the patient from falling over the edge of the operating bed. Untie the ties of the patient's gown, and take care not to allow the patient's gown or blanket to become lodged between the two surfaces.
5. Adequate assistance in lifting unconscious, obese, or weak patients is necessary to prevent injury. A minimum of four persons is recommended, and transfer devices and lifters may be used. The patient is moved on the count of three, with the anesthesia provider giving the signal. Sliding or pulling the patient may cause dermal abrasion or injury to soft tissues.
6. The anesthesia provider guards the head of the anesthetized patient at all times and supports it during movement. The head should be kept in a neutral axis and turned as little as possible to maintain the airway and cerebral circulation.
7. The physician assumes responsibility for protecting an unsplinted fracture during movement.
8. The anesthetized patient is not moved without permission of the anesthesia provider.
9. The anesthetized patient is moved slowly and gently to allow the circulatory system to adjust and to control the body during movement.
10. No body part should extend beyond the edges of the operating bed or contact metal parts or unpadded surfaces.
11. Body exposure should be minimal to prevent hypothermia and to preserve dignity.
12. Movement and positioning should not obstruct or dislodge catheters, intravenous (IV) infusion tubing, and monitors.
13. The armboard is protected to avoid hyperextending the arm or dislodging the IV cannula.
14. When the patient is supine (on the back), the ankles and legs must not be crossed. Crossing the ankles and legs creates occlusive pressure on blood vessels and nerves, and pressure necrosis may occur.
15. When the patient is prone (on the abdomen), the thorax is relieved of pressure by using chest rolls to facilitate chest expansion with respiration. In the event of cardiac arrest, a transport cart should be available

for immediate emergency repositioning into the supine position and subsequent resuscitation.

16. When patient is lateral (on the side), a pillow is placed lengthwise between his or her legs to prevent pressure on bony prominences, blood vessels, and nerves.

17. During articulation of the operating bed, the patient is protected from crush injury at the flex points of the operating bed.

18. When the operating bed is elevated, the patient's feet and protuberant parts are protected from compression by overbed tables, Mayo stands, and frames. An adequate clearance of 2 to 3 inches is maintained.

ANATOMIC AND PHYSIOLOGIC CONSIDERATIONS

A patient's tolerance of the stresses of the surgical procedure depends greatly on normal functioning of the vital systems. The patient's physical condition is considered, and proper body alignment is important. Criteria are met for physiologic positioning to prevent injury from pressure, obstruction, or stretching.

Respiratory Considerations

Unhindered diaphragmatic movement and a patent airway are essential for maintaining respiratory function, preventing hypoxia, and facilitating induction by inhalation. Chest excursion is a concern because inspiration expands the chest anteriorly. Some positions limit the amount of mechanical excursion of the chest. Some hypoxia is always present in a horizontal position; tidal volume, the functional residual capacity of air moved by a single breath, is reduced by as much as one third when a patient lies down. Therefore there should be no constriction around the neck or chest. The patient's arms should be at his or her side, on armboards, or otherwise supported—not crossed on the chest. Patients have additional respiratory compromise if they are obese, smoke, or have pulmonary disease.

Circulatory Considerations

Adequate arterial circulation is necessary for maintaining blood pressure, perfusing tissues with oxygen, facilitating venous return, and preventing thrombus formation. Occlusion and pressure on the peripheral blood vessels is avoided. Body support and restraining straps must not be fastened too tightly. Anesthetic agents alter normal body circulatory mechanisms, such as blood pressure. Some drugs cause constriction or dilation of the blood vessels, which is further complicated by positioning.

Peripheral Nerve Considerations

Prolonged pressure on or stretching of the peripheral nerves can result in injuries that range from sensory and motor loss to paralysis and wasting. The extremities, as well as the body, should be well supported at all times. Appliances, restraints,

and equipment are well padded if they will be coming into contact with skin. The most common sites of injury are the divisions of the brachial plexus and the ulnar, radial, peroneal, and facial nerves; the axons may be stretched or disrupted. Extremes of position of the head and arm greater than 90 degrees can easily injure the brachial plexus. If the patient is improperly positioned, the ulnar, radial, and peroneal nerves may be compressed against bone, stirrups, or the operating bed. Femoral nerve injury may be caused by retractors during pelvic procedures. Sciatic nerve injury may be caused by tissue retraction or manipulation during hip surgery. Facial nerve injury may result from a head strap that is too tight or from manually elevating the mandible too vigorously to maintain the airway.

Musculoskeletal Considerations

A strain on muscle groups results in injury and/or needless postoperative discomfort. An anesthetized patient lacks protective muscle tone. If the head is extended for a prolonged time, the patient may suffer more pain from the resulting stiff neck than from the surgical wound. Care is taken not to hyperextend a joint, which not only causes postoperative pain but also may contribute to permanent injury to an extremity. Proper body alignment is maintained.

Soft Tissue Considerations

Body weight is distributed unevenly when the patient lies on the operating bed. Weight that is concentrated over bony prominences can cause skin pressure ulcers and deep tissue injury. These areas should be protected from constant external pressure against hard surfaces, particularly in patients who are thin or underweight. In addition, tissue that is subjected to prolonged mechanical pressure (e.g., a fold in the skin under an obese or malnourished patient) will not be adequately perfused. Wrinkled sheets and the edges of a positioning or other device under the patient can cause pressure on the skin. Pressure injuries are more common after surgical procedures that last 2 hours or longer. During lengthy procedures, the head and other body parts should be repositioned if possible. Patients who are debilitated, poorly nourished, and diabetic are at particularly high risk for pressure ulcers.

Accessibility of the Surgical Site

The surgical procedure and patient condition determine the position in which the patient is placed. To minimize trauma and operating time, the surgeon must have adequate exposure of the surgical site.

Accessibility for Anesthetic Administration

The anesthesia provider should be able to attach monitoring electrodes, administer the anesthetic and observe its effects, and maintain IV access. The patient's airway is of prime concern and must be patent and accessible at all times.

Individual Positioning Considerations

If a patient is extremely obese (e.g., the torso occupies the width of the operating bed), his or her arms may be placed on armboards. Patients with arthritis or previous joint surgery may need special individualized care because of limited range of motion in their joints. A patient who has cardiac problems or is obese may experience orthopnea or dyspnea when lying flat.

EQUIPMENT FOR POSITIONING

Operating Bed

Many different operating beds with suitable attachments are available, and practice is necessary to master the adjustments. Operating beds are versatile and adaptable to a number of diversified positions for all surgical specialties; orthopaedic, urologic, and fluoroscopic tables are often used for specialized procedures. The patient's body habitus may preclude the use of some specialty operating beds. Most beds have a weight limit for safe use. The manufacturer's recommendations should be consulted for the operation of each model of operating bed.

Most operating beds consist of a rectangular metal top that rests on an electric or hydraulic lift base. Some models have interchangeable tops for various specialties. The surface of the operating bed surface is divided into three or more hinged sections: the head, the body, and the leg sections. The joints of the operating bed are referred to as breaks. Each hinged section can be manipulated, flexed, or extended to the desired position in a procedure called "breaking the operating bed."

Some operating beds have a metal crossbar or body elevator between the two upper sections, which may be raised to elevate an area for a gallbladder or kidney procedure. The head section is removable, which permits the insertion of special headrests for cranial procedures. An extension may be inserted at the foot of the operating bed to accommodate an exceptionally tall patient. A radiopaque cassette loading top extends the length of the bed and permits the insertion of an x-ray cassette holder at any area. A self-adhering, sectional, conductive rubber mattress (at least 3 inches [8 cm] thick) covers the surface of the operating bed.

Standard operating beds have controls for manipulation into desired positions. Some beds are electrically controlled by either remote hand or foot control switches or a lever-operated electrohydraulic system; other beds are controlled manually. The desired section(s) of the operating bed surface can be articulated by setting the selector control on "back," "side," "foot," or "flex." By activating other selector controls, the surface of the operating bed may be tilted laterally from side to side and raised or lowered in its entirety. A tiltometer indicates the degree of tilt between horizontal and vertical. All operating beds have a brake or floor lock for stabilization in all positions.

Special Equipment and Bed Attachments

The equipment used in positioning is designed to stabilize the patient in the desired position and thus permit optimal exposure of the surgical site. All devices are clean, free of sharp edges, and padded to prevent trauma or abrasion. Each operating bed has attachments for specific purposes. Many positioning devices to protect pressure points and joints are commercially available. If they are reusable, they are washable; some may be sterilized between uses.

Safety Belt (Thigh Strap)

To restrain leg movement during surgical procedures, a sturdy, wide strap of durable material (e.g., nylon webbing or conductive rubber) is placed and fastened over the thighs, above the knees, and around the surface of the operating bed. Some straps are attached at each side of the bed and fastened together at the center. This belt should be secure but not so tight that it impairs circulation; the circulator should be able to pass two fingers between the strap and the patient. Placement of the belt depends on body position. To prevent injury to underlying tissue, padding (e.g., a folded blanket) should be placed between the skin and the belt. The strap should be placed over, not under, this blanket for easy visualization.

The safety belt is used during surgical procedures except for certain positions (e.g., lithotomy). Belting across the patient's abdomen during the lithotomy position can cause compression of the abdominal structures. The safety belt is used before and after the procedure, when the patient's legs are in the down position.

Anesthesia Screen

A metal bar attaches to the head of the operating bed and holds the drapes from the patient's face. It is placed after the induction of anesthesia and the positioning of the patient and is used to separate the nonsterile from the sterile area at the head of the bed. The bar is adjustable and allows rotation or angling. Some facilities use two IV poles to secure the drapes at the head of the bed.

Lift Sheet (Draw Sheet)

A double-layer sheet of broad, heavy fabric that is stitched vertically through the middle is placed horizontally across the top of a clean sheet on the operating bed. (A smooth, folded bedsheet also may be used for this purpose.) After the patient is transferred to the operating bed, his or her arms are enclosed in the lower flaps of this sheet, with the palms against the sides in a natural position and the fingers extended along the length of the body. The upper flaps are brought down over the arms and tucked under the patient's sides. The sheet should not be tucked under the sides of the mattress because the combined weight of the mattress and the patient's torso may impair circulation or cause nerve torsion. The full length of each arm is supported at the patient's side, protected from injury, and secured. In addition, a plastic curved shield,

Figure 28-1 The patient's arms can be placed at sides with the lift sheet pulled over the length of the arm and tucked under the patient's body. **A,** Correct way to secure arm at patient's side. **B,** Incorrect placement of patient's arm results in ulnar nerve injury.

referred to as a "sled," can be used to protect and secure the arms from injury (Figure 28-1). The patient should be told that these methods are used to support the arms when he or she is anesthetized and relaxed. The word "restraint" is avoided. At the end of the surgical procedure, this sheet—if not soiled or wet—may be used to lift the patient from the operating bed.

Armboard

Armboard(s) are used to support the arm(s) if IV fluids are being infused, if the arm or hand is the site of the surgical procedure, if the arm at the side would interfere with access to the surgical area, if there is inadequate space on the operating bed for the arm to rest beside the body (as with an obese patient), or if the arm requires support (as in the lateral position). The armboard is padded to a height that is level with the operating bed. To prevent ulnar nerve pressure and abnormal shoulder rotation, the patient's arm is placed palm up (supinated), except when patient is in the prone position. The armboard has adjustable angles, but the arm is never abducted beyond an angle of 90 degrees from the shoulder, or nerve plexus injury may occur (Figure 28-2). A self-locking type of armboard is safest to prevent displacement.

Double Armboard With a double armboard, both arms are supported, with one directly above the other in lateral position. This type of armboard resembles the wings of a biplane and is sometimes called an airplane support or overbed arm support. Both levels of the armboard are padded.

Figure 28-2 Position of arm on armboard should not exceed 90 degrees or injury to the brachial plexus may result. **A,** Incorrect positioning. **B,** Correct positioning.

Wrist or Arm Strap

Narrow straps at least 1½ inches (3.8 cm) wide are placed around the wrists to secure the arms to the armboards. The straps are secured without pressure or a tourniquet effect to the hands or arms.

Upper Extremity Table

For a surgical procedure on an arm or hand, an adjustable extremity table may be attached to the side of the operating bed and used in lieu of an armboard. This attachment is sometimes referred to as a hand table. Some types of extremity tables slip under the mattress proximal to the surgical site and extend perpendicular to the patient's arm, with the distal end supported by a metal leg. Some models attach directly to the operating bed and require no additional floor support. A solution drain pan may fit into some extremity tables. After skin preparation or irrigation, the pan is removed and the top panel is reinserted. A firm foam rubber pad is placed on the table and draped to receive the arm, which is then draped. The upper extremity table provides a large, firm surface for the surgical procedure. The surgeon and sterile team usually sit for these types of procedures. If one team member sits, the entire team should sit to maintain the level of the sterile field.

Shoulder Bridge (Thyroid Elevator)

When a shoulder bridge is used, the head section is temporarily removed and a metal bar is slipped under the mattress between the head and body sections of the operating bed. The bridge can be raised to hyperextend the shoulder or thyroid area for surgical accessibility. This position can also be achieved by placing a towel or blanket roll transversely under the shoulders, which causes the neck to hyperextend. A perpendicular towel roll can be placed between the shoulders to cause the shoulders to fall back, which elevates the sternum.

Shoulder Braces or Supports

Adjustable, well-padded, concave metal supports are occasionally used to prevent the patient from slipping when the head of the operating bed is tilted down, such as in the Trendelenburg position. Braces should be placed equidistant from the head of the operating bed, with a ½ inch (13 mm) space between the shoulders and the braces to eliminate pressure against the shoulders. The braces are placed over the acromion processes, not over the muscles and soft tissues near the neck. To avoid nerve compression, a shoulder brace is not used when the arm is extended on an armboard; in such cases ankle straps may be used to stabilize the patient.

Body Rests and Braces

Body rests and braces are made of metal and have a foam rubber or gel pad covered with conductive, waterproof fabric. These devices are placed in metal clamps on the side of the operating bed and are slipped in from the edge of the operating bed against the body at various points to stabilize it in a lateral position.

Kidney Rests

Kidney rests are concave metal pieces with grooved notches at the base, and they are placed under the mattress on the body elevator part of the operating bed. They are slipped in from the edge of the operating bed and placed snugly against the body for stability in the kidney position. Even though the kidney rest is padded, care should be taken so that the upper edge of the rest does not press too tightly against the body. Some operating beds have built-in kidney rests that are raised and lowered electrically or by a hand crank.

Body (Hip) Restraint Strap

With a body restraint strap, a wide belt with a padded center portion (to protect the skin) is placed over the patient's hips and secured by hooks to the sides of the operating bed. This strap helps to hold the patient securely in the lateral position. Some surgeons prefer to use wide bands of adhesive tape to secure the shoulders and hips of patients in the lateral position. A towel can be placed over the patient's skin before the tape is applied. The ends of the long strips of tape are secured to the underside of the operating bed. Care is taken not to cause compression of the skin under the tape.

Positioning for Anal Procedures with Adhesive Tape

For anal procedures, the patient is placed in a prone position (Kraske position). To separate the buttocks, a piece of 3-inch (7.5-cm) adhesive tape is placed on each buttock, 4 inches (10 cm) lateral to the surgical site. For greater security of tape adhesion, benzoin or adhesive liquid is applied to each buttock before the tape strips are applied. Each end of the tape is fastened to the frame of the operating bed.

Adjustable Arched Spinal Frame

An adjustable arched spinal frame consists of two padded arches mounted on a frame that is attached to the operating bed. The patient is placed in the prone position with his or her abdomen over this device (referred to as a Wilson frame). The pads extend from the shoulders to the thighs, with the abdomen hanging dependently between the arches. The desired degree of flexion for spinal procedures is achieved by adjusting the height of the arch by means of a crank. Other types of frames are available (Figure 28-3).

Stirrups

Metal stirrup posts are placed in holders, one on each side rail of the operating bed, to support the legs and feet in the lithotomy position. The feet are supported by canvas or fabric loops, which suspend the legs at a right angle to the feet. These are sometimes called candy cane or sling stirrups (Figure 28-4).

During extensive surgery, special leg holders may be used to support the lower legs and feet. Also available are metal or high-impact-plastic knee-crutch stirrups that can be adjusted for knee flexion and extension. Even if well padded, these stirrups may create some pressure on the back of the knees and lower extremity and may jeopardize the popliteal vessel and nerve. Gel and foam pads are available for patient protection when stirrups are used (Figure 28-5).

Metal Footboard

The footboard can be left flat as a horizontal extension of the operating bed or raised perpendicular to the operating bed to support the feet, with the soles resting securely against it. It is padded when the patient is placed in the reverse Trendelenburg position.

Headrests

Padded headrests are used with supine, prone, sitting, or lateral positions. They attach to the operating bed to support

Figure 28-4 Legs should not rest on stirrup posts or nerve injury could result. Hands should be positioned away from bed flex points.

Figure 28-3 Frames for spinal surgery. **A,** Andrews. **B,** Wilson. **C,** 4-poster.

and expose the occiput and cervical vertebrae. The head is held securely but without the pressure that could cause injury to the ears or blindness. Headrests can be shaped like a doughnut or horseshoe for head and neck procedures; other styles are flat or concave to stabilize the head and neck in alignment. Nonpadded metal headrests have skull pins that are inserted into the patient's head for neurologic procedures.

Accessories

Various sizes and shapes of pads, pillows, and bead bags (bean bags) that fit various anatomic structures are used to protect, support, or immobilize body parts. Foam rubber, polymer pads, silicone gel pads, vacuum-shaped bags, and other accessories are covered with washable materials unless designed for single-patient use.

A donut (a ring-shaped foam rubber or silicone gel pad) may be used during procedures on the head or face to keep the surgical area in a horizontal plane. Donuts also are used to protect pressure points such as the ear, knee, heel, or elbow. Protectors made of foam rubber, polymers, silicone gel, or other material also may be used to protect the joints from pressure. For example, a hard plastic shell with a soft liner (sometimes referred to as a sled) is commercially available for the elbow. Many other types of protectors are available.

Bolsters are used to elevate a specific part of the body (e.g., to elevate the buttocks for anal procedures). Solid rolls of blankets or firm foam under each side of a patient's chest, referred to as chest rolls, raise the chest off the operating bed to facilitate respiration. Large 2- or 3-L water bags can also be used for this purpose. Commercially available bolsters and elevating pads are commonly used. Because patients may have a latex sensitivity, the manufacturer's literature should be checked for latex content (Figure 28-6).

Pressure-Minimizing Mattress

To minimize pressure on bony prominences, peripheral blood vessels, and nerves during prolonged surgical procedures (more than 2 hours), an alternating pressure mattress is put over the mattress on the operating bed before the patient arrives. This may be a positive-pressure air mattress, a circulating-water thermal mattress, a foam rubber mattress (with indentations similar to an egg crate), a gel pad, or a dry polymer pad. Unless designed to be placed next to a patient's skin, pressure mattresses and thermal blankets used to induce hypothermia or hyperthermia should be covered with an absorbent sheet or thin pad. Folds and creases in the covering should be avoided to prevent pressure indentations

Figure 28-5 Additional types of stirrups. **A,** Urologic stirrups. **B,** Stirrups used for abdominal/perineal and obstetric procedures.

in the skin. The manufacturer's instructions should be followed in using these devices.

Surgical Vacuum Positioning System

With the surgical vacuum positioning system, soft pads filled with tiny plastic beads are placed under or around the body part to be supported. Suction is attached to the vacuum port on the pad; as air is withdrawn, the pad becomes firm and molds to the patient's body. The suction is then disconnected. A vacuum is created inside the pad, causing the beads to press together. Friction between the beads prevents them from moving; this creates a solid mass that keeps its molded shape. Various sizes and shapes of pads provide firm support while relieving pressure points. To change the patient's position during the surgical procedure, the valve on the pad is squeezed until the pad is slightly soft. The patient is repositioned, and suction is applied to remold the pad.

Figure 28-6 Common positioning pads.

Figure 28-7 Supine position. Patient lies straight on back, face upward, with arms at sides, legs extended parallel and uncrossed, and feet slightly separated. Strap is placed above knees. Head is in line with spine. Note small pillow under ankles to protect heels from pressure.

SURGICAL POSITIONS

Many positions are used for surgical procedures; the most commonly used positions are discussed in the following sections. If IV fluids will be infused in the arm during the surgical procedure, the arm is placed on an armboard. This fact is assumed in the following discussion because IV fluids are usually given. If electrosurgery is used, the inactive dispersive electrode should be placed after the patient is in position for the surgical procedure.

Supine (Dorsal) Position

Figure 28-7 shows the patient in the supine position—the most natural position for the body at rest. The patient lies flat on the back with the arms secured at the sides with the lift sheet or wrist strap, and the palms extend along the side of the body. The elbows may be protected with plastic shells. The legs are straight and parallel and are in line with the head and spine; the hips are parallel with the spine. A safety belt is placed across the thighs 2 inches above the knees. Small pillows may be placed under the head, lumbar curvature, and popliteal area to relieve pressure on the spine. The heels are protected from pressure by a pillow, ankle roll, or donut. The feet must not be in prolonged plantar flexion. To prevent footdrop, the soles may be supported by a pillow or padded footboard.

The supine position is used for procedures on the anterior surface of the body, such as abdominal, abdominothoracic, and some lower extremity procedures. Modifications of the supine position are used for specific body areas:

1. *For procedures on the face or neck.* The neck may be slightly hyperextended by lowering the head section of the operating bed or by placing a shoulder roll. With the patient in the supine position, the head may be supported in a headrest or donut and/or turned toward the unaffected side. The eyes are protected from injury, laser light, or irritating solutions by shields, goggles, or tape. During skin preparation and the surgical procedure, the eyes should be kept closed with eye pads taped in place. The eyes should be inspected periodically and at the end of the surgical procedure.

2. *For shoulder or anterolateral procedures.* With the patient in the supine position, a small sandbag, roll, or pad is placed under the affected side to elevate the shoulder off the operating bed for exposure. The length of the body is stabilized to prevent the spine from rolling or twisting. Hips and shoulders should be kept in a plane. The operating bed can also be tilted laterally to elevate the affected part.

3. *Dorsal recumbent position.* For some vaginal or perineal procedures, the patient is in the supine position except that the knees are flexed upward and the thighs are slightly externally rotated. The soles of the feet rest on the operating bed. Pillows may be placed under the knees if needed for support.

4. *Modified dorsal recumbent (froglegged) position.* For some surgical procedures in the region of the groin or lower extremity, the patient is in the supine position except that the knees are slightly flexed with a pillow beneath each (Figure 28-8). The thighs are widely externally rotated, and the soles of the feet face each other.

5. *Arm extension.* For surgical procedures of the breast, axilla, upper extremity, or hand, the patient is placed in the supine position; the arm on the affected side is placed on an armboard or upper extremity table extension that locks into position at a right angle to the body. The affected side of body is close to the edge of the operating bed for access to the surgical area. If the axilla is involved, the arm is placed even with the lower edge of the armboard for accessibility. Hyperextension of the arm is avoided to prevent neural or vascular injury, such as brachial plexus injury or occlusion of the axillary artery. The armboard is well padded.

Trendelenburg Position

With the Trendelenburg position, the patient lies on his or her back in the supine position with the knees over the lower break of the operating bed (Figure 28-9). The knees must bend with the break of the operating bed to prevent pressure on the peroneal nerves and veins in the legs. Shoulder braces

Figure 28-8 Modified dorsal recumbent position. Patient lies on back with arms at sides. Knees are slightly flexed, with a pillow under each. Thighs are externally rotated.

Figure 28-9 Trendelenburg position. Note knees are over lower break in operating bed, with knee strap above knees.

may be applied. The entire operating bed is tilted downward approximately 45 degrees downward at the head, depending on the surgeon's preference. The foot of the operating bed is lowered to the desired angle.

The Trendelenburg position is used for procedures in the lower abdomen or pelvis when it is desirable to tilt the abdominal viscera away from the pelvic area for better exposure. Although surgical accessibility is increased, lung volume is decreased and the heart is mechanically compressed by the pressure of the organs against the diaphragm. Therefore the patient remains in this position for as short a time as possible. In returning to a horizontal position, the leg section should be raised first and slowly while venous stasis in the legs is reversed. The entire operating bed is then leveled.

A modification of this position may be used for patients in hypovolemic shock. Many anesthesia providers prefer to keep the trunk level and to elevate the legs by raising the lower part of the operating bed at the break under the hips. Others prefer to tilt the entire operating bed downward toward the head. Either position reduces venous stasis in the lower extremities and promotes venous return.

Figure 28-10 Reverse Trendelenburg position, with soft roll under shoulders for thyroid, neck, or shoulder procedures. (From Meeker MH, Rothrock JC: *Alexander's care of the patient in surgery,* ed 11, St Louis, 1999, Mosby.)

Figure 28-11 Lithotomy position. Patient is on back with foot section of operating bed lowered to right angle with body on operating bed. Knees are flexed and legs are on inside of metal posts with feet supported by canvas straps. Note that buttocks are even with edge of the operating bed.

Reverse Trendelenburg Position

With the reverse Trendelenburg position, the patient lies on his or her back in the supine position (Figure 28-10). The mattress is adjusted so the surgical area is over the elevator bridge on the operating bed. If the elevator bridge is not used, the surgical area may be hyperextended by a shoulder roll. The entire operating bed is tilted so the head is higher than the feet; a padded footboard is used to prevent the patient from sliding toward the tilt. Small pillows may be placed under the knees and the lumbar curvature. A small pillow or donut may stabilize the head.

This position is used for thyroidectomy to facilitate breathing and to decrease blood supply to the surgical site (blood will pool caudally). It is also used for laparoscopic gallbladder or biliary tract procedures to allow the abdominal viscera to fall away from the epigastrium, giving access to the upper abdomen.

Fowler's Position

With Fowler's position, the patient lies on his or her back with the buttocks at the flex in the operating bed and the knees over the lower break. The foot of the operating bed is lowered slightly, flexing the knees. The body section is raised 45 degrees, thereby becoming the back rest. Arms may rest on armboards parallel to the operating bed or on a large soft pillow on the lap. The safety belt is secured 2 inches above the knees. The entire operating bed is tilted slightly with the head end downward to prevent the patient from slipping toward the foot of the operating bed. Feet should rest on the padded footboard to prevent footdrop. For cranial procedures, the head is supported in a headrest.

In this position, the operating bed looks like a modified armchair. This position may be used for shoulder, nasopharyngeal, facial, and breast reconstruction procedures.

Sitting Position

With the sitting position, the patient is placed in Fowler's position except that the torso is in an upright position. The shoulders and torso should be supported with body straps but not so tightly that respiration and circulation are impeded. Pressure points (especially ischial tuberosities) are padded to reduce the risk of sciatic nerve damage. The flexed arms rest on a large pillow on the lap or on a pillow on an adjustable table in front of the patient. The head is seated forward in a cranial headrest for neurosurgical procedures.

This position is used on occasion for some otorhinologic and neurosurgical procedures. Air embolism is a potential complication. Antiembolic stockings or pneumatic counterpressure devices are used to counteract postural hypotension.

Lithotomy Position

The lithotomy position is used for perineal, vaginal, endourologic, or rectal procedures. Nonsterile cotton leggings may be put on the patient's legs before transfer to the operating bed. The patient's buttocks rest along the break between the body and leg sections of the operating bed. A padded metal footboard is used as an operating bed extension so the patient's legs do not extend over the foot of the operating bed.

Stirrups are secured in holders on each side of the operating bed at the level of the patient's upper thighs. They are adjusted at equal height on both sides and at an appropriate height for the length of the patient's legs to maintain symmetry when the patient is positioned (Figure 28-11). After the patient is anesthetized, the safety belt is removed and the patient's legs are raised simultaneously by two persons. Each person grasps the sole of a foot in one hand and supports the calf at the knee area with the other. The knees are flexed, and the legs are placed inside the posts of the stirrups. For loop stirrups, the feet are placed in the canvas slings of the stirrups at a 90-degree angle to the abdomen. One padded loop encircles the sole; the other padded loop goes around the ankle. Simultaneous movement as the knees are flexed is essential to avoid straining the lower back. If the legs are properly placed, undue abduction and external rotation are avoided. The lower leg or ankle must not touch the metal stirrup. Padding is placed as necessary. If the legs are put in stirrups before the induction of anesthesia, the patient can identify discomfort and pressure on the back and/or legs. The positioning procedure is similar for other types of stirrups.

After the patient's legs are placed in the stirrups, the lower section of mattress is removed, and the leg section of the operating bed is lowered. The buttocks must not extend beyond the edge of the operating bed, which would strain the lumbosacral muscles and ligaments as the weight of the body rests on the sacrum.

The hands should not extend along the operating bed, where they could be injured in the break during manipulation of the operating bed or movement of the patient. Hands have been crushed in the break as the leg section of the operating bed was raised at the conclusion of the surgical procedure. Arms may be placed on armboards or loosely cradled over the lower abdomen and secured by the lower end of the blanket. Arms must not rest on the chest, which would impede respiration. Lung compliance is decreased by pressure of the thighs on the abdomen, which hinders the descent of the diaphragm.

Blood pools in the lumbar region of the torso, especially during prolonged surgical procedures. Antiembolic stockings may be worn, or legs may be wrapped in sequential compression devices before the surgical procedure to prevent the formation of thrombi or emboli. The legs should be checked periodically for distal pulses, skin color, and evidence of edema. In the lithotomy position, nerve damage or compartment syndrome can occur from direct pressure and/or ischemia of the muscles, which compromises the viability of tissues.

At the conclusion of the surgical procedure, the leg section of the operating bed is raised, and the lower section of the mattress is replaced. The patient's legs are removed simultaneously from the stirrups and lowered slowly to prevent hypotension as blood reenters the legs and leaves the torso. To prevent wide abduction of the thighs, the legs are fully extended and brought together as they are lifted from the stirrups. The safety belt should be reapplied over the thighs during the patient's emergence from anesthesia.

Prone Position

When the prone position is used, the patient is anesthetized and intubated in the supine position, usually on the transport stretcher. When the anesthesia provider gives permission, the patient is slowly and cautiously turned onto his or her abdomen on the operating bed. The patient's body is rotated as if rolling a log; a team of at least four persons is needed to maintain body alignment during this transfer. Prone position is used for all procedures with a dorsal or posterior approach (Figure 28-12).

Chest rolls or bolsters under the axillae and along the sides of the chest from the clavicles to the iliac crests raise the weight of the body from the abdomen and thorax. The weight of the abdomen will fall away from the diaphragm and keep pressure off the vena cava and abdominal aorta. This facilitates respiration, although vital capacity and cardiac index are reduced. To ensure cardiac filling and to reduce hypotension, venous return from the femoral veins and inferior vena

Figure 28-12 Prone position. Patient lies on abdomen. Chest rolls under axillae and sides of chest to iliac crests raise body weight from chest to facilitate respiration; pillow under feet protects toes. Patient is anesthetized in supine position before being turned into prone position.

cava is uninterrupted. Female breasts should be moved laterally to reduce pressure on them. Male genitalia should be free from pressure.

The arms may lie supported along the sides of the body, with the palms up or inward toward the body. The prone position places more pressure on female breasts. An alternate position is to place the arms on angled armboards by lowering them toward the floor and rotating them upward in a natural range of motion. The elbows are padded and are slightly flexed to prevent overextension, and the palms are down. The arms may extend beyond the head.

The head is turned to one side and rests on a padded donut to prevent pressure on the ear, eye, and face. A pillow or padding under the ankles and the dorsa of the feet prevents pressure on the toes and elevates the feet to aid venous return. Donuts under the knees prevent pressure on the patellae. The safety belt is placed above the knees.

Modified Prone Positions

For surgical procedures on the spine, the mattress on the operating bed is adjusted so the hips are over the break between the body and leg sections. A large, soft pillow is placed under the abdomen. The upper break of the operating bed is flexed, and the operating bed is tilted so the surgical area is horizontal. Some surgeons prefer a special assembly for the orthopaedic operating bed, such as an adjustable arch (Wilson frame), a Hastings frame, or an Andrews frame for spinal surgery. The patient is carefully lifted and properly positioned on a special table or frame. The patient may be placed in a prone, sitting, or kneeling position with the torso at a right angle to the thighs. The lower legs, at right angles at the knees, rest on the foot extension, which is at a 90-degree angle. The midsection of the abdomen is allowed to hang free. This allows the anesthesia provider to use the hypotensive anesthetic technique for hemostasis.

For neurosurgical procedures, the head rests in a cranial headrest to expose the occiput and cervical vertebrae. The eyes are protected; ophthalmic ointment is applied to protect the corneas and to keep the lids closed before turning the patient onto the headrest. The ears are protected with foam support. When the patient is face down on a headrest, the head should be raised periodically to prevent pressure necrosis of the cheeks and forehead.

Figure 28-13   Kraske (jackknife) position. (From Meeker MH, Rothrock JC: *Alexander's care of the patient in surgery,* ed 11, St Louis, 1999, Mosby.)

Figure 28-14   Left lateral position. Note strap across hip to stabilize body. Pillow between legs relieves pressure on lower legs.

Kraske (Jackknife) Position

With the Kraske position, the patient remains supine until anesthetized and is then turned onto his or her abdomen (prone position) by rotation. The hips are positioned over the center break of the operating bed between the body and leg sections. Chest rolls or bolsters are placed to raise the chest if the patient is under general anesthesia. The arms are extended on angled armboards with the elbows flexed and the palms down. The head is to the side and is supported on a donut or pillow. The dorsa of the feet and toes rest on a pillow. The safety belt is placed below the knees. The leg section of the operating bed is lowered the desired amount (usually about 90 degrees), and the entire operating bed is tilted head downward to elevate the hips above the rest of the body. The patient is well balanced on the operating bed (Figure 28-13). For procedures in the rectal area (e.g., pilonidal sinus or hemorrhoidectomy), the buttocks are retracted with wide tape strips. Because of the dependent position, venous pooling occurs cephalad (toward the head) and caudad (toward the feet). It is very important to return the patient slowly to horizontal from this unnatural position.

Knee-Chest Position

The knee-chest position is used for sigmoidoscopy or culdoscopy. For this position, an extension is attached to the foot section. The operating bed is flexed at the center break, and the lower section is broken until it is at a right angle to the operating bed. The patient kneels on the lower section; the knees are thus flexed at a right angle to the body. The upper portion of the operating bed may be raised slightly to support the head, which is turned to the side. The arms are placed around the head with the elbows flexed, and a large soft pillow is placed beneath them. The chest rests on the operating bed, and the safety belt is placed above the knees. The entire operating bed is tilted head downward so the hips and pelvis are at the highest point—a modified jackknife position.

Lateral Positions

For lateral positioning, the operating bed remains flat. The patient is anesthetized and intubated in the supine position,

then turned to the unaffected side. In the right lateral position, the patient lies on the right side with the left side up (for a left-sided procedure); the left lateral position exposes the right side (Figure 28-14).

The patient is turned by no fewer than four people to maintain body alignment and achieve stability. The patient's back is drawn to the edge of the operating bed. The knee of the lower leg is flexed to prevent rolling and to aid in stabilization; the upper leg remains straight. The flexed knee may need to be padded to prevent pressure. In addition, a large soft pillow is placed lengthwise between the legs to take pressure off the lower leg and therefore prevent circulatory complications and pressure on the peroneal nerve. The ankle and foot of the upper leg should be supported to prevent footdrop. Bony prominences are padded. For added stability, a safety belt and/or a 3-inch (7.5-cm) wide tape is placed over the hip.

The patient's arms may be placed on a padded double armboard, with the lower arm palm up and the upper arm slightly flexed with the palm down. Blood pressure should be measured from the lower arm. As an alternative, the upper arm can be positioned on a padded Mayo stand. A small roll or pad under the axilla relieves pressure and protects neurovascular structures. The shoulders should be in alignment.

The patient's head is in cervical alignment with the spine. The head should be supported on a small pillow between the shoulder and neck to prevent stretching the neck and brachial plexus and to maintain a patent airway (Figure 28-15).

Referred to synonymously as the lateral, lateral decubitus, or lateral recumbent, this position is used for access to the hemithorax, kidney, or retroperitoneal space. This position contributes to physiologic alterations. Respiration is affected by differing gas exchange ratios in the lungs. Because of gravity, the lower lung receives more blood from the right side of the heart; the lower lung therefore has increased perfusion but less residual air because of mediastinal compression and the weight of the abdominal contents on the diaphragm. Positive pressure to both lungs helps control respiratory changes. Circulation is also compromised by pressure on the abdominal vessels. In the right lateral position, compression of the vena cava impairs venous return.

Figure 28-16 Right kidney position. Patient is in lateral position with kidney region over operating bed break. Note kidney strap across hip to stabilize body, raised kidney elevator for hyperextending surgical site, and pillow between legs. Patient's side is horizontal from shoulder to hip.

Figure 28-15 Proper alignment of spinal column in lateral position.

Kidney Position

In the kidney position, the flank region is positioned over the kidney elevator on the operating bed when the patient is turned onto the unaffected side (Figure 28-16). The short kidney rest is attached to the elevator at the patient's back. The longer rest is placed in front at a level beneath the iliac crest to minimize pressure on the abdominal organs. Both rests are well padded. In an obese patient, folds of abdominal tissue may extend over the end of the anterior rest and be bruised if caution is not taken. The operating bed is flexed slightly at the level of the iliac crest so the kidney elevator can be raised as desired to increase space between the lower ribs and iliac crest.

A body strap or wide adhesive tape is placed over the hip to stabilize the patient after the operating bed is flexed and the elevator is raised. The entire operating bed is tilted slightly downward toward the head until the surgical area is horizontal; the upper shoulder and hip should be in a straight line. A pillow may be used to support the chest and protect the breasts. A chest roll may be placed to take body weight off the deltoid muscle in the shoulder. Before closure, the operating bed is straightened to allow better approximation of tissues.

The kidney position is used for procedures on the kidney and ureter; this position is not well tolerated. Skin and underlying tissue can be damaged by excessive pressure during flexion of the operating bed. Operating bed flexion combined with use of the kidney elevator may cause cardiovascular responses. Blood tends to pool in the lower arm and leg. Circulation is further compromised by increased pressure on the abdominal vessels when the kidney elevator is raised.

Lateral Jackknife Position

For positioning in the lateral jackknife position, the patient is first placed in the lateral position, and then the operating bed is flexed at the level of the patient's flank or lower ribs. The operating bed is tilted so the torso is level; this drops the legs into a dependent position.

Similar to the kidney position already described, the lateral jackknife position is not well tolerated. Blood tends to pool in the legs. Extreme operating bed flexion into a lateral jackknife position may occlude the inferior vena cava, causing venous obstruction. Pulmonary compliance is reduced, making ventilation difficult.

Lateral Chest (Thoracotomy) Position

Modifications of the lateral position are used for unilateral transthoracic procedures with a lateral approach. After the patient is turned onto the unaffected side and positioned as described for the lateral position, a second strap may be placed over the shoulder for stability unless doing so would interfere with skin preparation. The arms may be extended on a double armboard, or the lower arm is extended on an armboard with the palm up while the upper arm is brought forward and down over a pad to draw the scapula from the surgical area. Position depends on site and length of the chest incision. A small, firm pillow or pad under the axilla and surgical area relieves pressure on the lower arm and assists in spreading the intercostal space for better exposure.

One body rest is placed at the lumbar area to facilitate respiratory movements and provide support. Another body rest is placed along the chest at the axillary level. This body rest is well padded to avoid bruising the breasts. Vacuum bags or bolsters may be used instead of body rests. The shoulders and hips should be level. Slightly lowering the head of the operating bed assists postural drainage during the surgical procedure. This position is restricting to the cardiopulmonary system, especially if used for a prolonged period.

Anterior Chest Position

For thoracoabdominal procedures with an anterior approach, the positioning is more supine than for the lateral chest position. After the patient is anesthetized, a small, firm pillow is placed under the shoulder; another pillow is placed under the buttocks on the affected side. The knee on the affected side is flexed slightly, and a large, soft pillow is placed beneath it to relieve strain on the abdominal muscles. The operating bed can be tilted laterally to raise the incisional site. The safety belt is placed above the knees, and the arm on the unaffected side is supported at the side. The arm on the affected side is padded well and bandaged loosely to the anesthesia screen. To avoid injury to the brachial plexus, the arm must not be hyperextended. The head of the operating bed is lowered slightly for postural drainage.

Sims Recumbent Position

In Sims recumbent position (a modified left lateral recumbent position), the patient lies on his or her left side with the upper leg flexed at the hip and knees; the lower leg is straight. The lower arm is extended along the patient's back, with the weight of the chest on the operating bed. The upper arm rests in a flexed position on the operating bed. This position may be preferred for an endoscopic examination performed via the anus in obese or geriatric patients.

MODIFICATIONS FOR INDIVIDUAL PATIENT NEEDS

As with everything else, the patient's individual needs are met during positioning. Anomalies and physical defects are accommodated. Whether the patient is unconscious or conscious, the avoidance of unnecessary exposure is an essential consideration for all patients. The patient's position should be observed objectively before skin preparation and draping to see that it adheres to physiologic principles. Protective devices, positioning aids, and padded areas should be reassessed before draping, because they could have shifted during the skin preparation procedure or during insertion of an indwelling urinary catheter. Careful observation of patient protection and positioning facilitates the expected outcome.

In the patient's record, the circulator should document any preoperative limitations in the patient's range of motion, the condition of the skin before and after the surgical procedure, and the position in which the patient was positioned during the surgical procedure—including the use of special equipment.

Bibliography

Daley MD: The best is yet to be: positioning and the geriatric surgical patient, *Todays Surg Nurse* 19(5):13-18, 1997.

Lawrence AM, Lebsack RS: Operating room 2010, *Semin Periop Nurs* 6(2):111-115, 1997.

Lewicki L et al: Patient risk factors for pressure ulcers during cardiac surgery, *AORN J* 65(5):933-936, 938-942, 1997.

Martin JT, Warner MA: *Positioning in anesthesia and surgery,* ed 3, Philadelphia, 1996, WB Saunders.

McEwen D: Intraoperative positioning of surgical patients, *AORN J* 63(6):1059-1063, 1066-1075, 1077-1079, 1996.

Michaels MJ et al: Patient positioning for radical retropubic prostatectomy, *Urology* 51(5):824-826, 1998.

St Clair JD: Intubating conditions, *Can J Anaesth* 45(1):93, 1998.

Steuer K: Patient positioning for laparoscopic procedures, *AORN J* 67(4):863-864, 1998.

Sunnel S, Maschak L: Positioning for clinical dental hygiene care: preventing back, neck, and shoulder pain, *Probe* 30(6):216-219, 1996.

Warner MA: Perioperative neuropathies, *Mayo Clin Proc* 73(6):567-574, 1998.

Williams H, Reeves F: Anesthetic techniques and positioning: implications for perioperative nurses, *Semin Periop Nurs* 7(1):14-20, 1998.

Yamanouchi Y et al: Venous dysfunction and the change of blood viscosity during head-up tilts, *Pacing Clin Electrophysiol* 21(3):520-527, 1998.

Chapter 29

Skin Preparation and Draping of the Surgical Site

After studying this chapter, the learner will be able to:

- Identify key elements of preoperative skin preparation of patients.
- Identify potential problems of inadequate skin preparation.
- Discuss the implications of chemical and mechanical action of prepping the patient.
- Describe how a patient is draped using sterile technique.

The type of surgical procedure to be performed, the age and condition of the patient, and the preferences of the surgeon will determine specific procedures to be carried out before the incision is made. Consideration must be given to control of urinary drainage, to skin antisepsis, and to establishment of a sterile field around the surgical site. Terms associated with prepping the surgical patient are defined in Box 29-1.

URINARY TRACT CATHETERIZATION

The patient should void to empty the urinary bladder just before transfer to the operating room (OR) suite unless an indwelling Foley catheter is in place. If the patient's bladder is not empty or the surgeon wishes to prevent bladder distention during a long procedure or following the surgical procedure, catheterization may be necessary after the patient is anesthetized. An indwelling Foley catheter may be inserted. This maintains bladder decompression to avoid trauma during a lower abdominal or pelvic procedure, to permit accurate

measurement of output during or following the surgical procedure, or to facilitate output and healing after a surgical procedure on genitourinary tract structures. Catheterization is performed before the patient is positioned, except for a patient who will remain in the lithotomy position.

Urinary tract infection can occur following catheterization from contamination or trauma to structures. Sterile technique must be maintained during catheterization. A sterile, disposable catheterization tray is used unless the patient is being prepared for a surgical procedure in the perineal or genital area. For these latter procedures, a sterile catheter and lubricant may be added to the skin preparation setup. For other surgical procedures the perineal and meatal areas should be cleansed (sterile gloves are worn) with an antiseptic agent to reduce normal microbial flora and remove gross contaminants before the catheterization procedure.

Urinary catheterization is an invasive procedure requiring sterile technique. Sterile gloves are worn to handle the sterile catheter. The catheter size should be small enough to minimize trauma to the urethra and prevent necrosis of the

Figure 29-1   Female urinary catheterization. (From Davis JH, Foster RS, Gamelli RL: *Essentials of clinical surgery,* St Louis, 1991, Mosby.)

Box 29-1

Terms Associated with Prepping the Surgical Patient

antiseptic solution   Topical cleansing chemical used to decrease the microbial count on the skin surface.

circumferential   The surface area of the patient's skin that encompasses a limb or other rounded tissue area.

degreaser   Topical chemical agent used to remove oils and non–water-soluble material from the surface of the patient's skin.

depilatory   Topical chemical agent used to remove hair from the patient's skin.

skin preparation   The process of chemical and mechanical cleansing of the skin.

meatus; usually a size 16 or 14 French catheter is inserted in a woman, and a 16 or 18 French catheter is inserted in a man. Care is taken to note whether the patient is sensitive to natural latex rubber. Many Foley catheters are composed of latex and could cause a reaction in susceptible patients. Silicone catheters are commercially available.

If an indwelling Foley catheter is to be inserted, check the integrity of the balloon by inflating it with the correct amount of sterile water or air before insertion. The solution is evacuated with the syringe before insertion of the catheter into the urethra. The balloon size may be 5 or 30 ml (5 ml is used most frequently); 10 ml of sterile water is needed to properly expand a 5-ml balloon to compensate for volume required by the expansion channel. Foley catheters have a Luer-Lok valve over the lumen to the expansion channel that is filled using a Luer-Lok syringe.

The hand used to spread the labia or stabilize the penis is considered contaminated and should not be used to handle the catheter (Figure 29-1). Sponges used to cleanse the labia minora or glans penis should be handled to avoid contaminating the gloved hand used to insert the catheter. To facilitate insertion and minimize trauma, the tip of the catheter is lubricated with a sterile, water-soluble lubricant. Urine will start to flow when the catheter has passed into the bladder. The balloon of a Foley catheter is expanded with sterile water, and the bladder is allowed to drain. If difficulty is encountered during catheter insertion, especially in a geriatric male patient with an enlarged prostate, the catheter should not be forced into the urethra. One should stop the catheterization procedure and

Figure 29-2 Secure the urinary catheter. (From Davis JH, Foster RS, Gamelli RL: *Essentials of clinical surgery,* St Louis, 1991, Mosby.)

request help from the surgeon. A firm catheter stylet may be needed to pass the catheter through the prostatic segment of the urethra to minimize trauma to the structures.

The catheter is attached to a sterile drainage system. The tubing is attached to the patient's leg with enough slack in it to prevent tension or pull on the penis or urethra (Figure 29-2). Drainage tubing should be positioned to enhance downward flow but should not fall below the level of the collection container. Attention is paid to the catheter and tubing during positioning of the patient for the surgical procedure to prevent compression or kinking. If the container must be raised above the level of the bladder during positioning, the tubing is clamped or kinked until the container can be lowered and secured under the operating bed to avoid contamination by retrograde, backward flow of urine. The drainage bag should be positioned in the view of the anesthesia provider for observation of output during the procedure.

If the catheter is to be removed at the end of the surgical procedure, a syringe is used to withdraw and measure the solution from the Foley balloon expansion port. Cutting the end off with scissors may cause the inflation port to collapse, trapping fluid within the expanded balloon. The urethra can be damaged by withdrawing the expanded balloon.

SKIN PREPARATION

Skin preparation (skin prep) begins before the patient arrives in the OR. Many surgeons prefer to have their patients bathe with antimicrobial soap the morning of the surgical procedure. The patient should be advised to avoid the use of body

emollients, oils, creams, and lotions after washing. Some products decrease the efficacy of the antimicrobial soap, and other products prevent adherence of electrodes to the skin.

The perioperative nurse should assess the patient's skin before, during, and after the prepping process. It is important to document the condition of the patient's tissues, noting lesions and other markings as appropriate. Patients who have been involved in accidents or injured during the commission of a crime may be bearing physical marks or materials important to the investigation. Objective description of injuries that may include sketches on the record is part of the chain of evidence. Any material on the patient's person could be evidence and should be handled according to facility policy.

Purpose of Skin Preparation

The purpose of skin preparation is to render the surgical site as free as possible from transient and resident microorganisms, dirt, and skin oil so that the incision can be made through the skin with minimal danger of infection from this source.

Preliminary Preparation of the Patient's Skin
Mechanical Cleansing

Bathing removes many microorganisms from the skin. This action can be enhanced to progressively reduce the resident microbial population with daily use of a skin-cleansing agent containing chlorhexidine gluconate or iodophor, or an antimicrobial bar soap. Bacteriostatic action takes place in the cumulative deposits of fatty acids in the skin. Many surgeons advise their patients to use such a product at home for several days before an elective surgical procedure.

Skin should be free of gross dirt and debris. The surgical site and surrounding area should be thoroughly cleansed with a rapid-acting, skin-degerming, antiseptic agent. The patient's history of allergies is obtained before applying any chemical agent to the patient's skin. Usually the surgeon is responsible for designating in the patient's preoperative orders the limits of the skin area and how it is to be prepped. The procedure book specifies anatomic areas that are mechanically cleansed and corresponding areas for hair removal, if ordered, for each type of surgical procedure (see Figures 29-3 to 29-8).

The patient's general skin condition is observed. Abnormal skin irritation, infection, or abrasion on or near the surgical site might be a contraindication to the surgical procedure and must be reported to the surgeon.

Hair Removal

Hair removal can injure skin. Breaks in the skin surface afford an opportunity for entry of microorganisms and are a potential source of infection. Hair surrounding the surgical site may be so thick that removal is necessary. Hair may be removed with clippers, by applying a depilatory cream, or by shaving with a razor. Hair may interfere with exposure, closure, or dressing. It may also prevent adequate skin contact with dispersive electrosurgical electrodes or electrocardiographic (ECG) leads.

Hair removal is carried out per the surgeon's order, either on the preoperative unit or in the OR suite as close to the scheduled time for the surgical procedure as possible. The patient is draped to expose the area to be prepped, but unnecessary exposure is avoided. Bath blankets also help prevent excess heat loss during the procedure.

Clippers Electric clippers with fine teeth cut hair close to the skin. The short stubble, usually about a millimeter in length, that remains does not interfere with antisepsis or exposure of the surgical site. Clipping can be done immediately before the surgical procedure or up to 24 hours preoperatively using short strokes against the direction of hair growth. The blade lies flat against the skin surface. After use, the blade assembly must be disassembled, cleaned, and disinfected if a disposable clipper blade assembly is not used. The clipper handle is cleaned and disinfected. Cordless handles with rechargeable batteries are available.

Depilatory Cream Hair can be removed by chemical depilation before the patient comes to the OR suite. A preliminary skin patch is tested on a forearm before general application. If the patient is not sensitive, a thick layer of cream is applied over the hair to be removed. Depilatories should not be used around the eyes or genitalia. After the cream has remained on the skin for the required time, usu-

ally about 20 minutes, it is washed off. The hair comes off in the cream. The skin is intact and free from cuts, but any evidence of irritation should be documented.

Razor Shaving should be performed as near the time of incision as possible if this method must be used. One should avoid making nicks and cuts in the skin. Nicks made immediately before the surgical procedure (i.e., up to 30 minutes) are considered clean wounds. However, nicks and abrasions made several hours before the procedure may present as infected wounds at the time of surgical incision. The surgeon should be notified if the skin is not intact at the surgical site. This may be cause for cancellation of the surgical procedure. The time lapse between the preoperative shave and the surgical procedure may increase the risk of postoperative infection.

Gloves should be worn to prevent cross-contamination even though this is a surgically clean procedure. Wet shaving is preferable. Soaking hair in lather allows keratin to absorb water, making hair softer and easier to remove. A sharp, clean razor blade should be used. The skin is held taut and is shaved by stroking in the direction of hair growth. Blades are discarded in the appropriate sharps container. If disposable razors are not used, the razor, minus the blade, is decontaminated and terminally sterilized between uses.

Skin Degreasing

The skin surface is composed of cornified epithelium with a coating of secretions that include perspiration, oils, and desquamated epithelium. These surface sebaceous lubricants are insoluble in water. Therefore a skin degreaser, or fat solvent, may be used to enhance adhesion of ECG electrodes. It may also be used before skin preparation to improve adhesion of self-adhering drapes or to prevent smudging of skin markings. Isopropyl alcohol and acetone are effective fat solvents. A fat-solvent emollient is incorporated into some antiseptic agents. Some solvents are flammable.

Patient's Skin Preparation on the Operating Bed

After the patient is anesthetized and/or positioned on the operating bed, the skin at the surgical site and an extensive area surrounding it is mechanically cleansed again with an antiseptic agent immediately before draping.

Setup

Prewarmed solutions may help reduce the patient's heat loss during the skin preparation procedure and are more readily tolerated by patients undergoing local anesthesia. Prep trays and/or solutions may be placed in a solution warmer for a few minutes to warm them if warming does not cause a change in the chemical composition or concentration of the solution. Solutions should not be warmed beyond 104° F (40° C). The manufacturer's recommendations should be consulted for warming.

Some disposable sterile skin preparation trays include applicators and/or containers of a premeasured amount of antiseptic solution. The solution of choice is added to other trays. If prepackaged trays are not used, a sterile table is prepared with the following sterile items:

- Two towels to define the upper and lower limits of the area to be prepped. Two absorbent towels are used to prevent pooling under body parts along the sides of the area.
- Small basins for solutions—usually at least two. One or two ounces of solution usually is sufficient.
- Gauze sponges (nonradiopaque)—may be 4 × 8 inches (10 × 20 cm) for large areas; 4 × 4 inches (10 × 10 cm) or 3 × 3 inches (7.5 × 7.5 cm) for small areas. These are not counted sponges from the instrument table. Textured foam sponges may be preferred.
- Cotton-tipped applicators as necessary.

Sterile gloves are worn, and a sterile setup is used to prep the skin around an open wound or to include urinary catheterization as part of the procedure. Studies have shown that a clean but unsterile setup may be used for intact skin without compromising antimicrobial activity. Skin cannot be sterilized; it is mechanically cleansed and chemically decontaminated to reduce skin flora.

Antiseptic Solutions

The infection control committee usually determines the chemical antiseptic or antimicrobial agent(s) to be used in the OR for skin preparation. The maximum concentration of a germicidal agent that can be used on skin and mucous membranes is limited by the agent's toxicity for these tissues. The ideal agent should have the following preferred qualities:

1. It has broad-spectrum antimicrobial action and rapidly decreases the microbial count. It should be virucidal and be active against protozoa and yeasts.
2. It can be quickly applied and remains effective against microorganisms.
3. It can be safely used without skin irritation or sensitization. It should be nontoxic.
4. It effectively remains active in the presence of alcohol, organic matter, soap, or detergent.   .
5. It should be nonflammable for use with laser, electrosurgical, or other high-energy devices.

Chlorhexidine Gluconate

Chlorhexidine gluconate was discovered in 1950 in England. A tincture of 0.5% chlorhexidine gluconate in 70% isopropyl alcohol (Hibitane Tincture) is a broad-spectrum, rapid-acting, nontoxic, antimicrobial agent. It binds to negative charges on microbial cell walls to produce irreversible damage and death. It has minimal activity against yeasts, spores, and tuberculosis. It is effective against most viruses.

Activity is adversely affected by traces of soap and is reduced in the presence of organic matter. If chlorhexidine is used in combination with personal soaps and shampoos for preoperative bathing, it is inactivated. The patient should be instructed to shampoo his or her hair with personal shampoo and thoroughly rinse before applying chlorhexidine. Body lotion should not be applied after bathing, since this will nullify the residual bacteriostatic properties of the compound.

This agent is not absorbed through intact skin. It significantly reduces and maintains a reduction of microbial flora, such as bacteria and yeasts, for at least 4 hours. The prolonged effect is inhibited if chlorhexidine is combined with iodine preparations. Its activity increases at elevated temperature because it binds with the stratum corneum. It is available either tinted for color demarcation of the skin area being prepped or nontinted to prevent skin staining if the surgeon needs to observe the skin color. Because it is an irritant to the eyes and ototoxic, it is contraindicated for facial antisepsis. If chlorhexidine gets on clothing, chlorine bleach is avoided because it will cause permanent staining of the fabric. Clothing should be rinsed with cold water until all traces of the product have been removed.

Iodine and Iodophors

Discovered in 1812, iodine was first used in wound care in 1839. A solution of 1% or 2% iodine in water or in 70% alcohol is an excellent antiseptic. However, potential hazards of skin irritations and burns led to a decline in its use. If used, iodine should dry and then be rinsed off with 70% alcohol to neutralize the damaging effect.

Iodophors are iodine compounds that may be combined with detergents. Povidone-iodine has a surfactant, a wetting and dispersive agent, in an aqueous solution such as Betadine surgical scrub, a commonly used detergent form of iodophor. The detergent form should be rinsed off. Iodophor solution without detergent can be used for rinsing. Iodophor in 70% alcohol also is available. Iodophors are excellent cleansing agents that remove debris from skin surfaces while slowly releasing iodine. They are broad-spectrum antimicrobial agents that have some virucidal and sporicidal activity. Iodophors are relatively nontoxic and virtually nonirritating to skin or mucous membranes.

The brown film left on the skin after application of the solution clearly defines the area of application. This should not be wiped off because microbial activity is sustained by the release of free iodine as the agent dries and color fades from the skin. It should remain on the skin for at least 2 minutes. To hasten drying of the skin, alcohol may be painted on the area without friction before a self-adhering drape is applied.

Iodophors should not be used to prep the skin of patients who are allergic to iodine or sea food. Shellfish, for example, contains iodine.

The type of preparation, concentration of iodine, and presence of surfactants affect the microbial activity of products. Povidone-iodine complexes are available in solution, spray, or gel forms. Tinctures are in solution. The manufacturer's instructions are strictly followed for the product in use. The concentration of povidone-iodine may be altered by evaporation if the solution is warmed. Skin irritation may be caused by an increase in iodine concentration. The manufacturer's recommendations should be followed.

Alcohol

Isopropyl and ethyl alcohols are broad-spectrum agents that denature proteins in cells. A 70% concentration with continuous contact for several minutes is satisfactory for skin antisepsis if the surgeon prefers a colorless solution that permits observation of true skin color. Because alcohol coagulates protein, it is not applied to mucous membranes or used on an open wound. Isopropyl alcohol is a more effective fat solvent than ethyl alcohol. Both are volatile and flammable. They must not pool around or under the patient, especially if an electrosurgical unit or laser will be used. Vapors can accumulate under the drapes and become an explosion hazard.

Triclosan

A solution of 1% triclosan is a broad-spectrum antimicrobial agent. It is incorporated into many over-the-counter products used by consumers, such as deodorants and bath soaps. It is blended with oils and lanolin in a mild detergent. Cumulative suppressive action develops slowly only with prolonged routine use. It is considered nontoxic and safe for use on the face around the eyes. Studies are underway to determine the efficacy of triclosan in dentifrice preparations as a plaque control agent.

Parachlorometaxylenol

Originally developed in 1948 in Europe as a hair conditioner, parachlorometaxylenol (PCMX) has bactericidal properties useful for skin antisepsis. It is effective against some fungi, tuberculosis, and viruses. PCMX has residual properties with repeated use. It is nontoxic to the skin, eyes, and ears.

Basic Prep Procedure

Skin preparation requires coordination of the hands, eyes, and body movements of the person doing the prep. Mechanical friction with an antiseptic agent is the basis for effective skin antisepsis. The procedure is as follows:

1. Double-check the surgical procedure. Expose only the skin area to be prepped by folding back the cotton blanket and gown to 2 inches (5 cm) beyond the limits of the prep area. If the surgical procedure is unilateral, be sure which side is the surgical site. Consult the chart (history and physical segment and consent form) and radiologic reports as applies. Ask the patient to verbally state the location, and point to and touch the site if possible. Some facilities require the correct site to be marked with an indelible ink before the patient is brought to the OR. Before amputation of an extremity, expose the opposite one also for comparison. Check with the surgeon.
2. Don gloves.
3. Place towels above and below the area to be cleansed to mark the limits of the area and also to protect the

gloved hands from touching the blanket or gown. Also place absorbent towels along each side of the area to act as an absorber of runoff solution. These two towels are removed after the prep is completed.

4. Wet the sponge with antiseptic agent but squeeze out excess solution. Solution should not run off the skin area onto the operating bed to pool under the patient. A patient lying in solution may develop skin irritation even though the solution itself is nonirritating. Waterproof pads or additional absorbent towels may be placed under the patient during the prep and then removed. Flammable solutions, such as alcohol or tinctures and solvents, must evaporate before drapes are applied to prevent accumulation of fumes under them.

5. Scrub the skin, starting at the site of incision, with a circular motion in ever-widening circles to the periphery. Use enough pressure and friction to remove dirt and microorganisms from the skin and pores. Effective skin antisepsis is achieved through mechanical and chemical action. Figure 29-3 shows abdominal preparation.

Some surgeons prefer to have the antiseptic agent applied over cancerous areas by painting rather than scrubbing. During vigorous scrubbing, cancer cells may be freed, picked up by blood and lymph streams, and carried to other parts of the body. To paint, secure a folded sponge in a sponge forceps, dip in the solution, squeeze out excess solution, and apply to the skin

Figure 29-3 Abdominal preparation. Area includes breast line to upper third of thighs, from table line to table line, with patient in supine position. Shaded area shows anatomic area to be prepared. Arrows within area show direction of motion for skin preparation on operating bed.

in circular motions from the incision site to the periphery. The same method can be used to prep the skin over an occluded blood vessel to prevent dislodging a clot or piece of plaque, causing an embolus.

No-touch technique may be used (i.e., an applicator device or a sponge forceps rather than the hands is used to apply the solution and scrub the skin).

Scrub brushes with bristles should not be used. Bristles might fall out and remain on the skin to become foreign bodies in the surgical wound. Bristles can be abrasive to the skin. Sponges or commercially prepared foam applicators should be used.

6. Discard the sponge after reaching the periphery. Never bring the sponge back toward the center of the area. Prep from clean to dirty.
7. Repeat the scrub with a separate sponge for each round.

Apply the antiseptic agent and scrub for the time recommended by the manufacturer of the agent(s) used. The recommended minimum time may be 2 to 5 minutes, but consideration should be given to the extent of the area being prepped. The prepped area needs to be large enough to provide a wide margin around the full length of the anticipated incision and to accommodate potential drain sites and openings in the draping material.

Contaminated Areas Within the Surgical Field

Umbilicus The umbilicus is considered a contaminated area in relation to the surface surrounding it because it may harbor microorganisms in the detritus that often accumulates there. Solution may be squeezed into the umbilicus to soften detritus while the remainder of the abdomen is scrubbed, or the umbilicus may be cleansed first with separate sponges and applicators to avoid runoff of dirty solution over the cleansed skin area. Then the abdominal prep begins with new sponges at the line of incision, moving with circular motions to the periphery and including the umbilicus again each round as it is approached within the area. The umbilicus is thoroughly cleansed with cotton-tipped applicators as the final step of the abdominal prep.

Stoma The external stoma (orifice) of a colostomy, ileostomy, etc., may be sealed off from the surgical site with a self-adhering towel drape or transparent adherent dressing. If this is not possible, the same rule applies for the use of sponges as for the umbilicus; that area should be scrubbed last, or a separate sponge should be used each round for the contaminated area only. The opening of the stoma may be packed with a prep solution–soaked sponge while the surrounding area is scrubbed.

Other Contaminated Areas Draining sinuses, skin ulcers, the vagina, the anus, etc., are considered contaminated areas also. In all of these, the general rule of scrubbing the most contaminated area last with separate sponges applies.

Foreign Substances Adhesive, grease, tar, and similar foreign materials are removed from skin before the area is mechanically cleansed with an antiseptic agent. A nonirritating solvent should be used to cleanse the skin. The solvent should be nonflammable and nontoxic. The solution should not be allowed to collect underneath the patient.

Traumatic Wounds In the preparation of an area in which the skin is not intact because of a traumatic injury, wound irrigation may be part of the skin preparation procedure. The wound may be packed or covered with sterile gauze while the area around it is thoroughly scrubbed and shaved if necessary. The extent and type of injury will determine the appropriate procedure.

Solutions irritating to a denuded area must not be used. Small areas may be irrigated with warm sterile solution, usually normal saline, in a bulb syringe. When a bulb syringe is used, care must be taken not to force debris and microorganisms deeper into the wound. The wound is irrigated gently to dislodge debris and flush it out. Soft nylon brushes are sometimes used.

Copious amounts of warm sterile solutions may be needed to flush out a large wound. A container of warm sterile normal saline or Ringer's lactate solution attached to intravenous (IV) tubing can be hung on an IV pole near the area to be copiously irrigated. If the area is on an extremity, a sterile irrigating pan with a wire screen fitted over the top is placed under the extremity. During irrigation, solution runs from the wound into the pan. A piece of tubing connected to an outlet on the pan carries the irrigating solution into a kick bucket on the floor near the table.

It may be necessary to place dry towels or sheets under the patient if the area has not been protected during irrigation. A moisture-proof pad placed under the wound before irrigation will help channel solutions into a drainage pan. Protective gloves, eyewear, and a mask should be worn during the irrigation procedure.

Debridement of the wound (excision of all devitalized tissue) usually follows irrigation. The surgeon may request to have sterile tissue forceps and scissors on the prep table for removal of nonviable tissue.

Areas Prepared for Grafts

Separate setups are necessary for skin preparation of recipient and donor sites before skin, bone, or vascular grafting procedures. The donor site is usually scrubbed first.

The donor site for a skin graft should be scrubbed with a colorless antiseptic agent so that the surgeon can properly evaluate the vascularity of the graft postoperatively. The recipient site for skin grafts is usually more or less contaminated (e.g., following a burn or other traumatic injury). Items used in preparation of the recipient site must not be permitted to contaminate the donor site. Also, microorganisms on the skin of the donor site must not be transferred to a denuded recipient site.

Skin Preparation
for Specific Anatomic Areas
Head and Neck
Eye

1. The eyebrows are never shaved or removed unless the surgeon deems this essential. Eyebrows do not grow back completely or evenly.
2. The eyelashes may be trimmed, if ordered by the surgeon, with fine scissors coated with sterile water-soluble lubricant to catch the lashes.
3. The eyelids and periorbital areas are cleansed with a nonirritating antiseptic agent, commonly triclosan detergent, and then rinsed with warm sterile water. The prep starts centrally and extends to the periphery (i.e., from the center of the lid to the brow and cheek).
4. The conjunctival sac is flushed with a nontoxic agent, such as sterile normal saline, with a bulb syringe. The patient's head is turned slightly to the affected side. The solution is contained with sponges or an absorbent towel. Care must be taken to prevent prep solution from entering the patient's eyes or ears.

Chlorhexidine is contraindicated for facial preps. Iodophors are used with caution around the eyes. Chlorhexidine gluconate and iodophors can cause corneal damage if accidentally introduced into the eyes or can cause sensorineural deafness if the agent enters the inner ear (e.g., through a perforated tympanic membrane).

Ears, Face, or Nose

1. Usually it is not possible to define the area with towels.
2. Protect the eyes with a piece of sterile plastic sheeting. If the patient is awake, ask that the eyes be kept closed during the prep.
3. As much of the surrounding area is included as is feasible and consistent with aseptic technique. Skin surfaces should be cleansed at least to the hair line.
4. Cotton applicators are used for cleansing the nostrils and external ear canals.

Neck

1. One sterile towel is folded under the edge of the blanket and gown, which are turned down almost to the nipple line.
2. The area includes the neck laterally to the table line and up to the mandible, tops of the shoulders, and chest almost to the nipple line.
3. For combined head and neck surgical procedures, include the face to the eyes; the shaved areas of the head, ears, and posterior neck; and the area over the shoulders.

Chest and Trunk
Lateral Thoracoabdominal Area

1. The gown is removed. The blanket is turned down well below the lower limit of the area to be prepared. A towel is folded under the edge of the blanket.

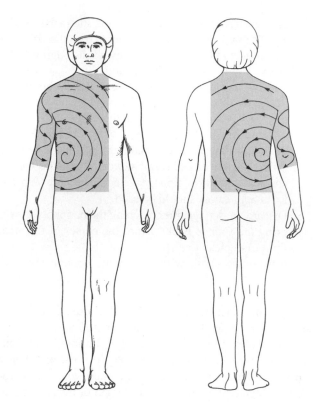

Figure 29-4 Lateral thoracoabdominal preparation. Area includes axilla, chest, and abdomen from neck to crest of ilium. Area extends beyond midline, anteriorly and posteriorly. Patient is in lateral position on operating bed.

2. The arm is held up during the prep.
3. Beginning at the site of incision, the area may include the axilla, chest, and abdomen from the neck to the crest of the ilium. For a surgical procedure in the region of the kidney, it extends up to the axilla and down to the pubis. The area also extends beyond midlines, anteriorly and posteriorly, and may include the arm to the elbow (Figure 29-4).

Chest and Breast

1. The anesthesia provider turns the patient's face toward the unaffected side.
2. One towel is folded under the blanket edge, just above the pubis. Another is placed on the operating bed under the shoulder and side.
3. The arm on the affected side is held up by grasping the hand and raising the shoulder and axilla slightly from the operating bed.
4. The area includes the shoulder, upper arm down to the elbow, axilla, and chest wall to the table line and beyond the sternum to the opposite shoulder (Figure 29-5).

Shoulder

1. The anesthesia provider turns the patient's face toward the opposite side.
2. A towel is placed under the shoulder and axilla.
3. The arm is held up by grasping the hand and elevating the shoulder slightly from the operating bed.

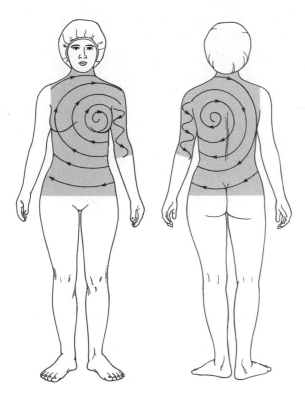

Figure 29-5 Chest and breast preparation. Area includes shoulder, upper arm down to elbow, axilla, and chest wall to table line and beyond sternum to opposite shoulder. If patient is in lateral position, back is prepped also.

4. The area includes the circumference of the upper arm to below the elbow, from the base of the neck over the shoulder, scapula, and chest to the midline.

Rectoperineal Area
1. One towel is folded under the edge of the blanket above the pubis. Another towel is placed under the buttocks.
2. The area includes the pubis, external genitalia, perineum and anus, and inner aspects of the thighs (Figure 29-6).
3. Begin the scrub over the pubic area, scrubbing downward over the genitalia and perineum. Discard the sponge after going over the anus.
4. The inner aspects of the upper third of both thighs are scrubbed with separate sponges.
5. The rectoperineal area is prepped first, with the patient in lithotomy position, followed by an abdominal prep, with the patient in supine position, for a combined abdominoperineal procedure. Two separate pairs of gloves and prep trays are used.

Vagina
1. Sponge forceps should be included on the preparation table for a vaginal prep because a portion of the prep is done internally. A disposable vaginal prep tray, with sponge sticks included, is available.
2. With the patient in lithotomy position, a moisture-proof pad is placed under the buttocks and extends to the kick bucket that receives solutions and discarded sponges.

Figure 29-6 Rectoperineal and vaginal preparation. Area includes pubis, vulva, labia, perineum, anus, and adjacent area, including inner aspects of upper third of thighs.

3. A towel is folded under the edge of the blanket above the pubis.
4. The area includes the pubis, vulva, labia, perineum, anus, and adjacent area, including inner aspects of the upper third of the thighs (see Figure 29-6). The vagina is prepped last.
5. Begin over the pubic area, scrubbing downward over the vulva and perineum. Discard each sponge after going over the anus.
6. The inner aspects of the thighs are scrubbed with separate sponges from the labia majora outward.
7. The vagina and cervix are cleansed with sponges on sponge forceps or disposable sponge sticks after external surrounding areas are scrubbed. The cleansing agent should be applied generously in the vagina because vaginal mucosa has many folds and crevices that are not easily cleansed.
8. After thoroughly cleansing the vagina, wipe it out with a dry sponge to prevent the possibility of the fluid entering the peritoneal cavity during the surgical procedure on pelvic organs.
9. Catheterize, if indicated.

Extremities
A moisture-proof pad should be placed on the operating bed under an extremity to retain drops of solution. This is removed after the prep so that the bed will be dry under the surgical site. The extremity remains supported and elevated until sterile drapes are applied under and around the prepped area.

A full extremity prep may be done in two stages to provide adequate support to joints and to ensure that all areas are scrubbed. It may include the foot for hip, thigh, knee, and lower leg procedures.

Caution must be taken to prevent solution from pooling under a tourniquet. If a pneumatic tourniquet is used, it is positioned before the prep. A towel tucked under the tourniquet cuff absorbs excess solution. This is removed before the tourniquet is inflated.

Upper Arm
1. A towel is placed under the shoulder and axilla.
2. The arm is held up by grasping the hand and elevating the shoulder slightly from the operating bed.

Figure 29-7 Hip preparation. Area includes abdomen on affected side, thigh to knee, buttock to table line, groin, and pubis.

Figure 29-8 Knee and lower leg preparation. Area includes entire circumference of affected leg and extends from foot to upper part of thigh.

3. The area includes the entire circumference of the arm to the wrist, the axilla, and over the shoulder and scapula.

Elbow and Forearm
1. A towel is placed under the shoulder and axilla.
2. The arm is held up by grasping the hand.
3. The area includes the entire arm from the shoulder and axilla to and including the hand.

Hand
1. Towels are omitted. The anatomy of the hand furnishes sufficient landmarks to define the area, and towels are apt to slip over the scrubbed area.
2. The arm must be held up by supporting it above the elbow so that the entire circumference can be scrubbed.
3. The area includes the hand and arm to 3 inches (7.5 cm) above the elbow.

Hip
1. One towel is placed under the thigh on the operating bed. Another towel is placed on the abdomen and folded under the edge of the gown, just above the umbilicus.
2. The leg on the affected side is held up by supporting it just below the knee.
3. The area includes the abdomen on the affected side, the thigh to the knee, the buttocks to the table line, the groin, and the pubis (Figure 29-7).

Thigh
1. One towel is placed under the thigh on the operating bed. Another towel is placed on the abdomen and folded under the edge of the gown, just below the umbilicus.
2. The leg is held up by supporting the foot and ankle.
3. The area includes the entire circumference of the thigh and leg to the ankle, over the hip and buttocks to the table line, the groin, and the pubis.

Knee and Lower Leg
1. A towel is placed over the groin.
2. The leg is held up by supporting it at the foot.
3. The area includes the entire circumference of the leg and extends from the foot to the upper part of the thigh (Figure 29-8).

Ankle and Foot
1. Towels are omitted.
2. The foot is held up by supporting the leg at the knee. A leg-holder device is useful.
3. The area includes the foot and entire circumference of the lower leg to the knee.

Skin Marking

Some surgeons use a staining solution or dye to mark the incision lines on the skin. This may be done before the patient is prepped. If so, the markings must withstand scrubbing without washing off. If the skin is marked after the prep, a sterile dye solution and applicator or a sterile marking pen is used. Methylene blue, brilliant green, or alcohol-based gentian violet are used for this purpose.

Documentation

Details of the preoperative skin condition and preparation should be documented in the patient's intraoperative record. These should include, but are not limited to, the following:

- The condition of the skin around the surgical site and placement sites of any electrodes
- Hair removal, if done, including the method and location, and areas for attachment of monitors or electrodes
- Antiseptic solutions, fat solvents, irrigating solutions, and any other agents used
- The skin area prepped and skin reaction, if any
- The name of the person who did the prep

DRAPING

Draping is the procedure of covering the patient and surrounding areas with a sterile barrier to create and maintain an adequate sterile field. An effective barrier eliminates or minimizes passage of microorganisms between nonsterile and sterile areas. Criteria to be met in establishing an effective barrier are that the material must be:

- Blood- and fluid-resistant to keep drapes dry and prevent migration of microorganisms. Material should be impermeable to moist microbial penetration (i.e., resistant to strike-through).
- Resistant to tearing, puncture, or abrasion that causes fiber breakdown and thus permits microbial penetration.
- Lint free to reduce airborne contaminants and shedding into the surgical site. Cellulose and cotton fibers can cause granulomatous peritonitis or embolize arteries.
- Antistatic to eliminate risk of a spark from static electricity. Material must meet standards of the National Fire Protection Association (NFPA).
- Sufficiently porous to eliminate heat buildup so as to maintain an isothermic environment appropriate for the patient's body temperature.
- Drapable to fit around contours of the patient, furniture, and equipment.
- Dull, nonglaring to minimize color distortion from reflected light.
- Free of toxic ingredients, such as laundry residues, and nonfast dyes.
- Flame resistant to self-extinguish rapidly on removal of an ignition source. This is a concern with use of lasers, electrosurgical units, and other high-energy devices, which provide an ignition source at the sterile field. Drapes become fuel for a fire. Some materials are more flammable than others; some are fire retardant.

Draping Materials
Self-Adhering Plastic Sheeting

Sterile, waterproof, antistatic, and transparent or translucent plastic sheeting may be applied to dry skin.

Incise Drape The entire clear plastic drape has an adhesive backing that is applied to skin. This may be applied separately, or the sheeting may be incorporated into the drape sheet. The skin incision is made through the plastic.

Antimicrobial incise drapes have an antimicrobial agent impregnated in the adhesive or the polymeric film. A film coated with an iodophor-containing adhesive, for example, slowly releases active iodine during the surgical procedure to effectively inhibit proliferation of organisms from the patient's skin. The antimicrobial may be triclosan or another agent that does not contain iodine. The skin may be prepped with alcohol and allowed to dry before the drape is applied. Time is a factor in microbial accumulation from resident bacteria. Antimicrobial incise drapes are used, particularly for procedures lasting more than 3 hours, to sustain suppression.

Towel Drape The plastic sheeting has a band of adhesive along one edge. Used as a draping towel, it will remain fixed on skin without towel clips. This is advantageous when clips might obscure the view of a part exposed to x-rays during the surgical procedure. It also is used to wall off a contaminated area, such as a stoma, from the clean skin area to prevent spilling contents and causing infection or chemical irritation.

Aperture Drape Adhesive surrounds a fenestration (opening) in the plastic sheeting. This secures the drape to the skin around the surgical site, such as an eye or ear. Caution is used in applying this type of drape around the face of a patient who is awake. The patient must have breathing space. Some patients experience claustrophobia. Fabric towels may not feel as confining.

Advantages of a self-adhering plastic drape include the following:

1. Resident microbial flora from skin pores, sebaceous glands, and hair follicles cannot migrate laterally to the incision.
2. Microorganisms do not penetrate through the impermeable material.
3. Landmarks and skin tones are visible through the transparent plastic.
4. Inert adhesive holds drapes securely, eliminating the need for towel clips and possible puncture of the patient's skin.
5. Plastic sheeting conforms to body contours and has elasticity to stretch without breaking its adhesion to skin.

Some self-adhering drapes have sufficient moisture-vapor permeability to reduce excessive moisture buildup that could macerate the skin and/or loosen adhesive. A nonporous material should not cover more than 10% of the body surface, since it may interfere with the patient's thermal regulatory mechanism of perspiration evaporation. The heat-retaining property of plastic causes the patient to perspire excessively, but its nonporous nature prevents evaporation.

This material is used in the following manner:

1. The usual skin preparation is done.
2. The scrubbed area must be dry. It may dry by evaporation, or excess solution may be blotted or wiped off with a sterile sponge or towel. Alcohol may be applied after an iodophor scrub to hasten drying by evaporation.
3. Transparent plastic material is applied firmly to the skin with the initial contact along the proposed line of incision. The drape is smoothed away from the incision area.
4. Regular fabric drapes are applied over the plastic sheeting unless plastic is incorporated into the fenestrated area of the drape.

Nonwoven Fabric Disposable Drapes

Most nonwoven disposable materials are compressed layers of synthetic fibers (i.e., rayon, nylon, or polyester) combined with cellulose (wood pulp) and bonded together chemically or mechanically without knitting, tufting, or weaving. This material may be either nonabsorbent or absorbent. Polypropylene and foil also are used. Those fabrics that comply with criteria for establishing an effective barrier have the following advantages as disposable drapes:

1. They are moisture repellent; they retard blood and aqueous fluid moisture strike-through to prevent contamination. Not all nonwoven fabrics have this characteristic; only nonabsorbent materials or those laminated with plastic are impermeable to moisture.
2. They are lightweight, yet strong enough to resist tears.
3. They are lint free unless cellulose fibers are torn or cut.
4. Contaminants are disposed of along with drapes.
5. They are antistatic and flame retardant for OR use.
6. They are prepackaged and sterilized by the manufacturer, which eliminates washing, mending, folding, and sterilizing processes.

Some drapes have a reinforced area of multiple layers surrounding the fenestration. The outer layer absorbs fluids, but the underneath layer is impermeable to strike-through. An antimicrobial may be incorporated into this reinforced area. Other drapes have an impermeable layer around the fenestration. Drapes that are completely laminated with a plastic layer may be used for an extremity or for instrument table covers. They are not used over the entire body of the patient because of their heat retention property.

Many nonwoven drapes have pouches or troughs incorporated close to the fenestration or along the sides of the drape to collect fluids, such as amniotic fluid. The pouch may have drainage ports, or fluid may be suctioned out. Some drapes also have pockets, skid-resistant instrument pads,

and/or devices for holding cords incorporated in them (see Figure 29-9).

Laser-Resistant Drapes Nonwoven drapes that contain cellulose ignite and burn easily. Polypropylene drapes will not ignite, but they can melt. An aluminum-coated drape may be safest for use with lasers, especially around the oxygen-enriched environment of the head and neck area.

Thermal Drape An aluminum-coated plastic body cover reflects radiant body heat back to the patient to reduce intraoperative heat loss. A sterile, nonconductive, radiolucent thermal drape may be used as the final drape. The patient may be wrapped in nonsterile reflective covers (Thermadrape) in the preoperative holding area. These may remain in place through the surgical procedure under standard sterile drapes and during postoperative recovery in the postanesthesia care unit (PACU). A reflective blanket or thermal drape is recommended when more than 60% of the body surface can be covered and when the surgical procedure will last more than 2 hours.

Nonwoven, disposable drapes are supplied prepackaged and presterilized by the manufacturer. A sterile package may contain a single drape, or it may have all of the drapes needed for a procedure, including towels, a Mayo stand and instrument table covers, and gowns. Unused disposable drapes and gowns should not be resterilized unless the manufacturer provides written instructions for reprocessing.

Woven Textile Fabrics

The thread count and finish of woven natural fibers determine the integrity and porosity of reusable fabrics. Tightly woven textile fabrics may inhibit migration of microorganisms. Cotton fibers swell when they become wet. This swelling action closes pores or interstices so that liquid cannot diffuse through tightly woven fibers. The fabric can be treated to further repel fluids (i.e., be impermeable to moisture strike-through). Reusable drapes may be made of 270- or 280-thread-count pima cotton with a Quarpel finish. This fluorochemical finish, combined with phenazopyridine or a melanin hydrophobe, produces a durable water-resistant fabric. However, this fabric has essentially the same heat-retaining qualities as plastic lamination, so it cannot be used for complete patient draping. This treated material can be used as reinforcement around fenestrations in otherwise untreated drapes.

Tightly woven 100% polyester reusable fabrics are hydrophobic (repel water droplets) but allow vapor permeation. Other reusable fabrics with different construction but similar barrier properties may be used.

Points about reusable woven textile drapes to consider:

1. Material must be steam penetrable and must withstand multiple sterilization cycles.
2. When packaged for sterilization, drapes must be properly folded and arranged in sequence of use. Drapes may be fanfolded or rolled.

3. Material must be free from holes and tears. The person who folds the drape is responsible for inspecting it for holes. Those detected may be covered with heat-seal patches. Tears or punctures (e.g., from towel clips or sharp instruments) compromise barrier qualities of drapes.
4. Drapes should be sufficiently impermeable to prevent moisture from soaking through them. Moisture has a wicking action that can cause migration of microorganisms.
5. Reusable fabrics must maintain barrier qualities through multiple launderings. Densely woven treated cotton will become moisture permeable after about 75 washings; untreated cotton will become moisture permeable after as few as 30 washings. Repeated drying, ironing, and steam sterilizing also alters fabric structure. The number of uses, washings, and sterilizing cycles should be recorded, and drapes that are no longer effective as barriers should be taken out of use.

Style/Type of Drapes

Towels

Disposable or reusable towels may be used to outline the surgical site. The folded edge of each towel is placed toward the line of incision. When reusable woven fabric is packaged, four towels intended for this purpose can be placed together with the folded edges graduated. Nonabsorbent disposable towels also are used for this technique. Towels usually are secured with nonperforating towel clips but may be sutured or stapled to skin. Some disposable types have adhesive strips to hold them in place.

Fenestrated Sheets

The drape sheet has an opening (fenestration) that is placed to expose the anatomic area where the incision will be made. Many styles of disposable nonwoven or reusable woven fabrics are available for specific uses. The size, direction, and shape of the fenestration vary to give adequate exposure of the surgical site. The sheet is long enough to cover the anesthesia screen at the head and extend down over the foot of the operating bed. Fenestrated sheets are usually marked to indicate the direction in which they should be unfolded. This may be an arrow or label designating the top or head, bottom or foot. It is wide enough to cover one or two armboards.

Reinforcement around the fenestration (Figure 29-9) for both nonwoven and woven fabrics provides an extra thickness to minimize the passage of microorganisms by capillary action to the sterile field. The reinforced area is usually 24 inches (60 cm) wide.

The drapes described are basic styles of fenestrated sheets.

Laparotomy Sheet The laparotomy sheet is often referred to as a lap sheet; the longitudinal fenestration is placed over the surgical site on the abdomen, back, or a comparable area (see Figure 29-9). The opening, about 40 inches (102 cm) from the top in the center of the sheet, is 9 × 4

Figure 29-9 Fenestrated laparotomy drape sheet with reinforcement around fenestration.

inches (23 × 10 cm), which is large enough to give adequate exposure in the usual laparotomy. The sheet is at least 108 × 72 inches (274 × 183 cm). It is unfolded toward the feet first (see Figure 29-11).

Thyroid Sheet The thyroid sheet is the same size as a laparotomy sheet. The fenestration is transverse and closer to the top of the sheet.

Breast Sheet The breast sheet is the same as a laparotomy sheet except that the fenestration is 11 × 11 inches (28 × 28 cm), which provides for a larger exposure. In addition to its use for breast procedures, it is used for surgical procedures within the chest cavity.

Kidney Sheet The kidney sheet is the same size as a laparotomy sheet. The fenestration is transverse to accommodate a transverse kidney incision.

Hip Sheet The hip sheet is the same as a laparotomy sheet except that it is somewhat longer to completely cover the orthopaedic fracture table.

Perineal Sheet The perineal sheet is of adequate size to create a sterile field with the patient in the lithotomy position. It has large leggings incorporated into it to cover the legs in stirrups. It has an opening 6½ to 7 inches (17 cm) in diameter with a 10-inch (25-cm) reinforcement around it.

Combined Sheet A combined sheet is a combination laparotomy and perineal sheet. It is used for combined abdominoperineal resection of the rectum when the entire procedure is done with the patient in the lithotomy position. Gynecologic laparoscopy is commonly performed using a combined sheet. It has two fenestrations.

Separate Sheets

Although fenestrated sheets are used for most surgical procedures, they are not always practical. The openings may be much too large for small incisions, such as taking specimens for biopsies or procedures on the hands or feet. Smaller, separate sheets may be used for these purposes, leaving exposed only the small surgical area, or for providing additional drapes on the surgical field. Many of these are disposable.

Split Sheet The split sheet is the same size as a laparotomy sheet. Rather than being fenestrated, one end is cut longitudinally up the middle at least one third the length of the sheet to form two free ends (tails). The upper end of this split may be in the shape of a U. Adhesive strips on each tail approximately 8 inches (20 cm) from the end of the split adhere together to snug the drape around an extremity or head. Shorter styles have adhesive strips the full length of the inner aspect of the tails for circumferential wrapping.

Minor Sheet The minor sheet is 36 × 45 inches (91 × 114 cm). It has many uses. Wrapped around an extremity, it permits the extremity to remain on the sterile field for manipulation during the surgical procedure. It is used under an arm to cover an armboard for shoulder, axillary, arm, or hand procedures.

Medium Sheet The medium sheet is about 36 × 72 inches (91 × 183 cm). It is used to drape under legs, as an added protection above or below the surgical area, or for draping areas in which a fenestrated sheet cannot be used.

Single Sheet The single sheet is 108 × 72 inches (274 × 183 cm). Folded lengthwise, it is placed above the sterile field to shield off the anesthesia provider and anesthesia machine or other equipment near the patient's head or operating bed. A single sheet also is used to cover the patient and operating bed below the surgical area around the face.

Leggings Leg drapes are supplied in pairs to cover the legs of a patient in the lithotomy position. A rectangle, approximately 36 × 72 inches (91 × 183 cm), is closed on two sides to form a tentlike pocket. One open edge is folded into a cuff to protect gloves from contamination during application.

Stockinette Stockinette is used to cover an extremity. This seamless tubing of stretchable woven material contours snugly to the skin. The material is very porous and absorbent, so it is not a microbial barrier. Therefore it may be covered with a layer of plastic. A two-ply tubular disposable drape is available that has an inner layer of stockinette and an outer layer of vinyl. An opening is cut through the material over the line of incision. Edges may be secured with a plastic incise drape before the incision is made, or it may be clipped to the wound edges after the incision. Rolled elastic bandage is sometimes used for this purpose. Care is taken to use nonlatex materials for patients sensitive to latex.

Draping Considerations

Because draping is a very important step in the preparation of the patient for a surgical procedure, it must be done correctly. The entire team should be familiar with the draping procedure. The scrub person must know it perfectly and be ready to assist with it. The scrub person should check beforehand to see that necessary articles are arranged in proper sequence on the instrument table.

The person responsible for draping the patient may vary, as do materials and styles of drapes used to create a sterile field. The surgeon or assistant usually places the self-adhering drape and/or towels and towel clips to outline the surgical site. The scrub person assists with placing the remainder of the drapes.

During any draping procedure the circulator should stand by to direct the scrub person as necessary and to watch carefully for breaks in technique. A contaminated drape or exposure of a nonsterile area is a potential source of infection for the patient.

Basic principles regarding draping are as follows:

1. Place drapes on a dry area. The area around or under the patient may become damp from solutions used for skin preparation. The circulator removes damp items or covers the area to provide a dry field on which to lay sterile drapes.
2. Allow sufficient time to permit careful application.
3. Allow sufficient space to observe sterile technique.
4. Handle drapes as little as possible.
5. Never reach across the operating bed to drape the opposite side; go around it.
6. Take towels and towel clips, if used, to the side of the operating bed from which the surgeon is going to apply them before handing them to him or her.
7. Carry folded drapes to the operating bed. Watch the front of the sterile gown; it may bulge and touch the nonsterile operating bed or blanket on the patient. Stand well back from the nonsterile operating bed.
8. Hold drapes high enough to avoid touching nonsterile areas, but avoid touching the overhead operating light.
9. Hold a drape high until it is directly over the proper area and then lay it down where it is to remain. Once a sheet is placed, do not adjust it. Be careful not to slide the sheet out of place when opening the folds. If a drape is incorrectly placed, discard it. The circulator peels it from the operating bed without contaminating other drapes or the prepped area.
10. Protect gloved hands by cuffing the end of the sheet over them. Do not let gloved hands touch the skin of the patient.
11. In unfolding a sheet from the prepped area toward the foot or head of the operating bed, protect the gloved hand by enclosing it in a turned-back cuff of sheet provided for this purpose. Keep hands at table level.

12. If a drape becomes contaminated, do not handle it further. Discard it without contaminating gloves or other items.
13. If the end of a sheet falls below waist level, do not handle it further. Drop it and use another.
14. If in doubt as to its sterility, consider a drape contaminated.
15. A towel clip that has been fastened through a drape has its points contaminated. Remove it only if absolutely necessary and then discard it from the sterile setup without touching the points. Cover the area from which it was removed with another piece of sterile draping material.
16. If a hole is found in a drape after it is laid down, the hole must be covered with another piece of draping material or the entire drape discarded.
17. A hair found on a drape must be removed, and the area covered immediately. Although hair can be sterilized, the source of a hair is usually unknown when it is found on a sterile drape. It would cause a foreign body tissue reaction in a patient if it got into the wound. Remove the hair with a hemostat and hand the instrument off the sterile field; cover the area with a towel or another piece of draping material.

Procedures for Draping the Patient

Draping procedures establish the sterile field. Standardized methods of application should be practiced using adequate draping materials. The most common procedures are discussed here merely to elaborate the principles. The following details procedures using only absorbent woven draping materials because it is more complex to establish a microbial barrier with them. The draping procedure is simplified when single-thickness, impermeable materials are used. A procedure book should be consulted for specific draping procedures.

Laparotomy

The term *laparotomy* refers to an incision through the abdominal wall into the abdominal cavity. All flat, smooth areas are draped in the same manner as the abdomen. These areas include the neck, chest, flank, and back. The draping procedure is as follows:

1. Hand up four towels and towel clips. With practice these can be held in the hands at the same time and separated one by one as the surgeon takes them. Go to the side of the operating bed on which the surgeon is draping to avoid reaching over the nonsterile table. The surgeon places these towels within the prepped area, leaving only the surgical area exposed.
2. Hand one end of a fanfolded medium sheet across the operating bed to the assistant, supporting the folds, keeping the sheet high, and holding it taut until it is

opened; then lay it down. Place this medium sheet below the surgical site with the edge of it at the skin edge, covering the draping towel. This sheet provides an extra thickness of material under the area from the Mayo stand to the incision, where instruments and sponges are placed, and closes some of the opening in the laparotomy sheet if necessary. This sheet may be eliminated if a self-adhering incise drape or impermeable drapes are used.
3. Place a laparotomy sheet with the opening directly over the prepped area outlined by the towels in the direction indicated for the foot or head of the operating bed. Drop the folds over the sides of the table. However, if an armboard is in place, hold the folds at table level until the sheet is opened all the way. Open it downward over the patient's feet and upward over the anesthesia screen (Figures 29-10 and 29-11).

    Sheets with appropriate fenestrations are used to expose the surgical site.
    a. For the neck, use a thyroid sheet.
    b. For the chest, with the patient in either the supine or lateral position, use a breast sheet.
    c. For the flank, with the patient in kidney position for transverse incision, use a kidney sheet.
    d. For the back, use a laparotomy sheet, the same as for the abdomen.
4. Place a large, single sheet crosswise on the operating bed above the fenestrated site. This sheet provides an extra thickness above the area and closes some of the opening in the laparotomy sheet if necessary. It also covers the armboard if one is in use. A single sheet may be needed for this latter purpose even if an impermeable laparotomy sheet is used.

Figure 29-10 Draping with sterile laparotomy sheet. Scrub person carries folded sheet to table. Standing far back from operating bed, with one hand, scrub person lays sheet on patient so that opening in sheet is directly over prepped skin area.

Figure 29-11 Unfolding upper end of laparotomy sheet over anesthesia screen. Note that hands approaching unsterile area are protected in cuff of drape and that sheet is stabilized with other hands.

Head

An overhead instrument table may be positioned over the patient for neurologic procedures. The table drape is extended down over the patient's shoulders to create a continuous sterile field between the instrument table and the surgical site. The draping procedure is as follows:

1. The surgeon places four towels around the head and secures them with towel clips or affixes them in place with sutures or skin staples. Towel clips and staples are not used if x-ray films will be taken during the surgical procedure.
2. Hand one end of a fanfolded medium sheet to the assistant. Holding it taut, unfold and secure it over the head end of the operating bed below the surgical site at the skin edge of the draping towel.
3. Place a fenestrated sheet with the opening over the exposed skin area of the head. Unfold the sheet across the front edge of the overhead table and secure it before allowing the remainder of the drape to drop over the head of the operating bed toward the floor. Some disposable fenestrated head sheets have transparent plastic adhesive sheeting to cover the incisional site. The plastic insert may be impregnated with iodophor for additional wound protection during the procedure.

Face

Even if the surgical site is unilateral, the surgeon may want the entire face exposed for comparison of skin lines. The draping procedure is as follows:

1. The surgeon places a drape under the head while the circulator or assistant elevates the head. This drape consists of an open towel placed on a medium sheet. The center of the towel edge is 2 inches (5 cm) in from the center of the sheet edge. The towel is drawn up on each side of the face, over the forehead or at the hairline, and fastened with a small, nonperforating towel clip. This leaves the desired amount of the face exposed.
2. Hand up three additional towels and four towel clips. These towels frame the surgical site.
3. Place a medium sheet just below the site. This sheet must overlap the one under the head.
4. A fenestrated drape may be placed to complete draping.
5. Cover the remainder of the foot of the operating bed, as necessary, with a single sheet.

If the patient is receiving inhalation anesthesia, use a minor sheet instead of a towel on a medium sheet for the first drape under the head. A minor sheet is large enough to draw up on each side of the face and to enclose the endotracheal tube and oropharyngeal monitoring probes from the anesthesia machine for a considerable distance, thus keeping them from contaminating the sterile field.

If the surgical procedure on the face is unilateral, the anesthesia provider may sit along the unaffected side, near the patient's head, with the anesthesia screen placed on the same side of the operating bed.

Skin staples or sutures may be used to affix towels around the contours of the face and neck. Each staple or stitch overlaps the skin and edge of the drape.

Eye

Following skin preparation, the unaffected eye is protected by covering it with a sterile eye pad before draping the patient. The draping procedure is as follows:

1. The surgeon places two towels and a medium sheet under the head while the circulator holds the head up,

as described for a face drape. One towel is drawn up around the head, exposing only the eyebrow and affected eye, and fastened with a clip without pressure on the eyes.

2. Hand up four towels and towel clips to isolate the affected eye. Some surgeons prefer a self-adhering aperture drape.
3. Cover the patient and remainder of the operating bed below the surgical area with a single sheet.

If local anesthetic will be administered, the drapes are raised off of the patient's nose and mouth to permit free breathing. A Mayo stand or anesthesia screen positioned over the lower face before the draping is one method used to elevate the drapes. Oxygen, 6 to 8 L/min, can be supplied under the drapes by tube or nasal cannula.

For a microsurgical procedure, a sterile, padded U-shaped steel wrist rest for the surgeon and assistant is fastened to the head of the operating bed after towels are put around the patient's head, before the rest of the draping is completed.

If irrigation will be used, a plastic fenestrated drape is placed over the four towels to keep them dry if an aperture drape is not preferred.

Ear

The basic draping procedure is the same as for draping a face or eye, except that only the affected ear is exposed. The head will be turned toward the unaffected side. Oxygen can be supplied under the drapes, as previously described. The anesthesia provider is usually positioned at the side of the operating bed near the patient's face.

Chest and Breast

While the arm is still being held up by the assistant following skin preparation:

1. Place a minor sheet on an armboard, under the patient's arm, extending the sheet under the side of the chest and shoulder. The prepped arm is lowered to the sterile draped armboard. The distal portion of the arm may be encased in sterile stockinette so that the arm can be manipulated during the surgical procedure.
2. The patient's body is draped with a sterile medium sheet.
3. Hand up towels and towel clips; five or six are required.
4. Apply a breast sheet so that the axilla is exposed for anticipated axillary dissection.

Shoulder

While the arm is still being held up by the assistant following skin preparation:

1. Place medium sheets over the chest and under the arm.
2. Place a minor sheet under the shoulder and side of the chest.
3. The surgeon outlines the surgical site with towels and secures them with clips.

4. Place a minor sheet over the patient's chest, covering the neck. Keep this sheet even with the edge of the towel that borders the surgical site laterally.
5. Wrap the arm in a minor sheet or encase it in sterile stockinette and secure it with a sterile gauze or elastic bandage. At this point, a sterile team member relieves the unsterile person who has been holding the arm.
6. Place a medium sheet above the area and secure these sheets together with towel clips.
7. A laparotomy or breast sheet may be used. Pull the arm through the opening. Or a single sheet may be placed above the area, and the foot of the operating bed covered with a medium sheet.

Elbow

While the arm is still being held up by the assistant following skin preparation:

1. Place a medium sheet across the chest and under the arm, up to the axilla.
2. The surgeon defines the surgical area on the upper arm by placing a towel around the arm and securing it with a clip.
3. Wrap the hand and lower the arm in a minor sheet or a double thickness of towel and secure it with a sterile bandage. At this point, a sterile team member relieves the unsterile person who has been holding the arm.
4. Draw stockinette over the exposed surgical site.
5. Place a medium sheet across the chest, on top of the arm, even with the towel on the upper arm and covering it. Secure this sheet around the arm with a towel clip.
6. Lay a laparotomy sheet over the hand and pull the arm through it, opening the sheet across the patient. Cover the foot of the operating bed with a medium sheet.

Hand

While the arm and hand are still being held up following skin preparation:

1. Place an impervious minor sheet, folded in half, on the armboard or extremity table.
2. The surgeon places a towel around the lower arm, limiting the exposed area to the affected hand, and secures it with a towel clip.
3. Pull stockinette over the hand. At this stage in draping, the unsterile person is relieved of holding the arm. The arm is laid on the armboard.
4. Place a minor sheet across the armboard just above the surgical site.
5. Place a laparotomy sheet on the hand with the foot end toward the patient. Do not drop folds below the level of the armboard. Open the laparotomy sheet across the patient's body.
6. Place a medium sheet below the laparotomy sheet to finish covering the patient.
7. Place a single sheet over the anesthesia screen.

Perineum

With the patient in the lithotomy position for a genital, vaginal, or rectal procedure:

1. Place a medium sheet under the buttocks. The circulator can grasp the underside and assist in placement. With the patient's legs elevated in stirrups, this drape hangs below the level of the operating bed and covers the lowered section of the operating bed.
2. Slide legging over each leg, protecting the gloved hands in the folded cuffs.
3. Hand up three or four towels and four towel clips for the surgeon to square off the perineum. The anus is covered if it is not part of the surgical site. An adhesive towel drape may be used for this purpose.
4. Place a medium sheet across the abdomen, from the level of the pubis, extending over the anesthesia screen.
5. A fenestrated perineal sheet may be used rather than a pair of leggings. After towels are placed, hand one end of the sheet to the assistant, opening out folds, and draw the leggings over the feet and legs simultaneously. The hands are kept on the outside of the sheet to avoid contaminating the gloves and gown.

Hip

If the leg will be manipulated during the surgical procedure, while the leg is still being held up following skin preparation:

1. Place a medium sheet on the operating bed under the leg, up to the buttock.
2. Place another medium sheet on the operating bed, overlapping the first one, to cover the unaffected leg.
3. The surgeon wraps a towel around the thigh, just below the surgical site, and clips or sews it in place if x-ray films will be taken.
4. Hand up additional towels to surround the surgical area, with towel clips to secure them.
5. The surgeon wraps the foot and leg, including a towel around the thigh, in a minor sheet and bandages it on. Some surgeons prefer to use stockinette. The leg, held up to this point, is laid on the operating bed.
6. Place a minor sheet lengthwise of the operating bed on each side of the exposed area, even with the skin. The sheets under the leg and above the site do not overlap. Some surgeons prefer to draw the leg through the opening of a hip sheet or place a split sheet under the leg with the tails crossed over it toward the patient's head.
7. Place a medium sheet above the exposed area. Secure these last three sheets with towel clips.
8. Place a single sheet above the surgical area and over the anesthesia screen.

If manipulation of the leg is not necessary during the surgical procedure, drape the same as for a laparotomy, using a hip sheet instead of a laparotomy sheet.

Knee

While the leg is still being held up following skin preparation:

1. Place a medium sheet lengthwise on the operating bed, under the leg, up to the buttock.
2. Place another medium sheet on the operating bed, overlapping the first sheet, to cover the unaffected leg.
3. The surgeon limits the sterile field above the knee by placing a towel around the leg and securing it with a towel clip.
4. Lay a minor sheet on the sterile sheets under the leg. The person who has been holding the leg lays it on this minor sheet. The surgeon wraps the leg in the minor sheet and secures it with a sterile bandage. Stockinette may be preferred for this step.
5. Place a medium sheet above the exposed area, at the skin edge, over the draping towel and fasten it with a towel clip.
6. Place a laparotomy sheet, with the opening on the foot and the longer part of the sheet toward the head of the operating bed. Open it and draw the leg through the opening. A split sheet may be used.

Lower Leg and Ankle

While the leg is still being held up following skin preparation:

1. Place a medium sheet under the leg and over the unaffected leg to above the knees.
2. The surgeon limits the sterile field by placing a towel around the leg above the area of the intended surgical site and securing it with a towel clip.
3. Put stockinette over the foot and draw it up over the leg to above the skin edge of the towel. The person who has been holding the leg is relieved, and the leg is held by a sterile team member.
4. Place a medium sheet above the surgical area and secure it around the leg with a towel clip.
5. Place a laparotomy sheet or split sheet with the leg drawn through the opening.
6. Cover the remainder of the operating bed over the anesthesia screen with a single sheet as necessary.

Foot

The general method of draping a foot is the same as that for the hand. While the foot is still being held up following skin preparation:

1. Place a medium sheet on the operating bed under the foot.
2. The surgeon limits the exposed area to the foot by placing a towel around the ankle and securing it with a towel clip.
3. Enclose the foot in stockinette. A sterile team member relieves the unsterile person who has been holding the leg.
4. Place a medium sheet above the foot and secure it around the ankle with a towel clip.

5. Place a laparotomy sheet with the opening over the foot and longer part of the sheet toward the head of the operating bed.

Draping of Equipment

A pneumatic tourniquet frequently is used to control bleeding during surgical procedures on the upper and lower extremities. A nonsterile tourniquet cuff is placed around the extremity before skin preparation. It is enclosed within (i.e., covered by) the draping material. The towel that delineates the upper limit of the surgical area is placed around the extremity below the tourniquet cuff.

Equipment that is brought into the sterile field but cannot be sterilized must be draped before it is handled by sterile team members. The following applies to draping of equipment:

1. Tailored disposable drapes are available to cover equipment, such as the operating microscope, so that it can be manipulated in the sterile field by the surgeon.
2. If x-ray films are to be taken during the surgical procedure, a cassette holder may be placed on the operating bed, under the patient, before the patient is positioned, prepped, and draped. The circulator raises the drape for the radiology technician to place and remove the cassette. The holder and/or cassette may be covered with a sterile Mayo stand cover or specially designed disposable cover and placed on sterile drapes when a lateral view is needed.
3. Cords, attachments, or tubings that are not sterile must be inserted into sterile coverings before they are placed on the sterile field.

Nonsterile equipment that must stand near the sterile field must be excluded from the sterile area by a drape shield. IV poles frequently are used to attach drapes to shield off power-generating sources of mechanical and electrical equipment, such as electrosurgical and cryosurgical units, fiberoptic lighting units, and air-powered or electrical instruments. The drape over the patient or a separate single sheet is extended from the operating bed upward in front of or over the nonsterile equipment. The circulator fastens the drape to IV poles on each side of the equipment that stands above the level of the sterile field or near it.

Heat-generating equipment must have adequate ventilation to dissipate heat. Impermeable, heat-retaining materials cannot completely encase these units. Ends of fiberoptic light cables should not make prolonged contact with drapes, or a fire may result.

Some nonsterile equipment, of necessity, will be moved over the sterile field. The sterile field is protected by additional draping material, as follows:

1. Sterile disposable drapes are available to cover x-ray equipment, image intensifiers, and the like.
2. When ready to move an x-ray tube or image intensifier over the sterile field, cover the field with a minor sheet. Discard this sheet after use.
3. Photographic equipment and video cameras should be draped as much as feasible when used over the sterile field.

PLASTIC ISOLATOR

A plastic isolator (a shield around the patient's bed or the operating bed) may be used to exclude microorganisms from the environment immediately surrounding the patient. It may isolate a patient who is highly susceptible to infection, such as a burned or immunosuppressed patient, or it may isolate a patient with a gross infection and provide protection for others. In the OR, plastic isolators are used to isolate the sterile field from both room air and the OR team and thus exclude microorganisms normally in the OR environment.

The portable, lightweight, optically transparent surgical isolator forms a bubble over the patient when inflated. This surgical isolation bubble system (SIBS) has two elements: a filter/blower unit and a prepackaged sterile, disposable bubble. Its floor provides a sterile drape that adheres to prepped skin around the incision site. Built into the sides are ports (armholes) through which the team works and a port for passing sterile supplies from the circulator.

A patient isolation drape may be used that is a modification of the total isolator. It isolates the sterile field from equipment, such as the C-arm image intensifier used for hip procedures. The drape is suspended from a steel frame but does not enclose the patient. The incise portion of the drape may be impregnated with a time-release iodophor. Storage and irrigation pouches are incorporated into the side.

Bibliography

Association of Operating Room Nurses: *Standards, recommended practices, and guidelines,* Denver, 1998, The Association.
Belkin NL: More on squaring off . . . elimination of squaring off with towels, *AORN J* 64(5):685-686, 1996.
Belkin NL, Koch FT: OR barrier materials . . . necessity or extravagance? *AORN J* 67(2):442-445, 1998.
Bhargava HN, Leonard PA: Triclosan: applications and safety, *Am J Infect Control* 24(3):209-218, 1996.
Christianson C: Total hip arthroplasty: positioned, prepped, and draped, *Orthop Nurs* 16(1):43-48, 1997.
Coyne MA: Squaring off with cloth towels, *AORN J* 64(1):21, 1996.
Hagen KS, Treston-Aurand J: A comparison of two skin preps used in cardiac surgical procedures, *AORN J* 62(3):393-402, 1995.
Lavanchy C: Surgical drapes, *Infect Control Today* 2(4):49, 1998.
Leaper D: Antiseptics in wound healing, *Nurs Times* 92(39):63-64, 66-68, 1996.
Michels M: Wound cleansing versus skin antisepsis, *Infect Control Today* 2(4):54-58, 1998.
Patterson P: Reusable textiles with a new look make OR comeback, *OR Manager* 10(3):1, 6-9, 1994.
Pearce BA et al: Efficacy of clean vs. sterile surgical prep kits, *AORN J* 66(3):464-470, 1997.
Smith CD: Clinical issues: combined vaginal/abdominal preps; seated personnel, *AORN J* 59(6):1313-1318, 1994.

Section

X

Surgical Site Management

Chapter 30

Hemostasis and Wound Closure

 Chapter Objectives

After studying this chapter, the learner will be able to:

- Describe mechanical methods of hemostasis.
- Describe chemical methods of hemostasis.
- Describe thermal methods of hemostasis.
- Identify several absorbable sutures.
- Identify several nonabsorbable sutures.
- List several different types of needles.

The story of hemostasis and sutures, in some measure, is the story of surgery itself. Many kinds of materials were used in the past, and many are used today, to close or cover wounds. Terms associated with hemostasis and wound closure are defined in Box 30-1.

HISTORICAL BACKGROUND

The first written description of sutures, which were probably made of linen, to approximate wound edges is in the Edwin Smith papyrus from the sixteenth century BC. The *Shusruta Samhita,* an ancient Indian classic written between 600 and 1000 BC, refers to plaited horsehair, cotton, strips of leather, and fibers from tree bark for use as sutures. These and other writings dating back to 2000 BC refer to strings and animal tendons for ligating and suturing. In 30 AD Celsus referred to the use of twisted sutures.

Galen (130-220 AD) mentioned the use of animal gut sutures for the primary closure of wounds in Roman gladiators, although he recommended silk when it could be obtained. Previous knowledge of ligatures seems to have been lost un-

til Galen wrote of using them to stop bleeding after trying all other methods known at the time.

Mohammedan religious laws required caravan leaders to carry sutures and needles to care for injuries. Sometimes camel hair was used for sutures. Arabian surgeons used harp strings. Rhazes (circa 854-930 AD) of Persia is credited with first employing kitstrings to suture abdominal wounds. In Arabic a *kit* is a fiddle. The fiddle strings, referred to as kitgut, were made from sheep intestines (ovine source), which were twisted and dried in the sun. The term *catgut* is believed to have evolved from its origin as *kitgut.* Suture material is still made from sheep or beef intestine but is more accurately called surgical gut today.

Sutures fell into disuse during the Middle Ages, accompanying a general regression in surgical technique. Their use was revived by Ambroise Paré (1510-1590), a French army surgeon. He ligated arteries to stop the bleeding following amputations.

Early in the nineteenth century Dr. Philip Syng Physick (1768-1837) found that the body absorbs sutures made from animal tissue. Probably the first surgeon to realize this,

523

hematoma Accumulation of blood and fluid in the wound that can promote infection and delay wound healing.

hemostasis Control of arterial and/or venous bleeding in the surgical site.

ligature A strand of material used to tie or bind. The act of ligating.

suture A strand of material used for joining tissue together or ligating a structure. To suture.

Physick was the first American to use catgut extensively. He also fashioned a curved needle for circumventing an artery.

Catgut sutures were used in the early nineteenth century by English surgeons. However, Joseph Lister (1827-1912) is credited with sterilizing and chromicizing them. Only since Lister's time have wound closure techniques been brought to an advanced state of development.

Many materials have been used as ligatures and sutures through the centuries, including gold, silver, and tantalum wire; silk; silkworm gut; horsehair; kangaroo tendon; cotton; and linen. The synthetic polymers developed in the twentieth century resulted in the demise of many of these materials for use as surgical sutures. Polymer chemistry has revolutionized the manufacture of sutures, although silk and surgical gut continue to be widely used. Needles were first swaged (i.e., permanently attached to the suture material) in 1928. Today more than a hundred shapes, sizes, and types of surgical needles are swaged to the suture materials that are in common use.

Although surgical stapling is considered to be an innovation of the twentieth century, the concept of mechanically holding tissues together dates back to antiquity. The *Shusruta Samhita* describes the use of termites to hold wound edges in apposition. The termite would bite through the skin at the wound site and, with subsequent beheading, would hold the wound edges together with its pincers. Ancient Egyptians and some modern South American tribes used ant jaws. East Africans closed wounds with acacia thorns. These insects and plants were the forerunners of the skin staplers used today.

The first internal stapler was introduced in Budapest by Professor Hamer Hültl in 1908 for closing the stomach. This was followed in 1924, also in Hungary, by a mechanical device for gastrointestinal anastomosis developed by Aladar von Petz. Although cumbersome and heavy, weighing over 7 pounds (5 kg), the von Petz clamp received worldwide acceptance. The Russians subsequently became the leaders in the field of stapling tissue with their refinements in instrumentation during the 1950s. Most of the reusable staplers currently in use are available through patents licensed from the former Soviet Union. A disposable skin stapler was introduced in 1978, and disposable internal staplers have been available since 1980.

HEMOSTASIS

Hemostasis, the arrest of a flow of blood or hemorrhage, is essential to successful wound management. The mechanism is coagulation, or the formation of a blood clot. The clotting of blood takes place in several stages by enzyme reaction.

HEMOSTATIC PROCESS

When severed by incision or traumatic injury, a blood vessel constricts and the ends contract somewhat. Platelets rapidly clump and adhere to connective tissue at the cut end of a constricted vessel. Interaction with collagen fibers causes platelets to liberate adenosine diphosphate (ADP), epinephrine, and serotonin from their secretory granules. In turn, ADP causes other platelets to clump to the initial layer and to each other, forming a platelet plug. This may be sufficient in small vessels to provide primary hemostasis.

The reaction of plasma from vessels with connective tissue cells at the site of injury activates clotting factors and causes a series of other reactions. Prothrombin, normally present in blood, reacts with thromboplastin, which is released when tissues are injured. Prothrombin and thromboplastin, along with calcium ions in the blood, form thrombin. This requires several minutes. Thrombin unites with fibrinogen, a blood protein, to form fibrin, which is the basic structural material of blood clots. This last reaction is very rapid.

The fibrin strands reinforce the platelet plug to form a resilient hemostatic plug capable of withstanding arterial pressure when the constricted vessel relaxes. Massive thrombosis within the vessels would occur once coagulation were initiated, if it continued. However, fibrin is digested during the process. The products of this digestion, as well as antithrombins normally present in blood, act as anticoagulants. The coagulation mechanism rapidly and efficiently inhibits excessive blood loss so that excessive coagulation does not occur (Figure 30-1).

Basically, two types of bleeding occur during surgical procedures: gross bleeding from transected or penetrated vessels and diffuse venous oozing from denuded or cut surfaces. Although the need to control gross bleeding is obvious, insidious but continuous loss of blood from small vessels and capillaries can become significant if oozing is uncontrolled. Complete hemostasis, gentle tissue handling, elimination of dead space, precise wound closure, and a protective wound dressing are essential to minimize trauma to tissue and to enhance healing without complication. Incomplete hemostasis may cause the formation of a hematoma. A hematoma is a collection of extravasated blood in a body cavity, space, or tissue caused by uncontrolled bleeding or oozing. It may be painful and firm to the touch. Some hematomas require evacuation to prevent infection; others reabsorb with time.

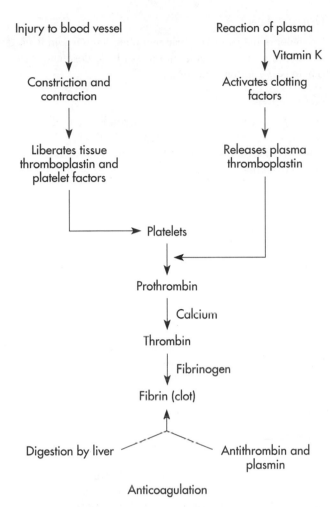

Figure 30-1 Mechanism of hemostasis.

METHODS OF HEMOSTASIS

Numerous agents, devices, and sophisticated pieces of equipment are used to achieve hemostasis and wound closure. These various methods can be classified as chemical, mechanical, or thermal.

Chemical Methods
Absorbable Gelatin

Available in either powder or compressed pad form, gelatin (Gelfoam) is an absorbable hemostatic agent made from purified gelatin solution that has been beaten to a foamy consistency, dried, and sterilized by dry heat. As a pad, it is available in an assortment of sizes that can be cut as desired without crumbling. When it is placed on an area of capillary bleeding, fibrin is deposited in the interstices and the sponge swells, forming a substantial clot. The sponge is not soluble; it absorbs 45 times its own weight in blood. It is denatured to retard absorption, which takes place in 20 to 40 days. It is frequently soaked in thrombin or epinephrine solution, although it may be used alone. Before a gelatin sponge is

handed to the surgeon, it is dipped into warm saline, if used without thrombin or epinephrine, and pressed between the fingers or against the sides of the basin to remove air from it. The same procedure is used with thrombin or epinephrine solution, but then the sponge is dropped back into the solution and allowed to absorb solution back to its original size.

In powder form, gelatin is mixed with sterile saline to make a paste for application to cancellous bone to control bleeding or to denuded areas of skin or muscles to stimulate growth of granulation tissue.

Absorbable Collagen

Hemostatic sponges (Collastat, Superstat, Helistat) or felt (Lyostypt) of bovine collagen origin are applied dry to oozing or bleeding sites. The collagen activates the coagulation mechanism, especially the aggregation of platelets, to accelerate clot formation. The material dissolves as hemostasis occurs. Any residual will absorb in the wound. Because of an affinity for wet surfaces, it must be kept dry and should be applied with dry gloves or instruments. Absorbable collagen is contraindicated in the presence of infection or in areas where blood or other fluids have pooled. It is applied directly to the bleeding surface as supplied from the sterile package.

Microfibrillar Collagen

Available in compacted nonwoven web form or in loose fibrous form, microfibrillar collagen (Avitene, Instat) is an absorbable topical hemostatic agent. It is produced from a hydrochloric acid salt of purified bovine corium collagen. It is applied dry. When it is placed in contact with a bleeding surface, hemostasis is achieved by adhesion of platelets and prompt fibrin deposition within the interstices of the collagen. Tissue cohesion is an inherent property of the collagen itself. It functions as a hemostatic agent only when it is applied directly to the source of bleeding from raw, oozing surfaces, including bone and friable tissues, or directly to active bleeding from irregular contours, from crevices, and around suture lines. Firm pressure is applied quickly with a dry gauze sponge, which is held either by the fingers in accessible areas or by a sponge forceps in less accessible areas. It is important that the material be compressed firmly against the bleeding surface before excessive wetting with blood can occur. Effective application is evidenced by a firm, adherent coagulum with no break-through bleeding from either the surface or edges. Excess material should be removed from around the site without recreating bleeding. The remaining coagulum absorbs during wound healing.

Oxidized Cellulose

Absorbable oxidation products of cellulose are available in the form of a pad of oxidized cellulose (Oxycel) similar to absorbent cotton or oxidized regenerated cellulose in a knitted fabric strip that is of low density (Surgicel) or high density (Surgical Nu-Knit). These products may be sutured to, wrapped around, or held firmly against a bleeding site or laid dry on an oozing surface until hemostasis is obtained. When oxidized cellulose comes into contact with whole blood, a clot forms rapidly. As it reacts with blood, it increases in size to form a gel and stops bleeding in areas in which bleeding is difficult to control by other means of hemostasis. Except in situations in which packing is required as a lifesaving measure, only the minimal amount required to control capillary or venous bleeding is used. If left on oozing surfaces, it will absorb with minimal tissue reaction. It is not recommended for use on bone unless it is removed after hemostasis because it may interfere with bone regeneration. Oxidized regenerated cellulose has some bactericidal properties, but it is not a substitute for antimicrobial agents.

Oxytocin

Oxytocin is a hormone produced by the pituitary gland. It can be prepared synthetically for therapeutic injection. During cesarean section, oxytocin (10 units) may be directly injected into the uterine muscle to cause contraction after delivery of the baby and placenta. It is a systemic agent used to control hemorrhage from the uterus, rather than a local hemostatic agent per se. Oxytocin is sometimes used to induce labor. It also causes contraction of the uterus after delivery of the placenta.

Phenol and Alcohol

Some surgeons use a cotton-tipped swab dipped in 95% phenol to cauterize tissue when cutting across the lumen of the appendix. Phenol coagulates proteins and in high concentration is so caustic that it can cause severe burns. It is neutralized with 95% alcohol.

Styptics

A styptic is an agent that checks hemorrhage by causing vasoconstriction. Styptics have the disadvantage of being rapidly carried away by the bloodstream.

Epinephrine

A hormone of the adrenal gland, epinephrine (Adrenalin) is prepared synthetically for use as a vasoconstrictor to prolong the action of local anesthetic agents or to decrease bleeding. Used in some local anesthetic agents to constrict the vessels locally, epinephrine keeps the anesthetic concentrated within the area injected and reduces the amount of bleeding when the incision is made. It is rapidly dispersed, leaving little local effect. Within the incision, gelatin sponges soaked in 1:1000 epinephrine may be applied to bleeding surfaces. These are especially useful in ear and microsurgical procedures in which localized hemostasis is critical.

Silver Nitrate

Crystals of silver nitrate in solution or mixed with silver chloride and molded into applicator sticks are applied topically. Both an astringent and an antimicrobial, silver nitrate is commonly used in the treatment of burns. It may be used to seal areas of previous surgical incisions that fail to heal with time.

Tannic Acid

A powder made from an astringent plant, tannic acid is used occasionally on mucous membranes of the nose and throat to help stop capillary bleeding.

Thrombin

An enzyme extracted from bovine blood is used therapeutically as a topical hemostatic agent in 5000-U or 10,000-U solutions. Thrombin accelerates coagulation of blood and controls capillary bleeding. It unites rapidly with fibrinogen to form a clot. Topically it may be used as a dry powder to sprinkle on an oozing surface or as a solution, alone or to saturate a gelatin sponge. Topical thrombin may be sprayed on areas of capillary bleeding that do not lend themselves to other means of hemostasis, such as sealing a skin graft onto a denuded area. It should not be allowed to enter large vessels.

Thrombin is used for topical application only. It is never injected. It is recommended that thrombin be mixed just before use because it loses potency after several hours. Thrombin solution should be labeled with the name of the drug and the concentration and kept separate from any other solutions on the instrument table. The manufacturer's instructions should be followed for mixing solution. Thrombin is contraindicated if the patient is allergic to bovine products.

Sclerotherapy

A caustic sclerosing solution may be injected into veins, as in the mucosal lining of the esophagus or anus, to stop or prevent bleeding. The solution may be sodium morrhuate or a mixture of equal parts of dehydrated alcohol, bacteriostatic saline, and sodium tetradecyl. Other sclerosants are mixtures of absolute ethanol or ethanolamine.

External Mechanical Methods

Mechanical hemostasis is achieved by occluding severed vessels until normal forces of blood have time to form a clot. During the surgical procedure the surgeon uses many mechanical devices to apply pressure or to create a mechanical barrier to the flow of blood. Pressure also is used prophylactically preoperatively and postoperatively.

Mechanical external pressure devices may be applied before the patient arrives in the OR or after the patient is transferred to the operating bed. The intended purpose may be prophylactic to prevent venous stasis, deep vein thrombosis (DVT), or pulmonary embolus intraoperatively and postoperatively. Or the function may be therapeutic to control internal hemorrhage preoperatively or hematoma postoperatively. A bloodless surgical field also can be created by external pressure devices.

Antiembolic Stockings

Elastic stockings may be applied to the lower extremities to prevent thromboembolic phenomena. Static compression on the legs helps prevent venous stasis. Stockings are available in knee- or groin-length sizes. To apply, the circulator rolls the stocking from top to toe. After being placed over the patient's toes, the stocking is gently unrolled over the leg from foot to ankle to calf.

Sequential Compression Device

Inflatable, double-walled vinyl or woven fabric leg wraps use alternating compression and relaxation to reduce the risk of DVT in the legs of high-risk patients undergoing general anesthesia or experiencing extremes of intraoperative positioning. The leg wraps may be used over antiembolic stockings on each leg, although the compression device alone is sufficient in the prevention of DVT. The patient's foot is not encased within the wrap. The circulator should measure the patient's thigh or calf for the correct size selection (i.e., small, medium, large, or extra large) for either full-leg (thigh-high) or knee-high leg wraps. Proper selection and application are essential for effective compression. Disposable leg wraps are commercially available.

A motorized pump, attached by tubing to each wrap, sequentially inflates leg wraps at the ankles, then at the calves, and then at the thighs for full-leg compression. The pressure of this wavelike action is greatest at the ankles. The leg wraps are divided into chambers so that pressure can be regulated by preset or adjustable gauges. Pressure between 40 and 50 mm Hg applied for 12 seconds and then released for 48 seconds empties blood from deep leg venous sinuses. The action prevents venous stasis and accumulation of clotting factors in deep veins. The pumping action is started before induction of anesthesia because general anesthesia reduces venous return and causes vasodilation.

The circulator should check operation of the pump regularly and periodically inspect the leg wraps and tubing. Care is taken to ensure that the patient is not lying on the tubing. The type of device, time started, pressure and cycle settings, and time discontinued must be documented on the intraoperative record. If the surgeon wants leg wraps to remain on the patient postoperatively, the device is transported to the postanesthesia care unit (PACU) or intensive care unit (ICU) with the patient. Frequently, sequential compression is continued for 24 hours postoperatively or until the patient is fully ambulatory following an abdominal, hip, or neurosurgical procedure.

MAST Pneumatic Counterpressure Device

Although the concept dates back to 1903, external counterpressure was not a popular medical device until the Vietnam War. There it was used to control hemorrhagic shock until definitive hemostasis became available to casualties. Circumferential pneumatic compression counteracts postural hypotension, maintains venous pressure, and controls hemorrhage. Several types of pneumatic antishock garments (PASGs) are used, primarily to treat hypovolemic shock. The acronym *MAST* can refer to medical antishock trousers, military antishock trousers, or a military antigravity suit. An inflatable, waterproof garment is fastened around the patient from ankles to rib cage. The trouser chambers are inflated first to prevent venous stasis in the legs. The entire suit or only specific chambers of it can be inflated from the feet up. Each chamber is inflated separately with a foot pump. By increasing pressure on vessel walls of the legs and abdomen, systemic vascular resistance of peripheral vessels increases blood flow to the heart, lungs, and brain. Compression of torn vessel walls reduces the size of the laceration and diminishes blood loss.

The MAST device may be in place when the trauma patient arrives in the operating room (OR). Deflation begins after induction of anesthesia, beginning with the abdominal chamber. Leg chambers may remain inflated for counterpressure if blood pressure remains unstable. Deflation must be slow and gradual. The MAST suit is never cut off the patient. Rapid deflation reduces cerebral and cardiopulmonary circulation, with resultant shock. Blood pressure is monitored; it should not drop more than 5 mm Hg.

Pneumatic counterpressure devices may be used to prevent air embolism during some head and neck procedures performed with the patient in a sitting position. The increased venous filling produced decreases the possibility of an air embolus. Also, these devices may be used postoperatively to reduce bleeding or to stabilize the patient following massive blood loss during the surgical procedure.

Tourniquets

A tourniquet is a device used to provide hemostasis by constricting the flow of blood in an extremity. It is frequently used on the proximal aspect of an extremity to keep the distal surgical site free of blood. A bloodless field makes dissection easier and less traumatic to tissues and reduces surgical time. Bleeding must be controlled before pressure is released.

Precautions for tourniquet application and use are observed. A tourniquet should is not used when circulation in an extremity is impaired or when an arteriovenous access fistula for dialysis is present. A tourniquet can cause tissue, nerve, and vascular injury. Paralysis may result from excessive pressure on nerves. Prolonged ischemia can cause gangrene and loss of the extremity. Tourniquet time should be kept to a minimum. Metabolic changes may be irreversible after 1 to 1½ hours of tourniquet ischemia. Consideration for latex sensitivity may be an issue for some devices used as tourniquets. Rubber materials should be latex free if the patient is sensitive to latex products.

A tourniquet is dangerous to apply, to leave on, and to remove. A tourniquet may be applied by the surgeon, assistant, or the circulator on the surgeon's orders.

Pneumatic Tourniquet   Similar to a blood pressure cuff, although heavier and more secure, the pneumatic cuff consists of a rubber bladder shielded by a plastic insert inside a fabric cover with a hook-and-loop (Velcro) closure. Many different types of cuffs are available. Some are straight and cylindric in shape; others are contoured. A cuff of appropriate length and width must be used; various sizes are available. Cuffs are inflated automatically with compressed gas (air or oxygen) by means of tubing interconnected between the cuff and a pressure cartridge, piped-in system, or battery-powered unit. The desired pressure is uniformly maintained by a pressure valve and registered on a pressure gauge. The tourniquet console, a pressure regulator with a gauge, may be contained in a unit mounted on a portable stand or hung on an IV pole. An automated tourniquet with a computerized microprocessor control signals both audible alarms and visual indicators for deviations from preset pressure and for elapsed time of inflation.

Correct pressure is the minimum amount required to produce a bloodless field. The calculation of tourniquet cuff pressure is according to the systolic blood pressure. An exact pressure to which the cuff should be inflated has not been determined. In a healthy adult, upper extremity pressure 30 to 70 mm Hg higher than the systolic value of the blood pressure may be sufficient to suppress arterial circulation. Tourniquet pressure on an average adult arm usually ranges from 250 to 300 mm Hg (up to 6 pounds). In the lower extremity, cuff pressure should be higher than the systolic pressure by one half the value. This may require 350 mm Hg on the thigh. Thin adults and children require less pressure; muscular and obese extremities may require more. Inflation time should also be kept to a minimum. If needed for more than 1 hour on an arm or 1½ hours on a leg, the tourniquet may be deflated at intervals periodically at the discretion of the surgeon.

A pneumatic tourniquet should be used and maintained according to the manufacturer's written instructions. These and institutional policies and procedures should be available to users of this complex equipment. The cuff, tubing, connectors, gauges, and pressure source should be maintained in working order. Precautions to be taken when using a pneumatic tourniquet include the following:

1. Inspect and test the pneumatic tourniquet equipment before each use.
   a. Inspect the inflatable cuff, connectors, and tubing for cleanliness, integrity, and function.
   b. Ensure that the cuff and tubing are intact and that the connectors are securely fastened to the tourniquet pressure source.
   c. Check the pressure gauge for accuracy. An aneroid pressure gauge can be checked by comparing it with a mercury manometer. Pressure drifts can be detected by wrapping the cuff around a rigid cylinder, inflating it to 300 mm Hg, and observing for pressure variations.
2. Protect the patient's skin under the tourniquet cuff.
   a. Place wrinkle-free padding around the extremity. A length of stockinette or lint-free cotton sheet wadding may be used (Webril). Disposable padded covers are commercially available.
   b. Keep the padding and cuff dry. Antiseptic solutions and other fluids should not contact or accumulate under the cuff. Skin maceration or burns could re-

sult. Placing an impervious drape around the cuff prevents the pooling of fluids.
3. Position the cuff at the point of maximum circumference of the extremity.
   a. Avoid vulnerable neurovascular structures. Nerves and blood vessels may be compressed against bone when the cuff is inflated. Soft tissue provides padding for underlying structures. The cuff should be placed on the upper arm or proximal third of the thigh.
   b. Select a cuff of appropriate width for the size and shape of the extremity. A wide cuff occludes blood flow at a lower pressure than a narrow cuff.
   c. Select a cuff with adequate length to overlap at least 3 inches (7.5 cm) but not more than 6 inches (15 cm).
   d. Apply the cuff smoothly and snugly over padding, if used, before prepping the extremity.
   e. Apply a sterile cuff, if used, after prepping and draping. A sterile cuff may be used for an immunocompromised patient.
4. Preset pressure gauges. The surgeon determines the pressure setting according to the patient's age, limb size, and systolic blood pressure and the width of the cuff to be used.
5. Exsanguinate the extremity after prepping and draping, but before cuff inflation, to prolong the tourniquet time.
   a. Wrap a rubber Esmarch's bandage around the extremity to compress superficial vessels.
   b. Elevate the arm or leg for 2 minutes to encourage venous drainage by gravity if a rubber Esmarch's bandage is contraindicated (e.g., for latex-sensitive patients).
   c. Deflate the cuff completely and exsanguinate again if the cuff inflates either excessively or insufficiently. Reinflation over blood-filled vessels may cause intravascular thrombosis.
6. Inflate the cuff rapidly to occlude arteries and veins simultaneously to predetermined minimum pressure.
7. Monitor safety parameters during use of the pneumatic tourniquet.
   a. Monitor the pressure gauge to detect pressure fluctuations within the bladder of the cuff.
   b. Monitor the duration of inflation. Inform the surgeon when the cuff has been inflated for 1 hour and every 15 minutes thereafter. In some ORs the circulator posts the tourniquet time on a tally board in view of the surgeon.
8. Document the use of a tourniquet on the intraoperative record.
   a. Record the times the tourniquet is applied, inflated, deflated, and removed. The anesthesia provider also records the inflation time on the anesthesia sheet when a tourniquet is used with a Bier block for regional anesthesia.
   b. Record the location of the cuff, who placed it, and the pressure setting.
   c. Record the model and serial number of the tourniquet used.

d. Document assessment of the skin condition of the extremity preoperatively and evaluation of skin and tissue integrity after removal of the cuff.
9. Clean and inspect the pneumatic tourniquet after each patient use.
   a. Wash the reusable cuff and bladder according to the manufacturer's instructions. An enzymatic detergent should be used if blood or body fluid came in contact with the cuff. A disposable cuff cover facilitates cleaning.
   b. Rinse and dry the cuff and bladder. Water droplets inside the bladder can damage the pressure mechanism if forced backward during subsequent deflation. Care should be taken to prevent water from getting into the bladder during washing.
   c. Wipe the connecting tubing with a disinfectant.
   d. Test the cuff, tubing, connectors, and gauges before storage between uses. A malfunctioning device must be removed from service until repaired and tested by appropriate personnel.

A pneumatic tourniquet is used most frequently to produce a bloodless surgical field. Other types of tourniquets include the following:

- *Blood pressure cuff.* The cuff is inflated with ambient air. The surgeon determines the amount of pressure to be sustained. The regulator valve is tightened. The pressure gauge or sphygmomanometer must be monitored for pressure deviations.
- *Rubber band.* This may be used as a tourniquet for a finger or toe. The surgeon will put a sterile rubber band on the digit after draping. This method is not used for latex sensitive patients.
- *Rubber bandage (Esmarch's bandage).* Friedrich von Esmarch, a German military surgeon, introduced an elastic bandage for the control of hemorrhage on the battlefield in 1869. Known today as Esmarch's bandage, a 3-inch (7.5-cm) latex rubber roller bandage is used to compress superficial vessels to force blood out of an extremity. An Esmarch's bandage is not used, however, to empty vessels of blood preoperatively in a patient who has sustained traumatic injury or if the patient has been in a cast. Danger exists that thrombi might be present in vessels because of injury or stasis of blood. These could become dislodged and result in emboli. An extremity with active infection or a malignant tumor also is not wrapped with an Esmarch's bandage.

  Starting at the distal end of the extremity, the surgeon wraps a sterile Esmarch's bandage tightly, overlapping it spirally, to the level of the blood pressure cuff or a pneumatic tourniquet. (An elastic Ace bandage may be used.) The circulator tightens the tourniquet. Then the rubber bandage is removed. Or, starting from the distal end of the extremity, the rubber bandage can be partially removed, leaving the last three rounds, which constitute a tourniquet.

After terminal cleaning of a reusable Esmarch's bandage, a layer of gauze bandage is rolled between layers of the rubber bandage to ensure sterilization of all surfaces. The gauze must be removed and the bandage rerolled before use. Disposable sterile Esmarch's bandages are commercially available.

- *Rubber tubing.* When an intravenous (IV) infusion is started, a small length of rubber tubing is tied around the extremity, usually an arm, while the needle is being inserted. This stops venous return and makes the vein more visible for venipuncture. A Penrose drain is commonly used as a tourniquet.

Pressure Dressings

Pressure on the wound in the immediate postoperative period can minimize the accumulation of intercellular fluid and decrease bleeding by eliminating dead space. Pressure dressings are used on some extensive wounds to decrease edema and potential hematoma or seroma formation. They may be used as an adjunct to wound drainage to distribute pressure evenly over the wound.

Packing

Packing is used with or without pressure to achieve hemostasis and to eliminate dead space in an area where mucosal tissues need support, such as the vagina, rectum, or nose. Packing impregnated with an antiseptic agent, such as iodoform gauze, may be used to ensure closure of an incision from the wound base toward the outside (i.e., healing by second intention), as in a large abscess cavity. The surgeon inserts sterile packing as the final stage of the surgical procedure. It is usually removed in 24 to 48 hours. The intraoperative record and patient's chart should reflect the type and location of packing.

Internal Mechanical Methods

Meticulous hemostasis during the surgical procedure is essential to control bleeding and to minimize blood loss. The surgeon uses many mechanical tools to achieve hemostasis.

Hemostatic Clamps

Clamps for occluding vessels are used to compress blood vessels and to grasp or hold a small amount of tissue. The hemostat is the most frequently used surgical instrument and the most commonly used method of hemostasis. This instrument has either straight or curved jaws that narrow to a fine point. Often the pressure of clamping an instrument is sufficient to constrict and seal a vessel with minimal trauma or adjacent tissue necrosis. A wide variety of hemostatic clamps are used for vessel occlusion, including noncrushing vascular clamps that do not damage large vessels.

Ligating Clips

When placed on a blood vessel and pinched shut, clips occlude the lumen and stop the vessel from bleeding. Metallic clips, such as stainless steel or titanium clips, are small pieces of thin, serrated wire that are bent in the center to an oblique angle. Absorbable polymer clips are similar in configuration. Clips are most frequently used on large vessels or those in anatomic locations difficult to ligate by other means. Many surgeons use clips for ligating vessels, nerves, and other small structures. A specific forceps is required for the application of each type available. Single clips may be mounted in a sterile plastic cartridge that can be secured in a heavy stainless steel base to facilitate loading the applier forceps. Disposable manual and powered appliers preloaded with multiple clips also are available. Some disposable clip appliers ligate as they apply the clip to a vessel.

Ligating clips were devised in 1917 by Dr. Harvey Cushing for use in brain surgery. Cushing clips are made of silver. Titanium clips are more common today because they cause less interference with computed tomography (CT) and magnetic resonance imaging (MRI) examinations. The serrations across the wire prevent their slipping off the vessels. Polymeric clips have a locking device to secure them on vessels.

Metallic clips may also be used to mark a biopsy site or other anatomic areas to permit x-ray visualization and thus detect postoperative complications. For example, migration of a marker clip could indicate the presence of a hematoma in the wound. The artifacts (i.e., distortion) caused by stainless steel clips may be a disadvantage in future radiologic studies or magnetic MRI. Titanium and absorbable polymeric clips are used to eliminate or decrease image distortion of CT and MRI scans.

Ligature

A ligature, commonly called a tie, is a strand of material that is tied around a blood vessel to manually occlude the lumen and prevent bleeding. Frequently the ligature is tied around a hemostat and slipped off the point onto the vessel and pulled taut to effect hemostasis. Vessels are ligated with the smallest-size strand possible and include the smallest amount of surrounding tissue possible. Ends are cut as near the knot as possible.

Large and pulsating vessels may require a transfixion suture. A ligature on a needle (stick tie) is placed through a "bite" of tissue and brought around the end of the vessel. This eliminates any possibility of its slipping off the vessel. All bleeding points should be ligated before the next layer of tissue is incised.

Pledgets

Small pieces of Teflon felt are used as a buttress under sutures when bleeding might occur through the needle hole in a major vessel or when friable tissue might tear, such as cardiac muscle during cardiomyotomy. Placed over an arteriotomy site, they exert pressure to seal off bleeding. Pledgets are used most frequently in cardiovascular surgery.

Packs

Packs are used to sustain pressure on raw wound surfaces and keep viscera from becoming injured during a procedure. The application of sponges or laparotomy tapes effectively controls capillary ooze by occluding the capillaries. The surgeon usually wants these moistened, often with room temperature but sometimes with warm normal saline solution. Warm packs promote hemostasis by accelerating the coagulation mechanism.

Compressed Absorbent Patties

Compressed absorbent radiopaque patties (cottonoids) are used for hemostasis when placed on the surface of brain tissue and to absorb blood and fluids around the spinal cord or nerves. These patties are available in an assortment of sizes. Before use, the scrub person counts and moistens them with normal saline solution, presses out excess solution, and keeps them flat. Some surgeon prefer antibiotics, thrombin, or epinephrine when moistening the patties for hemostasis.

Bone Wax

Composed of a sterile nonabsorbable mixture of beeswax, isopropyl palmitate, and a softening agent, bone wax provides a mechanical tamponade barrier to stop oozing from cut bone surfaces. Each packet contains 2.5 g of wax and is opened just before use to minimize drying. The scrub person can warm wax to the desired consistency by manipulating it with the fingers or by immersing the unopened packet in warm solution. Small pieces can be rolled into 1-cm balls and placed around the rim of a medicine cup. When needed, the cup can be presented to the surgeon.

Bone wax is used in some orthopaedic and neurosurgical procedures and when the sternum is split (sternotomy) for cardiothoracic procedures. Bone wax should be used sparingly and is contraindicated when rapid bone regeneration is desired. The wax is mechanical and may impede ossification as a foreign body reaction. The product is cobalt sterilized, and the expiration date should be checked before use. It should not be stored in areas that exceed 77° F (25° C).

Digital Compression

When digital pressure is applied to an artery proximal to the area of bleeding, such as in traumatic injury, hemorrhage is controlled. The main disadvantage of digital pressure is that it cannot be applied permanently. Firm pressure is applied on the skin on both sides as the skin incision is made, to help control subutaneous bleeding until vessels can be clamped, ligated, or cauterized. Pressure is applied while the surgical area is sponged to locate a bleeding vessel.

Suction

Suction is the application of pressure less than atmospheric either continuously or intermittently. It is used during surgical procedures for removal of blood and tissue fluids from the surgical field, primarily to enhance visibility. An appropriate diameter and style of tip for locating bleeding is attached to sterile disposable suction tubing. The scrub person hands the end of the tubing to the circulator, who attaches it to a suction collection container.

A powered suction/irrigation system may be used to simultaneously irrigate the wound and evacuate solution. The irrigation may be pulsed (i.e., intermittent to remove debris and clots) or continuous with gravity flow. The surgeon adjusts the flow of irrigation and suction with controls on the disposable tip assembly. Spatter screens that fit around the tip of the irrigator like a cone to minimize splashes are commercially available.

Drains

Postoperatively, drains aid in removal of blood, fluid, and air from the surgical site to obliterate dead spaces and to enhance approximation of tissues, thus preventing hematoma and seroma formation. Drains usually are placed through a stab wound in the skin adjacent to the primary incision.

Thermal Methods

Hemostasis may be achieved or enhanced by application of either cold or heat to body tissues.

Cold Methods

Cryosurgery   Cryosurgery is performed with the aid of special instruments for local freezing of diseased tissue without harm to normal adjacent structures. Extreme cold causes intracapillary thrombosis and tissue necrosis in the frozen area. Frozen tissue may be removed without significant bleeding during or after the surgical procedure. Cryosurgery is also used to alter cell function without removing tissue. It tends to be hemostatic and lymphostatic, particularly in highly vascular areas.

Extreme cold is delivered to extract heat from a small volume of tissue in a rapid manner. Liquid nitrogen is the most commonly used refrigerant; however, Freon or carbon dioxide gas may be used. The liquid or gas is in a vacuum container and comes through an insulated vacuum tube to a probe. All but the tip of the probe is insulated. Freezing of tissue at this tip is a result of the liquid nitrogen at the lowest temperature of $-320°$ F ($-196°$ C) becoming gaseous. In the process, heat is removed from the tissue. A ball of frozen tissue gradually forms around the uninsulated tip. The extent of tissue destruction is controlled by raising or lowering the temperature of cells surrounding the lesion to $-46°$ to $-40°$ F ($-20°$ to $-40°$ C).

The machines vary in range of temperatures obtained according to their design and type of refrigerant used. Some are nonelectric with foot switch–operated probes. Special miniature, presterilized, disposable models for single-patient use are particularly suitable for ophthalmic applications.

Because the process is rapid, involves less trauma to destroy or remove tissue, controls bleeding, and minimizes local pain, cryosurgery is used to alter the function of nerve cells and to destroy otherwise unapproachable brain tumors. Other techniques for which it is used include removal of superficial tumors in the nasopharynx and the skin, destruction of the prostate gland, removal of highly vascular tumors and some otherwise nonresectable liver tumors, removal of lesions from the cervix and anus, cataract extraction, and retinal detachment. The amount of tissue destroyed is influenced by the size of the tip of the probe, temperature used, duration of use, kind of tissue and its vascularity, and skill of the surgeon.

Hypothermia   Cooling of body tissues to a temperature as low as $78.8°$ F ($26°$ C) in adults and large children and $68°$ F ($20°$ C) in infants and small children, well below normal limits, decreases cellular metabolism and thereby decreases the need for oxygen by tissues. The decreased requirement for oxygen decreases bleeding. Hypothermia lowers blood pressure to slow the circulation and increases the viscosity of blood. This process results in hemoconcentration, which contributes to capillary sludging and microcirculatory stasis to provide an essentially dry field for the surgeon. Hypothermia may be localized or generalized (systemic). Hypothermia is used as an adjunct to anesthesia, particularly during heart, brain, or liver procedures.

Hot Methods

Diathermy   Oscillating, high-frequency electric current generates enough heat to coagulate and destroy body tissues. Heat is generated by resistance of tissues to passage of alternating electric current. A short-wave diathermy machine produces a high frequency of 10 to 100 million cycles per second. The machine should not be activated until the surgeon is ready to deliver this current. Diathermy is useful in stopping bleeding from small blood vessels. It is used primarily to repair a detached retina and to cauterize small warts, polyps, and other small, superficial lesions.

Electrocautery   A small battery-operated pencil with a loop heated by a steady, direct electric current to red heat will coagulate or destroy tissue on contact. Heat is transferred to tissue from the preheated wire. These cautery pencils are commonly used for eye procedures and vasectomies. The hot point of the cautery should be at least 24 inches (60 cm) from the anesthesia machine and face mask, which is an oxygen-rich environment. Cautery should not be used in the mouth, around the head, or in the pleural cavity. Cautery should not be used when any flammable agent is present. To prevent fire, only moist sponges should be permitted on the field while cautery is in use.

Electrosurgery   High-frequency electric current provided from an electrosurgical unit (ESU) frequently is used to cut tissue and to coagulate bleeding points. The concentration and flow of current generates heat as it meets resistance in passage through tissue. Because air has low electrical conductivity, an active electrode tip delivering radiofrequency energy must be in direct contact with tissue. Both cutting and coagulating currents are used in many open and minimally invasive surgical procedures. Some surgeons prefer electrosurgery to other methods of cutting and ligating vessels.

Coagulated tissue is devitalized and causes a foreign body reaction that must be resorbed by the body during healing. If a large amount of coagulated tissue is present, sloughing may result, so the wound may not heal by primary intention.

Because the high-frequency electric current goes through tissues, a dispersive electrode is applied to the patient and plugged into the grounded generator. Smoke, or plume, from use of the ESU should be removed from the air with a smoke evacuator.

Fulguration

Sparks of high-voltage electric current char the surface of tissue, producing a thin, coagulated crust (eschar) without damaging underlying tissues. Fulguration uses a spark-gap generator that emits a higher-frequency current than does electrocoagulation. This high-voltage arcing, described as spray coagulation, is used primarily for transurethral bladder and prostate procedures. A grounding pad is used on the patient.

Argon Beam Coagulator

Argon gas effectively delivers radiofrequency energy to tissue in a directional noncontact white light beam for the purpose of rapid hemostasis by coagulation. The argon beam coagulator directs a gentle flow of ionized argon gas from a generator to a pencil-shaped handpiece. The gas flow over tissues clears blood and fluid from the target site and allows creation of a superficial eschar directly on tissue. Less necrotic tissue is produced than with the high-current density of electrocoagulation because the temperature never exceeds 230° F (110° C), and penetration is approximately half the depth, which minimizes tissue destruction. The depth of penetration depends on the power, duration of application, and electrical characteristics of the tissue. Coagulation occurs through the arcing effect of electrical energy, not through the action of argon gas. The coaxial flow of gas delivers monopolar current that coagulates the surface with practically no smoke or odor. A dispersive electrode is applied to the patient to complete the electrical circuit.

The argon beam coagulator is used to control hemorrhage from vascular structures, surface bleeding, and diffuse oozing and to achieve hemostasis of bone marrow. Handpieces and electrodes are available for use through endoscopes, but they are not used in fluid environments, such as joints.

Hemostatic Scalpel

The sharp steel blade of the hemostatic scalpel seals blood vessels as it cuts through tissue. The disposable blade, size No. 10, 11, or 15, has a heating and sensing microcircuitry between the steel and a layer of copper coated with electrical insulation and a nonstick surface. The blade fits into a reusable handle that contains control switches. The scrub person hands the end of the electrical cord attached to the handle to the circulator, who plugs it into the controller unit. When the surgeon activates it at the handle, the blade transfers thermal energy to tissues as the sharp edge cuts through them. An audible sound is emitted to signal the activation of the device. The temperature can be adjusted between 230° and 518° F (110° and 270° C). The surgeon can raise or lower the temperature in increments of 50° F (10° C). After use, it remains hot to the touch for 30 to 40 seconds. The blade also can be used cold, like any other scalpel.

The hemostatic scalpel can be used to incise skin, soft tissues, and muscle in a long, smooth stroke. This is particularly advantageous in vascular areas, such as the scalp, head and neck, and breast. The blade is kept clean by wiping. Scraping the surface of the blade will decrease its efficiency. Care is taken not to touch the hemostatic scalpel blade to an active ESU tip; the circuitry will be damaged.

This scalpel may be used to debride burns. Blood flow into the incised area is minimal, providing the surgeon with a clear, dry field, thus shortening surgical time. The rapid hemostasis with minimal tissue damage promotes wound healing and may eliminate a need for blood replacement. It is not effective in a bloody field or for vessels larger than 1.5 mm. Because electric current from the microcircuitry does not pass through tissue, a grounding pad or dispersive electrode is not required. This also prevents muscle contractions.

Plasma Scalpel

The plasma scalpel vaporizes tissues and stops bleeding as it simultaneously cuts and coagulates tissue. Within the instrument, which looks like a large ballpoint pen, argon or helium gas passes through an electric arc that ionizes it into a high thermal state. These gases are inert and noncombustible. As the instrument moves over tissue, the gas that flows from the tip is visible, allowing the surgeon to see the depth and extent of the incision. Tissue damage, with resultant inflammatory response during wound healing, is greater than that caused by a steel knife blade but less than that caused by other electrosurgical instruments and lasers. Because it will coagulate blood vessels up to 3 mm in diameter, the plasma scalpel is useful in highly vascular areas.

Ultrasonic Scalpel

The titanium blade of the scalpel moves by a rapid ultrasonic motion that cuts and coagulates tissue simultaneously. The portable generator, a microprocessor with piezoelectric disks, converts electrical energy into mechanical energy. This energy is transmitted through a handpiece to a single-use blade. All three parts of the system lock into a frequency of 55,500 movements per second. When this happens, the system is said to be in harmony, thus the name Harmonic scalpel. The scalpel can be used for sharp or blunt dissection without damage to adjacent tissues. Vibrations from the blade denature protein molecules as it cuts through tissue, producing a coagulum that seals bleeding vessels. The continuous vibration of the denatured protein generates heat within the tissue to cause deeper coagulation. This action does not raise tissue temperature above 176° F (80° C), so that char or smoke is not produced. A fatty particulate mist may be generated. The vibrating blade also produces a cavitation effect, as it cuts through tissue with high water content, that disrupts cell walls and separates tissue, which aids in dissection.

The ultrasonic scalpel is used primarily for laparoscopic and thoracoscopic procedures. Blades and accessories for open procedures make this technology available to all surgical specialties. Because electricity is not required for effects on tissue, a grounding pad is not necessary.

Laser Laser light is used for control of bleeding or for ablation and excision of tissues in organs that can be exposed or are accessible endoscopically. The laser furnishes an intense and concentrated light beam of a single wavelength from a monochromatic source of nonionizing radiation. Thermal energy of this beam may simultaneously cut, coagulate, and/or vaporize tissue. The laser wound is characterized by minimal bleeding and no visible postoperative edema. The amount of tissue destruction is predictable by adjusting the width and focus of the beam. Different lasers have selective uses.

Photocoagulation The photocoagulator uses an intense multiwavelength light furnished by a xenon tube to coagulate tissue. Its use is limited to ophthalmology.

WOUND CLOSURE

Closure of a surgical site or other wound is performed after necessary hemostasis has been achieved. Wounds include deep and superficial structures. Methods of wound closure include sutures, staples, clips, tapes, and glues.

SUTURES

The noun *suture* is used for any strand of material used for ligating or approximating tissue; it is also synonymous with *stitch*. The verb *to suture* denotes the act of sewing by bringing tissues together and holding them until healing has taken place.

If the material is tied around a blood vessel to occlude the lumen, it is called a ligature or tie. A suture attached to a needle for a single stitch for hemostasis is referred to as a stick tie or suture ligature. A free tie is a single strand of material handed to the surgeon or assistant to ligate a vessel. A tie handed to the surgeon in the tip of a forceps is referred to as a tie on a passer.

Suturing Techniques
Halsted's Suture Technique
The education a physician receives during postgraduate surgical training exerts a lasting influence on his or her surgical techniques. The classic example of the influence of a professor on his students is that of Dr. William Stewart Halsted (1852-1922). Halsted, a professor of surgery at Johns Hopkins Hospital in Baltimore from 1893 to 1922, perfected and brought into use the fine-pointed hemostat for occluding vessels, the Penrose drain, and rubber gloves. He is best known for his principles of gentle tissue handling. The silk suture technique he initiated in 1883, or a modification of it, is in use today. Its features are as follows:

1. Interrupted individual sutures are used for greater strength along the wound. Each stitch is taken and tied separately. If one knot slips, all the others hold. Halsted also believed that interrupted sutures were a barrier to infection, for he thought that if one area of a wound became infected, the microorganisms traveled along a continuous suture to infect the entire wound.
2. Sutures are as fine as is consistent with security. A suture stronger than the tissue it holds is not necessary.
3. Sutures are cut close to the knots. Long ends cause irritation and increase inflammation.
4. A separate needle is used for each skin stitch.
5. Dead space in the wound is eliminated. Dead space is that space caused by separation of wound edges that have not been closely approximated by sutures. Serum or blood clots may collect in a dead space and prevent healing by keeping the cut edges of tissue separated.
6. Two fine sutures are used in situations usually requiring one large one.
7. Silk is not used in the presence of infection. The interstices (braid pattern) can harbor microorganisms.
8. Tension is not placed on tissue. Approximation vs. strangulation preserves the blood supply.

Halsted's principles were based on use of the only suture materials available to him: silk and surgical gut. With the advent of less reactive synthetic materials, wound closure may be safely and more quickly performed with different techniques without complications.

Principles of Suturing
The strength of the wound is related to the condition of the tissue and the number of stitches in the edges. Care is taken not to place more sutures than necessary to approximate the edges. The amount of tissue incorporated into each stitch directly influences the rate of healing. The adequacy of the blood supply to the tissue needs to be preserved for healing to take place.

Methods of Suturing The edges of the wound are intentionally directed by the placement of sutures during closure. Suturing techniques are depicted in Figure 30-2. Examples of suturing techniques that direct the wound edges for specific healing mechanisms include, but are not limited to, the following:

1. *Everting sutures.* These interrupted (individual stitches) or continuous (running stitch) sutures are used for skin edges.
   a. Simple continuous (running). This suture can be used to close multiple layers with one suture. The suture is not cut until the full length is incorporated into the tissue (Figure 30-2, *A*).
   b. Simple interrupted. Each individual stitch is placed, tied, and cut in succession from one suture (Figure 30-2, *C*).
   c. Continuous running/locking; also known as a blanket stitch. A single suture is passed in and out of the tissue layers and looped through the free end before the needle is passed through the tissue for another stitch. Each new stitch locks the previous stitch in place (Figure 30-2, *B*).

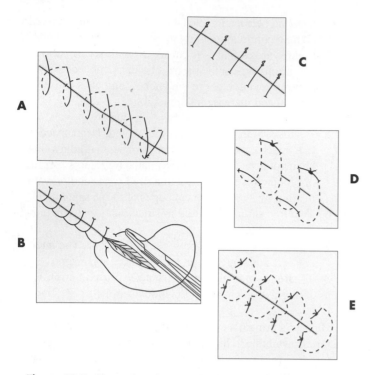

Figure 30-2 Examples of suturing techniques. **A,** Simple continuous. **B,** Continuous locking. **C,** Simple interrupted. **D,** Horizontal mattress. **E,** Vertical mattress.

d. Horizontal mattress. Stitches are placed parallel to wound edges. Each single bite takes the place of two interrupted stitches (Figure 30-2, *D*).

e. Vertical mattress. This suture uses deep and superficial bites, with each stitch crossing the wound at right angles. It works well for deep wounds. Edges approximate well (Figure 30-2, *E*).

2. *Inverting sutures.* These sutures are commonly used for two-layer anastomosis of hollow internal organs, such as the bowel and stomach. Placing two layers prevents passing suture through the lumen of the organ and creating a path for infection. A single layer is placed for other structures, such as the trachea, bronchus, and ureter. The edges are turned in toward the lumen to prevent serosal and mucosal adhesions. The number of layers is proportional to the quality of the blood supply. Stitches can be interrupted or continuous.

a. Halsted's suture is a two-layer modification of the horizontal mattress suture used for friable tissue.

b. Connell's suture is a continuous single-layer suture of gut used for hemostasis in the inner layer of bowel with a separate outer inverting layer of alternating horizontal and vertical mattress sutures.

c. Cushing's suture is a continuous vertical mattress suture that unites one half of the lumen followed by a second continuous vertical mattress suture that completes the second half of the circumference.

d. A Grey-Turner suture is a series of inverted interrupted horizontal or vertical mattress stitches.

e. A purse-string suture is a continuous stitch that encircles and closes a lumen while inverting the edges.

Knot Placement   Each suture placed in tissue usually requires the placement of a knot to secure the ends. Interrupted stitches require individual knots, and therefore placement of each knot can influence how well the wound heals and the cosmetic result. Principles concerning knots and knot tying include the following:

1. The knot should be tied away from:
   a. Vital structures, such as the eye
   b. Sources of contamination, such as the mouth
   c. Potential irritants, such as the nares
   d. Potential sources of increased inflammation, such as the incision line
2. The knot should be tied toward:
   a. The better blood supply
   b. The area that provides the best security of the knot
   c. If possible, where the mark would be less noticeable

Cutting Sutures   Care is taken to prevent excess suture from remaining in the wound. Suture tails are trimmed close to the knot. Considerations for cutting suture include the following:

1. Scissors should be stabilized by the index finger on the screw (tripod stance), the blades are angled slightly and slide down to the area just above the knot, and the suture is cut with the tips of the scissors.
2. The tips of the scissors must be visible to ensure that other structures are not injured by the cutting motion.
3. A hemostat and/or a second suture should be available in the event that the knot is inadvertently cut, releasing the sutured tissue.
4. A hemostat may be placed on one of the suture ends to stabilize the suture to be cut.
5. If removing a suture, a forceps is used to grasp the suture at the knot. Cut the suture between the knot and the skin. Extract the cut suture with the forceps.

Retention Sutures

Interrupted nonabsorbable sutures are placed through tissue on each side of the primary suture line, a short distance from it, to relieve tension on it. Heavy strands are used in sizes ranging from 0 through 5. The tissue through which retention sutures are passed includes skin, subcutaneous tissue, and fascia and may include rectus muscle and peritoneum of an abdominal incision. Following abdominal surgical procedures, retention sutures are used frequently in patients in whom slow healing is expected because of malnutrition, obesity, carcinoma, or infection; in geriatric patients; in patients receiving cortisone; or in patients with respiratory problems. Retention sutures may be used as a precautionary measure to prevent wound disruption when postoperative stress on the primary suture line from distention, vomiting, or coughing is anticipated. Retention sutures should be removed as soon as

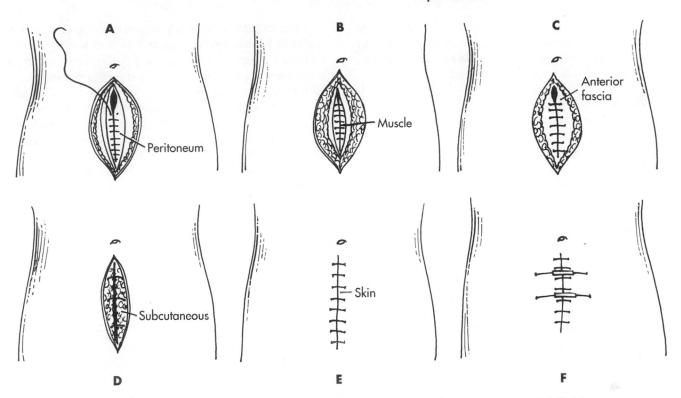

Figure 30-3   Suturing incised tissue layers. **A,** Peritoneum (continuous stitch, taper-point needle). **B,** Muscle (interrupted stitch). **C,** Anterior fascia (interrupted stitch, cutting needle). **D,** Subcutaneous (not always sutured, taper-point needle). **E,** Skin (interrupted stitch, cutting needle). **F,** Retention sutures. Note bumpers to protect skin.

the danger of sudden increases in intraabdominal pressure is over, usually on the fourth or fifth postoperative day. Retention sutures are also used to support wounds for healing by second intention and for secondary closure following wound disruption for healing by third intention.

Retention Bridges, Bolsters, and Bumpers

To prevent heavy retention suture from cutting into skin, several different types of bridges, bolsters, or bumpers are used, as follows:

1. Bridges are plastic devices placed on the skin to span the incision. The retention suture is brought through the skin on both sides of the incision and through holes on each side of the bridge and is fastened over the bridge. One type allows adjustment of tension on the suture during the postoperative healing period.
2. Bolsters and bumpers—the names are used interchangeably—are segments of plastic or rubber tubing. One end of the suture is threaded through the tubing before the suture is tied. It covers all of the retention suture strand that is on the skin surface (Figure 30-3, *F*). Compression bolsters are made from polyethylene foam held in place with malleable aluminum buttons to secure and distribute tension of retention sutures.
3. Buttons and beads are used as bolsters and bumpers to prevent the suture from retracting or cutting into skin or friable tissue. The suture is pulled through holes and

tied over a button (e.g., with pull-out tendon sutures). Beads may be placed on the ends of pull-out subcuticular skin sutures. The devices are used most frequently in plastic and orthopaedic surgery.

Traction Suture

A traction suture may be used to retract tissue to the side or out of the way, such as the tongue in a surgical procedure in the mouth. Usually a nonabsorbable suture is placed through the part. Other materials may be used to retract or ligate vessels, including the following:

- *Umbilical tape.* Aside from its original use for tying the umbilical cord on a newborn, umbilical tape may be used as a heavy tie or as a traction suture. It may be placed around a portion of bowel or a great vessel to retract it. These should be counted and accounted for at the end of the procedure.
- *Vessel loop.* A length of flat silicone can be placed around a vessel, nerve, or other tubular structure for retraction. It can be tightened around a blood vessel for temporary vascular occlusion. These should be counted and accounted for at the end of the procedure.
- *Aneurysm needle.* An aneurysm needle is an instrument with a blunt needle on the end. The eye is on the distal end of the needle. The needle forms a right or oblique angle to the handle, which is one continuous unit with the needle. The needles are made in symmetric pairs

right and left. The surgeon uses them to place a ligature around a deep, large vessel, such as in a thyroidectomy or in thoracic surgery. These should be counted and accounted for at the end of the procedure.

Endoscopic Suturing

Endoscopic sutures are available as ligatures and preknotted loops or with curved or straight, permanently swaged needles for use through an endoscope. The ligatures are fashioned into loosely knotted loops before being passed through the endoscope to tie off vessels and tissue pedicles. After the loop is placed around the target site, the knot is slid into position and tightened. The ends are cut with endoscopic scissors and removed through the endoscope. Suture with a permanently swaged needle is placed through either a 3-mm suture introducer for a straight needle or an 8-mm suture introducer for a curved needle. Used to suture vessels, reconstruct organs, approximate opposing tissue surfaces, and anastomose tubular structures, the technique varies according to the method used for knot tying. The methods of endoscopic knot tying are as follows:

1. *Extracorporeal method.* The swaged needle and both ends of the suture are brought outside the body through the trocar. The needle is cut off, and the knot is loosely fashioned. The knot is reintroduced into the body through the trocar by means of a knot-sliding cannula. It is snugged into position and tightened against the tissue. The ends of the suture are cut close to the knot with endoscopic scissors. Excess suture ends are removed through the endoscope.
2. *Intracorporeal method.* The needle and suture are passed through the tissue with an endoscopic needleholder. Endoscopic instruments are used to tie the knot and cut the suture inside the body.

Specifications for Suture Material

1. It must be sterile when placed in tissue. Sterile techniques must be rigidly followed in handling suture material. For example, if the end of a strand drops over the side of any sterile surface, discard the strand. Almost all postoperative wound infections are initiated along or adjacent to suture lines. Affinity for bacterial contamination varies with the physical characteristics of the material.
2. It must be predictably uniform in tensile strength by size and material. Tensile strength is the measured pounds of tension or pull that a strand will withstand before it breaks when knotted. Minimum knot-pull strengths are specified for each basic raw material and for each size of that material by the U.S. Pharmacopeia (USP). Tensile strength decreases as the diameter of the strand decreases.
3. It must be as small in diameter as is safe to use on each type of tissue. The strength of the suture usually need be no greater than the strength of the tissue on which it is used. Smaller sizes are less traumatic during placement in tissue and leave less suture mass to cause tissue reaction. The surgeon ties small-diameter sutures more gently and thus is less apt to strangulate tissue. A small-diameter suture is flexible, easy to manipulate, and leaves minimal scar on skin.
4. USP-determined sizes range from heavy 10 (largest) to very fine 12-0 (smallest); ranges vary with materials. Taking size 1 as a starting point, sizes increase with each number above 1 and decrease with each 0 added. The more 0s in the number, the smaller the size of the strand. As the number of 0s increases, the size of the strand decreases. In addition to this system of size designation, the manufacturer's labels on boxes and packets may include metric measures for suture diameters. These metric equivalents vary slightly by types of materials. Box 30-2 shows how suture gauge is measured in numeric descriptions from smallest to largest.
5. It must have knot security, remain tied, and give support to tissue during the healing process. However, sutures in the skin are always removed 3 to 10 days postoperatively, depending on the site of incision and cosmetic result desired. Because they are exposed to the external environment, skin sutures can be a source of microbial contamination of the wound that inhibits healing by first intention.
6. It must cause as little foreign body tissue reaction as possible. All suture materials are foreign bodies, but some are more inert (less reactive) than others.

Choice of Suture Material

Surgical sutures are classified as either absorbable or nonabsorbable:

1. Absorbable sutures are sterile strands prepared from collagen derived from healthy mammals or from a synthetic polymer. They are capable of being absorbed by living mammalian tissue but may be treated to modify resistance to absorption. They may be colored by a dye approved by the Food and Drug Administration (FDA).

Box 30-2	**Suture Gauge Diagram**																		
	Smaller Gauge								**Zero**				**Larger Gauge**						
10-0	9-0	8-0	7-0	6-0	5-0	4-0	3-0	2-0	0	1	2	3	4	5	6	7	8	9	10

2. Nonabsorbable sutures are strands of natural or synthetic material that effectively resist enzymatic digestion or absorption in living tissue. During the healing process, suture mass becomes encapsulated and may remain for years in tissues without producing any ill effects. They may be dyed with a color additive approved by the FDA. They may be modified with respect to body, texture, or capillarity. Capillarity refers to a characteristic of nonabsorbable sutures that allows the passage of tissue fluids along the strand, permitting infection, if present, to be drawn along the suture line. These suture materials may be untreated or may be treated to reduce capillarity. Noncapillarity is the characteristic of some nonabsorbable sutures in which the nature of the raw material or specific processing meets USP tests that establish them as resistant to wicking transfer of body fluids.

The two classifications of suture materials are subdivided into monofilament and multifilament strands:

1. Monofilament suture is a strand consisting of a single threadlike structure that is noncapillary.
2. Multifilament suture is a strand made of more than one threadlike structure held together by braiding or twisting. This strand is capillary unless it is treated to resist capillarity or is absorbable.

The surgeon selects the type of suture material best suited to promote healing. Factors that influence choice include the following:

- Biologic characteristics of the material in tissue (e.g., absorbable vs. nonabsorbable, capillary vs. noncapillary, or inertness).
- Healing characteristics of tissue. Tissues that normally heal slowly, such as skin, fascia, and tendons, usually are closed with nonabsorbable sutures. Absorbable suture placed through the skin may cause a stitch abscess to develop because it is inclined to act as a culture medium for microorganisms in the pores of the skin. Tissues that heal rapidly, such as stomach, colon, and bladder, may be closed with absorbable sutures.
- Location and length of the incision. Cosmetic results desired may be an influencing factor.
- Presence or absence of infection, contamination, and/or drainage. If infection is present, sutures may be the origin of granuloma formation with subsequent discharge of suture and sinus formation. Foreign bodies in potentially contaminated tissues may convert contamination to infection. Foreign bodies in the presence of some body fluids may cause stone formation, as in the urinary or biliary tract.
- Patient problems such as obesity, debility, advanced age, and diseases, which influence the rate of healing and time desired for wound support.
- Physical characteristics of the material such as ease of passage through tissue, knot tying, and other personal preferences of the surgeon.

Absorbable Sutures
Surgical Gut

Surgical gut is collagen derived from the submucosa of sheep intestine or serosa of beef intestine. The intestines from these freshly slaughtered animals are sent to processing plants. There they undergo many elaborate mechanical and chemical cleaning processes before intestinal ribbons of collagen are spun into strands of various sizes, ranging from the heaviest (size 3) to the finest (size 7-0). Although the larger sizes are made from two or more ribbons, the behavior of surgical gut is that of a monofilament suture.

Surgical gut is digested by body enzymes and absorbed by tissue so that no permanent foreign body remains. The rate of absorption is influenced by the following:

- *Type of tissue.* Surgical gut is absorbed much more rapidly in serous or mucous membrane. It is absorbed slowly in subcutaneous fat.
- *Condition of tissue.* Surgical gut can be used in the presence of infection; even knots are absorbed. However, absorption takes place much more rapidly in the presence of infection.
- *General health status of the patient.* Surgical gut may be absorbed more rapidly in undernourished or diseased tissue, but in geriatric or debilitated patients it may remain for a long time.
- *Type of surgical gut.* Plain gut is untreated, but chromic gut is treated to provide greater resistance to absorption. Surgical gut may be made pliable to enhance its handling characteristics, but the process significantly reduces tensile strength.

Plain Surgical Gut Plain surgical gut loses tensile strength relatively quickly, usually in 5 to 10 days, and is digested within 70 days because collagen strands are not treated to resist absorption. Plain surgical gut is used to ligate small vessels and to suture subcutaneous fat. It is not used to suture any layers of tissue likely to be subjected to tension during healing. It is available in sizes 3 through 6-0. Usually used in its natural yellow-tan color, it may be dyed blue or black.

Fast absorbing plain surgical gut is specially treated to speed absorption and tensile strength loss. It may be used for epidermal suturing where sutures are needed for no more than a week. These sutures are used only externally on skin, not internally, particularly for facial cosmetic surgery.

Chromic Surgical Gut Chromic surgical gut is treated in a chromium salt solution to resist absorption by tissues for varying lengths of time depending on the strength of the solution and duration and method of the process. The chromicizing process either bathes each ribbon of collagen before it is spun into strands or applies solution to the finished strand. This treatment changes the color from the yellow-tan shade of plain surgical gut to a dark shade of brown. Chromic surgical gut is used for ligation of larger vessels and for suture of tissues in which nonabsorbable materials are not usually recommended because they may act as a nidus for stone formation, as in the urinary or biliary tracts. In closure of muscle or fascia, it has the disadvantage of rapidly declining tensile strength. If the absorption rate is normal, chromic surgical gut will support the wound for about 14 days, with some strength up to 21 days, and will be completely absorbed within 90 days. Sizes range from 3 through 7-0. Chromic surgical gut may be dyed blue or black.

Collagen Sutures

Collagen sutures are extruded from a homogeneous dispersion of pure collagen fibrils from the flexor tendons of beef. Both plain and chromic types are similar in appearance to surgical gut and may be dyed blue. Sizes range from 4-0 through 8-0. These sutures are used primarily in ophthalmic surgery.

Handling Characteristics of Surgical Gut and Collagen

1. Most surgical gut and collagen sutures are sealed in packets that contain fluid to keep the material pliable. This fluid is chiefly alcohol and water but may be irritating to ophthalmic tissues. Hold the packet over a basin and open carefully to avoid spilling fluid on the sterile field or splashing it into your own eyes. Rinsing is necessary only for surgical gut or collagen sutures to be implanted into the eye.
2. Surgical gut and collagen sutures should be used immediately after removal from their packets. When the material is removed and not used at once, the alcohol evaporates and the strand loses pliability. Many surgeons prefer that the scrub person quickly dip the strand into water or normal saline solution to soften it slightly. Do not soak. Excessive exposure to water will reduce the tensile strength. Before unwinding, the strand can be dipped momentarily in water or normal saline solution at room temperature; heat will coagulate the protein.
3. Unwind the strand carefully. Handle it as little as possible. Never jerk or stretch surgical gut; this weakens it. Do not straighten suture by running fingers down the length of the strand; excessive handling with rubber gloves can cause fraying. Grasp the ends and tug gently to straighten.

Synthetic Absorbable Polymers

Polymers, either dyed or undyed, are extruded into absorbable suture strands. These synthetic sutures are absorbed by a slow hydrolysis process in the presence of tissue fluids. They are used for ligating or suturing except when extended approximation of tissues under stress is required. They are inert, nonantigenic, and nonpyrogenic and produce only a mild tissue reaction during absorption. They may be monofilament or multifilament, coated or uncoated.

Polydioxanone (PDS Suture) Monofilaments extruded from polyester poly (p)-dioxanone (polydioxanone)

PDS and PDS II sutures are particularly useful in tissues in which slow healing is anticipated, as in the fascia, or where extended wound support is desirable, as in geriatric patients, but an absorbable suture is preferable. They may be used in the presence of infection; they will not harbor bacterial growth because of their chemical and monofilament construction. PDS II suture is more pliable than PDS suture. Absorption is minimal for about 90 days, then complete within 6 months. Approximately 50% of the tensile strength is retained for 4 weeks, and 25% is retained for 6 weeks. PDS suture retains its breaking strength longer than any other synthetic absorbable suture. Violet PDS suture is available in sizes 2 through 9-0, blue PDS suture is available in sizes 7-0 through 10-0 for ophthalmic tissues, and clear PDS suture is available in sizes 1 through 7-0.

Poliglecaprone 25 (Monocryl Suture) Prepared from a copolymer of glycolide and epsilon-caprolactone, Monocryl suture is the most pliable of the monofilament synthetic sutures. It retains approximately 50% to 60% of its tensile strength in tissue for 7 days, retains approximately 20% to 30% at 14 days, and loses all tensile strength by 21 days. Absorption is essentially complete between 91 and 119 days. Because of its strength retention and absorption profiles, it is indicated for use in all types of soft tissue approximation and/or ligation, especially in general, gynecologic, urologic, and plastic surgery, but it is not indicated for use in cardiovascular, neural, or ophthalmic tissues. Undyed and natural golden in color, it is available in sizes 2 through 6-0.

Polyglyconate (Maxon Suture) A monofilament is prepared from a copolymer of glycolic acid and trimethylene carbonate. It is indicated for approximation of soft tissue except in cardiovascular, neural, and ophthalmic tissues. Absorption is minimal for about 60 days, then is complete within 6 months. Approximately 70% of tensile strength remains at 2 weeks, and 55% remains at 3 weeks. Clear or dyed green, this suture is available in sizes 2 through 7-0. Maxon CV monofilament absorbable suture is available for pediatric cardiovascular and peripheral vascular procedures.

Polyglactin 910 (Vicryl Suture) The precisely controlled combination of glycolide and lactide results in a copolymer with a molecular structure that maintains tensile strength longer than surgical gut, but not as long as polydioxanone. Approximately 30% of original strength is retained at 3 weeks. Absorption is minimal for about 40 days; then it absorbs rapidly within 90 days. The acids of both glycolide and lactide exist naturally in the body and are readily excreted in urine. Polyglactin 910 sutures are available in two forms: uncoated monofilament and coated multifilament:

1. Uncoated monofilament polyglactin 910 (Vicryl suture) is available dyed violet in sizes 9-0 and 10-0 for ophthalmic procedures.
2. Coated multifilament polyglactin 910 (Coated Vicryl suture) is a braided strand coated with a mixture of

equal parts of a copolymer of glycolide and lactide (polyglactin 370) and calcium stearate. The coating provides a nonflaking lubricant for smooth passage through tissue and precise knot placement. This absorbable coating does not affect the absorption rate or tensile strength of the suture. It absorbs with the suture. Coated Vicryl suture is available dyed violet in sizes 2 through 9-0 and undyed in sizes 1 through 8-0.

Polyglycolic Acid (Dexon Suture)   The homopolymer of glycolic acid loses tensile strength more rapidly and absorbs significantly more slowly than polyglactin 910. Strands are smaller in diameter than surgical gut of equivalent tensile strength. Polyglycolic acid suture loses approximately 45% of its tensile strength by 14 days and absorbs significantly by 30 days. It is a braided suture material available in two forms: uncoated and coated:

1. Uncoated polyglycolic acid (Dexon S suture) is available dyed green in sizes 2 through 8-0 and undyed natural beige in sizes 2 through 7-0. (A 9-0 monofilament suture, dyed green, is also available.)
2. Coated polyglycolic acid (Dexon Plus suture) has a surfactant, poloxamer 188, on the surface that becomes slick in contact with body fluids for smooth passage through tissue. This suture requires two or three extra throws in knot tying, and the ends must be cut longer than for uncoated material. The coating virtually disappears from the suture site within a few hours, which may strengthen knot security. Sutures are available in the same sizes as uncoated polyglycolic acid sutures.

Handling Characteristics of Synthetic Absorbable Polymers

1. Synthetic absorbable sutures have an expiration date on the package. Therefore rotate stock. "First in, first out" is a good rule to follow.
2. Sutures are packaged and used dry. Do not soak or dip in water or normal saline solution. The material hydrolyzes in water, so excessive exposure to moisture will reduce the tensile strength. It is smooth, soft, and will retain its pliability.

Nonabsorbable Sutures
Surgical Silk

Surgical silk is an animal product made from the fiber spun by silkworm larvae in making their cocoons. From the raw state, each fiber is processed to remove natural waxes and gums. Fibers are braided or twisted together to form a multifilament suture strand. The braided type is used more frequently because surgeons prefer its high tensile strength and better handling qualities. Surgical silk is treated to render it noncapillary. It also is dyed, most commonly black, but it is also available in white. Sizes range from 5 through 9-0. Silk sutures are used dry. They lose tensile strength if wet. Therefore they should not be moistened before use.

Silk is not a truly nonabsorbable material. It loses much of its tensile strength after about 1 year and usually disappears within 2 years. It gives good support to wounds during early ambulation and generally promotes rapid healing. It causes less tissue reaction than surgical gut, but it is not as inert as most of the other nonabsorbable materials. It is used frequently in the serosa of the gastrointestinal tract and to close fascia in the absence of infection.

Virgin Silk   Virgin silk suture consists of several natural silk filaments drawn together and twisted to form 8-0 and 9-0 strands for tissue approximation of delicate structures, primarily in ophthalmic surgery. It is white or dyed black.

Dermal Silk   Dermal suture is a strand of twisted silk fibers encased in a nonabsorbing coating of tanned gelatin or other protein substance. This coating prevents ingrowth of tissue cells and facilitates removal after use as a skin suture. Because of its unusual strength, it is used for suturing skin, particularly in areas of tension. It is black and comes in sizes 0 through 5-0.

Surgical Cotton

Cotton is a natural cellulose fiber. Suture is made from individual, long-staple cotton fibers that are cleaned, combed, aligned, and twisted into a smooth multifilament strand. Sizes range from 1 through 5-0. Usually white, it may be dyed blue or pink.

Cotton is one of the weakest of the nonabsorbable materials; however, it gains tensile strength when wet. It should be moistened before it is handed to the surgeon. Tensile strength is increased 10% by moisture. Also, moisture prevents clinging to the surgeon's gloves. Like silk, cotton suture may be used in most body tissues for ligating and suturing, but it offers no advantages over silk. It is rarely used, with the exception of umbilical tape.

Surgical Stainless Steel

Stainless steel sutures are drawn from 316L-SS (*L* for low carbon) iron alloy wire. This is the same metal formula used in the manufacture of surgical stainless steel implants and prostheses.

Two different kinds of metal should not be embedded in the tissues simultaneously. Such a combination creates an unfavorable electrolytic reaction. Some implants and prostheses are made of Vitallium, titanium, or tantalum. Suture material in the wound must be compatible with these metals.

Before the availability of surgical stainless steel from suture manufacturers, commercial steel was purchased by weight, using the Brown and Sharpe (B&S) scale for diameter variations. Many surgeons still refer to surgical stainless steel size by the B&S gauge from 18, the largest diameter, to 40, the smallest. One manufacturer labels surgical stainless steel with both B&S gauge and equivalent USP diameter classifications from 7 through 6-0. Both monofilament and twisted multifilament stainless steel strands are available.

Surgical stainless steel is inert in tissue and has high tensile strength. It gives the greatest strength of any suture material to a wound before healing begins and supports a wound indefinitely. Some surgeons use stainless steel for abdominal wall or sternal closure or for retention sutures to reduce the danger of wound disruption in the presence of contributing factors. It may be used in the presence of infection or in patients in whom slow healing is expected. It is used for secondary repair or resuture following wound disruption.

Unlike most other suture materials, steel lacks elasticity. A suture tied too tightly may act as a knife and cut through tissue. Stainless steel sutures are harder to handle than any other suture material. A painstaking knot-tying technique is required. For most surgeons this disadvantage more than outweighs the advantages for routine use. However, in selected situations it fills an important need. It is used in the respiratory tract, in tendon repair, in orthopaedics and neurosurgery, and for general wound closure.

Handling Characteristics of Surgical Stainless Steel

1. Surgical stainless steel strands are malleable and kink rather easily. Kinks in the strand can make it practically useless. Therefore care must be taken in handling to keep the strand straight.
2. Use wire scissors for cutting stainless steel sutures. Barbs on the end of a strand can tear gloves, puncture the skin, or traumatize tissue.
3. If surgical stainless steel must be threaded through a needle, some surgeons prefer one or two twists of the end around the strand just below the eye of the needle to prevent unthreading during suturing.

Synthetic Nonabsorbable Polymers

Although silk is the most frequently used nonabsorbable suture material, synthetic nonabsorbable materials are used because they offer unique advantages in many situations. They have higher tensile strength and elicit less tissue reaction than silk. They retain their strength in tissue. Knot tying with most of these materials is more difficult than with silk. Additional throws are required to secure the knot. The surgeon may sacrifice some handling characteristics and ease of knot tying for strength, durability, and nonreactivity of the synthetics. These advantages may outweigh the disadvantages.

Surgical Nylon
Nylon is a polyamide polymer derived by chemical synthesis from coal, air, and water. It produces minimal tissue reaction. Nylon has high tensile strength, but it degrades by hydrolysis in tissue at a rate of about 15% to 20% per year. It may be used in all tissues where a nonabsorbable suture is acceptable, except when long-term support is critical. It is available in three forms: monofilament, uncoated multifilament, and coated multifilament:

1. Monofilament nylon (Ethilon suture and Dermalon suture) is a smooth single strand of noncapillary material, clear or dyed black, blue, or green. The smaller the diameter becomes, the stronger the strand becomes proportionately. Sizes range from 2 through 11-0; the latter is the smallest of all sutures manufactured for use in microsurgery. Monofilament nylon is also used frequently in ophthalmic surgery because it has a desirable degree of elasticity. Larger sizes are used for skin closure, particularly in plastic surgery, where cosmetic results are important, and for retention sutures. Wet or damp monofilament nylon is more pliable and easier to handle than dry nylon. A limited line of sutures is supplied in a moisturized state; most are supplied dry.
2. Uncoated multifilament nylon (Nurolon suture) is very tightly braided and treated to prevent capillary action. Usually dyed black but also available in white, nylon looks, feels, and handles similarly to silk, but it is stronger and elicits less tissue reaction. Sizes range from 1 through 7-0. It may be used in all tissues in which a multifilament nonabsorbable suture is acceptable.
3. Coated multifilament nylon (Surgilon suture) is a braided strand of nylon treated with silicone to enhance its passage through tissue. Otherwise its characteristics are similar to silk and uncoated multifilament nylon.

Polyester Fiber
A polymer of terephthalic acid and polyethylene, Dacron polyester fiber is braided into a multifilament suture strand that is available in two forms: uncoated and coated fibers:

1. Uncoated polyester fiber suture (Mersilene suture and Dacron) is closely braided to provide a flexible, pliable strand that is relatively easy to handle. However, uncoated braided polyester fiber suture has a tendency to drag and exert a sawing or tearing effect when passed through tissue. It may be used in all tissues in which a multifilament nonabsorbable suture is indicated. It is especially useful in the respiratory tract and for some cardiovascular procedures. Available white or dyed green or blue, sizes range from 2 through 11-0.
2. Coated polyester fiber suture has a lubricated surface for smooth passage through tissue. It is widely used in cardiovascular surgery for vessel anastomosis and placement of prosthetic materials because it retains its strength indefinitely in tissues. Sutures are available with different coating materials:
   a. Polybutilate is the only coating developed specifically as a surgical lubricant. This polyester material adheres strongly to the braided polyester fiber. Polyester fiber coated with polybutilate (Ethibond suture) provides a strand superior to any other braided material, coated or uncoated, in decreasing drag through tissue. Colored green or white, sizes range from 5 through 7-0.
   b. Polytetrafluoroethylene, a commercial product of DuPont named Teflon, is used as a coating bonded to the surface (Polydek suture) or impregnated into spaces in the braid of the polyester fiber strand (Tevdek suture). Minute particles of this coating can flake off the strand. Because these particles are insoluble and resistant to enzymes, foreign body granulomas may be produced. Sutures with this material on them are white or dyed green and are available in sizes 5 through 10-0.

c. Silicone, a commercial lubricant, provides a slippery coating but does not bond well to polyester fiber. It can become dislodged in tissues as the strand is tied. Sutures with this coating (Ti-Cron sutures) are available white or dyed blue in sizes 5 through 7-0.

Polybutester (Novafil Suture)   A copolymer of poly (glycol)–terephthalate and poly (butylene)–terephthalate is extruded into a monofilament strand. It is more flexible and elastic than other synthetic polymers, which may be a physiologic advantage in limited circumstances for apposing wound edges. It is available clear or dyed blue in sizes 2 through 10-0.

Polyethylene (Dermalene Suture)   A long-chain polyethylene polymer is extruded into a monofilament strand. It is available dyed blue in sizes 0 through 6-0 for use in some situations in which a monofilament material is desirable.

Polypropylene (Prolene Suture and Surgilene Suture)   A polymerized propylene is extruded into a monofilament strand. It is the most inert of the synthetic materials and almost as inert as stainless steel. Polypropylene is an acceptable substitute for stainless steel in situations in which strength and nonreactivity are required, and it is easier to handle. The suture may be left in place for prolonged healing. It can be used in the presence of infection. It has become the material of choice for many plastic surgery and cardiovascular procedures because of its smooth passage through tissues, as well as its strength and inertness. It is frequently used for continuous abdominal fascia closure, as a subcuticular pull-out suture, and for retention sutures. It is available dyed blue in sizes 2 through 10-0 and clear in sizes 4-0 through 6-0.

Handling Characteristics of Synthetic Nonabsorbable Polymers

1. Physical damage to suture materials can occur from the time the suture is removed from a packet if the strand is mishandled. Handle all sutures and needles as little as possible. Avoid pulling or stretching. Sutures should be handled without using instruments except when grasping the free end during an instrument tie. Clamping instruments, especially needleholders and forceps with serrations, on strands can crush, cut, and weaken them.
2. All synthetic materials require a specific knot-tying technique. Knot security requires additional flat and square ties. Multifilament materials are generally easier to tie than monofilament sutures.

SURGICAL NEEDLES

Except for simple ligating with free ties, surgical needles are needed to safely carry suture material through tissue with the least amount of trauma. The best surgical needles are made of high-quality tempered steel that is:

- Strong enough so that it does not break easily
- Rigid enough to prevent excessive bending, yet flexible enough to prevent breaking after bending

- Sharp enough to penetrate tissue with minimal resistance (yet it need not be stronger than the tissue it penetrates)
- Approximately the same diameter as the suture material it carries to minimize trauma in passage through tissue
- Appropriate in shape and size for the type, condition, and accessibility of the tissue to be sutured
- Free from corrosion and burrs to prevent infection and tissue trauma

Because needles are made of steel, they are theoretically detectable by x-ray if inadvertently lost in tissue. The location in tissue may preclude the needle from appearing on an x-ray film. For example, the angle of the needle or its position behind bone may obstruct detection. The smaller the size of the needle, the more likely the image is to be obstructed. All needles should be accounted for so that they do not become foreign bodies in tissue.

Many shapes and sizes of surgical needles are available. Names vary from one manufacturer to another; general classification only, not nomenclature, is standardized. They may be straight like a sewing needle or curved. All surgical needles have three basic components: the point, the body (or shaft), and the eye. They are classified according to these three components.

Point of the Needle

Points of surgical needles are honed to the configuration and sharpness desired for specific types of tissue. The basic shapes are cutting, tapered, or blunt (Figure 30-4).

Figure 30-4   Configurations of needle points. **A,** Conventional cutting and reverse cutting. **B,** Side cutting. **C,** Cutting edge at end of tapered body with, **D,** trocar point. **E,** Taper. **F,** Blunt.

| TABLE 30-1 | Select Examples of Common Taper-Point Needles (Alphanumeric Codes) and Representative Manufacturers |

Purpose	Ethicon	Davis and Geck	U.S. Surgical	Configuration
General closure	CT	T 25	GS 24	½ circle taper 40 mm
General closure	CT 1	T 12	GS 21	37 mm
Cardiovascular	RB	T 31	EV 23	17 mm
Gastrointestinal	SH	T 5	EV 20	25 mm
Multilayer closure	CTX	T 20	GS 25	48 mm
Cardiovascular	BB	TE 7	CV 15	⅜ circle taper 17 mm
Urologic	UR 6	TT 2	GU 46	⅝ circle taper 27 mm

Cutting Point

A razor-sharp honed cutting point may be preferred when tissue is difficult to penetrate, such as skin, tendon, and tough tissues in the eye. These make a slight cut in tissue as they penetrate. The location and degree of sharpness of cutting edges vary.

Conventional-Cutting Needles Two opposing cutting edges form a triangular configuration with a third edge on the body of the needle. Cutting edges are on the inside curvature of a curved needle. Cutting edges may be honed to precision sharpness to ensure smooth passage through tissue and a minute needle path that heals quickly.

Reverse-Cutting Needles A triangular configuration extends along the body of the needle. The edges near the point are sharpened or honed to precision points. The two opposing cutting edges are on the outer curvature of a curved needle.

Side-Cutting Needles Relatively flat on the top and bottom, angulated cutting edges are on the sides. Used primarily in ophthalmic surgery, they will not penetrate underlying tissues. They split through layers of tissue.

Trocar Points Sharp cutting tips are at the points of tapered needles. All three edges of the tip are sharpened to provide cutting action with the smallest possible hole in tissue as it penetrates.

Taper Point

These needles are used in soft tissues, such as intestine and peritoneum, which offer a small amount of resistance to the needle as it passes through. They tend to push the tissue aside as they go through rather than cut it. The body tapers to a sharp point at the tip.

Blunt Point

These tapered needles are designed with a rounded blunt point at the tip. They are used primarily for suturing friable tissue, such as liver and kidney. Because the blunt point will not cut through tissue, it is less apt to puncture a vessel in these organs than is a sharp-pointed needle. Blunt needles may also be used in some tissues to reduce the potential for needle sticks, especially in general and gynecologic surgery.

Body of the Needle

The body, or shaft, varies in wire gauge, length, shape, and finish. The nature and location of tissue to be sutured influences the selection of needles with these variable features. Most manufacturers have designated a specific alphanumeric code to describe each needle they produce. Examples of alphanumeric codes for taper-point needles can be found in Table 30-1.

Considerations relating to the body of the needle are as follows:

1. Tough or fibrosed tissue requires a heavier-gauge needle than the fine-gauge wire needed in microsurgery.
2. The depth of the bite (placement) through tissue determines the appropriate needle length.
3. The body of the needle may be round, oval, flat, or triangular. The point determines the shape: round or oval bodies have trocar, taper, or blunt points; flat or triangular bodies have cutting edges. The shape may also be straight or curved (Figure 30-5).
   a. Straight needles are used in readily accessible tissue. They have cutting points for use in skin, which is their most frequent use, or tapered points for use in intestinal tissue.
   b. Curved needles are used to approximate most tissues because quick needle turnout is an advantage. The curvature may be ¼, ⅜, ½, ⅝, circle, half-curved with only the tip curved, or compound curved. Curved needles always are armed in a needleholder before being handed to the surgeon.
   c. J-shaped needles range from 15.5 cm to 17.5 cm in length. The width of the J bend at the tip is available

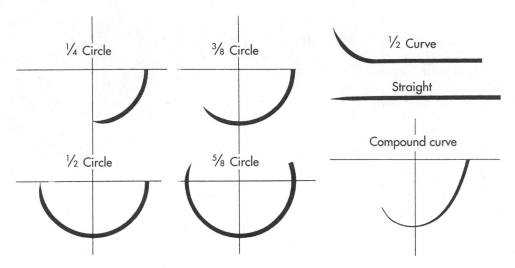

Figure 30-5 Shapes of needle bodies.

in 7- to 9-mm curvature. They are used for 10- to 14-mm fascial incisions created for trocar use during laparoscopy. They are multiuse needles that can be threaded with the suture of the surgeon's choice at the point of use. Their unique shape enables the surgeon to close the deep layers of the wound without perforation of underlying organs while visualizing closure of the accessory ports with the laparoscopic camera.

4. Curved needles that have longitudinal ribbed depressions or grooves along the body on the inside and outside curvature can be cross locked in the needleholder. This feature virtually eliminates twisting or turning of the needle in any position in the needleholder.

5. In all needles the body must have a smooth finish. Many needles have a surface coating of microthin plastic or silicone to enhance smooth passage through tissue. Others have a black surface finish to enhance visibility at the surgical site.

Eye of the Needle

The eye is the segment of the needle where the suture strand is attached. Surgical needles are classified as eyed, French eye, or eyeless (also known as swaged or atraumatic) (Figure 30-6).

Eyed Needle

The closed eye of an eyed surgical needle is like that of any household sewing needle. The shape of the enclosed eye may be round, oblong, or square. The end of the suture strand is pulled 2 to 4 inches (5 to 10 cm) through the eye so that the short end is about one sixth the length of the long end.

French Eye Needle

Sometimes referred to as spring eye or split eye, a French eye needle has a slit from the inside of the eye to the end of the needle through which the suture strand is drawn. To thread a French eye after arming the needle in a needleholder, 2 to 3 inches (5 to 7.5 cm) of the strand is secured between the fin-

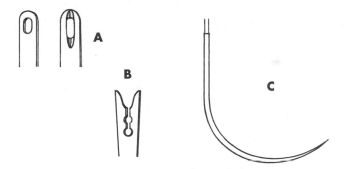

Figure 30-6 Eyes of needles. **A,** Oblong eyes. **B,** French eye. **C,** Eyeless (swaged).

Figure 30-7 To thread French eye needle, pull strand taut across center of V-shaped area and draw down through slit into eye.

gers holding the needleholder. The strand is pulled taut across the center of the V-shaped area above the eye and drawn down through the slit into the eye (Figure 30-7). French eye needles as a general rule are used with pliable braided materials, primarily silk and cotton, of medium or fine size. These needles are not practical for surgical gut; the strand may fray, or the eye may break because the diameter is usually too large for the slit.

Handling of Eyed and French Eye Needles

Eyed and French eye needles have the following disadvantages for the scrub person, surgeon, and patient:

1. Each needle must be carefully inspected by the scrub person before and after use for dull or burred points, corrosion, and defects in the eye.
2. Care must be taken to avoid puncturing gloves with the needle point when threading.
3. If the scrub person must choose an appropriate needle to thread, the needle should be the same approximate diameter as the suture size requested by the surgeon.
4. Needles can unthread prematurely. This is an annoyance to the surgeon and prolongs operating time for the patient. To avoid this, the surgeon may prefer the suture strand threaded double with both ends pulled the same length through the eye; the ends may be tied together in a knot, if desired. Or the scrub person may lock the suture strand by threading the short end through the eye twice in the same direction.
5. Two strands of suture material are pulled through tissue when threaded needles are used. The bulk of the double strand through the eye creates a larger hole than the size of the needle or suture material, causing additional trauma to tissue.

Eyeless Needle

An eyeless needle is a continuous unit with the suture strand. The needle is swaged onto the end of the strand in the manufacturing process. This eliminates threading at the operating bed and minimizes tissue trauma because a single strand of material is drawn through tissue (Figure 30-8). The diameter of the needle matches the size of the strand as closely as possible. The surgeon uses a new sharp needle with every suture strand. Usually referred to as swaged needles, four types of eyeless needle-suture attachments are available.

Single-Armed Attachment   One needle is swaged to a suture strand.

Double-Armed Attachment   A needle is swaged to each end of the suture strand. The two needles are not necessarily the same size and shape. These are used when the surgeon wishes to place a suture and then continue to approximate surrounding tissue on both sides from a midpoint in the strand.

Permanently Swaged Needle Attachment This attachment is secure, so the needle will not separate from the suture strand under normal use. The needle is separated by cutting it from the strand.

Controlled-Release Needle Attachment   This attachment is secure, so the suture strand will not separate

Figure 30-8   Tissue effects of needle penetration. **A,** Threaded. **B,** Swaged atraumatic.

from the needle inadvertently, but it will release rapidly when pulled off intentionally. The surgeon grasps the suture strand just below the needle, pulling the strand taut, and releases the needle with a straight tug of the needleholder on the needle. This facilitates fast separation of the needle from the suture when desired. This type of needle is referred to as a "pop-off" needle.

Placement of the Needle in the Needleholder

Needleholders have specially designed jaws to securely grasp surgical needles without damage if they are used correctly. The scrub person should observe the following principles in handling needles and needleholders:

1. Select a needleholder with appropriate-size jaws for the size of the needle to be used. An extremely small needle requires a needleholder with very fine tipped jaws. As the wire gauge of the needle increases, the jaws of the needleholder selected should be proportionately wider and heavier. Curved jaws or angulated handles may be needed for placement of the needle in tissues.
2. Select an appropriate-length needleholder for the area of tissue to be sutured. When the surgeon works deep inside the abdomen, chest, or pelvic cavity, a longer needleholder will be needed than in superficial areas.

Figure 30-9 Correct position of curved needle in needleholder, about one third down from swage or eye.

3. Clamp the body of the needle in an area one fourth to one half of the distance from the eye to the point (Figure 30-9). Never clamp the needleholder over the swaged area. This is the weakest area of an eyeless needle because it is hollow before the suture strand is attached. Pressure on or near the needle-suture juncture may break the needle.

4. Place the needle securely in the tip of the needleholder jaws and close the needleholder in the first or second ratchet. If the needle is held too tightly in the jaws or the needleholder is defective, the needle may be damaged or notched in such a manner that it will have a tendency to bend or break on successive passes through tissue.

5. Pass the needleholder with the needle point up and directed toward the surgeon's thumb when grasped so that it is ready for use without readjustment. If a hand-free technique is preferred, place the needleholder on a tray or magnetic mat with the needle point down.

6. Hand the needleholder to the surgeon so that the suture strand is free and not entangled with the needleholder. Hold the free end of the suture in one hand while passing the needleholder with the other hand. Protect the end of the suture material from dragging across the sterile field. The assistant may take hold of the free end to keep the strand straight for the surgeon and to keep it from falling over the side of the sterile field.

7. Hand the needleholder to an assistant to pull the needle out through tissue. A hemostat or other tissue forceps is not used for this purpose because the instrument may be damaged or may damage the needle. The needle should be grasped as far back as possible to avoid damage to the taper point or cutting edges.

CONSIDERATIONS IN THE CHOICE OF NEEDLE AND SUTURE

The surgeon chooses from available types and sizes of sutures and needles the ones that best suit each purpose. In general, fine sizes are used for plastic, ophthalmic, pediatric, and vascular surgery; medium sizes are used for all other kinds of surgery; heavy sizes are used for retention and for anchoring bone. In general, cutting needles are used in tough tissue such as skin, fascia, tendon, and mucous membranes, including the cervix, palate, tongue, and nose. Medium tissue calls for round taper-point or cutting needles. Round taper-point needles usually are used for nerve, peritoneum, muscle, and other soft tissue, such as lung and intestine, subcutaneous tissue, and dura.

It is almost impossible to learn the needle-tissue-suture-surgeon combinations by memory alone because of the unlimited number of combinations. Learning the general classification of needles, sutures, and tissues is the first step; practical experience is necessary to remember the combinations. One should not feel discouraged by not being able to anticipate the surgeon's wishes and should not hesitate to ask if uncertain of the proper combination at the proper time.

The preference card usually lists the surgeon's usual suture-and-needle routine by tissue layer. Some cards list swaged sutures by order number. Others list sutures by size and materials and needles by size and shape. Suture and needle sizes are as variable as patient sizes. Therefore the surgeon may unexpectedly request a smaller or larger size out of routine for a particular patient's situation. Each manufacturer produces different needle styles. Most types have a comparable counterpart in another brand name. Table 30-1 describes cross-referencing of needle types by alphanumeric codes between different manufacturers.

SUTURES AND NEEDLES: PACKAGING AND PREPARATION

Most suture material is individually packaged and supplied sterile by the manufacturer. It is sterilized by cobalt-60 irradiation or ethylene oxide gas. A few materials can be steam sterilized, but most cannot. Protein in absorbable materials derived from animals will coagulate; synthetic absorbable materials are affected by moisture and heat. Only stainless steel can be repeatedly steam sterilized. Nylon, polyester fiber, and polypropylene can be steam sterilized a maximum of three times without loss of tensile strength. The manufacturer's recommendations should be followed for sterilization of nonsterile suture materials.

Swaged needles come in sterile packets with the suture material. They eliminate the labor and expense of cleaning, packaging, and sterilizing needles. Disposable eyed and French eye needles are packaged and sterilized by the manufacturer. Needles are counted when dispensed to the sterile field.

Preparation of Reusable Needles

Standard sets of reusable eyed and French eye needles may be prepared for each surgical procedure. This necessitates preparing many more needles in a set than any one surgeon uses if each surgeon's preferences are to be accommodated. An alternative may be to choose needles for each procedure on the surgical schedule according to each surgeon's preferences as listed on the preference card.

Eyed needles can be loaded on a metal rack with a spring to hold them. The rack can be steam sterilized with the instruments for that surgical procedure, or it may be wrapped, labeled, and sterilized separately. Needles are counted before and after use.

Packaging of Suture Materials

A strand of sterile suture material is supplied with as many as four coverings.

Box

Each box contains one, two, or three dozen packets of sterile suture material. The label on the box may be color coded by suture material (e.g., light blue for silk, yellow for plain surgical gut). Most boxes fit into a suture cabinet rack. Competing manufacturers frequently select similar colors as their competitors for box labels and suture material identification.

Overwrap

Each packet has a sealed outer overwrap. The overwrap is peeled back to expose the inner primary packet for sterile transfer to the sterile table. The circulator must not contaminate the sterile inner primary packet as the overwrap is peeled apart and the packet is transferred onto the sterile table or presented to the scrub person.

Primary Packet

Suture material, with or without swaged needles, is sealed in a primary inner packet that is opened by the scrub person. The primary packet may be made of foil, paper, plastic, or combinations of these. Labels may be color coded by material, the same as the box. If a swaged needle is enclosed, a silhouette of the needle is included on the label, along with the size and type of suture material. A single strand of material or multiple strands may be in the primary packet. The packet may be designed for dispensing individual strands from a multiple suture packet. Packaging configurations and considerations include the following:

1. Suture packets, both overwrap and primary, should be opened only as needed to minimize waste.
2. Custom kits with multiple suture packets within a single package facilitate dispensing sutures to and organizing them on the sterile table. The kit may have appropriate sutures, with or without swaged needles, to meet the requirements of a particular surgeon or procedure. The packets are organized in order of use. The contents are listed on the cover of the package to facilitate counts.
3. Sterile suture packets are labeled "Do Not Resterilize." Component layers of the packaging materials cannot withstand exposure to the heat of steam sterilization without potential physical damage to the contents and packets. The manufacturer will not guarantee product

Figure 30-10 Scrub person preparing one-third length sutures. One free end of full-length strand is passed from right to left hand. At same time loop is caught around third finger of right hand. Other loop is caught around third finger of left hand while each end is held and suture is adjusted to equal lengths (thirds). Then each loop is cut with scissors.

stability or sterility for packets resterilized in the hospital or in secondary processors, or for strands removed from packets and sterilized.
4. Some suture materials have an expiration date stamped on the box and primary packet to indicate the shelf life of the material. Oldest sutures should be used first.

Inner Dispenser

Suture material is contained within the primary packet in a manner that facilitates removing or dispensing it. This may be a folder, reel, organizer, or tube that may or may not be removed with the suture strands.

Preparation of Suture Material

The length of each strand of suture material within the primary packet varies; the shortest is 5 inches (approximately 13 cm), and the longest is 60 inches (150 cm). The most commonly used lengths range from 18 to 30 inches (45 to 75 cm). The length the surgeon prefers should be noted on the preference card. The scrub person may have to cut the strands to the desired length, depending on the lengths available.

Standard Length

The term *standard length* refers to a 60-inch (150-cm) strand of nonabsorbable material or a 54-inch (135-cm) strand of absorbable material without a swaged needle. It is never handed to the surgeon in this length. The scrub person may cut it into a half-length, third-length, or fourth-length for use as a free tie or thread it for a stick tie or suture as shown in Figures 30-10 and 30-11.

Ligating Reels

Twelve-foot (approximately 4-m) lengths of nonabsorbable or 54-inch (135-cm) lengths of absorbable suture are wound on plastic reels. These reels are color coded by material and have size identification. The surgeon keeps the reel in the palm of the hand for a series of free ties. The reel is radi-

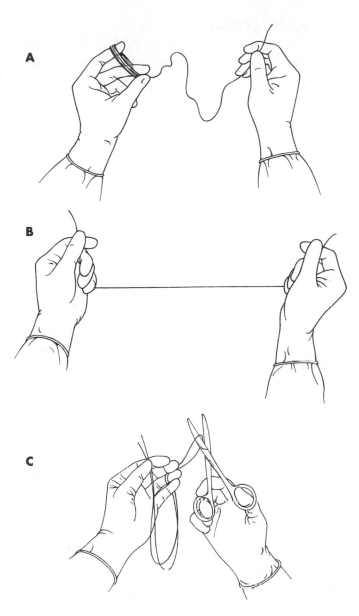

Figure 30-11 Sequence of scrub person preparing half-lengths. **A,** Suture loops are separated by fingers of left hand while unwinding. **B,** Full length is gently unwound and straightened before cutting. Scrub person does not pull hard or test strand, but keeps firm grasp on both ends to prevent suture from snapping away and possibly becoming contaminated. **C,** Suture is bent in half, and loop is cut.

opaque in case it is inadvertently dropped in a body cavity. If reels are not stocked, the surgeon may ask the scrub person to wind a standard length onto a rod or other device for this purpose.

Precut Lengths

Most suture materials are supplied in precut lengths of 12 to 18 inches and are ready for use as free ties or for threading. These facilitate handling for the scrub person. They are dispensed individually from some primary packets or may be removed and placed in a fold of the suture book. Packets contain from 3 to 17 strands, depending on the material.

Swaged Needle-Suture

Lengths of sutures are predetermined by the manufacturer; however, the surgeon has a wide variety of choices to meet all suturing needs. The scrub person must remember that a strand can be shortened but not extended. An appropriate length for location of tissue must be handed to the surgeon. A packet may contain one suture strand armed with a single or double needle(s) or multiple strands with swaged needles. The needle may be armed in a needleholder and withdrawn from the inner dispenser of some packets.

SURGICAL STAPLES

Surgeons can join many tissues with staples. This involves inserting stainless steel or titanium staples through tissues with a stapler, a device specifically designed for this purpose. Some surgical procedures have become simplified or feasible since the advent of surgical stapling techniques. As Hültl recognized in 1908, for stapling to be successful, fine wire as the basic material must form a B shape. This shape allows blood to flow through tissues, preventing necrosis secondary to devascularization beyond the staple line. Sufficient pressure must be exerted, however, to provide hemostasis of cut tissues. The length and width of the staples must accommodate tissue being approximated or transected. The number of staples varies with the length of the staple line.

Advantages of Using Staples

Staples can be used safely in many types of tissues and have a wide range of applications:

1. Stapling is a rapid method of ligating, anastomosing, and approximating tissues. The time saved, as compared with suturing techniques, reduces blood loss and the total operating and anesthesia time for the patient.
2. Wound healing may be accelerated because of minimal trauma and the nonreactive nature of metallic staples.
3. Staples produce an even surface and an airtight, leakproof closure.
4. Staples can be placed through an endoscope.

Stapling Instruments

Each stapler is designed for stapling specific tissues (i.e., skin, fascia, bronchus, gastrointestinal tract, or vessels). The surgeon selects the correct instrument for the desired application. The consequences of an erroneous staple application, however, are much more difficult to correct than those of manually placed sutures. The surgeon must learn when and how to use each instrument. Whether the stapler is reusable or a single-use disposable, the basic technical mechanics of stapling are the same.

Staplers either fire a single staple or simultaneously fire straight or circular rows of staples. A different instrument must be used for each type of firing.

Skin Stapler

To approximate skin edges, the stapler fires a single staple with each squeeze of the trigger. Edges of both cuticular and subcuticular layers are aligned with the edges slightly raised in an everted direction, as close to their original configuration on the horizontal plane as possible. The stapler is positioned over the line of incision so that the staple will be placed evenly on each side. The staple forms a rectangular shape over the incision. As many staples are placed as needed to close the incision. Skin staplers are supplied preloaded with different quantities of staples in varying widths (i.e., crown span). The most appropriate stapler should be chosen for the selected use. For example, an average range of 28 to 35 staples is needed to close most abdominal incisions. More may be needed to close the chest; fewer may be needed for an inguinal herniorrhaphy.

Skin staples are removed 5 to 7 days postoperatively. Extractors are used for this purpose. As it heals, the skin flattens out to form an even surface with excellent cosmetic results if the staples have been properly placed lightly over the skin. Imbedded staples are difficult to remove, and results may be less than desired.

Linear Stapler

Two staggered or side-by-side straight double rows of staples are placed simultaneously in tissue with a linear stapler. This stapler is used throughout the alimentary tract and in thoracic surgery for transection and resection of internal tissues. The tissue is positioned in the straight jaws, of appropriate length, of the stapler. The gap between the jaws must be adequate for the thickness of tissues. A tissue-measuring device may be used for this determination in the gastrointestinal tract in conjunction with a disposable stapler so that the instrument can be adjusted to the appropriate settings for the desired staple height.

When formed, each staple is shaped like a capital B. This shape allows staples to hold tissues together without crushing so that tissue perfusion is maintained. The number of staples that will be fired depends on the length of the stapler jaws.

Intraluminal Circular Stapler

With the circular stapler a double row of staggered staples is placed in a circle for intraluminal anastomosis of tubular hollow organs in the gastrointestinal tract. Because the diameter of the lumen of organs in the alimentary tract varies, the surgeon must choose a stapler with an appropriate head size. The number of staples the instrument fires depends on its head size. A circular knife within the head of the stapler trims tissue to produce a proper lumen as the stapler is fired. As with the linear stapler, staples form a B.

Ligating and Dividing Stapler

A double row of two staples each ligates tissue that is then divided simultaneously between the staple lines with a cutting knife incorporated in the stapler. This stapler is used primarily to ligate and divide omental vessels or other soft tubular structures.

Endoscopic Stapler

Endoscopic staplers are available for ligating and dividing and for linear stapling. The stapling device is passed through an 11- or 12-gauge laparoscopic trocar. It may be reloaded several times with staple cartridges for multiple firings. The stapler is discarded after single-patient use.

Reusable Staplers

Reusable, manually operated, heavy mechanical stapling instruments have many moving and detachable parts. They are not always mechanically reliable. They must be precisely aligned to fire accurately. The scrub person is responsible for correctly assembling instruments. The manufacturer's instructions for use and care must be followed to avoid technical failures.

Reusable staplers are supplied with presterilized, disposable cartridges that contain six or more staples. Quantities vary according to the stapler they fit. The number of cartridges needed varies with the procedure and/or design of the instrument. Cartridges are color coded by the size of the staples.

Reusable staplers must be disassembled and cleaned after use. They should be terminally sterilized and then cleaned in an ultrasonic cleaner. They should be steam sterilized completely disassembled, according to the manufacturer's recommendations.

Disposable Staplers

Preassembled, sterile disposable staplers eliminate assembling, cleaning, and sterilizing processes. These self-contained, lightweight instruments with integral or reloadable staple cartridges are discarded after single-patient use. To avoid unnecessary contamination of a sterile instrument, the package should not be opened until the surgeon determines the correct size for the intended use of the stapler. The number and size of staples in cartridges vary; the length of the linear jaws or the diameter of the circular head varies for internal use. Internal staplers are available with either stainless steel or titanium staples. The surgeon may prefer titanium because it creates less distortion when CT and MRI scans are used.

TISSUE ADHESIVES

Conventional suturing and stapling hold tissues in apposition during the healing process. Sutures and staples will not fuse or bond tissues. Ancient Egyptians used resins and gums to hold tissue surfaces together. Research is ongoing for an ideal tissue adhesive that will bond tissue, effect hemostasis, promote regeneration of cells, and serve as a barrier to microbes, fluid, and air. Biologic and synthetic tissue adhesives have extensive potential applications for wound closure and reconstruction.

Biologic Adhesives

Fibrin sealants, most commonly called fibrin glue, act as biologic adhesives and hemostatic agents. The components are

<table>
<tr><td>

Box 30-3 **Sample Fibrin Glue Compound and Supplies**

Sterile specimen cup
Two 20-ml disposable syringes
Two 14-gauge intravenous (IV) catheters
6 units thawed cryoprecipitate
One ampule calcium chloride (CaCl) (10%, 1 g)
50,000 U thrombin

Instructions

Mix CaCl and thrombin in the specimen cup. Draw into the 20-ml syringe and attach a 14-gauge IV catheter. Draw cryoprecipitate into the second syringe with a 14-gauge IV catheter on the end. Both syringes are discharged over the wound at the same time. The fibrin glue will form a clot over the wound.

</td></tr>
</table>

fibrinogen, cryoprecipitated from human plasma, calcium chloride, and reconstituted thrombin of bovine origin. When applied directly to tissues, thrombin converts fibrinogen to fibrin to produce a clot. Fibrin sealants can be applied to deeper tissues as a liquid, gel, or aerosol spray to control bleeding and approximate tissues technically difficult to approximate by suturing, especially following resections or traumatic injuries of friable or highly vascular tissues, such as liver, spleen, and lung. Each component is applied simultaneously with separate syringes to prevent congealing before application to the tissue site. A sample formula and supplies for fibrin glue compound are found in Box 30-3.

Fibrin glue may also be used for microsurgical anastomoses of blood vessels, nerves, and other structures such as fallopian tubes; for reconstruction of the middle ear; to fix ocular implants; to close superficial lacerations and fistula tracts; and to secure some skin grafts. It may be used as a carrier for demineralized bone powder to promote osteoregeneration.

In 1998 the FDA approved Tisseel, a fibrin glue produced by Baxter Healthcare Corporation. Tisseel is derived from the blood proteins fibrin and thrombin and is applied in the same manner as earlier forms of fibrin sealant.

Autologous or Homologous Plasma

Plasma collected from the patient (autologous) or a single donor (homologous) is processed into a cryoprecipitate containing clotting factor XIII to produce fibrinogen. Autologous plasma is obtained preoperatively and prepared either in the blood bank or in the OR. A single donor must be tested for human immunodeficiency virus (HIV) and hepatitis before plasma is processed.

Autologous or homologous fibrinogen is warmed to 98.6° F (37° C) immediately before use. Thrombin is reconstituted to 1000 U/ml. Equal volumes of fibrinogen and thrombin are applied simultaneously.

Pooled-Donor Plasma Fibrin glue commercially prepared from pooled-donor plasma (i.e., blended from multiple donors) has significantly greater bonding strength than autologous or single-donor plasma. The fibrinogen must undergo purification and viral inactivation, however, to prevent transmission of blood-borne pathogens. Used extensively in Europe, this product has not been approved by the FDA for use in the United States.

Synthetic Adhesives

Synthetic gluelike adhesive substances that polymerize in contact with body tissues effect hemostasis and hold tissues together.

Cyanoacrylate

Butyl cyanoacrylate and cyanoacrylate derivatives may be used for skin closure. In 1998 the FDA approved Dermabond, a topical skin adhesive marketed by Ethicon. Dermabond is a synthetic product for skin closure that is derived from cyanoacrylate and applied with an applicator along approximated, clean wound edges. The glue dries after 2½ minutes and remains on the wound for 5 to 10 days. It is contraindicated in the presence of infection and for patients allergic to cyanoacrylate or formaldehyde. Additional information is available at **www.ethiconinc.com.**

Methyl Methacrylate

Methyl methacrylate is used to augment fixation of pathologic fractures and to stabilize prosthetic devices in bone. It is an acrylic, cementlike substance commonly referred to as bone cement. It is a drug supplied in two sterile components that must be mixed together immediately before use. One component is a colorless, highly volatile, flammable, liquid methyl methacrylate monomer in an ampule. This powerful lipid solvent must be handled carefully. The other component is a white powder mixture of polymethyl methacrylate, methyl methacrylate–styrene copolymer, and barium sulfate in a packet. The barium sulfate provides radiopacity to the substance. When the powder and liquid are mixed, an exothermic polymeric reaction forms a soft, pliable, doughlike mass. This reaction liberates heat as high as 230° F (110° C). As the reaction progresses, the substance becomes hard in a few minutes. The mixing and kneading of the entire contents of the liquid ampule and powder packet must be thorough and should continue for at least 4 minutes. The substance must be adequately soft and pliable for application to bone. The completion of polymerization occurs in the patient. After it hardens, it holds a prosthesis firmly in a fixed position.

A hazard to OR personnel has been reported in regard to the use of methyl methacrylate in the OR. Some personnel have experienced dizzy spells, difficulty breathing, and/or nausea and vomiting following mixing of methyl methacrylate. The fumes can cause severe eye irritation in persons wearing contact lenses during the use of this chemical compound. The monomer and several of its ingredients are potent allergenic sensitizers when vapor is inhaled. A suitable means of local exhaust should be provided that will collect vapor at the source of mixing at the sterile field and will discharge it into outside air or absorb the monomer on activated charcoal.

TISSUE REPAIR MATERIALS

Tissue deficiencies may require additional reinforcement or bridging material to obtain adequate wound healing. Sometimes edges of fascia, for example, cannot be brought together without excessive tension. In obese or older persons the fascia cannot withstand this tension because of weakness caused by the infiltration of fat. Biologic or synthetic mesh materials are used to fill congenital, traumatic, or acquired defects in fascia or a body wall and to reinforce fascia, as in hernia repair.

Biologic Materials
Cargile Membrane

A thin membrane is obtained from the submucosal layer of cecum of the ox. Cargile membrane is rarely used, although it is still commercially available in a 4 × 6 inch (10 × 15 cm) sheet, to cover peritoneum to prevent adhesions, for isolating ligations, as a covering for packing in submucous nasal resections, and as a dural substitute.

Fascia Lata

Strips of fascia lata are obtained from the fibrous connective tissue that covers thigh muscles of beef cattle. In lieu of commercial fascia lata—a heterogeneous graft—the surgeon may strip a piece of fascia from the patient's thigh—an autogenous graft. Fascia lata also is obtained from cadavers and freeze-dried—an allograft. Fascia lata contains collagen. It increases the amount of tissue already present and becomes a living part of the tissue it supports. It is used to strengthen weakened fascial layers or to fill in defects in fascia. Since the advent of allografts and synthetic meshes, heterogenous strips are used infrequently.

Synthetic Meshes

Synthetic meshes offer several advantages for reinforcing or bridging fascial or other tissue deficiencies:

1. They are easily cut to desired size for the defect.
2. They are easily sutured underneath the edges of tissue to create a smooth surface.
3. They are pliable to preclude erosion into major structures.
4. They are inert to avoid inflammatory response and to minimize foreign body tissue reaction.
5. They are porous to allow free drainage of exudate.
6. Fibrous tissue easily grows through openings to incorporate mesh into tissue to maximize tensile strength.

The manufacturer's instructions must be followed for each type of mesh product. Unused mesh should be discarded.

Polyester Fiber Mesh (Mersilene Mesh)

Mesh remains soft and pliable in tissue but has limited elasticity. It is the least inert of the synthetic meshes. It is not preferred in the presence of infection or in contaminated wounds because of its multifilament construction. Polyester fibers are knitted by a process that interlocks each fiber juncture to prevent unraveling when cut. However, a minimum of ¼ inch (6.5 mm) of mesh should extend beyond the suture line. Sterile sheets are available in sizes 2½ × 4½ inches (6 × 11 cm) and 12 × 12 inches (30 × 30 cm).

Polyglactin 910 Mesh (Vicryl Mesh)

Mesh is knitted fibers of undyed and uncoated polyglactin 910. Because it is absorbed by hydrolysis, this mesh is intended for use as a buttress to provide temporary support during healing. The mesh acts as a scaffold for ingrowth of connective tissue. It may be used to support a traumatized spleen, kidney, or abdominal wall and to support facial fascia. Absorption is essentially complete in 60 to 90 days. Sterile sheets are available in sizes 10½ × 13½ inches (26.5 × 34 cm) and 5 × 6½ inches (13 × 17 cm).

Polypropylene Mesh (Prolene Mesh, Marlex Mesh)

Knitted mesh of polypropylene has high tensile strength and good elasticity. However, Marlex mesh is stiffer and exhibits greater fiber fatigue than Prolene mesh. Because polypropylene is inert, it may be used in the presence of infection or during healing by second intention. Mesh is used to span and reinforce traumatic abdominal wall defects, incisional ventral hernias, large inguinal hernias, and other fascial deficiencies. It stimulates rapid tissue ingrowth through interstices of mesh. Mesh remains soft and pliable in tissues. It will not unravel when cut. Sterile sheets are available in sizes 2½ × 4½ inches (6 × 11 cm), 6 × 6 inches (15 × 15 cm), and 12 × 12 inches (30 × 30 cm).

Polytetrafluoroethylene (Gore-Tex Soft Tissue Patch)

A sheet of expanded polytetrafluoroethylene (PTFE) may be used to repair hernias and tissue deficiencies that require prosthetic material. This material is flexible, soft, and porous to allow tissue ingrowth. It is not used in the presence of infection. It must be handled only with clean gloves or rubber-shod forceps. Nonsterile patches may be sterilized by steam or ethylene oxide gas according to the manufacturer's instructions.

Stainless Steel Mesh

Available in nonsterile sheets 6 × 12 inches (15 × 30 cm) and 12 × 12 inches (30 × 30 cm), steel is the most inflexible and difficult of the meshes to handle. The sharp edges may puncture gloves. Wire scissors, not dissecting scissors, should be used to cut it. Steel is opaque to x-rays, which may be a disadvantage for the patient in later life. Also, the mesh may fragment and cause patient discomfort.

TISSUE REPLACEMENT MATERIALS

For centuries surgeons have sought materials to replace parts of anatomy. Tissue may be absent or distorted because of congenital deformity, traumatic injury, degenerative disease, or surgical resection. Replacement or substitution of tissue may be possible with biologic dressings or implanted materials, or with synthetic prosthetic materials implanted in the body. An overview of the types of biologic and synthetic tissue replacement materials is given here. Their uses are referenced in other chapters by surgical specialty or procedure.

Biologic Wound Cover

A biologic dressing temporarily covers an open surface defect in skin and underlying soft tissues. Although defects are usually the result of trauma such as burns, vascular or pressure necrosis can cause skin ulcers. Open wounds quickly become contaminated. The dressing arrests loss of fluid, reduces or eliminates microbial growth, and minimizes scarring. It promotes production of granulation tissue and epithelialization before healing by second or third intention. A fibrin-elastin biologic bonding adheres the dressing to exposed surfaces. Biologic dressings are dermal replacements. The source determines the type of dressing.

Autograft

Skin is grafted from one part of the patient's body to another part.

Allograft

Human tissue obtained from one genetically dissimilar person (i.e., unmatched donor) is grafted to another person. This is referred to as an allograft. Negative HIV and hepatitis B virus (HBV) status of donor and recipient should be determined and documented before use. Any natural body tissue transferred from one human to another must be infection free.

Cryopreserved Skin Allograft skin provides a protective covering that initially acquires, then eventually loses, vascular connection with underlying tissue. A cadaver usually is the source of skin for a dermal allograft. Cryopreservation maintains viability of skin during prolonged storage. Skin is frozen by cooling at a rate of 1.8° to 9° F (1° to 5° C) to −94° F (−70° C) and then stored in a liquid nitrogen freezer. Immediately before use, skin is warmed by immersion in sterile water at 107.6° F (42° C), the maximum compatible with cellular viability. Skin should be warmed at a rate of 90° to 126° F (50° to 70° C) per minute. (The patient's own skin can be cryopreserved for prolonged storage for later use as an autograft.) Allografts may be obtained from a skin bank.

For storage of allografts or autografts up to 14 days, skin may be placed in isotonic saline solution or tissue nutrient medium and refrigerated at 33.8° to 50° F (1° to 10° C).

Amniotic Membrane Prepared from human placenta, amniotic membranes can be used as biologic dressings to promote the healing of burns, skin ulcers, and infected wounds and to cover defects such as spina bifida. The placenta has two loosely connected membranes: amnion is used for partial-thickness wounds, and chorion is used for full-thickness defects. Membranes are harvested by cleaning blood and clots from the placenta immediately after delivery, placing the placenta in an iodophor solution, and refrigerating it at 39° F (4° C). Membranes should be stripped from the placenta within 36 hours after delivery. Amnion can be used fresh or preserved frozen or dried. It may be obtained from a tissue bank that prepares and stores amniotic membranes.

Xenograft

Skin obtained from a dissimilar species may be placed on human tissue as a temporary dressing.

Porcine Dermis Porcine (pig) skin is used to cover body surfaces denuded of full-thickness skin until permanent skin grafting can be accomplished. Vascularization does not occur, but the xenograft adheres tightly while reepithelialization proceeds underneath it. It may remain in place for as long as 2 weeks before it dries up and peels off spontaneously. Porcine biologic dressings are available in rolls or strips. They may be prepared fresh for refrigeration, fresh frozen, irradiated and then frozen, or dried. Some dressings are soaked in an iodophor and should not be placed on a patient allergic to iodine. Dressings must be prepared and used according to the manufacturer's instructions.

Artificial Skin A skin substitute may be prepared from a layer of collagen obtained from the dermis of a calf or pig and coated with autogenous epithelium obtained from the recipient. Another type is synthesized from a bilayered polymeric membrane. The top layer is silicone elastomer. The bottom layer is a porous cross-linked network of collagen and glycosaminoglycan. This artificial skin is biodegradable, but it can be used as a temporary covering that is similar to porcine xenografts.

Biologic Materials

Autogenous tissues may be grafted or transferred from one part of the patient's body to another. Allograft tissues or organs may be transplanted from another human. Xenograft biomaterials may be used to supplement tissues.

Standards are set by the American Association of Tissue Banks for screening donors and retrieving, processing, and preserving homogenous tissues, including skin, cartilage, bone, and blood vessels. Potential donors of allografts are tested for HIV and HBV. Excluded from donating are persons who are HIV positive, have a history of hepatitis, have an active infection, or have an immune disorder.

Bone Grafts

A bone graft affords structural support and a pattern for regrowth of bone within a skeletal defect. Cancellous bone is porous. Its porosity permits tissue fluid to reach deeper into it than into cortical bone, and thus most of the bone cells live. Cortical bone is used for bridging large skeletal defects because it gives greater strength. It may be fixed in the recipient site by means of metallic suture or screws. Bone obtained from the crest of the ilium or a rib is cancellous and cortical bone; cortical bone is obtained from the tibia. The main purpose of a bone graft is to stimulate new bone growth.

Autogenous bone, which is obtained from the patient, usually is taken from the ilium, tibia, or rib cage at the time of the surgical procedure. Calvarial bone from the frontal, parietal, or occipital cranial bones may be harvested for maxillofacial bone grafts. A free bone graft with its vascular pedicle, such as a free fibular graft, may be obtained for revascularization by microvascular anastomosis after removal of dead (avascular) bone. A separate small sterile table may be prepared for the instrumentation required for the donor site. If the recipient area is potentially contaminated, the donor site must not be cross-contaminated from the recipient site.

Homogenous bone, which is obtained from a cadaver, is dead bone. This bone is weaker than autogenous bone, thus requiring a longer time of immobilization. Union occurs from bone regeneration in the recipient with this type of bone graft. It may be desirable, however, to spare the patient the added operating time and trauma of removing an autogenous graft.

Composite bone grafts are freeze-dried allografts combined with autogenous particulate cancellous bone and marrow. A crib formed from a cadaver bone (e.g., rib) is packed with the patient's bone particles and marrow. When implanted to reconstruct bony defects, the composite graft induces bone regeneration in the recipient site. The freeze-dried allograft is biodegradable by slow resorption. Eventually it is replaced by mature, functional bone.

Decalcified bone and demineralized bone chips or powder, prepared from homogenous bone, also are used to stimulate bone regeneration or to fill defects in bone. This material is sterilized and stored at room temperature. For use, it is soaked in Ringer's lactate solution. The powder then becomes a paste that can be used to fill a depressed area or to caulk an irregularity (e.g., in craniofacial reconstruction).

Bone Bank   Bone may be preserved and stored in a bone bank until needed. Autogenous bone may be preserved following the surgical procedure by storage in a bone bank for subsequent grafting into the same patient. Bone such as a rib or femoral head may be salvaged from patients (i.e., living donors) who are free of malignancy or infection for a homogenous graft into another person. Bone may also be obtained from cadavers (i.e., nonliving donors).

Bone used for allografts must be clean and sterile. Immediately after removal, bone marrow, fat, and blood are rinsed out with sterile distilled water or normal saline solution. The bone may be put in sterile nested glass jars or double plastic or metal containers. If it is to be used for a homogenous graft, a small piece of bone is put into a sterile Petri dish and sent to the laboratory for culture tests. Bone should never be used until negative results of culture and serology are received. Several methods are used to preserve bone:

1. Freezing is the most common method of preserving bone. Bone is quick frozen in a freezer at $-94°$ F ($-70°$ C) or in liquid nitrogen. If bone will be used within 6 months, it can be stored in a refrigerator freezer at $-4°$ to $-5°$ F ($-15°$ to $-20°$ C). For prolonged storage of more than 6 months, the freezer temperature must be maintained below $-4°$ F ($-20°$ C) to avoid damage from a buildup of ice crystals. Bone frozen by liquid nitrogen is stored in vapor at about $-238°$ F ($-150°$ C). The container initially is placed on a shelf labeled not ready for use. It is labeled sterile and moved to the freezer compartment labeled ready for use when negative results of culture and serology tests are recorded on the identification card. Bone is thawed rapidly immediately before grafting.
2. Freeze-drying requires specialized equipment that removes moisture as the freezing process takes place in a condenser with a vacuum cycle.
3. Ethylene oxide sterilization ensures safety of bone. It must be aerated for 72 hours before storage at room temperature or in a refrigerator. When protected from air and contamination, sterilized bone can be stored indefinitely, although a 1-year expiration date is recommended if bone is placed in a heat-sealed peel-apart package. In lieu of ethylene oxide sterilization, packaged bone may be shipped in dry ice to a center equipped to sterilize it by irradiation.
4. Formaldehyde solution, 0.25% to 1% concentration, may have a bacteriostatic effect around the graft site in infected or contaminated wounds, such as in osteomyelitis. During storage, temperature is maintained at 35.6° to 39° F (2° to 4° C) in a refrigerator freezer.

The container must be labeled with donor information and not used until laboratory reports are available. The donor must be seronegative for hepatitis B surface antigen and HIV. Bone from a living donor is quarantined for 90 days, awaiting results of a repeat test for HIV.

Heterologous Bone Implant   Coraline hydroxyapatite, which is composed of skeletons of sea coral, and collagen may be used to replace facial or cranial bone. This material has hardness, mineral content, and porosity similar to that of human bone. These implants stimulate bone growth into the porous architecture of the coral.

Organ Transplants

Some whole body organs can be transplanted from one human to another. This is done in an effort to sustain life by compensating for physiologic deficits or inadequate function of vital organs.

Tissue Transplants

Skin and blood vessels are frequently transplanted from one part of the body to another. These are referred to as autografts because the patient is both donor and recipient. The transplanted tissue becomes a part of the living tissue in the recipient site.

Some tissues can be transplanted from one person to another to restore function, such as the cornea, or to provide support in structures, such as cartilage in nasal reconstruction. These are referred to as allografts. Some allografts are commercially prepared, such as lyophilized human dura mater and human umbilical cord vein graft.

Human Dura Mater   A trimmed and measured piece of cadaver dura mater is freeze-dried, sterilized by exposure to ethylene oxide, and stored in a vacuum container. It may be stored at room temperature indefinitely, provided that the vacuum is maintained. The graft is reconstituted by the addition of normal saline solution to the container for a minimum of 30 minutes. Most of these grafts are used for closure of dural defects, but they may also be used to repair abdominal and thoracic wall and diaphragmatic defects. Neurologic tissue for transplant may harbor the prion responsible for the development of Creutzfeldt-Jacob disease (CJD). Routine sterilization does not render this material safe for use in the presence of CJD. Routine testing does not reveal CJD contamination.

Human Umbilical Cord Vein Graft   A glutaraldehyde tanning process converts an umbilical vein into an inert, antithrombogenic graft. A polyester mesh covering over the outer surface allows tissue ingrowth and provides added strength. Commercially supplied, a biograft modified human umbilical vein graft is an acceptable graft material for arterial reconstruction when an autogenous saphenous vein is not available. The glutaraldehyde must be thoroughly irrigated from the graft with sterile heparinized saline or Ringer's lactate solution before implantation. After rinsing, the graft should remain in sterile heparinized saline solution to keep it moist until implanted. Only noncrushing clamps should be used to avoid damage to the graft during handling.

Xenograft Biomaterials

In addition to porcine skin used as biologic dressings, artificial skin derived from the collagen of a calf or pig, heterologous bone, and other materials derived from animals are commercially prepared for tissue replacement.

Arteriovenous Shunts   Enzymatically treated bovine carotid artery xenografts are used for blood access in patients on hemodialysis therapy who have poor blood vessels or in whom it is difficult to create either fistulas or shunts. Femoral arteriovenous bovine shunts can be punctured innumerable times with a low incidence of thrombus formation.

Collagen   Collagen is used in its natural form, such as a processed bovine graft and microfibrillar hemostatic powder, and restructured into membranes or films. It can be injected into middle to deep dermis to fill and smooth nasolabial furrows and facial creases. It is implanted to correct soft tissue defects and contours. The duration of effect is 4 to 6 months. Collagen can be altered by a variety of techniques to change its physical properties and duration of action in tissue.

Corium   Corium implants are prepared from porcine dermis to replace tissue loss or to support tissues. They can be used as a fascia lata substitute or dural replacement or to repair tympanic membrane, hernia, or bladder sling. Corium will form a collagen matrix to close a defect in soft tissues around teeth. Available in sterile sheets of several sizes, corium implant (Zenoderm) is freeze-dried or air dried before sterilization by gamma irradiation. It should not be resterilized.

Human Skin Equivalent   In 1998 the FDA approved a new bioengineered skin product referred to as Apligraf and derived from bovine collagen and human tissue taken from discarded foreskins of circumcised newborns. The mixture takes 5 days to generate and grow under sterile conditions in the laboratory. It is specially ordered for each patient and cannot be stored for additional uses. The cell culture mixture is applied to nonhealing wounds, such as venous stasis ulcers after debridement.

Synthetic Materials

A prosthesis is a permanent or temporary replacement for a missing or malfunctioning structure. Some implants replace vital structures, such as diseased heart valves and blood vessels. Devices such as pacemakers assist the function of vital organs. Other materials are used to repair or replace defects. Prosthetic materials implanted into the body must:

- Be compatible with physiologic processes
- Produce no or minimal tissue reaction
- Be sterile so they will not cause infection or become a culture medium
- Be noncarcinogenic or other disease causative
- Have viable and adequate tissue coverage unless used as a biologic dressing over denuded skin surfaces
- Have adequate blood supply through or around them
- Be stable so that they will not degenerate or change shape if used for permanent function
- Contour or conform to normal tissue configuration as desired

Permanently implanted devices can provide support, restore function, and augment or restore body contour. Inorganic substances cannot unite with tissue, however. Their physiologic responses may be predictable. All synthetic materials implanted in contact with blood will activate coagulation and promote the process of thrombosis. The surface of some materials is less thrombogenic (i.e., less likely to form clots) than others. The magnitude of the inflammatory response they stimulate varies in patients. An immune response may cause chronic inflammation from bacterial adhesion. Infection that develops around a prosthesis usually necessitates its removal. Most infections arise from microorganisms inoculated into the wound at the time of implantation. Therefore meticulous sterile technique is mandatory. Prosthetic implants should not be flash sterilized in steam. They must be sterilized in a standard cycle for the agent used (see Chapter 17). The cycle should be monitored with a biologic indicator, and a negative spore test result should be confirmed before the implant is used. Many implants are sterilized by the manufacturer.

Carbon Fiber

Pure carbon fibers braided into a strip are used for ligament replacement and articular resurfacing. Inert in tissue, carbon fiber stimulates regrowth of connective tissue and cartilage. The fibers may be braided with polypropylene or coated with a resorbable gelatin or lyophilized dura. The prosthesis should be soaked in normal saline solution before implantation to facilitate handling.

Metal

Stainless steel, a cobalt alloy (with the trade name Vitallium), and titanium are manufactured into prosthetic implants. Used primarily for stabilization of bone, metal implants must be strong enough to withstand the stress of weight bearing or muscular action and must not corrode in body tissues. They are never reused because of the weakening that can occur with use.

Special care must be taken in handling metal implants to protect the surfaces. A simple scratch on a metal implant can lead to its corrosion in the body. The implant will be bathed continuously by weakly chloride body fluids. If corrosion begins, the implant may fail and have to be removed. It is very important, therefore, that all metal implants be protected from scratches. This can be accomplished by:

1. Wrapping each implant individually, or wrapping sets with each size implant in a separate compartment, for both storage and sterilization. Most prostheses come from the manufacturer in protective coverings or cases. Some of these are suitable for adequate sterilization, with subsequent placement in the sterile field to minimize handling before implantation.
2. Preventing implants from coming in contact with other hard surfaces of metal or glass, either during storage and sterilization or on the instrument table.
3. Not handling or transferring an unprotected implant with any type of forceps.

Implants of one metal should not come in contact with those of another metal because an electrochemical reaction occurs between metals. Two different metals are not implanted in the same patient for this reason. Instruments used for insertion also should be of the same metal as the implant (e.g., a stainless steel screwdriver and screw).

Methyl Methacrylate

A highly refined methyl methacrylate mixture can be molded and shaped to fit a defect in bone. When it hardens, this material looks and feels very much like bone. It is used to repair a skull.

Polyester Fiber

Polyester fibers (Dacron) woven or knitted into seamless cylinders are used to replace major arteries.

Polyethylene

Polyethylene tubing may be inserted into structures such as fallopian tubes or ureters to give support during healing or to bridge a defect in tissue continuity. Polyethylene may be combined with silicon to produce a thromboresistant coating for vascular grafts and artificial hearts.

A polyethylene sliding rail, as on a reclosable plastic bag, affixed to polypropylene mesh is used in the manufacture of a surgical zipper. A zipper may be used for temporary abdominal wound closure in the presence of extensive sepsis to allow repeated access to the abdomen.

Implants of porous polyethylene are used for anatomic reconstruction, such as of the external ear. The porosity of the implant encourages both soft tissue and vascular ingrowth. Collagen deposited along the framework adds strength. Porous polyethylene is a strong, flexible material that can be molded or shaped to the desired configuration. When dipped into boiling normal saline solution, the material becomes pliable for molding by hand. An implant can be shaped by cutting with a scalpel blade. Glove powder, lint, and dust particles must not adhere to the implant because they can cause a foreign body reaction around the implant.

Polytetrafluoroethylene (Teflon)

Some prostheses or parts of prosthetic devices are made of the polymer PTFE. It may be woven into a fabric for arterial grafts, extruded into tubing for struts, or molded into a solid configuration for valves or joints. Its lubricity makes it a useful replacement for tissues when motion is desirable.

Silicone

Silicone is one of the most inert of the synthetic polymers used for implantation. It has a durable and nonthrombogenic surface. It is used in many forms: gel, sponge, film, tubing, liquid, and preformed molded anatomic structures. It may be coated with polyurethane or polyester or used as an elastomer to coat polyester. A medical-grade silicone elastomer (Silastic) in one form or another is used in virtually every surgical specialty for tissue reconstruction or replacement. Silicone may migrate from a ruptured or leaking gel- or liquid-filled implant and cause systemic illness.

Complete instructions for cleaning and sterilizing silicone implants before use are supplied by the manufacturer with each type of prosthesis. These instructions must be followed meticulously. Implants are not handled with bare hands, and care must be taken to ensure that they do not pick up lint and dust. Gloves worn during handling must be entirely free of powder. Skin oil, lint, dust, powder, and other surface contaminants can evoke foreign body reactions around the implant in tissue.

SKIN CLOSURE

In addition to sutures and staples, other materials may be used to hold skin edges in approximation.

Wound Zipper

Patients requiring multiple open abdominal procedures may benefit from a simple method of regaining entry to the peritoneal cavity. Commercially prepared sterile nylon wound zippers (Woundmate) are available from Wound Care International for repeated wound opening and closure. This method can be used for other body areas, such as facial wounds or extremities. The self-adherent zipper should be 2 to 4 cm longer than the surgical site and placed over clean, dry skin edges. Available sizes range from 4 to 50 cm. The zipper can be opened under sterile conditions for irrigation, repeated debridement, or additional tissue sampling. The resultant scar is minimal, and cosmetic effects can be achieved. More information is available from the manufacturer at (800) 361-4693.

Skin Closure Strips

Adhesive-backed strips of microporous nylon (Proxi-Strip) or polypropylene (Steri-Strip) or rayon acetate are placed at intervals across the line of incision. They may be used to approximate skin edges of superficial lacerations, as the primary closure of skin in conjunction with subcuticular suture, or in conjunction with interrupted skin sutures or staples. Often they are used following early suture or staple removal to support the wound during healing. A skin tackifier, such as tincture of benzoin, may be recommended by the manufacturer for ensuring adhesion to skin.

Sterile strips are available in widths of ⅛, ¼, and ½ inch (3, 6, and 12.7 mm) and in lengths from 1½ to 4 inches (3.7 to 10 cm). They are ethylene oxide gas sterilized in peel-apart packets. Skin closure strips have the following advantages:

1. They may be used in the emergency department on superficial lacerations to eliminate the need for sutures that would require local anesthesia for placement and subsequent return of the patient for suture removal.
2. They eliminate foreign body tissue reaction of suture material in skin.
3. They have enough porosity to permit adequate ventilation of clean or contaminated wounds.

4. They permit removal of sutures within 32 to 48 hours postoperatively. Crosshatch scarring and the possibility of infection are reduced when sutures are removed early. Skin closure strips provide long-term wound reinforcement and support.
5. They permit visibility of the healing wound so that the surgeon can see how well the wound edges have coapted. Some strips are translucent; others have a color tone or opacity that does not afford this advantage.
6. They minimize skin irritation because they are hyporeactive.
7. They can be applied and removed rapidly.
8. They can be easily cut to meet exact length requirements.

Bibliography

Bardaxoglou E et al: Oesophageal perforation: primary suture repair reinforced with absorbable mesh and fibrin glue, *Br J Surg* 81(3):399, 1994.

Blust JB et al: Suture conversion without the knots, *AORN J* 65(1):116-118, 1998.

Chang LY, Yang JY: Clinical experience of postage stamp autograft with porcine skin onlay dressing in extensive burns, *Burns* 24(3):264-269, 1998.

Clark HC: An improved ligator in operative laparoscopy, *Obstet Gynecol* 83(2):299-301, 1994.

Cohn SM et al: Recipe for poor man's fibrin glue, *J Trauma* 44(5):907, 1998.

Curry J: Human fibrin makes effective tissue adhesive, *OR Manager* 10(6):18-19, 1994.

Davis MS: Blunt-tipped suture needles, *Infect Control Hosp Epidemiol* 14(1):224-225, 1994.

Device tracking: questions and answers about tracking program; internal tracking system eases employee burden; hospital expands tracking system to comply with law, *OR Manager* 10(4):13-17, 1994.

Fahey C: Experience with a new human skin equivalent for healing venous leg ulcers, *J Vasc Nurs* 16(1):11-15, 1998.

Furst E: The safe medical device act, *J Cardiovasc Nurs* 8(2):79-85, 1994.

Geis WP, Malago M: Laparoscopic bilateral inguinal herniorrhaphies: use of a single giant preperitoneal mesh patch, *Am Surg* 60(8):558-563, 1994.

Hagen L: Surgical wound closure, *Infect Control Today* 2(10):44, 46, 49-50, 1998.

Kearney JN: Quality issues in skin banking: a review, *Burns* 24(4):299-305, 1998.

Kessler DA: Introducing medWatch: a new approach to reporting medication and device adverse effects and product problems, *Gen Hosp Psychiatry* 16(2):96-102, 1994.

O'Connor JJ: Single-operator ligation, *Dis Colon Rectum* 37(7):733, 1994.

Pomahac B et al: Tissue engineering of skin *Crit Rev Oral Biol Med* 9(3):333-334, 1998.

Tian F et al: The disintegration of absorbable suture materials on exposure to human digestive juices: an update, *Am Surg* 60(4):287-291, 1994.

Trott A: *Wounds and lacerations: emergency care and closure,* ed 2, St Louis, 1997, Mosby.

US Department of Health and Human Services: *Medical device tracking: questions and answers based on the final rule,* USDHSS Pub No FDA 93-4259, Washington, DC, 1993, US Government Printing Office.

Ward-English L: Suture materials: the surgeon's selection, *Surg Technol* 26(5):16-18, 1994.

Wound closure manual, Somerville, NJ, 1994, Ethicon.

Chapter 31

Wound Healing

 Chapter Objectives

After studying this chapter, the learner will be able to:

- Identify tissue layers specific to the anatomic site of a wound.
- List several factors that affect wound healing.
- Describe the process of wound healing.

The skin contributes to the health and well-being of the patient. Intact skin is an effective barrier to most harmful elements. Wounded, nonintact skin is an open avenue for microbial entry. Wounds occur intentionally or unintentionally. Most wounds, when treated properly, heal without incident. Unfavorable outcomes occur when wound healing is disrupted by poor circulation, infection, or immune dysfunction.

As a multifunction body cover, skin assessment is an important measurement of generalized wellness. Skin color, texture, and condition can be the best predictor of how well a surgical site will heal. The most intricate procedure can be done in deep tissue layers, but the superficial layers are what the patient sees and measures the outcome against. Durability and viability of the skin of the perioperative patient is influenced by many factors. Within reasonable limits, in the absence of hemorrhage and sepsis, wound healing is predictable. Disregard for the principles of tissue handling and wound management can lead to complications. The intent of this chapter is to provide an overview of body tissues, mechanisms of wounding, healing influences, and postoperative wound care. Terms associated with wound healing are defined in Box 31-1.

HISTORICAL BACKGROUND

Historically, warfare has necessitated that there be some means of controlling hemorrhage, closing intentional and nonintentional wounds, and promoting healing. Egyptian papyri dating back to 2100 BC describe how various injuries, including head injuries and fractures, were treated.

Wound management techniques improved slowly and sporadically. Two schools of surgical wound management taught clearly opposite theories and approaches. Fourteenth-century French surgeon Guy de Chauliac (1300-1368) and other followers of Galen's technique believed that a wound needed to suppurate, or generate laudable pus, before it could heal. Followers of Theodoric, such as Henri de Mondeville (1260-1320), stressed the need for clean wounds and healing by first intention.

Sixteenth-century French battle medic Ambroise Paré (1510-1590) found that treating gunshot wounds with a mixture of egg yolk, rose or lily oil, and turpentine was more beneficial than pouring boiling oil into the wound. His methods openly challenged the practices of his day yet eventually became the standard of care. He never attended medical school, but he taught that observation of the patient was more important than blind adherence to dogma. In his 1547 text,

Box 31-1

Terms Associated with Wound Healing

dead space   Space caused by separation of wound edges or by air trapped between layers of tissue.

debridement   Removal of damaged tissue and cellular or other debris from a wound to promote healing and to prevent infection.

dehiscence   Partial or total splitting open or separation of the layers of a wound.

edema   Abnormal accumulation of fluid in interstitial spaces of tissues.

evisceration   Protrusion of viscera through an abdominal incision.

extravasation   Passage of blood, serum, or lymph into tissues.

hematoma   Collection of extravasated blood in tissue.

seroma   Collection of extravasated serum from interstitial tissue or a resolving hematoma in tissue.

exudate   Fluid, cells, or other substances that have been discharged from vessels or tissues. It contains white blood cells, lymphokines, and growth factors that stimulate healing.

granulation tissue   Formation of fibrous collagen to fill the gap between the edges of a wound healing by contraction (i.e., second intention).

granuloma   Inflammatory lesion that forms around a foreign substance, such as glove powder or a suture knot.

hemostasis   Arrest of blood flow or hemorrhage; the mechanism is by coagulation (formation of a blood clot).

incision   Intentional cut through intact tissue (synonym: *surgical incision*).

ischemia   Decrease of blood supply to tissues.

necrosis   Death of tissue cells.

scar   Deposition of fibrous connective tissue to bridge separated wound edges and to restore continuity of tissues.

adhesion   Band of scar tissue that holds or unites surfaces or structures together that are normally separated.

contracture   Formation of extensive scar tissue over a joint.

tensile strength   Ability of tissues to resist rupture.

tissue reaction   Immune response of the body to tissue injury or foreign substances.

wound disruption   Separation of wound edges.

The Method of Treatment for Wounds Caused by Firearms, he described how, when he ran out of boiling oil, he dressed the patient's wounds with lard. He observed that the patients treated with boiling oil were feverish and the ones treated with lard were afebrile.

Research in wound healing did not occur before the eighteenth century. John Hunter (1728-1793), a Scottish surgeon, recorded observations of inflammation and healing patterns for the first time. He differentiated healing by first intention from healing by second intention by calling the first type of healing adhesive inflammation and second type suppurative inflammation. He also distinguished between epithelialization and granulation in healing wounds. He was the first to demonstrate that inflammation could be the cause of wound infection but was also necessary for wound healing.

In the late nineteenth century, French physician Alexis Carrel (1873-1944) studied the growth of tissues for transplantation. He grew several types of tissues in laboratory flasks. His studies provided the ground work for tissue and skin cell transplantation as it is today. He developed the triangulation method for anastomosis of blood vessels, for which he won the Nobel Prize in 1912.

ANATOMY AND PHYSIOLOGY OF BODY TISSUES

Structure and Function of Tissue

Tissue structure and function varies according to location in the body. Basic tissue types are described in Table 31-1.

Structure and Function of the Skin

The skin is the largest and heaviest organ of the body. The two main skin layers are the epidermis and the dermis. The thickness of the skin and its layers is determined by its location. The combined thickness of the epidermis and dermis ranges from 4 mm on the back to 1.5 mm of scalp. Figure 31-1 shows a cross section of the skin and its layers. The two basic types of skin are glabrous skin and hairy skin. Glabrous, smooth skin is very thick and is found on the palms and soles. The surface is marked by ridges and sulci arranged in unique configurations referred to as dermatographics, or fingerprints. These ridges first appear in the fingertips during the thirteenth week of fetal life. Sweat glands are present in the dermal layer, but a marked absence of hair follicles and oil glands is characteristic of this tissue.

Hairy, thin skin has hair follicles, sweat glands, and oil glands. Other types of sweat glands are found in the axilla and groin.

Epidermis

The epidermis is the outermost layer. It is organized into five levels of stratified squamous epithelium and contains no organs, glands, nerve endings, or blood vessels. It renews itself every 15 to 30 days, depending on the body surface area, the age of the individual, and the individual's generalized condition. The basic anatomy and physiology of epidermal layers are as follows:

- *Strata corneum.* Keratinized cells make up 75% of the epidermal thickness. Cells are shed from this level,

TABLE 31-1	Four Basic Histologic Tissue Types	
Histologic Tissue Type	**Description**	**Implications to Surgical Team**
Epithelial Tissue		
A. Types		
1. Simple	Single layer of cells (endothelium) that lines the blood vessels, heart, and lymphatics	Delicate tissue that is easily damaged by rough handling
2. Stratified	Several layers of cells that form the skin, gastrointestinal tract, genitourinary (GU) tract, reproductive tract, and oropharynx; lines area that serves as a passage; reduces friction with mucus; can convert into keratin	Superficial layer of body cover; surface modifications are performed here; forms hair and nails
3. Transitional	Combination of simple and stratified layers found in ureters and bladder	Encountered during GU reconstruction and neoconstruction
B. Cellular surface structure		
1. Squamous	Flat	
2. Columnar	Tall, cylindric	
3. Cuboidal	Square shaped	
Connective Tissue		
A. Fluid	Blood, lymph, chyle, cerebrospinal fluid, synovium vitreous and aqueous, and mucinous material	Care with body substance isolation and provision of hemostasis
B. Fibrous		
1. Areolar	Loose network forming the frame for subcuticular tissue	Reorganized during liposuction and fat transplantation procedures
2. Adipose	Fat that fills the loose network; visible in fetus at 14 weeks' gestation; not found in eyelid, penis, scrotum, labia minorum, cranium, and lung tissue	
3. Reticular	Forms firmer framework for organs and vessels	
C. Supportive		
1. Cartilage	Avascular, no lymphatics or nerves	Structural integrity is altered during rhinoplasty and otoplasty; cartilage may be used as graft material; radical neck reconstruction may involve tracheal rings or laryngectomy for multidisciplinary treatment
a. Hyaline	Translucent, articular, and rubs against other articular surface; forms the epiphyseal line in long bone, portions of the nose, and tracheal rings	
b. Costal elastic	Becomes fibrous with age; found in ribs, nose, trachea, and larynx	
c. White fibrocartilage	Forms circular menisci in joints and between vertebrae	
d. Yellow elastic	Found in auricle of ear, eustachian tubes, and epiglottis	
2. Erectile	Found in corpus cavernosa, clitoris, and nose	
D. Hard	Bony surfaces covered with periosteum except at articulations and cartilaginous areas of circulatory insertion points	Reconstruction requires framework of underlying bone or graft material; autologous bone may be harvested from graft site for neoconstruction; donor bone may be used as transplant material
1. Cancellous bone	Spaces are filled with red marrow; erythroblasts and smaller vessels	
2. Compact bone	Hollow center filled with yellow marrow (higher fat content) and larger vessels	
Muscle Tissue		
A. Visceral	Smooth, involuntary muscle; hollow organs, vessels, glands, areola, scrotum, iris of eye	Skeletal muscle may be used to replace bulk lost to debridement; vascularized flaps replace radical tissue excisions
B. Skeletal	Cylindric, striated, voluntary cells	
C. Cardiac	Branching cells, nonnucleated, less fibrous connective tissue	
Nerve Tissue		
A. Types		
1. Neuron	Cells generate and conduct nerve impulses; has multiple cytoplasmic fibers on one side (dendrites) and a single myelinated extension from the other side (axon)	Nerves may be injured during any procedure
2. Neuroglia	Insulate and support neurons in central nervous system	
B. Classification by activity type		
1. Afferent	Sensory	
2. Efferent	Motor	

From Fortunato NM, McCullough SM: *Plastic and reconstructive surgery,* St Louis, 1998, Mosby.

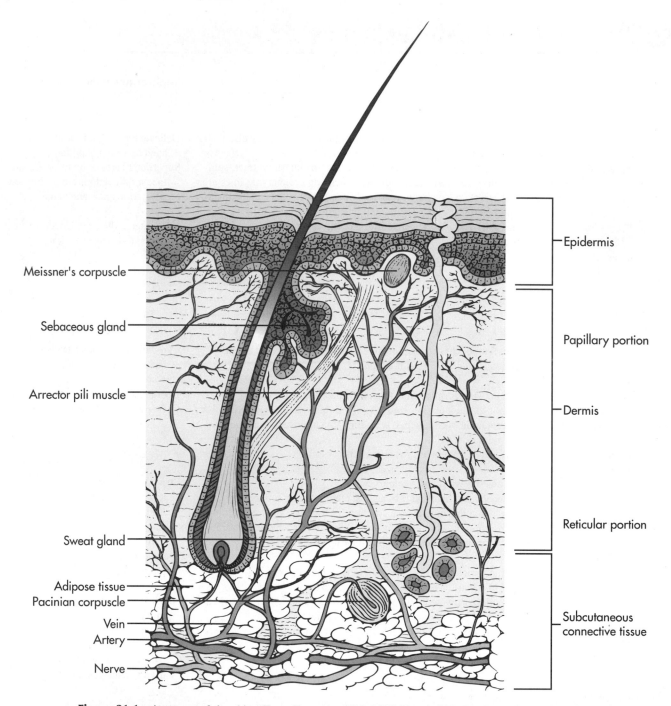

Meissner's corpuscle

Sebaceous gland

Arrector pili muscle

Sweat gland

Adipose tissue
Pacinian corpuscle

Vein

Artery

Nerve

Epidermis

Papillary portion

Dermis

Reticular portion

Subcutaneous
connective tissue

Figure 31-1 Anatomy of the skin. (From Fortunato NM, McCullough SM: *Plastic and reconstructive surgery,* St Louis, 1998, Mosby.)

which is referred to as the horny layer. It is thinner in hairy, thin-skinned areas.

- *Strata lucidum.* Cells are flattened. Organelles and nuclei are absent.
- *Strata granulosum.* This level is arranged in three to five layers. Mitotic activity creates cells for renewal of epidermal layers.
- *Strata spinosum.* This layer creates cells for renewal of epidermal layers.
- *Stratum basale.* A single cell layer that lies between the junction of the epidermis and the dermis. Intense mitosis in this layer in combination with the basal layer and

the spinosum causes epidermal regeneration. As cells are generated, they migrate upward, toward the surface. Melanocytes, located between basal cells and in hair follicles, create melanin, which causes skin pigmentation. Melanin enters and accumulates in keratocytes, causing superficial skin tone and providing ultraviolet protection. Exposure to sunlight causes darkening of existing melanin and accelerated generation of new melanin.

Each epithelial layer consists of keratin-producing cells (keratinocytes). Keratin is modified into functional components such as hair and fingernails on select body surfaces. Overactivity of the spinosum and basal levels can increase epidermal thickness in normally thin areas, causing psoriasis.

Dermis

The dermis is composed of papillary and reticular layers of flexible connective tissue. Superficially, the dermis has an irregular surface of papilla-like fingers that project into the strata basale of the epidermal layers. The dermis, regardless of location, is a loose areolar connective tissue that contains pain and touch receptors, glands, blood vessels, and lymphatics. It is the key layer in wound repair and tissue healing.

Glandular Structures and Ducts

Oil Glands (Sebaceous Glands) Sebaceous and sudoriferous glands are found within the dermal layers of the skin. Sebaceous glands are referred to as holocrine glands because the oily secretion, sebum, also carries cellular debris. The sebaceous duct empties into a hair follicle or, on nonhairy areas, directly onto the surface of the skin. Sebum is a lubricant with minor antibacterial and antifungal properties. The palms and soles lack sebaceous glands, but these glands are numerous on the scalp and face, and around natural body orifices.

Sweat Glands (Sudoriferous Glands) Sudoriferous glands are found on every area except the lips, nipples, and glans penis. Eccrine and apocrine glands are two types of sudoriferous glands. Eccrine glands are widely distributed over the entire surface of the body and are responsible for producing 700 to 900 g of sweat per 24 hours. These simple structures are embedded in the dermis and have a funnel-shaped exit path (pore) leading directly to the skin's surface. Secretions are produced in response to physical activity and cool the body by evaporation. These glands are most numerous on the palms, soles, and forehead.

Apocrine glands are located only in the axillary, perineal, and areolar areas in combination with eccrine glands. Apocrine glands are larger than eccrine glands and are embedded in subcutaneous tissue. These glands secrete a viscous fluid and have ducts that open into hair follicles. Initially the secretion is odorless, but it quickly develops an odor caused by bacterial decomposition. These glands secrete in response to stress or excitement. In animals, apocrine and sebaceous glands are thought to release pheromones, which are hormones thought to cause sexual attraction. Modified apocrine glands are found in the ear canals and secrete cerumen (earwax).

Blood Supply and Innervation

The dermis contains a rich blood and lymph supply. In some areas arterial and venous communication is by direct shunting, without using a capillary mechanism. Arteriovenous shunts allow for thermoregulation and blood pressure control. Capillary networks are located in the papillary layer to nourish the epidermis. Effector innervation of the dermis is derived from postganglionic fibers of the sympathetic ganglia. Affector innervation is a superficial dermal network of free nerve endings, hair follicles, and encapsulated sensory organs.

Subcutaneous Adipose Layer

Below the dermis is a loose, fatty layer that is referred to as the subcutaneous layer. Beneath the subcutaneous tissue is a layer of striated muscle. The looseness of this structure allows for movement of the skin over supporting musculature. In males the distribution is through the nape of the neck, deltoids, triceps, abdomen, lumbosacral region, and buttocks. In females the fatty layer extends through the breasts, abdomen, buttocks, epitrochanteric area, and anterior thighs.

Fascia

The fascia is a fibrous areolar tissue that supports the superficial skin layers and encases the muscle. The superficial fascia is directly below the integument and is the point to which injection of local anesthetic should extend for the best effect. Sensory nerve fibers run through this area, and anesthetic is easily absorbed. Adipose cells occupy areolar spaces, rendering the fascia soft and pliable and permitting vessels, nerves, and lymphatics to pass through the layers.

The deep fascia is tough and less pliable. It runs the length of the muscle bundle and terminates in fibrous tendons that attach to bones beneath the periosteum. Incisions greater than 10 mm are sutured meticulously to prevent herniation of underlying structures. This includes laparoscopic trocar punctures.

Accessory Appendages to the Skin

Modifications in the epidermal layer cause varied degrees of keratin deposition. Thickness and durability are functionally related to the location of keratinization. Hair and fingernails are modified keratin.

Other skin appendages include glands, blood vessels, and sensory organs. Glands arise in the dermis, and some exit the body through ducts that penetrate the epidermis. Other glands empty into the superior segment of hair follicles.

Hair Follicles

Hair follicles are keratinized epidermal epithelium that terminates in the dermal layers. The follicle is nourished by a capillary bed. Loss of this blood supply results in death of the follicle. Small bundles of smooth muscle cells, referred to as arrector pilli, form attachments to the surrounding connective tissue in a diagonal fashion. As arrector pilli contract, the shaft of the hair is straightened to an upright position. This contraction causes the superficial skin to dimple and pucker, creating "goose bumps."

Nails (Ungues)

The dorsal tip of each phalanx is tipped with a plate of specialized keratinized cells. Proximally, the nail root is covered by stratum corneum, which is referred to as the eponychium or cuticle. The nail plate rests on a bed of epidermis (nail bed). Nails are chemically similar to the surface epidermis. Peripheral blood supply may be assessed through the translucent nail plate but should not be the sole determinant of oxygenation of the patient.

MECHANISM OF WOUND HEALING

Interruption of tissue integrity, either intentionally or nonintentionally, requires understanding of the mechanism and factors that cause wounding and influence wound healing. When tissue is cut, the body's inherent defense mechanisms respond immediately to begin repair. Three types of wound healing are recognized: first/primary intention, second intention, and third intention/delayed primary closure. Each has practical applications in making and closing incisions or traumatic wounds. The degree of contamination and the amount of viable tissues are factors in the determination of which method of healing is used.

First Intention/Primary Union

Healing by first intention is desired following primary union of an incised, aseptic, accurately approximated wound. Key elements of first-intention closure include the following:

- No tissue loss
- Well-approximated edges with suture, wound sealant, or wound closure strips
- Minimal or no postoperative swelling
- No serous discharge or local infection
- No separation of wound edges
- Minimal scar formation

The rate and pattern of wound healing differ in various tissues. In general, first-intention wound healing consists of three distinct phases:

1. *Lag phase of acute inflammatory response.* Tissue fluids containing plasma, proteins, blood cells, fibrin, and antibodies exude from the tissues into the wound, depositing fibrin, which weakly holds the wound edges together for the first 5 days. Fibrin and serum protein dry out, forming a scab that seals the wound from further fluid loss and microbial invasion. At the same time, fibroblasts, fibrous tissue germ cells, and epithelial cells migrate from the general circulation. Subsequent adhesion of these cells, a process known as fibroplasia, holds the wound edges together. Leukocytes and other white blood cells produce proteolytic enzymes to dissolve and remove damaged tissue debris. Macrophages and neutrophils ingest foreign material, cellular debris, and bacteria.
2. *Healing or proliferative phase of fibroplasia.* After the fifth postoperative day, fibroblasts multiply rapidly, bridging wound edges and restoring the continuity of body structures. Collagen, a protein substance that is the chief constituent of connective tissue, is secreted from

the fibroblasts and formed into fibers. Reepithelialization causes the rapid gain in tensile strength and pliability of the healing wound. Tensile strength is the ability of the tissues to resist rupture. The healing phase begins rapidly, diminishes progressively, and terminates on about the fourteenth day. It may continue for up to 20 days.
3. *Maturation or differentiation phase.* From the fourteenth postoperative day until the wound is fully healed, scar formation occurs by deposition of fibrous connective tissue. The collagen content remains constant, but the fiber pattern re-forms and cross-links to increase the tensile strength. Wound contraction occurs over a period of weeks up to 6 months. As collagen density increases, vascularity decreases, and the scar grows pale. The scar tissue is only 80% as strong as the original tissue.

Second Intention

The mechanism of second-intention healing is by granulation, eventual reepithelialization, and wound contraction rather than by suturing it closed by first intention. The wound will heal spontaneously if the dermal base is preserved. The following are considerations with this type of healing:

1. Infection, excessive trauma, loss of tissue, or poorly approximated tissue is common. Inflammatory response is exaggerated.
2. The wound is left open and allowed to heal from the inner toward the outer surface. Devitalized tissue is debrided, and the wound is packed with moist packing material.
3. Healing is delayed. The wound may need grafting.
4. Healing may produce a weak union, which may be conducive to incisional herniation (rupture) later.
5. The risk of secondary infection is proportional to the amount of necrotic tissue present in the wound and to compromised immune response in the patient. Repeated debridement may be necessary.
6. Scar formation is excessive.
7. Contracture of skin is pronounced. After healing is complete, the scar may need revision or release.

Third Intention/Delayed Primary Closure

Suturing is delayed or secondary for the purpose of walling off an area of gross infection or where extensive tissue was removed (e.g., in a debridement or by a traumatic injury). The edges are closed 4 to 6 days postoperatively. The following are considerations in healing by third intention:

1. The wound is cleaned and debrided.
2. The defect is packed with moist gauze to promote drainage and granulation.
3. Antibiotic therapy is implemented.
4. The wound may be an old traumatic or septic wound.

5. The area should not be devascularized, and deep sutures should be avoided. Granulomas can form.
6. Two clean surfaces of granulation tissue are brought together for later closure.
7. A deeper and wider scar usually results.

TYPES OF WOUNDS

A wound is an injury, either intentional or unintentional, that disrupts the continuity of body tissues with or without tissue loss. Wounds may be surgical, traumatic, incidental, or chronic.

Intentional Wounds
Surgical Site Incision and/or Excision

An incision is a cut or an opening into intact tissue. An excision is removal of tissue. A sterile sharp scalpel, scissors, curette, or other cutting instrument may be used to separate skin and underlying tissues. Thermal instruments that both cut or vaporize tissue and coagulate surrounding blood vessels are used for incision and excision. The location, length, and depth of an incision must be planned.

The surgeon spreads the skin taut between the thumb and index finger in preparation for making the skin incision. With one stroke of evenly applied pressure on the scalpel, a clean incision is made through the epidermis and dermis into the subcutaneous layers. A number of factors influence the ease with which a primary skin incision is made:

- Sharpness, shape, and size of the knife blade
- Resistance of self-adhering plastic drapes
- Toughness of skin or scar tissue
- Thickness of subcutaneous tissue

A clean stroke with a sterile surgical scalpel, followed by attention to all of the principles of sterile technique and tissue handling, is the best insurance for healing by first intention. The line of direction of the incision in relation to the natural lines of direction of the skin may be a factor in wound healing. Figure 31-2 depicts natural lines of skin tension (Langer's lines). Excess tension on the healing wound can delay wound healing. Wounds heal side to side, not end-to-end.

Other Types of Intentional Wounds
Occlusion Banding Hemorrhoid ligation results in ischemia and degeneration of a hemorrhoid. A Silastic band is placed around the hemorrhoid, using a special spring-loaded applicator. Other types of occlusion banding are performed on fallopian tubes with ligatures, Silastic bands, or plastic clips through a laparoscope. Portions of tissue distal to the occlusion point separate from perfused tissues, interrupting the continuity of the lumen of the part in the banding process.

Chemical Wounds Chemicals can intentionally be applied to skin or other tissue surfaces to denude the area.

These chemicals cause inflammation and reepithelialization of the surface. This procedure is common in facial peels used in plastic or dermatologic surgery.

Unintentional Wounds: Traumatic Injuries

Following traumatic injury, preservation of life is the first critical concern. The patient's general condition is of prime consideration, and the plan of care is individualized to meet the patient's needs. Injuries are evaluated, and those that pose the greatest hazards to life or to return to normal function are cared for first. The primary objective following life support is wound closure with minimal deformity and functional loss. Minor injuries are cared for in the emergency department. Patients with major injuries receive treatment in the emergency department before going to the operating room (OR) as quickly as their condition warrants it. Traumatic wounds can be considered closed or open, simple or complicated, clean or contaminated. Wound closure is predicated on the type, location, severity, and extent of injury.

Closed Wounds

Skin is intact in a closed wound, but underlying tissues are injured. A blister filled with serum or a hematoma of blood and serum may form under the epidermis. Torn ligaments and simple fractures are closed wounds.

Open Wounds

The skin is broken by abrasion, laceration, or penetration.

Simple Wounds Continuity of skin is interrupted in simple wounds, but without loss or destruction of tissue and without implantation of a foreign body. These lacerations are usually caused by a sharp-edged object cutting or penetrating at a low velocity. These wounds can be closed by first intention unless underlying structures or organs have been injured.

Complicated Wounds In complicated wounds, tissue is lost or destroyed by crush or burn, or a foreign body is implanted by high-velocity penetration. If a penetrating wound was made by an object, such as a knife or bullet, this is not removed until the surgeon explores the wound in the OR. The device should be stabilized to prevent additional injury. Movement of a foreign object may cause further trauma. The depth of a penetrating wound is irrigated and may be excised. The wound may be closed by second or third intention. Skin grafting may be required if the dermis has been destroyed. Any object removed from the patient's wound may be forensic evidence. The hospital's policy and procedure manual should be consulted for guidance on handling potential police evidence.

Clean Wounds Clean wounds will heal by first intention after closure of all tissue layers and wound edges. The cosmetic care of lacerated areas is important, as is treatment to provide normal function and satisfactory appearance of a part.

Figure 31-2 Langer's lines. **A,** Anterior view. **B,** Posterior view. **C,** Forearm. **D,** Relaxed skin tension lines of face. (From Fortunato NM, McCullough SM: *Plastic and reconstructive surgery,* St Louis, 1998, Mosby.)

Contaminated Wounds When dirty objects penetrate skin, microorganisms multiply rapidly. Within 6 hours contamination can become infection. Debridement is performed to remove devitalized tissue, and the wound is irrigated. Devitalized tissue is removed because it acts as a culture medium. The wound may be left open to heal by second or third intention. Closure may be delayed for several days.

The patient's history should be assessed for tetanus bacillus immunization. Tetanus is most likely to occur in deep wounds contaminated by soil or animal feces. Adsorbed tetanus toxoid (0.5 ml) may be given as an initial immunizing dose or as a booster if the patient has been immunized within the previous 5 years. Tetanus immune globulin (human, 250 to 500 U) also should be given to any patient who has a severe wound or who has had the wound for more than 24 hours and has not been immunized within the previous 10 years.

Delayed Full-Thickness Injury Industrial accidents commonly include crush injury or deep injection of substances, such as paint or printer's ink, beyond the level of the dermis. The full extent of the tissue damage may not be apparent for several days following the event as the effects of the injury cause increasing tissue loss. The patient may have occlusive dressings or casting for the initial apparent injuries but should be continually assessed for signs of increasing tissue necrosis or full-thickness tissue loss. Electrocution or lightning strikes act similarly by causing deep tissue necrosis several days after the initial wounding.

Incidental and Chronic Wounds

Pressure sores and decubitus ulcers may result from compromised circulation over bony prominences or other pressure points for extended periods of time. Positioning and padding considerations in the plan of care can help prevent incidental pressure-related injuries in the perioperative environment.

Ulcers

Venous stasis or arterial insufficiency in the legs may cause chronic skin ulcers. Tissue necrosis may occur following radiation therapy. These chronic wounds have tissue loss and usually have heavy bacterial contamination. Topical application of fibronectin (a platelet-derived wound-healing formula) or some other preparation of growth factors from the patient's own blood may help control infection and promote healing. Growth factors stimulate the growth of tissue, capillaries, and skin. If a wound fails to heal by second intention with formation of granulation tissue, debridement and skin grafting may be required.

FACTORS INFLUENCING WOUND HEALING

Each patient has internal and external forces that influence healing. Most wounds will progress to healing unless the closure is poor, an infection ensues, or the tissue is devitalized by other forces. Hemostatic and inflammatory responses must be intact for healing to take place.

The degree of wound contamination is evaluated, and the potential risk for postoperative wound infection is taken into consideration.

Surgical Wound Classification

The surgical site may be clean or contaminated when the surgeon makes the initial incision. A clean site may become contaminated depending on the type of wound, the pathologic findings or circumstances creating the need for the surgical procedure, the anatomic location, or the techniques of the OR team. After completion of wound closure, the circulator should verify the wound classification with the surgeon. This is documented in the patient's intraoperative records.

Surgical wounds are classified by the degree of microbial contamination or exposure that may predispose a patient to a postoperative wound infection. According to the Centers for Disease Control and Prevention (CDC), risk of infection increases in proportion to contamination of the incision and surrounding tissues exposed during the course of the surgical procedure. The true extent of risk cannot be evaluated until the procedure is completed. The wound is classified at the end of the surgical procedure as one of four types (Box 31-2):

1. Clean
2. Clean-contaminated
3. Contaminated
4. Dirty and infected

Generalized Health Condition of the Patient

Chronic diseases alter normal physiology. Diseases such as diabetes, uremia, fibrocystic disease, cirrhosis, active alcoholism, and leukemia can delay wound healing.

Circulatory Status

Cardiovascular and respiratory insufficiency inhibit tissue perfusion. Oxygenation is essential to wound healing and to inhibit growth of anaerobic microorganisms.

Smoking Vasoconstriction caused by smoking decreases blood supply to the wound. Carbon monoxide in smoke binds with hemoglobin (forming carboxyhemoglobin) and further diminishes oxygenation. Smoking contributes to respiratory complications. This can cause forceful coughing that can raise intraabdominal pressure and create increased strain on an abdominal wound and impair healing.

Age

Loss of skin turgor and muscle tone and elasticity is a natural characteristic of the aging process. Thickened connective tissue, decreased subcutaneous fat, diminished capillary blood flow, and reduced vascularity are age-related factors that may delay wound healing. The tension of sutures on aged skin can further inhibit tissue perfusion. Sutures or skin

Clean Wound (Expected Infection Rate: 1% to 5%)

Elective procedure with wound made under ideal OR conditions

Primary closure, wound not drained

No break in sterile technique during surgical procedure

No inflammation present

Alimentary, respiratory, and genitourinary tracts or oropharyngeal cavity not entered

Clean-Contaminated Wound (Infection Rate: 8% to 11%)

Primary closure, wound drained

Minor break in technique occurred

No inflammation or infection present

Alimentary, respiratory, and genitourinary tracts or oropharyngeal cavity entered under controlled conditions without significant spillage or unusual contamination

Contaminated Wound (Infection Rate: 15% to 20%)

Open, fresh traumatic wound of less than 4 hours' duration

Major break in technique occurred

Acute nonpurulent inflammation present

Gross spillage/contamination from gastrointestinal tract

Entrance into genitourinary or biliary tracts with infected urine or bile present

Dirty and Infected Wound (Infection Rate: 27% to 40%)

Old traumatic wound of more than 4 hours' duration from dirty source or with retained necrotic tissue, foreign body, or fecal contamination

Organisms present in surgical field before procedure

Existing clinical infection: acute bacterial inflammation encountered, with or without purulence; incision to drain abscess

Perforated viscus

staples should be reinforced with wound closure strips. Newborn infants, especially those who are preterm, and geriatric patients are especially prone to infection.

Nutritional Status

Wound healing is impaired by deficiencies in proteins, carbohydrates, zinc, and vitamins A, B, C, and K. Protein provides essential amino acids for new tissue construction. Carbohydrates are necessary energy sources for cells, preventing excessive metabolism of amino acids to meet caloric requirements. Vitamin B complex is necessary for carbohydrate, protein, and fat metabolism. Vitamin C permits collagen formation. Although vitamin A and zinc are known to be important in collagen synthesis, their mechanism in wound healing is not well understood. Vitamin K is involved in the synthesis of prothrombin and other clotting factors. Copper and iron assist in collagen synthesis. Calcium and magnesium are important in protein synthesis. Manganese serves as an enzyme activator.

Malnutrition, whether primary or secondary to disease, can be a major factor in wound healing and infection. Impairment of physiologic functions associated with a body weight loss that is greater than 10% and protein energy malnutrition increase the risk of postoperative complications. Liver function, skeletal and respiratory muscle function, overall physical and mental activity, and inflammatory response to wound healing are altered in the malnourished patient. Protein and fat deficiency is especially significant in patients with extensive burns or multiple injuries, who have greatly increased caloric requirements. Malnutrition caused by anorexia or cachexia has a deleterious effect on wound healing. Hyperalimentation with vitamin, trace element, and mineral supplements preoperatively and postoperatively usually is indicated for malnourished patients.

Obesity The bulk and weight of adipose tissue cause difficulty in confining excess fat and securing good wound closure in obese patients. To minimize dead space, the surgeon may place drains and sutures in subcutaneous fat; both may actually potentiate infection. Of all tissues, fat is the most vulnerable to trauma and infection because of its poor vascularity. Many morbidly obese patients, more than 100 pounds (45.4 kg) over ideal body weight, have cardiac decompensation and respiratory insufficiency.

Fluid and Electrolyte Balance

The body's system for balancing fluids and electrolytes is extremely complex. As a result of illness, injury, or infection, the patient may not be able to maintain normal fluid and electrolyte balance. Fever associated with infection, for example, can raise fluid requirements as much as 15% for each 1.5° F (1° C) rise in body temperature. Body fluid is intracellular (ICF)—within cells—and extracellular (ECF)—outside cells as intravascular plasma and interstitial fluid between cells. The electrolyte content differs. ECF contains more sodium than ICF; ICF has more potassium than ECF. Changes in this balance can affect kidney function, cellular metabolism, oxygen concentration in the circulation, and hormonal function. Adequate ECF volume is necessary for circulation of blood to tissues.

Hematology

The presence of an abnormal or pathologic condition affecting the blood should be carefully evaluated preoperatively. A low hemoglobin level (red blood cell count) associated with anemia can result in tissue hypoxia, which alters synthesis of collagen and epithelialization. A hematocrit value below 20% lowers oxygen tension in tissues, which disrupts cell regeneration. An elevated leukocyte level (white blood cell count) indicates the presence of infection in the body.

Inflammatory and Immune Responses

The body repairs tissues at the cellular level in response to injury or exposure to foreign substances. It triggers an inflammatory response in order to mobilize cellular components associated with healing. Some foreign materials cause more inflammatory reaction than others. Extremes of inflammation may result in response to allergy, infection, or chronic irritation and may delay wound healing.

Allergic Response Hypersensitivity to substances inhaled, ingested, injected, or in contact with skin causes an acute allergic reaction. Consideration should be given to the type of allergic response displayed by the patient. A localized response may appear as a rash or hives. A systemic response may be more severe and include signs of airway obstruction and cardiac dysrhythmia.

Immunosuppression The patient's immunologic response may be deficient because of a congenital or acquired immunologic disease, drugs, or radiation therapy. Immunosuppressed patients are easily infected with potentially pathogenic flora within their own bodies. They may not present the usual signs and symptoms of infection, such as initial inflammatory response. Lack of integrity of the immune system, such as leukopenia or defective immunoglobulin synthesis, can be life threatening.

Drug Therapy

Wound healing occurs basically through collagen synthesis. Agents that interfere with cellular metabolism have a potentially deleterious effect on the healing process. Prolonged high dosage of steroids such as cortisone preoperatively inhibits fibroplasia and collagen formation. Some antineoplastic agents used as chemotherapeutic adjuvants to surgery also may delay systemic wound healing or cause localized tissue necrosis from extravasation at the site of injection. Immunosuppressants are given to transplant patients to prevent organ or tissue rejection. Leukopenia and susceptibility to infection are common sequelae to administration of these drugs. Other drugs that interfere with wound healing include anticoagulants, antiinflammatories, and colchicine.

Radiation Therapy

Healing is delayed if the patient has had radiation in large doses preoperatively. The blood supply in irradiated tissue is decreased. However, little change from the normal healing pattern occurs if radiation has been given in low doses and the surgical procedure is performed within 4 to 6 weeks of radiation.

Surgical Technique

Devitalized tissue caused by laser or electrosurgery is unable to regenerate. Interruption of blood supply and innervation decrease circulation and prevent epithelialization. Excess tension on the suture line that inhibits tissue perfusion prolongs healing time.

Aseptic Technique

Healthy tissues are able to combat a certain amount of contamination. Microorganisms are normally present in skin and air. Devitalized tissues have little power of resistance. Infec-

tion may occur from any one of a variety of causes that result in a breakdown of the wound postoperatively. The surgeon gives meticulous attention to sterile technique throughout the surgical procedure to minimize contamination of the surgical site. The entire OR team carefully carries out aseptic and sterile techniques. In addition, many precautions are taken by all OR personnel. Strict adherence to housekeeping techniques, air engineering, sterilization procedures, and all of the principles of aseptic technique is necessary. Infection may be caused by a break in the chain of asepsis.

Method of Hemostasis

Complete hemostasis must be achieved to prevent loss of blood and prevent hematoma (blood clot) formation. Blood loss is caused by tissue trauma. The method of dissection and coagulation of bleeders can cause devitalization of tissue. Devitalized tissue cannot heal; it only necroses. Delivery of oxygen to healing tissues is affected. Any condition that lowers circulatory flow and the delivery of oxygen to the tissues impairs healing.

Tissue Handling

All tissues should be handled very gently and as little as possible throughout the surgical procedure. The surgeon makes an incision that is just long enough to afford sufficient operating space. Careful consideration is given to underlying blood vessels and nerves to preserve as many as possible. Retractors are placed to provide exposure without causing undue pressure on tissues and organs or tension on muscles. Trauma to tissue in dissecting, handling with instruments, ligating, or suturing may cause edema and necrosis (death of tissue cells) with resultant slow healing. The body must rid itself of necrotic cells before the healing phase of fibroplasia takes place.

Tissue Approximation

Tissue edges are brought together with precision, avoiding strangulation and eliminating dead space, to promote wound healing. Too tight a closure or closure under tension causes ischemia, a decrease of blood supply to tissues.

Dead space is caused by separation of wound edges that have not been closely approximated or by air trapped between layers of tissue. Serum or blood may collect in a dead space and prevent healing by keeping cut edges separated. Wound edges not in close contact cannot heal. A drain may be inserted to aid in removal of fluid or air from the surgical site postoperatively, or a pressure dressing may be applied over a closed wound to help obliterate dead space.

The choice of wound closure materials and the techniques of the surgeon are prime factors in the restoration of tensile strength to the wound during the healing process.

Wound Security

The quality of approximated tissue and the type of closure material are two factors that determine the strength of the wound. Tensile strength of the tissues themselves varies; some are more friable than others. Drains or catheters may be placed in the wound to evacuate serum or fluid and prevent it from accumulating in the dead space postoperatively. Drainage tubes may cause a weak spot in the incision, and underlying tissue may protrude. Also, drains may provide an inlet for microorganisms, as well as an outlet for drainage. When possible, drains are placed through a stab wound in the skin rather than through the surgical incision.

When sutures are used, the suture material provides all of the strength of the wound immediately after closure. Closely spaced sutures give a stronger suture line. The strength of a suture should not be greater than the strength of the tissue in which it is placed. To minimize tissue reaction to sutures, the fewest and the smallest sutures consistent with the holding power of the tissues should be used. Inert surgical staples are used to approximate some tissues.

Immediately after closure, tissue along the incision is at about 40% of its original strength. It reaches its greatest strength in 7 to 15 days. The wound is about one-third healed on the sixth postoperative day and two-thirds healed on the eighth day. The condition of the patient, the type of surgical procedure, and many other factors may cause variance from the average patient response. As tensile strength of the wound increases, reliance on other support for wound security gradually lessens.

Postoperative Complications

Edema, vomiting, or coughing can place stress on the healing wound before fibroplasia takes place. Complications in other parts of the body, far from the surgical site, such as pneumonia, thrombus, or embolus, can inhibit oxygen supply to the wound site. Collagen synthesis is partly a function of the oxygenation of tissues. Therefore oxygen perfusion to tissues contributes to the rate of healing, tensile strength of the wound, and resistance to infection. This is particularly important in arterialized and microvascular tissue grafts and flaps used to cover soft tissue defects and in organ transplantation. Ischemic tissue is more susceptible to infection than well-vascularized tissue.

Physical Activity

Early ambulation postoperatively is one of the most important factors in recovery for the surgical patient. Ambulation may be started immediately after recovery from anesthesia if the patient's condition does not contraindicate it. Some surgeons exempt only the patient whose blood pressure is not stable, the patient who has a cardiac problem, or the patient whose general condition is poor. If the patient's physical condition does not safely permit ambulation, the surgeon orders otherwise.

Ambulation is started gradually, with the patient first turning onto one side. The patient then sits up with the feet over the side of the bed and then stands on the floor for a minute before returning to bed. After repeating this several times, the patient takes a few steps and finally increases the distance walked. Sitting in a chair for prolonged periods is discouraged because this contributes to stasis of blood. The patient must understand the value of early ambulation, which includes the following:

1. Early ambulation improves circulation, which aids in the healing process and eliminates stasis of blood, which may result in thrombus and embolus formation.
2. The patient is better able to cooperate in deep-breathing exercises to raise bronchial secretions; thus pulmonary complications are reduced.
3. Early ambulation decreases gas pain, distention, and the tendency toward nausea and vomiting. It helps prevent constipation. Bodily functions return to normal more readily.
4. Increased exercise aids digestion. Thus the patient's oral intake progresses sooner after the surgical procedure, so that less supplementary intravenous fluid is necessary for hydration and nutrition.
5. Early ambulation eliminates the general muscle weakness that follows bed rest.
6. Fewer pain-relieving drugs are necessary.
7. It boosts patients' morale to know that they will be out of bed early after the surgical procedure, able to care for themselves, and soon ready to go home. This helps the mental outlook and, through it, the physical recovery.
8. Early ambulation shortens hospitalization.

WOUND MANAGEMENT

Providing appropriate conditions for wound healing has been a quest through the ages. In ancient mythology the Greek god Hermes carried a staff entwined with two snakes. This signified the snake's ability to repeatedly shed and regenerate its skin. Although humans do not shed their skin, they can regenerate tissue cells if the wound is protected from accumulations of blood and serum, mechanical injury, impaired circulation, and infection.

Drains

The use of devices to drain fluids and pus from the body dates back to the writings of Hippocrates. He wrote of insertion of a hollow tin tube with flushings of wine and tepid oil to treat empyema (Figure 31-3). This was the first wound

Figure 31-3 Early reusable metal drains.

drainage system. In the nineteenth century, glass tubes, to be replaced by rubber catheters, were commonly used for gravity drainage. In 1897 Dr. Charles Penrose described a tubular drain made of gutta-percha, the coagulated latex from rubber trees, with a gauze wick inserted through the length of the lumen. This latex drain, which still bears his name, is in use today to maintain a vent for the escape of fluid or air or to wall off an area of exudate in the wound. Sump drains, commercially introduced in 1932, offered advantages, such as use with suction apparatus. Suction drainage has been used since 1947. Closed wound drainage systems, first introduced in 1952, are used to enhance wound healing.

The use of gravity drainage through various types of tubes vs. capillary drainage through wicking devices historically has been a controversial issue. Even today, surgeons do not universally agree on the use of systems currently available. The location and purpose of the drain determine the surgeon's selection from the many types available. Drains may be used prophylactically or therapeutically during the surgical procedure and/or postoperatively.

Intraoperative Drainage

Used prophylactically to evacuate gastric contents, intestinal fluids, or urine, intraoperative drainage and decompression help prevent tissue trauma and restore organs to normal function.

Gastrointestinal Decompression A plastic or rubber nasogastric tube inserted through a nostril down into the stomach or small intestine removes flatus, fluids, or other contents. The tube has holes in several locations near the tip to permit withdrawal of the contents. Several types of nasogastric tubes are used; the most common are the Levin tube into the stomach and the Miller-Abbott tube into the small intestine. A vented tube, such as the Salem sump tube, is preferable for use with nasogastric suction.

To prevent aspiration of stomach contents, the anesthesia provider may insert a nasogastric tube preoperatively to empty the stomach before an emergency surgical procedure. The surgeon may ask the anesthesia provider to insert a tube during an intraabdominal procedure for one of the following purposes:

- Decompression of the gastrointestinal tract
- Relief of distention that obstructs the view of the surgical site
- Measurement of blood loss from gastric hemorrhage
- Evacuation of gastric secretions during intestinal anastomosis

The nasogastric tube may remain in place postoperatively to prevent vomiting and distention caused by decreased peristalsis following anesthesia, manipulation of the viscera during the surgical procedure, or obstruction from edema of tissues at the surgical site. For this purpose the tube is connected to a suction apparatus. The tube may also be used for nasogastric feeding during the healing process after a surgical procedure on the upper alimentary canal.

Urinary Drainage Urethral or ureteral catheters inserted preoperatively provide constant drainage from the bladder or kidneys during the surgical procedure. The purpose may be to keep the bladder decompressed or to prevent extravasation of urine into the tissues around the surgical site during and after genitourinary procedures. Postoperatively the inflated balloon of an indwelling Foley catheter maintains an even pressure on the bladder neck, which may help control bleeding following prostatectomy, for example. An indwelling Foley catheter may be connected to a bladder irrigation or gravity drainage system until the bladder resumes normal function postoperatively.

Postoperative Drainage

Drains are used therapeutically in the presence of purulent or necrotic material. Prophylactically they may be inserted to evacuate fluids, including blood, or air from a wound or body cavity postoperatively. Drains are usually placed in a separate small stab wound adjacent to the surgical incision and secured with a nonabsorbable monofilament suture. Drains can stimulate a walling-off process around a surgical site in which subsequent drainage may accumulate. This enhances wound healing by:

- Eliminating fluid accumulation
- Obliterating dead space
- Allowing apposition of tissues
- Preventing formation of hematomas or seromas
- Preventing tissue devitalization or wound margin necrosis
- Minimizing a potential source of wound contamination
- Decreasing postoperative pain
- Minimizing scarring

The action of drains may be either passive or active.

Passive Drains Passive drains provide the path of least resistance to the outside. They function by overflow and capillary action through the drain to the absorbent dressing. They are influenced by pressure differentials and may be assisted by gravity.

PENROSE DRAIN A Penrose drain is a thin-walled cylinder of radiopaque latex. The diameter may be ¼ to 2 inches (6 mm to 5 cm), depending on the surgeon's preference. The drain is usually supplied to the sterile field in a 6- to 12-inch (15- to 30-cm) length for the surgeon to cut as desired. Penrose drains are commercially available prepackaged and sterilized. However, if they are prepared for on-site steam sterilization, a gauze wick is inserted to permit steam penetration of the lumen.

Although Penrose drains are usually used without a wick, the surgeon may prefer that the wick of gauze packing be left in the lumen to absorb drainage from the wound. This is referred to as a cigarette drain. For use without a wick, the drain is moistened in normal saline solution before it is handed to the surgeon. After it is placed into the surgical area and brought out through a stab wound in the skin, the drain is secured with a skin suture, or a sterile safety pin is attached on the outside close to the skin to keep the drain from retracting into the wound. The head of the safety pin should be crimped closed with a large forceps to prevent it from opening and piercing the patient.

CONSTANT GRAVITY DRAINAGE A drain may be inserted for drainage by gravity flow from the gallbladder, bladder, or kidney. Each OR suite has a supply of sterile rubber and/ or silicone tubes and catheters. Those used for drains, such as a T-tube, should be radiopaque. Some have inflatable balloons like Foley catheters or enlarged bulbous ends (mushroom, Malecot, Pezzer catheter) to help hold them in place.

A closed or semiclosed system is used to collect drainage. The scrub person keeps the end of the tube or catheter sterile until it is connected to the sterile end of the constant drainage tubing. Tubing should be connected or clamped as soon as the drain is brought through a stab wound in the skin or a tube or catheter is inserted into an organ. The circulator connects tubing to a drainage bag. Constant drainage bags are marked in gradations from 500 to 2000 ml. The bag must be in a dependent position, lower than the site of the drain, to avoid retrograde reflux.

Active Drains
Active drains are attached to an external source of vacuum to create suction in the wound. A constant, gentle, negative pressure vacuum evacuates tissue fluid, blood, and air through a silicone, polyvinyl chloride, or polyurethane drain. Suction levels vary, depending on the system, to create the negative pressure (less than atmospheric).

CLOSED WOUND SUCTION SYSTEMS These systems are used when it is necessary to apply suction to an uninfected closed wound site in the chest wall (e.g., after mastectomy), in the upper part of the abdomen, and in areas of joint replacement. They also are placed under large tissue flaps or in subcutaneous spaces in obese patients to eliminate dead space and to hold tissues in apposition.

The sterile plastic drain with tubing connected to a stainless steel trocar is placed in the surgical area. The trocar makes a small stab wound in the skin as it is brought through the underlying tissues. The drain, either round or flat, has several perforations along the length placed in tissues. It also is radiopaque or has radiopaque markings to aid in checking its location on an x-ray film, if desired. The tubing is connected to a sterile, self-contained portable container, such as a Hemovac (Figure 31-4). Several different units are available with containers of different capacities, as well as sizes of tubings. Calibrations on the side of the container measure the drainage, and a line designates when it should be emptied or changed. These units are made entirely or partially of clear plastic so that the surgeon can inspect drainage.

The drainage container can be attached immediately after placement of the tubing or after wound closure; then the vacuum is activated. Directions printed on each unit must be followed to activate the vacuum. The amount of suction in these systems varies depending on the method of creating the vacuum. Manually activated spring-loaded devices (Hemovac) and grenade-type or bulb evacuators (Relia-Vac, Jackson Pratt) have variable preset suction levels between 30 and 125 mm Hg. A portable battery-powered device (VariDyne) can pro-

Figure 31-4 Hemovac drain reservoir.

vide a constant and continuous vacuum at any setting between 10 and 350 mm Hg. With the latter system, the surgeon can determine the suction level on the basis of the material and area to be evacuated. The drainage container does not need to be in a dependent position with closed wound suction systems. An antireflux valve guards against backflow of fluids.

SUMP DRAINS Sump drains may be used for aspiration, irrigation, or introduction of medication. Either flat or round, a sump drain has a double or triple lumen. Usually made of radiopaque silicone, it has large lateral openings to minimize clogging. The drain is brought out through a separate stab wound. Sump drains create equalized negative pressure at the site to be drained, usually in the abdomen. They are connected to a constant drainage system, with or without suction. Irrigation of the surgical site and connection to suction as soon as possible enhance function. Levels of suction between 80 and 120 mm Hg are desirable. The tubing may be attached to a piped-in (wall) or portable vacuum system. The drain must be clamped when not attached to suction or connected to a closed container. It functions as a passive drain if suction is not used and must be in a dependent position.

CHEST DRAINAGE Drainage of the pleural cavity ensures complete expansion of the lungs postoperatively. Air and fluid must be evacuated from the pleural space following surgical procedures within the chest cavity. One or more chest tubes are inserted. If the surgeon inserts two, the upper tube evacuates air, and the lower tube drains fluid. After the chest tube is inserted during closure, the end is covered with a sterile gauze until it can be connected to a sterile closed water-seal drainage system. The drainage system must prevent outside air from being drawn into the pleural space during expiration. Water in the collection unit seals off outside air to maintain a negative pressure within the pleural cavity.

Two tubes vent the leakproof top of the collection unit. A short air-outlet tube extends 1 inch (2.5 cm) or more above the stopper to about 3 inches (7.5 cm) below it into the collection unit. The long inlet tube extends from above the stopper, through it, to about 1 inch (2.5 cm) from the bottom of the collection unit. Sterile water is poured into the collection unit to a level 1 to 2 inches (2.5 to 5 cm) above the end of the long inlet tube. The circulator marks the water level on the outside of the collection unit. Clear sterile tubing connects the inlet tube to the tube placed into the pleural space. On the patient's initial expiration, water rises a short distance up into the inlet tube. With each subsequent inspiration-expiration the water level in the tube fluctuates. If the water level in the tube remains stationary, the chest tube or connecting tubing may be clogged or kinked. The collection unit must be kept well below chest level to prevent water from entering the chest and to keep the tubing free of kinks.

Fluid drains by gravity from the chest into the water. The collection unit should be calibrated so that drainage can be measured. Air bubbles through the water and escapes through the outlet tube.

If gravity drainage is not adequate for reexpansion of the lungs, suction may be applied at 15 to 20 cm water pressure to ensure evacuation of air and fluid. This requires the addition of one or two collection units to the system to act as a pressure regulator and the addition of a suction machine to maintain negative pressure. Disposable chest drainage units are available commercially, as a single unit or in a series of two or three. Some units have modifications based on the principle described for a closed water-seal system. The manufacturer's directions should be followed for use. The unit must be properly connected before the patient leaves the OR.

With some units the chest tube may be clamped during transportation as a safety measure. The surgeon should be consulted as to whether or not clamping is contraindicated.

Patient Care Considerations

Drains, tubes, catheters, drainage tubing, and adapters are used for one patient only; they are never reused for another patient. If not properly handled by the scrub person and circulator, a drain can be a source of wound contamination or irritation. When the surgeon inserts a drain, the following considerations should be kept in mind:

1. Drains, tubes, and catheters are kept sterile, ready for the circulator to open if needed. They are available in many styles and sizes. They are patient charge items. Do not open until the surgeon specifies the style and size.
2. If patient has a sensitivity to latex, do not use a drain, tube, or catheter with any latex components.

3. The scrub person keeps the end of the drain sterile until it is connected to the sterile end of the drainage tubing.
4. Tubing connections must be physically tight and secured. Do not completely obscure connections by wrapping tape around them.
5. The drain site is dressed separately from the incision site. A nonadherent dressing can be used as the contact layer around the drain. Gauze dressings can be slit in a Y shape to fit around the base of the drain.
6. Avoid tension on the drain and kinks in the drain and tubing. A gentle loop can be made and secured with tape at the time of dressing application.
7. Collection bags or containers connected to passive drains, including chest tubes, must be kept well below the level of the body cavity where the drain is inserted and below the level of the drainage tubing to prevent retrograde flow. The amount of drainage should be recorded.
8. The circulator must check the suction level to be certain it is consistent with the surgeon's orders or should activate the suction as appropriate for the system being used.
9. An x-ray film may be taken to verify placement of the drain or tube.
10. The type of drain and its location are documented on the intraoperative record and reported to the postanesthesia care unit (PACU) nurse.

Dressings

Most skin incisions and surgical wounds are covered with a sterile dressing for at least 24 to 48 hours to provide an optimal physiologic environment for wound healing. The dressing serves several functions:

- To keep the incision free of microorganisms, both exogenous and endogenous
- To protect the incision from outside injury, especially in children
- To absorb the drainage of exudates and secretions from the wound
- To maintain a moist environment that supports healing
- To give some support to the incision and surrounding skin or to immobilize surrounding tissue
- To provide pressure to reduce edema or prevent hematoma
- To conceal the wound aesthetically

The function of a dressing is determined by its structure. The overall dressing should be:

- Large enough to cover and protect the wound site and tissue around it
- Permeable to gas and vapor, allowing circulation of air to the skin
- Secure to prevent slippage
- Comfortable for the patient

Types of Dressings

In considering the components to assemble for the dressing, the needs of the particular wound should be kept in mind. One wound may require a dressing that provides a function different from that needed for another type of wound. The dressing materials should be tailored to the location and condition of the wound site.

One-Layer Dressing   A clean incision that is primarily closed with sutures, staples, or skin closure tapes in which no or slight drainage is expected may be covered with an adhering occlusive dressing (such as Bioclusive or Op-Site). These sterile, transparent polyurethane film dressings are available in various sizes. The patient can bathe or shower with these in place. They usually are removed in 24 to 48 hours. Liquid collodion or an aerosol adhesive spray may be used.

Skin Closure Dressing   A transparent plastic film with an adhesive backing (Op-Site) can be placed over the entire length of the incision to hold the skin edges in apposition. The film is vented to allow the escape of exudate. An additional wound dressing may be overlaid to further splint and reinforce approximation of the skin edges. These dressings are available in various sizes.

Dry Sterile Dressing   A single- or multilayered dressing is applied dry over a clean incision from which no or slight drainage is expected. Dry gauze is not used on a denuded area because it adheres and acts as a foreign body. Granulation tissue will grow into it; bleeding can be reactivated when it is removed. A dry sterile dressing can be applied over a dry wound. It is secured with adhesive tape. A circumferential wrap may be preferred on an extremity, but it must not compromise circulation.

Three-Layer Dressing   When moderate to heavy drainage is expected, a complete dressing consists of at least three layers.

CONTACT LAYER   The contact layer acts as a passageway for the secretion and exudates that emanate from a draining wound. It has a wicking action to help reduce the risk of infection and skin maceration. It must conform to body contours regardless of the site and extent of the wound and must stay in intimate contact with the wound surface for at least 48 hours yet be nonadherent for painless removal. The contact layer may be:

- *Nonocclusive.* Nonadherent materials, such as gauze sponges or compressed material on a thin plastic or aluminum film, draw secretions from the wound but remain air permeable. The looser the weave of the material, the more nonocclusive it is.
- *Semiocclusive.* Hydroactive materials, such as foams, hydrogels, and hydrocolloids, provide a mechanical surface with permeability properties. Some of these agents actually help debride the wound.

- *Occlusive.* An airtight seal prevents drying of the wound. The dressing is impermeable to air and water but allows passage of exudates. This is usually a fine mesh gauze dressing impregnated with an oil emulsion, such as petrolatum, Xeroform, iodophor, antibiotic ointment, or scarlet red. It is nonadherent to the skin or wound.

INTERMEDIATE LAYER   This layer absorbs secretions passing through the contact layer. To provide adequate capacity, it should be layered (e.g., with gauze sponges) to the thickness required by the particular wound. It should not be excessively bulky. It must not unnecessarily apply pressure that could compromise circulation.

OUTER LAYER   This layer holds the contact and intermediate layers in proper position. It should be conforming, stretchable to avoid constriction if edema develops, and capable of clinging to itself so that it will stay in position without telescoping if mobility is desired. The following materials are used for this purpose:

1. Nonallergenic tape is used most frequently.
2. An elastic bandage provides gentle, even pressure to hold bulky dressings in place or to bind a splint onto an extremity. It stretches to conform to body contours, does not constrict, yet gives firm support. The types available include:
   a. Four-ply crinkled-gauze bandage
   b. Cotton elastic bandage
   c. Cotton elastic bandage with adhesive on one side, which is especially useful in holding dressings on the chest, because it is firm yet permits chest expansion
3. Montgomery straps are used to hold bulky dressings that require frequent changes or wound inspections. These are pairs of adhesive straps in assorted widths with strings attached to one folded end of each strap. The other end of each strap is secured to the skin on each side of the dressing. The strings are tied across the dressing to hold it in place, usually on the abdomen.
4. Stockinette is put over the dressing on an extremity before application of a rigid cast used for immobilization. Available in several widths, stockinette is a seamless tubing of stretchable knitted cotton.

Pressure Dressing   Bulky dressings are added to the intermediate layer of a three-layer dressing following many extensive surgical procedures, especially in plastic surgery and surgical procedures on the knee or breast. Pressure dressings are used for the following purposes:

- To eliminate dead space and prevent edema or hematoma
- To distribute pressure evenly
- To absorb extensive drainage
- To encourage wound healing and minimize scarring by influencing wound tension

- To immobilize a body area or support soft tissues when muscles are moved
- To help provide comfort to the patient postoperatively

Materials used for pressure dressings include the following:

- Fluffed gauze
- Combine pads, which are gauze-covered absorbent cellulose
- Single-piece bulk dressings, which are available for use on the trunk and extremities and save time in application
- Cotton rolls, which are used, for example, to apply pressure on each side of a knee following a surgical procedure on that joint
- Foam rubber

Stent Dressing   Stent fixation is a method of applying pressure and stabilizing tissues when it is impossible to dress an area, such as the face or neck. A form-fitting mold may be taped over the nose. Long suture ends can be crisscrossed over a small dressing and tied.

Bolster/Tie-Over Dressing   Dressing materials may be sutured in place to exert an even pressure over autografted wounds to prevent hematoma or seroma formation. Sterile gauze may be rolled into a tubular shape and tied with the ends of the wound closure suture.

Wet-to-Dry Dressing   Dressing materials soaked in sterile normal saline solution are applied to the wound and allowed to dry thoroughly. The dried dressing is then removed, taking adhering tissue layers with it. This process is used to facilitate new tissue growth and is commonly used on burn wounds. Because this method of debridement is extremely painful, it is frequently performed in the OR with the patient under general anesthesia.

Wet-to-Wet Dressing   Dressing materials are soaked in sterile normal saline solution or other medicated solution and applied wet. This method provides little mechanical debridement and is less painful for the patient. The dressing material may be changed in the OR or under sterile conditions on the nursing unit.

Application of Dressings

Applying sterile dressings is regarded as part of the surgical procedure. The scrub person and circulator assist the surgeon or first assistant in dressing the wound properly. The procedure is as follows:

1. The circulator opens sterile dressings after the final sponge count is completed. Radiopaque sponges are not used because they could distort a postoperative x-ray film or cause an incorrect count if the patient's incision must be reopened.
2. Skin surrounding the incision is cleaned of blood with a sterile saline–dampened sponge.

3. The incision and wound drainage sites are dressed separately unless the drain comes out through the incision. The scrub person cuts a Y-shaped slit in dressings to go around the drain.
4. Sterile dressings are applied before drapes are removed.
5. Benzoin or some other adhesive substance may be applied on the skin around the intermediate layer before adhesive tape is applied to increase its adhesion.
6. The circulator applies tape or Montgomery straps firmly but not tightly to avoid wrinkling and traction on skin. Traction and wrinkling can cause skin irritation.

   If a patient has a known sensitivity to regular adhesive tape, hypoallergenic tape should be used. It is lightweight, yet strong, sticks well, is porous, and allows skin to breathe.
7. The surgeon or first assistant applies elastic bandages, pressure dressings, stockinette and casts, and splints. The circulator provides the necessary supplies and assists as appropriate. A patient care assistant may help hold the patient's torso or extremity during application of an elastic bandage or cast.

COMPLICATIONS OF WOUND HEALING

The surgeon gives meticulous attention to sterile technique, hemostasis, tissue handling and approximation, and selection of wound closure materials, including drains and dressings. The entire OR team carries out strict aseptic and sterile techniques to prevent infection and other possible complications of wound healing.

Hematoma/Seroma

Collections of blood or serum in a wound can act as a mechanical barrier to margination of the wound. Circulation can be interrupted, and neovascularization cannot take place. Studies have shown that biochemical action of the collection causes tissue destruction and promotes bacterial growth. Hematomas in deep tissue can lead to abscess formation.

Scar/Surgical Cicatrix

Following the natural process of wound healing, a scar (cicatrix) will remain on the skin surface. To achieve a cosmetically acceptable scar, the surgeon attempts to make the surgical incision along natural creases or within natural skin folds or hairlines. The location and direction of the incision affect scarring. Tension needed for approximation of wound edges during closure and subsequent movement of underlying tissues can affect wound healing and scar formation. Wounds in mobile skin will contract, resulting in a smaller scar.

Hypertrophic scars, which are a result of excessive fibrin formation within the borders of the scar, can develop from too much tension on the wound, poor approximation of wound edges, or infection. Some suture materials may contribute to hypertrophy. Burn wounds are also conducive to excessive scarring. The patient may wish to have an unsightly scar revised at a future time.

Keloids develop when the inflammatory response and fibroblast proliferation are overactive during wound healing. This is an inherited trait, most common among Africans, Asians, and people with dark skin tones or those who freckle. Keloids extend beyond the borders of the scar and can continue to grow and become very large over a prolonged period after the surgical procedure. They may be painful, itchy, and prone to bleeding. They can be excised, leaving a small border of scar tissue. The edges are approximated using skin staples or fine monofilament nonabsorbable suture. If a patient is known to form keloids, an antiinflammatory agent may be injected into tissue before closure. A pressure dressing is useful in minimizing keloid formation. Application of silicone gel sheeting placed over healed bulky tissue scars for 24 hours over a period of 2 weeks can reduce the size of the scar.

Nodules and granulomas may form in the scar if excess suture material is used. Scar tissue hypertrophies around the suture, particularly the knot. Some patients will extrude suture pieces through their incision line for several months or years postoperatively. This may represent a sensitivity to the suture material.

Adhesions

An adhesion is a fibrous scar band that binds together two surfaces or structures that normally are separate. Fibrous bands that develop in the peritoneal cavity can hold viscera together, sometimes causing bowel obstruction or female infertility. The most common cause is previous abdominal or pelvic surgery, but acute appendicitis or peritonitis can cause adhesion formation. Serosal injury caused by abrasion from sponges or gloves, tissue handling, infection, and tissue ischemia may be precipitating factors. Other substances, such as blood and biologic debris, can contribute to adhesion formation. Granulomas that form from powder on gloves, lint on sponges, or other foreign material left in the wound also predispose the patient to adhesion formation.

Techniques to prevent peritoneal adhesions include gentle tissue handling, careful irrigation with sterile saline or Ringer's lactate solution, and prevention of foreign body introduction, such as glove powder and lint. Placing a flap of omentum over the affected organ before closure is another acceptable method.

A single-layer knitted absorbable adhesion barrier sheet, such as Interceed (TC7), can be placed over abdominal organs after attaining hemostasis and before closure. It is composed of oxidized regenerated cellulose and absorbs in about 4 weeks. This product is contraindicated in the presence of known infection. Other barrier sheets composed of sodium hyaluronate and carboxymethylcellulose (HA/CMC) can be used over organs at risk for adhesion formation. Once moistened, it adheres to the surface of the organ. No suturing is

necessary. It converts to a gel form and is absorbed by the body in 7 days.

Postoperative Wound Disruption

Failure of a wound to heal or closure material to secure it during the healing process leads to wound disruption, a separation of wound edges. Disruption usually occurs between the fifth and tenth postoperative day. This is the lag period in healing, the time when the wound is not yet strong. Wound disruption is caused not by a single factor but by a combination of predisposing factors that influence healing.

Although it may occur in any body area, acute wound disruption most frequently follows abdominal laparotomy, surgical incision into the peritoneal cavity. It starts with a small opening in the peritoneum, which allows a wedge of omentum to slip through it. This omentum becomes edematous and extends the opening along the line of incision and upward through other layers of the abdominal wall. Disruption is usually precipitated by distention or a sudden strain, such as vomiting, coughing, or sneezing. Terms used to describe abdominal wound disruption include the following:

- *Dehiscence.* Partial or total separation of the superficial layers of the wound. The strength of the tissues and extent of separation determine whether or not the wound must be reclosed. Strangulated sutures can cause devitalized wound edges that may fail to heal. Wound infection can cause dehiscence.
- *Evisceration.* Protrusion of viscera through the full thickness of the abdominal incision. Although wound disruption of any degree calls for emergency care, an evisceration requires immediate replacement of viscera and reclosure of the incision.
- *Herniation.* The surface layers remain intact, but the deep layers separate, permitting the underlying muscles or organs to bulge.
- *Fistula.* Draining tunnels may form between two organs, such as between loops of bowel and the bladder.
- *Sinus tract.* An abscess may form in deeper tissues and form a tunnel to the outside of the body.

Symptoms

Patients who subsequently experience wound disruption often do not have a smooth course immediately after surgery. They may have undue pain, discomfort, nausea, drainage, slight fever, vomiting, or hiccups. Acute symptoms of wound disruption include the following:

- Tachycardia
- Vomiting
- Abnormal serosanguineous discharge
- Change in contour of the wound
- Sudden pulling pain during straining (the patient feels something give)

Any seepage of serosanguineous fluid is suspicious and should be sent for culture and sensitivity. A swab culture for both aerobic and anerobic microorganisms should be obtained. If the patient has had antibiotic therapy, this should be noted on the laboratory request. The patient's wound, rather than the eschar, should be swabbed. Gloves should be worn when culturing a patient's wound or handling dressing material.

Any of these symptoms should be investigated at once. Examination of the wound may show it gaping somewhat, or viscera may appear at the skin surface.

Treatment at the Bedside

1. Place an emergency call for the surgeon. Have a nasogastric tube ready for insertion to relieve distention.
2. Reassure the patient.
3. Apply sterile, moist saline dressings over the wound and a loose binder.
4. Give drugs according to the surgeon's order.
5. Do not give the patient anything by mouth.
6. Prepare the patient for return to the OR. Treatment in the OR consists of secondary wound closure. Grossly infected wounds may require delayed primary closure.

Wound Infections

Wound healing can be interrupted by infection at almost any phase. Infection results from introduction of virulent microorganisms into the receptive wound of a susceptible host. Moisture and warmth in the wound create an environment conducive to bacterial growth. Wound infections warrant special attention because many occur in clean wounds as a result of microorganisms introduced at the time of the surgical procedure. Secondary contamination is uncommon because fibrin seals the wound within hours after the surgical procedure.

POSTOPERATIVE WOUND INFECTIONS

A postoperative wound infection may occur in the incision or in deep structures that were entered or exposed. Its nature and severity vary because of local, systemic, technical, or environmental factors. Each factor is important; all are interrelated in clinical infection. Usually a postoperative infection is localized, but severe systemic reaction is possible. The specific pathogen and site of infection determine its gravity. Postoperative wound infections are classified as follows:

- *Incisional infection.* An infection occurs at the site of the incision within 30 postoperative days. It involves skin, subcutaneous tissue, or muscle. The incisional area is usually inflamed and sore. Purulent drainage or an organism identified by culture is present. The surgeon usually must open and drain the wound.
- *Deep wound infection.* An infection occurs at the surgical site within 30 postoperative days if a prosthesis was not implanted or within 1 year around the site of an im-

plant. The infection involves tissues or spaces at or beneath the fascia. Pus may be present. The wound may spontaneously dehisce. The surgeon may need to open and drain the wound or remove an implant. Infection involving an implant or gross necrotic tissue is prone to serious sequelae.

Compromised patients and geriatric patients are highly likely to develop endogenous infection. Procedures on potentially contaminated areas, such as the gastrointestinal tract, are more apt to result in postoperative infections. Wound infections can progress to septicemia and multisystem organ failure.

Nosocomial Infections

Infections that were not present or incubating when the patient was admitted are hospital-associated infections or are acquired (i.e., nosocomial) during the course of health care. Nosocomial infections may occur as complications of surgical or other procedures performed on uninfected patients. The term also refers to complicating infections in organs unrelated to the surgical procedure, occurring with or as a result of postoperative care. Wound infection is the second most common infection. Nosocomial infections may be exogenous or endogenous.

Exogenous Infections

An exogenous nosocomial infection is acquired from sources outside the body, such as personnel or the environment. Cross-contamination occurs when organisms are transferred to the patient from another individual or inanimate object.

Endogenous Infections

An endogenous infection develops from sources within the body. Most postoperative wound infections result from seeding by endogenous microorganisms. Disruption of the balance between potentially pathogenic organisms and host defenses permits invasion of microorganisms for which the patient is the primary reservoir. For example, abdominal sepsis may result from enteric flora if the intestine is perforated or transected.

Prevention of Wound Infections

Prevention of wound infection and a successful outcome of surgical intervention are goals of the team administering perioperative care to surgical patients. In summary, preventive measures should focus on the following:

- Adherence to aseptic and sterile techniques and standard precautions with all patients
- Control of endogenous infection
- Meticulous surgical technique and wound closure
- Reduction of exogenous or environmental sources of contamination, such as airborne microorganisms

- Thorough, prompt cleansing and debridement of traumatic wounds
- Prevention of intraoperative contamination of a wound
- Appropriate use of prophylactic antibiotics
- Frequent handwashing
- Sterile technique for dressing changes

Serious sequelae, such as wound disruption or septicemia, may follow wound infection. Therefore they must be assiduously prevented so that wound healing can occur naturally.

WOUND ASSESSMENT

The stages of wound healing will vary among individuals according to generalized health and age. Other factors influence the mechanism and should be taken into consideration when assessing the progress of healing postoperatively.

Objective Inspection of the Postoperative Wound

The perioperative nurse should inspect the patient's wound and document its condition. The nurse should have a basic understanding of the mechanism of the injury or the source of the wound, such as a surgical incision, and should be able to assess the wound for complications. All complaints of pain should be investigated and referred to the physician. Gloves should be worn during wound assessment. Sterility should be maintained as appropriate. Assessment of the wound should include the following:

1. Location of single or multiple sites.
   a. Laparoscopy can yield multiple puncture sites.
   b. Trauma can cause multiple wounds varying in type.
   c. Some injuries can be unseen, such as organ trauma.
   d. Incidental wounds, such as pressure sores, may not be obvious for several days postoperatively.
2. Color of the wound and surrounding tissue. It may be a combination of one or all colors. Estimate the volume of each color in percentages of the total wound.
   a. A red wound bed indicates healing, granulating tissue. Pink indicates epithelialization.
   b. Yellow to yellow-white indicates exudate caused by microorganisms. The color can range from greenish to beige, depending on which organism is present and if antibiotic therapy is in place.
   c. Black indicates necrotic tissue that can interfere with healing and supports the growth of microorganisms.
   d. Redness combined with swelling surrounding the edges of the wound may indicate infection.
   e. Macerated tissue around a wound may indicate the need for thicker dressing material or a pouch to collect drainage.
3. Perfusion of the patient's tissues.
   a. Capillary refill should be assessed.
   b. Blanching of surrounding tissues may indicate lack of blood flow.

4. Size in length, width, and depth.
   a. The wound should be measured in centimeters.
   b. The depth can be measured with a sterile cotton-tipped swab.
   c. Tunneling should be noted for direction and depth.
   d. Anatomic description pertaining to lines of direction should be described like the face of a clock. The direction of the patient's head should be considered as 12 o'clock.
5. Temperature of the site(s) and the patient.
   a. Hot to warm tissue surrounding the wound may indicate infection.
   b. Elevated body temperature may indicate systemic sepsis.
6. Dressing type and condition.
   a. Is the dressing wet or dry?
   b. Is the dressing constrictive?
   c. Is the dressing effective for its intended purpose?
7. Drainage and/or drainage device.
   a. Odors usually indicate drainage and infection.
   b. The presence of embedded material may become obvious as the wound bed sloughs. Traumatic or industrial wounds may entrap foreign material that could be extruded in exudate.
   c. Drainage of more than 50 ml/day should be pouched for collection.
   d. Gastrointestinal contents, such as bile, stool, or pancreatic enzymes, should not be permitted to contact surrounding skin. An ostomy appliance should be used.

BASIC WOUND CARE

Gloves are worn for all dressing change procedures. Eye protection or full face shields should be worn if syringes are used for irrigation. The wound should be cleansed before replacing the dressing. Rinsing with sterile normal saline provides a moist environment for healing and promotes granulation formation. Some antiseptics, such as povidone-iodine, hydrogen peroxide, or acetic acid, can cause tissue injury and delay wound healing. The wound should be cleaned before the surrounding area to prevent contamination of the open site. Gauze used for cleansing surrounding tissue should not drag across the open wound.

Debridement may be necessary. Nonsurgical methods of debridement include chemical autolysis and mechanical packing materials. Autolysis involves placing proteolytic enzymes in the wound to break down necrotic tissue. The viable tissue is unaffected. Mechanical debridement is accomplished by the use of wet-to-dry dressings as described earlier under Dressings. The results of debridement are fresh, granulation tissue and a clean wound bed. Surgical debridement may be performed with dissection instruments, such as scissors or a scalpel. A laser is sometimes used, although it can cause devitalization of tissue by charring.

Dressing material and wound care products are determined by physicians' orders. Types, advantages, and disadvantages of various wound care materials can be found in Table 31-2.

TABLE 31-2	Wound Care Materials				
Dressing Material	**Composition and Properties**	**Indications for Use**	**Advantages**	**Disadvantages**	**Notes**
Alginate	Originates from brown seaweed; highly absorbent; becomes a gel when exposed to exudate, creating a moist environment	Used for infected and noninfected wounds with moderate to heavy drainage; some are used for tunneling wounds	Can absorb 20 times its own weight in fluid; rehydrates wound and facilitates debridement; requires secondary dressing cover	Contraindicated for use with light exudate or dry eschar; can promote bacterial growth if used with occlusive dressing cover; not used with third-degree burns	Packaged as ropelike fibers or pad; do not use with alkaline solutions; packaged sterile; remains in place 2 to 4 days
Composite	Composed of two or more moisture-enhancing materials in combination with absorbent material	Used for partial- or full-thickness wounds with moderate to heavy exudate; can also be used over fresh granulation or necrotic tissue	Facilitates debridement and allows for moisture/vapor exchange; safe for use over healthy or infected tissue; easy to apply and remove	Should be placed in area with border of healthy intact tissue for anchoring; should not be used for light exudate; may cause excess moisture loss; can become very adherent	Check manufacturer's recommendations about use with adjunct topical medications
Exudate absorber	Added to wound surface to eliminate dead space and absorb exudate; minimizes odors	Used for full-thickness wounds with moderate to heavy exudate; can be used with necrotic wounds; some can be used as lining material before packing and surface dressing	Can absorb five times its own weight in fluid; rehydrates wound and facilitates debridement; requires secondary dressing cover	Contraindicated for use with light exudate or dry eschar	Supplied in bottles or packets; clean wound and irrigate before use; fill the wound cavity to eliminate dead space and line the defect
Foam	Semipermeable, either hydrophilic or hydrophobic	Creates a moist environment and affords thermal insulation	Nonadherent; repels contaminants and is easy to apply and remove; absorbs light to moderate exudate; can be used with compression dressings; requires secondary dressing cover	Not used for dry wounds; can cause maceration of adjacent skin	Some erythema or itching may occur during the first 24 hours; not used with occlusive dressings; change more frequently if exudate is heavy
Gauze	Composed of woven or nonwoven materials; can be impregnated; used as primary or secondary dressing; can be natural or synthetic material; nonocclusive	Used for wound protection, wicking, and absorption; can be used wet or dry; packaged in rolls, pads, or strips	Moderately absorbent; less expensive to use and can be used in combination with other material; can be used as packing	Needs to be changed frequently; can leak or strike through; can dry out, causing injury to healing tissue	If applied wet and allowed to dry, gauze can be used as debridement agent; may be saturated with oils, iodophor, bismuth, petroleum jelly, scarlet red

From Fortunato NM, McCullough SM: *Plastic and reconstructive surgery,* St Louis, 1998, Mosby.

Continued

TABLE 31-2	Wound Care Materials—cont'd				
Dressing Material	**Composition and Properties**	**Indications for Use**	**Advantages**	**Disadvantages**	**Notes**
Hydrocolloid	Occlusive, adhesive wafer; the contact layer may differ in composition; creates a moist environment; supplied in packets, tubes (paste), oral discs, and wafers; can be cut to fit	Clean wounds will granulate and necrotic wounds will debride autolytically	Impermeable to contaminants; self-adhesive and can remain in place for 3 to 5 days without tissue damage; slight to moderate absorption	Not used with heavy exudate, sinus tracts, or infection; not intended for full-thickness wounds exposing bone; unable to visualize the wound; occlusive properties inhibit air exchange; can injure fragile tissue at wound edges	Safe to use under compression devices and wraps; can be used at ostomy sites or areas affected by incontinence
Hydrogel	Water or glycerin-based gel, gauze, or sheet dressing that has high moisture content; supplied in tubes, packets, spray, liquid	Used for partial- and full-thickness wounds; good for burns, necrosis, and radiated tissue	Very soothing; can rehydrate dried tissues; used to fill dead space and facilitate debridement	Not used for absorption of exudate because of inherent moisture content; can dry out easily; not a bacterial barrier; may be difficult to secure to wound	Keep covered after application to prevent evaporation of the gel
Transparent film	Adhesive, semi-permeable membrane; bacterial and water barrier; permeable to oxygen	Waterproof, but permeable to air and moisture vapors; bacterial barrier	Promotes a moist environment for new granulation and autolysis of necrotic tissue	Not used for infected wounds; periphery of wound needs to be intact to apply the film; may be hard to apply	Used for superficial and partial-thickness wounds with minimal exudate
Skin sealant	Barrier film applied in liquid form that dries to form a plasticlike barrier coating; supplied in liquid form and individual wipettes	Used on intact skin surrounding a wound, ostomy site, or over a surgical incision closed by primary intention	Waterproof barrier	Can sting raw skin when applied; has alcohol base to cause drying by evaporation	Some have vapors that may be harmful to inhale as product evaporates

From Fortunato NM, McCullough SM: *Plastic and reconstructive surgery,* St Louis, 1998, Mosby.

Bibliography

Bane CL, Jennings C: Adhesion reduction as a new treatment innovation, *AORN J* 67(4):774, 776-778, 781-782, 1998.

Brown-Etris M et al: Case studies: considering dressing options, *Ostomy Wound Manage* 40(5):50-52, 1994.

Department of Health and Human Services: Draft guideline for the prevention of surgical site infection, part 3, *Fed Register* 63(116):33168-33179, 1998.

Erwin-Toth P, Hocevar BJ: Wound care: selecting the right dressing, *Am J Nurs* 95(2):46-51, 1995.

Fortunato NM, McCullough SM: *Plastic and reconstructive surgery,* St Louis, 1998, Mosby.

Giadani MB, Grabski WJ: Cutaneous candidiasis as a cause of delayed surgical wound healing, *J Am Acad Dermatol* 30(6):981-984, 1994.

Goodman T: Preventing surgical site infections, *Infect Control Today* 2(11):36, 38, 1998.

Holmadahl L: Mechanisms of adhesion development and effects on wound healing, *Eur J Surg Suppl* 579:7-9, 1997.

Katz BE: Silicone gel sheeting in scar therapy, *Cutis* 56(1):65-67, 1995.

Lazarus GS et al: Definitions and guidelines for assessment of wounds and evaluation of healing, *Arch Dermatol* 130(4):489-493, 1994.

Michie DD, Hugill JV: Influence of occlusive and impregnated gauze dressings on incisional healing: a prospective, randomized, controlled study, *Ann Plast Surg* 32(1):57-64, 1994.

O'Hanlon-Nichols T: Clinical savvy: commonly asked questions about wound healing, *Am J Nurs* 95(4):22-24, 1995.

Ondrey FG, Hom DB: Effects of nutrition on wound healing, *Otolaryngol Head Neck Surg* 110(6):557-559, 1994.

Ovington LG: Infection control issues in chronic wound management, *Infect Control Today* 2(8):20, 22, 24, 1998.

Pryor F, Messmer PR: The effect of traffic patterns in the OR on surgical site infections, *AORN J* 68(4):649-655, 657-660, 1998.

Sawyer RG, Pruett TL: Wound infections, *Surg Clin North Am* 74(3):519-536, 1994.

Wound care handbook, *Nursing* 26(8):42-45, 1996.

Section
XI

Postoperative
Patient Care

Chapter 32

Postoperative Patient Care

 Chapter Objectives

After studying this chapter, the learner will be able to:

- List several functions of a postanesthesia recovery unit.
- Discuss the role of the perianesthesia nurse.
- Define the differences in postanesthesia phases as compared to patient condition.

Surgical procedures are performed in many diverse settings, including surgeons' offices, ambulatory surgery centers, and hospital-based surgical suites and specialty units. In general, the selection of the surgical setting is influenced by the anticipated complexity of the procedure, the patient's health status, available technology, and financial resources. Regardless of the surgical setting or procedure, the patient should be observed and monitored postoperatively for physiologic condition in a controlled postsurgical/postanesthesia environment before being transferred to a patient care unit or discharged from the facility. The postoperative phase of the surgical patient's perioperative experience begins after the surgical procedure is completed and the patient is admitted to a post-procedural area (usually a postanesthesia care unit [PACU] or an intensive care unit [ICU]) or discharged to his or her home. An on-line postanesthesia patient care scenario is available for practice at **nursing.about.com/library/weekly/ aa061798.htm.** Terms associated with postoperative patient care are defined in Box 32-1.

HISTORICAL BACKGROUND

The concept of a PACU (formerly referred to as a "postanesthesia recovery room") has been popular since the early 1940s, when postoperative mortality and morbidity studies demon-

strated that appropriate observation and monitoring could have prevented death in a significant number of postsurgical patients. Prior to this, patients were sent to various patient care areas and did not have the benefit of appropriate monitoring. Causes of death documented within the first 24 hours of anesthetic administration and surgical procedure were obstruction of airway, laryngospasm, hemorrhage, cardiac arrest, and inappropriate administration of medication. Contributing factors included inadequate postoperative patient care, a lack of standardized observation parameters, and an absence of medical supervision. Postoperative patient care was inconsistent and inefficient. The need for postoperative care performed by appropriately educated registered nurses in a controlled environment was identified in these studies.

The 1950s were years of great progress in postanesthesia recovery. Blood pressure monitoring and mechanical respirators improved quality of care. Many facilities expanded to include specialized departments designed to accommodate patient admission directly from the operating room (OR). By 1960, most hospitals had a recovery room near the OR suite.

Instrumentation and monitoring equipment increased the efficiency of postoperative recovery during the 1970s. Many surgical procedures required prolonged intensive recovery. Personnel hours increased, and recovery room activities extended beyond an 8-hour shift. Disposable supplies were

Box 32-1   Terms Associated with Postoperative Patient Care

dermatome   Unilateral segment of skin and subcutaneous tissue supplied by a single sensory nerve root. Level is named for the area of the spine from which the afferent nerve originates.

dermatome map   Topographic outline of bilateral sensory nerve root distribution beginning with the cervical spinal nerves and ending at the sacral spinal nerves.

perianesthesia nursing   Providing patient care before and after the administration of anesthesia for a surgical procedure.

TABLE 32-1   American Society of Anesthesiologists Physical (P) Status Classification

Status*	Definition
P1	A normal healthy patient
P2	Mild systemic disease without functional limitations
P3	Severe systemic disease associated with definite functional limitations
P4	Severe systemic disease that is an ongoing threat to life
P5	Patient is unlikely to survive 24 hours without the surgical procedure
P6	Patient is brain dead and being prepared as an organ donor

From American Society of Anesthesiologists: *Manual for anesthesia departments,* Park Ridge, Ill, 1997, The Society.
*With P2, P3, and P4, the systemic disease may or may not be related to the cause for surgery. If a patient (P1 through P5) requires emergency surgery, an E is added to the physical status (e.g., P1E, P2E). ASA 1 through ASA 6 or I-VI is often used for physical status.

more readily available and made the job much easier. By the 1980s, the use of computerized equipment was becoming the standard of care. Ambulatory surgery was more common, and the average length of stay in recovery was 1 hour.

The PACU of the 1990s has increased the capability for invasive and noninvasive monitoring. Patient care standards are integral to perianesthesia care. The outcomes are more readily evaluated when all perioperative caregivers participate in the plan of care.

POSTANESTHESIA CARE

Ideally, an area is designated for the care of postoperative/postprocedural patients. The area may vary in name or location according to its specific function within the health care facility. In some settings in which only local anesthetics are used, the patient has a brief postoperative observation period in the room where the procedure was performed. When this patient is determined to be physiologically stable, he or she is discharged from the facility. Dental, podiatric, and dermatologic offices often function in this capacity.

Immediate postoperative patient care is usually provided in a designated area of the hospital or ambulatory care facility. This area may be called the recovery room (RR) or postanesthesia recovery unit (PAR). In this text the term *postanesthesia care unit* is used to describe a specialized area for patient care during recovery from anesthesia. Institutional policies and procedures guide patient care activities in the PACU according to protocol established by the anesthesia and surgical services departments. The American Society of Anesthesiologists (ASA) has devised a scale of physical assessment ratings by which patients are categorized by perioperative/perianesthesia risk and outcome (Table 32-1).

Organized in 1980, the American Society of PeriAnesthesia Nurses (ASPAN), formerly known as the American Society of Post Anesthesia Nurses, has established standards of practice for the postoperative care of diverse populations, such as pediatric, adult, and geriatric patients. ASPAN has identified specific phases of care:

- *Preanesthesia phase:* Focuses on the emotional and physical preparation of patients before a surgical procedure. The patient is assessed to establish the nursing diagnoses for the perianesthesia period.
- *Postanesthesia phase I:* Focuses on providing immediate postoperative care from an anesthetized state to a condition requiring less acute intervention. The patient may be ASA III or IV. Nurses in this realm of care should be certified in advanced cardiac life support (ACLS) or have equivalent education. Registered nurses who care primarily for pediatric patients should be certified in pediatric advanced life support (PALS).
- *Postanesthesia phase II:* Focuses on preparing the patient for self-care or care in an extended-care setting.
- *Remote postanesthesia phase III:* Focuses on the patient who is eminently preparing for discharge.

The goal of postanesthesia/postprocedural care is to assist the patient in returning to a safe physiologic level after having received an anesthetic or after having undergone a surgical procedure. In some settings, perianesthesia nurses follow the patient to phase III, with a phone call to the patient's home within 24 to 28 hours of discharge. More information about ASPAN position statements concerning patient care is available at **www.aspan.org.**

Postanesthesia Care Unit

Located in close proximity to the OR, the basic PACU design consists of a large room (approximately 80 square feet) divided into a series of individual cubicles that are separated by privacy curtains. The beds should be a minimum of 4 feet apart, and there should be equivalent spacing between the bedside tables and walls. Each cubicle has a cardiac monitor, pulse oximeter, blood pressure measurement device, suction apparatus, and oxygen administration equipment. Additional supplies that are available include warming devices, airway management equipment, intravenous fluids and administration sets, dressing reinforcement materials, medications, indwelling Foley catheters and drainage systems, emesis basins, and bedpans. Lead screens should be available when x-ray studies are performed. Other equipment, including cardiac arrest carts with defibrillators, should be positioned strategically throughout the room for easy accessibility when needed. More than one emergency setup should be immediately available in case the other is in use. Foot- or elbow-controlled handwashing stations should be in close proximity to patient care areas.

Some facilities include isolation rooms for patients who are highly contagious or highly susceptible to infection. If the PACU does not have a partitioned isolation area, these patients may be placed at one end of the room and separated from other patients by screens or curtains. Isolation procedures should be used in handling bedding and equipment per institutional policy. All patients have the right to receive the same level of care regardless of extenuating circumstances.

Ideally, the amount of cubicle space is allotted according to the number of ORs in the OR suite. This allotment may vary between one and one-half to two cubicles per OR and is based on the case load, duration of surgical procedures, and room turnover time in the OR. A rapid succession of short procedures could easily fill the PACU and leave no vacancy for additional postoperative patients. This scenario is more common in facilities in which the PACU doubles as a special procedure care unit for ambulatory patients who are receiving nerve blocks for pain therapy. Some institutions allow an uncomplicated endoscopy to be performed in the PACU. The rationale behind this practice is that patients having special procedures need to be monitored by experienced personnel for a short time after a treatment or test. For some procedures the PACU nurse monitors a patient receiving intravenous conscious sedation and may assist the physician, thus depleting the staff available for postoperative care.

In larger institutions in which prolonged and complex surgical procedures are performed (e.g., transplantation or multiple trauma), postoperative patients may remain in the PACU for more than 24 hours because of the potential need to return to the OR for an additional surgical procedure. In such cases the PACU doubles as a surgical ICU. Increased patient load and acuity increases the need for adequate staffing, space allocation, education of personnel, and management of resources. The consolidation of facilities and personnel should not jeopardize the delivery of safe postoperative patient care. Use of the PACU as an overflow ICU depletes the resources intended for the adequate care of postsurgical patients.

Postoperative Observation of the Patient

The duration and type of postoperative observation and care will vary according to the following:

- Patient's condition (e.g., alert and oriented vs. unresponsive)
- Need for physiologic support (e.g., ventilator-dependent vs. awake and extubated)

Box 32-2	Dermatome Sensory Somatic Landmarks		
C2	Occiput	L1	Groin to dorsum of foot
C5	Shoulder	L5	Dorsum of foot
T1	Little finger	S1	Heel, lateral foot to sole of foot
T4	Nipple line	S3	Genitalia
T6	Xiphoid process	S5	Perianal area
T12	Iliac crest		

- Complexity of the surgical procedure (e.g., open laparotomy vs. laparoscopy)
- Type of anesthesia administered (e.g., a general inhalation agent vs. local infiltration)
- Need for pain therapy (e.g., intermittent analgesic administration vs. continuous epidural infusion)
- Prescribed period for monitoring parameters to evaluate physiologic status (e.g., stable vs. unstable vital signs)

Perianesthesia Patient Care Personnel

Adequate personnel should be available to monitor patients and to provide appropriate care as needed. The education and training of PACU nurses should include knowledge of the following:

- Airway management techniques, including positioning, chin lift, jaw thrust, suctioning, bagging, and placement of an airway
- Circulatory assessment, including hemodynamics, neurovascular condition, and renal function
- Neurologic condition, such as level of consciousness or dermatome level associated with epidural infusion (Box 32-2 and Figure 32-1)
- Anesthetic agents and their actions (e.g., physiologic depression associated with general anesthesia)
- Medications and their actions (e.g., narcotics and tranquilizers)
- Most invasive and minimally invasive surgical procedures (e.g., open laparotomy and laparoscopy)

PACU nurses should demonstrate competency in the following:

- Physical assessment (e.g., heart and lung sounds)
- Recognition of physiologic complications (e.g., airway obstruction, hypothermia, malignant hyperthermia, pain, nausea or vomiting, and/or oropharyngeal aspiration)
- Management of physiologic emergencies (e.g., airway obstruction, hemorrhage, cardiac arrest)
- Interpretation of monitoring data from electrocardiogram (ECG) and oximetry devices

Additional competencies should include certification in cardiopulmonary resuscitation (CPR)—both basic cardiac life support (BCLS) and ACLS. If pediatric patients are involved, credentials should include PALS.

Figure 32-1   Dermatome levels.

Professional Activities

In 1986, ASPAN developed specialty certification for perianesthesia nurses. Eligibility for certification includes current licensure as a registered nurse and 1800 hours of perianesthesia nursing experience as a caregiver, manager, educator, or researcher. A nurse specializing in the care of phase I postanesthesia patients in hospital-based or extended-recovery care facilities may attain certification as a certified postanesthesia care nurse (CPAN) by taking and passing a written examination. In ambulatory surgery settings, nurses who specialize in the postanesthesia care of patients who move rapidly from phase I to phase II to phase III can attain certification in ambulatory postanesthesia care (CAPA). The certification for both CAPAs and CPANs is valid for 3 years and can be renewed by passing a written examination or by obtaining 90 contact hours of continuing education credits. ASPAN has produced a core curriculum as an additional reference for perianesthesia nurses who plan to take the certification examination.

Other personnel in the PACU may include licensed practical/vocational nurses (LPNs/LVNs) and other unlicensed patient care personnel. These caregivers are supervised by the registered nurse, who is responsible for their training and use within the PACU. Their duties will vary according to the needs of the department.

ADMISSION TO THE POSTANESTHESIA CARE UNIT

Before the phase I or phase II patient leaves the OR the circulator should call the PACU nurse to give the estimated time of arrival in the PACU and to advise of a need to have special life support equipment on "standby" for immediate use. As the patient enters the PACU, his or her immediate physiologic and psychologic status is reported to the PACU nurse by the accompanying personnel (usually the circulating nurse, first assistant, or resident). Any necessary life support equipment, such as a ventilator, is connected. The PACU nurse connects the ECG electrodes, attaches a pulse oximeter lead, and places a blood pressure cuff on the patient. Many PACUs are supplied with automatic or computerized equipment that provides an immediate display of vital signs and physiologic data. The PACU nurse simultaneously assesses the patient and assimilates the data. The flow of activity is fast paced but directed toward the immediate physiologic needs of the patient.

Postoperative Report

The postoperative report provides information from the anesthesia provider (if one was in attendance), the surgeon (or appropriate designee, such as the first assistant), and the circulator. Much of the report is delivered verbally, but postoperative orders and pertinent information regarding the patient's condition and intraoperative care are reinforced in writing. If the surgeon gives a verbal order, he or she should co-sign the chart within 24 hours. The content of the postoperative report to the PACU nurse should include, but is not limited to, the information discussed in the following sections.

Anesthesia Provider's Report

- Patient's name, sex, age, preoperative and postoperative diagnosis, surgical procedure, and surgeon
- Type of anesthesia and the patient's response(s)
- Baseline preoperative vital signs and summary of vital sign flow during the surgical procedure up to the point of discharge from the OR
- Allergies and reaction to allergen
- Any physiologic changes or existing conditions and interventions to counteract them (e.g., diabetes, chronic obstructive pulmonary disease, previous myocardial infarction, hypertension)
- Medications administered preoperatively, intraoperatively, and postoperatively (e.g., preoperative sedation, intraoperative antibiotic, or continuous infusion of medication)
- Intravenous fluid administration and body fluid output (e.g., blood products, urine, and gastric contents)
- Specific patient care orders to be performed in the PACU or in the immediate postoperative period (e.g., aerosol or mist mask)

Surgeon's Report

- Postoperative orders pertaining to immediate treatments or therapies to be performed in the PACU or in the immediate postoperative period (e.g., passive-range-of-motion device or x-ray study to check placement of central line catheter)
- Serial diagnostic tests that are to be initiated in the PACU and continued through the immediate postoperative period (e.g., blood counts at specified intervals)
- Specific interventions pertaining to care of the surgical site (e.g., dressing change or reinforcement)

Circulator's Report

- Baseline assessment data
- Positioning and skin preparation
- Condition of dispersive electrode site
- Use of specialized surgical equipment (e.g., laser or endoscope)

- Intraoperative irrigation fluids
- Administration of medication or dyes in the surgical field
- Any implants, transplants, or explants
- Type of dressings and the presence of drains and/or stents
- Any pertinent information not reported by the anesthesia provider or surgeon
- Location of family member or significant other who may be waiting

• • •

The postoperative report will vary according to the type of anesthesia and the surgical procedure, the preferences of the anesthesia provider and surgeon, and institutional policy and procedure. The main emphasis is the patient's needs in the immediate postoperative period. This continues until the patient is discharged from the PACU.

Patient Care Activities

The application of physiologic and psychosocial knowledge, principles of asepsis, and technical knowledge and skills are necessary to promote, restore, and maintain the patient's physiologic processes in a safe, comfortable, and effective environment. Particular attention is given to monitoring oxygenation, ventilation, and circulation. PACU care includes maintaining adequate ventilation, preventing shock, and alleviating pain. Postoperative medical orders are coordinated by the anesthesia provider and the surgeon and include monitoring requirements, oxygen and fluid therapies, pain medications, and other special considerations. Patients are evaluated continually by appropriate monitoring methods and frequent observations by registered nurses. Clinical evaluation of each patient's status through listening, watching, and feeling is augmented by electronic monitoring devices.

As in all other patient care areas, standard precautions are carried out for the disposal of needles and the handling of any item contaminated by blood and body fluids. Handwashing is essential after each patient contact to prevent cross-contamination.

Family members are notified when a patient is admitted to the PACU. This lets them know the surgical procedure is complete, which helps to relieve the anxiety experienced during the hours of waiting. Depending on institutional policy, some facilities allow parents or other visitors in the PACU.

Documentation

Institutional policies and procedures should be followed in documenting PACU care. Observations of respiratory and circulatory functions and level of consciousness are recorded at frequent intervals. Postoperative physiologic and psychologic status is documented at the time of any significant event (e.g., the administration of medication), as well as routinely at 5- to 7-minute intervals for the first hour and at 15- to 30-minute intervals for the second hour and thereafter. Pertinent observations are recorded as appropriate or necessary.

DISCHARGE FROM THE POSTANESTHESIA CARE UNIT

Most patients remain in the PACU at least 1 hour or until they have sufficiently recovered from anesthesia so that their vital signs have stabilized and they are capable of reasonable self-care. The patient's condition is scored according to vital signs, activity level, and consciousness; several standardized formats are available for this purpose. The anesthesia provider assesses the patient as necessary and may determine when the patient is stable enough for discharge from the PACU. After discharge from the PACU, the patient is transported to a patient care unit or an ICU or is released from the ambulatory care facility.

A physician is responsible for the patient's discharge from the PACU. The anesthesia department and medical staff may approve discharge criteria for the PACU nurse to use in determining readiness for discharge. These criteria should be consistent with the standards of the ASA and the accreditation standards of the Joint Commission on Accreditation of Healthcare Organizations (JCAHO) and/or the Accreditation Association for Ambulatory Health Care.

Postoperative Evaluation of Expected Outcomes

Ideally, the perioperative nurse who preoperatively assessed the patient and intraoperatively developed and implemented the plan of care will have the opportunity to assess and/or interview the patient postoperatively and evaluate patient care outcomes. An assessment is performed in person if possible, or the patient may be interviewed by a follow-up telephone call within 24 to 48 hours of discharge.

The plan of care should be evaluated in terms of the attainment of expected outcomes. The identification of influencing factors provides a foundation for ongoing improvement of perioperative patient care services. Considerations for the design of the postoperative evaluation include, but are not limited to, the following:

1. Was a preoperative visit made and was it helpful to the patient?
2. Were the patient and family adequately prepared for the surgical procedure physically, psychologically, emotionally, and spiritually? Did the patient receive written preoperative instructions?
3. What could have been improved?
4. Were all pertinent patient needs, problems, or health status considerations identified in the nursing diagnoses?
5. Did the plan of care address the nursing diagnoses?
6. Did the patient experience any complications?
7. Was preoperative teaching used? Was it adequate and helpful?
8. What were the patient's perceptions of the surgical experience?
9. Were the expected outcomes achieved to the patient's satisfaction?
10. To what degree do the patient's observable physiologic and psychosocial responses indicate the attainment of expected outcomes?
11. Was the patient given a postage-paid, follow-up survey of satisfaction to complete and return to the department?

The evaluation of patient outcomes helps to identify environmental influences and procedural activities that may need to be modified by the OR staff. For example, if the patient has developed a reddened pressure area over a bony process, was the positioning equipment at fault, or was the area unpadded? A reevaluation of products currently being used may be indicated. Injury to skin may be caused by the pooling of prep solutions under the patient, inadequate padding of body prominences, or faulty electrical equipment.

The subjective data received from the patient will help evaluate how much discomfort the patient is experiencing, especially paresthesia (a numb, tingling sensation). Neurovascular injuries may be related to positioning on the operating bed. The perioperative nurse may suggest comfort measures to help this patient, but an adverse outcome indicates a need to improve positioning procedures for subsequent patients.

The postoperative assessment or follow-up telephone call terminates the direct perioperative nurse-patient relationship. The evaluation of the degree of attainment of expected outcomes completes the perioperative nursing process.

To be successful, a postoperative evaluation program requires the cooperative effort of and input from all personnel involved with patient care, including registered nurses, technicians, and physicians. Administrative personnel may seek specific information and should be consulted for input. They should participate in structuring the program at its inception to avoid duplication of action and to promote a collegial effort. Postoperative evaluation data may be collected through the following measures:

- Interview and assessment of the patient
- Conferences with physicians, nurses, and other caregivers
- Review of responses on the patient evaluation form

The postoperative evaluation program should be reviewed periodically and revised as necessary. An interdisciplinary conference is an effective medium for the accomplishment of these objectives. An effective perioperative evaluation program and positive patient experiences promote good public relations and demonstrate a caring image to the public it serves.

DEATH OF A PATIENT IN THE OPERATING ROOM

Although it is an uncommon occurrence, a patient may die while on the operating bed or shortly after reaching the PACU or ICU. When this happens, the perioperative manager should be notified immediately. Ideally, the family or significant others are informed by the surgeon or the surgeon's designee. It may be appropriate to discuss organ donation with the family at this time and to request permission to proceed with organ procurement. If circumstances warrant, an autopsy may be necessary.

In the event of a high profile accident or event, the facility's public relations personnel should be the contacts with the press or news media. Perioperative/perianesthesia personnel should not provide information about any patient to any person not authorized in the patient's care. A breech of confidentiality is a serious ethical consideration, especially in the event of a police investigation or medical malpractice suit.

Forensic Issues and Coroner's Cases

In some states the body of a patient who dies in the OR or does not awaken from general anesthesia automatically becomes the property of the coroner; a consent for autopsy is not necessary in this situation. The coroner must give approval for organ procurement and has the right to overrule the wishes of the family.

Individual state law and institutional policy determine the postmortem care of the patient's body. For example, all drainage tubes, implants, and catheters may need to be left in place for removal and examination at autopsy. All medication vials and intravenous solution containers should remain with the body.

In a life-threatening emergency, a patient may be admitted directly to the OR without being undressed or prepared for a surgical procedure. The body of a patient who dies under these circumstances is also considered the property of the coroner, but postmortem care is more complex. Critical medicolegal issues should be taken into consideration if the patient was a suspected victim or perpetrator of violence or was injured in a suspicious manner. All information about the patient's condition, personal effects and attire, and materials discovered during the surgical procedure are considered forensic evidence. Forensic evidence is critical for the reconstruction of events involved in a crime or suspected illegal activity. All forensic evidence is preserved according to institutional policy and procedure and is relinquished only to the appropriate authorities. The documentation of handling and disposition of evidence is referred to as a chain of evidence. This chain is maintained by requiring the signatures of all persons who come in contact with forensic evidence. The goal is to attempt to validate that the evidence has not been tampered with before reaching the appropriate law enforcement agency.

Intraoperative documentation, another form of evidence, should include a written account of the patient's physical appearance on arrival in the OR, as well as a hand-drawn diagram of any physical markings present before skin preparation (e.g., penetrating wounds or bruises on the body). Other pertinent data might include unusual odors, such as chemicals, gasoline, or alcohol. Clothing, undergarments, and shoes should be allowed to air dry before being placed in paper containers for release to the authorities. Items placed in airtight containers or plastic bags may decay and destroy vital evidence. Bullets, knife fragments, or other weaponlike implements are handled according to institutional policy for transport to the appropriate law enforcement agency. They are packaged dry and in an impervious container to prevent injury. Gloves are worn in handling evidence. Nothing is washed, wiped clean, or discarded. A clear, documented chain of evidence is often difficult to maintain in a crisis, but every attempt is made to document the disposition of evidence and the location from which it was taken.

Surgical interventions for the perpetrator and the victim of the same crime are a challenge for the OR team. It may be difficult to deliver objective care to the perpetrator if the victim has died within moments of reaching the OR. Regardless of the personal feelings or beliefs of team members, both patients have rights and are entitled to professional care at all times.

Postmortem Patient Care

A death may be anticipated, such when a patient is brought to the OR on mechanical life support for organ procurement. A death may occur as a result of shock following extensive traumatic injuries, exsanguination after rupture of an aortic aneurysm, unsuccessful cardiopulmonary resuscitation following cardiac arrest, or other causes. The circulator's responsibilities after intraoperative death include the following:

1. Provide after-death care for the body as appropriate, or ensure that forensic protocol is followed before releasing the body to authorities or the morgue.
   a. Follow institutional policy and procedure.
   b. Be sure identification is correct.
   c. Secure the patient's personal effects.
   d. Do not wash the body if it is considered part of forensic evidence.
2. Arrange for transportation from the OR to the morgue, or release it to an appropriate authority.
   a. Release the body from the OR according to institutional policy and procedure.
   b. Avoid exposing other patients, visitors, and family to removal of the body.
   c. If the religious or cultural preference of a patient and/or family is known, an appropriate member of the clergy or a spiritual advisor may be consulted concerning postdeath practices.
3. Complete the intraoperative chart and additional documentation as required by institutional policy.

Policy may allow the family to view a loved one before the body is transported to the morgue. The room in which the viewing takes place should be clean, presentable, and private. The perioperative/perianesthesia nurse (or designee) should accompany the family and lend support. This person must remain in attendance if the body will be involved in a forensic investigation.

Following a death in the OR, from whatever cause, team members should be given time to express and deal with their feelings about the event.

Bibliography

American Society of Anesthesiologists: *Standards for postanesthesia care,* Park Ridge, Ill, 1988 (date of adoption), The Society.

American Society of PeriAnesthesia Nurses: *Standards of perianesthesia nursing practice,* Thorofare, New Jersey, 1998, The Society.

Badgewell JM: The postanesthesia care unit: a high-risk environment for blood borne and infectious respiratory pathogens, *J Post Anesth Nurs* 11(2):66-70, 1996.

Calhoun MJ et al: Nurses find solution to postoperative leg and back pain, *AORN J* 68(6):1013-1015, 1998.

Dester F, Rittenmeyer H: Quantification of phase I postanesthesia nursing activities in the phase II postanesthesia unit, *Nurs Outlook* 45(2):86-88, 1997.

Einhorn GW, Chant P: Postanesthesia care unit dilemmas: prompt assessment and treatment, *J Post Anesth Nurs* 9(1):28-33, 1994.

Litwack KL: *Core curriculum for post anesthesia nursing practice,* ed 3, Philadelphia, 1995, WB Saunders.

Litwack KL: *Post anesthesia care nursing,* ed 2, St Louis, 1995, Mosby.

Muro GA, Easter CR: Clinical forensics for perioperative nurses, *AORN J* 60(4):585-593, 1994.

VanRiper S, Luciano A: Basic cardiac arrhythmias: a review for postanesthesia care unit nurses, *J Post Anesth Nurs* 9(1):2-13, 1994.

Whitis G: Visiting hospitalized patients, *J Adv Nurs* 19(1):85-88, 1994.

Zickuhr MT, Atsberger DB: *Pre- and postanesthesia nursing knowledge base and clinical competencies,* Philadelphia, 1995, WB Saunders.

Chapter 33

Potential Perioperative Complications

 Chapter Objectives

After studying this chapter, the learner will be able to:

- Describe several respiratory complications that are possible in the perioperative period.
- Identify three potential dysrhythmias that may complicate the patient's perioperative course.
- Demonstrate the procedure for weighing surgical sponges in the OR.
- List the primary drugs used in the management of an acute malignant hyperthermic crisis.
- Identify three methods for preventing hypothermia in the perioperative patient.

The anesthesia provider must be constantly aware of the surgeon's actions. He or she must do everything possible to ensure the safety of the patient and reduce the stress of surgery. Continuous appraisal of the patient's overall condition helps prevent complications. Some complications may occur as a direct result of anesthesia; others may have additional contributing factors. Some conditions may occur during the procedure; others may appear in the postoperative period. Tragically, catastrophic emergencies may sometimes arise when least expected. Minutes can make the difference between life and death for the patient. Anticipation and preparedness may determine that difference. Terms associated with perioperative complications are defined in Box 33-1.

HISTORICAL BACKGROUND

From early times, it was known that loss of blood meant loss of life, although the circulation of blood was not clearly understood. The writings of Aristotle (384-322 BC) reveal that veins were thought to contain all or most of the blood. Arteries were thought to contain air, with only a small amount of blood. This doctrine continued until the physiologist Galen (130-200 AD) demonstrated that arteries, like veins, contain blood, which he believed just ebbed and flowed. This theory held for about 1500 years, until William Harvey (1578-1657), an English anatomist, realized that blood circulated and could flow only in one direction. His hypothesis that it passed from arteries to veins through capillaries was proved under the microscope in 1661 by Marcello Malpighi (1628-1694), an Italian anatomist.

Before the advent of anesthesia in 1846, surgical skill was based on speed. Most surgical procedures were done for major injuries or life-threatening conditions, such as gangrene or infection in an extremity. Amputations were swift and guillotine style. Blood dripped onto the floor or into a box of sawdust. Loss of blood was one of the most dangerous complications of surgery.

The first attempt to transfuse blood in humans occurred in 1818 when English physician James Blundell transfused

Terms Associated with Perioperative Complications

allogenous   Having different genetic constitution although same species.

anemia   Reduction of the number of functioning red blood cells capable of containing enough hemoglobin to transport oxygen.

anoxia   Absence of oxygen. Not synonymous with hypoxia.

anticholinergic   Blocks the impulses of parasympathetic nerve fibers, causing dry mouth or blurred vision.

aspiration   Entry of gastric, oropharyngeal, or other substance into the lungs.

atelectasis   Collapsed or airless lung.

autologous   Originating from self.

cardiotonic   Drug that increases the tone of the heart, such as digitalis.

dysrhythmia   Abnormal, disordered, disturbed rhythm.

embolism   Obstruction of a vessel or a lumen caused by a blood clot or other substance, such as plaque.

hemoglobinopathy   Any one of a group of blood diseases that are characterized by abnormal forms of hemoglobin in the blood.

hemorrhage   Abnormal internal or external loss of blood from an arterial, venous, or capillary source.

hypertension   Elevated blood pressure. If on several occasions the systolic pressure is above 140 or the diastolic pressure is above 90, the patient is considered hypertensive.

hypotension   Low blood pressure. If on several occasions the systolic pressure is lower than 100, the patient is considered hypotensive. This should be compared with other assessment parameters.

hypoventilation   Reduced rate and depth of breathing that causes an increase in carbon dioxide.

hypoxia   Decreased concentration of oxygen.

metabolic crisis   Physical and chemical changes that cause catabolic or anabolic activity that may be life threatening to the organism.

   anabolism   Buildup of tissues or properties.

   catabolism   Breakdown of tissues or properties.

thrombosis   Formation, existence, or development of a blood clot within the vascular system.

vasoconstrictor   A drug that causes narrowing of a blood vessel.

vasodilator   A drug that causes relaxation of a blood vessel or causes opening (dilation).

venospasm   Contraction of a vein that may follow the infusion of a cold or irritating substance.

---

blood by syringe from a husband to his wife, who was dying of postpartum hemorrhage. He developed transfusion instrumentation and successfully performed this procedure on five other patients between 1825 and 1830. American physicians attempted volume expansion between 1873 and 1880 using cow, goat, and human milk, with many adverse reactions. Later in the century saline was used for this purpose, and in 1886 John Duncan transfused autologous blood directly from the surgical field into a trauma patient by femoral injection.

In 1901 Karl Landsteiner (1868-1943), an Austrian-American pathologist, discovered the blood groups A, B, and O. Other researchers discovered group AB the following year. In 1930 Landsteiner was awarded the Nobel prize for his work in transfusion research. The knowledge of blood groups led to the feasibility of donor (allogenous) blood transfusions. Plasma was first used during World War I to combat shock.

The development of blood banking superseded previous attempts at autotransfusion. The first blood bank was established in 1936 at the Mayo Clinic in Rochester, Minnesota. Interest in allogenous blood prospered during World War II because a large donor pool collected by the Red Cross, along with improved methods of typing and crossmatching, made banked blood easier to obtain and safer to use. Resurgence of interest in autologous blood occurred, however, with direct salvage devices during the Vietnam War. The first technically safe commercial autologous blood recovery equipment was marketed in 1971.

Although blood loss is a serious concern for the surgical patient, other systemic complications can cause problems with other vital functions. The perioperative caregiver should be aware of the potential for respiratory, cardiac, vascular, and metabolic complications and be prepared to assist in supportive care.

RESPIRATORY COMPLICATIONS

One of the primary areas of postoperative complications is the respiratory system. The patient's potential for developing pulmonary problems depends on several factors. Any preexisting lung disease, such as emphysema, infection, or asthma, predisposes the patient. Smokers have the highest risk of succumbing to postoperative pulmonary problems because of chronic irritation of the respiratory tract with consequent production of excess mucus. Chest wall deformities, obesity, and extremes of age are other pertinent preoperative influences. Intraoperative factors include the following:

- Type of preoperative medications
- Type and duration of anesthesia
- Type and duration of assisted ventilation
- Position of the patient during the surgical procedure
- Extent of the surgical procedure

Postoperatively, one of the most critical factors is the patient's ability to mobilize secretions by deep breathing, coughing, and ambulation. Patients undergoing chest and abdominal surgery are likely to breathe shallowly because of pain and therefore may not adequately raise accumulated secretions. Development of one pulmonary complication often predisposes the patient to development of another. Acute respiratory distress syndrome (ARDS), also known as progressive pulmonary insufficiency or shock lung, may develop in the first 24 to 48 hours following a traumatic injury.

Aspiration

Aspiration of gastric contents into the lungs may occur because of decreased throat reflexes when the patient is unconscious or is conscious with the throat anesthetized, as for bronchoscopy. Residual effects impede lung function and blood-gas exchange. A chemical pneumonitis results from aspiration of highly acidic gastric juices. Edema forms, alveoli collapse, ventilation-perfusion mismatch occurs, and hypoxemia results. Aspiration of solids in emesis results in edema, severe hypoxia, and respiratory obstruction. Bronchospasm and atelectasis may be followed by pneumonitis or bronchopneumonia. Most aspiration is irritative, but it can be infectious if nasopharyngeal or gastric flora are aspirated. Pneumonia or lung abscess may result with necrosis of the pulmonary parenchyma.

Etiology

Every patient who has food in the stomach is a poor risk for anesthesia. Increased intragastric pressure is an aspiration hazard and may result from conditions such as pylorospasm, diaphragmatic hernia, gastrointestinal bleeding, intestinal obstruction, or gas forced into the stomach by application of positive pressure ventilation without use of a cuffed endotracheal tube.

Symptoms

Symptoms include central cyanosis, dyspnea, gasping, and tachycardia, followed by cardiac embarrassment, lung collapse, and consolidation.

Treatment

Most effective treatment occurs during the first minutes after aspiration. The strategy is to remove as much aspirate as possible and limit the spread of what is left in the lung. The head of the operating bed is lowered with a right lateral tilt for postural drainage; the right mainstem bronchus bifurcates slightly higher than the left mainstem bronchus. The oropharynx and tracheobronchial tree are suctioned. If the patient has aspirated particulate matter that causes obstruction of the airways, bronchoscopy must be performed to remove it. Suctioning must be interrupted every 10 to 15 seconds to give oxygen. Oxygenation and carbon dioxide removal are high priorities.

Aspiration of acid gastric content injures the alveolar capillary interface, resulting in intrapulmonary shunting and pulmonary edema. Intensive pulmonary care is aimed at improving ventilation-perfusion ratios and decreasing abnormal gas exchange. This may require endotracheal intubation for mechanical ventilation with continuous positive pressure. Most cases of severe hypoxemia occur rapidly within the first 30 to 60 minutes after aspiration. Careful cardiovascular monitoring and frequent blood-gas and acid-base determinations guide therapeutic measures to maintain intravascular volume. Prophylactic antibiotics may be given for aspiration of bowel-contaminated fluid to prevent infection, and a bronchodilator may be used to treat spasm. Most cases of permanent injury or death result from the initial hypoxemia.

Prevention

Prevention involves adequate preoperative preparation (withholding oral intake 8 to 10 hours before induction) and careful administration of anesthetic agents. The anesthetic is decreased near the end of the surgical procedure, hastening the return of throat reflexes. All trauma and obstetric patients receiving general anesthesia should be treated as if they have full stomachs and should be intubated using cricoid pressure. The cricoid pressure should be released after verification of endotracheal tube placement. Gastric evacuation is delayed during labor and by analgesic medications. A nasogastric tube may be inserted preoperatively or intraoperatively.

Laryngospasm and Bronchospasm

Laryngospasm is a partial or complete closure of the vocal cords as an involuntary reflex action. Bronchospasm is contraction of smooth muscle in the walls of the bronchi and bronchioles, causing narrowing of the lumen. Spasms or abnormal narrowing is produced by a marked increase in smooth muscle tone of the airway walls. Marked elevation of airway resistance profoundly alters gas flow into and out of the lungs. Accompanying changes result in a decreased ventilation-perfusion ratio with a subsequent reduction in PaO_2 and rise in $PaCO_2$. Many factors can precipitate spasm.

Etiology

Etiologic factors include mechanical airway obstruction, use of certain anesthetics and drugs, allergic conditions such as asthma, vagal reflex, stimulation of the pharynx and larynx with the patient under light anesthesia, traction on the peritoneum, foreign material in the tracheobronchial tree, movement of the head or neck or traction on the carotid sinus, and painful peripheral stimuli. The degree of spasm varies from mild to severe.

Symptoms

Symptoms include wheezing respirations or stridor, reduced compliance, central cyanosis, and respiratory obstruction.

Treatment

Treatment depends on the precipitating factor. Methods generally used include positive pressure ventilation, oxygen, tracheal intubation, and neuromuscular blockers for relaxation. Bronchodilator drugs such as aminophylline, isoetharine, and metaproterenol sulfate are given with caution because they act as cardiac stimulators and, in the presence of hypoxia, may contribute to cardiac dysrhythmia and cardiac arrest. Patients may be refractory (unresponsive) to bronchodilators because of acid-base abnormalities. Correction can reduce the side effects and augment the beneficial effects of bronchodilators. If the etiologic factor is an allergy, steroids and antihistamines may be given. Vagal reflexes are inhibited by atropine. If reflex is the cause, anesthesia is deepened. Drying agents are given for excessive secretions. Immediate effective treatment is mandatory to counteract hypoxia and prevent cardiac arrest.

Prevention

Prevention involves maintenance of a patent airway, appropriate premedication such as glycopyrrolate, avoidance of factors stimulating the vagal reflex, and treatment of the predisposing pulmonary condition.

Airway and Respiratory Obstruction

An airway is maintained with an oral airway or endotracheal tube. Airway obstruction is the most frequent cause of respiratory difficulty in the immediate postoperative period. The patient may exhibit paradoxical respiration (i.e., downward movement of the diaphragm occurring with contraction rather than expansion of the chest), resulting in hypoxia and carbon dioxide retention. As the condition worsens, the patient becomes restless, diaphoretic, cyanotic, and finally unconscious. If not relieved within seconds, this serious complication may lead to cardiac arrest.

Etiology

Etiologic factors include blocking of the airway by the tongue, soft tissue, excessive secretions, or a foreign body; laryngospasm or bronchospasm; or positioning of the head with the chin down.

Symptoms

Symptoms of respiratory obstruction include increased respiratory effort with inadequate ventilatory exchange, visible use of accessory muscles, and respiratory motion of the chest and abdomen without audible air movement at the airway. If the airway is totally obstructed, breath sounds will be absent; if it is partially obstructed, a snoring sound will be elicited. The pulse is rapid and thready.

Assessment of oxygenation is essential if the patient's airway patency is in question. Visual inspection of the patient may reveal *peripheral cyanosis*—pallor, duskiness, or bluish color of the nailbeds and extremities. This is caused by a decrease in capillary oxygen levels. Peripheral cyanosis is not always indicative of impending danger to the patient. It can be caused by hypothermia, stress, medications, or other physiologic factors that cause peripheral vasoconstriction.

If the patient is in an arterial hypoxemic state, he or she will exhibit *central cyanosis*—pallor, duskiness, or bluish color of the lips, face, and generalized body surface. Central cyanosis is a serious sign that requires immediate airway and ventilatory assessment followed by emergent treatment. Central cyanosis may develop more slowly if the patient has been breathing a high concentration of oxygen.

Treatment

The cause of obstruction may be eliminated by suctioning blood, mucus, or emesis; gently hyperextending the neck; and elevating the chin. Oxygen is administered by positive pressure; a nasal airway or endotracheal intubation may be necessary. If the anesthesia provider has been unable to manually ventilate or intubate the patient in two or three attempts, it may be necessary to establish an indirect airway by opening the patient's anterior neck; a needle is inserted through the cricoid cartilage for a cricothyrotomy or, if time permits, a tracheotomy.

Hypoventilation

The ability to oxygenate depends on the condition of the lungs, hemoglobin concentration, cardiac output, and oxygen saturation. Inadequate or reduced alveolar ventilation can cause a deficit in oxygenation. This can lead to hypoxia (a decreased level of oxygen in arterial blood and tissues), hypoxemia (a decreased level of oxygen in arterial blood), and hypercapnia, also known as hypercarbia (an elevated level of carbon dioxide in arterial blood). The body compensates for mild hypoxia with increased heart and respiratory rates, bringing oxygen to the blood and tissues at a faster rate. If hypoxia progresses, this compensation is inadequate. If hypoxia is prolonged, cardiac dysrhythmia or irreversible brain, liver, kidney, and heart damage results. Retention of carbon dioxide also leads to acidosis.

Etiology

Contributing factors to hypoventilation include alveolar impairment, pain, faulty positioning, a full bladder, or a short, thick neck. Inadequate pulmonary ventilation from depression of the medullary center in the brain by narcotics or anesthetics, neurologic effects of spinal or epidural drug administration, reduced cardiac output, severe blood loss, obstruction to the respiratory passages, or abnormality of the ventilation-perfusion ratio also can contribute to hypoxia and hypercapnia.

Symptoms

Symptoms of hypoventilation and hypoxia include an increased pulse rate; pallor or central cyanosis from hypoxia or a flushed or reddened appearance from hypercapnia; decreased volume of respirations; stertorous or labored respirations; and dark blood in the surgical field. The acid-base balance can be affected.

Treatment

The immediate administration of oxygen in the proper dosage is the treatment of choice for hypoventilation and hypoxia. Oxygen is a medication requiring proper dosage for safe, effective administration. In the healthy patient, changes in the concentration of carbon dioxide in the blood stimulate the primary central chemoreceptor (respiratory center) in the medulla of the brain. In response to this stimulation, the patient takes a breath to increase oxygenation. Patients with chronic obstructive pulmonary disease (COPD) have higher than normal levels of circulating carbon dioxide and have a decreased primary chemoreceptor response. They rely on secondary chemoreceptors in the carotid and aortic bodies to sense the changes in carbon dioxide levels in the blood. High concentrations of oxygen decrease the sensitivity of the secondary chemoreceptors in patients with COPD, causing respiratory depression. To minimize the risk for respiratory arrest in these patients, a 2- to 3-L flow of oxygen per nasal cannula is recommended postoperatively. An endotracheal tube may be left in place postoperatively to support assisted ventilation in select patients.

Patients are encouraged to cough and breathe deeply postoperatively. If a patient received naloxone hydrochloride (Narcan) to reverse the respiratory depressant effect of a narcotic, the patient may awaken rapidly and cough, inadvertently causing extubation. The patient must be watched closely during recovery.

Prevention

A patent airway, appropriate oxygenation, and proper positioning help prevent hypoventilation. Intraoperative measurements of arterial pH, Pco_2, and Po_2 enable the anesthesia provider to evaluate oxygenation and carbon dioxide gas exchange. To prevent hypoventilation and hypoxia, patients may be given oxygen and assisted ventilation during transport to the recovery area.

Pulmonary Embolism

Pulmonary embolism is a major cause of death during a surgical procedure and in the immediate postoperative period. Some intraoperative problems may extend into postoperative recovery.

Pulmonary embolism is an obstruction of the pulmonary artery or one of its branches by an embolus, most often a blood clot. The most important factor leading to pulmonary emboli is stasis of blood, particularly in deep veins of the legs and pelvis, where the majority of thrombi arise. These become detached and are carried to the lungs. Changes in vessel walls and coagulative changes in blood are also important factors. A prolonged period on the operating bed may decrease blood flow to the lower extremities by more than 50%. Blood flow is impaired further if the knees are raised on a pillow, putting pressure on the vessels. Venous stasis also is correlated with obesity, congestive heart failure, and atrial fibrillation. Local trauma to a vein or venous disease enhances the chance of thrombus formation. Hypercoagulability may coexist with conditions such as pregnancy, fever, myocardial infarction, and some malignancies and after abrupt cessation of anticoagulant therapy. Prevention consists of a regimen of prophylactic anticoagulants or antiplatelets for high-risk patients and routine measures to prevent venous stasis, such as intermittent compression or antiembolic stockings.

Because of the origin of thrombi in deep veins, it is important to observe the patient postoperatively for thrombophlebitis, evidenced by heat, edema, redness, pain in the calf, or a positive Homans' sign, which is pain in the calf on forceful dorsiflexion of the foot. Nonspecific symptoms depend on whether the embolism is mild or massive. The patient may have dyspnea, pleural pain, hemoptysis, tachypnea, crackles, tachycardia, mild fever, or persistent cough. Patients with massive emboli have air hunger, hypotension, shock, and central cyanosis. Treatment of pulmonary emboli consists of bed rest, oxygen therapy, anticoagulant therapy, thrombolytic agents, and sometimes a surgical procedure to remove the emboli or to place a vena cava filter to prevent their recurrence.

Fat embolism occurs primarily following fracture of a long bone, pelvis, or ribs. However, it sometimes occurs after a blood transfusion, cardiopulmonary bypass, or renal transplant. Fat globules enter the bloodstream. Symptoms develop when globules block pulmonary capillaries, causing interstitial edema and hemorrhage. Frequently, ARDS ensues 24 to 48 hours after injury, with hypoxia and decreased surfactant production, resulting in collapse of the alveolar membrane and microatelectasis. The syndrome develops most frequently in patients older than 10 years of age, especially those who have traveled long distances with an immobilized fracture. Symptoms include disorientation, increased pulse and temperature, tachypnea, dyspnea, crackles, and pleuritic chest pain. Other significant signs are fat in the sputum and urine and a petechial rash on the anterior chest. Treatment is supportive. Mortality is high.

Air embolism may follow incidental injection of air into a body cavity or a bolus of air in an intravenous (IV) or intraarterial infusion. Another means of entry is during transection of large veins with the patient in a sitting or prone position. The pull of gravity on the venous drainage exerts a significant negative pressure that sucks air into the veins and into the heart. This can be a complication in handling central venous catheters and using syringes to obtain blood for gas analysis.

Intrauterine fetal death, abruptio placenta, or placenta previa may precipitate an embolism of amniotic fluid. Also, tumors may cause emboli from primary or metastatic sites.

Pneumothorax

Although it is rare, insertion of a needle into the thoracic cage can occur during a nerve block or subclavian catheter insertion. The primary symptoms are pain and shortness of breath. Confirmation is made by x-ray study. If the pneumothorax is extensive and the lung fails to reexpand, a chest tube with an underwater seal is required.

Intercostal Muscle Spasm

A "rigid chest" may occur after large doses of IV fentanyl or on emergence from general anesthesia. It may reverse itself, or neuromuscular blockers may be needed.

Atelectasis (Pulmonary Collapse)

Partial collapse of a lung is one of the most common postoperative problems. If mucus obstructs a bronchus, air in the alveoli distal to the obstruction is resorbed. That segment of lung then collapses and consolidates. Retained mucus becomes contaminated by inhaled bacteria; the patient may develop bronchopneumonia.

Etiology

Factors that promote increased production of mucus, such as certain irritating anesthetics, and decreased mobilization of mucus, such as from a tight abdominal dressing, predispose the patient to pulmonary collapse. Furthermore, normal respiration includes a deep sigh several times an hour to help keep the lungs expanded. This natural sigh is inhibited by anesthetics, narcotics, and sedatives. Oxygen and carbon dioxide are absorbed into the pulmonary blood flow, and the alveoli collapse. Low tidal volume intensifies the problem. High concentrations of oxygen remove nitrogen from the lungs, leaving oxygen, carbon dioxide, and water in the alveoli.

Symptoms

Atelectasis increases the temperature, pulse, and respiratory rate. The patient may appear cyanotic and uncomfortable, with shallow respirations and pain on coughing. Breath sounds are diminished, with fine crackles. Chest x-ray study reveals collapsed areas of the lungs as patch opacities, generally involving the lung bases.

Treatment and Prevention

Measures to help prevent or treat atelectasis are abstention from smoking, a regimen of coughing and deep breathing, and early ambulation. An upright position allows for better lung expansion. Medication for pain, when appropriate, before breathing exercises or ambulation improves the ability to breathe deeply and cough effectively. Splinting the thoracic or abdominal incision with a pillow also helps decrease the pain of coughing. Repeated vigorous coughing is contraindicated in some patients (e.g., following cataract extraction, craniotomy, or herniorrhaphy).

Pulmonary Edema

Pulmonary edema may be defined as an abnormal accumulation of water in extravascular portions of the lungs, including both alveolar and interstitial spaces. In surgical patients the cause is most probably increased microvascular pulmonary capillary permeability or capillary endothelial injury. Blood stagnates in the pulmonary circulation. Fluid exudes from capillaries into the alveoli and interstitial spaces. Reduction of capillary membrane perfusion leads to hypoxia. Symptoms, usually seen postoperatively in the postanesthesia care unit (PACU) or intensive care unit (ICU), may include a bounding rapid pulse, crackles, dyspnea, and engorged peripheral veins.

CARDIOVASCULAR COMPLICATIONS

The emotional and physical stresses to which a surgical patient is subjected may lead to cardiovascular complications. The patient who fears dying while under anesthesia runs a greater risk of cardiac arrest on the operating bed than patients with known cardiac disease. Psychologic stress can have physiologic manifestations. Extreme preoperative anxiety predisposes the patient to a difficult induction and intraoperative period and to postoperative discomfort. Patients with a history of cardiovascular problems are prone to develop complications. These may include dysrhythmias, hypotension, thromboembolism and/or thrombophlebitis, myocardial infarction, or congestive heart failure. Cerebral thrombosis or embolism may result in prolonged coma. Patients must be closely monitored for symptoms of cardiovascular complications. Anoxia, the complete or almost total absence of oxygen from inspired gases, arterial blood, or tissues, is a precursor to cardiovascular collapse. Cardiac arrest can result in death in the OR.

Hypotension

Reduced blood pressure, with resultant inadequate circulation, may accompany depression of the myocardium, depression of the vasomotor center in the brain, a decline in cardiac output, or dilation of the peripheral vessels. Hypotension may occur also when positive pressure is applied to the airway. Progressive deepening of general anesthesia usually produces peripheral vasodilation and diminished myocardial contractility. Adequate blood flow to the brain and heart, the two most vulnerable vascular beds because of their high metabolic demand, must be maintained. If arterial hypotension is uncontrolled, it may cause a cerebrovascular accident, myocardial infarction, or death.

Etiology

Overdosage of general anesthetic or rapid vascular absorption of local agents may result from the patient's receiving an amount of the agent that exceeds his or her tolerance. Tendency for overdosage occurs during prolonged anesthesia with large amounts of drugs absorbed, in age-extreme patients, or with unrecognized hypothermia during lengthy abdominal or thoracic procedures. Circulatory effects of spinal or epidural anesthesia, such as diminished cardiac output or reduced peripheral resistance, also produce hypotension.

Other causes of hypotension include the following:

- Volume depletion; hemorrhage
- Circulatory abnormalities such as cardiac tamponade, heart failure
- Cerebral or pulmonary embolism (fat embolism from fracture sites, amniotic fluid emboli during delivery, or air emboli from introduction of air into the circulation during an infusion or procedure)
- Myocardial ischemia or infarction
- Changes in position, especially if executed rapidly or roughly
- Excessive preanesthetic medication (postural hypotension may follow narcotic administration)
- Epidural or spinal anesthesia above the level of T6 (sympathetic block)
- Potent therapeutic drugs (tranquilizers, adrenal steroids, antihypertensives) given before the anesthetic
- Hypoxia

Surgical manipulation may induce hypotension mechanically by obstructing venous return to the heart with packs, retractors, or body rests. Or hypotension and bradycardia may result from a vagal-induced reflex precipitated by intraperitoneal traction, manipulation in the chest or neck area, rapid release of either increased intraabdominal pressure or overdistention of the bladder, anorectal stimulation, or stimulation of the periosteum or joint cavities. Other causes are transfusion reaction (suggested by accompanying cyanosis and oozing at the surgical site), septic shock, severe hyperthermia, and anaphylactic reaction.

Symptoms

Early reversible shock is accompanied by unstable blood pressure, vasoconstriction, elevated serum pH, and elevated catecholamine levels. Late manifestations are pallor or central cyanosis, clammy skin, dilated pupils, decreased urinary output, tachycardia, decreased bleeding in the surgical field or pallor of organs caused by compensatory vasoconstriction, nausea, vomiting, sighing respirations, or air hunger in conscious patients.

Diagnosis

Determination of arterial blood pressure and pulse rate and estimation of pulse volume are indicative of the volume of cardiac ejection. Arbitrary figures of measured blood pressure are not as important as individual circulatory status. A specific measurement in a healthy adult may be relatively insignificant, whereas the same figure in an geriatric patient could be hazardous. In critically ill patients, direct arterial pressure, central venous pressure (CVP), and urinary output are monitored.

Treatment

Treatment must be prompt to avoid circulatory collapse. The aim is to increase perfusion of the vital organs and to treat any specific cause while giving general supportive therapy. Supportive measures include oxygen by mask with assisted respiration; elevation of the legs to increase blood pressure by draining pooled blood, especially after sympathetic blockade; and rapid IV fluid therapy to increase blood volume. Because the volume of fluid is more vital than its composition, various solutions are applicable for early treatment in an emergency. If whole blood is not available, crystalloid solutions (e.g., Ringer's lactate), 5% dextrose in water, physiologic saline solution, plasma or serum albumin, or 6% dextran (plasma expander) may be given. Rapid infusion under pressure may be necessary. Vasoactive drugs are given as necessary; these are usually vasopressors to constrict arterioles and veins while increasing the myocardial contractile force. Blood gases should be monitored.

Prevention

The causes must be reversed or avoided. Therefore the patient should be observed constantly throughout anesthesia; in suspected individuals the cardiovascular response to the desired surgical position should be tested before induction. Overdosage of premedication and anesthetic drugs is avoided. The patient's position is changed slowly, tissue is manipulated gently, and blood and fluid loss are replaced promptly. The anesthesia provider administers a minimal amount of the anesthetic and takes adequate time to induce and deepen anesthesia so as not to raise the blood level of the anesthetic too rapidly. Positive pressure is applied to the airway prudently.

Some narcotics and anesthetic agents, surgical trauma, anoxia, and blood loss can lead to postoperative hypotension. When combined, these factors interfere with the complex physiologic mechanisms that support blood pressure. Peripheral vessels dilate. A degree of cardiovascular collapse ensues. Vasoconstriction reduces renal blood flow, causing decrease or failure of kidney function. Patients must be monitored postoperatively for sudden drops in blood pressure or other signs of shock. Vasoactive drugs and oxygen may be administered. Fluid management is critical during the recovery phase of renal function following restoration of systemic blood pressure to avoid hypertension.

Hypertension

Abnormal elevation of the blood pressure may occur, especially in a hypertensive or arteriosclerotic patient. Even mildly hypertensive patients are prone to myocardial ischemia (inadequate blood flow to heart) during induction of and emergence from anesthesia. Intubation stimulates the sympathetic nervous system. Other predisposing factors include pain, shivering, hypoxia, hypercapnia, effects of vasopressor drugs, or hypervolemia from overreplacement of fluid losses. Treatment consists of administration of oxygen, diuretics, and antihypertensive beta-blocker drugs as indicated. If not controlled, hypertension may precipitate a cerebrovascular accident or myocardial infarction. It may cause bleeding from the surgical site or may threaten the integrity of a vascular bypass.

Venospasm

If caused by cold IV fluid infusion, venospasm may manifest as very slow flow. It may result from pressure infusion or extravasation. IV procaine relieves spasm. Thrombophlebitis may follow venospasm.

Coronary Thrombosis

Coronary thrombosis can occur from severe hypoxia and lack of oxygen to coronary vessels. Sometimes its occurrence is the reason for a patient's never regaining consciousness following a surgical procedure.

Air Embolism

Air embolism may occur intraoperatively with the patient in a sitting position for a craniotomy or posterior cervical operation. Cerebral diploic veins are noncollapsible; venous sinuses in the skull remain open. Air entering a vein is carried rapidly to the right side of the heart and pulmonary circulation, obstructing ventricular flow. Cardiac dysrhythmias and unexplained hypotension are prime symptoms. A characteristic heart murmur may be audible with a precordial stethoscope or Doppler device. Air embolism may also occur during cardiopulmonary bypass, thyroidectomy, or laparoscopy.

Preoperative placement of a central venous catheter allows immediate aspiration of air. To relieve ventricular obstruction if no catheter is in place, the patient is placed in a steep head-down position with the right side up. If cardiac arrest occurs, cardiopulmonary resuscitation (CPR) is begun. Closed heart massage may move an embolus obstructing the coronary artery.

Venous Stasis

Venous return of blood from the lower extremities can be slowed by the effects of general or spinal anesthesia and by the position of the legs during prolonged surgical procedures. The venous stasis that develops in most patients during a surgical procedure can be effectively counteracted. To prevent thrombophlebitis and thrombosis in patients with thromboembolic disease, anticoagulants may be administered. Antiembolic stockings, with or without a sequential pneumatic compression device, augment venous flow from the legs. Elevation of the legs as little as 15% above horizontal can assist in venous return.

Postoperatively the patient may be placed in the Trendelenburg position with the legs elevated. Flexion and extension of the legs and feet, frequent turning, and early ambulation, unless contraindicated, aid circulation.

Deep Vein Thrombosis

Venous stasis, changes in clotting factors in the blood, and damage to vessel walls are the primary causes of deep vein thrombosis (DVT) in the lower extremities. Age, obesity, immobility, and a history of thromboembolic or other cardiovascular disease are predisposing factors. The type, location, and extent of the surgical procedure can contribute also. Preoperative prophylactic interventions, including anticoagulants, sequential compression devices, or antiembolic stockings, can reduce the risk of postoperative pulmonary embolism, which is a life-threatening complication of DVT.

Disseminated Intravascular Coagulation

Although it occurs rarely, disseminated intravascular coagulation (DIC) is a life-threatening syndrome. It is a complex derangement of clotting factors. The hemostatic process involves vasoconstriction with platelet aggregation and clotting. In DIC the normal clotting mechanisms do not function. Instead, a repetitive, overactive cycle of clot formation and simultaneous clot breakdown (fibrinolysis) occurs. This leads to consumption of platelets and coagulation factors and release of fibrin degradation products that act as potent anticoagulants. DIC can follow hemorrhage, thrombi, emboli, infection, or allergic reaction to an incompatible blood transfusion. It may be precipitated by septic shock, abruptio placentae during pregnancy, or massive soft tissue damage of extensive trauma or burns. As blood becomes depleted of platelets and major clotting factors, coagulation is initiated throughout the bloodstream, especially in microcirculation. Prolonged bleeding may be noted; hematomas and cutaneous petechiae may appear. Massive hemorrhage and ischemia of vital organs may ensue. Bleeding may be noted from various sites, such as through the nasogastric tube. The patient may have hypotension and oliguria. Postoperatively the patient may have nausea and vomiting, severe muscular pain, and convulsions and may lapse into a coma. Diagnosis is based on laboratory blood studies. Treatment begins with control of the primary condition. Blood, plasma, and dextran can be administered IV. Heparin and clotting factors, if given early, may prevent hemorrhage.

Cardiac Dysrhythmias

An alteration of normal cardiac rhythm may decrease cardiac output, exhaust the myocardium, and lead to ventricular fibrillation or cardiac arrest. Bradycardia is the slowing of the heart or pulse rate. Tachycardia is an excessive rapidity of the heart's action. Ventricular tachycardia and ventricular fibrillation are the dysrhythmias of most serious consequence and thus most feared.

Etiology

Etiologic factors include hypoxia; hypercapnia; acidosis; electrolyte imbalance; coronary disease; myocardial infarction; vagal reflexes; anesthetic agents; toxic doses of digitalis, epinephrine, or other drugs; and laryngospasm and coughing initiated by the presence of secretions in the airway following induction. Other causes may be hypotension, hemorrhage, hypovolemia, pneumothorax, and mechanical injuries.

Ventricular Dysrhythmias

An impulse originating in the ventricles must travel to the rest of the myocardium from one ventricle, proceeding then to the other ventricle. Because the impulse does not travel via the rapid, specialized conduction system, depolarization of both ventricles takes longer and is not simultaneous. The complexes of dysrhythmias have an abnormal appearance on an electrocardiogram (ECG) as compared with normally initiated and conducted impulses.

Premature Ventricular Contraction   An ectopic focus in the ventricles stimulates the heart to contract or beat prematurely before the regularly scheduled sinoatrial impulse arrives (Figure 33-1). Primary precipitating factors are electrolyte or acid-base imbalance, myocardial infarction, digitalis toxicity, and caffeine. The premature ventricular contraction (PVC) must be distinguished from a premature atrial contraction (PAC). Isolated PVCs may not require treatment, but those occurring in clusters of two or more or over five or six per minute require therapy. The aim is to quiet the irritable myocardium and restore adequate cardiac output.

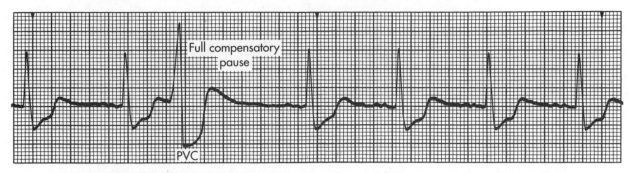

Figure 33-1 Premature ventricular contractions. (From Huszar RJ: *Basic dysrhythmias: interpretation and management,* ed 2, St Louis, 1994, Mosby.)

Figure 33-2 Ventricular tachycardia. (From Phipps WJ et al: *Medical-surgical nursing: concepts and clinical practice,* ed 5, St Louis, 1995, Mosby.)

Figure 33-3 Ventricular fibrillation. (From Phipps WJ et al: *Medical-surgical nursing: concepts and clinical practice,* ed 5, St Louis, 1995, Mosby.)

Treatment consists of a lidocaine bolus followed by a continuous drip by infusion, correction of the cause (e.g., hypoxia), and other antidysrhythmic drugs if indicated (e.g., procainamide or quinidine). Temporary pacing may be used for severe bradycardia. Paired PVCs pose an increased danger of ventricular tachycardia.

Ventricular Tachycardia A rapid heart rate (100 to 220 beats per minute) may be caused by ventricular ischemia or irritability, anoxia, or digitalis intoxication. The heart rate does not allow time for ventricular filling (Figure 33-2). The resultant reduced cardiac output predisposes the patient to ventricular fibrillation or cardiac failure. Ventricular tachycardia is treated by prompt IV administration of lidocaine, procainamide, or intramuscular quinidine.

Synchronized cardioversion of 10 to 200 joules may be used if the blood pressure is palpable. This is the application of a high-intensity, short-duration electric shock to the chest wall over the heart to produce total cardiac depolarization. This countershock is timed to interrupt an abnormal rhythm in the cardiac cycle, thereby permitting resumption of a normal one. Cardioversion is usually applied in instances of nonarrest for a nevertheless dangerous ventricular tachycardia. It may be an elective or emergency treatment. Asynchronous cardioversion is used if the patient is pulseless. Treatment includes correction of the underlying cause.

Ventricular Flutter Often called fine ventricular fibrillation, the flutter appears as a transient state between ventricular tachycardia and ventricular fibrillation. The patient will show signs of poor cardiac output.

Ventricular Fibrillation The most serious of all dysrhythmias, fibrillation is characterized by total disorganization of ventricular activity (Figure 33-3). There are rapid and irregular, uncoordinated, random contractions of small myocardial groups without effective ventricular contraction or cardiac output. Circulation ceases. The patient in fibrillation is unconscious and possibly convulsing from cerebral hypoxia.

TREATMENT   Because respiratory and cardiac arrest quickly follow, ventricular fibrillation is rapidly fatal unless successful defibrillation is effected as follows:

1. *Precordial thump.* In a monitored patient a fast, sharp, single blow to the midportion of the sternum (using the nipple line as a landmark) may be delivered with the bottom fleshy part of a closed fist struck from 8 to 12 inches (20 to 30 cm) above the chest. The blow generates a small electrical stimulus in a heart that is reactive. It may be effective in restoring a beat in cases of asystole or recent onset of dysrhythmia.
2. *Asynchronous cardioversion.* Prompt defibrillation by short-duration electric shock to the heart produces simultaneous depolarization of all muscle fiber bundles, after which spontaneous beating (conversion to spontaneous normal sinus rhythm) may resume if the myocardium is oxygenated and not acidotic. Defibrillation of an anoxic myocardium is difficult. The time fibrillation is started should be noted. The electric shock is coordinated with controlled ventilation and cardiac compression. CPR begins as soon as fibrillation is identified. Many variables may affect defibrillation, such as body weight, paddle position, electrical waveform, and resistance to electric current flow. Procedures follow an established protocol.
3. *Adjunct drug therapy.* Drugs are given as necessary: vasopressor, cardiotonic, and myocardial stimulant drugs to maintain a useful heartbeat; vasodilator or antidysrhythmic drugs to prevent recurrence; and sodium bicarbonate to combat acidosis. Continuous monitoring of the heart and laboratory analysis of arterial blood gases are essential.

Defibrillation: Equipment and Technique

Necessary equipment for defibrillation includes a defibrillator machine and two paddle electrodes. Defibrillators use direct electric current. Most have integrated monitors; monitor and defibrillator switches may be separate or combined. An operational monitor does not always indicate that the fibrillation power is on. Many monitor-defibrillator units can monitor the ECG from the paddle electrodes, as well as from separate patient leads. These paddles and patient leads cannot operate simultaneously, however. Depending on the type of defibrillator, the electrical cord must be plugged in or batteries charged. All defibrillators should be checked regularly with suitable test equipment. Paddles must be cleaned immediately and prepared for reuse. This is emergency equipment and must be available at all times.

External Defibrillation   External defibrillation of the heart is used unless the chest is already open, as for intrathoracic surgery. Standard electrode paste or jelly, or saline-soaked 4×4 inch gauze pads reduce the resistance of the skin to passage of the electric current. If paste is used on paddles, it should not extend beyond the electrodes or onto any part of the handles. Gel pads between the paddles and the patient's skin provide the advantage that if external cardiac compression is resumed after defibrillation, hands will not slip on the chest. The large diameter of the paddles increases the area of skin contact, thus reducing the possibility of skin burns by spreading of the current. The paddles must be held flat against the skin and more than 2 inches (5 cm) apart to prevent electrical arcing. They must be kept scrupulously clean because foreign material reduces the uniformity of the shock. The electrodes must be pressed firmly against the chest wall for good contact. One of two external paddle positions may be used:

1. *Standard position.* One electrode is placed just to the right of the upper sternum below the clavicle. The other is positioned to the left of the cardiac apex (i.e., left of the nipple at the fifth intercostal space along the left midaxillary line). The delivered current flows through the long axis of the heart.
2. *Anterior-posterior position.* One electrode is placed anteriorly over the precordium between the left nipple and the sternum. The other is positioned posteriorly behind the heart immediately below the left scapula, avoiding the spinal column. This allows for more energy passage through the heart, but placement is more difficult.

Internal Defibrillation   For internal defibrillation, sterile electrodes are placed on the myocardium, one over the right atrium, the other over the left ventricle. If these electrodes are gauze covered, they are dipped in sterile saline solution before use. Minimal current is needed when paddles are placed directly on the heart.

Perioperative team members must understand the functioning of the defibrillator for the patient's safety and their own. The person holding the electrode paddles delivers the electric charge by pressing a switch on the handle or a foot switch. The safest method is to activate both paddles simultaneously for discharge of electrical energy. The operator should have dry hands and stand on a dry floor. To avoid possible self-electrocution when using a defibrillator, neither the person holding the electrodes nor anyone else should touch the metal frame of the operating bed or the patient while the current is being applied. No part of the operator's body should touch the paste or the uninsulated electrodes. Loud verbal warning is given before discharge. Countershock is repeated at intervals if fibrillation persists. Transthoracic impedance falls with repetitive, closely spaced electrical discharges. After each countershock, the ECG and pulse should be reassessed.

Myocardial damage resulting from defibrillation efforts is in direct proportion to the energy used; therefore maximal settings, when not required, may increasingly impair an already-damaged myocardium. The energy level delivered through a specific ohm load should be indicated on the front panel of the defibrillator. Delivery output ranges vary among machines. The strength of the countershock is expressed in energy as joules or watt-seconds, the product of power and duration. If the patient's chest muscles do not contract, no current has reached the patient. The defibrillator's connection to the electrical source and the "off" button to the synchronizer circuit should be checked. If the machine is battery operated, the battery must be charged enough to energize the capacitor. Personnel must be familiar with and follow operating instructions for the defibrillator in use.

Prevention

Appropriate preoperative sedation and skillfully administered anesthesia help to prevent hazardous cardiovascular reflexes. Since PVCs are precursors to ventricular fibrillation, in itself a precursor to cardiac arrest, any cardiopulmonary emergency in a prearrest phase requires the following:

1. *Monitoring of the heart rhythm and rate.* The ability to recognize the rhythms that precede arrest permits intervention that may prevent arrest. If the cardiac status is not under constant monitoring, hypoxia and acidosis may be present and require correction before other therapeutic modalities can be used effectively.
2. *Establishment of an IV lifeline.* Venous cannulation provides access to peripheral and central venous circulation for administering drugs and fluids, obtaining venous blood specimens for laboratory analysis, and inserting catheters into the right side of the heart and pulmonary arteries for physiologic monitoring and electrical pacing. If cardiac arrest appears imminent or has occurred, cannulation of a peripheral or femoral vein should be attempted first so as not to interrupt CPR. To keep the infusion open, the rate should be kept low. The usual complications to all IV techniques should be guarded against.

Cardiac Arrest

In cardiac arrest there is cessation of circulatory action; the pumping mechanism of the heart ceases. Cardiac standstill represents total absence of electrical cardiac activity (asystole), reflected as a straight line on an ECG rhythm strip. It may occur as primary cardiac failure or secondary to failure of pulmonary ventilation. The types of circulatory arrest are profound cardiovascular collapse, electromechanical dissociation, ventricular fibrillation, and ventricular asystole or standstill. Cardiac arrest may precede or follow failure of the respiratory system because the systems are interrelated.

Incidence

Arrest may occur during induction of anesthesia, intraoperatively, or postoperatively. Occurrence during cardiac surgery or following massive hemorrhage is not uncommon. Patients more prone to arrest include those at age extremes and those with previously diagnosed paroxysmal dysrhythmias, primary cardiovascular abnormalities, myocarditis, heart block, or digitalis toxicity. An unexpected arrest is one that happens in a patient of general good health who is undergoing a low-risk or relatively routine procedure. These arrests are associated with major morbidity and mortality.

Etiology

A single factor or combination of factors may precipitate arrest, but the general cause is inadequate coronary arterial blood flow. Defective respiratory function produces systemic hypoxemia, causing myocardial hypoxia and depression. It also increases myocardial irritability and the heart's susceptibility to vagal reflexes. Some of the specific precipitating factors are dysrhythmias, emboli, extreme hypotension or hypovolemia, respiratory obstruction, aspiration, effects of drugs, anesthetic overdosage, excessively rapid or unsmooth induction, sepsis, pharyngeal stimulation, metabolic abnormalities (acidosis, toxemia, electrolyte imbalance), poor cardiac filling caused by positioning, manipulation of the heart, central nervous system trauma, anaphylaxis, and electric shock from ungrounded or faulty electrical equipment.

Symptoms

Symptoms include loss of heartbeat and blood pressure; sudden fixed, dilated pupils; sudden pallor or cyanosis; cold, clammy skin; absence of reflexes; unconsciousness or convulsions in a previously conscious patient; respiratory standstill; and dark blood or absence of bleeding in the surgical field.

Diagnosis

Arrest is readily detected by the ECG monitor during anesthesia, with absence of blood pressure and precordial heart sounds and the lack of a palpable carotid pulse. The onset of pupillary dilation is within 45 seconds after cerebral anoxia; full dilation is reached about 90 to 110 seconds after cessation of cerebral circulation.

Treatment

CPR is initiated immediately to restore oxygenation to vital organs. Defibrillation may be needed for ventricular fibrillation. IV drugs usually are used to improve cardiopulmonary status.

Prevention

Optimal psychologic preoperative assessment to identify the level of anxiety and testing for abnormalities and sensitivities are important preoperative preparations. Intraoperative precautions include the following:

- ECG and temperature monitoring
- No stimulation during induction
- Maintenance of an adequate airway
- Oxygen and carbon dioxide monitoring
- Arterial blood pressure monitoring
- Medications
- Appropriate positioning and slow position changes with the patient under anesthesia; no weight on the patient
- Gentle handling of tissues with minimal traction and manipulation
- Skillful anesthetic administration

INTRAVENOUS CARDIOVASCULAR DRUGS

An important factor in optimal anesthesia management is prompt recognition of the causes of hypotension, shock, and other complications that could lead to cardiac arrest. Prompt correction of reversible precipitants is critical. Many IV drugs are used to correct hypoxia and metabolic acidosis, manipulate cardiovascular variables, or treat pulmonary edema.

Pharmacodynamics

Uptake, movement, binding, and interactions of drugs vary at the tissue site of their biochemical and physiologic actions. Drug action is determined by how the drug interacts in the body. Some drugs alter body fluids; others, such as anesthetics, interact with cell membranes; most act through receptor mechanisms.

Receptor Mechanisms

Most drugs mimic naturally occurring compounds and interact with specific biologic molecules to produce biologic responses. For example, some cardiovascular drugs are sympathomimetics. They evoke physiologic responses similar to those produced by the sympathetic nervous system. A receptor is a structural protein molecule on a cell surface or within cytoplasm that binds with a drug to produce a biologic response. Three types of receptors are noteworthy in understanding the drugs used to counteract complications that may occur during anesthesia.

Adrenergic Receptors Adrenergic receptors are innervated by sympathetic nerve fibers and activated by epinephrine or norepinephrine secreted at the postganglionic nerve endings. These receptors are classified as alpha or beta, depending on their sensitivity to specific adrenergic activating and blocking drugs. Alpha$_1$ and alpha$_2$ receptors are located primarily in peripheral and renal arteriolar muscles; beta$_1$ receptors predominate in the heart; beta$_2$ receptors are primarily in smooth muscle of the lungs and blood vessels.

Cholinergic Receptors Cholinergic receptors are sites where acetylcholine exerts action to transmit nerve impulses through the parasympathetic nervous system to regulate the heart rate and respirations.

Opiate Receptors Opiate receptors are regions in the brain capable of binding morphine in areas related to pain.

Drug Interactions

No drug has a single action. Each modifies existing functions within the body by interactions to stimulate or inhibit responses. The desired action may be accompanied by side effects or an exaggerated response. An allergic reaction may occur immediately after exposure or may be delayed.

Anaphylaxis is a life-threatening, acute allergic reaction in which cells release histamine or a histamine-like substance. Anaphylaxis, a form of vasogenic shock, causes vasodilation, hypotension, and bronchial constriction. Within seconds, the patient will exhibit edema, wheezing, cyanosis, and dyspnea. Treatment includes epinephrine and antihistamines to control bronchospasm. Isoproterenol, vasopressors, corticosteroids, and aminophylline may also be administered.

In combination with local, regional, or general anesthetics, drugs must be carefully administered and monitored. The action of one drug may counteract another. Patients who do not respond to one drug (e.g., a catecholamine) may respond to another. Physicians do not always agree on the use of potent drugs. For example, a vasoconstrictor used to treat hypotension may possibly cause ischemic damage to organs. The physician's orders should be followed for all drugs.

Intravenous Administration

The speed of administration and dosage will depend on the drug and its intended action. Dosages given in this text vary according to individual patient circumstances. The technique of IV administration also varies.

Continuous Intravenous Drip The drug is diluted in a volume of dextrose or normal saline solution. The rate of administration is regulated by adjusting the number of drips per minute from the solution container into the IV tubing. A drug that might be absorbed by plastic should not be added to solution in a plastic infusion bag.

Bolus A bolus is a single rapid injection of the full dosage of a drug that cannot be diluted. It is usually given through an existing IV line. It may be injected directly into a vein or an intrathecal catheter. Some drugs can be given via an endotracheal tube for absorption through the alveoli or mucous membranes. The drug quickly reaches peak level in the bloodstream.

Intravenous Push A drug may be injected slowly into an IV line or through an intermittent infusion pump over a period of minutes. The total dose may be diluted and given in repeated doses over a period of hours. An infusion pump may be used to control the rate of delivery precisely.

Titration Dosage is calculated on the basis of body surface area (BSA) and hemodynamic parameters. Cardiac output is evaluated in terms of BSA. This may be determined by the ratio of the patient's height and weight on the BSA scale or by thermodilution. The patient's physiologic responses also will determine total dosage.

Considerations for Drug Administration

Some drugs are inactivated by others. The IV tubing should be flushed or changed to avoid precipitation, such as can occur with sodium bicarbonate. Many potent drugs should be infused through an IV catheter, which is safer than a needle to prevent extravasation. If a drug extravasates at the site of injection, the area must be promptly infiltrated with phentolamine (Regitine) to prevent the necrosis that can result from some vasoactive drugs.

Drugs by Classification

Pharmacokinetics includes the mechanisms of absorption, distribution, and metabolism of drugs in the body and elimination from the body. Nurses must have knowledge of drug actions and of how to prepare and administer drugs. The following drugs are classified by their pharmacodynamics to counteract adverse cardiovascular and pulmonary status.

Sympathomimetics are most often used for the following purposes:

- To increase force (inotropic effect), maintain contractility (noninotropic effect), or decrease the stroke volume of myocardial contractions
- To increase the pulse rate
- To increase or decrease arterial blood pressure
- To correct dysrhythmias
- To increase renal blood flow
- To stimulate the central nervous system
- To treat bronchospasm
- To prolong the effect of local anesthetics
- To manage life-threatening emergencies

Patients receiving any of the following drugs must be carefully monitored.

Antidysrhythmics

Antidysrhythmics control the heart rate and rhythm. They may induce a decreased rate and cardiac output. They may reduce cardiac conduction and increase dilation of peripheral vessels.

Lidocaine Hydrochloride (Xylocaine) Lidocaine increases the threshold for ventricular irritability by exerting a focal anesthetic effect on the myocardial cell membrane. It is used for ventricular tachycardia and fibrillation, especially if resistance to defibrillation effort occurs. It can be given IV, intrathecally, or by endotracheal tube. DOSAGE: 1 mg/kg or 75 to 100 mg by IV push over 30 to 60 seconds, followed by half the initial dose every 8 to 10 minutes to a total of 3 mg/kg if ectopic heartbeats continue. After conversion, a maintenance dose of 2 to 4 mg/min can be given by IV drip. Half these dosages are used to treat shock or pulmonary edema.

Bretylium Tosylate (Bretylol) Bretylium lowers the defibrillation threshold, permitting otherwise refractory rhythms to be electrically converted. It is indicated for ventricular tachycardia and fibrillation unresponsive to other therapy. DOSAGE: 5 mg/kg by rapid IV bolus, followed by defibrillation. If fibrillation continues, the dose can be doubled and repeated as necessary. For ventricular fibrillation 300 to

600 mg may be required. The drug may be diluted for continuous IV drip at a dosage of 1 to 2 mg/min for ventricular tachycardia and to prevent fibrillation. Some degree of hypotension may occur.

Procainamide Hydrochloride (Pronestyl) Procainamide suppresses PVCs and recurrent tachycardia. This drug may be used if lidocaine is contraindicated or has not controlled ventricular tachycardia. DOSAGE: 100 mg by IV push every 5 minutes until dysrhythmia ceases, or to a total of 1 g. Maintenance IV drip is 1 to 4 mg/min. Marked hypotension may occur if infusion is too rapid.

Adenosine Triphosphate (Adenocard) Adenosine slows atrioventricular (AV) node conduction. This action converts supraventricular tachycardia to normal sinus rhythm. DOSAGE: 6 to 12 mg by IV bolus followed immediately by a saline bolus. Incremental doses of 0.05 mg/kg can be given as necessary. This drug is contraindicated for patients with asthma.

Verapamil Hydrochloride (Isoptin, Calan) A calcium channel blocker, verapamil inhibits calcium ions to slow myocardial contractility, the heart rate, and the demand for oxygen. It is used as an antidysrhythmic to treat paroxysmal supraventricular tachycardia, acute atrial flutter, and atrial fibrillation. DOSAGE: 5 to 10 mg (0.075-0.15 mg/kg adult body weight) by slow IV push over 2 minutes; may be repeated after 30 minutes. This drug is not given to patients with severe hypotension or cardiogenic shock, nor is it given concurrently with an IV beta-adrenergic blocker, such as propranolol.

Propranolol Hydrochloride (Inderal) A beta-adrenergic receptor blocking agent, propranolol is used to control supraventricular dysrhythmias and to treat hypertension. It reduces myocardial oxygen consumption by blocking catecholamine-induced increases in the heart rate, blood pressure, and cardiac contractions. It may be used if control of ventricular fibrillation is not achieved with lidocaine or other drugs. DOSAGE: 1 to 3 mg by IV push, not to exceed 1 mg/min, titrated for heart rate and rhythm. This drug is contraindicated for patients with asthma, bronchospasm, or cardiac depression.

Isoproterenol Hydrochloride (Isuprel) A beta-adrenergic receptor stimulant, isoproterenol stimulates the sympathetic tone, rate, and strength of myocardial contractions and cardiac output. It increases the myocardial demand for oxygen. It may be used for ventricular dysrhythmias, but it may produce tachycardia or dysrhythmia. It is indicated to control hemodynamically significant bradycardia in a patient who has a pulse but who is unresponsive to atropine. It is a vasodilator and bronchodilator. DOSAGE: IV drip of 1 mg to 500 ml of dextrose or saline solution at the rate of 1.25 ml/min, titrated according to the heart rate and rhythm.

Antimuscarinics/Anticholinergics

Antimuscarinics/anticholinergics block passage of impulses through the parasympathetic nerves to the heart and smooth muscles. When both the sympathetic and parasympathetic components of the autonomic nervous system are stimulated, the parasympathetic dominates to slow the heartbeat and respirations. An anticholinergic allows desired sympathetic action.

Atropine Sulfate   Atropine reduces cardiac vagal tone, enhances AV conduction, and increases cardiac output. It accelerates the cardiac rate in sinus bradycardia with severe hypotension or in bradycardia associated with hypoxia and reduced cardiac output. It may restore cardiac rhythm in AV block or ventricular asystole. It is a primary drug used in cardiopulmonary arrest. Atropine may be given IV, intrathecally, or via an endotracheal tube. DOSAGE: 1 mg by IV bolus for asystole, 0.5 mg for bradycardia, at 5-minute intervals until the desired rate is achieved or to a total dose of 2 mg. Full vagal blockage could result from overdosage.

Vasodilators

Vasodilators are noninotropic drugs that relax smooth muscle in the capillaries and cause peripheral dilation. They dilate arteries and veins almost equally without increasing myocardial contractility. This reduces venous return to heart. They are used to alter blood flow and lower blood pressure in patients with severely reduced cardiac output or in hypertensive crisis.

Sodium Nitroprusside (Nipride, Nitropress)
Sodium nitroprusside acts rapidly as a direct peripheral vasodilator to increase cardiac output and redistribute cardiac work in patients with pump failure. It increases tissue perfusion without reflex tachycardia. DOSAGE: IV drip, not to exceed 10 µg/kg/min, of 50 mg dissolved in 2 to 3 ml of dextrose added to 250 to 1000 ml of 5% dextrose in water for infusion. An infusion pump or microdrip-regulating system ensures a precise flow rate. The solution deteriorates in light, so it must be protected by opaque material such as aluminum foil. No other drug should be injected into the IV line while sodium nitroprusside is running.

Nitroglycerin (Nitrostat IV, Nitrol IV, Tridil)
Nitroglycerin decreases venous return to the heart and reduces preload and afterload, thus lowering myocardial oxygen demands. It is used for control of blood pressure in hypertension associated with cardiovascular procedures or endotracheal intubation, or in the immediate postoperative period. DOSAGE: Up to 50 µg/min by IV push. The drug should be titrated to increase the dose and the time intervals between infusions should be adjusted, depending on lowering of the blood pressure. This potent drug must be diluted in dextrose or saline solution. It is absorbed by polyvinyl chloride (PVC) plastic, so glass solution bottles and tubing that is not made of PVC should be used. The drug is also light sensitive.

Trimethaphan Camsylate (Arfonad)   A ganglionic blocking agent, trimethaphan camsylate is used to produce controlled hypotension during surgical procedures and to lower blood pressure in patients with hypertension or in patients with an acute hypertensive crisis. DOSAGE: 500 mg diluted in 500 ml of 5% dextrose in water (1 mg/1 ml) IV drip. Initially the drug is infused slowly at the rate of 1 to 2 mg/min and increased gradually to an average dose range of 3 to 6 mg/min.

Cardiotonics

Cardiotonics combine inotropic effect on the contractility of muscle with vasodilation of blood vessels. They stimulate myocardial function. Vasodilation reduces cardiac afterload, thereby improving cardiac performance and correcting peripheral vascular compensations.

Amrinone (Inocor)   Amrinone possesses significant vasodilator activity to improve tissue perfusion, especially to the kidneys, and to improve cardiac output. It is used for short-term effect in patients with ischemic heart disease and severe heart failure. The blood pressure and heart rate remain unchanged, whereas peripheral arteriolar resistance falls. DOSAGE: 0.5 to 3.5 mg/kg by IV bolus followed by IV drip of 5 to 10 µg/kg/min. Titrated to hemodynamic response, a second bolus can be given after 30 minutes.

Dobutamine Hydrochloride (Dobutrex)   A synthetic derivative of dopamine, dobutamine increases myocardial contractility while producing little systemic arterial constriction. It is used for short-term treatment of refractory heart failure, cardiogenic shock, and hemodynamically significant hypotension. DOSAGE: 2.5 to 10 µg/kg/min IV drip. Tachycardia or dysrhythmia may result from a larger dose. It is incompatible with alkaline solutions and drugs such as sodium bicarbonate.

Catecholamines

Catecholamines are vasoconstrictors that improve tissue perfusion by maintaining perfusion pressure, preventing or diminishing blood loss, decreasing tissue vascularity, and improving coronary blood flow. Among indications for their use are anesthesia overdose, hypotension associated with blood loss, and adrenergic insufficiency. They raise the blood pressure. They are antispasmodic.

Epinephrine Hydrochloride (Adrenalin)   An endogenous catecholamine and alpha-adrenergic receptor stimulant, epinephrine plays an essential role in restoration of spontaneous circulation in asystole; therefore it is the first drug administered in cardiac arrest. By increasing systemic vascular resistance, it improves coronary perfusion pressure and cardiac output produced by cardiac compression during CPR. It improves myocardial contractility and tone and causes vasoconstriction of arteries. It may be given IV, intrathecally, via endotracheal tube, or by intracardiac injection. DOSAGE: 0.5 to 1.0 mg by IV bolus, repeated every

5 minutes as necessary. It is available in preloaded syringes of 1:10,000 dilution (1 mg/10 ml). It may be added to an IV infusion of 250 ml of 5% dextrose in water. It is inactivated by alkaline solutions. Continuous infusion may increase the heart rate, blood pressure, and cardiac output. Side effects include elevated myocardial oxygen demand and possible PVCs or ventricular fibrillation.

Norepinephrine Bitartrate (Levophed)   An endogenous catecholamine, norepinephrine restores and maintains blood pressure. It may be given following peripheral vascular collapse as a result of severe hypotension or cardiogenic shock. It constricts renal and mesenteric vessels and may cause severe peripheral vasoconstriction. DOSAGE: 16 mg/L (16 μg/ml) IV drip in 5% dextrose in water, titrated to the desired blood pressure; average dose range is 2 to 4 μg/min. The drug is toxic if extravasation occurs. Hypotension from hypovolemia is a contraindication.

Diuretics

Diuretics increase the amount of urine excreted. Potent diuretics are used to treat pulmonary edema and postarrest cerebral edema. They inhibit reabsorption of sodium. They are used with caution, since they may have a direct venodilating effect or may lead to fluid and electrolyte depletion. The most commonly used diuretics are the following:

- Furosemide (Lasix), 0.5 to 2.0 mg/kg injected slowly over 1 to 2 minutes by IV push; the dose can be repeated in 2 hours
- Ethacrynate sodium (Sodium Edecrin), 40 to 50 mg or 0.5 to 1.0 mg/kg injected slowly by IV push

Vasopressors

Vasopressors exert an inotropic vasoconstriction action on arterioles and veins through stimulation of alpha-adrenergic receptors, and they increase the heart rate, blood pressure, and myocardial contractility by activation of beta-adrenergic receptors. These drugs cause vasomotor depression of the peripheral circulation but increase coronary flow. They may increase ventricular contractile force, alter sinoatrial nodal activity, constrict smooth muscles, and dilate renal and mesenteric blood vessels. They may produce ventricular dysrhythmia, which can be intensified by hypoxia or hypercapnia. Drug effectiveness is reduced in the presence of respiratory or metabolic acidosis.

Dopamine Hydrochloride (Intropin)   In high dosage (greater than 10 μg/kg/min IV drip), dopamine causes peripheral vasoconstriction to increase cardiac output and blood pressure. It may be used during cardiogenic shock, severe hypotension, and asystole and then be titrated to the desired blood pressure. Discontinuance should be gradual. A low dose, 1 to 2 μg/kg/min IV drip, dilates renal and mesenteric blood vessels to maintain urinary output but may not increase the heart rate or blood pressure. The drip rate may be increased until organ perfusion is evidenced by the blood pressure and urinary output. Tachydysrhythmias are an indi-

cation for reduction in dose or discontinuation. Dopamine is inactivated in alkaline solution and by sodium bicarbonate. It is caustic if it extravasates. It should be diluted immediately before use.

Metaraminol Bitartrate (Aramine)   Metaraminol produces marked vasoconstriction and increases cardiac output and blood pressure, which may be useful to treat severe hypotension. It may be given IV or via endotracheal tube. DOSAGE: 0.4 mg/min IV drip in 5% dextrose in water.

Other Vasopressors   These drugs have various actions. Selection will depend on the action needed. Drugs that may be used include the following:

- Isoproterenol hydrochloride (Isuprel)
- Methoxamine hydrochloride (Vasoxyl)
- Mephentermine sulfate (Wyamine)
- Norepinephrine bitartrate (Levophed)
- Phenylephrine hydrochloride (Neo-Synephrine)

Other Drugs

The foregoing list is not intended to be all-inclusive. Other drugs are used for specific problems. Life-threatening acid-base or electrolyte imbalances associated with cardiovascular or pulmonary complications may need to be corrected (e.g., following CPR). The following two drugs may be used with caution; they are not recommended for routine administration at the onset of CPR.

Calcium Salts   Calcium should be avoided unless the patient has hyperkalemia, hypocalcemia, or calcium channel blocker toxicity. It may be administered by IV bolus as calcium chloride, 2 ml of 10% (1 g/10 ml) solution repeated as necessary at 10-minute intervals; calcium gluconate, 5 to 8 ml; or calcium gluceptate, 5 to 7 ml.

Sodium Bicarbonate   Metabolic acidosis secondary to accumulation of lactic acid produced by respiratory metabolism may need to be corrected. Bicarbonate binds with hydrogen ion from lactic acid to produce carbonic acid that breaks down into carbon dioxide and water. Sodium bicarbonate may be given after other resuscitation measures to reverse acidosis. DOSAGE: 1 mEq/kg by IV bolus initially, titrated according to blood gas analyses for subsequent doses, usually no more than 0.5 mEq/kg at 10- to 15-minute intervals. An excessive dose can produce metabolic alkalosis. Sodium bicarbonate should not be mixed in an IV line with any other drug; it will precipitate calcium salts and inactivate catecholamines.

CARDIOPULMONARY RESUSCITATION

CPR is aimed at rapidly restoring oxygen delivery to vital organs to reverse the processes that lead to death. CPR is an emergency procedure requiring special training to recognize cardiac or respiratory arrest and to perform artificial ventilation and circulation. To prevent irreversible brain damage, resuscitative measures must be instituted immediately, within 3 to 5 minutes after the arrest. The combination of anoxia and acidosis can make restoration of normal function impossible. Resuscitation is not a one-person job. The team must be completely familiar with the preplanned routine before the necessity for its use arises. Success depends on prompt diagnosis and immediate effective treatment. Outcome is directly related to the rapidity with which a functional, spontaneous heart rhythm can be restored. Patients who experience arrest in an operating room (OR) may be on monitors with an IV line already in place and resuscitation equipment on hand. These arrests are referred to as witnessed arrests. The time of onset of arrest should be noted and the time-elapsed clock started. Basic life support is instituted at once to reestablish oxygenation and restore the heartbeat.

Basic Life Support

Basic life support (BLS) is that particular phase of emergency cardiac care that either prevents circulatory or respiratory arrest or insufficiency through prompt recognition and intervention or externally supports circulation and respiration of a victim of cardiac or respiratory arrest through CPR. BLS can and should be initiated by any person present when cardiac arrest occurs.

The ABCs of resuscitation are as follows:

A *Airway:* patent and free of secretions or foreign body for effective pulmonary ventilation
B *Breathing:* prompt restoration and maintenance of oxygenation through artificial ventilation
C *Circulation:* provision of oxygen to vital tissues by means of cardiac compression (artificial circulation)

These steps should be started immediately and performed in the order given except when the patient is already intubated. Advanced cardiac life support should be instituted without delay to restore circulation. Resuscitation continues until the patient can resume normal, spontaneous respiration and circulation or until its discontinuation is warranted by diagnosis of brain death.

When the arrested patient is in the OR, anesthesia providers and other team members are present. In a witnessed arrest, the carotid pulse is palpated. The carotid artery is located in the groove between the trachea and muscles of the side of the neck. Palpation of the femoral artery is an acceptable option. If the patient has respiratory arrest, two quick, full lung inflations are given without allowing for full lung deflation between breaths. Maintenance of positive pressure in the lungs more effectively fills, ventilates, and prevents collapse of alveoli. If pulse and breathing are not immediately restored, CPR is begun.

If ventricular fibrillation or tachycardia without a pulse is evident, countershock is delivered as soon as possible (DC 200 to 300 joules delivered energy in an adult; 2 joules/kg or 1 joule/lb in an infant or child). If this is unsuccessful, additional countershocks and medications are given as ordered or per written protocol. In open heart defibrillation, between 5 and 40 joules are delivered, beginning with lower energy levels.

In infants and small children a hand is placed over the precordium to feel the apical beat, or the brachial pulse is checked in lieu of a carotid pulse. The brachial pulse is on the inside of the upper arm midway between the elbow and the shoulder. The index and middle fingers are used. A precordial thump is not given to an infant or child. In infants and children, bradydysrhythmias and heart block lead to cardiac arrest more commonly than does ventricular fibrillation.

Artificial Respiration

Immediate opening of the airway is mandatory to combat respiratory failure. If respiratory obstruction is present, it must be cleared. During general anesthesia either an oropharyngeal or nasopharyngeal airway or endotracheal tube may be in place to maintain a patent air passage. Oxygen (100%) can be delivered at once under positive pressure by manual ventilation. Otherwise, ventilation by other means, such as an esophageal obturator airway or expired-air technique, should be initiated to sustain oxygenation, followed by tracheal intubation as soon as possible. A cuffed endotracheal tube permits continual delivery of high oxygen concentration without the hazard of stomach distention or aspiration. It facilitates adequate ventilation since, with its use, interposed breaths are not necessary, thereby permitting a faster, uninterrupted cardiac compression rate of 80 beats per minute. When a tube or airway is lacking, the most rapid means of reestablishing oxygenation is by an expired-air technique or mouth-to-mouth or mouth-to-nose artificial ventilation. When artificial ventilation is combined with cardiac compression, tissues receive oxygen. In the OR the anesthesia provider manages artificial ventilation. The following principles apply to artificial respiration:

1. If attempts to ventilate the patient are unsuccessful despite proper opening of the airway, further attempts to remove the obstruction should be made. Laryngoscopy, cricothyrotomy, or tracheotomy may be indicated.
2. Tracheal suctioning should last no longer than 5 seconds at a time without ventilation to prevent hypoxia.
3. If spinal injury is suspected or present, extension of the neck is avoided and a modified jaw-thrust technique is employed. The head, neck, and chest are kept aligned.
4. Ventilation is assessed by seeing the chest rise and fall and hearing and feeling air escape during the patient's exhalation.

Artificial Circulation

Cardiac compression must accompany ventilation in a pulseless patient to maintain adequate blood pressure and circulation, thereby keeping tissues viable, preserving cardiac tone and reflexes, and preventing intravascular clotting. This may be accomplished by external closed chest cardiac compression, the rhythmic application of pressure over the lower half of the sternum above the xiphoid process (Figures 33-4 and 33-5). Because the heart occupies most of the space between the sternum and the thoracic spine, intermittent sternal compression 1½ to 2 inches raises intrathoracic pressure and produces cardiac output (Figure 33-6). Blood is forced from the heart into the pulmonary artery and aorta. During

Figure 33-4 Cross indicates correct spot to place hands for performing closed chest cardiac compression: over lower half of sternum and above xiphoid process.

Figure 33-6 Manual depression of sternum raises intrathoracic pressure and produces cardiac output. Blood is sent from heart into pulmonary artery and aorta.

Figure 33-5 Closed chest cardiac compression. Patient is supine on hard, flat surface. Resuscitator places heel of one hand over lower half of sternum with heel of other hand on top. Fingers are arched upward to avoid exerting force on ribs. Elbows are straight and locked with shoulders straight over hands.

Figure 33-7 Releasing pressure on sternum allows heart to fill with venous blood.

relaxation of pressure, negative intrathoracic pressure causes venous blood to flow back into the heart from the pulmonary and systemic circulatory systems (Figure 33-7). Blood moves in the arterial direction through the heart valves. Carotid artery blood flow from this technique usually is only one quarter to one third of normal (mean blood pressure 40 mm Hg), although systolic blood pressure is raised. It may peak at 100 mm Hg, but diastolic pressure is low. Artificial ventilation is always required when external cardiac

compression is employed because oxygenation of the circulating blood is inadequate. The brain and myocardium must be perfused effectively for survival. External cardiac compression must be instituted immediately on cessation of circulation. Any interruption in compression causes cessation of blood flow and a drop in blood pressure.

Cardiac compression must be performed with knowledge and care. All physicians and patient care personnel must be trained and certified in CPR at the minimal BLS level. Basic principles are the same for infants and children. Differences in technique are related to the position of the heart in the chest, small chest size, and faster heart rate.

BLS should not be interrupted for more than 5 seconds at a time except for endotracheal intubation. If intubation is difficult, the patient must be ventilated between short attempts. CPR is never suspended for more than 30 seconds, such as during defibrillation. Preferably, the patient should not be moved until stabilized and ready for transport or until arrangements are made for uninterrupted CPR during movement.

Elevation of the legs to a 60-degree angle with the trunk aids venous return and augments artificial circulation. Cardiac compression is successful only if the heart fills with blood between compressions and the resuscitator can move an adequate volume of oxygenated blood. The carotid or femoral pulse is checked every few minutes to indicate compression effectiveness or return of a spontaneous, effective heartbeat.

Manual external cardiac compression causes fatigue leading to variation in cardiac output; therefore it is advisable to have additional relief personnel available. Commercially available, manually operated mechanical chest compressors or automatic compressor-ventilators that provide simultaneous compression and ventilation eliminate this problem. When such devices are used, compression must always be started with the manual method first. Compressor-ventilators should be used only with a cuffed endotracheal tube, esophageal obturator airway, or mask, and only by experienced operators. Use should be limited to adult patients.

Complications of external compression are minimized by careful attention to detail. Compression must be performed with extreme caution to prevent injuries such as rib or sternal fracture, costochondral separation, fat embolism, laceration of the liver, lung contusion, pneumothorax, and hemothorax. To prevent fractures, the xiphoid process at the tip of the sternum is never compressed and pressure is never exerted on the ribs.

Internal Cardiac Compression   Internal cardiac compression is instituted if the patient's chest is already open, such as during a cardiothoracic procedure. Thoracotomy may be performed and internal compression administered in instances where external compression may be ineffective (e.g., internal thoracic injuries, such as penetrating wounds of the heart; flail chest; pericardial tamponade caused by hemorrhage; chest or spinal deformities). The advantages of internal compression are more complete ventricular emptying with greater outflow of blood into the circulation and rapid diastolic filling for a faster stroke rate than with external compression. Less blood flows in a retrograde manner. The disadvantages are delay in compression, potential trauma to the lungs and myocardium, and possible infection.

If the chest is not open, the incision is made through the left fifth or sixth intercostal space. The pericardial sac is opened for direct manual compression of the myocardium. A rib spreader is placed to avoid strangulation of the operator's hands. By cradling the heart in both hands, the operator compresses the ventricles between the thumb and fingers of one hand, or the fingers of both hands, 80 times per minute. Venous filling is necessary for adequate ventricular stroke volume.

Checking the Effectiveness of Cardiopulmonary Resuscitation

Signs suggestive of effective compression are constricted, reactive pupils; a palpable peripheral pulse; an audible heartbeat; and improvement in color of the mucous membranes, skin, and blood. Additional signs indicative of potential re-

covery are prompt return of spontaneous respiration and consciousness. Continuous compression is stopped when arterial blood pressure remains above 70 to 90 mm Hg and a strong spontaneous pulse is resumed. CPR may be performed intermittently as necessary to assist the restored heart.

Persistent dilation of the pupils and lack of reaction to light are ominous signs usually indicative of brain damage. Cell destruction is also manifested by convulsions, hyperpyrexia, and persistent coma. Survival in relation to these symptoms is usually accompanied by tragic consequences such as decerebration or paralysis.

Advanced Cardiac Life Support

Advanced cardiac life support (ACLS) consists of definitive therapy intended to reinstitute spontaneous oxygenation. It includes BLS; use of adjunctive equipment and special techniques for establishing and maintaining effective ventilation and circulation; cardiac and supplemental monitoring; recognition and control of dysrhythmias; defibrillation; establishing and maintaining an IV infusion route; drug administration; and postresuscitative care. It requires the supervision and direction of a physician. It should be initiated within 8 minutes of arrest to improve long-term functional survival. Subsequent insertion of an arterial line supplies access for direct pressure monitoring and arterial blood gases.

Intravenous Drugs

Compression is usually accompanied or followed by judicious use of drugs, administered IV, to manipulate cardiovascular variables, such as hypoxia and acidosis. These drugs may improve the patient's cardiopulmonary status by increasing the perfusion pressure during cardiac compression, stimulating spontaneous or more forceful myocardial contractions, accelerating the cardiac rate, and suppressing abnormal ventricular activity.

Oxygen, epinephrine, and atropine are the mainstays of pharmacologic management in CPR. Used in combination with basic life support, lidocaine, and defibrillation, they correct most CPR oxygen delivery problems. Each additional drug serves as a vital adjunct in definitive therapy and postresuscitative care.

Emergency Arrest/Crash Cart

An emergency arrest cart should be available at all times in all critical care areas (i.e., OR, emergency department [ED], PACU, and ICU). Specific drugs and equipment vary depending on how well equipped the anesthesia provider is for emergencies. Equipment on a portable cart usually includes the following:

- Oxygen and resuscitation equipment: oxygen cylinder, tubing, mask, Ambu bag or bag-valve-mask
- Laryngoscope tray, blades; endotracheal equipment and tubes; assorted airways—oral and nasal; stylet; padded tongue blades
- Tracheotomy tray

- Sterile gloves, sterile gauze sponges, prep swabs or spray, adhesive tape, tourniquets, sutures, armboard, drapes
- Suction machine and catheters
- IV infusion solutions and sets, IV needles and catheters (14 and 16 gauge), tubing stopcocks, infusion pump, additive labels
- Cutdown tray, venous cannulas, wire-guided catheters
- Assorted sterile syringes: 3, 5, 10, 20, and 50 ml
- Assorted sterile needles: 25 gauge × ⅝ inch, 20 gauge × 1½ inches, 18 gauge × 1½ inches, 20 gauge × 3 inches (intracardiac), and spinal needles
- Arterial blood sampling kit with needles, heparinized syringes; arterial line tray
- Disposable scalpels, hemostats
- Emergency thoracotomy set: scalpel with No. 20 blade, rib retractor, self-retaining retractor
- ECG monitor, leads, recording sheets
- Cardiac arrest board
- Defibrillator with paddles (adult, pediatric, external, internal), electrode jelly or paste, saline pads
- Cardiac arrest record for treatment documentation/flow sheets
- Cardiac pacemaker
- Drugs: mainly vasoconstrictors, cardiotonics, vasopressors, cardiac depressants, anticholinergics, cerebral dehydrating agents, pulmonary dehydrating agents (Many frequently used emergency drugs are available in sterile commercially prefilled syringes to avoid delay in preparation. They are routinely checked for expiration dates.)
- CVP manometer
- Nasogastric tube and bulb syringe
- Flashlight

Personnel Responsibilities

During CPR, team members must remain calm but react quickly and act efficiently as follows:

1. *Director:* One person, the most knowledgeable, usually the anesthesia provider, commands resuscitation efforts. He or she is assisted by surgeons, nurses, surgical technologists, and other available personnel. A cardiologist is usually summoned. Resuscitation teams are multidisciplinary. The person in charge directs lifesaving interventions that entail minute-to-minute decisions such as medications and defibrillation. To avoid confusion, the director issues orders for others to follow. Every circulator should be prepared to be a team captain.
2. *Circulator:*
   a. Start the time-elapsed clock (if available) and record the time of arrest.
   b. Activate the emergency alarm to alert the OR manager and summon assistance.
   c. Help reposition the patient as necessary into the supine position for CPR. Lower the operating bed and provide the resuscitator with a standing platform to facilitate cardiac compression. The circulator

must be able to perform chest compressions if an additional resuscitator is not immediately available.
   d. Obtain and prepare necessary equipment, such as medications, the defibrillator, and the ECG if it is not already in use.
   e. Help with and observe IV and monitoring lines, such as an arterial line. Assist in collection of blood samples.
   f. Maintain accuracy of sponge, needle, and instrument counts and sterility to best of ability if wound closure progresses (but sterility is secondary to resuscitation efforts).
   g. Supervise termination of the procedure as necessary.
   h. Delegate duties to assisting personnel.
   i. Control traffic. Exclude unauthorized personnel from the room. Students should be either instructed to stand back or enlisted to obtain supplies as able. Provide an optimal environment for successful resuscitation.
   j. Document all medications given, the time and amount, and the sequence of procedures performed. Documentation is important in guiding therapy and providing legal protection.
   k. Assist where needed most.
   l. In unsuccessful resuscitation, follow protocol regarding notification of family, care of the deceased, specimens to be saved, and forms to be filled out after a death in the OR.
3. *Scrub person:*
   a. Remain sterile and keep the tables sterile if possible. If arrest occurs during a noncardiac surgical procedure, when the chest is not open, the surgical site is packed with saline-soaked sponges and covered with sterile drape, and the patient is repositioned as necessary for CPR. If the surgical site is in an area that can be closed rapidly during resuscitation, this may be done.
   b. Keep track of sponges, needles, and instruments. Counts are completed, and the surgical site is closed as soon as possible despite the outcome. In a life-threatening emergency, the surgeon may order that counts be aborted. Follow the written institutional policy and procedure for counts during emergency situations.
   c. Give attention to the field and the surgeon's needs. If the patient is hemorrhaging, keep suction tubing clear and tapes available.
   d. If the circulator is performing chest compressions, obtain the emergency cart and assist as required.
4. *OR manager/head nurse:*
   a. Assign professional and assistive support personnel to augment the team (e.g., an extra circulator, medication nurse, personnel to obtain supplies or handle laboratory samples).
   b. Notify the attending physician, if not present, and appropriate administrative personnel.
   c. Have the patient placed on the critical list. Alert the ICU of a potential patient admission.

d. Reassign subsequent patients' scheduling.
e. Keep track of resuscitation progress.
f. Evaluate the arrest procedure and emergency equipment; verify the documentation.
g. Support the team as necessary. Keep the surgical suite running smoothly during the emergency.

Duration of Cardiopulmonary Resuscitation

CPR may be done as long as necessary to restore circulatory function if adequate ventilation and a good peripheral pulse have been restored. It is not uncommon for a second arrest to occur following successful resuscitation. The time frame for survival is shortened drastically if the arrest is unwitnessed. When the patient's condition is adequately stabilized and the surgical site is closed, he or she is transferred to the ICU.

The decision to discontinue resuscitative efforts in the OR is made by a physician. However the resuscitation team is included in this decision. The decision is based on assessment of cerebral and cardiovascular status. The end point of cardiovascular unresponsiveness is suggested as the most reliable basis for this decision.

Appropriate administrative personnel and services, such as the nursing unit, ICU, and clergy, as well as the patient's family, are notified of the cardiac arrest as required. In case of death, the surgeon notifies the family.

Postresuscitation Care

Postarrest supportive therapy depends on the cause and duration of arrest. Care centers on cardiac and cerebral preservation, maintenance of circulation and ventilation, and minimizing of sequelae such as cerebral edema. The patient must be carefully monitored and closely observed for 48 to 72 hours postarrest. In select patients, hypothermia may be used to reduce oxygen needs. Vital signs, acid-base and electrolyte balances, and urinary output are closely watched. Seizures should be controlled to prevent further anoxia. The patient is observed for signs of embolism, pulmonary edema, fractured ribs caused by chest compressions, or hemopericardium. A chest x-ray film is taken as soon as feasible after the arrest. An IV fluid lifeline must be left in place. If there is evident cerebral damage, the prognosis is guarded.

Staff Education

Practice sessions of a cardiac arrest emergency and CPR with subsequent evaluation and revision are valuable to review the protocol and prepare the OR staff before need for implementation. Current CPR/BLS certification is required of all OR personnel. Many ORs require yearly BLS review, with recertification every 2 years. ICU personnel are required to be ACLS certified.

FLUID AND ELECTROLYTE IMBALANCE

Fluid and electrolyte imbalances may be caused by many different factors and may be manifested by numerous symptoms. Maintenance of correct balance, which greatly influences the outcome of surgical intervention, is a very relevant aspect of intraoperative and postoperative care.

Fluid loss is replaced by IV infusion. Usually normal saline or dextrose (5% or 10% in water or saline) solution is started initially. Electrolytes may be added to the solution as needed. Two other IV solutions are commonly used to maintain balance:

1. Mannitol, an osmotic diuretic agent, has an effect on renal vascular resistance. Depending on the percentage of drug in solution, it can either increase or decrease renal blood flow. It may be given prophylactically to prevent renal failure. It also is used to decrease intracranial and intraocular pressure. It is rapidly excreted by the kidneys.
2. Ringer's lactate solution, a physiologic salt solution, may be infused when the body's supply of sodium, calcium, and potassium has been depleted or for improvement of circulation and stimulation of renal activity. Its electrolyte content is similar to that of plasma.

Changes in fluid and electrolyte balance affect renal function, cellular metabolism, and oxygen concentration in the circulation.

Acid-Base Balance

For enzyme systems to function, a normal balance must be maintained between acidity and alkalinity of body fluids located within intracellular and extracellular compartments. The symbol *pH* represents the hydrogen ion concentration that determines acidity or alkalinity of a solution; neutral pH is 7.0, below 7 is acid, and above 7 is alkaline. Urine is usually acid, with a pH range between 4.6 and 8.0. Normal serum pH is 7.40, within a range of 7.35 to 7.45.

Hydrogen ions do not exist as separate electrolytes in body fluids but are maintained in balance with other electrolytes to ensure neutrality. Because most metabolic processes produce acids, chemical buffers interact with hydrogen ions. Carbonic acid and a hydrogen ion form bicarbonate (HCO_3), the most important buffer. The kidneys and lungs regulate this system by excreting or retaining needed ions in body fluids. Abnormal acid-base balance results from the following:

1. Respiratory malfunction in handling carbon dioxide produced from carbonic acid
   a. *Acidosis:* pH less than 7.35 with carbon dioxide above 45 torr
   b. *Alkalosis:* pH more than 7.45 with carbon dioxide below 35 torr
2. Metabolic abnormality in balance between hydrogen and serum HCO_3
   a. *Acidosis:* pH less than 7.35 with HCO_3 less than 22 mEq/L
   b. *Alkalosis:* pH more than 7.45 with HCO_3 more than 26 mEq/L

Electrolytes

Compounds that separate into ions, which are charged particles capable of conducting electrical impulses, are essential in maintaining fluid and acid-base balance and in regulating cell functions. The primary electrolytes in the body (Table 33-1) are as follows:

1. *Sodium.* A key regulator in water balance, sodium is necessary to the normal function of muscles and nerves. Large amounts are in extracellular fluid in concentrations of 136 to 145 mEq/L; intracellular concentration is 10 mEq/L. This balance is necessary for normal metabolism.
   a. Hyponatremia, insufficient serum sodium, usually accompanies excessive fluid loss or adrenal insufficiency. Muscle twitching, hypovolemia, hypotension, and tachycardia may be symptoms.
   b. Hypernatremia, elevated serum sodium, may be caused by hyperglycemia or administration of mannitol. Diaphoresis (sweating) may be the only obvious symptom. Convulsions can occur.
2. *Chloride.* Essential to electrochemical reactions for acid-base regulation, chloride is in extracellular fluids in large amounts. Chlorides are retained or excreted by the kidneys to offset HCO_3 excretion. Sodium tends to carry chloride with it.
   a. Hypochloremia, loss of chloride, may occur from vomiting, suctioning, sweating, and diuresis. It produces symptoms of metabolic alkalosis: slow, shallow respirations and muscle tightening.
   b. Hyperchloremia, excessive chloride, can result in renal failure. Acidosis develops, and breathing becomes labored.
3. *Potassium.* One of the main constituents of cell protoplasm, potassium is primarily (98%) in intracellular fluid. It is essential for electrochemical reactions for cellular functions.
   a. Hypokalemia, a shift of potassium from the blood to the cells or depletion of potassium from the body, can be associated with metabolic alkalosis. Cardiac dysrhythmias can occur when the serum potassium level falls.
   b. Hyperkalemia, an increase in serum potassium, may be caused by renal failure and may lead to respiratory and/or cardiac arrest. Metabolic or respiratory acidosis can occur.
4. *Calcium.* Essential to normal muscle physiology, calcium also is an integral part of the blood-clotting mechanism.
   a. Hypocalcemia, decreased calcium intake or absorption, may be a result of increased excretion. This can cause cardiac dysrhythmias.
   b. Hypercalcemia, increased serum calcium, may be a result of a shift of calcium from the bones to plasma, decreased excretion, or increased uptake and absorption. It causes neuromuscular depression and cardiac dysrhythmias.
5. *Magnesium.* Essential to electrochemical reactions for normal body functions, magnesium is primarily in intracellular fluid. An imbalance may be accompanied by calcium and/or potassium imbalances.
   a. Hypomagnesemia, a low magnesium level, usually is associated with hypokalemia. This may be the most undiagnosed electrolyte deficiency in geriatric patients or in patients who have illnesses associated with malabsorption in the intestine or kidneys. It may cause cardiac dysrhythmias and nervous system and muscular irritability, and it may exaggerate drug toxicities.
   b. Hypermagnesemia, elevated serum magnesium, can inhibit nerve and muscle responses. It may lead to respiratory depression and cardiac arrest.
6. *Phosphate.* Normally in intracellular fluid, phosphate allows electrochemical reactions for metabolic functions. Phosphate and calcium vary inversely; thus phosphate will buffer acidosis from a rising calcium level.
   a. Hypophosphatemia, a low serum phosphate level, may produce tissue hypoxia.
   b. Hyperphosphatemia, an increase in phosphate, usually occurs in renal failure. It is associated with hypocalcemia.

Disturbances in fluid and electrolyte balance can result from the following:

- *Acid-base imbalances associated with chronic disease or organ dysfunction.* Acidosis increases serum chloride,

TABLE 33-1	Normal Blood Chemistry Laboratory Values

Parameter	Normal Values for Adult
Base excess of blood	0 ± 2 mmol/L
Bicarbonate (HCO_3)	22-26 mEq/L
Bilirubin (total)	0.1-1.0 mg/dl
Blood urea nitrogen (BUN)	5-20 mg/dl
Calcium (Ca)	9.0-10.5 mg/dl
Carbon dioxide (CO_2) in serum	23-30 mEq/L
Chloride (Cl)	90-110 mEq/L
Creatinine	0.7-1.5 mg/dl
Creatine phosphokinase (CPK)	12-80 U/L
Glucose	70-115 mg/dl
Magnesium (Mg)	1.6-3.0 mEq/L
pH of serum	7.35-7.45
Phosphate (P)	2.5-4.5 mg/dl
Potassium (K)	3.5-5.0 mEq/L
Sodium (Na)	136-145 mEq/L
Serum glutamic oxaloacetic transaminase (SGOT)	5-40 IU/L
Serum glutamic pyruvic transaminase (SGPT)	5-35 IU/L

potassium, and calcium; alkalosis decreases chloride, potassium, calcium, and phosphate.

- *Cell destruction leading to hyperkalemia.* Cellular potassium is depleted, with serum potassium increase.
- *Shift of potassium from blood into cells, causing hypokalemia.* This may be caused by the effects of epinephrine, insulin, bicarbonate, hypothermia, or cardiopulmonary bypass.
- *Changes in blood lipids.* Calcium and magnesium are depleted by poor absorption.
- *Fever.* Metabolic rate is increased; water and electrolytes are lost.
- *Stress.* Glucose tolerance is diminished, and blood glucose and serum potassium levels are increased.
- *Gastric drainage.* Sodium and chlorides are lost.
- *Fluid loss from drainage tubes, diaphoresis, vomiting, or diarrhea.* Sodium, chloride, and potassium are lost.
- *Maxillofacial injury.* Oral intake is inhibited.
- *Radiation enteritis.* Magnesium and potassium are diminished.
- *Disease of the bowel, liver, or biliary tract; intestinal tract obstruction; or gastrointestinal fistula.* Calcium and phosphate are poorly absorbed.
- *Loss of muscle mass as a result of preoperative malnutrition.* Nitrogen loss is increased.
- *Drugs.* Metabolic balance can be adversely affected; losses of potassium, magnesium and chloride from diuretics are examples.
- *Inadequate oxygen/carbon dioxide exchange.* Acid-base balance is disrupted.

Hypovolemia

Hypovolemia is a decreased circulating blood volume from loss of blood and plasma or a deficit of extracellular fluid volume commonly referred to as dehydration. When excessive fluid loss is greater than absorption of interstitial fluid into the circulation, the patient may go into hypovolemic shock.

Etiology

Etiologic factors include reduced fluid intake; hemorrhage; plasma loss (e.g., through extensive burns and wound drainage); and dehydration from loss of gastrointestinal fluids (e.g., by vomiting, from diaphoresis due to fever, or from diuresis). Impaired renal function and metabolic acidosis are predisposing factors. Prolonged cardiopulmonary bypass can cause hypovolemic shock.

Symptoms

Symptoms include dry skin and mucous membranes, depressed blood pressure, elevated pulse, oliguria, decreasing CVP and blood volume determinations, and deep, rapid respirations.

Treatment

Hypovolemic shock resulting from hemorrhage or underestimated blood loss is most often seen in the OR. This is usually reversed by prompt restoration of circulating blood volume. The extent of hypovolemia will determine treatment:

1. *Fluid volume replacement.* Whole blood, plasma expander, or infusion of Ringer's lactate or other IV fluid is indicated to increase blood volume. Hypervolemia must be avoided in replacement.
2. *Position.* Elevation of the legs may aid venous return and cardiac output except in severe oligemia (low total blood volume [TBV]).
3. *Temperature.* The patient is kept warm but not overheated. Perspiration increases fluid loss. Shivering can cause hypothermia.
4. *Oxygen.* Oxygen is administered when Po_2 is low because the circulation is not delivering enough oxygen to tissues.
5. *Drugs.* Drugs are administered as needed to maintain blood pressure, correct acidosis, or protect the kidneys from failure.

Prevention

Decreased blood volume, if present preoperatively, increases surgical risk and morbidity. It should be treated, and the electrolyte imbalance should be corrected. Fluids, blood gases, and blood loss must be monitored intraoperatively.

Hypervolemia

Hypervolemia is an excess of extracellular fluid in the blood, commonly referred to as edema. IV infusions given too rapidly or in excessive amounts, especially isotonic saline solution, can cause hypervolemia. Prolonged administration of adrenocorticosteroids is also a predisposing factor. Hypervolemia may progress to pulmonary edema.

Dyspnea, coarse crackles, an elevated pulse and respiratory rate, and diminished urinary output are symptomatic of hypervolemia. Increasing CVP may indicate fluid overload with venous distention. Diuretics and fluid restriction ameliorate hypervolemia and prevent pulmonary edema.

BLOOD VOLUME COMPLICATIONS

Blood Loss Considerations

Some blood loss is inevitable whenever tissues are severed by intent or traumatic injury. Blood loss is computed as a percentage of TBV. TBV averages from 6% to 8% of total body weight. This equals about 75 ml/kg in the average healthy adult man and 60 to 70 ml/kg in the average woman. Calculation of TBV depends on the venous hematocrit value. Normal hematocrit, the volume of red blood cells expressed as a percentage of the volume of whole blood, is 42% to 52% in men and 37% to 47% in women. An infant reaches these blood volume levels at approximately 3 months of age. An increase in hematocrit indicates a decrease in plasma volume, normally by dehydration and loss of sodium. A decrease in hematocrit indicates a decrease in the number of red blood cells, but this does not necessarily reflect blood loss; it may be caused by overhydration. Fluid and electrolyte balance is important for maintenance of blood volume. Inadequate fluid replacement can lead to a decrease in cardiac output and cardiovascular collapse.

A decrease in red blood cells (erythrocytes) and in hemoglobin, the chief oxygen-carrying component of these cells, causes hypoxia if values fall below normal (Table 33-2). Therefore determination of intraoperative blood loss may be critical to physiologic functions. The extent of blood loss will depend on the location and magnitude of the surgical procedure. Blood loss can be categorized as follows:

- *Minor.* Loss of 500 to 700 ml is about 15% of TBV.
- *Moderate.* Loss of 750 to 1500 ml is about 15% to 30% of TBV. A resultant decrease in pulse pressure and slight tachycardia (rapid heart rate) may progress to tachycardia, tachypnea (rapid breathing), and postural hypotension (reduced blood pressure).
- *Major.* Loss of 1500 to 2250 ml is about 30% to 45% of TBV. The blood pressure drops, the skin becomes cold and clammy, and urinary output decreases.
- *Catastrophic.* Loss of over 2250 ml is greater than 45% of TBV. Hypoxia (decrease in oxygen level) develops from loss of hemoglobin (red blood cells). Prolonged hypoxia leads to irreversible heart, brain, liver, and kidney damage.

Hemorrhage

Severe bleeding into or from a wound is a major contributing factor to intraoperative and postoperative morbidity and mortality. If uncontrolled, exsanguination can occur. Massive hemorrhage may cause hypovolemic shock, ventricular fibrillation, or death as a result of marked decrease in cardiac output. Common symptoms are arterial hypotension, pale or cyanotic moist skin, oliguria, bradycardia from hypoxia or tachycardia after moderate to marked blood loss, restlessness, and thirst in the conscious patient.

In the OR, hemorrhage is readily visible. Meticulous hemostasis during every step of the surgical procedure and good nutritional status of the patient preoperatively are cru-

cial to prevention. Preoperative evaluation of the patient's clotting time and history of bleeding (personal and familial), type and crossmatch of blood, and insertion of an IV line before incision are necessary precautions.

In treating hemorrhage the surgeon locates the source of bleeding and applies digital compression to severed or traumatized blood vessels until noncrushing vascular clamps can be placed to occlude the vessel proximally and distally to the site of bleeding. The vessel is then ligated, clipped, electrocoagulated, or sutured. Circulating blood volume must be restored promptly. If allogenous blood is transfused, it must be fresh and warmed to limit electrolytic changes. Sodium bicarbonate may be given IV to reduce acidosis. Multiple IV infusion routes can be used, by cutdown if necessary, to infuse blood under pressure. Ringer's lactate solution or other plasma expanders are used when blood is contraindicated (e.g., for religious reasons). Oxygen is administered to combat hypoxia. Accurate measurement of blood and fluid losses intraoperatively, followed by adequate replacement, will help prevent hypovolemic shock. Autotransfusion may be feasible.

Hemorrhage can be detected postoperatively by observation of blood-soaked dressings. The patient must be checked frequently for both observable and nonobservable symptoms of hemorrhage. Internal bleeding can be caused by slipping or sloughing of a ligature or by the passage of clots from ligated or coagulated vessels.

Estimation of Blood Loss

An accurate determination of TBV involves measuring plasma and red blood cell volumes separately and then adding these values together. This may be done rapidly by an electronic counting device In lieu of this, blood loss is estimated in all surgical procedures in which a major loss is anticipated. This can be done by:

- Visual inspection of blood on drapes and the floor by the anesthesia provider.
- Estimation of blood in the suction container. Allowance must be made for the presence of other body fluids and irrigating solution, if used. The scrub person must estimate the amount of solution suctioned into the container

TABLE 33-2	Normal Values of Blood*		
	Males	**Females**	**Children**
Red blood cells (RBCs)	4.7-6.1 million/mm^3	4.2-5.4 million/mm^3	3.8-5.5 million/mm^3
Hemoglobin (Hgb)	14-18 g/dl	12-16 g/dl	11-16 g/dl
Hematocrit (Hct)	42%-52%	37%-47%	31%-43%
Prothrombin time (PT)	11.0-12.5 seconds	Same	Same
Platelets	150,000-400,000/mm^3	Same	Same after 1 week of age
Partial thromboplastin time (PTT)	30-40 seconds	Same	25-35 seconds

*Values vary depending on calibration of testing equipment in the laboratory that services the health care facility.

through irrigation of the wound and/or tubing. This can be done by knowing the capacity of the irrigation syringe in use and keeping track of the number of times it is used. The circulator subtracts these amounts to estimate the volume of blood in the container.

- Visual inspection of blood in sponges by the anesthesia provider.
- Measurement of blood in sponges by weighing them. Sponges are weighed after use as they are discarded from the surgical field.

Weighing Sponges

Some anesthesia providers and surgeons prefer to have sponges weighed for blood loss rather than visually estimating the loss. A scale calibrated in grams is used. The dry and wet weights of each type of sponge must be known. Wet weight is that of a sponge soaked in normal saline solution and wrung out until almost dry. A chart of these weights should be available; often it is attached to the scale. The number of sponges being weighed is multiplied by the appropriate dry or wet weight. Each type must be weighed separately, with the dry sponges separated from the wet ones. To allow for (i.e., by subtracting) dry or wet weights and the weight of a moisture-proof cover on the scale platform or a container, the scale is adjusted to register at zero. When blood-soaked sponges are weighed, the reading on the scale equals the blood loss; 1 g equals 1 ml. The scale is checked at each use for readjustment to zero. Some scales are controlled by a microprocessor that automatically makes calculations.

The circulator must weigh sponges before they dry out. Blood loss is recorded each time sponges are weighed, adding new weight to previous ones to keep a current total. A tally board for this purpose may be mounted on the wall where the anesthesia provider and surgeon can read it. The estimated blood in the suction container can be recorded here also. Irrigation solutions used for moistening sponges should be carefully measured and documented.

Reduction of Blood Loss

When significant bleeding can be anticipated, several techniques are used to reduce red blood cell loss during the surgical procedure or to eliminate blood transfusion requirements.

Hemodilution

Acute normovolemic or isovolemic hemodilution reduces red blood cells but maintains normal or equal blood volume. After induction of anesthesia, a physician, usually the anesthesia provider, withdraws blood through an arterial or venous catheter. The blood is drawn into bags containing anticoagulant, usually citrate. Citrate metabolizes rapidly, thus minimizing the risk of systemic anticoagulation when blood is reinfused. The amount withdrawn depends on the anticipated blood loss and the patient's estimated TBV and hematocrit. A plasma volume expander is given by IV infusion while blood is removed to restore blood volume. This hemodilution technique reduces red blood cell loss during the surgical proce-

dure because the hematocrit has been lowered. The surgical procedure begins when the hematocrit is between 27% and 30%. Adequate intravascular volume and oxygenation are maintained. Urinary output must be measured.

Each bag of blood must be labeled with the patient's name and identifying number and the time of withdrawal. Blood may be stored at room temperature for 6 hours or in a refrigerator for 24 hours. At the conclusion of the surgical procedure, or sooner if indicated, the blood is reinfused IV to raise the hematocrit back to the preoperative level. Units are reinfused in reverse order of withdrawal (i.e., last one first) so that the unit with the highest concentration of red blood cells and coagulation factors is infused last. More information is available at the Web site of the American Association of Blood Banks (**www.aabb.org**).

Blood Volume Expanders

Crystalloid or colloid solutions are administered IV for fluid replacement and plasma volume expansion. They are not sole replacements for blood loss. They must be used with caution. The following are the most commonly used plasma volume expanders:

- *Dextran.* This crystalloid polymer of glucose acts by drawing fluid from tissues to decrease blood viscosity. It remains in circulation for several hours. It interferes with the crossmatching of blood; thus a blood sample for this purpose must be drawn before dextran is infused. It may be used until blood or blood products are available or for hemodilution. As a 6% or 10% solution, it may be mixed in water with glucose or sodium chloride.
- *Ringer's lactate solution.* This crystalloid physiologic salt solution is infused for the improvement of circulation and stimulation of renal activity and in patients in whom the body's supply of sodium, calcium, and potassium has been depleted.
- *Hetastarch (Hespan).* This colloid polymer expands plasma volume slightly in excess of the volume infused. It approximates the action of serum albumin. Large volumes may alter coagulation factors. It can be used for hemodilution.

Pharmacologic Agents

The action of specific pharmacologic agents either stimulates or retards the coagulation mechanism. This action may reduce blood loss and help to provide hemostasis in patients with hematologic disorders. Some of these disorders are associated with cardiovascular disease or end-stage renal disease. Others are congenital or acquired coagulopathies. Three types of agents affect bleeding.

Desmopressin Acetate   Desmopressin promotes hemostasis in patients with von Willebrand's disease and shortens the bleeding time in patients with uremia. When given prophylactically, this synthetic vasopressin analogue can decrease surgical blood loss in patients undergoing spinal surgery and reduce blood loss after cardiac surgery.

Vasodilators Vasodilators lower systemic blood pressure, thus decreasing bleeding. Sodium nitroprusside, nitroglycerin, and trimethaphan camsylate are the most commonly used.

Anticoagulants Anticoagulants minimize the tendency of blood to clot yet do not lead to excessive bleeding during or following the surgical procedure. These agents provide adequate anticoagulation with a minimum of hemorrhagic complications. They help prevent venous stasis to reduce the incidence of DVT and pulmonary embolus. They may be given orally, subcutaneously (SQ), or IV, beginning preoperatively, especially in patients who have a history of thromboembolic disease. The action of each anticoagulant is different and is described as follows:

1. Heparin acts to inhibit conversion of prothrombin to thrombin. This prolongs clotting time. It may be administered SQ to keep activated partial thromboplastin time in the high normal range between 30 and 40 seconds. Given IV, heparin is effective immediately. It may be used as a flush to keep IV lines open or to flush the lumen of a blood vessel (1 ml of heparin in 100 ml of normal saline solution). Heparin does not dissolve a thrombus, but it will prevent a clot from becoming larger.
2. Coumarin derivatives depress blood prothrombin and decrease the tendency of blood platelets to cling together, thus decreasing the normal tendency of blood to clot. They also interfere with action of vitamin K to prevent the synthesis of prothrombin and fibrinogen. Warfarin sodium is the most commonly used coumarin derivative.
3. Low-molecular-weight dextran reduces platelet adhesiveness and aggregation to prevent sludge from forming in the bloodstream. It coats blood platelets to keep them from massing together.
4. Aspirin diminishes clumping of platelets by inhibiting the release reaction of platelet factors and action of vitamin K.

Vitamin K enables the liver to produce clotting factors in blood, including prothrombin. To reduce the possibility of intraoperative hemorrhage, patients who have been receiving anticoagulant therapy and those who have faulty metabolism or absorption of vitamin K are given it preoperatively. It also is given to geriatric or debilitated patients before intraocular surgery, to newborns preoperatively, and to mothers just before delivery. The latter helps prevent postdelivery hemorrhage and ensures that the baby has an adequate prothrombin level until a sufficient amount is produced by the liver.

Hypotensive Anesthesia

In selected situations when excessive blood loss is anticipated or encountered, arterial blood pressure may be deliberately lowered to produce an essentially bloodless field. When induced, hypotension is carefully controlled by the anesthesia provider.

Hematologic Disorders

Some hemolytic and hemorrhagic disorders require special consideration during perioperative care to minimize risks of surgical intervention. Concern is for the maintenance of adequate tissue perfusion and oxygenation and for hemostasis and coagulation in patients at risk. Patients at risk for intraoperative bleeding or who have a known hematologic disorder should have a complete blood count, SMA-18 (sequential multichannel autoanalyzer) test, and urinalysis done preoperatively. Hemoglobin, hematocrit, and red blood cell counts are critical determinants for blood replacement requirements preoperatively and intraoperatively. Precautions can be taken to minimize the risks of surgical intervention with adequate blood replacement.

Anemia

Anemia is a symptom of a deficiency in either the quantity or quality of red blood cells (erythrocytes). Hemoglobin, the chief component of these cells, delivers oxygen to tissues. Normal hemoglobin values are 14 to 18 g/dl of blood in males, 12 to 16 g/dl in females, and 11 to 16 g/dl in children. These values are lower in anemic patients. Thus anemia may result in tissue hypoxia. The various types of this disorder may be caused by the following:

- Blood loss from massive bleeding (e.g., from a traumatic injury) or chronic blood loss (e.g., from a gastric or intestinal ulcer). This blood loss can be replaced by transfusion of blood products.
- Dietary deficiency of sufficient iron, protein, vitamins, and minerals to form red blood cells or produce hemoglobin. Dietary supplements are given to correct the deficiency.
- Diseases or drugs that inhibit the bone marrow from producing blood cells, such as tumors or chronic renal disease. The cause must be diagnosed and treated.
- Destruction of red blood cells by an overactive reticuloendothelial system in the spleen or liver. A splenectomy may be indicated for hypersplenism or hereditary spherocytosis, for example.
- Destruction of red blood cells by foreign substances entering the circulatory system (e.g., through an incompatible blood transfusion). Neonatal anemia may necessitate an exchange transfusion.
- Abnormal blood cells produced by the bone marrow, usually by genetic or hereditary factors.

The average normal life span of red blood cells is 120 days. In patients with any one of the many forms of hemolytic anemia, red blood cells have a shortened life span. Hemolytic anemias may be acquired or inherited. All must be adequately assessed preoperatively.

Sickle Cell Hemoglobinopathies A severe chronic inherited hemolytic disorder, sickle cell anemia is most prevalent among blacks of African descent. It may be found in other ethnic groups, particularly people of Mediterranean descent. Pairing of identical abnormal recessive genes causes substitution of a single amino acid for glutamic acid in the polypeptide chain, which alters the hemoglobin. These abnormal cells, known as hemoglobin S, become distorted in shape when exposed to low oxygen tension in the venous circulation. Dehydration, cold, infection, and physical or emotional stress may precipitate crisis periods that vary in duration and intensity when sickling occurs. A crisis may also occur spontaneously without apparent cause. The resultant sickle-shaped red blood cells occlude the microcirculation through the capillaries, arterioles, and venules. Occlusion results in blood stasis, hypoxia, vasospasm, ischemia, and necrosis, which causes pain and ultimately permanent damage to tissues and organs. Stasis ulcers and biliary tract disease are common complications that may require surgical intervention. Elective surgical procedures are performed when the patient is not in crisis, but these patients are always at risk of crisis.

Sickle cell trait is present when one abnormal gene is inherited. The red blood cells have both hemoglobin A (normal) and hemoglobin S (sickle cell). Persons with this trait usually are asymptomatic and tolerate routine anesthesia and surgical intervention well. However, when they are stressed by hypothermia, acidosis, or hypoxemia, local or regional sickling can occur during the surgical procedure.

Sickle cells have a life span of 15 to 30 days. The severity of the hemolytic process is proportional to the amount of hemoglobin S in the blood. Hemoglobin in patients with sickle cell anemia usually ranges from 6 to 9 g, with a hematocrit of 25% to 30%. Patients of African descent and other susceptible persons should be tested preoperatively. Electrophoresis is the standard laboratory test for hemoglobin S. Consideration must then be given to the following in the perioperative management of patients with sickle cell anemia or sickle cell trait:

1. Transfusion of whole blood, packed cells, or low-molecular-weight dextran may be administered preoperatively, especially if the patient's hemoglobin is 5 g or less.
2. Urea may be given orally or IV prophylactically to prevent a sickle cell crisis. It may also be used to reverse a crisis.
3. Systemic antibiotics are initiated preoperatively because these patients are susceptible to postoperative infection.
4. Normal body temperature must be maintained. Any lowering increases the requirement for oxygen. The patient must be kept warm to avoid hypothermia.
   a. Add extra blankets during transport to the OR suite.
   b. Avoid drafts from the air-conditioning system in the holding area, OR, and PACU.
   c. Cover the patient's head for warmth.
   d. Raise the temperature in the OR to 80° to 85° F (27° to 29° C).
   e. Place the patient on a hyperthermia blanket on the operating bed.
   f. Monitor the patient's temperature intraoperatively with an electronic probe.
   g. Place warm blankets over the patient before transfer to the PACU.
5. Oxygen is administered during induction of anesthesia, intraoperatively, and following extubation to prevent deoxygenation of the sickle cells and subsequent ischemic infarction in tissues.
6. Blood gases are monitored to avoid hypoxia, acidosis, hypotension, and hypovolemia. Fluid and blood replacement intraoperatively reduces the risk of crisis from dehydration.
7. Scheduling an elective surgical procedure early in the morning minimizes dehydration following a period of nothing by mouth (NPO).

Hemorrhagic Disorders

Patients with a disorder in the mechanism of blood coagulation have abnormal bleeding tendencies. These may be related to the following:

- Hemorrhagic diseases, such as a type of purpura in which spontaneous bleeding occurs under the skin, through mucous membranes, or in the gastrointestinal tract, that is idiopathic (cause unknown) or secondary to a systemic or an infectious disease or to exposure to chemical agents
- Platelet deficiency in the blood, such as thrombocytopenia as a result of decreased production of platelets by bone marrow or excessive destruction of platelets in the peripheral circulation
- Abnormal clotting factors, such as in hemophilia and von Willebrand's disease, which are inherited genetic disorders

A baseline of blood values should be established preoperatively. The baseline consists of a complete blood count, including platelets, plasma clotting time, bleeding time, prothrombin time, and partial thromboplastin time. Adequate blood replacement of the deficient factors must be available during the surgical procedure and postoperatively.

Hemophilia   The term *hemophilia* refers to a group of genetic bleeding disorders characterized by abnormal clotting factors.

Hemophilia A, the classic disorder, is caused by a deficiency of functional factor VIII, the antihemophilic globulin in plasma. Hemophilia B, also known as Christmas disease, is caused by a lack of functional factor IX, the plasma thromboplastic cofactor. A carrier mother transmits to her son this sex-linked recessive trait of the specific clotting factor. Hemophilia occurs most commonly in males of Russian-Jewish descent.

The severity of the disorder depends on the percentage of functional vs. nonfunctional factor in the blood. Partial thromboplastin times or thromboplastin generation times are the standard tests for this determination. These patients have normal vasculature and platelets (150,000 to 400,000/mm^3

of blood); thus bleeding time (1 to 3 minutes by the Duke method) and prothrombin time (11 to 12.5 seconds) test results are normal.

Severely affected hemophiliacs have spontaneous bleeding episodes into the skin, muscles, and joints, most commonly the ankles, knees, wrists, and elbows. If untreated, joint deformities can result. Bleeding will be excessive from even a minor wound such as a bruise or cut.

For hemostasis during a severe bleeding episode, replacement therapy must be initiated to raise the clotting factor to between 60% and 100% (normal individuals have clotting factor levels of 60% to 120%). In hemophiliacs fibrin clots do not form and bleeding continues. The missing clotting factor must be raised temporarily to control hemorrhage. This is started preoperatively for elective surgery. Concentrates available for replacement therapy include the following:

1. Factor VIII for hemophilia A
   a. Lyophilized concentrate products, such as Hemofil CT and Koate HT or HS reconstituted with diluent provided by the manufacturer
   b. Cryoprecipitate
   c. Fresh frozen plasma or concentrate
2. Factor IX for hemophilia B
   a. Lyophilized concentrate products, such as Konyne and Profilnine reconstituted with diluent provided by the manufacturer
   b. Fresh frozen plasma
3. Lyophilized concentrate with inhibitors to neutralize the antibody that prevents clotting

Lyophilized concentrates are made from pooled normal human plasma obtained by plasmapheresis, a process of separating red blood cells by centrifugation. The circulator should obtain factor concentrate from the blood bank and must be familiar with how to prepare it. The dosage for factor deficiency is calculated on the basis of the plasma volume, half-life of the factor, and percentage of the deficit. It is given by IV infusion intraoperatively and postoperatively.

Blood Loss Replacement

Despite meticulous hemostasis and methods to reduce blood loss, blood replacement is necessary during many extensive surgical procedures, particularly cardiovascular, orthopaedic, organ transplantation, and trauma surgery. Surgeons limit the use of transfused blood whenever possible. However, to compensate for blood loss of more than 1200 ml or a hematocrit value below 30% and to prevent shock, transfusions of whole blood, fresh frozen plasma, packed red blood cells, platelets, serum albumin, or blood substitutes must be carried out according to policy. Transfusions may be allogenous, autologous, or a blood substitute.

Allogenous Blood

Allogenous blood is that drawn from one individual for transfusion into another. It must be compatible (i.e., not cause a reaction). Therefore blood typing and crossmatching are es-

sential to determine compatibility between donor and recipient. The four main blood types are A, B, O, and AB. In addition, many subgroups of antigens exist in red blood cells. Also, agglutinogens, known as Rh factor positive, may be present. If these are not present in red blood cells, the blood is Rh negative. A recipient must receive donor blood of the same type and Rh factor. In extreme emergency situations, O-negative blood, referred to as universal donor blood, may be given until the patient's blood can be typed and crossmatched or until compatible blood can be obtained. Conversely, type AB is considered to be the universal recipient, being compatible with A, B, O, and AB.

A transfusion of the wrong blood type can be fatal. Transmission of hepatitis B or C, human immunodeficiency virus (HIV), and other viruses and infections is a potential danger, even with current testing of all donor blood. According to the American Association of Blood Banks, in 1998 the Transmissible Spongiform Encephalopathy Advisory Committee of the Food and Drug Administration (FDA) recommended deferral of potential donors who have traveled to or resided in the United Kingdom. This exclusion is intended to prevent the risk of new-variant Creutzfeldt-Jacob disease (nvCJD) transmission. Other diseases that require deferral of blood donation include the following:

- Syphilis
- Hepatitis B, C
- HIV
- HTLV I and II
- Cytomegalovirus (CMV)
- Malaria
- Babesiosis
- Toxoplasmosis
- Chagas disease
- Lyme disease
- Creutzfeldt-Jakob disease (and patients who have had injections of human pituitary hormone)

Consequently, because of many transmissible disease issues, many patients prefer "directed donors." When blood replacement is anticipated before a surgical procedure, a family member or friend with a compatible blood type can be asked to donate blood to be held in the blood bank for the patient. Directed donations are not necessarily safer than nondirected voluntary donations supplied from the blood bank, however. When multiple units of blood must be transfused, packed cells, fresh frozen plasma, and platelets usually are given to supplement units of whole blood. These components are not part of whole blood replacement.

All established measures must be strictly observed for the patient's safety. The following basic rules apply to the transfusion of all allogenous blood products:

1. Blood products are obtained from the blood bank by a person responsible for signing them out to a specific patient.
2. To have blood nearby, a refrigerator with controlled temperature may be installed in the OR suite. Blood

products for transfusion are kept at a constant temperature between 34° and 43° F (1° and 6° C), verified by a recording thermometer on the outside and a standard one inside. Both audible and visible alarms are activated if a dangerous temperature is reached. Fluctuations in temperature cause red blood cells to deteriorate. Microorganisms can multiply in unrefrigerated blood. If blood is brought into the OR and not needed, it should be returned to the refrigerator in the suite or blood bank immediately. Do not allow whole blood or its derivatives to stand unrefrigerated in the OR. Before use, each blood product should be checked for the expiration date. Each product has a specific shelf life (Table 33-3).

3. Blood products are administered by a physician or nurse after a careful comparison of the label on the bag with the identity of the patient. A second professional person confirms the data. The label stays on the container while the blood product is being transfused.

4. Cold, refrigerated blood may induce hypothermia. Blood should be warmed as it is transfused by immersion of administration tubing in a controlled water bath or through coils in a temperature-modifying device. The temperature must be maintained between 89° and 105° F (32° and 41° C). Hemolysis may occur if the temperature exceeds 110° F (43° C).

5. Another solution may be infused immediately before a blood product is administered. In changing to the blood product, avoid the possibility of air entering tubing. A blood filter must be used for transfusion. The filter should be changed after the second or third unit of whole blood because the filter can become clogged with microaggregates.

6. The anesthesia provider records on the anesthesia record the following information for each unit transfused:
   a. The name of the person who started the transfusion.
   b. The type and amount of product transfused (i.e., whole blood, plasma, packed cells, platelets, or albumin).
   c. The time started and drops per minute.
   d. Information on the label, including the blood group, Rh factor, and number.

7. The patient is observed closely for any type of reaction. This probability increases in direct proportion to the number of units transfused. The most common type of reaction is allergic; febrile is almost as common, and hemolytic reactions are possible. Transfusion reactions with the patient under anesthesia may be accompanied by profound hypotension, temperature change, blood in urine, and/or skin rash. The common physical reactions and chills are not seen in an anesthetized patient. If any suspicious reactions occur:
   a. Stop the transfusion. Keep the IV line patent with IV solution as directed by the physician.
   b. Return unused blood to the blood bank along with a sample of the patient's blood.
   c. Send a urine sample to the laboratory as soon as possible.
   d. Take vital signs (temperature, pulse, respirations, blood pressure) every 5 to 10 minutes until the patient is stable.
   e. Have emergency medications and resuscitation equipment available.
   f. Document on the patient's chart the type of reaction, action taken, patient's response, and other documentation as required by the institution.

Autologous Blood

Autologous blood is blood recovered from the patient and reinfused. Referred to as autotransfusion, this process is the preferred method of replacement for either elective or emergency procedures. The patient's own blood is the safest form of transfusion; it eliminates concerns about compatibility/reactions and transmission of exogenous organisms. Autologous blood is equal or superior in quality to allogenous blood. It may be obtained preoperatively from patients and returned to them intraoperatively or postoperatively as needed.

Some patients who, because of religious beliefs, will not accept allogenous blood may accept autotransfusion. Jehovah's Witnesses, for example, believe that receiving blood or blood products violates a biblical prohibition against consumption of blood. They have the right to refuse transfusion. Written informed consent should be obtained from all patients for whom autotransfusion is contemplated.

Preoperative Blood Donation One or more units of whole blood or blood components can be obtained by phlebotomy from the patient preoperatively and stored in the blood bank. Blood may be donated as often as every seventh day for a period of 6 weeks if the hemoglobin remains at least 11 g/dl or the hematocrit is 33%, with the final unit donated no less than 72 hours before the scheduled surgical procedure. If two or more units are donated, an oral or intramuscular iron supplement may be prescribed because as much as 10% of iron stores are lost with each donation. Epoetin alfa, a glycoprotein, can be administered SQ or IV for up to 6 weeks preoperatively to stimulate red blood cell pro-

TABLE 33-3	Shelf Life of Blood Products According to the American Association of Blood Banks
Blood Products	**Shelf Life**
Red blood cells	42 days refrigerated
Frozen red blood cells	10 years
Platelets	5 days at room temperature
Fresh frozen plasma	1 year
Cryoprecipitated antihemophiliac factor	Frozen 1 year
Granulocytes	Transfuse within 24 hours of collection

duction. Red blood cell stimulation can be continued post-operatively and is effective if iron stores are adequate. The patient's body replenishes the fluid lost in donation within 24 hours.

Autologous blood is usually stored in a liquid state as whole blood or packed red blood cells. Whole blood, with anticoagulant, can be stored for 35 days and red blood cells, with preservative, for 42 days. Red blood cells and plasma can be frozen for prolonged storage. The same protocol is used in the OR for reinfusing autologous blood as described for allogenous transfusions. If the patient does not need reinfusion, the blood is discarded. It is not given to another patient.

Intraoperative Autotransfusion Recovery of blood as it is lost requires sterile equipment that suctions blood from the surgical site, filters and anticoagulates it, and contains it for IV reinfusion to the patient with minimal damage to cells. Intraoperative blood salvage is widely used when potential blood loss may exceed 20% of the patient's blood volume. Blood can be suctioned directly from a body cavity or the wound. Any plastic devices, including suction tubing and pouches, used for blood recovery must be approved by the FDA.

Blood is not salvaged if microfibrillar collagen (Avitene) has been used for hemostasis. This may not wash out when red blood cells are processed and can predispose the patient to DIC or ARDS. Also, blood contaminated with enteric organisms or amniotic fluid is not salvaged. If a malignant tumor can be resected intact, autotransfusion may benefit the patient with cancer. Most cancer cells will filter out of processed blood. Autologous blood is not collected from patients with known systemic infections or from open traumatic wounds. Other patients, of all ages, are candidates for autotransfusion.

The autotransfusion unit must be easily and quickly assembled, since it may be lifesaving for a trauma patient in an emergency situation. All fluid paths should be disposable and must be sterile. Three basic systems are used for intraoperative autotransfusion:

1. *Automated cell salvage processor.* Blood is suctioned through double-lumen tubing. An anticoagulant solution of heparinized saline or citrated dextrose mixes with blood at the tip end of the tubing. The aspirate passes through a 140-μm filter before entering the collection reservoir. This filter removes fat and debris. When a sufficient quantity to be processed has accumulated, the blood is pumped into a centrifuge bowl. The centrifugal force separates red blood cells from plasma, platelets, white blood cells, and other debris, including anticoagulant. These red blood cells are washed with normal saline solution. A suspension of red blood cells in saline solution is pumped into a reinfusion bag. Each bag contains about 250 ml of washed packed red blood cells with a hematocrit of 50% to 55%, ready for IV reinfusion. The entire cy-

cle takes 3 to 7 minutes. Some autotransfusion units have automatic, programmed cycles, including process air and foam detectors; others operate manually. Platelet-rich plasma suitable for autotransfusion can be sequestered from some units.

2. *Canister collection method.* Blood is suctioned and anticoagulated as described for the cell processor. From the tubing, the blood collects in a reservoir with a disposable liner. When the reservoir becomes full, or at the end of the surgical procedure, the liner is removed. The contents are washed in a standard red blood cell washer before being reinfused. This equipment may be located in the blood bank. The liner must be labeled with the patient's name and identifying number if it leaves the OR for washing. Autologous blood obtained using this technique has a high hematocrit level and is almost free of protein, anticoagulant, and debris.

3. *Salvage collection bag.* An anticoagulant, usually citrate, is added to blood collected directly into a single-use, self-contained transfusion bag. The blood is not washed. It is reinfused through a blood filter. This simple method is most appropriate when profuse bleeding occurs in areas that form pools that can be easily suctioned, such as the abdominal or chest cavities.

All three methods are safe when used according to the manufacturer's instructions. The automated cell salvage devices are the most sophisticated and complex. Only properly trained personnel should operate them. OR personnel may be trained to set up the sterile suction and containers.

Postoperative Autotransfusion Autologous blood may be collected, processed, and bagged during a surgical procedure for reinfusion postoperatively. Bags must be labeled with the name and identifying number of the patient and the time of processing. Autologous blood can also be salvaged postoperatively from a drainage tube placed into the surgical wound, most commonly a chest tube. The tube may be connected to a cell washer in a portable unit that attaches to wall suction in the PACU or ICU. Another method collects wound drainage by suctioning it directly into a filtered collection bag. With both of these methods blood is anticoagulated. It may be collected for a maximum of 6 hours. The concentrated red blood cells, either washed or unwashed, are reinfused IV. Whether obtained intraoperatively or postoperatively, unwashed blood can be kept at room temperature for 4 hours, and washed blood can be kept for 6 hours at room temperature or refrigerated for 24 hours at 39.2° F (4° C).

Blood Substitutes

Oxygen-carrying blood substitutes offer another alternative for transporting oxygen. Oxygenation of body tissues is a serious issue when the patient's blood volume or hemoglobin level is decreased because of blood loss. These substitutes may be used in anemic patients, in persons who refuse blood or blood products for religious reasons, or when compatible allogenous blood is not available. Examples of blood substitutes under investigation include the following:

- *Fluorovent.* Oxygen-carrying perfluorocarbon (PFC) can be used for preterm infants with underdeveloped lungs and in both adults and children with ARDS. It is a liquid instilled directly into the lungs to act as a surfactant. It encourages the exchange of oxygen and carbon dioxide. Patients with COPD may benefit from its use as well.
- *Oxycyte.* This IV form of PFC carries five times the amount of oxygen carried in hemoglobin. The oxygen-hemoglobin exchange ratio is extremely efficient because the molecules are one seventieth the size of a red blood cell and can reach tiny capillary surfaces. It can be stored at room temperature and requires no crossmatching.
- *Hemopure.* This bovine hemoglobin–based polymer solution has been used in clinical trials in the United States and Europe. It is stable for 2 years at room temperature and requires no crossmatching. It is given by IV infusion and is compatible with all blood types.
- *PolyHeme.* Human polymerized hemoglobin is processed from outdated human red blood cells. The product is screened for infectious disease, pasteurized, and polymerized. It is safe for use with any blood type. The shelf life is 12 months.
- *Oxyglobin.* This red blood cell alternative for veterinary services is compatible with all blood types.

Complications of Blood Loss or Replacement

The patient is constantly monitored to detect any complications that might be developing as a result of blood loss or replacement or as a compromise of the cardiovascular system. Hemorrhage can cause shock and DIC.

Earlier PFC emulsions caused pulmonary complications, such as hyperinflated, noncollapsible lungs. Traces of older PFC emulsions can persist systemically and cause the threat of accumulation in fatty tissue. Accumulation could compromise developing neonatal nervous tissue, which has a high fatty content. Newer PFCs have been refined to have a shorter persistence period.

Early blood substitute products have been associated with gastrointestinal problems, coagulopathies, kidney and liver dysfunction, fever, and vasoconstriction. More information is available at **www.biopure.com or at www.sybd.com.**

SHOCK

Shock is a state of inadequate blood perfusion to parts of the body. If untreated, it will become irreversible and result in death. All forms of shock carry high mortality.

Hemorrhagic shock results from a decrease in circulating blood volume caused by loss of blood, plasma, or extracellular fluid. Fluid loss is excessive when it is greater than compensatory absorption of interstitial fluid into the circulation. Shock resulting from hemorrhage or inadequate blood volume replacement, as seen in the OR and PACU, usually is reversed by prompt restoration of circulating blood volume.

Shock is a complex phenomenon, a life-threatening condition in which circulation fails for one or several reasons. Loss of circulating blood volume, loss of the pumping power of the heart, or loss of peripheral resistance can result in insufficient flow of blood for adequate tissue perfusion or oxygenation. If it is prolonged, inadequate organ blood flow with deficient microcirculation profoundly depresses vital processes. Because the objective of circulation is achieved in the capillaries, defective cellular metabolism derived from shock interferes further with the body's inherent defenses and metabolic acidosis occurs. Normal defense mechanisms are reflex vasoconstriction and increased pulse rate, which tend to redistribute the flow of blood to the heart and brain at the expense of the other vital organs. If shock is promptly recognized, treated, and reversed, permanent damage is avoided. If it progresses to irreversibility, death ensues from cellular dysfunction and organ hypoperfusion.

Multiple types and causes of shock present problems in relationships among the heart, circulatory system, and blood volume. Circulatory inadequacy may originate from a marked decrease in cardiac output, venous return to the heart, or peripheral vascular resistance. All forms of shock carry high mortality rates. The best treatment is prevention. Shock is classified according to the cause of inadequate tissue perfusion.

Hypovolemic Shock

Fluid loss is greater than compensatory absorption of interstitial fluid into the circulation.

Hemorrhagic Shock

Shock results from hemorrhage or inadequate blood volume replacement.

Cardiogenic Shock

The pumping action of the left ventricle is insufficient to pump enough blood to vital organs. Cardiogenic shock may be precipitated by congestive heart failure, myocardial contusion or infarction, coronary air embolism, mechanical venous obstruction, or hypothermia. In addition to drugs, various mechanical devices may be used, such as an auxiliary ventricle or counterpulsation with an intraaortic balloon pump (IABP) to temporarily increase left ventricular function.

Neurogenic Shock

Loss of vasomotor tone in peripheral blood vessels leads to sudden vasodilation and pooling of blood. Vasodilation produces hypotension. Peripheral resistance is too great for compensation by increased cardiac output, increasing the risk for congestive heart failure and pulmonary edema. Causes may be brain damage, deep anesthesia, emotional trauma, vagal reflex from pain or surgical manipulation, or spinal cord injury.

Traumatic Shock

Damage to the capillaries caused by soft tissue trauma increases capillary permeability, with loss of blood volume into the tissues. This state is aggravated by pain, which inhibits the vasomotor center, leading to vasodilation and hypovolemia. Toxic factors associated with intravascular coagulation lead to pulmonary, renal, and/or multiple organ failure.

Vasogenic Shock

Anaphylaxis and septic shock are the most common types of vasogenic shock.

METABOLIC CRISES

Convulsions

Convulsions occur most often in patients with a hyperactive metabolic rate, especially in dehydrated or febrile children. Anoxia and death can occur.

Etiology

Etiologic factors include severe hypoxia and carbon dioxide retention, hypernatremia, hyperthermia, overdose of regional anesthetic drugs, air embolism, and epilepsy.

Symptoms

Symptoms include muscular twitching, dilated pupils, rapid snorting respirations, rapid pulse, grimacing, and cyanosis.

Treatment

Oxygen is administered to maintain respiration, and diazepam, a rapid-acting barbiturate, or a neuromuscular blocker is given to stop muscular activity. Mechanical ventilation may be needed for apnea or to support circulation.

Prevention

Metabolic crises are prevented by maintaining normal body temperature and fluid and electrolyte balance.

Inadvertent Hypothermia

A decrease in the patient's core body temperature to below 96° F (35° C) can affect vasoconstriction and vasodilation, cardiac output, and renal function. Depending on the degree of body heat loss, hypothermia is categorized as follows:

- Mild (down to 90° F [32° C])
- Moderate (down to 85° F [30° C])
- Deep (down to 80° F [27° C])

If core temperature falls below 68° F (20° C), brain activity ceases. Patients can emerge from anesthesia with a body temperature below normal. Inadvertent hypothermia occurs spontaneously intraoperatively; it not to be confused with induced hypothermia. Age-extreme, thin, and debilitated patients are most susceptible, as are patients undergoing neurosurgical, cardiovascular, thoracic, and abdominal procedures.

Etiology

Anesthesia inhibits the protective reflexes that generate body heat (i.e., shivering). It also depresses the thermoregulating center in the hypothalamus, decreases the basal metabolic rate, and increases vasodilation for heat loss by radiation and conduction. Core body heat is lost by exposure to a cool external environment (e.g., during skin preparation) and through the surgical incision. Other factors include preoperative sedation, use of general vs. regional anesthesia, adjunctive drugs, the length of the surgical procedure, blood and fluid loss and replacement, the room temperature, and evaporative loss through the respiratory tract. General anesthesia commonly causes a 1° to 1.5° F decrease in core temperature during the first hour, extending the action of propofol by 30%. The greatest risk for hypothermia is in the patient who has had combined general and epidural anesthesia. Protective central inhibition of the thermoregulatory center and peripheral nervous system is delayed.

Symptoms

Hypothermia can cause adverse cardiovascular, hematologic, immunologic, metabolic, and neurologic effects. Cardiac dysrhythmias, hypoxia, metabolic acidosis, hyperglycemia, and dilated pupils may be a result. A depressed central nervous system, which can lead to coma, may not be evident until the postoperative period. Shivering, impaired speech, muscle rigidity, peripheral or central cyanosis, a weak pulse, falling blood pressure, and dysrhythmias seen in the PACU may be symptoms of hypothermia. The incidence of ventricular tachycardia is doubled, causing an increased incidence of postoperative myocardial infarction.

Treatment

The hypothermic patient must be rewarmed as soon as possible. However, postanesthesia shivering during the rewarming process can be hazardous. Shivering is an involuntary rhythmic contraction of muscle groups with irregular and intermittent relaxation. This physiologic response to cold is activated when the hypothalamus senses that the core temperature has dropped. Some postanesthesia shivering is caused by anesthetic agents. Untreated shivering leads to increased oxygen consumption as a result of muscular activity and to increased cardiac stress as a result of hypoxia. In the PACU a forced-air skin surface warmer (Bair Hugger) or an ultraviolet or infrared heat lamp directed at the lightly covered patient are effective means for raising the body temperature. A temperature-regulating hypothermia/hyperthermia machine, set at 104° to 107° F (40° to 42° C), may be used with a heated blanket beneath the patient. If warmers are not available, warm blankets placed over and underneath the patient should be changed at 15-minute intervals. Blankets can be heated to 105° F (40.5° C) for an adult or 100° F (38° C) for a small child or infant. The patient should wear a cap. Warmed humidified oxygen and IV fluid should be administered. Clonidine (an alpha$_2$-adrenergic agonist) or analgesics such as meperidine or morphine derivative may suppress shivering.

Prevention

Prevention of hypothermia is the best treatment. Prevention begins before the patient arrives in the OR and continues during the procedure:

1. Place a hypothermia/hyperthermia mattress or reflective blanket on the operating bed. A radiant heat source can be placed over an infant.
2. Check the room temperature and humidity.
3. Apply warmed blankets as soon as the patient arrives in the OR and immediately after drapes are removed. A warm blanket can be put on the stretcher under the patient.
4. Limit skin exposure during positioning and skin preparation (i.e., keep the patient covered as much as possible).
5. Minimize the time of exposure between skin antisepsis and draping.
6. Keep the sheet under and the drapes over the patient and around the surgical site dry to provide insulation, prevent heat loss, and maintain asepsis. Dry the area following skin preparation.
7. Warm antiseptic, irrigating, and IV solutions, including blood, before administration. Anesthetic gases, including oxygen, can be warmed also.
8. Monitor body temperature.
9. Leave a cap on the patient; a plastic head covering retains more heat than other materials.

Malignant Hyperthermia

Malignant hyperthermia (MH) is a fulminant hypermetabolic crisis in susceptible persons. It is triggered by potent halogenated anesthetic agents and depolarizing skeletal muscle relaxants. MH, a potentially fatal complication of anesthesia, is characterized by uncontrolled acceleration of muscle metabolism accompanied by tremendous oxygen consumption and production of heat and carbon dioxide. The body temperature can rapidly rise at a rate of 1.8° F (1° C) every 5 minutes if MH is untreated. A temperature as high as 117° F (47° C) has been recorded, but 111.2° F (44° C) is probably highest with survival. The survival rate with appropriate treatment is between 80% and 90%. The mortality rate without appropriate treatment is around 10%; thus MH is of significant concern.

Etiology

The exact cause of MH is unknown. It is understood that certain patients are susceptible, and some anesthetic agents may trigger this crisis.

Susceptible Patients   A familial genetic transmission exists as an autosomal dominant trait with variable multifactorial inheritance patterns. The genetic defect manifests by increasing calcium levels in skeletal muscles. The crisis results from a hereditary inability of the sarcoplasmic reticulum, a skeletal muscle cell membrane, to control intramyoplasmic levels of calcium. Skeletal muscle undergoes contraction as a result of release of calcium ions in response to drugs or stress. A rapid increase of calcium in muscle fiber leads to generalized catabolism. As biochemical reactions occur, the body produces heat and carbon dioxide.

Susceptible patients also include those with any type of myopathy or acquired muscle disease, such as ptosis, strabismus, hernia, muscle weakness or hypertrophy, or muscular dystrophy. The incidence of MH is higher in children than in adults. Patients, especially children, with rheumatoid arthritis are particularly susceptible to MH. MH may occur in a patient's first exposure to anesthesia or in a later one; one third of reported cases of MH have occurred in a second or subsequent anesthesia.

Triggers   Several agents may trigger this abnormal hypermetabolic response in susceptible individuals. Succinylcholine, halothane, enflurane, desflurane, and isoflurane are the main triggers of MH.

Symptoms

Clinical signs and symptoms occur according to the swiftness of onset. The onset may be rapid, occurring immediately after induction, or occur after several hours of general anesthesia or even in the postoperative recovery period.

Spasm of the jaw muscles with rigidity of the masseter muscles (trismus) or severe fasciculation following succinylcholine administration may suggest MH development to the anesthesia provider, although this activity is not uncommon in pediatric patients.

The most common presenting sign of MH is unexplained ventricular dysrhythmia, primarily tachycardia or PVCs. This is associated with an unexplained increase in end-tidal carbon dioxide, tachypnea, cyanosis, skin mottling, and unstable blood pressure. Blood in the surgical field may appear dark as a result of central venous desaturation.

When a sudden, generalized hypermetabolic state is produced, the temperature rises rapidly as more heat is produced than the body can eliminate. Elevated temperature may be a late sign or may be absent in MH syndrome. Fever, hot skin or tissues, and diaphoresis are symptoms of heat buildup. A favorable prognosis decreases when excessive heat in the tissues is noted through the surgeon's gloves or when the anesthesia provider senses heat in the reservoir bag or soda lime canister on the anesthesia machine. The body tries to adjust by vasodilation and increased cardiac output. If rapidly increasing tissue demands are not met, hypoxia, central venous hypercapnia, and severe respiratory and metabolic acidosis occur, progressing to cardiovascular collapse. Blood tests will reveal increased serum levels of potassium, magnesium, creatine phosphokinase (CPK), and myoglobin. Excessive myoglobin release caused by rapid muscle destruction (rhabdomyolysis) can cause renal failure and lead to anuria.

Late clinical findings include hyperkalemia; acute renal failure; left-sided heart failure; disseminated intravascular coagulopathy; skeletal muscle swelling or necrosis from hypoxia and acidosis; pulmonary edema; neurologic sequelae, including paraplegia and decerebration; and coma from ischemia secondary to hypoxia. Recurrence of MH crisis can occur 24 to 72 hours postoperatively.

Monitoring   Parameters and studies to be monitored routinely in patients at risk for MH who undergo general anesthesia are heart rate and rhythm, blood pressure, core temperature by esophageal probe, pulse oximetry, capnometry, nerve stimulation to measure the level of muscle relaxation, and precordial stethoscopy. A rise in temperature greater than ½° F/hr should raise suspicion of MH.

Treatment

Success is contingent on complete preparedness (preplanned action, written protocol, immediate equipment supply), early diagnosis, and vigorous therapy. The following treatment outline is the suggested protocol established by the Malignant Hyperthermia Association of the United States (MHAUS). The 1999 wall chart describing accepted protocol is shown in Figure 33-8. The emergency therapy wall chart can be ordered from the organization by calling the nonemergency telephone number (800) 986-4287 or on-line at **www.mhaus. org.** Institutional policies and procedures should be in place as follows to guide the perioperative team in caring for a patient in MH crisis:

1. Discontinue anesthesia and stop the surgical procedure immediately. The anesthesia provider immediately institutes hyperventilation with 100% oxygen at a high flow rate of at least 10 L/min. Research has shown that the breathing circuit and anesthesia delivery machine need not be changed because the high concentration of oxygen delivery clears the machine of anesthetic gases very rapidly. If the surgical procedure cannot be interrupted, safe agents may be employed to maintain anesthesia during the stabilization period.
2. Immediately start drug therapy. Administer:
   a. Dantrolene sodium (Dantrium IV), 2 to 3 mg/kg in an initial IV bolus and repeat every 5 to 10 minutes until the maximum dose of 10 mg/kg is given or the MH episode is controlled. Patients generally respond to the drug quickly. The onset of action is usually 2 to 3 minutes. Occasionally doses higher than 10 to 20 mg/kg are needed.

Dantrolene is a specific drug for treatment of MH. It directly blocks accumulation of calcium within the muscles by preventing its release from the sarcoplasmic reticulum and by uncoupling excitation-contraction, thus relaxing skeletal muscle. It has no effect on cardiovascular or respiratory functions. Calcium channel blockers may not be given with dantrolene because they may cause hyperkalemia, myocardial depression, and cardiovascular collapse.

Given IV, dantrolene is supplied in 70-ml vials as a sterile, lyophilized powder that contains 20 mg of dantrolene and 3 g of mannitol. Each vial must be reconstituted before use with 60 ml of sterile water for injection without a preservative agent. The large quantities of sterile water that are needed would contain the preservative agent in toxic amounts. A semiautomatic fluid-dispensing syringe expedites mixing. If this is not available, additional personnel should help with the reconstitution process because large quantities of the diluted drug will be needed and each vial will require vigorous shaking to mix. The solution will be yellow-orange when mixed. In extreme circumstances the drug may be given through a filter to remove particulates from the solution. Once reconstituted, dantrolene must be used within 6 hours and must be protected from exposure to light.

If other IV solutions have been running, the line should be flushed with sterile water before dantrolene is injected; this will prevent precipitation. Do not use Ringer's lactate solution because it will increase the level of acidosis. An additional IV site should be established to infuse iced normal saline solution at the rate of 15 ml/kg every 15 minutes for at least 45 minutes.

Dantrolene is continued postoperatively at a minimum of 1 mg/kg every 6 hours for 24 to 72 hours postepisode. After the initial 48 hours, 1 mg/kg every 6 hours may be given orally for 24 hours. No serious side effects have been reported with short-term use, but muscle weakness may be evident for 24 to 48 hours after administration. A few isolated reports of nausea, vomiting, and fatigue have been documented. Prolonged administration may lead to hepatotoxicity.

   b. Procainamide (Pronestyl), 15 mg/kg diluted in 500 ml physiologic saline solution IV over 60 minutes. Procainamide treats cardiac dysrhythmia if required.
   c. Sodium bicarbonate, 1 to 2 mEq/kg IV stat and repeat as guided by blood gas analysis. An alkali, sodium bicarbonate raises pH temporarily. It combats acidosis and antagonizes hyperkalemia by lowering the plasma potassium level. It can cause rebound acidosis. Monitoring of arterial pH and P_{CO_2} is necessary to determine subsequent doses.

LOOK FOR • elevated end-tidal CO_2 • rigidity • tachycardia • hypercarbia • tachypnea • cardiac dysrhythmia • respiratory and/or metabolic acidosis • fever • unstable/rising blood pressure • cyanosis/mottling • myoglobinuria

Emergency Therapy for
Malignant Hyperthermia
❖ Revised 1999 ❖

ACUTE PHASE TREATMENT

1. **GET HELP. GET DANTROLENE.** Immediately discontinue all volatile inhalation anesthetics and succinylcholine. Hyperventilate with 100% oxygen at high gas flows; at least 10 L/min. The circle system and CO_2 absorbent need not be changed.
2. Administer dantrolene sodium 2.5 mg/kg bolus rapidly. Continue bolus administration as needed until signs of MH (e.g., tachycardia, rigidity, increased end-tidal CO_2, and temperature elevation) are controlled. Occasionally, a total dose greater than 10 mg/kg may be needed. Each vial of dantrolene contains 20 mg of dantrolene and 3 grams mannitol. Each vial should be mixed with 60 ml of sterile water for injection USP without a bacteriostatic agent.
3. Administer bicarbonate to correct metabolic acidosis as guided by blood gas analysis. In the absence of blood gas analysis, 1-2 mEq/kg should be administered.
4. Simultaneous with the above, actively cool the hyperthermic patient. Use IV cold saline (not Ringer's lactate) 15 ml/kg q 15 min × 3.
   a. Lavage stomach, bladder, rectum, and open cavities with cold saline as appropriate.
   b. Surface cool with ice and hypothermia blanket.
   c. Monitor closely since overvigorous treatment may lead to hypothermia.
5. Dysrhythmias will usually respond to treatment of acidosis and hyperkalemia. If they persist or are life threatening, standard anti-arrhythmic agents may be used, with the exception of calcium channel blockers (may cause hyperkalemia and CV collapse).
6. Determine and monitor end-tidal CO_2, arterial, central, or femoral venous blood gases, serum potassium and other electrolytes, urine output, PT/PTT, and calcium for baseline values. Repeat as clinically indicated.
7. Hyperkalemia is common and should be treated with hyperventilation, bicarbonate, intravenous glucose, and insulin (10 units regular insulin in 50 ml 50% glucose titrated to potassium level or 0.15 U/kg regular insulin in 1 cc/kg 50% glucose). Life-threatening hyperkalemia may also be treated with calcium administration (e.g., 2-5 mg/kg of $CaCl_2$). Check blood glucose every two hours if insulin has been given.
8. Ensure urine output of greater than 2 ml/kg/hr by hydration and/or administration of mannitol or furosemide. Consider central venous or PA monitoring because of fluid shifts and hemodynamic instability that may occur.
9. **Sudden Unexpected Cardiac Arrest in Children:** Children less than about 10 years of age who experience sudden cardiac arrest after succinylcholine in the absence of hypoxemia and anesthetic overdose should be treated for acute hyperkalemia first. In this situation calcium chloride should be administered along with other means to reduce serum potassium. They should be presumed to have subclinical muscular dystrophy and a neurologist should be consulted.

POST ACUTE PHASE

A. Observe the patient in an ICU setting for at least 24 hours since recrudescence of MH may occur.
B. Administer dantrolene 1 mg/kg or more q 4-6 hours for 24-48 hours post episode.
C. Follow ABG, CK, potassium, urine and serum myoglobin, clotting studies, and core body temperature until such time as they return to normal values (e.g., q 6 hours). Central temperature (e.g., rectal, esophageal) should be continuously monitored until stable.
D. Counsel the patient and family regarding MH and further precautions. Refer the patient to MHAUS. Fill out an Adverse Metabolic Reaction to Anesthesia (AMRA) report available through MHAUS. A letter to the patient's primary care doctor is advised.

CAUTION: This protocol may not apply to every patient and may require alteration according to specific patient needs.

Names of on-call physicians available to consult in MH emergencies may be obtained 24 hours a day through the

MH Emergency HOTLINE
1 800 MH HYPER
(1 800 644-9737)

For Non-Emergency or Patient Referral Calls:
MHAUS
(800) 986-4287
PO Box 1069
Sherburne NY 13460-1069
E-mail: mhaus@norwich.net
Web site: www.mhaus.org
MH INFO-BY-FAX:
1 800 440-9990

Publication of this poster has been made possible by an educational grant from Augustine Medical, Inc.

(ORPO-3) 7/98/15K

Figure 33-8   1999 wall chart distributed by the Malignant Hyperthermia Association of the United States (MHAUS), which describes the protocol for managing a malignant hyperthermia crisis. (Reprinted with permission of the Malignant Hyperthermia Association of the United States, Sherburne, NY.)

d. Regular insulin, 10 U in 50 ml of 50% dextrose in water IV. Insulin offsets the high glucose metabolic demands and improves glucose uptake. It shifts potassium back into the cells to help treat hyperkalemia. Blood glucose and potassium levels must be monitored.

e. Calcium chloride, 2.5 mg/kg, to treat severe cardiac toxicity caused by hyperkalemia.

f. Mannitol, 0.25 g/kg IV, and furosemide (Lasix), 1 mg/kg IV, up to four doses each. These drugs dislodge myoglobin from the renal tubules and sustain urinary flow. Urinary output greater than 2 ml/kg/hr must be maintained to prevent renal failure. The dose is calculated in consideration of the mannitol contained in the dantrolene solution.

3. Begin active cooling. Administer refrigerated or iced normal saline IV. Lavage the stomach and rectum. Avoid irrigating the bladder, because accurate measurement of urinary output is important. If the peritoneal or thoracic cavity is open, cool sterile saline may be poured into the opening. Cool the body surface by placing the patient on a plastic sheet and applying ice bags and ice water, or use a hypothermia blanket. If readily available, use extracorporeal perfusion apparatus for partial (femoral-to-femoral) cardiopulmonary bypass to cool the viscera. Body temperature must be carefully monitored to avoid accidental cooling to dysrhythmic levels. Medication may be given to limit shivering, normally a heat-retaining mechanism that also increases oxygen consumption. Surface cooling is considered more effective in children because of their high ratio of surface area to body volume. Too vigorous cooling can result in inadvertent hypothermia and cardiac arrest. To avoid hypothermia, cooling should be discontinued when the core temperature reaches 100° F (38° C).

4. Correct the electrolyte imbalance on the basis of blood sampling of electrolytes, pH, and blood gases. After the presumed onset of MH, an arterial line must be established if one is not already in place. Blood samples are taken at 10-minute intervals for pH, Pco_2, Po_2, sodium, potassium, chlorides, calcium, magnesium, and phosphate. Hypocalcemia and hyperkalemia followed by hypokalemia may be expected.

   Also measured are CPK, serum glutamic oxaloacetic transaminase, alkaline phosphatase, and lactate dehydrogenase for indication of muscle destruction. Blood urea nitrogen for kidney function, bilirubin for liver function, coagulation studies, blood lactate and pyruvate, and serum thyroxine levels may be ordered.

5. CVP should be monitored. A CVP line may need to be inserted if one is not already in place.

6. Urinary output is monitored via an indwelling Foley catheter. In addition to the measurement of volume, urine is sampled for hemoglobin and myoglobin. The urine may be brown as the amount of hemoglobin and myoglobin increases.

Supplies for Malignant Hyperthermia Supplies should be kept in a specific location and must be immediately available for both adult and pediatric patients. A cart marked for use in MH is convenient. Supplies that may be needed include the following:

1. Monitors: ECG, electronic temperature probes, and recorder
2. IV equipment: blood administration sets and pumps; CVP line setup; IV solutions—12 bags, 1000 ml each, of physiologic saline kept in a refrigerator
3. Arterial line setup
4. Intubation equipment
5. Ice chips and plastic bags; hypothermia blankets
6. Gastric lavage set; three-way indwelling catheter for insertion into the rectum; 50-ml syringes
7. Blood sampling and arterial blood gas equipment
8. Indwelling Foley catheter and urometer bag
9. Drugs:
   a. Thirty-six 20-mg vials of dantrolene sodium (the quantity needed to treat and stabilize a 70-kg adult)
   b. Thirty-six 60-ml vials of sterile water without a preservative agent to reconstitute dantrolene (the quantity needed for a 70-kg adult is 2100 ml)
   c. Five 100-ml prefilled syringes of sodium bicarbonate 5%
   d. Six 1-g ampules of procainamide
   e. Ten 50-ml vials of 20% mannitol
   f. Four 2-ml (20-mg) prefilled syringes of furosemide
   g. One 100-U vial of regular insulin
   h. Two 50-ml vials of 50% dextrose in water
   i. Three 1000-U vials of heparin
   j. Ten 250-mg vials of hydrocortisone sodium succinate (Solu-Cortef)
10. Associated needles and syringes
11. Extracorporeal perfusion apparatus, if available
12. Defibrillator machine and electrodes

Prevention

Identification of susceptible patients is the best prevention. The preoperative history should routinely include questions about the patient's previous anesthesia experiences, unexplained incidents or death of family members who underwent anesthesia, and known muscular abnormalities or episodes of heat stroke in the patient or relatives. Hereditary predisposition has been detected in three generations; however, the patient's family history frequently is not known. The most prominent clue to identification of a patient susceptible to MH is a family history of unexplained death while under general anesthesia. Genetic counseling of the patient and family is advised. Although the crisis usually occurs when the patient is under general anesthesia, it can occur during periods of emotional or physical stress. Susceptible persons should wear a medical-alert bracelet or tag.

Diagnosis of susceptibility to MH can be accomplished by preoperative muscle biopsy. A 1-g specimen of skeletal muscle is excised from the thigh with the patient under local anesthesia. The specimen is removed from the muscle as a strip and outstretched between the prongs of a double-tipped clamp. Evaluation of the muscle response to caffeine-induced contracture during exposure to halothane reveals sensitivity. Although a local anesthetic is used to obtain the muscle biopsy, dantrolene should be readily available in the unlikely event of an episode of MH.

The blood CPK level may be elevated in susceptible patients, but it can also be influenced by alcohol consumption or strenuous exercise. A normal CPK level does not ensure absence of the MH trait. Nuclear magnetic resonance imaging using phosphorus also may detect susceptibility, but it is not always a reliable indicator.

Prophylaxis   Dantrolene may be given preoperatively to susceptible patients. The suggested dose is 1 mg/kg increments every 4 to 6 hours orally up to a total dose of 4 mg/kg, followed by 2.5 mg/kg IV 30 minutes before induction of general anesthesia. Intraoperative monitoring is mandatory. When nontriggering anesthetic agents are used, prophylactic dantrolene therapy may be unnecessary. Each patient should be evaluated individually. Some indications for dantrolene prophylaxis may include the following:

- Previous history of suspected MH episode
- Family history of MH (actual or suspected)
- Known MH susceptibility
- Prolonged procedure anticipated in an MH-susceptible patient
- Underlying disease or physiology causing suspicion of MH susceptibility

Nontriggering anesthetic agents should be administered to MH-susceptible individuals. Barbiturates, benzodiazepines, and narcotics are considered safe. Nitrous oxide by inhalation or IV propofol or ketamine hydrochloride can be administered for general anesthesia. Most of the synthetic nondepolarizing neuromuscular blockers are safe muscle relaxants. Amino amide and ester agents can be used safely for local anesthesia.

Postoperatively the patient should be continuously monitored in the ICU for 24 to 48 hours. If the vital signs remain stable during this time, the patient may be discharged. More information is available from MHAUS at **www.mhaus.org.**

PHYSIOLOGIC INJURY

Physiologic injuries are many and varied. The anesthesia provider may inadvertently loosen teeth or damage dental work during endotracheal intubation. Nerves can be injured from faulty positioning, such as hyperabduction or extension of the arm. Pressure sores may develop on poorly padded areas. Fingers and body parts can be pinched in table flexures. Careless handling of an anesthetized patient can result in paralysis, fractures, or postoperative pain.

Eyes can be injured from irritating anesthetics or face masks, or from drying or scratching of the cornea if the eyelids are not closed. Patients with protruding eyes, faces cov-

ered by drapes, or those in prone positions are at high risk for eye injury. Use of an ocular lubricant protects the cornea from drying, and taped eyelids prevent corneal abrasions.

Extravasation, thrombophlebitis, and air emboli are associated with IV infusions. IV cannulas should be visible and not entirely hidden beneath drapes; infusions should be checked frequently. Precaution is the best prevention of injuries.

Bibliography

Beck CF: Malignant hyperthermia: are you prepared? *AORN J* 59(2):367-390, 1994.

Bright LD, Georgi S: How to protect your patient from DVT, *Am J Nurs* 94(12):28-32, 1994.

Craig V, Bower JO: Blood administration in perioperative settings, *AORN J* 66(1):133-136, 138, 140-142, 1997.

Donnelly AJ: Malignant hyperthermia: epidemiology, pathophysiology, treatment, *AORN J* 59(2):393-405, 1994.

Dreger V, Tremback T: Blood and blood product use in perioperative patient care, *AORN J* 67(1):154, 156, 158, 160, 162-164, 166, 169, 171-174, 176, 178, 181-184, 187-188, 1998.

Ferguson KJ et al: Physician recommendation as the key factor in patients' decisions to participate in preoperative autologous blood donation programs, *Am J Surg* 168(1):2-5, 1994.

Figueredo E, Canosa L: Can hypothermia be evidenced during laparoscopic cholecystectomy? *Surg Laparosc Endosc* 7(5):378-383, 1997.

Gould SA et al: The first randomized trial of human polymerized hemoglobin as a blood substitute in acute trauma and emergent surgery, *J Am Coll Surg* 187(4):113-120, 1998.

Gruen GS et al: The acute management of hemodynamically unstable multiple trauma patients with pelvic ring fractures, *J Trauma* 36(5):706-711, 1994.

Haskell RM, et al: Hypothermia, *AACN Clin Issues* 8(3):368-382, 1997.

Huntington TR, LeMaster CB: Laparoscopic hypothermia: heat loss from insufflation gas flow, *Surg Laparosc Endosc* 7(2):153-155, 1997.

Huston CJ: Disseminated intravascular coagulation, *Am J Nurs* 94(8):51, 1994.

Lenhardt R et al: Mild intraoperative hypothermia prolongs postanesthetic recovery, *Anesthesiology* 87(6):1318-1323, 1997.

Leslie K et al: Mild hypothermia alters propofol pharmacokinetics and increases the action of atracurium, *Anesth Analg* 80(5):1007-1014, 1995.

Malignant Hyperthermia Association of the United States: *Managing malignant hyperthermia: drugs and equipment,* Westport, Conn, 1998, The Association.

Maness CP et al: Bloodless medicine and surgery, *AORN J* 67(1):144-148, 150-152, 1998.

Mathias JM: No heat surgical device uses ultrasonic motion for cutting, *OR Manager* 10(2):16-17, 1994.

Moss R: Inadvertent perioperative hypothermia, *AORN J* 67(2):460, 462-463, 1998.

Nash CA, Jensen PL: When your surgical patient has hypertension, *Am J Nurs* 94(12):38-44, 1994.

O'Neal PV: How to spot early signs of cardiogenic shock, *Am J Nurs* 94(5):36-40, 1994.

Pasero C, McCaffery M: Avoiding opioid-induced respiratory depression, *Am J Nurs* 94(4):24-30, 1994.

Phillips GR et al: Massive blood loss in trauma patients: the benefits and dangers of transfusion therapy, *Postgrad Med* 95(4):61-72, 1994.

Saver CL: Decoding the ACLS algorithms, *Am J Nurs* 94(1):27-35, 1994.

Saver CL: Your guide to first- and second-line code drugs, *Am J Nurs* 94(2):15, 1994.

Smith EA, Kilpatrick ES: Intraoperative glucose measurements: the effect of hematocrit on glucose monitoring strips, *Anaesthesia* 49(2):129-132, 1994.

Tappen RM, Andre SP: Inadvertent hypothermia in elderly surgical patients, *AORN J* 63(3), 1996.

Trovarelli T et al: Transfusion-free surgery is a treatment plan for all patients, *AORN J* 68(5):773-776, 778, 780-784, 1998.

Wilson BA et al: *Nurse's drug guide,* Norwalk, Conn, 1994, Appleton & Lange.

Section XII

Surgical Specialties

Chapter 34

General Surgery

Chapter Objectives

After studying this chapter, the learner will be able to:

• Identify the pertinent anatomy of the abdominal organs within the peritoneal cavity.
• List six common surgical incisions used in general surgery.
• Describe the method of preparing a patient for an abdominal procedure.
• Describe patient care during laparoscopy.

The discipline of general surgery provides the fundamentals for surgical practice, education, and research. The definition of general surgery agreed on by the American Board of Surgery and the Residency Review Committee for Surgery serves as the basis of graduate education and certification as a specialist in surgery. The following principles are inherent in general surgery:

1. A central core of knowledge and skills common to all surgical specialties (e.g., anatomy, physiology, metabolism, pathology, immunology, wound healing, shock and resuscitation, neoplasia, and nutrition)
2. The diagnosis and preoperative, intraoperative, and postoperative care of patients with diseases of the alimentary tract; the abdomen and its contents; breast; head and neck; endocrine system; and vascular system (excluding intracranial vessels, the heart, and vessels intrinsic and immediately adjacent thereto)
3. Responsibility for the comprehensive management of trauma and critically ill patients with underlying surgical conditions

In a rural community hospital, the practice of general surgery usually encompasses many aspects of surgical care. In larger facilities, general surgery services are commonly specialized (e.g., breast, biliary tract, gastrointestinal, or colon and rectal surgery). The introduction of surgical specialties was the outgrowth of increased knowledge of the etiology of disease and specialized treatment of all parts of the body. General surgery, the basis for all specialties, has decreased in breadth as specialization has increased. The anatomic parts not specifically delegated to specialists have remained in the realm of the general surgeon. Other surgical disciplines depend on general surgeons for clinical collaboration in reconstruction involving the gastrointestinal and vascular systems. The scope of this chapter focuses on procedures commonly categorized as general surgery.

HISTORICAL BACKGROUND

The earliest time in which surgical procedures were performed is not exactly known. Artifacts documenting brain and bone surgery have been found in archaeologic excavations of ancient civilizations. The Egyptians had extensive knowledge of surgical anatomy, which they acquired through the art of embalming and preserving abdominal organs. This practice allowed them to observe the position and natural appearance of the internal organs. The cases of earliest human dissection were performed by Egyptian priests, who later translated these acts into surgical procedures on the living. Organ structures became part of the written hieroglyphic language.

Documented historical surgical procedures include those performed in the sixteenth century by Ambroise Paré (1510-1590), a French barber turned military surgeon. The seventeenth century saw the publication of *A Discourse in the Whole Art of Chirgurie* by Peter Lowe (1550-1613)—the first surgical textbook written in English. (In this era, all books for physicians were written in Latin.) Strides in the eighteenth century included the addition of pathologic study associated with the art of surgery. Scottish anatomist John Hunter (1728-1793) was considered the father of experimental surgery because he emphasized that surgical wounds would not heal without the inflammatory process. Records indicate the removal of an ovarian tumor by Ephraim McDowell in 1809. Crowds gathered outside the patient's home in Kentucky where the surgical procedure was taking place, and they threatened to hang the physician if he failed in his task. Fortunately, the patient survived.

The first recorded successful appendectomy was performed in 1885 by William West Grant, an American surgeon. He was the first to open the abdomen, isolate the cecum, and amputate the appendix. The patient, a 22-year-old female from Iowa, survived the procedure without any serious complications. Most surgeons of this time considered the abdomen an area not to be opened unless by accident.

The nineteenth century did not see an increase in the number of surgical procedures until developments in anesthesia permitted surgeons to operate with greater precision on anesthetized patients. Although complex surgical procedures were becoming increasingly common, fewer procedures were performed in one year than are currently performed in one day at any given facility.

SPECIAL CONSIDERATIONS FOR GENERAL SURGERY

Technologic advances characterize many aspects of surgical practice. The general surgery team of today should be familiar with endoscopic techniques for diagnosis and treatment. Electrosurgery, lasers, and surgical staplers are part of the setup for standard general surgery. Patients are best cared for when the entire perioperative team understands the principles of available technologies and has clinical experience in the safe use of these technologies. The following are examples of technologic applications and the associated aspects of patient care:

1. Malignant lesions, especially those of the breast, thyroid, and gastrointestinal tract, account for a large percentage of surgical interventions. The extent of the surgical excision of a lesion may be determined only after thorough exploration during a surgical procedure, sometimes scheduled as a diagnostic laparoscopy or as a biopsy and frozen section.

a. Although the patient has been informed preoperatively of an anticipated procedure, the unknown factor is cause for apprehension. The circulator should provide comfort while the patient is awake. A biopsy or endoscopic procedure may be performed with the patient under local anesthesia and with or without intravenous conscious sedation (IVCS).

b. A definitive open or laparoscopic surgical procedure may be performed on the basis of results of the biopsy and frozen section or endoscopic examination while the patient is under anesthesia. The scrub person should be prepared with two draping and instrument setups, depending on the diagnosis established and the surgeon's plan for the surgical procedure. Anticipated equipment and supplies should be available without delay.

2. The types of anesthesia administered are as varied as the types of surgical procedures. Blood pressure, pulse, respiration, electrocardiogram (ECG), and pulse oximetry should be monitored for all patients regardless of the anesthetic used. Personnel responsible for monitoring patients should be qualified to interpret data, assess the patient, and effect corrective action in the event of an untoward reaction.

3. Patients are placed in the supine position for many general surgical procedures. Extra padding and accessory positioning aids should be available for other positions.

4. Draping for abdominal incisions is usually standardized. Modifications are necessary for other sites, such as the breast or neck.

5. Instrumentation is quite varied and suited to function in a specific anatomic area. For example, gastrointestinal procedures require crushing clamps (e.g., Péan clamps to occlude the intestinal lumen before resection) and atraumatic clamps (e.g., Bainbridge clamps to protect delicate tissues). Included in all procedures are instruments for exposing, dissecting, grasping, holding, clamping, occluding, and suturing. For atraumatic retraction, various lengths of umbilical tape, hernia tape, or vessel loops may be placed around vessels or other structures to retract them. These materials should be included in the count.

6. Some procedures require minimal access and are adaptable to ambulatory surgery; others are extremely extensive. More complex procedures, such as colectomy and cholecystectomy, are often performed endoscopically and require less in-house hospitalization.

7. The electrosurgical unit (ESU), argon beam coagulator, laser, endoscope, laparoscope, and/or ultrasound transducer may be used during the procedure.

8. In complex open and laparoscopic abdominal and pelvic procedures, the following should be noted:
a. Indwelling Foley or ureteral catheters may be inserted preoperatively.
b. Nasogastric tubes may be passed before or during the surgical procedure.

---

c. After the abdominal cavity is entered, single, free 4 × 4 sponges should be removed from the field. They are used only while folded and secured on a sponge stick. Wet or dry tapes (laparotomy packs) are used in the abdominal cavity. A small dissector (peanut or Kitner) is always clamped in a forceps before being handed to the surgeon.

d. Before the peritoneum is incised, suction should be available and ready for immediate use, especially in biliary or intestinal procedures or when fluid or blood may be anticipated in the peritoneal cavity.

e. Drains may be exteriorized through a stab wound in the adjacent abdominal wall before closure.

f. Contaminated items, such as those used to anastomose intestinal segments, are isolated in a basin on the back table.

g. Before closure, the wound is irrigated with warm, sterile, normal saline solution to remove blood and debris.

h. Retention sutures may be used to give additional strength to wound closure.

9. Assorted sizes of drains, tubes, drainage bags, and wound suction systems should be available.

10. Irrigating solutions should be at body temperature when they are used. All radiopaque dyes, anticoagulants, and solutions on the instrument table are clearly labeled to avoid any error in administration.

11. Blood loss and urinary output are recorded on the perioperative record.

BREAST PROCEDURES

The mammary glands are bilateral organs lying in the superficial fascia of the pectoral area (Figure 34-1). They are attached to the underlying muscles by loose areolar tissue. The breasts extend from the border of the sternum to the anterior axillary line (tail of Spence) and from approximately the first to the seventh rib. The breasts are highly vascular. The blood supply is derived laterally from the thoracic branches of the axillary, intercostal, and internal mammary arteries. Venous drainage forms an anastomotic circle around the base of the nipple, with branches draining the circumference of the gland into the axillary and internal mammary veins. Lymphatic drainage follows the same path as the venous system and empties into the thoracoabdominal and lateral thoracic vessels. Innervation arises from the anterior and lateral cutaneous nerves of the thorax.

General surgery on the breast includes diagnostic procedures and those performed for known pathologic disease, such as cancer. Diagnostic techniques include mammography, xeroradiography, ultrasonography, and thermography, as well as the traditional tissue biopsy.

The desired surgical procedure should be determined on an individual basis after careful diagnostic studies and histologic diagnosis. Size, location, and type of diseased tissue or stage of malignancy are important considerations. No single surgical procedure is suitable for all patients.

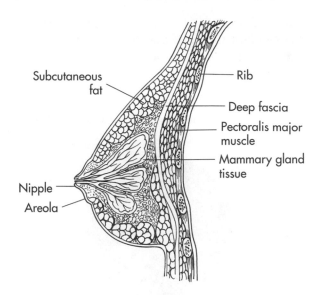

Figure 34-1 Sagittal section of normal breast in relation to chest wall and rib cage.

Incision and Drainage

Surgical opening of an inflamed and suppurative area is most often carried out because of infections in the lactating breast. The cavity is usually irrigated, and the wound is packed and allowed to heal by granulation. The causative organism is often staphylococcus.

Breast Biopsy

Figure 34-2 illustrates the average size of lumps found by women practicing breast self examination. All breast masses are considered malignant until proved benign. To determine the exact nature of a mass in the breast, tissue is removed for pathologic examination. The size and location of the lesion influence the type of biopsy:

- *Fine-needle aspiration (FNA).* A 22- or 25-gauge needle attached to a syringe is inserted into the tumor mass. A few cells are aspirated and sent to the pathology laboratory for cytologic studies. This may be performed in conjunction with a mammogram (mammographic breast biopsy) or as an office procedure. FNA also may be used to evacuate fluid from benign cysts.

- *Core biopsy.* For this type of incisional biopsy, a large-bore trocar needle, such as a Tru-cut or Vim-Silverman biopsy needle, is inserted into the mass for this type of incisional biopsy. A core of suspected tissue is withdrawn for histologic examination. Any retrieved fluid is also sent to the pathology laboratory.

- *Stereotactic breast biopsy.* The patient is placed prone on a special radiographic table, and her breast is placed in an opening in the table. A computer guided system is used to digitally locate and pinpoint nonpalpable breast lesions. The biopsy is obtained with a mammotome while the patient is under local anesthesia.

- *Incisional biopsy.* The mass is incised and a portion is removed for histologic examination.
- *Excisional biopsy.* The entire mass is removed for pathologic study.

Preoperatively, the surgeon discusses with the patient possible findings and treatment options. The patient may agree to

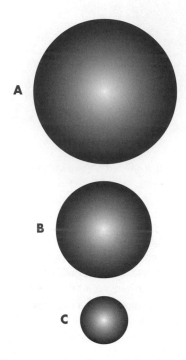

Figure 34-2 Average size of breast lumps found by women practicing breast self-examination. **A,** Woman not practicing BSE. **B,** Woman practicing occasional BSE. **C,** Woman practicing monthly BSE. (From Fortunato NM, McCullough SM: *Plastic and reconstructive surgery,* St Louis, 1998, Mosby.)

an immediate definitive surgical procedure if warranted by the biopsy and frozen section results. Two separate prepping, draping, and instruments sets are necessary.

To minimize disfigurement, many women with early operable breast cancer (a mass less than 5 cm) opt for limited resection followed by radiation and chemotherapy. The difference between tumor and deep tumor-free resection margin remains an important consideration in determining the most appropriate type of mastectomy (Table 34-1).

Lumpectomy

Lumpectomy, a partial mastectomy, consists of removal of the entire tumor mass along with at least 1 to 2 cm of surrounding nondiseased tissue. This procedure is recommended for peripherally located tumors that measure less than 5 cm. Lumpectomy is contraindicated if breast size precludes postoperative radiation or if negative margins around the tumor cannot be obtained.

Breast conservation, the surgical treatment of choice for many women with breast cancer, includes a lumpectomy to excise a primary tumor and axillary node dissection followed by radiation therapy. This approach maintains the appearance and function of the breast. The surgeon may prefer to perform the lumpectomy first, followed by the axillary dissection. The patient should be reprepped and redraped between procedures. A separate set of instruments is used for each procedure to avoid possible tumor cell implantation in the axilla. A transverse incision for axillary dissection, approximately 1 cm below the axillary hairline, extends from the pectoralis major muscle anteriorly to the latissimus dorsi muscle posteriorly. Lymphoareolar tissue between these muscles is removed—usually at least 10 lymph nodes.

TABLE 34-1	**Stages of Breast Cancer**		
Stage I	**Stage II**	**Stage III**	**Stage IV**
Size			
≤1-2 cm	2-5 cm	≥5 cm	Large and fully integrated with surrounding tissue
Location			
Confined to breast	Breast mass with or without suspicious axillary lymph nodes	Breast mass with palpable, fixed axillary and/or subclavicular lymph nodes	Distant metastasis; extension to skin
	May or may not extend to pectoral fascia or muscle	Mass may be adherent to surrounding tissue	Lymphedema above or below the clavicle
	No distant metastasis	No distant metastasis	
Surgical Options			
Segmental mastectomy	Total mastectomy	Modified or radical mastectomy	Radical or extended radical mastectomy
Breast conservation surgery for stages I and II Lumpectomy with axillary node dissection and radiation therapy			

Segmental Mastectomy

In a segmental mastectomy, a wedge or quadrant (quadrantectomy) of breast tissue is removed; this wedge includes the tumor mass and the lobe in which it is growing. Some surgeons explore the axilla and take a few lymph nodes for histologic studies.

Simple Mastectomy (Total Mastectomy)

In a simple mastectomy, the entire breast is removed without lymph node dissection. A simple mastectomy may be performed for a malignancy that is confined to breast tissue with negative nodes, as a palliative measure for an advanced ulcerated malignant tumor, or for the removal of extensive benign disease. Skin grafting may be necessary if the primary closure of skin flaps would create unacceptable tension. Skin flaps are then loosely approximated, and grafts taken from the thigh are applied to the remaining defect. A latissimus dorsi or rectus abdominis myocutaneous flap may be preferred for reconstruction.

A subcutaneous mastectomy may be performed for patients with chronic cystic mastitis who have had multiple previous biopsies, for patients with multiple fibroadenomas or hyperplastic duct changes, and for patients with central tumors that are noninvasive in origin. All breast tissue is removed, but the overlying skin and nipple remain intact. A prosthesis may be inserted at the time of the surgical procedure, depending on the surgeon's decision and the patient's wishes.

Modified Radical Mastectomy

A modified radical mastectomy is usually performed for infiltrating ductal and localized small malignant lesions. The term *modified* encompasses various techniques, but all include removal of the entire breast (total mastectomy). In addition, all axillary lymph nodes are resected. The underlying major pectoral muscle is left in place; the minor pectoralis muscle may or may not be removed. In patients with small lesions and no metastases, breast reconstruction may be performed immediately or a few days after the procedure.

Radical Mastectomy

A radical mastectomy is performed to control the spread of malignant disease from large infiltrating cancers. Following a positive finding on the tissue biopsy, the entire involved breast is removed along with the axillary lymph nodes, the pectoral muscles, and all adjacent tissues. During the surgical procedure, skin flaps and extensive exposed tissue are covered with moist packs for protection. The chest wall and axilla are irrigated before closure.

Extended Radical Mastectomy

Cancer is a disease that grows both deeply and laterally. An extended radical mastectomy is indicated when malignant disease is present in the medial quadrant or subareolar tissue because it tends to spread to the internal mammary lymph nodes. The involved breast is removed en bloc along with the underlying pectoral muscles, axillary contents, and upper internal mammary (mediastinal) lymph node chain. This procedure is more difficult than a classic radical mastectomy.

Considerations for Female Breast Procedures

For a breast procedure, the patient is placed in the supine position; the involved side is positioned close to the edge of the operating bed, and the arm on the affected side is extended on an armboard. The affected side is elevated with a small pillow. The anterior part of the chest is prepped from the chin to the umbilicus and from the axilla on the affected side to the nipple line of the opposite breast. The entire arm on the affected side is included in this preparation. General anesthesia is usually preferred for a mastectomy because local infiltrate may obscure a tumor.

Because of the vascularity of breast tissue, a laser or electrocoagulation is commonly used for hemostasis. Larger vessels may require a tie. Patients undergoing a mastectomy should be watched for excessive bleeding. Some surgeons prefer to irrigate the mastectomy wound with sterile water instead of sterile normal saline solution to crenate (shrivel or shrink) cancerous cells. The circulator should check with the surgeon about the care of the specimen for the pathologist. The specimen is placed in sterile normal saline solution if estrogen or progesterone receptor studies are to be performed. Formalin is used for permanent sections.

A bulky compression dressing may be applied in the OR. Depending on the amount of tissue resected, a closed-wound suction system may be inserted to remove extravasation of blood and serum and to prevent pressure necrosis of skin flaps.

Patients who have undergone a mastectomy are often referred to the Reach to Recovery rehabilitative program. In this program, volunteers who have had mastectomies visit patients, share information with them, and give them encouragement.

Reduction of the Male Breast

Reduction of the male breast is carried out for gynecomastia, a pathologic lesion that consists of bilateral or unilateral enlargement of the male breast. Gynecomastia occurs primarily after 40 years of age or during puberty and is usually related to alterations in the normal hormonal balance. All subareolar fibroglandular tissue is removed, followed by reconstruction of the resultant defect. Some surgeons perform liposuction-assisted procedures to debulk the male breast. Carcinoma can also occur in the male breast.

ABDOMINAL SURGERY

A laparotomy involves surgically opening the abdominal wall and entering the peritoneal cavity (Figure 34-3). In this procedure, the skin and subcutaneous tissue are incised, and

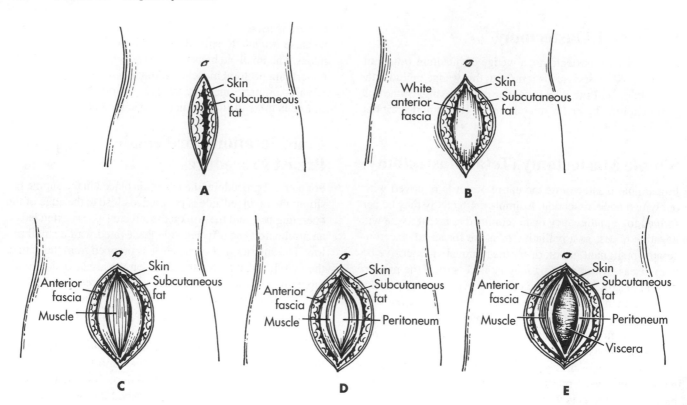

Figure 34-3 Dissecting tissue layers of the abdomen. **A,** Subcutaneous fat (yellow). **B,** Anterior fascia (white). **C,** Muscle (red). **D,** Skin through muscle dissected. Thin white peritoneum is shown for dissection. **E,** Open peritoneum with viscera beneath.

the blood vessels are ligated or electrocoagulated. Fascia covers the muscles anteriorly and posteriorly. The anterior fascia is incised and each muscle layer is separated and/or divided; bleeding vessels are ligated or electrocoagulated. The layers are retracted. Lying beneath the posterior fascia is the peritoneum—the thin serous membrane that lines the interior of the abdominal cavity (parietal peritoneum) and surrounds the organs (visceral peritoneum). Both the posterior fascia and the peritoneum may be cut at the same time, thus exposing the contents of the abdominal cavity (see Figure 34-3).

Various types of incisions are used in a laparotomy, but each follows essentially the same technique. Before the procedure begins, the surgeon chooses the most suitable incision for the procedure being performed. All incisions incorporate, with varying degrees of success, certain characteristics that include the following:

- Ease and speed of entry into the abdominal cavity
- Maximum exposure
- Minimum trauma
- Least postoperative discomfort
- Maximum postoperative wound strength

Types of Abdominal Incisions

Direction and location are the two main factors governing the type of abdominal incision. Incisions may be vertical, horizontal, or oblique and may occur in various areas of the torso (Figure 34-4). The incisions discussed in the following sections are applicable to open abdominal or pelvic procedures. Laparoscopy is performed through multiple incisions that are smaller, separate, and distinct.

Paramedian Incision

The paramedian incision is a vertical incision made approximately 4 cm (approximately 2 inches) lateral to the midline on either side in the upper or lower abdomen. After the skin and subcutaneous tissue are incised, the rectus sheath is split vertically and the muscle is retracted laterally. This incision allows quick entry into and excellent exposure of the abdominal cavity. It limits trauma, avoids nerve injury, is easily extended, and gives a firm closure. Examples of use include access to the biliary tract or pancreas in the right upper quadrant and access to the left lower quadrant for resection of the sigmoid colon.

Longitudinal Midline Incision

A longitudinal midline incision can be upper abdominal, lower abdominal, or a combination of both going around the umbilicus. Depending on the length of the incision, it begins in the epigastrium at the level of the xiphoid process and may extend vertically to the suprapubic region. After incision of the peritoneum, the falciform ligament of the liver is divided. An upper midline incision offers excellent exposure of and rapid entry into the upper abdominal contents.

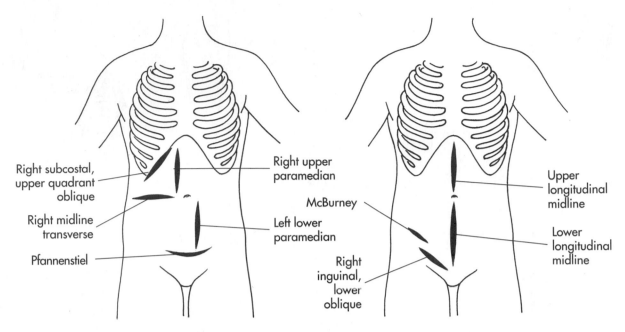

Figure 34-4 Abdominal incisions.

Subcostal Upper Quadrant Oblique Incision

A right or left oblique incision begins in the epigastrium and extends laterally and obliquely just below the lower costal margin. It continues through the rectus muscle, which is either retracted or transversely divided. Although this type of incision affords limited exposure except for upper abdominal viscera, it provides good cosmetic results because it follows skin lines and produces limited nerve damage. Although painful, it is a strong incision postoperatively. Examples of use include biliary procedures and splenectomy.

Bilateral incisions that join in the midline may be preferred for procedures that involve the stomach and/or pancreas. A bilateral modified subcostal incision (Chevron incision) is made for increased visibility during a liver transplantation or resection.

McBurney Incision

McBurney's point is located in the right lower quadrant, just below the umbilicus and 4 cm (approximately 2 inches) medial from the anterior superior iliac spine. A McBurney incision involves a muscle-splitting incision that extends through the fibers of the external oblique muscle. The incision is deepened, the internal oblique and transversalis muscles are split and retracted, and the peritoneum is entered. This is a fast, easy incision, but exposure is limited. Its primary use is for appendectomy.

Thoracoabdominal Incision

For a thoracoabdominal incision, the patient is placed in a lateral position. Either a right or a left incision begins at a point midway between the xiphoid process and umbilicus and extends across the abdomen to the seventh or eighth costal interspace and along the interspace into the thorax. The rectus, oblique, serratus, and intercostal muscles are divided in the line of incision down to the peritoneum and pleura. This converts the pleural and peritoneal cavities into one main cavity, thus allowing excellent exposure for the upper end of the stomach and lower end of the esophagus (see Figure 42-5). Examples of use include esophageal varices and the repair of a hiatal hernia.

Midabdominal Transverse Incision

The midabdominal transverse incision starts on either the right or left side and slightly above or below the umbilicus. It may be carried laterally to the lumbar region between the ribs and crest of the ilium. The intercostal nerves are protected by cutting the posterior rectus sheath and peritoneum in the direction of the divided muscle fibers. The advantages are rapid incision, easy extension, a provision for retroperitoneal approach, and a secure postoperative wound. Examples of use include choledochojejunostomy and transverse colostomy.

Pfannenstiel Incision

A Pfannenstiel incision is a curved transverse incision across the lower abdomen and within the hairline of the pubis. The rectus fascia is severed transversely and the muscles are separated. The peritoneum is incised vertically in the midline. This lower transverse incision provides good exposure and strong closure for pelvic procedures. Its primary use is for an abdominal hysterectomy.

Inguinal Incision (Lower Oblique)

An oblique incision of the right or left inguinal region extends from the pubic tubercle to the anterior crest of the ilium, slightly above and parallel to the inguinal crease. Incision of the external oblique fascia provides access to the cremaster muscle, inguinal canal, and cord structures. Its primary use is for inguinal herniorrhaphy.

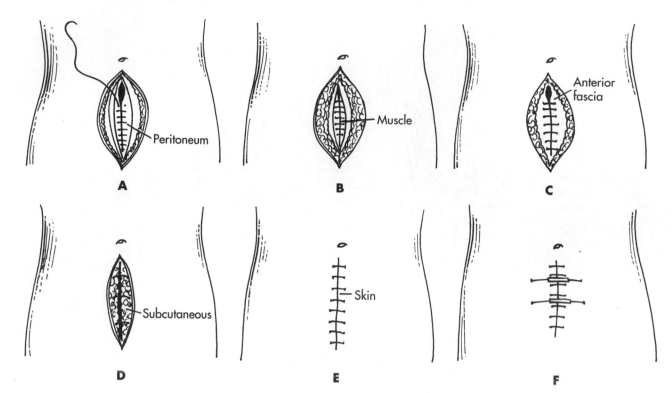

Figure 34-5 Suturing incised tissue layers. **A,** Peritoneum (continuous stitch, taper point needle). **B,** Muscle (interrupted stitch). **C,** Anterior fascia (interrupted stitch, cutting needle). **D,** Subcutaneous (not always sutured, taper point needle). **E,** Skin (interrupted stitch, cutting needle). **F,** Retention sutures. Note bumpers to protect skin.

Wound Closure

Wound closure is performed in reverse order of the incision. Each layer is closed with interrupted or continuous sutures (Figure 34-5). Separation of tissues produced by a failure to closely approximate wound edges results in dead space, which delays healing. Absorbable material is usually used if the peritoneum is sutured, and either absorbable or nonabsorbable material is used on muscle and fascia. It may be necessary to place a few absorbable sutures in the subcutaneous layer. Skin edges are approximated with nonabsorbable sutures, skin clips, or staples. The suture line is sometimes supported by retention or stay sutures.

Many surgeons prefer the Smead-Jones far-and-near technique for abdominal wound closure (Figure 34-6). This technique involves a single-layer closure through both layers of fascia, the abdominal muscles, and the peritoneum with interrupted sutures of either monofilament stainless steel or polypropylene. These sutures resemble a figure-of-eight when placed. This closure is rapid and strong.

An abdominal wound closure must provide tensile strength to the incision until the wound is healed. It should not inhibit wound healing or promote wound infection, and it should be well tolerated by the patient. Care is taken not to suture the bowel or other organ structures to the abdominal wound. More information about wound closure can be found in Chapter 30.

Figure 34-6 Smead-Jones figure-of-eight abdominal wound closure technique.

Laparoscopy

Instead of incising the abdominal wall to enter the peritoneal cavity, a rigid laparoscope can be introduced through a sharp trocar and sheath for video-guided, minimal access, intraabdominal surgical procedures. The lysis of adhesions or the inspection of organs may eliminate the need for a laparotomy. Needle biopsies, wedge resections, and the ablation of some tumors can be performed. Specialized graspers, scissors, sutures, staplers, and ligating clips can be manipulated through trocars strategically located through the abdominal wall. Laser, electrical, and thermal energy can be directed through secondary ports for cutting and coagulating tissues. Care is taken not to burn unintended tissues with the hot ends of instrumentation.

Laparoscopic Procedure

After the patient has been anesthetized, intubated, prepped, and draped, the operating bed may be tilted approximately 10 degrees into a slight Trendelenburg position. A Verres insufflation needle or blunt Hasson trocar is inserted into the peritoneal cavity through a small infraumbilical incision. The anterior abdominal wall is thinnest at the lower edge of the umbilicus, which makes this area easiest for penetration of and extraction through a single layer of fascia and peritoneum with minimal interruption of skin and dermal blood vessels. The peritoneal cavity is insufflated with carbon dioxide to an intraoperative pressure of 12 to 15 mm Hg. The circulator monitors this pressure during insufflation; it should not fall below 8 mm Hg. After sufficient pneumoperitoneum is established, the patient is placed in a slight reverse Trendelenburg position for upper gastrointestinal procedures. A padded footboard should be in place to prevent the patient from sliding downward on the operating bed.

If an insufflation needle is used to fill the peritoneal cavity with carbon dioxide gas, then it is replaced by a trocar and sheath, which is inserted straight into the peritoneal cavity. The sharp obturator is then removed from the trocar sheath. The telescope is introduced into the abdomen through the trocar sheath. The sheath matches the size of the rigid laparoscope. A 7- or 10-mm, 0-degree telescope is inserted through the sheath for direct visualization within the peritoneal cavity. Secondary 5-, 7-, or 10-mm trocars are inserted through the abdominal wall under direct vision through the laparoscope. If 10-mm trocars are used, sizing caps or lumen reducers can be used to reduce the opening of the sheath for the use of smaller endoscopic instruments and probes. The use of size-reducing caps prevents the escape of pneumoperitoneum. A sterile camera attached to the laparoscope transmits images on video monitor(s). Two monitors, one on each side of the operating bed, are usually used. Without straining their necks, the surgeon and the team can view the manipulation of instruments inserted through secondary ports in the direct line of vision.

BILIARY TRACT PROCEDURES

The gallbladder is located in the right upper quadrant in a fossa under and immediately adjacent to the right lobe of the liver (see Figure 34-8). The gallbladder is a thin-walled sac and has a normal capacity of 50 to 75 ml of bile. Bile secreted by the hepatic cells enters the intrahepatic bile ducts and progresses to the common bile duct. When not needed for digestion, bile is diverted through the cystic duct into the gallbladder, where it is stored. When bile is needed, the gallbladder contracts and empties bile into the cystic duct; the bile flows into and through the common duct into the duodenum.

Gallstones are concretions of elements of bile, particularly cholesterol, and may be found in the gallbladder or in any portion of the extrahepatic biliary duct system. The incidence of stones, referred to as cholelithiasis, increases with age and is more prevalent in women and in persons who are obese. Acute or chronic inflammation of the gallbladder, common

duct stones (choledocholithiasis), carcinoma, or the congenital absence of bile ducts (biliary atresia) are the most common indications for a surgical procedure. Obstructive jaundice, which is potentially fatal, may be a sign of ductal cholelithiasis or the presence of a neoplasm. The cause of jaundice should be determined and the condition relieved to spare the patient irreversible progressive liver damage.

The greatest hazards of biliary tract surgery are associated with the anatomic relationships of the ducts and the cystic artery and with pathologic changes in the gallbladder. Complications include hemorrhage and injury to the extrahepatic biliary duct system.

Ultrasonography, nuclear imaging such as hepatic intraductal assay (HIDA scan), and computed tomography (CT) scanning are used for the diagnosis of gallbladder disease. Oral and IV cholecystography may be used for visualization of the gallbladder in the initial evaluation of patients with biliary symptoms. Endoscopic retrograde cholangiopancreatography also may be performed, usually by a gastroenterologist, to identify stones, tumors, inflammatory lesions, or an obstruction. A flexible fiberoptic duodenoscope is introduced with the patient under IV sedation and with the use of a topical anesthetic to control the gag reflex.

Dye is injected to opacify the entire biliary tract and pancreatic duct under fluoroscopy. Some definitive therapy is possible during this procedure, such as stone retrieval (endoscopic papillotomy), stent insertion, and sphincterotomy. A percutaneous transhepatic puncture is used to biopsy tumors, dilate strictures, place stents in the bile duct, and to establish temporary drainage through ducts. A contrast medium can be injected for a cholangiogram.

Cholecystectomy

Gallbladder disease is cured by removal of the gallbladder in a procedure referred to as a cholecystectomy—the most common surgical procedure performed on the biliary tract. A cholecystectomy is performed to relieve the gastrointestinal distress common in patients with acute or chronic cholecystitis (with or without gallstones); it also removes a source of recurrent sepsis. Persistent infection in the biliary tract may cause recurrent stones.

For a cholecystectomy, the patient is placed in the supine position. As requested by the surgeon, the right upper quadrant may be slightly elevated on a gallbladder rest or pillow after the induction of general anesthesia. The operating bed may be tilted slightly into a reverse Trendelenburg position so the abdominal viscera gravitates downward, away from the surgical area.

Laparoscopic Cholecystectomy

With a laparoscopic cholecystectomy, a rigid fiberoptic laparoscope is inserted into the peritoneal cavity. Trocars are inserted through three or four puncture wounds in the right upper quadrant: one or two just right of midline, with the uppermost trocar slightly below the xiphoid and costal margin and the other midway to the umbilicus; one laterally in an anterior axillary line above the iliac crest at the costal margin; and another in a midclavicular line slightly above the level of the umbilicus and 2 cm below the rib. (The location of puncture sites will vary according to patient size and surgeon preference.) A camera attached to the laparoscope allows the surgeon to view the manipulation of instruments through the sheaths of these trocars. Viewing monitors are positioned on each side of the head of the operating bed.

With this procedure, the fundus of the gallbladder is grasped through lateral port(s) and held by the assistant. After careful dissection, the surgeon ligates and divides the cystic duct and artery with suture loops or clips. A laser, an ESU, or microscissors may be used to transect these structures. The gallbladder is freed, most often by using an ESU or argon, KTP, contact Nd:YAG, or Ho:YAG laser. The gallbladder is usually aspirated to remove bile and collapse the sac. It may then be removed in one piece or cut into sections and withdrawn through the periumbilical incision.

Open Abdominal Cholecystectomy

With an open abdominal cholecystectomy, the gallbladder is usually exposed through a right subcostal incision that may be extended over the midline. The incision should be adequate for good exposure of the gallbladder and bile ducts. Following exploration of the abdominal cavity, laparotomy packs are used to wall off the surrounding organs for exposure. The contents of the gallbladder may be aspirated to prevent bile from spilling into the peritoneal cavity—a potential source of peritonitis, especially if the gallbladder is tightly distended. The cystic duct, cystic artery, hepatic ducts, and common bile duct are accurately identified.

After palpation of the ducts for stones, the cystic duct and artery are ligated with hemostatic clips and divided. Using blunt dissection, the gallbladder is freed and removed from the liver and its fossa. Some surgeons use ESU and/or Nd:YAG or a Ho:YAG laser for sharp dissection and coagulation. Stones removed as part of the specimen should be sent to the pathology department for analysis and documentation. If bile leakage or hemorrhage has been excessive, a sump drain or closed wound suction drain may be placed in the subhepatic space and brought out through a stab wound after intraabdominal irrigation.

Common Duct Exploration

Concomitant exploration of the common duct is often but not routinely performed during cholecystectomy. Curved stone forceps, small malleable scoops, dilators of various sizes, balloon catheters, stone baskets, and nylon brushes are useful in clearing the hepatic and biliary ducts of stones to prevent them from lodging in the duct and causing subsequent obstructive jaundice. Palpable stones, jaundice with cholangitis, and dilation of the common bile duct are indications for exploration. A T-tube may be inserted to stent the duct and provide postoperative drainage. The surgeon may choose other intraoperative techniques to identify unsuspected stones, pathologic conditions, or anatomic variations in the hepatic duct system.

Intraoperative Cholangiograms

X-ray films are obtained during either open abdominal or laparoscopic procedures. The radiology department is notified in advance if a cholangiogram is anticipated. To check for patient position, scout films should be obtained when the patient is initially positioned on the operating bed—before the procedure is started. The perioperative nurse should assess the patient for allergies or sensitivities to contrast media and should ensure that the operating bed has a radiographic top or can be equipped for x-ray studies or fluoroscopy.

The radiology technician returns to the OR when the surgeon is ready for films. Cholangiograms may be obtained after the gallbladder is removed or before the cystic duct and artery are ligated. A radiopaque contrast medium, usually diatrizoate sodium (Hypaque or Renografin), is injected into the cystic duct or common bile duct with a 50-ml syringe. Unless fluoroscopy is used, a series of three or four x-ray films are obtained. The surgeon injects dye before each exposure through a cholangiocath (a plastic catheter inserted into cystic or common duct), cannula, or direct needle puncture in the common duct. Instruments are removed from the field to the extent possible to minimize the obstruction of structures on the x-ray films. The field is covered with a sterile barrier before the x-ray tube or C-arm is positioned over the patient. Sterile x-ray tube and C-arm covers are commercially available. All other radiologic precautions for patient and personnel safety should be observed.

Ultrasonography

Ultrasonography, a noninvasive technique, takes less time and does not have the radiation hazards of intraoperative cholangiograms. A sterile ultrasound probe is manipulated along the common bile duct from the liver to the duodenum. The probe transmits high-frequency sound waves back to the ultrasound unit in the form of echoes, which are displayed on a screen as black-and-white, real-time images. To enhance the transmission of ultrasound waves, the abdominal cavity is irrigated with warm normal saline solution. Density in tissue causes sound waves to echo in altered patterns and directions. Gallstones appear as bright echoes, often with an acoustic shadow. Photographs or a videotape can be obtained to document the findings of ultrasonography.

Choledochoscopy

Intraoperative biliary endoscopy provides image transmission and illumination, thus allowing the surgeon visual guidance in exploring the biliary system. Intrahepatic and extrahepatic bile ducts can be visualized with a flexible fiberoptic choledochoscope introduced into the common duct. To provide distention of the biliary tract, normal saline solution must continuously flow through the irrigation channel. Stones are easily seen and are usually free-floating under the pressure of the irrigating solution. A flexible stone forceps or a basket or a balloon-tipped biliary catheter may be inserted through the instrument channel of either a rigid or flexible scope to allow manipulation of a stone under direct vision. A biopsy forceps may be inserted to obtain a tissue sample. An Nd:YAG laser fiber may be used through the choledochoscope to crush bilirubin stones in the distal common hepatic duct; this allows easy removal of the stones.

Cholelithotripsy

Cholelithotripsy is a noninvasive procedure in which high-energy shock waves are used to fragment cholesterol gallstones. The procedure is performed under IV sedation or general anesthesia. The patient is usually placed in the prone position but may also be in the supine or lateral position, on a lithotripter table, or submerged in a water bath. Spark-gap shock waves generated from an electrode pass through a fluid medium into the body until they reach the stone, which is focused with an ultrasound probe and computer. The shock waves are synchronized with the R waves of the patient's cardiac rhythm, which is monitored by ECG to avoid dysrhythmias. Each shock pulverizes the stone(s) into small fragments, which then pass through the bile duct. This passage may be aided by oral administration of deoxycholic acid (ursodiol) taken daily after lithotripsy to dissolve the fragments.

Choledochostomy, Choledochotomy

With choledochostomy, a T-tube is used to drain the common bile duct through the abdominal wall. A choledochotomy is the incision of the common bile duct for the exploration and removal of stones. Intraoperative cholangiography may be performed before and after exploration and/or stone removal. The duct is irrigated after calculi are removed. Patency of the duct and of the ampulla of Vater is investigated, often through a choledochoscope. If a neoplasm is found during exploration, resectability is determined; many tumors of the liver or pancreas are inoperable.

Cholecystoduodenostomy, Cholecystojejunostomy

Either a cholecystoduodenostomy or cholecystojejunostomy is performed to relieve an obstruction in the distal end of the common duct. Through anastomosis, these procedures establish continuity between the gallbladder and either the duodenum or jejunum. Careful evaluation precedes the surgical procedure. Cholecystoduodenostomy and cholecystojejunostomy are bypass procedures to avoid further obstructive jaundice, but they do not solve the problem. Common causes of the obstruction are calculi, stricture of the duct, or neoplasms of the duct, ampulla of Vater, or pancreas.

Choledochoduodenostomy, Choledochojejunostomy

Choledochoduodenostomy and choledochojejunostomy are side-to-side anastomoses between the duodenum or jejunum and the common duct. These procedures are carried out for difficult or recurrent biliary or pancreatic obstruction as a result of benign or malignant disease.

LIVER PROCEDURES

The liver, the largest gland in the body, is divided into left and right segments (or lobes) and is located in the upper right abdominal cavity beneath the diaphragm (Figures 34-7 and 34-8). Part of the stomach and duodenum and the hepatic flexure of the colon lie directly beneath the liver. A tough fibrous sheath, Glisson's capsule, completely covers the organ; the tissue within this capsule is very friable and vascular. The hepatic artery, a branch of the celiac axis, maintains the arterial supply. Blood from the stomach, intestine, spleen, and pancreas is carried to the liver by the portal vein and its branches.

The many functions of the liver include forming and secreting bile, which aids digestion; transforming glucose into glycogen, which it stores; and helping to regulate blood volume. The liver is vital for the metabolic functioning of the body. It metabolizes fats, proteins, and carbohydrates;

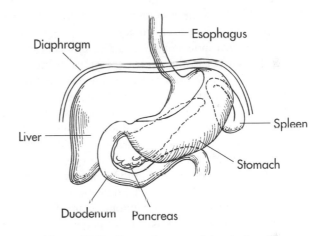

Figure 34-7 Organs in upper abdominal cavity.

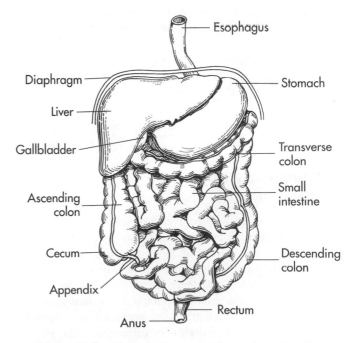

Figure 34-8 Abdominal organs within peritoneal cavity.

synthesizes cholesterol; excretes bilirubin; and secretes hormones. This organ has remarkable regenerative capacity, and up to 80% of it may be resected with little or no alteration in hepatic function. Liver function tests are used to assess the degree of functional impairment and to evaluate liver activity and reserve. Most of these tests involve taking a series of blood samples from the patient for specific studies. Ascites may result from impaired liver function.

Liver Needle Biopsy

A percutaneous needle biopsy may help establish a diagnosis of liver disease. Because the procedure is performed with the patient under local anesthesia or monitored anesthesia care, the patient should be instructed to take several deep breaths and then hold his or her breath and remain absolutely still while the needle is inserted. Failure of the patient to cooperate can cause needle penetration of the diaphragm or hepatic injury and result in hemorrhage, a serious complication. Leakage of bile into the abdominal cavity may produce chemical peritonitis, an additional hazard.

After skin preparation and the induction of local anesthesia (with the patient in the supine position), a Franklin-Silverman or Tru-cut biopsy needle is introduced into the liver via a transthoracic intercostal or transabdominal subcostal route. The needle is rotated to separate a small core of tissue, and it is then withdrawn to remove the specimen. As soon as the needle is removed, the patient is told to resume normal breathing and is assisted to turn onto his or her right side to compress the chest wall at the penetration site and prevent the seepage of bile or blood. Slight bleeding may follow a liver biopsy; the patient's prothrombin time is checked. This method of biopsy is not used if the patient has a blood abnormality.

In certain patients under local anesthesia, a laparoscopic-assisted approach may be used to enhance visualization of the biopsy site. The anterior abdominal wall is elevated with a low volume of carbon dioxide insufflation or a planar lift device without insufflation. The biopsy needle is inserted through the abdominal wall as described previously. A topical hemostatic gelatin sponge or other topical chemical hemostatic agent is laparoscopically applied to the biopsy site on the liver. The patient remains supine following this procedure.

Drainage of Subphrenic and Subhepatic Abscesses

Abscesses in and around the liver may be caused by a variety of microorganisms or as a result of secondary infections from abdominal organs. In general, these abscesses are treated by incision and drainage. A catheter may be introduced into the abscess cavity, which has been localized on a CT scan. The location of the abscess determines the percutaneous approach (i.e., transpleural, subpleural, transperitoneal, or retroperitoneal). Care must taken to avoid contamination of the pleural or peritoneal cavity.

Intraoperative Hepatic Ultrasound

Intraoperative ultrasound can be used to identify anatomic structures or liver densities associated with a primary tumor or metastasis. Before rotating the liver forward and excising diseased or injured lobes or segments, it is necessary to divide the appropriate ligamentous attachments and to ligate the veins and arteries. Lesions that are not accessible for resection may be treated with cryosurgery or a Cavitron ultrasonic aspirator. These techniques may also be used in conjunction with resection. An ultrasonic aspirator permits the precise removal of tissue and controls bleeding during resection.

Hepatic Resection

The standard anatomic resections of the liver are right or left lobectomy, right or left trisegmentectomy, and left lateral segmentectomy. Because it is a vital organ, the entire liver cannot be removed without liver transplantation. Lobectomy or segmental resection is indicated for cysts, benign or malignant tumors, or severe penetrating or blunt trauma. Depending on the location of the lesion to be resected, a right or bilateral subcostal incision or an upper midline incision is made and can be extended as needed for exposure and exploration. The liver is the most commonly injured abdominal organ. Hepatic parenchymal injuries usually cause intraperitoneal hemorrhage and shock.

Liver tissue is very friable. The prevention or arrest of hemorrhage is a prime concern. Omental flaps, falciform ligament, or Gerota's fascia flap may be used for coverage and tamponade of bleeding surfaces in conjunction with local hemostatic substances. Microfibrillar collagen or oxidized cellulose is often used to control bleeding. Large, blunt, noncutting needles are used to suture the liver. Drains are usually placed in the wound and brought out through stab wounds. Equipment for blood replacement, portal pressure measurement, and chest drainage should be available.

Portosystemic Shunts

Portal hypertension, bleeding esophageal varices, or massive gastrointestinal hemorrhage may necessitate an emergency surgical procedure for decompression of the portal venous system. Often the patient is alcoholic, with cirrhosis, poor nutrition, and unstable blood volume, or generally is a poor surgical risk. A portosystemic shunt is a vascular anastomosis between the portal and systemic venous systems. The surgeon may select one of several techniques for a portacaval or mesocaval shunt. In patients with portal hypertension and hypersplenism, a splenorenal shunt may be performed in conjunction with a splenectomy for portal decompression.

SPLENIC PROCEDURES

The highly vascular spleen is located in the upper left abdominal cavity and lies beneath the dome of the diaphragm; it is protected by the lower portion of the rib cage (see Figure 34-7).

The capsule of the spleen is covered with peritoneum and is held in place by numerous suspensory ligaments. The splenic artery furnishes the arterial blood supply, and the splenic vein drains into the portal system. As the largest lymphatic organ of the body, the spleen has an intimate role in the immunologic defenses of the body and acts as a blood reservoir. The main functions of the spleen involve the formation of blood elements. Radionuclide scanning and other radiographic studies provide information for analysis.

Splenectomy

The most common reason for removal of the spleen is hypersplenism—overactivity that causes a reduction in the circulating quantity of red cells, white cells, platelets, or a combination of them. Splenectomies are often scheduled at specific times because patients often require the administration of whole blood immediately before a surgical procedure. Often these patients are also receiving steroid treatment, and provisions are made to maintain therapy during the surgical procedure and postoperatively. Hematologic disorders, tumors, or accessory spleens may also necessitate surgical intervention. A splenic rupture requires an immediate surgical procedure to prevent fatal hemorrhage and may require a splenectomy. In certain patients with benign disease, a laparoscopic approach has been successfully used for splenectomy.

In performing a splenectomy, a left rectus paramedian, midline, or subcostal incision is used to enter the peritoneal cavity, and the spleen is displaced medially by careful manual manipulation. The splenorenal, splenocolic, and gastrosplenic ligaments are ligated and divided. Great care should be exercised in ligating the splenic artery and vein because these vessels are often friable. Hemorrhage is the principal intraoperative hazard. After removal of the spleen and before closure, careful inspection for bleeding from the splenic pedicle and retroperitoneal space is essential.

Splenorrhaphy

After a splenectomy, patients—especially children—are immunologically impaired (i.e., more susceptible to infection), which sometimes can produce catastrophic results. To protect the patient's immune competence, surgeons attempt to salvage splenic tissue following splenic trauma. Splenorrhaphy, or splenic repair, can be accomplished in several ways. Once the spleen is mobilized, actively bleeding vessels are ligated, and devitalized tissues are debrided. The spleen can then be sutured or stapled along the edge of a partial splenectomy. Microfibrillar collagen or absorbable gelatin sponges can be placed over a small laceration or capsular tear to effect hemostasis. The splenic artery may be ligated. The spleen may be wrapped in omentum or synthetic mesh. Segments can be reimplanted into an omental pouch in the intraperitoneal space to preserve splenic function. In patients with extensive trauma, a drain that is exteriorized through a stab wound may be inserted in the left subdiaphragmatic space.

PANCREATIC PROCEDURES

The pancreas is both an endocrine gland and an exocrine gland. The islets of Langerhans form the endocrine division and secrete the hormones insulin and glucagon, both of which are essential to the metabolism of carbohydrates and the storage of calories. Acini and the ducts leading from them constitute the exocrine portion, which secretes pancreatic juice into the duodenum. Pancreatic juice neutralizes stomach acid; the loss of pancreatic juice results in severe impairment in the digestion and absorption of food.

The pancreas lies transversely across the posterior wall of the upper abdomen behind the stomach. The head, or right extremity of the pancreas, is attached to the duodenum; the tail, or left extremity of the pancreas, is in proximity to the spleen (see Figure 34-7).

Disorders of the pancreas generally include acute and chronic inflammation, cysts, and tumors. The head of the pancreas is the most common site of a malignant pancreatic tumor. Accuracy in the diagnosis of pancreatic problems is difficult, but evaluation by ultrasonography, endoscopic retrograde cholangiopancreatography, and scanning has led to significant improvements in planning surgical treatment. An exploratory laparotomy is the most reliable means of diagnosing and evaluating pancreatic trauma. Pancreatitis is most often associated with pancreatic duct stones, gallstones, or alcoholism. Corrective biliary tract procedures usually alleviate gallstone pancreatitis.

Pancreaticojejunostomy

Pancreaticojejunostomy may be performed for relief of pain associated with chronic alcoholic pancreatitis and pseudocysts of the pancreas. There are several types of procedures for the drainage of obstructed ducts or pseudocysts. These methods involve anastomosing a loop of the jejunum (Roux-en-Y loop) to the pancreatic duct. Hemorrhage and leakage of bile are complications to be avoided.

Pancreaticoduodenectomy (Whipple Procedure)

Pancreaticoduodenectomy is an extensive procedure performed on patients with carcinoma of the head of the pancreas or the ampulla of Vater. A gastrointestinal setup is used for this procedure. The abdominal cavity is exposed through one of several possible anterior incisions, but a long right paramedian incision is usually made. The abdominal and pelvic cavities are explored for distant metastases. Because many vital structures and organs are involved in resecting the diseased portion of the pancreas, careful dissection of vessels is necessary to prevent hemorrhage, which complicates the procedure. Resection includes the distal stomach, the duodenum distal to the pylorus, the distal end of the common bile duct, and all but the tail of the pancreas. Several methods of reconstructing the digestive tract are possible, but all include anastomosis of the pancreatic duct, common bile duct, stomach, and jejunum. Most surgeons reestablish biliary-intestinal continuity by end-to-side chole-dochojejunostomy. The stomach and pylorus may be preserved in patients with benign disease or localized, small tumors. After pancreatic and biliary reconstruction, the divided end of the duodenum is anastomosed to the side of the jejunal limb used for the reconstruction. A watertight seal of all anastomoses is essential to prevent peritonitis or pancreatitis. Drains are inserted.

Improvements in preoperative and postoperative care and the refinement of technical details have increased the survival rate of patients who undergo this potentially hazardous radical surgical procedure. The most common postoperative complications of pancreaticoduodenectomy are shock, hemorrhage, renal failure, and pancreatic or biliary fistula. If a fistula should occur, wound suction is continued until the fistula closes. In general, the fistula will close spontaneously if adequate nutrition and electrolyte balance are maintained.

Pancreatectomy

Subtotal distal pancreatectomy is usually performed to resect a benign tumor or for chronic pancreatitis. The distal tail is resected to the head of the pancreas. A splenectomy is usually performed with this procedure because the blood supply to the tail of the pancreas comes from splenic vessels that are sacrificed.

A total pancreatectomy allows a wide resection of a primary malignant tumor and its multifocal sites in the pancreas. A patient who has undergone a total pancreatectomy will have some endocrine and pancreatic insufficiency.

Pancreatoduodenal Trauma

Combined injuries of the pancreas and duodenum from penetrating wounds or blunt trauma are among the most complicated to treat. A midline incision is used to explore the abdomen. Suturing to control bleeding, debriding of devitalized tissue, and draining are the initial therapies. Pancreatic fistulas and abscesses are potential complications. Extensive injury of the head of the pancreas and duodenum may require pancreaticoduodenal resection with gastrojejunostomy.

ESOPHAGEAL PROCEDURES

The esophagus is the musculocutaneous canal between the pharynx in the throat and the stomach in the abdomen. It passes through the thoracic cavity and enters the abdominal cavity through the esophageal hiatus (opening) in the right crus of the diaphragm; it joins the right medial surface of the stomach. Within the abdominal cavity the esophagus lies between the liver anteriorly and the aorta posteriorly and slightly to the left (with the spleen on the left), and between the right and left branches of the vagus nerve (see Figures 34-7 and 34-8).

Esophageal Hiatal Herniorrhaphy (Nissen Fundoplication)

When intraabdominal pressure exceeds pressure in the chest, the abdominal esophagus and a portion of the stomach may slide through the esophageal hiatus and into the thoracic cavity. Although this condition (referred to as hiatal or diaphragmatic hernia) is quite common, a surgical procedure is indicated when the resultant esophagitis causes ulceration, bleeding, stenosis, or chest and back symptoms. Reflux esophagitis and sphincter incompetence may also have other causes that necessitate a surgical procedure.

The abdominal approach to correct the problem involves a midline or left subcostal incision. Because visualization of the hiatal area may be difficult, the incision may be extended over the lower rib cage. The patient may be placed in a slight Trendelenburg position. Organs and vital structures should be protected with moist tapes and gently retracted to expose the hiatus. Long-handled clamps are needed. Following mobilization, the hiatus is narrowed with heavy sutures, and the fundus of the stomach is anchored against the diaphragm to prevent recurrent herniation and gastroesophageal reflux.

Prevention of reflux is one of the prime objectives of Nissen fundoplication because it was the cause of the patient's previous esophagitis. Lengthening the intraabdominal esophagus and increasing pressure on the lower esophageal sphincter also help control reflux. Pressure is augmented by wrapping the proximal stomach around the gastroesophageal junction—the Nissen fundoplication procedure. The fundus of the stomach acts as a flap valve to create pressure around the distal esophagus, thus decreasing reflux. As an alternative to fundoplication, some surgeons insert an antireflux collarlike prosthesis around the esophagus just above the gastroesophageal junction.

A laparoscopic Nissen fundoplication, which may be performed in select patients, has similar advantages to laparoscopic cholecystectomy. The procedure involves mobilizing the esophagogastric junction and repairing the hiatal defect with a continuous suture technique. This is followed by a total fundoplication to fix the anterior margin of the diaphragmatic hiatus proximally and the esophagogastric junction distally. The laparoscopic approach has been successful in treating gastroesophageal reflux as a minimally invasive procedure.

Esophagogastrectomy

Removal of the lower portion of the esophagus and proximal stomach may be indicated to resect malignant tumors, benign strictures, or perforations at or near the esophagogastric junction. A left thoracoabdominal or upper midline incision is made. After the esophagus and stomach are mobilized and divided, an end-to-end esophagogastric anastomosis may be completed with staples and/or sutures. An end-to-side anastomosis with plication of the stomach around the distal part of the esophagus may be preferred. Depending on the extent of esophageal resection, other options for restoring continuity of the alimentary tract may be necessary.

Surgical Procedures for Esophageal Varices

Esophageal varices are tortuous dilated veins in the submucosa of the lower esophagus that may extend up into the esophagus or down into the stomach. This condition is caused by portal hypertension and is usually associated with obstruction within a cirrhotic liver. The rupture of esophageal varices can cause massive hemorrhage. The patient may come to the OR with a Sengstaken-Blakemore tube in place to control bleeding by the use of pressure from the inflated balloon in the tube.

During the surgical procedure, varices may be sclerosed through an esophagoscope. A sclerosant is injected via a needle puncture into each varix. Several injections may be necessary to achieve complete hemostasis. Sclerotherapy is usually attempted before more radical procedures are performed. The lower esophagus may be transected and the distal segment anastomosed with a circular stapler just proximal to the stomach. A portosystemic shunt procedure may be performed for portal decompression.

GASTROINTESTINAL SURGERY

Advances in the surgical management of patients with gastrointestinal problems have lessened the mortality rate. Interference with the gastrointestinal tract affects its functioning; specific deficiencies may result from gastrointestinal surgery depending on the site and extent of the surgical procedure. Massive resection of the small intestine can produce long-term nutritional problems such as weight loss and malabsorption of most nutrients. Metabolic bone disease may follow gastric surgery because of poor absorption of calcium and vitamin D. Patients who have undergone extensive gastrointestinal procedures should have a periodic nutritional evaluation. Biochemical tests monitor nutritional status and include serum proteins, albumin-globulin ratio, and blood urea nitrogen. Body weight is also significant. If caloric intake is inadequate, protein is converted to carbohydrates for energy and, as a result, protein synthesis suffers.

Considerations for Gastrointestinal Surgery

The separation of instruments used for resection and anastomosis and for abdominal closure is a matter of preference of the surgeon and institution. Two distinct setups may be used, but the single setup is most commonly used. The single setup consists of identifying and using only selected instruments and supplies for resection, anastomosis, and abdominal closure and discarding contaminated instruments and equipment from the field after use. Acid secretions from the gastric resection site are very irritating and may cause peritonitis. In addition, the intestinal tract harbors many microorganisms. Leakage into the peritoneal cavity can be a source of generalized peritoneal sepsis. Gloves should be changed after anastomosis is completed; gowns may also be changed.

A nasogastric tube is often inserted for the aspiration of gastric contents or for decompression of the intestinal tract. A variety of gastrointestinal tubes should be available for aspiration and irrigation.

Normal saline solution, not sterile water, should be used in abdominal procedures to moisten laparotomy packs. Normal saline is an isotonic solution and has the same osmotic pressure as blood serum and interstitial fluid. It will not alter sodium, chloride, or fluid balance because it does not cross cellular membranes. (Hypotonic solutions cause cells to swell; hypertonic solutions cause them to shrink.) Normal saline is used for intraperitoneal irrigation unless the surgeon prefers to use a solution such as Ringer's lactate. Antibiotic solutions may also be needed for irrigation.

ESUs are used routinely by many surgeons for electrocoagulation of bleeding vessels in the abdominal wall, omentum, and mesentery. Ligating clips or suture ligatures are used for large vessels. To reduce tissue trauma, the jaws of intestinal forceps should be protected with soft covers made of rubber or fabric. Stapling devices are preferred by most surgeons for mechanical anastomosis of organs. An intraluminal circular stapler can be used for end-to-end, end-to-side, or side-to-side anastomoses from the esophagus to the rectum. A straight linear stapler may be preferred for some gastrointestinal anastomoses and resections. Because the size of the lumen varies in different organs of the gastrointestinal tract, the circulator should not open a sterile disposable stapler until the surgeon determines the appropriate head size or cartridge length for the instrument to be used.

The technical principles that guide the surgeon for all gastrointestinal anastomoses include the following:

- Good blood supply
- No tension
- Adequate lumen
- Watertight and leakproof
- No distal obstruction

A sutured anastomosis produces an inverted suture line with serosa-to-serosa approximation. A stapled anastomosis results in anastomosed mucosa-to-mucosa apposition.

GASTRIC PROCEDURES

The stomach, a hollow muscular organ, is situated in the upper left abdomen between the esophagus and duodenum (see Figures 34-7 and 34-8). Anatomically, it is divided into the fundus, body, and pyloric antrum. The two borders of the stomach, the lesser and greater curvatures, are important surgically because of their relation to the major vascular and lymphatic systems that supply the stomach. Omentum, a double fold of peritoneum attached to the lesser and greater curvatures, loosely covers the stomach and small intestine. The autonomic nervous supply from the vagus nerve controls the reflex activities of movement and the secretions of the alimentary canal and is significant in rhythmic relaxation of the pyloric sphincter.

Food entering the stomach is reduced to chyme, a semiliquid, and then passes through the duodenum and small intestine. The interference of gastric activity or muscular contractions results in gastrointestinal complaints of abdominal pain, nausea, vomiting, hemorrhage, and dyspepsia. Some diseases, such as cancer, may not produce symptoms until the condition is far advanced. A surgical procedure is indicated when the presence of disease is established following laboratory tests such as gastric analysis, gastroscopy, and/or radiographic studies.

Following gastric surgery, the dumping syndrome may be experienced by patients shortly after eating; this complication occurs when food and fluids empty rapidly into the jejunum. It is characterized by nausea, vomiting, weakness, dizziness, pallor, sweating, palpitations, and diarrhea, and it may persist for 6 months to 1 year.

Gastroscopy

Gastroscopy involves the passage of a flexible fiberoptic gastroscope. This procedure is usually performed while the patient is sedated, with a topical anesthetic applied in the oropharynx to control the gag reflex. The operator visually inspects the mucosal walls of the stomach, and tissue specimens are sometimes obtained. Bleeding points may be coagulated with a laser beam, electrocoagulation, or a sclerosing agent.

Gastrostomy

Establishment of a temporary or permanent opening in the stomach may be indicated for gastrointestinal decompression or to provide alimentation for a prolonged period when nutrition cannot be maintained by other means. A gastrostomy tube eliminates the incidence of aspiration that may occur around a nasogastric tube. Often the patient is too debilitated to tolerate a major surgical procedure or may have an inoperable esophageal tumor or oropharyngeal trauma. A Foley, Malecot, Pezzer, or mushroom catheter may be inserted percutaneously into the stomach.

Simple Gastrostomy

With the patient under general anesthesia, the stomach is exposed through a small upper left abdominal or midline incision. The catheter is inserted into the anterior gastric wall and is held in place with purse-string sutures; it is brought out through a separate stab wound in the left upper quadrant. The stomach is sutured to the abdominal wall at the exit site of the catheter. Following an abdominal procedure on a critically ill patient, the surgeon may prefer to place a small-bore catheter into the jejunum rather than the stomach for enteral hyperalimentation.

Percutaneous Endoscopic Gastrostomy

With percutaneous endoscopic gastrostomy, the patient is placed under IV sedation, and an endoscopist introduces a fiberoptic gastroscope and insufflates the stomach with air. Light from the scope is directed anteriorly for transillumination through the abdominal wall. The surgeon infiltrates the skin with a local anesthetic at a selected gastrostomy site, usually approximately one third of the distance along the left costal margin at the midclavicular line. The catheter is introduced through a small incision and secured with sutures.

Gastric Resections

The stomach may be totally or partially resected for removal of a malignant tumor or for benign chronic ulcer disease. Although surgical resection is the only cure, gastric carcinomas are often inoperable because of metastases to the liver or extension into surrounding tissues. In such cases, palliative procedures may be performed. The appropriate procedure is determined after thorough exploration of the abdominal cavity by the surgeon. Circular staplers are commonly used for anastomosis following resection. Leakage at the site of anastomosis leads to peritonitis. Some surgeons oversew the staple line.

Total Gastrectomy

With a total gastrectomy, the entire stomach is excised for malignant lesions through a bilateral subcostal, long transrectus, or thoracoabdominal incision. A total gastrectomy necessitates reconstruction of esophagointestinal continuity by establishing an anastomosis between a loop of jejunum and the esophagus. This anastomosis may be end-to-side with a lateral jejunojejunostomy or end-to-end with a Roux-en-Y jejunojejunostomy. The purpose of the jejunojejunostomy is to prevent the reflux of bile and pancreatic fluids into the esophagus. Some surgeons create a jejunal pouch for this purpose.

Subtotal Gastrectomy

Partial resections of the stomach, originally described by Theodor Billroth (1829-1894), are often referred to as Billroth procedures. A benign lesion (usually an ulcer) or a malignant lesion located in the pyloric half of the stomach requires removal of the lower half to two thirds of the stomach. In a patient with a gastric or duodenal ulcer, a partial resection limits gastric acidity and relieves pain, bleeding, vomiting, and weight loss.

In this procedure, the peritoneal cavity is entered through a right paramedian or upper midline abdominal incision. A variety of surgical procedures may be used to reestablish gastrointestinal continuity. Anastomosis of the remaining portion of the stomach to the duodenum (gastroduodenostomy, or Billroth I [Figure 34-9]) or to a loop of the jejunum (gastrojejunostomy, or Billroth II [Figure 34-10]) is often performed. A truncal vagotomy, which is discussed in the following section, is performed to eliminate the possibility of postoperative peptic ulceration.

Common modifications of the Billroth I procedure are the Schoemaker and von Haberer–Finney techniques. The Schoemaker procedure involves end-to-end anastomosis of the stomach and duodenum after the lesser curvature of the stomach is sutured to make the anastomosis site the same size as the duodenum. With the von Haberer–Finney method, the lat-

Figure 34-9 Billroth I gastroduodenostomy. End-to-end anastomosis of duodenum to stomach may be sutured (**A**) or stapled with an intraluminal circular stapler (**B**).

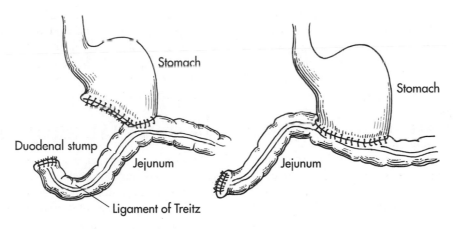

Figure 34-10 Billroth II gastrojejunostomy with end-to-side sutured anastomosis of stomach to loop of jejunum.

eral wall of the duodenum is brought up to the stomach so that the entire end of the stomach is open for direct anastomosis.

Popular modifications of the Billroth II procedure include the Polya and Hofmeister techniques, both of which involve variations of end-to-side gastrojejunostomy.

Vagotomy

Chronic gastric, pyloric, and duodenal ulcers that do not respond to medical treatment cause patients severe pain and difficulty in eating and sleeping. Vagotomy, the division of

the vagus nerves, may be recommended to interrupt vagal nerve impulses, thus lowering the production of gastric hydrochloric acid and hastening gastric emptying. Proximal gastric vagotomy, also known as parietal cell vagotomy, divides the vagal nerve fibers to the proximal stomach but maintains the entire stomach and vagal nerves to the antrum. These sections of the vagal nerve inhibit the release of gastrin, a stimulant of gastric secretion.

Truncal vagotomy and selective vagotomy require a concomitant drainage procedure because these procedures denervate the stomach. A gastroenterostomy is performed with a truncal vagotomy, which divides the vagal trunks at the distal esophagus. An antrectomy is performed with a selective vagotomy, which transects the gastric branches. Vagotomy with drainage is a compromise procedure and is restricted to high-risk patients or those with severe duodenal deformity.

Pyloroplasty, enlarging the pyloric opening between the stomach and duodenum, may be performed in patients with an obstructing pyloric ulcer or in conjunction with vagotomy to treat bleeding duodenal ulcers. Duodenal dilation or duodenoplasty may be indicated.

Vagotomy procedures, which are conservative surgical therapies compared with gastrectomy, decrease the surgical risk for select patients with chronic ulcers. It is now known that ulcers caused by the *Helicobacter pylori* organism can be cured with antibiotics.

Gastrojejunostomy (Roux-en-Y Gastroenterostomy)

A procedure may be necessary to reestablish continuity between the stomach and intestinal tract, such as following a partial gastrectomy or when the lower end of the stomach is obstructed by an ulcer or a nonresectable tumor. A gastrojejunostomy may be performed to treat alkaline reflux gastritis, postgastrectomy syndromes such as postvagotomy diarrhea, and dumping syndromes. Except in geriatric patients, a concomitant vagotomy is necessary to prevent a postoperative gastrojejunal ulcer when the acid-forming portion of the stomach is not resected.

In this procedure, a loop of jejunum may be anastomosed to either the anterior or the posterior wall of the stomach; both approaches have advantages and disadvantages. In a Roux-en-Y gastrojejunostomy, the jejunum is divided. The distal end is anastomosed to the side of the stomach, and the proximal end is anastomosed to the side of the jejunum at a lower level. The result is a Y-shaped double anastomosis that diverts the flow of bile and pancreatic enzymes directly into the jejunum, bypassing the created gastric stoma. An adaptation of a Roux-en-Y anastomosis is also used to drain the biliary tract or other organs, such as the pancreas or esophagus, directly into the jejunum to bypass the stomach and prevent the reflux of intestinal contents.

Bariatric Surgery

An interest in the study of morbid obesity, or bariatrics, has led to the development of a subspecialization in general surgery—bariatric surgery. Persons who weigh 100 pounds (45.4 kg) more than their ideal weight, who have no serious disease, and who have failed to lose weight despite years of medical treatment are potential candidates for bariatric surgery.

The physical size of a patient who is obese presents special needs with respect to transporting and positioning, selecting instrumentation, and providing psychologic and physiologic support. Many morbidly obese patients have medical complications such as hypertension, peripheral vascular disease, cardiac disease, degenerative arthritis, gallbladder disease, or diabetes mellitus. Routine OR procedures for obese or large patients usually include the application of antiembolic stockings and the insertion of nasogastric, indwelling Foley urinary, IV infusion, and monitoring catheters. Because respiratory distress is a potential complication during the induction of anesthesia, intubation while the patient is awake may be the technique of choice. Bariatric procedures for gastric restriction are not without risks. Nutritional deficiencies, anemia, wound infection, and a failure of staple lines have occurred postoperatively. The capacity of the stomach is reduced to approximately 50 ml to restrict food absorption or intake.

Gastric Bypass

In a gastric bypass the size of the stomach is reduced by creating a small pouch in the fundus (the proximal segment of the stomach). The stomach is transected horizontally with a linear stapler, and the proximal jejunum is divided. A Roux-en-Y gastrojejunostomy is constructed between the pouch and the jejunum, bypassing the remainder of stomach, to establish intestinal continuity for the passage of gastric contents. The proximal jejunal segment is anastomosed end-to-side to the distal segment for drainage of gastric, biliary, and pancreatic fluids.

Gastroplasty

In gastroplasty, which is usually referred to as a vertical banded gastroplasty, four linear staple lines are placed vertically on the lesser curvature side of the stomach just left of the gastroesophageal junction. This creates a channel for the passage of gastric contents from the proximal to the distal segments. The stomach is divided between staple lines and oversewn with sutures. To prevent dilation, the outlet at the end of the staple line is usually reinforced with silicone tubing, a Silastic ring, polypropylene mesh, or a soft rubber drain.

INTESTINAL PROCEDURES

The term *intestines* is an inclusive term that refers to the continuous muscular tube of the bowel, which extends from the lower end of the stomach to the rectum (see Figure 34-8). Food and the products of digestion pass through this section of the alimentary canal during digestion, absorption, and the elimination of waste products. Anatomically, the intestines are divided into the small (upper) and large (lower) intestine, and there are subdivisions of each.

The small intestine extends from the pylorus to the ileocecal valve. The three sections include the duodenum (proximal portion), the jejunum (middle section), and the ileum (distal portion that joins the large intestine). The ileocecal valve, a sphincter muscle, lessens the back flow of material that has been discharged to the large intestine.

The large intestine, or colon, extends from the ileum to the rectum and is generally divided into the ascending, transverse, descending, and sigmoid colon. The cecum is the pouch formed where the large intestine joins the small intestine.

The mesentery, a peritoneal fold, attaches the small and large intestines to the posterior abdominal wall and contains the arteries, veins, and lymph nodes that supply the intestines.

Inflammation, intestinal obstruction, and disruption in absorption and motility are disorders that may lead to surgical intervention. Etiologic factors determine the surgical procedure.

Resection of the Small Intestine

Tumors, as well as strangulation from adhesions, volvulus, obstruction, and regional ileitis, usually are treated by resection of the involved segment. An abdominal incision is made over the suspected or known site of disease. After exposure, clamps are placed above and below the diseased segment of the bowel and mesentery to avoid spillage. The involved area is resected, and an end-to-end, end-to-side, or side-to-side anastomosis is performed to restore continuity (Figure 34-11). Variations of this technique are used for other related problems of the small intestine, such as extensive perforation. Bowel strangulation and obstruction necessitate an immediate surgical procedure to prevent necrosis, peritonitis, and death.

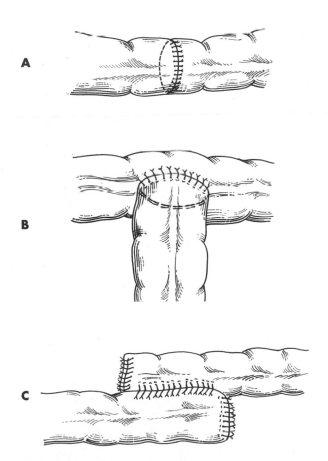

Figure 34-11 Intestinal anastomoses. **A,** End-to-end. **B,** End-to-side. **C,** Side-to-side. Intestinal anastomoses can be performed with sutured anastomoses, as shown here, or with circular or linear staplers.

Hemicolectomy, Transverse Colectomy, Anterior Resection, Total Colectomy

Colitis, diverticulitis, obstruction, and neoplasms are the most common reasons for surgical intervention to remove a diseased segment of the colon. Most surgical procedures involve opening the abdomen, walling off the peritoneal cavity, incising and clamping at the points where resection is to be carried out and, finally, reestablishing continuity by anastomosis. In select patients, a laparoscopic approach may be used to mobilize the segment of the large or small bowel to be resected. The resected bowel is removed through a small minimal-access incision in the abdominal wall. Stomas can also be created with the laparoscopic technique.

The perioperative plan of care includes preoperative administration of intestinal antibiotics, bowel-cleansing methods, and diet restrictions (e.g., a clear liquid diet). Intraoperatively, separate instrument technique should be used during the procedure. A nasogastric tube may be inserted before the surgical procedure and may remain in place until partial healing of anastomosis occurs and effective peristalsis returns. Fluid and electrolyte balance is maintained.

Intestinal Stomas

An intestinal *-ostomy* is a surgically created opening, or stoma, that extends from a portion of the bowel to the exterior via the abdominal wall. This procedure may be performed to divert intestinal contents so that inflamed bowel can heal, to decompress pressure caused by an obstructive lesion, or to bypass an obstruction such as a benign or malignant tumor. The type and level of the lesion determine whether an ileostomy, cecostomy, or colostomy is indicated. The opening may be permanent or temporary depending on the cause and course of the disease or obstruction. In patients with a temporary stoma, intestinal continuity is reestablished following healing through closure of the opening in the bowel and anastomosis of the previously separated ends.

A patient's acceptance of these procedures is as varied as an individual's emotional reactions. Each patient requires a rehabilitation plan based on personal needs. These plans should include care of the pouching system, maintenance of skin integrity, proper diet, odor control, and comfortable clothing. Patient participation is an integral part of the preparation for self-care and enhances self-confidence.

Ileostomy

An ileostomy is performed for conditions such as chronic ulcerative colitis or following removal of the colon (colectomy). In this procedure the proximal end of the transected ileum is exteriorized through the abdominal wall. The usual stoma site is the midportion of the right rectus sheath, approximately 3 cm below the level of the umbilicus. First, a disk of skin is excised. The anterior and posterior sheaths are then incised, and the rectus sheath is divided with a muscle-splitting incision. The proximal end of the ileum is brought out through the peritoneum and muscle to the skin; here the end is everted and sutured to the skin (Figure 34-12). Liquid or semisolid discharge is collected in an ileostomy bag placed over the stoma. The surrounding skin requires special care to prevent excoriation and irritation.

The entire cecum and colon, as well as the rectal mucosa (mucosal proctectomy), are resected in the endorectal-ileoanal pull-through procedure. The ileum is anastomosed to the anus, and the rectal and anal muscles are preserved for anal continence. A pouch is constructed from the terminal ileum proximal to the anal anastomosis to serve as a reservoir for intestinal contents. A temporary diverting loop or double-barreled ileostomy is brought to the skin for drainage during

the healing of the anastomoses; after the anastomoses have healed, this stoma is closed. Although not without complications, these procedures offer acceptable alternatives to a permanent ileostomy stoma, especially in children and young adults.

In the Kock pouch, a nipple valve is created by inverting an intestinal stoma to maintain continency. The patient intubates the valve regularly through the stomal nipple valve to empty the bowel of mucus and fecal matter.

Cecostomy

With a cecostomy, an opening is created in the cecum and a tube is inserted for decompression of the massive distention caused by colonic obstruction. The tube is placed into the cecum through the lower right side of the abdomen. Less severe distention may be relieved by suction and irrigation through a colonoscope and the insertion of an intestinal tube through the anus to the cecum. Cecostomy or colonoscopic decompression may precede subsequent colon resection.

Colostomy

An opening anywhere along the length of the colon to the exterior skin surface creates an artificial anus (Figure 34-13). The section of colon to be exteriorized depends on the location of the lesion to be resected or treated. For example, a low anterior bowel resection necessitates a sigmoid colostomy. Either a double-barreled or loop colostomy may be performed. In a double-barreled colostomy (Figure 34-13, *B*), the transverse colon is divided and both ends are brought out to the margins of the skin incision. The proximal stoma serves as an outlet for feces, and the distal opening leads to the nonfunctioning bowel. In a loop colostomy (Figure 34-13, *C*), a loop of colon is brought out onto the abdominal wall. A plastic rod or ostomy bridge is placed under the loop

Figure 34-12 Ileostomy. Proximal end of transected ileum is brought out through peritoneum and muscle. The end is everted and sutured to skin. Stoma site is in midportion of right rectus sheath below level of umbilicus.

A **B** **C**

Figure 34-13 Colostomy. **A,** Permanent colostomy. Terminal end of descending or sigmoid colon is brought out through peritoneum and muscle and sutured to skin. **B,** Double-barreled colostomy. Both ends of transected colon are brought out to skin. **C,** Loop colostomy. Loop of colon is exteriorized over plastic rod for temporary fecal diversion.

to hold it out on the exterior abdominal wall. The peritoneum is closed, and the wound around the colostomy is sutured.

A permanent colostomy in the sigmoid colon forms an artificial anus following a combined abdominoperineal resection for rectal carcinoma. A collection device for fecal material is not needed after a patient's bowel evacuation becomes regulated. Most patients wear a stoma cap even when they are in the process of regulation.

Appendectomy

Appendicitis can occur at any age but is seen most often in adolescents and young adults. It may imitate other conditions such as a ruptured ovarian cyst or ureteral calculus. Some appendices are retrocecal, which makes diagnosis more difficult. Classic symptoms of early appendicitis include pain in the right lower quadrant, rebound tenderness, nausea, and moderate elevations in temperature and white blood count.

An emergency appendectomy is necessary to prevent a progression to gangrene and the perforation of friable tissue, with subsequent peritonitis. The abdominal approach involves a muscle-splitting incision in the right lower quadrant, over McBurney's point. The blood supply to the appendix is ligated and severed. A crushing clamp is applied to the appendiceal base, which is then ligated and severed from the cecum. Following amputation, the surgeon may elect to cauterize the stump with phenol and alcohol or wipe it with a sponge soaked with an iodophor (Betadine) to reduce contamination. The stump is then inverted into the cecum as a purse-string suture is tightened around the stump.

Drainage is indicated in the presence of an abscess, appendix rupture, or any gross contamination of the wound. An appendectomy is usually an uncomplicated procedure with rapid convalescence unless life-threatening peritonitis results.

Laparoscopic Appendectomy

After peritoneal insufflation and insertion of a laparoscope through the periumbilical incision, trocars are inserted in the suprapubic area and left lower quadrant. The appendix is elevated and hemostatically freed from the mesoappendix with a laser or endoscopic clips or staples. Endoloop ligatures are placed at the base of the appendix, and endoscopic scissors or lasers transect it. Grasping forceps are used to place the appendix into an endopouch reservoir to prevent the extrusion of contents during withdrawal through the periumbilical trocar.

COLORECTAL PROCEDURES

Colorectal carcinoma is one of the most common abdominal malignancies, with the highest incidence in persons over 60 years of age. Resection of the carcinoma is the surgical procedure of choice; radiation and chemotherapy are adjuvant therapies or palliative therapies for advanced disease. Early diagnosis and prompt treatment of asymptomatic carcinoma improve the survival rates.

Diagnostic procedures are routinely performed in patients with bowel or rectal bleeding, chronic diarrhea, or a history of intestinal polyps and/or carcinoma of the colon. Serial guaiac stool tests may detect the presence of occult blood. A barium enema provides a complete radiographic study of the colon; an endoscopic examination is routine. Some therapeutic procedures may be accomplished with laser or electrocoagulation through endoscopes.

Sigmoidoscopy

Sigmoidoscopy is direct visual inspection of the sigmoid and rectal lumens by means of a flexible fiberoptic or rigid lighted sigmoidoscope. The flexible scope is more comfortable for the patient and gives the surgeon better visualization of the mucosal surface to evaluate the left colon and rectosigmoid. It may be used intraoperatively or for preoperative diagnosis.

The patient is prepared preoperatively with enemas. Placing the patient in the knee-chest or Kraske position allows the sigmoid colon to fall forward into the abdomen. The Sims or lithotomy position may be used for an extremely obese or extremely ill patient. The surgeon may inflate air to better visualize the mucosal walls. This insufflation stimulates the stretch receptors of the bowel, causing a feeling of desire to defecate, which necessitates reassurance of the patient.

Colonoscopy

Colonoscopy provides visual inspection of the lining of the entire colon. The scope is flexible and consists of two channels: one for suctioning and irrigating and one for operating. Its greatest uses are to examine the lumen of the colon, to biopsy tissues, and to search for and excise or ablate polyps. Other indications are for the study of inflammatory bowel or diverticular disease, the passage of blood in the feces (hematochezia), or a change in bowel habits; as a preoperative screen before colostomy closure; for confirmation of x ray findings; and as a follow-up for patients who have undergone intestinal procedures. Argon and Nd:YAG lasers or ESUs are used through a colonoscope to ablate some tumors and to treat polyps, arteriovenous malformations, and bleeding disorders.

Because the presence of stool in the rectum prevents adequate examination with the scope, the patient should have a complete preoperative bowel evacuation prep. Colonoscopy is contraindicated if the patient is precariously ill or uncooperative. If perforation is likely, relative contraindications may include acute, severe, or radiation-caused inflammatory disease or complete obstruction.

Complications of colonoscopy include electrical burn during polypectomy, tearing or perforation of the colon by tip pressure, tearing of the liver or spleen by air pressure, and tearing of diverticula resulting from the introduction of air into them.

Polypectomy

Most surgeons and pathologists agree that adenomatous mucosal polyps in the colon are potentially malignant and should be removed. A polypectomy is usually performed through a fiberoptic colonoscope. Polyps, which are often familial, may be single or multiple and are easily excised at the base. The colonoscope may be used intraoperatively to locate polyps. If the polyps are pedunculated, they are cauterized and retrieved for microscopic examination. Electrocoagulation or lasing of the base provides hemostasis. Some polyps or the involved segment of colon are removed by laparotomy or laparoscopy. Following a polypectomy, patients should have annual colonoscopic examinations.

Abdominoperineal Resection

Abdominoperineal resection is an extensive procedure for carcinoma. This procedure is performed mainly in the lower third of the rectum, but it may extend into the anal canal. Preoperative preparation is meticulous to verify diagnosis, to search for metastasis, and to optimize the condition of the patient. Before the surgical procedure, an indwelling Foley catheter is attached to a closed-drainage system.

With an abdominoperineal resection, two approaches—abdominal and perineal—are required; this necessitates the preparation and draping of both areas, and two sets of instruments are necessary. Because the colon is a reservoir for bacteria, contaminated instruments are removed from the field after resection of the sigmoid. With the patient in the Trendelenburg position, the peritoneal cavity is entered through a lower abdominal incision. Preliminary exploration is performed to seek metastases. If the tumor is resectable, the sigmoid colon is mobilized, clamped, and divided. The proximal end of the sigmoid is exteriorized through a stab wound in the left lower quadrant to create a permanent colostomy. The mesentery may be sutured to the abdominal wall to prevent internal hernias. The distal end of the sigmoid is tied to prevent contamination and is placed deep in the presacral space for ultimate removal. The pelvic floor is reperitonealized, and the abdomen is closed. Dressings are placed on the abdominal incision and on the colostomy.

The second phase of the surgical procedure is closure of the anus with a purse-string suture to prevent contamination and removal of the anus, rectum, rectosigmoid, and surrounding nodes and lymphatics through a perineal incision. Drains are placed, and the perineum is closed.

Two teams are used when the abdominal and perineal procedures are performed simultaneously. The patient is initially positioned supine in a modified lithotomy position. This approach reduces operating time and blood loss and provides simultaneous exposure of the abdominal and perineal fields.

Because of the great amount of blood loss from vascular areas and the length of the procedure, patients are carefully monitored to prevent hypovolemic shock.

Low Anterior Colon Resection

The sigmoid colon and rectum lie within the bony pelvis, which makes the resection of tumors in the lower sigmoid colon, rectosigmoid, and rectum technically difficult. The objective is to achieve wide local excision with en bloc resection of the lymphatics and perirectal mesentery. Intraluminal and linear staplers facilitate colorectal anastomosis in a low anterior colon resection. The distal colon is transected after closure with a linear stapler. The intraluminal stapler, with the anvil removed, is introduced through the anus and rectal stump either through or adjacent to the linear staple line. After the anvil is replaced, an intraluminal end-to-end or end-to-side anastomosis with the proximal segment of colon is completed. Total excision of the mesorectum is necessary to prevent recurrence of the tumor in the pelvis or at the staple line; a distal tumor clearance of at least 2 cm is necessary. With this technique for low anterior colorectal anastomosis, colorectal continuity is restored and anal sphincter control is maintained without necessitating a permanent colostomy; with an abdominoperineal resection, a permanent colostomy is necessary.

ABDOMINAL TRAUMA

Trauma is the major cause of death in persons under 40 years of age. Bleeding from the disruption of solid organs or major vessels in the abdomen (including the pelvis) and infection from perforation of a hollow viscus are life-threatening injuries. Blunt and penetrating trauma have different mechanisms of injury. Blunt trauma caused by direct impact, rapid deceleration, shearing forces, and/or increased intraluminal pressure can rupture or sever multiple structures, including those that are retroperitoneal. Penetrating injuries involve structures within the path of the weapon; gunshot wounds may also injure adjacent structures through the blast effect or cavitation. A stab or gunshot wound of the abdomen can penetrate across the diaphragm into the chest or vice versa. Ultrasonography, angiography, CT scan, and peritoneal lavage are useful diagnostic tests to assess the extent of abdominal injuries and to determine indications for surgical intervention. Injuries to the great vessels require an immediate surgical procedure to control bleeding and restore vascular continuity. Major organ injuries mandate a laparotomy for repair or reconstruction or to resect severely damaged tissues. Time is a critical factor that significantly influences survival.

Many patients have multiple injuries that affect more than one body system. These patients require a comprehensive approach to diagnosis and treatment by a multidisciplinary team. The philosophy of trauma management has changed from that of an individual surgeon treating an injured patient in the emergency department and operating room (OR) to a system that begins at the site of the accident with stabilization by trained personnel and continues with definitive care, including rapid surgical intervention and rehabilitation.

COMPLICATIONS OF ABDOMINAL SURGERY

Patients are particularly prone to pulmonary complications following abdominal surgery. They are also subject to a variety of fluid and electrolyte imbalances because they generally have an NPO status (nothing by mouth) postoperatively.

They may also lose sodium, potassium, chloride, and water through nasogastric suction. If great quantities of alkalotic pancreatic secretions are lost through decompression of the small bowel, metabolic acidosis may result. The loss of acidic stomach secretions may lead to metabolic alkalosis.

Peritonitis and wound infection may result after gastrointestinal surgery because of spillage of contaminants from the lumen of the gastrointestinal tract. *Escherichia coli* and *Bacteroides fragilis* are the most common organisms; *Clostridium perfringens,* the chief cause of gas gangrene, can also be found in the intestinal tract. Wound infection can cause wound disruption and/or the formation of scar tissue; the latter is enhanced by peritonitis or postoperative radiation therapy. Even years after an abdominal procedure, increased intraabdominal pressure may induce an incisional hernia through an old scar that has weakened.

Adhesions are the most common cause of postoperative intestinal obstruction. They are caused by an outpouring of fibrin from traumatized tissues, which causes intestinal surfaces to stick together and thus limits mobility. Foreign bodies in the peritoneal cavity can produce granulomas that stimulate fibrin. Glove powder, lint from sponges, and some powerful antibiotics also can produce granulomas. Some patients must return to the OR for lysis of adhesions. Adhesions may present a contraindication for future laparoscopic surgery.

ANORECTAL PROCEDURES

Hemorrhoids, abscesses, fissures, and fistulas are often indications for surgical intervention. The anal region is well supplied with nerves, and these procedures often cause much discomfort. Patients are also sensitive and embarrassed because of the surgical site. Following rectal surgery, patients may have an initial difficulty voiding and usually experience considerable pain, which requires medication and sitz baths.

Anoscopy, Proctoscopy, Sigmoidoscopy

Endoscopic diagnostic procedures such as anoscopy, proctoscopy, and sigmoidoscopy are used for visual examination of the mucosa of the anus, rectum, and sigmoid. Sigmoidoscopy is routinely performed before rectal surgery. Fiberoptic equipment has aided in the early detection and treatment of tumors, polyps, and ulcerations.

Hemorrhoidectomy

Hemorrhoidectomy is the surgical removal of varicosities of veins or prolapsed mucosa of the anus and rectum that do not respond to conservative treatment. Hemorrhoids are classified as internal (occurring above the internal sphincter and covered with columnar mucosa), or external (appearing outside the external sphincter and covered with skin). Often both types are present in the patient. External hemorrhoids cause pruritus and pain, whereas the internal type often bleed and may become thrombosed and edematous. Rectal bleeding cannot be assumed to be a result of hemorrhoids; a thorough investigation is required to rule out gastrointestinal disease.

The usual procedure for a hemorrhoidectomy consists of dilating the sphincter, ligating the hemorrhoidal pedicle with suture ligatures, and excising each hemorrhoidal mass with a sharp dissection, laser, ESU, or cryosurgical unit. The Kraske position is usually used, with the patient's buttocks retracted by hemorrhoid straps that are fastened to the edges of the operating bed. Some surgeons prefer to position female patients in the lithotomy position to avoid contamination of the vagina with bloody anal fluid. Petrolatum gauze packing may be inserted in the anal canal, or a compression dressing and perineal binder are applied at completion of the surgical procedure.

As an alternative to a surgical procedure, McGivney rubber-band ligation of internal hemorrhoids is a popular office procedure. After infiltration of a local anesthetic, the hemorrhoid is visualized with an anoscope and grasped with the ligating instruments. Two bands are placed around the base of each hemorrhoid. Sloughing of the avascularized hemorrhoid occurs in 7 to 10 days.

Incision and Drainage of an Anal Abscess

Localized infection in tissues around the anus results in abscess formation. Early incision and drainage are essential to prevent spreading of the infection.

Fistulotomy, Fistulectomy

An anal fistula often develops after incision and drainage or the spontaneous drainage of an anorectal abscess. A fistulous tract may be opened (fistulotomy) to allow drainage and healing by granulation, or the tract may be excised (fistulectomy). Injection of a dye or the use of a probe and grooved director aids in identifying the tract. Fistulas can be excised with a laser beam.

Fissurectomy

When a benign ulcerative lesion occurs in the lining of the anal canal, the anus is dilated and the infected tissue is excised. Some fissures can be vaporized with a laser. Fecal incontinence caused by damage to the anal sphincter is a potential complication that the surgeon tries to avoid.

Treatment of Rectal Tumors

Surgeons prefer to resect a small rectal cancer instead of performing a radical surgical procedure. Many cancers within 20 cm of the anal verge are amenable to local treatment with endoscopic, laser, or cryosurgical techniques. Electrosurgical cutting and coagulating can also be combined to remove superficial anorectal and pararectal lesions. For electrosection, the lesion should be small, mobile, and polypoid, with no palpable lymph nodes. The procedure may be performed for palliation to relieve bleeding, painful sphincter spasms (tenesmus), or severe constipation. Interstitial radiation therapy is sometimes used for small anorectal squamous cell carcinomas. The protocol may include external radiation, but bleeding lesions do not respond well to radiation.

In a procedure called transanal endoscopic microsurgery (TEM), tumors in the upper half of the rectum may be excised through an operating rectoscope. This long, tubular instrument improves the surgeon's visual image by incorporating a binocular stereoscope. With TEM, carbon dioxide is insufflated to hold open the walls of the rectum. Tissue graspers, a high-frequency knife, suction, needleholders, and other instruments can be inserted through ports in the airtight eyepiece on the rectoscope. TEM may be used to remove benign lesions and some malignant tumors.

EXCISION OF PILONIDAL CYSTS AND SINUSES

A painful draining cyst with fistulous tract(s) may occur in the soft tissues of the sacrococcygeal region. When the cyst becomes infected, drainage is necessary to relieve pain, swelling, and suppuration. The cyst and sinus tracts are excised or marsupialized to prevent recurrence. Marsupialization is the suturing of cyst walls to the edges of the wound following evacuation; this permits the packed cavity to close by granulation. A Z-plasty may be preferred for primary closure to produce a strong transverse scar, or the wound may be closed with a rotational pedicle flap. Surgical judgment determines whether primary closure or healing by granulation is chosen.

HERNIA PROCEDURES

A hernia is the protrusion of an organ or part of an organ through a defect in the supporting structures that normally contain it. A hernia may be congenital, acquired, or traumatic. Most occur in the inguinal or femoral region, but umbilical, ventral, and hiatal hernias also occur. A hernia is usually composed of a sac (covering), hernial contents, and an aperture (opening), but in some locations the sac is absent.

A hernia is called reducible when the hernial contents can be returned to the normal cavity by manipulation. If this cannot be done, the hernia is called irreducible or incarcerated. Bowel present in an incarcerated hernia may not only lack adequate blood supply but also may become obstructed. This is referred to as a strangulated hernia, and an immediate surgical procedure is necessary to prevent necrosis of the strangulated bowel.

Inguinal Herniorrhaphy

An inguinal hernia is often repaired with the patient under local anesthesia. An oblique inguinal incision on the affected side is extended through external oblique aponeurosis. The hernia sac is emptied of its contents, ligated, and excised, and the floor of the inguinal canal is reconstructed. Prosthetic mesh is sometimes needed to reinforce a large or recurrent defect.

Repair depends on whether the inguinal hernia is indirect or direct. In both indirect and direct inguinal herniorrhaphy in male patients, the spermatic cord and blood supply to the testis are protected from injury. If herniorrhaphies are performed bilaterally, severance of the cords will cause sterility. Infarction of a testis can occur if the blood supply is compromised.

Indirect Hernia

With an indirect hernia, the peritoneal sac containing intestine protrudes through the internal inguinal ring and passes down the inguinal canal. It may descend all the way into the scrotum. An indirect inguinal hernia, more common in male patients, originates from a congenital defect in the fascial floor of the inguinal canal.

Direct Hernia

A direct hernia protrudes through a weakness in the abdominal wall in the region between the rectus abdominis muscle, inguinal ligament, and inferior epigastric artery. This hernia is the most difficult type to repair and is more common in men. An acquired weakness of the lower abdominal wall, a direct inguinal hernia often results from straining, such as heavy lifting, chronic coughing, or straining to urinate or defecate. Prompt surgical repair prevents possible discomfort and the threat of later complications.

Laparoscopic Repair

A laparoscopic procedure may be used to repair either an indirect or a direct reducible inguinal hernia. This procedure is particularly advantageous for repairing bilateral or recurrent hernias. A transabdominal preperitoneal or intraperitoneal approach may be used, or an extraperitoneal procedure can be performed. Polypropylene mesh is inserted to reinforce the wall of the inguinal canal; this is stapled in place.

Femoral Herniorrhaphy

Femoral herniorrhaphy involves repairing the defect in the transversalis fascia below the inguinal ligament, as well as removing the peritoneal sac protruding through the femoral ring. The transversalis fascia is normally attached to Cooper's ligament, which prevents the peritoneum from reaching the femoral ring. To repair this defect it is necessary to reconstruct the posterior wall and close the femoral ring. These hernias are more common in women.

Umbilical Herniorrhaphy

Repair of an umbilical hernia consists of closing the peritoneal opening and uniting the fasciae above and below the defect to reconstruct the abdominal wall surrounding the umbilicus. This type of hernia is seen most often in children and represents a congenital defect of protrusion of the peritoneum through the umbilical ring. It may also be acquired by women following childbirth.

Ventral (Incisional) Herniorrhaphy

Impaired healing of a previous surgical incision, usually a vertical abdominal incision, may cause an incisional hernia. Often the result of a weakening of abdominal fasciae, projections of peritoneum carrying segments of bowel protrude through fascial perforations. It is necessary to reunite the tissue layers to close the defect. After excising the old scar, the peritoneal sac is opened, the hernia is reduced, and the layers are firmly closed. If existing tissue is not sufficient for repair, synthetic mesh may be used to reinforce the repair. Incisional hernias are sometimes the aftermath of postoperative hematoma, infection, or undue strain.

Ventral hernias have a high recurrence rate when mesh is placed on the outside of a large repair. Through an intraabdominal laparoscopic approach, omentum can be placed over the mesh, or the peritoneum can be put back over the mesh.

Hiatal (Diaphragmatic) Herniorrhaphy

A hiatal hernia results when a portion of the stomach protrudes through the hiatus of the diaphragm. The hiatus is the opening for the esophagus through the diaphragm, the chief muscle of respiration. A weakening in the hiatus permits violation of the muscular partition between the abdomen and the chest. Symptoms are caused mainly by inflammation and ulceration of the adjacent esophagus, which results from the reflux of gastric juices from the herniated stomach. Symptoms include pain, blood loss, and difficulty in swallowing (dysphagia). Diagnosis is made by radiologic and endoscopic studies.

Surgical treatment is appropriate when medical therapy fails to alleviate the problem. The surgical approach may be thoracoabdominal or via the abdomen or chest; each approach offers certain advantages. The abdominal approach is generally preferred, but opening the chest may provide a better view of the hiatal region and thus may be preferred.

AMPUTATION OF EXTREMITIES

Amputation is the total or partial removal of any extremity. The need for amputation is associated most often with massive trauma, a malignant tumor, extensive infection, and vascular insufficiency. Orthopaedic or vascular surgeons may perform these procedures.

In preparing the patient for a lower extremity amputation, the patient's chart is checked, and both legs are exposed for comparison before skin preparation. It must be made absolutely certain that the correct leg is prepared.

Many lower extremity amputations are performed with the patient under spinal anesthesia. It must be ensured that the specimen is never, at any time, within the patient's sight. Policy is followed in regard to the patient's permission for disposal of an extremity.

In general, two types of amputation are performed: open (guillotine) and closed. The guillotine procedure is regarded as an emergency procedure and is rarely performed. Patients who are severely ill or toxic or who experience severe trauma (e.g., an extremity caught under an immovable object) are candidates for this procedure. In the guillotine procedure, tissues are cut circularly with the bone transected higher to allow soft tissues to cover the bone end. Blood vessels and nerve endings are ligated, but the wound is left open. The surgical procedure is often followed by prolonged drainage and healing, muscle and skin retraction, and excessive granulation tissue. A second procedure is often required for final repair.

The conventional flap or closed type of amputation is more desirable. Fashioning curved skin and fascial flaps before amputation of the bone allows deep and superficial fasciae to be approximated over the bone end before closure of the loose skin. Drainage by catheter or suction apparatus may or may not be required. The wound usually heals in approximately 2 weeks.

Amputations of the Lower Extremity

Amputations of the lower extremity are classified as above-knee (AK), below-knee (BK), toe, transphalangeal, transmetatarsal, and the Syme amputation. The level of amputation is determined by the patient's general health, vascular status, and potential for rehabilitation.

Above-Knee Amputation

Amputation at the lower third of the thigh is selected when gangrene or arterial insufficiency extends above the level of the malleoli. A mid-thigh amputation involves making a circular incision over the distal femur, creating large anterior and posterior skin flaps, and transecting fascia and muscles. Vessels and nerves such as the femoral and sciatic nerves, respectively, are ligated and severed. Sharp bone edges of the stump are smoothed by filing. The wound is irrigated with sterile normal saline solution before closure of tissue layers. Hemostasis is important to prevent massive hemorrhage or painful hematoma. Drains may be used depending on the surgeon's preference. A noncompressive dressing is applied. AK amputation is a more extensive procedure than BK amputation, and thus a longer time is required for rehabilitation. In general, a prosthesis is fitted 4 to 6 weeks after amputation.

Below-Knee Amputation

Amputation at the middle third of the leg provides for more functional prosthesis fitting and the reduction of phantom limb pain; it also permits a more natural gait. An immediate postoperative prosthesis (IPOP) can be applied in the OR. The IPOP dressing requires a stump sock, felt and lamb's wool for padding, twill Y-straps that are attached to a fitted corset, and a rigid plaster dressing. This dressing not only protects the stump but aids in controlling the weight placed on it. The prosthesis is metal and provides a pull on the stump. The pylon (foot) may be attached before the patient returns to the unit. If the patient is obese or debilitated, weight bearing may be delayed for several days.

Toe and Transmetatarsal Amputations

Toe and partial foot amputations are generally performed for gangrene and osteomyelitis.

Syme Amputation

A Syme amputation is usually performed for trauma and involves the distal part of the foot. The amputation is above the ankle joint. The skin of the heel is used for the flap.

Hip Disarticulation and Hemipelvectomy

Hip disarticulation and hemipelvectomy involve total removal of the right or left pelvis, including the innominate hipbone, along the ipsilateral lower extremity. The division of bone may be carried through the sacroiliac joint, or a portion of iliac bone and crest may be preserved. An internal hemipelvectomy includes the removal of innominate bone with adjacent muscles. The large defect created may be covered by a myocutaneous flap of the quadriceps femoris muscle and the overlying skin and subcutaneous tissue. The neck of the femur rests against the soft tissues. These radical procedures are indicated for malignant bone or soft tissue tumors and extensive traumatic injuries. Specialized prosthetic devices are available to permit ambulation.

Amputations of the Upper Extremity
Amputations of the Hand

Hand amputations usually result from trauma and include part or all of the distal phalanges of the digits. Attention is directed to keeping the hand as a working unit when one or more fingers are removed. Every effort should be made to save the thumb—the smallest stump is better than a prosthesis.

Forearm and Forequarter Amputation

Wrist, elbow, and humerus disarticulations are radical procedures performed for malignant tumors or extensive trauma.

Rehabilitation

Postoperative considerations for any amputation include control of bleeding and phantom limb sensations, stump care, immediate fitting of a functional terminal prosthesis, exercises to prevent flexion contractures, and ambulation or use of a hand or arm.

The loss of an extremity involves major psychologic and physical adjustments. The rehabilitative process is very important and is often affected by the emotional reactions of the patient. Patients with an early postoperative prosthesis have a more positive outlook about their loss. Morale is boosted by being able to walk the first postoperative day or soon thereafter (which, in the case of a leg amputation, depends on the surgeon's orders for the weight-bearing program). This in turn aids in ambulation.

Phantom limb pain is particularly distressing to many patients. The nerves have been severed, but the patient has the sensation that the amputated part is still present. This sensa-

tion is often associated with painful paresthesia (i.e., tingling, prickling, tickling, or burning). The pain is real. It usually responds to aspirin, acetaminophen (Tylenol), or a similar agent, but narcotics may be necessary to control pain. The combined efforts of the patient, family, and interdisciplinary professional personnel are needed for successful rehabilitation.

Bibliography

Boshaw DL: New instrumentation allows for removal of nonpalpable breast lesions, *AORN J* 66(2):296, 298, 300, 302, 1997.

Butler RW: Managing the complications of cirrhosis, *Am J Nurs* 94(3):46-49, 1994.

Buyske J et al: Breast cancer in the nineties, *AORN J* 64(1):64-65, 67-72, 1996.

Chin AK et al: Gasless laparoscopy using a planar lifting technique, *J Am Coll Surg* 178(4):401-403, 1994.

Clark GJ et al: Laparoscopic distal pancreatectomy procedures in a rural hospital, *AORN J* 65(2):334-343, 1997.

Collins LG: Laparoscopic extraperitoneal herniorrhaphy, *AORN J* 63(6):1089-1098, 1996.

Cooperman AM: *Laparoscopic cholecystectomy: difficult cases and creative solutions,* St Louis, 1992, Quality Medical Publishing.

Deane KA et al: Determining the information needs of women after breast biopsy procedures, *AORN J* 65(4):767-768, 770-772, 775-777, 1997.

Deane KA: The role of the breast clinic nurse, *AORN J* 66(2):304-307, 309-310, 1997.

Geis WP, Malago M: Laparoscopic bilateral inguinal herniorrhaphies: use of a single giant preperitoneal mesh patch, *Am Surg* 60(8):558-563, 1994.

Gonzalez-Cortes SB, Procuniar CE: Laparoscopic inguinal herniorrhaphy, *AORN J* 60(3):419-430, 1994.

Graling PR et al: Managing the patient with perforated intrathoracic esophagus, *AORN J* 68(7):56-67, 1998.

Hashizume M et al: Laparoscopic splenectomy, *Am J Surg* 167(6):611-614, 1994.

Hilmer DM: Technical considerations of bariatric surgery in the superobese, *Surg Technol* 26(7):8-12, 1994.

Lyerly HK, Mault JR: Laparoscopic ileostomy and colostomy, *Ann Surg* 219(3):317-322, 1994.

McEwen DR et al: Managing patients with pancreatic cancer, *AORN J* 64(5):716-735, 1996.

McGinnis C, Matson SW: How to manage patients with a Roux-en-Y jejunostomy, *Am J Nurs* 94(2):43-45, 1994.

McKernan JB, Laws HL: *Laparoscopy and the general surgeon,* Somerville, NJ, 1990, Ethicon.

Payne JH et al: Laparoscopic or open inguinal herniorrhaphy? A randomized trial, *Arch Surg* 129(9):973-979, 1994.

Phillips E et al: Laparoendoscopy and partial resection of the small bowel, *Surg Endosc* 8(6):686-688, 1994.

Rogers MA, Cox JA: Laparoscopic paraesophageal hernia repair with Nissen fundoplication, *AORN J* 67(3):536-551, 1998.

Shoaf BA, Apelgren KN: Intraoperative endoscopy of the small bowel, *AORN J* 51(3):776-782, 1990.

Stengel JM, Dirado R: Laparoscopic Nissen fundoplication to treat gastroesophageal reflux, *AORN J* 61(3):483-489, 1995.

Wyman A et al: Surgery for gastric cancer, *Dig Dis* 12(2):117-126, 1994.

Chapter 35

Gynecologic and Obstetric Surgery

Chapter Objectives

After studying this chapter, the learner will be able to:

- Identify the organs of the female genitourinary system.
- Describe the physiology of the female reproductive system.
- Describe the pertinent considerations when caring for a pregnant patient.

From its inception in 1930 the American Board of Obstetrics and Gynecology has emphasized the inseparability of gynecology and obstetrics because of their anatomic and physiologic relationships. Gynecology, commonly referred to as "gyn" (GYN), is the science of health and diseases of the female reproductive organs. Gynecologic surgery includes certain problems of the female genitourinary tract. Obstetrics (OB) concerns the care of women during pregnancy, labor, and the puerperium (period from delivery to the time the uterus regains normal size, usually about 6 weeks). Although all surgeons certified by the American Board of Obstetrics and Gynecology are competent in both disciplines, some limit their practice to either obstetrics or gynecology. Specialty certification boards have also been established in gynecologic oncology, endocrinology and infertility, and perinatal medicine. This text limits discussion to the most common surgical procedures performed by gynecologists and/or obstetricians in the perioperative environment.

HISTORICAL BACKGROUND

Obstetric care, left to the mother herself or to a midwife, was neglected until the Renaissance. In prehistoric cultures the woman squatted on a bed of leaves, delivered, chewed off or cut the umbilical cord, bathed the infant in a stream, wrapped

the infant in an animal hide, and resumed her womanly duties in the field. Up through the Dark Ages, based on the Biblical decree, "In sorrow shalt thou bring forth children," it was believed that pregnant women should suffer. Some were attended by untrained midwives. The first book on obstetric care was written by the German physician Eucharius Rösslin in 1513, but it was the treatise of François Mauriceau (1637-1709), published in Paris in 1668, that became the basis of obstetrics. Mauriceau's writings described how the mother's pelvic bones did not separate but remained intact during delivery. He is known as the founder of modern obstetrics and gynecology.

The practice of gynecology was limited, bound by tradition, and even regressed during medieval times. New interest developed in the Renaissance. In 1663 the Dutch surgeon Hendri von Roonhuyze (1622-1672) published the first book on surgical obstetrics and gynecology having modern connotations. He described extrauterine pregnancy, uterine rupture, and vesicovaginal fistula. He also performed cesarean sections.

In the eighteenth century, progress was made, particularly in England. Practitioners advocated the treatment of ovarian cysts. However, surgical gynecology did not become an independent specialty until the early nineteenth century. Early male gynecologists fought public prejudice against exposure of female organs, even for examination. Clergy, midwives, and physicians attempted to deter their practice. Opposition to the progress of surgery in general eventually was overcome.

In 1809 Ephraim McDowell of Kentucky successfully removed an ovarian cyst by an abdominal approach without benefit of modern anesthesia or aseptic techniques. The 22-year-old patient survived without complication. A limited variety of gynecologic procedures, such as oophorectomy and salpingectomy, were developed by succeeding pioneers. The first successful vaginal hysterectomy was performed in 1818. Use of the speculum was a notable advance for gynecologists.

The practice of dilating the cervix for a variety of purposes was known since the days of Hippocrates. Many instruments were used. In 1879 Alfred Hegar (1830-1914) developed graduated metal cervical dilators that bear his name and are still commonly used. Softening of the lower uterine segment is a recognized sign of early pregnancy that was named for him.

ANATOMY AND PHYSIOLOGY OF THE FEMALE REPRODUCTIVE SYSTEM

The female genitourinary system comprises the organs, glands, secretions, and other elements of reproduction. Components of the female reproductive system are both external and internal organs.

Female External Genitalia

The term *vulva* is used collectively for the female external genitalia. This sensitive, delicate area is highly vascular, with an extensive superficial and deep lymph supply and rich cutaneous sensory innervation. It includes the following.

Labia Majora

The labia majora are two large folds, or lips, containing sebaccous and sweat glands embedded in fatty tissue covered by hair-bearing skin. They join together anteriorly in a fatty pad, the mons veneris, which overlies the pubic bone (symphysis pubis). In the adult female this area is covered with hair. Sebaceous secretions of the labia lubricate the proximal area. The labia majora atrophy and hair follicles decrease in number after menopause, making the labia minora more prominent.

Labia Minora

The labia minora, or small lips, lying within the labia majora, are flat folds of connective tissue containing sebaceous glands. Anteriorly these labia split into two parts. One part passes anteriorly over the clitoris to form a protective prepuce, or foreskin. The other passes behind the clitoris to shape a frenulum, a fold of mucous membrane. Posteriorly they join across the midline behind the vagina to form the fourchette, or fold of skin just inside the posterior vulvar commissure.

Clitoris

The clitoris, an erectile organ, is the female homologue of the penis. The mucous membrane covering the glans contains many nerve endings and is a source of sexual stimulation for the female. The blood supply is derived from a terminal branch of the pudendal artery, which is a terminal division of the internal iliac artery. The venous drainage is continuous with the labiae plexae. Innervation is from the sacral plexus.

Vestibule

The vestibule is the space, or shallow elliptic depression posterior to the clitoris, enclosed by the labia minora. The urethral opening is located in this region posterior to the clitoris and anterior to the vagina. The fourchette forms the posterior boundary.

Bartholin Glands

Small bilateral Bartholin glands lie deep in the posterior third of the labia majora, within the bulbocavernosus muscle. The mucus secretion is a vaginal lubricant.

Hymen

The hymen is a thin, vascularized connective tissue membrane that surrounds and may partially or completely occlude the vaginal orifice. It varies among individuals in thickness and elasticity. The central aperture permits passage of menstrual flow and vaginal secretions. This structure will vary according to individual anatomy and physical activity. In some patients the aperture may be imperforate or divided by a septum, requiring surgical intervention. The presence or absence of a hymenal ring is not an indicator of sexual activity.

Perineum

The perineum is a diamond-shaped wedge of fibromuscular tissue between the vagina and the anus. It is divided by a transverse septum into an anterior urogenital triangle and a posterior anal triangle. It consists of the perineal body and perineal musculature. With fibers of six muscles converging at its central point, the perineum forms the base of the pelvic floor and helps support the posterior vaginal wall. These muscles are the bulbocavernosus (vaginal sphincter), the two superficial transverse perineal muscles, the two levator ani muscles, and the external anal sphincter. The levator ani muscles are the largest muscles and, in contrast to the other superficial muscles, are deep. The most important muscles in the pelvis, the levator ani muscles form a hammock-type suspension (pelvic diaphragm) from the anterior to the posterior pelvic wall, beneath the pelvic viscera. These muscles retain the organs within the pelvis by offering resistance to repeated increases in intraabdominal pressure, such as coughing, bearing down in labor, and straining at stool.

Internal Female Reproductive Organs

The internal female reproductive organs (Figure 35-1) lie within the pelvic cavity, protected by the bony pelvis. Bones

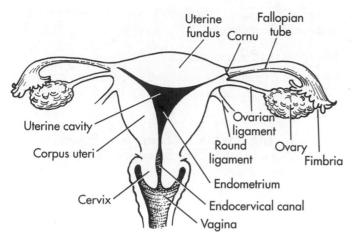

Figure 35-1 Female reproductive system.

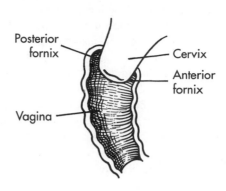

Figure 35-2 Cervix in vaginal vault.

and ligaments form the pelvic outlet. The dilated cervix of the uterus and the vagina constitute the birth canal.

Vagina

The vagina is a thin-walled, 8-cm, fibromuscular tube extending from the vestibule obliquely backward and upward to the uterus, where the cervix projects into the top of the anterior wall. The vagina is elastic and capable of distention during intercourse and parturition. The bladder lies anteriorly to it; the rectum lies posteriorly to it. It is lined with mucous membrane and contains glands that produce a cleansing acid secretion.

The anterior vaginal wall is shorter than the posterior wall. The upper third of the posterior wall is covered by peritoneum reflected onto the rectum. Normally the anterior and posterior walls relax and are in contact. However, the lateral walls remain rigid because of the pull of the muscles and therefore are in close contact with pelvic tissues.

A rich venous plexus in the muscular walls makes the vagina highly vascular. Uterine and vaginal arteries supplying the area are branches of the internal iliac artery. Branches of the vaginal artery extend to the external genitalia and the adjacent bladder and rectum. Lymphatic drainage is extensive. The upper two thirds of the vagina drains into the external and internal iliac nodes; the lower third drains into the superficial inguinal nodes.

The vault (dome, or upper part of the vagina) is divided into four fornices, or arches (Figure 35-2). During digital pelvic examination, pelvic organs can be palpated through the thin walls of the vault. The anterior fornix, in front of the cervix, is adjacent to the base of the bladder and distal ends of the ureters.

The pouch of Douglas (retrouterine cul-de-sac) directly behind the larger posterior fornix lies behind the cervix. This pouch separates the back of the uterus from the rectum: anteriorly by the uterine peritoneal covering, which continues down to cap the posterior vaginal fornix, and posteriorly by the anterior wall of the rectum. Lateral uterosacral ligaments embrace the lower third of the rectum. The floor of the pouch, about 7 cm above the anus, is formed by reflection of

the peritoneum from the rectum to the upper vagina and uterus. The posterior cul-de-sac is the route of entry for a number of diagnostic or surgical procedures because the pouch of Douglas, the lowest part of the peritoneal cavity, is separated from the vagina only by the thin vaginal wall and peritoneum.

The lateral fornices lie on either side of the cervix, in contact with anterior and posterior sheets of the broad ligaments surrounding the uterus. Proximal structures are the uterine artery, ureters, fallopian tubes, ovaries, and sigmoid colon.

Uterus

The uterus is the female organ of gestation. It receives and holds the fertilized ovum during development of the fetus and expels it during childbirth. Resembling an inverted pear in shape, this hollow muscular retroperitoneal organ is situated in the bony pelvis. It lies between the bladder anteriorly and the sigmoid colon posteriorly. The uterus is divided transversely by a slight constriction into a wider upper part—the body or corpus uteri—and a narrower lower part—the 2- to 3-cm cervix uteri or ectocervix that protrudes into the vagina (see Figure 35-2). The corpus meets the cervix at the internal os. Peritoneum covers the corpus externally; the endometrium, ranging in thickness from 2 to 10 mm, lines it internally. This mucous membrane is uniquely adapted to receive and sustain the fertilized ovum. The fundus, or dome-like portion of the uterus, lies above the uterine cavity.

The uterine cavity, flattened from front to back, is roughly triangular in shape in the nonpregnant female. The upper lateral angles extend out toward openings of the fallopian tubes, which enter bilaterally through the uterine walls at the cornua. The apex of the triangle is directed downward to the cervix. The cavity within the cervix, the endocervical canal, narrows to a slit at the distal orifice where the cervix communicates with the vagina via the external os. The endocervix is the glandular mucous membrane of the cervix. The corpus of the uterus and the cervix are considered individually in relation to disease and therapy because they differ in structure and function.

As the incubator and nurturer of the developing embryo, the uterus is capable of expansion. Much of the bulk of the corpus consists of involuntary muscle, the myometrium, composed of three layers. The inner layer prevents reflux of menstrual flow into the tubes and peritoneal cavity, which could result in endometriosis. It also contributes to the competency of the internal os sphincter to prevent premature expulsion of the fetus. The middle layer encloses large blood vessels. These muscle fibers act as living ligatures for hemostasis after delivery. The outer layer has expulsive action, ejecting menstrual flow and clots, an aborted embryo, or the fetus at term.

Usually the uterus lies forward at a right angle to the vagina and rests on the bladder. Although the cervix is anchored laterally by ligaments, the fundus may pivot about the cardinal ligaments widely in an anterior-posterior plane. Mobility rather than position is the criterion for normality.

Fallopian Tubes (Salpinges)

The fallopian tubes, small, hollow musculomembranous tubes, sometimes called oviducts or uterine tubes, run bilaterally like arms from each side of the upper part of the uterus to the ovaries. Near each ovary the open end of each tube expands into the infundibulum, which divides into fimbriae—fingerlike projections that sweep up the ovum (the female reproductive cell) as it is expelled from the ovary. Ciliated cells move the ovum toward the uterus. The lumen of the tube becomes very narrow where it penetrates the uterine wall to reach the uterine cavity. Contractions in the muscular walls change the shape and position of the tubes. At ovulation they move the fimbriated ends into close apposition with ovarian surfaces. The fallopian tubes serve as a continuous passage from the external environment into the abdominal cavity via the vagina, cervix, and uterine body. Infectious diseases and other substances can enter the peritoneal cavity through this route.

Ovaries

The ovaries are oval-shaped glandular gonads located in shallow peritoneal fossae on the lateral pelvic walls, from which they are suspended by the infundibulopelvic ligaments. They are attached to the posterior layer of the broad ligament by the mesovarium (a peritoneal fold) and to the uterus by the ovarian ligament (a fibromuscular cord).

The ovaries, the counterpart of the male testes, contain ova. Each ovary measures 2×3 cm and consists of a center of cells and vessels surrounded by the cortex. This main portion contains the stroma or fibrous framework in which the ovarian follicles are embedded. Of the approximately 200,000 primordial follicles present at birth, less than 400 are likely to produce a mature ovum (graafian follicle) during the reproductive years. A serous covering derived from peritoneum surrounds the ovaries. In addition to protecting maturing ova, the ovaries, which atrophy after menopause, produce female sex hormones.

The ureters course along the retroperitoneum bilaterally and lie close to the ovarian blood supply just anterior to the common iliac arteries. The ovaries, when diseased, may be adherent to the ureters.

Muscles and Ligaments

Muscles and ligaments support and suspend the uterus and fallopian tubes in the normal position in the center of the pelvic cavity.

Broad Ligaments Bilateral broad ligaments are composed of a broad double sheet of peritoneum extending from each lateral surface of the uterus outward to the pelvic wall. Between these two layers of peritoneum, the fallopian tubes are enclosed in the free upper borders (mesosalpinges), with the tubal ostia opening directly into the peritoneal cavity.

Round Ligaments The round ligaments are fibromuscular bands that extend from the anterior surface of the lateral borders of the fundus to the labia majora. They run beneath the peritoneum and anterior sheet of the broad ligament down, outward, and forward through the inguinal canal to the labia.

Cardinal Ligaments The lower portion of the broad ligaments, the cardinal ligaments are attached to the lateral vaginal fornices and supravaginal portion of the cervix. They act as a supportive pivot.

Uterosacral Ligaments The uterosacral ligaments are peritoneal folds containing connective tissue and involuntary muscle. They arise on each side from the posterior wall of the uterus at the level of the internal os, pass backward around the rectum, and insert on the sacrum at the level of the second sacral vertebra. They pull on the cervix to keep the uterus anteverted and, through the cervix, the vagina in position as well.

Physiology

The function of the female reproductive organs is to conceive, nurture, and produce offspring. The development and function of these organs are influenced by the hormonal secretions of the ovaries and adrenal, thyroid, and pituitary glands. These hormonal relationships also affect primary and secondary sex characteristics.

The physiologic hormonal cycle prepares the uterus for the fertilized ovum. Hormone production stimulates the endometrium and breasts, resulting in thickening of tissue and increased blood supply.

Each month during the years from puberty to menopause, one (or both) of the ovaries matures a follicle from within. When the matured graafian follicle ruptures, it discharges the enclosed ovum, which enters the fallopian tube at the fimbriated end. The process of maturation and discharge of the egg is called ovulation, resulting in a fertile period that lasts several days. Changes in cervical mucus and vaginal epithelium also accompany ovulation. Union of the ovum with a viable mature male germ cell (spermatozoon), which has ascended to the fallopian tube from the vagina, results in fertilization within 12 hours of ovulation. The union takes place in the outer third of the tube and travels toward the uterus over a period of 3 days. The fertilized ovum normally proceeds to the cornu of the uterus, where it enters to implant in the endometrium within 14 days of fertilization. By day 17 the blood supply of the fetal and maternal blood vessels are functional. The placental circulation is established. The ensuing pregnancy will last approximately 266 days, or 9 calendar months, if carried to full term.

The ovarian hormone estrogen, together with progesterone, causes a sequence of changes in the endometrial lining of the uterus to prepare for implantation of the fertilized ovum. Estrogen also produces the development of secondary sexual characteristics. Progesterone is responsible for maintaining pregnancy until hormones from the placenta assume this role.

Menstruation is the periodic discharge of blood, mucus, disintegrated ovum, and uterine mucosa formed during the hormonal cycle if pregnancy does not take place. The duration of the menstrual period varies but averages 3 to 5 days. The amount of blood lost varies greatly. The menstrual cycle, the time between the onset of each period, is approximately 28 days. Regularity of menstruation can be disturbed by disease conditions and emotions in addition to the onset of pregnancy. This physiologic cycle continually recurs throughout the reproductive life of the woman. Assessment of the female patient should include documentation of the age of menarche (first menses), the date of the last menstrual period (LMP), use of contraception, and sexual history. The possibility of pregnancy should be taken into consideration if the female patient is within childbearing age, regardless of status or vocation. A surgical procedure and/or the administration of anesthetic agents could be hazardous to a developing embryo.

GYNECOLOGY: GENERAL CONSIDERATIONS

The emotional preparation of gynecologic patients presents a special challenge to the operating room (OR) team. Anticipation of physical exposure, potential loss of sexual function, infertility problems, or termination of pregnancy can create severe anxiety. Some surgical procedures terminate reproductive capability and produce menopause. Patients must be able to express concerns, ask questions, and receive reassurance and support.

Examination with the Patient Under Anesthesia

Bimanual examination of the pelvis with the patient in the lithotomy position and relaxed from anesthesia usually precedes vaginal and abdominal gynecologic surgical procedures. This allows the surgeon to thoroughly assess the size, outline, consistency, position, and mobility of the uterus, fallopian tubes, and ovaries. This examination also helps the surgeon determine or confirm the approach for the procedure

and whether a lesion is resectable. This is helpful in evaluating women experiencing pain or nervous tension or those who are obese. The vaginal vault and perineum are prepped and the examination is performed before prepping the abdomen for laparotomy.

Special Features of Gynecologic Surgery

Diagnostic and surgical procedures may be carried out through a vaginal or abdominal approach, or the two approaches may be combined. Each requires a different position and different preparation, drapes, and setup. Surgical techniques for general abdominal procedures apply to gynecologic surgery. Diagnostic and surgical procedures are often combined and done in one surgical procedure.

The following applies to both vaginal and abdominopelvic procedures:

1. Spinal, epidural, or more commonly, general anesthesia is used. An epidural catheter may be inserted preoperatively for postoperative pain control.
2. A Foley catheter may be inserted after the administration of anesthesia to prevent the bladder from becoming distended during the procedure and to record urinary output. The circulator should check the urinary drainage bag frequently and report urine volume or evidence of blood. This could indicate injury to the bladder or ureters. Insertion of a cannula directly into the bladder through the abdominal wall (suprapubic cystostomy) provides an alternative indwelling drainage system in selected patients.
3. An electrosurgical unit (ESU), with either monopolar or bipolar electrodes, is frequently employed.
4. Argon, CO_2, and Nd:YAG lasers are used, usually in conjunction with a colposcope or laparoscope and the operating microscope.
5. Closed wound suction drainage, or another type of drain, may be used to prevent hematoma or serum accumulation in the pelvis and/or the wound.
6. Prophylactic preoperative anticoagulation with subcutaneous heparin, antiembolic stockings, sequential compression devices, and early ambulation are especially important in pelvic surgery because of the potential for deep vein thrombosis.

Vaginal Approach

1. The patient is in the lithotomy position.
2. Instrumentation must be of sufficient length for use within the vaginal canal and uterine cavity. In addition to retracting, cutting, holding, clamping and suturing instruments, vaginal setups include dilation and curettage (D&C) instruments for intrauterine procedures (Table 35-1).
3. A laser, ESU, or cryosurgical unit may be used to remove hypertrophied tissue or certain benign neoplasms.
4. A suction system, including a Poole suction tip with guard, tubing, and collection canister, is part of the setup.

TABLE 35-1 Instruments for Dilation and Curettage

Purpose	Instruments
To expose	Vaginal speculum Posterior retractor Weighted posterior retractor Narrow lateral Heaney retractors
To grasp and hold	Single- and double-toothed tenaculi
To measure uterine cavity	Uterine sound (graduated probe)
To dilate cervix	Graduated dilators Goodell dilator
To scrape tissue	Sharp and blunt, large and small uterine curettes
To obtain specimen	Endometrial biopsy suction curette
To carry sponges	Sponge forceps
To remove polyps and biopsy tissue	Polyp and biopsy forceps
To insert packing	Uterine dressing forceps

5. Sponges may be secured on sponge forceps in deep areas (also referred to as sponge sticks). Long, narrow, 4 × 18 inch sponges with radiopaque markers on the end are used for packing off abdominal viscera in vaginal procedures. All counts are very important in these procedures.
6. Vaginal packing is inserted following certain procedures. Antibiotic or hormone cream may be applied to the packing during insertion. Impregnated vaginal packing is commercially available. The packing should be recorded on the patient's chart and removed at the surgeon's order.
7. At the completion of the surgical procedure, a sanitary pad is placed against the perineum between the patient's legs.

Abdominal Approach

1. The supine or Trendelenburg position is used for abdominopelvic procedures. Preparation and drapes are the same as for abdominal laparotomy.
2. When a large abdominal mass is present or the pelvic organs are pushed from their normal relationships, ureteral catheters may be inserted via cystoscopy before the surgical procedure to facilitate identification of the ureters to prevent inadvertent dissection. Severing of the ureters during the procedure greatly increases postoperative morbidity and mortality if the injury is not immediately detected and corrected.
3. Instrumentation includes the basic laparotomy setup with the addition of long instruments for deep manipulations within the pelvis.

Abdominal Complications   Injuries to ureters, which can lead to loss of renal function if unrecognized, can occur during the surgical procedure because of their rela-

tionship to pelvic structures. The surgeon must identify and isolate the ureter(s) on the affected side(s) to prevent accidental crushing or kinking.

Adhesions following pelvic surgery can cause infertility, intestinal obstruction, and/or chronic abdominal pain. The surgeon may place a biodegradable fabric (Interceed Absorbable Adhesion Barrier) over tissues and pelvic organs before closing the peritoneal cavity. This satinlike, knitted fabric acts as a physical barrier to prevent adhesion formation during the healing process. Within 8 hours the fabric becomes a gelatinous protective coating. This is completely absorbed within 28 days.

Combined Vaginal-Abdominal Approach

If vaginal and abdominal surgery is indicated, a combined procedure is planned. For example, the patient may be scheduled for a total abdominal hysterectomy with anterior vaginal colporrhaphy. In such instances the vaginal procedure is performed first. The patient is then removed from the lithotomy position and repositioned in the supine position, and the abdominal preparation and surgical procedure are carried out.

The following considerations apply:

1. Because of the possibility of infection, separate sterile setups are used for vaginal and abdominal procedures performed concurrently.
2. Vaginal preparation precedes exploratory pelvic laparotomy in readiness for the unexpected or for a D&C scheduled to precede an abdominal procedure. A separate sterile prep table is used for the external genitalia and vagina. Another sterile setup is used for the abdominal preparation.

DIAGNOSTIC TECHNIQUES

The gynecologist employs both noninvasive and invasive diagnostic techniques. Some are performed as office or ambulatory procedures, especially those using the vaginal approach.

A pelvic examination includes inspection and palpation of the external genitalia; bimanual abdominovaginal and abdominorectal palpation of the uterus, fallopian tubes, and ovaries; and speculum examination of the vagina and cervix. This inspection is augmented by a cytologic study of smears of cervical and endocervical tissue obtained by scrapings. The Papanicolaou (Pap) smear has significantly facilitated diagnosis of cervical cancer and premalignant lesions. Characteristic cellular changes in cervical epithelial cells are identified. Cytologic aspiration from within the endocervical canal may reveal unsuspected carcinoma of the endometrium, fallopian tubes, or ovaries and occult cervical cancer.

Schiller's test involves staining the vaginal vault and cervical squamous epithelium with Lugol's solution. Glycogen in normal epithelium takes up the iodine. Abnormal tissues, with little or no glycogen, do not stain brown and thereby pinpoint sites for biopsy. Abnormal cytologic findings are an indication for further evaluation by histologic tissue study. Use of iodine products is contraindicated in patients with systemic iodine allergy.

Uterine cancer consists of two entities: cervical cancer and endometrial cancer. These differ by age-groups, types, and consequences. Cancer of the cervix appears most often in association with coitus at an early age, multiple partners, nonbarrier contraceptives, poor sexual hygiene, a chronically infected cervix, or a history of sexually transmitted diseases. These include infection with herpes simplex virus (HSV), human papillomavirus (HPV), cytomegalovirus (CMV), *Chlamydia trachomatis,* and *Trichomonas vaginalis.* A higher frequency of abnormal Pap smear findings are associated with these infections. HPV produces condylomas (venereal warts), which have been identified as a possible cause of cervical carcinoma. Cancer of the endometrium, more common than cervical cancer, occurs primarily in postmenopausal women. It is often associated with obesity, low parity, late menopause, hypertension, and diabetes mellitus.

Biopsy of the Cervix

Cervical cancer may not present symptoms in the early stage and may progress to invasion before discovery. Spotting, postmenopausal bleeding, or chronic cervicitis may be the first visible signs. The condition may be suspected by results of cytologic examination or visual inspection, but diagnosis is made by biopsy.

Excisional Biopsy

In excisional biopsy an attempt is made to excise the entire cervical lesion by sharp dissection. Sutures or ESUs are used for hemostasis. Packing may be needed.

Incisional Biopsy

Incisional biopsy involves the use of a scalpel, punch biopsy, or other instrument to obtain tissue for diagnosis but not to remove the lesion. If a malignancy is diagnosed, additional evaluation and further treatment is carried out by additional surgery and/or radiation therapy.

Cone Biopsy

Patients diagnosed by Pap smear as having severe cervical dysplasia or intraepithelial carcinoma of the cervix require conization to remove the lesion and rule out invasive carcinoma. The biopsy, obtained with a laser, scalpel, or cervitome (cold knife conization), includes the squamocolumnar junctions of the ectocervix (transformation zone) and is tapered to include the endocervical canal to the level of the internal os. Most of the lesions categorized as cervical intraepithelial neoplasia (CIN), dysplasia, or carcinoma in situ are found in this area. Conization of the cervix provides the most comprehensive specimen to diagnose a premalignant or malignant lesion. Multiple blocks and sections are examined by the pathologist to determine the extent of invasive disease.

Complications include hemorrhage, infection, cervical stenosis, an incompetent cervix, and infertility. The cutting beam of the CO_2 laser used for conization minimizes these risks. Hemostasis is secured with sutures as needed.

Fractional Curettage

Tissue is obtained for histologic examination by scraping the uterine cavity. Fractional curettage differentiates specimens between the endocervix and the endometrium. A biopsy specimen may be taken from the cervix, if indicated by Schiller's test, in association with curettage. A small curette is introduced into the endocervical canal, which is scraped from the internal to the external os. The specimen is placed on a Telfa pad, and both are put into a container. This scraping precedes cervical dilation to avoid dislodging tissue from above. After dilation, a curette is inserted into the uterine cavity for curettage of the endometrium. The endometrial specimen is placed in a separate container from those obtained by endocervical curettage.

Colposcopy

Illumination and binocular magnification afforded by the colpomicroscope permit identification of abnormal epithelium to target for biopsy. The colposcope has a cool, intense white light that can be fitted with a green filter to improve visualization of the vascular pattern. With the colposcope positioned in front of the vulva, without touching the patient, the colposcopist can focus light through a speculum on the ectocervix, the lower part of the cervical canal, and the vaginal wall. The cervix is wiped with 3% acetic acid to eradicate mucus and to facilitate viewing the surface and vasculature. Biopsies are taken for histologic confirmation of the diagnosis. Endocervical curettage may also be performed. A video or still camera can be attached to a colposcope to photograph lesions.

Vaginal condylomas and adenoses, preinvasive lesions of the cervix, cervical dysplasia, CIN, and other vaginal and cervical lesions can be treated by laser with the colpomicroscope. Visualization, unobstructed by instruments, is excellent. Condylomas appear as white raised areas when exposed to acetic acid. The laser permits selective destruction of large areas of vaginal epithelium without vaginal or cervical stenosis. It cuts, coagulates, seals, and sterilizes simultaneously. This results in less blood loss, a shorter period of vaginal discharge after treatment of the cervix, and a lower incidence of infection than in other surgical treatment modalities. Electrosurgery and cryosurgery are other options to ablate lesions.

Culdocentesis and Colpotomy
Culdocentesis

In culdocentesis blood, fluid, or pus in the cul-de-sac is aspirated by needle via the posterior vaginal fornix for suspected intraperitoneal bleeding, ectopic pregnancy, or tubo-ovarian abscess.

Posterior Colpotomy

In posterior colpotomy a transverse incision is made through the posterior vaginal fornix into the posterior cul-de-sac to facilitate diagnosis by intraperitoneal palpation, inspection of the pelvic organs, or determination of free fluid, blood, or pus in the pouch of Douglas. Pus from a pelvic abscess or blood, possibly a sign of ectopic pregnancy or a ruptured ovarian cyst, is evacuated. Tubes and ovaries are inspected. If they are normal, the incision is closed. A drain may be inserted.

Some surgical procedures, such as aspiration of an ovarian cyst or reproductive sterilization by tubal ligation, can be performed through the incision, although exposure and visualization are limited. A tube or ovary is sometimes removed through the vagina.

Fallopian Tube Diagnostic Procedures
Tubal Perfusion
To test tubal patency, methylene blue or indigo carmine dye in a solution of sterile normal saline is introduced into the uterine cavity via a 50-ml syringe or intravenous (IV) tubing attached to a cervical cannula. The surgeon views the ends of the fallopian tubes through a laparoscope. Dye seen coming from one or both tubes indicates patency.

Tubal Insufflation
Uterotubal insufflation may be used to test the patency of the fallopian tubes. It usually is done as an office procedure to study infertility. The test may be therapeutic in relieving minor obstructions. Contraindications include genital tract infection, possible pregnancy, and uterine bleeding.

A cannula with an airtight seal is inserted into the cervicouterine canal and connected to an insufflation apparatus. Carbon dioxide is introduced slowly under controlled flow. A relationship exists between tubal patency and the pressure required to force gas through the fallopian tubes into the peritoneal cavity. Resistance to flow (i.e., back pressure) is measured on a mercury manometer. To prevent gas embolism, Rubin's test is done before, never following, curettage. Intraabdominal irritation before total absorption of carbon dioxide from the peritoneal cavity causes referred pain in the shoulders. The patient may refer to the feeling as "gas pains."

Hysterosalpingography
Radiologic study of the uterus and tubes may afford further evaluation of infertility following repeated negative Rubin's test findings. The patient is placed in the lithotomy position. The vagina is prepped. The cervix is grasped with a single-tooth tenaculum. A cannula is inserted into the cervical canal, and 10 ml of a water-soluble radiopaque contrast media is instilled with a syringe through the cannula. This contrast medium ascends into the corpus uteri and fallopian tubes to yield information about structure and function. Serial x-ray films may be taken to assess postprocedural tubal spillage. In some patients tubal spasms prevent immediate passage of the contrast media through the tubes. Iodine-based contrast media is contraindicated in a patient with iodine allergy.

Pelvic Endoscopy
Pelvic endoscopy (also known as laparoscopy) is an established part of the gynecologist's diagnostic and therapeutic regimen. It permits detailed intraperitoneal inspection of the pelvic organs without laparotomy. These procedures are not without danger, however. Inadvertent perforation of vessels, a hollow viscus, and/or infection are major hazards. Operator expertise, careful patient selection, adequate anesthesia, and safe equipment are essential. Pelvic endoscopy is a sterile procedure.

Vaginal and abdominal approaches are employed for direct visualization of pelvic organs and adjacent structures.

Culdoscopy
A culdoscope is introduced into the peritoneal cavity via the posterior vaginal fornix and pouch of Douglas. Some gynecologists prefer culdoscopy to investigate ovaries or posterior surfaces in the lower pelvis. Local or caudal anesthesia is used. The patient is placed in the knee-chest or lithotomy position. With the posterior lip of the cervix held by a tenaculum and retracted anteriorly, the uterus is elevated while counterpressure is applied to the posterior vaginal wall by the speculum. This maneuver stretches the posterior vaginal fornix while a trocar and cannula or sheath penetrate the thin wall and enter the pelvis between the uterosacral ligaments. When the trocar is removed with the cannula in place, air enters the cul-de-sac because of the negative intraabdominal pressure produced by the knee-chest position. Air displaces the bowel, and the scope may be inserted through the cannula.

At the completion of the procedure the culdoscope is removed. Before the cannula is removed, the operating bed is straightened and the patient is flattened while as much air as possible is evacuated by hand pressure on the abdomen. Some surgeons place a suture in the puncture site.

Hysteroscopy
A rigid fiberoptic hysteroscope, introduced vaginally, provides direct inspection of the interior of the uterus to diagnose disease or treat conditions such as menorrhagia and uterine fibroids. The hysteroscope may also be used to identify and remove polyps, lost intrauterine devices (IUDs), or intrauterine adhesions. Adequate dilation of the uterine cavity is a prerequisite for viewing endometrial surfaces and tubal orifices. High-viscosity fluid, such as prewarmed 1.5% glycine or dextran 10 or dextran 70, is instilled to provide uterine distention. Hysteroscopy systems have been developed that use sterile normal saline as expansion media. The fluid should be delivered through a pressure-controlled infusion pump. Intrauterine pressures should be maintained at or below the mean arterial pressure. Use of a continuous flow pump makes it difficult to monitor intrauterine pressures.

The circulator monitors inflow and outflow of the uterine expansion fluid medium and informs the surgeon and the anesthesia provider of any discrepancy in excess of 1500 ml. Visibility is further enhanced with a video camera and monitor screen. The procedure may be videotaped.

Hysteroscopy is used to perform endometrial ablation using a laser (Nd:YAG, argon, or KTP) or ESU to stop or decrease uterine bleeding. The Nd:YAG laser is the laser of choice for deep photocoagulation, causing endometrial destruction and scarring the uterine lining. The entire endometrial lining is treated from the fundus to about 4 cm above the external cervical os. The tip of the laser fiber can be held away from tissue (blanching technique) or in contact with endometrium (dragging technique). A specialized electrosurgical rollerball electrode is an alternative method to using a laser. This can provide relief from menorrhagia (i.e., excessively heavy menses).

Air or gas is not used for uterine insufflation or laser fiber cooling during hysteroscopy because of the risk of air or gas embolism. Also, 32% dextran 70 in dextrose (Hyskon) is not used as an irrigant or uterine expansion media for endometrial laser ablation because of the systemic effects of fluid absorption through open capillaries. Precise measurements of intake and output are critical to patient safety.

Hysteroscopy can be performed as an ambulatory surgery or office procedure.

Laparoscopy

Procedures using a 10- or 12-mm fiberoptic laparoscope with a 0- or 30-degree-angle lens inserted into the peritoneal cavity permits direct observation of pelvic and abdominal organs and peritoneal surfaces. This technique may be used to diagnose and treat ectopic pregnancy; inspect the ovaries for evidence of follicular activity and retrieve ova for in vitro fertilization; visualize and reduce pelvic masses; and determine the cause of infertility, endocrinopathies, or amenorrhea. Many pelvic diseases, such as endometriosis, adhesions, and ovarian cysts, may be identified and treated through the laparoscope and its accessory instrumentation. The gynecologist can perform myomectomy, salpingectomy, oophorectomy, hysterectomy, and other procedures such as tuboplasty and incidental appendectomy without the need for a large abdominal incision. Surgical procedures such as tubal sterilization by electrocoagulation with or without partial resection, placement of a clip or silicone ring on the tube, or biopsy can be performed.

The argon laser will pass through the working channel of the sheath to ablate endometrial implants. The CO_2 laser may be used to vaporize tissue in conjunction with the operating microscope attached to the laparoscope. Special instrumentation may be needed for microsurgical procedures.

Procedure The increasing popularity of minimally invasive and minimal access surgery has led to the expansion of laparoscopy to pelviscopy. The technique for using both types of scopes is essentially the same. The surgeon and assistant manipulate instruments through trocar sheaths. A video camera and monitor are used for optimal visualization. Frequently, procedures are recorded as part of the permanent record. Most equipment is capable of taking still photographs also. Both sterile and nonsterile equipment is needed.

Sterile endoscopic equipment includes the following:

- D&C instrument tray, including uterine manipulator/cannula (Hulka tenaculum, Cohen/Jarcho cannula, or Humi inflatable uterine cannula).

- 20-ml Luer-Lok syringe.
- Endoscope.
- Verres needle, 80- or 120-mm needle for insufflation through an abdominal puncture; 150-mm needle for insufflation through the cul-de-sac in an obese patient.
- Appropriate-size trocars and insulated sheaths with sealing caps to prevent gas leakage.
- Insufflation tubing with an in-line filter.
- Aspiration cannula, biopsy forceps, and graduated probe. Most are insulated and compatible with a monopolar ESU.
- Bipolar grasping forceps (Kleppinger forceps).
- Suction/irrigation tubing.
- Endoscopic needleholders, sutures, clip appliers, and staplers. These may be needed for more complex procedures.
- Electrosurgical probe or endocoagulator, and/or laser fiber.

Nonsterile endoscopic equipment includes the following:

- Insufflator with full tank of carbon dioxide and a compatible disposable hydrophobic filter.
- Fiberoptic light source.
- Video camera and monitor(s).
- Laser and/or ESU. Only a solid-state electrical generator should be used with the endoscope. High peaks of voltages from spark-gap generators may cause excessive tissue destruction.

Usually, general anesthesia is administered. The patient is placed in a modified lithotomy position with the stirrups adjusted so that the legs are at 45-degree angles to the axis of the operating bed. The abdomen is prepped, followed by perineal and vaginal preparation. An indwelling Foley catheter is inserted. The patient is draped for a combined abdominovaginal procedure. The sterile drapes must provide two exposures (i.e., an abdominal opening and a perineal opening) and cover the legs.

A tenaculum is placed on the cervix. A cannula is inserted for instillation of dye and for manipulation of the uterus during the procedure to provide greater visibility. A D&C may be performed as part of the procedure after the injection of dye (Figure 35-3).

Insertion of the scope is preceded by a pneumoperitoneum to produce abdominal distention. The infraumbilical midline area is most commonly used if no scars, with possible adherent viscera beneath, are present. This area is preferred because it has no abdominal wall vessels that might be injured. The firm attachment of the fascia to the peritoneum facilitates entry. Great care is taken to avoid injury to the great vessels or intraabdominal organs.

To produce a pneumoperitoneum, a Verres needle may be introduced percutaneously into the peritoneal cavity. This spring-loaded needle has an outer sharp hollow cannula with an inner blunt retractable stylet with a two-way stopcock at the base for control of gas flow. Some surgeons prefer to incise the infraumbilical margin through the fascial and peritoneal layers and insert a blunt Hasson trocar and sleeve for

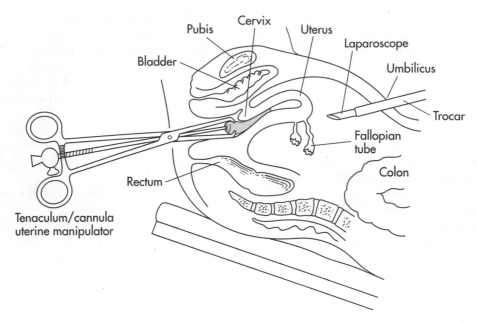

Figure 35-3 Uterine manipulation during laparoscopy. Shown in cross section.

insufflation. This method decreases the risk of a perforated viscus. Sterile insufflation tubing is attached to convey carbon dioxide from the insufflation apparatus to the patient. Carbon dioxide is used as the insufflation medium because it is nontoxic, highly soluble in blood, and rapidly absorbed from the peritoneal cavity. The gas is introduced into the cavity under a controlled high flow with a pressure of 12 to 14 mm Hg until the volume insufflated ranges between 2.5 and 4.5 L. The flow rate and volume are monitored by the circulator and surgeon. Overdistention must be avoided to prevent respiratory impairment and subcutaneous emphysema. After the desired pneumoperitoneum is established, the insufflator is switched to a maintenance flow of 3 to 4 L at a pressure of 14 mm Hg. Electronic sensors in the device maintain the pneumoperitoneum at a constant level during periods of irrigation and suction.

The patient is placed in a 15-degree Trendelenburg position to shift the abdominal organs cephalad. A small infraumbilical skin incision is made in the anterior abdominal wall. Through it a trocar and sheath are introduced into the peritoneal cavity via puncture. The sharp tip of the trocar must be carefully guided to avoid inadvertent perforations. Some trocars and sheaths have spring-loaded end guards that cover the sharp tip and protect the underlying structures after penetration of abdominal tissue layers, although studies have not shown this to be an advantage. The sharp trocar is removed, and the scope of the same caliber is inserted through the trocar sheath, which remains in the cavity.

Before use, warming the tip of the fiberoptic scope in warm towels or normal saline solution can prevent fogging of the distal lens of the endoscope by the intraperitoneal temperature and moisture. (Sterile antifog solution is commercially available.) The fiberoptic cable is connected to the en-

doscope and the light source. Because of the potential fire hazard to drapes, the light source is not activated until it is attached to the scope. The gas tubing is connected to the inflow valve. The video camera is draped and connected to the endoscope.

Although an operating scope permits insertion of accessory instruments, these may be introduced through one or two additional 3-, 5- or 7-mm insulated trocar(s) and sheath(s) inserted through small incision(s) in the lower and/or lateral abdomen. These trocars may be inserted into the peritoneal cavity under direct vision through the endoscope, which offers good transillumination for the puncture when the room lights are dimmed, or visualization on the video monitor. The suction/irrigation tubing is attached to a side port on an accessory sheath.

Intraabdominal ligation is achieved with loops of chromic or plain surgical gut (Endoloop ligatures). After the applicator is passed through the scope, the loop is placed around the tissue and pulled taut. An endoscopic swaged needle-suture is passed in a needleholder for suturing. Intracorporeal (inside body) and extracorporeal (outside body) knotting techniques are used to secure sutures. Endoscopic ligating clips and staples also are used for ligation and tissue approximation. Hemostasis may also be accomplished with a laser fiber, an electrosurgical probe, or an endocoagulator. The endocoagulator uses directed heat at a temperature of about 212° F (100° C) for coagulation of protein by thermal conduction rather than high-frequency current.

At the completion of the surgical procedure, the carbon dioxide, video monitor, and light source are turned off, accessory instruments and sheaths are removed, and the patient is returned to the supine position. Hemostasis is surveyed before the scope is removed from the primary puncture site. The valve of its sheath closes to prevent escape of intraperitoneal gas into the room air. The pneumoperitoneum contains aerosolized blood and body fluids and should be evacuated through the suction tubing into the suction canister. Electrosurgical plume also should be suctioned from the peritoneal cavity because it binds with hemoglobin and causes the arterial oxygenation to decrease. The patient can become hypoxic. The skin incisions are sutured, and small dressings or adhesive bandages (Band-Aids or Steri-Strips) are applied.

The patient requires close monitoring by the anesthesia provider because increased intraabdominal pressure may lead to cardiovascular disturbances from vagal reflex. This reflex is caused by stretching of the peritoneum, retention of carbon dioxide, or compression of the inferior vena cava.

Postoperative shoulder pain may follow the use of a pneumoperitoneum. This is referred pain caused by pressure on the diaphragm, which is somewhat displaced by carbon dioxide during the procedure. Slight elevation of the head after recovery from anesthesia relieves this pain. Although numerous complications have been reported, the most common are perforation of the intestine or major blood vessel, hemorrhage from a biopsy site, gas embolism from intravascular injection, and burns of the abdominal wall and bowel. Some injuries, such as viscus puncture or thermal damage, may not be immediately apparent. Symptoms may not be present until 48 to 72 hours postoperatively, when tissue necrosis or sloughing occurs.

VULVAR PROCEDURES

Benign growths, although rare, consist mainly of fatty and fibrous tumors. These are excised if large. Suspicious lesions should be removed for pathologic examination. Cancerous lesions may be multicentric, with the majority found on the labia majora and a lesser percentage on the labia minora, vestibule, clitoris, and posterior commissure. Vaginal smears should be taken to determine the presence of metastatic growth to the vaginal wall. Treatment depends on the size of the primary lesion, involvement of nodes, and extent of metastasis. Mutilative procedures require emotional adjustment to permanent change.

Vulvectomy

Wide local excision of a single, well-localized area with no premalignant changes elsewhere may be done. Punch biopsies may be obtained. Leukoplakia and preinvasive lesions of the vulva may be treated with a laser or ultrasonic aspirator.

Simple Vulvectomy Without Node Dissection

The labia majora and minora, part of the mons veneris, and the hymenal ring, including the clitoris, may be removed for premalignant lesions and early microinvasive cancer of limited penetration. The clitoris and perianal region are spared if the lesion is small. The incision must be wide to avoid local recurrence.

Total Vulvectomy

Basal cell carcinoma usually does not metastasize but is often locally extensive and prone to recur. Treatment consists of wide total vulvectomy, also without node dissection.

Radical Vulvectomy with Bilateral Inguinal-Femoral Lymphadenectomy

Radical vulvectomy is performed for invasive vulvar cancers or melanoma and is usually done in one stage. Resection lines may vary depending on the location and size of the lesion. Because the procedure involves abdominal and perineal dissection, both areas, including the thighs to the knees, are prepped. Structures generally removed include all of those from the anterior surface of the pubis to the perianal region posteriorly, with wide lateral excision beyond the vulva, to fascial depth. More specifically, large areas of abdominal and groin skin, the labia majora and minora, the mons, the clitoris, Bartholin and periurethral glands, and bilateral inguinal lymph nodes are removed en bloc. Inguinal skin flaps are retained for closure. Deep pelvic node dissection is carried out if frozen sections determine that these nodes are cancerous. If the vagina, urethra, and/or anus are involved, they are also removed. Anal involvement may require a colostomy.

Lymphadenectomy is carried out with the patient in the supine position. Two teams may perform bilateral dissection. The patient is then placed in the lithotomy position for vulvectomy. Reconstruction of the pelvic floor and vaginal walls may be necessary. The legs are abducted for easier approximation of subcutaneous tissue during primary closure with sutures or staples. Closed wound suction drainage is used postoperatively to avoid fluid collection beneath skin flaps. A pressure dressing is applied.

Bartholin Glands

Obstruction of the secretory duct of Bartholin gland may be caused by inflammation. A cyst may be prone to secondary infection or abscess formation.

Marsupialization of Bartholin Cyst

A cyst enlarges as mucus secretions accumulate. Marsupialization establishes drainage from within the vagina by creation of a new, enlarged ductal opening. The cyst is incised linearly in the region of the normal opening and evacuated. The edges of the vaginal mucosa and cyst wall are sutured together to produce epithelialization so that the cyst cannot recur. An abscess may be drained.

VAGINAL PROCEDURES

The vaginal wall, cervix, and uterus may be approached with the patient in the lithotomy position. Tumors, benign or malignant, may be confined to any one of these structures or may involve adjacent tissues. Herniation or fistula formation may require repair of the vaginal wall and adjacent structures. Excision or repair may require a combined vaginal-abdominal procedure.

Vaginal Wall
Excision of a Vaginal Lesion

A biopsy taken from an epithelial tumor should be studied histologically to rule out adenocarcinoma. Vaginal adenosis and gross cervical abnormalities, as well as clear cell adenocarcinoma of the vagina, have occurred in female offspring of women who received diethylstilbestrol (DES) or similar synthetic estrogen during the first trimester of pregnancy to avoid spontaneous abortion. Adenosis may be treated with a laser.

Vaginectomy

Vaginectomy (partial or complete) is performed for carcinoma in situ or carcinoma of the vagina. Vaginoplasty is necessary for reconstruction. External radiation and radium, with possible eventual pelvic exenteration, are the treatment for advanced invasive malignancy. The proximity of the bladder and rectum makes therapy difficult.

Radical vaginal or abdominal hysterectomy and vaginectomy with extraperitoneal lymphadenectomy sometimes are combined for carcinoma of the upper and middle thirds of the vagina if the bladder or rectum is not involved.

Vaginoplasty

A vagina may be constructed in patients with congenital absence of an entire vagina or, more commonly, those with stenosis after radiation therapy or after surgical removal of the vagina. Care must be taken to avoid damage to the urethra, bladder, or rectum. The vaginal space is created by blunt and sharp dissection. If a large part of the surface of the space is denuded, a skin or amnion graft is shaped around a vaginal mold. The mold is placed in such a way that the graft will take. With the use of dilators to prevent stenosis and estrogen cream to assist in epithelization of the cavity, an adequate functional vagina can be created in many patients. A pseudovagina is created for transsexual surgery.

Procedures for Repair of the Pelvic Outlet

Injury to muscles and fascial layers of the perineum and/or genital tract, usually during childbirth, may result in extensive vaginal relaxation. Manifestation of perineal hernias may be delayed until later years, when generalized loss of elastic tissue develops. Downward pressure is exerted on other structures, such as the bladder. Moderate to severe degrees of herniation of viscera require surgical intervention to restore pelvic floor integrity and sphincter competency. Vaginal plastic procedures for genital prolapse consist of narrowing and reconstructing the damaged pelvic floor. Vaginal repairs are referred to as vaginal plastic procedures.

Anterior Colporrhaphy (Kelly Procedure)
Anterior colporrhaphy is performed for prolapse of the anterior vaginal wall to repair a urethrocystocele (herniation of the bladder into the vaginal canal). The wall is incised, and a strip of redundant vaginal mucosa is excised, the extent of which depends on the severity of the prolapse. The bladder is dissected free from the vaginal septum and returned to normal position by suturing the pubocervical ligaments beneath it. Approximation of the pubococcygeus muscles provides further suburethral support. The vaginal wall is closed with sutures. By improving support to the bladder neck region, restoring the posterior urethrovesical angle, and narrowing the urethral opening, stress incontinence (urine leakage with coughing, sneezing, or laughter) is relieved. The surgical procedure also prevents voiding difficulty and the recurrent cystitis that accompanies retention of urine caused by a cystocele bulging below the bladder neck.

Posterior Colpoperineorrhaphy   Repair of the posterior vaginal wall for rectocele, a herniation of the rectum into the vagina, consists of a triangular excision of redundant vaginal mucosa and separation of the vagina from the rectum. Support is reestablished by suturing together rectovaginal fascia, as well as the levator ani, as high as possible. Perineal muscles are reconstructed to restore continuity of support. A lacerated perineum may also be sutured. The surgical procedure relieves fecal incontinence and/or constipation.

Repair of an Enterocele   An abnormally deep hernial sac may contain a segment of intestine, referred to as an enterocele or cul-de-sac hernia. Repair consists of opening the sac, reducing its contents, excising the sac, closing the aperture or weakness that allowed the sac to descend into the rectovaginal septum, and strengthening the normal anatomic coverings. Approximation of the uterosacral ligaments and levator ani in the midline removes the cul-de-sac defect.

Repair of a Prolapsed Uterus, or Procidentia
Various surgical procedures correct and restore support. Correction of prolapse anteverts the uterus and shortens an elongated cervix and cardinal ligaments. In a Manchester colpoperineorrhaphy, for example, the cervix is amputated and the cardinal ligaments united in front of it. The anterior vaginal wall is plicated, and the posterior pelvic floor is reconstructed. Often cystocele and rectocele are present and are simultaneously repaired. In complete prolapse both the cervix and the uterine body protrude through the vaginal aperture and the vaginal canal is inverted. Bleeding ulceration of exposed tissues may ensue. Vaginal hysterectomy is done for severe prolapse or prolapse accompanied by stress incontinence when childbearing is no longer desired. A vaginal pessary to support a retrodisplaced or prolapsing uterus may be inserted in a woman who presents a poor surgical risk.

Repair of Vaginal Eversion   Outward protrusion of the vagina can occur following obstetric or surgical trauma or from inherent weakness in vaginal muscle tone, particularly in postmenopausal years. The fascia of the vagina is attached to the sacrospinous ligament, located within the coccygeus muscle. The resultant scarring and fibrosis fixates the vagina in a normal anatomic position.

Colpocleisis (Le Fort Procedure) Colpocleisis (obliteration of the vagina by denuding and approximating the anterior and posterior walls) is generally reserved for geriatric patients or those who present a poor surgical risk.

Procedures for Repair of Genital Fistulas

A fistula is an abnormal communication between a part of the genital canal and either the urinary or the intestinal tract. Various dye tests, cystoscopy, and pyelography help pinpoint a urinary tract fistula. Injury during parturition, surgical trauma (especially radical procedures for cancer), penetrating extension of cervical carcinoma, and radiation necrosis are common etiologic factors.

Repair of a Vesicovaginal Fistula A vesicovaginal fistula, which develops between the bladder and vagina, is the most common type of genital fistula. A small opening permits seepage of urine, although the patient may void normally. Total incontinence may result from a large fistulous aperture and cause irritation of the vagina, vulva, and thighs. Through a vaginal approach, the anterior vaginal wall is dissected free. The fistula to the bladder is closed, and the attachment of the bladder to the vagina is reestablished. The repair should be made with at least three layers of tissue. The bladder should be decompressed by an indwelling Foley catheter postoperatively. Antibiotics may be administered judiciously to prevent infection in the healing site.

If the vesicovaginal fistula is high in the vagina, a better result will be obtained by entering the bladder via suprapubic incision for direct repair rather than using a vaginal approach. Care must be taken not to occlude ureteral orifices. This is accomplished by insertion of ureteral catheters, which can be removed following the procedure. Attention is given to excision of any infected tissue, closure with multiple layers, and bladder decompression by the Foley catheter.

Repair of a Rectovaginal Fistula A fistula between the rectum and vagina may follow episiotomy or obstetric perineal lacerations, vaginal or rectal surgery, radiation therapy, trauma, or infection. Fecal incontinence and fecal material in the vagina are characteristic, although the anal sphincter is intact. Preoperative bowel preparation, including prophylactic antibiotic therapy, is important because of the contaminated surgical area. A temporary colostomy may be advisable before the surgical procedure to divert the fecal stream from the repair site. With a vaginal approach, a plastic repair of the perineum is done. Scar tissue and the fistulous tract are excised, and the edges of the perineal muscles and fascia are approximated.

Cervix

Surgical treatment of an abnormal cervix should be preceded by tests, such as a Pap smear, to rule out early malignant change.

Cauterization

The cervix may be cauterized by laser or electrocautery to treat chronic inflammation and/or leukorrhea (i.e., vaginal discharge).

Trachelorrhaphy

Lacerations of the cervix may result from childbirth. Repair (i.e., trachelorrhaphy) involves reconstruction of the cervical canal as necessary. A vaginal plastic setup is used.

Conization

Cervical dysplasia can occur in females age 15 years and older; the peak incidence is between ages 25 and 35. Employed therapeutically for chronic inflammation and for premalignant lesions in women of childbearing age, conization may be performed by scalpel, electrosurgery, or laser. Laser conization is used to treat severe dysplasia and carcinoma in situ. Loop electrosurgical excision procedures (LEEP) use a stainless steel or tungsten loop electrode to excise a central core of tissue from the transformation zone of the endocervical canal. Large loop excision of the transformation zone (LLETZ) is performed with minimal bleeding and few complications. These procedures may be performed in the OR or office setting with local anesthesia. Future childbearing is unaffected. Although the specimen is comparable in size to that obtained with cold knife conization, the specimen has superficial dessication and may be inferior in quality. Wide conization may result in scaring and obstruction of the os.

Amputation

The cervix may be amputated to remove an intraepithelial cancer. Most surgeons prefer total hysterectomy to cervical amputation, because the remaining uterine component may become cancerous.

Uterus
Dilation and Curettage

The most frequently performed gynecologic procedure, dilation of the cervix and curettage of the uterus (D&C), is done for diagnostic and/or therapeutic purposes. The main purpose of a D&C is to establish the cause of abnormal uterine bleeding so that the gynecologist can plan definitive treatment. The procedure is performed for women with postmenopausal bleeding or symptoms suggestive of endometrial cancer, even when cytologic smear findings are negative. It may be performed in infertility studies or to confirm preoperative diagnosis before amputation of the cervix or hysterectomy. D&C is performed therapeutically to relieve dysmenorrhea by cervical dilation only, to remove polyps or benign endometrial pathologic conditions, to remove residual tissue and arrest bleeding following incomplete abortion, or to perform voluntary or therapeutic abortion before the thirteenth week of pregnancy. A regional paracervical block or general anesthesia is required.

With the anterior lip of the cervix held in a tenaculum and the posterior vaginal wall retracted, a uterine sound is introduced into the uterus to determine the length and direction of the intrauterine cavity. It is important that the surgeon know the shape and position of the uterus to avoid perforation. The cervical os is sequentially dilated with graduated metal probes. A small curette is introduced into the endocervical canal, which is scraped from the internal to the external os. Submucous fibroids are usually discernible as the curette passes over them. Exploration of the fundus with a polyp or placental forceps usually extracts any polyps present in the endometrium.

Intrauterine Thermal Balloon Ablation

A specialized electrically heated latex balloon probe can be introduced into the uterine cavity through the cervical os to treat menorrhagia. The intrauterine probe is attached to a cable system controlled by a microprocessing unit that measures temperature, pressure, and time. The thermal balloon is expanded by the computer to fill the capacity of the uterine cavity and heated to 188° F (87° C). A depth of approximately 3 to 5 mm of endometrium is ablated within 8 minutes of contact. This procedure is suitable for patients who have regularly shaped uterine cavities with a capacity of less than 30 cc or 10 cm in depth. A larger or irregularly shaped uterine cavity would not evenly accommodate the expansion of the balloon.

Intrauterine thermal balloon therapy is contraindicated for women who wish to have future pregnancies. The thermal process destroys the endometrial lining that supports the placental attachment during pregnancy. As per all latex devices, use of a latex balloon is contraindicated for patients sensitive to latex products.

Vaginal Hysterectomy

Vaginal hysterectomy is performed for severe uterine prolapse or prolapse accompanied by stress incontinence and for patients with pelvic relaxation or a history of myomas, irregular uterine bleeding, or a treated premalignant lesion.

The uterus is removed through the vagina, with incision of the vaginal wall and the pelvic cavity. Urinary incontinence caused by an enterocele and/or a rectocele may be simultaneously repaired by anterior and posterior colporrhaphies and with reconstruction of the pelvic floor. Advantages of the procedure include restoration of normal anatomic relationship and preservation of vaginal function. The ovaries are not always removed. Contraindications are immobility of pelvic organs, a large uterus, a pathologic condition such as an ovarian mass, or pelvic cancer.

The vaginal wall is incised anteriorly, and the bladder is separated from the cervix. The incision is continued around the cervix. The peritoneal cavity is entered through the posterior cul-de-sac and the anterior uterovesical pouch. Ligaments supporting the uterus and uterine vessels are ligated and cut. The fundus is delivered, the upper pedicles are sutured, the uterus is removed, and the peritoneum is closed. Suturing the cardinal and uterosacral ligaments together and to the vaginal vault supports the vault and prevents prolapse of the vagina. Potential complications include injury to the

ureters, bowel, or bladder and massive hemorrhage from the uterine vessels. An unopened laparotomy setup should be available.

Radical Vaginal Hysterectomy (Schauta's Procedure)

A surgical approach to early carcinoma of the cervix, radical vaginal hysterectomy does not permit pelvic lymph node dissection but is useful in selected patients (e.g., obese patients). It includes vaginal removal of the uterus, upper third of vagina, fallopian tubes, and ovaries. Damage to the ureters or bladder is a potential complication.

Laparoscopic-Assisted Vaginal Hysterectomy

In laparoscopic-assisted vaginal hysterectomy (LAVH), an abdominal endoscopic approach is used to dissect the uterus from its supporting ligaments and vasculature. Endoscopic clips, linear staplers, sutures, electrosurgery, or a laser may be used to enhance hemostasis. Once the intraperitoneal attachments of the uterus are ligated and divided, a vaginal approach is used to separate the bladder from the anterior aspect of the uterus as in a standard vaginal hysterectomy. Direct visualization of the bladder flap dissection through the endoscope from above enables the surgeon to avoid damage to adjacent structures. The uterine vascular pedicles are ligated vaginally. In the Heaney technique the uterus is inverted and removed fundus first through a posterior colpotomy. The uterosacral ligaments are sutured to the posterior aspect of the vaginal cuff, and the colpotomy is closed. This method is used in moderate prolapse of the uterus. In Döderlein's technique a nonprolapsed uterus is inverted and removed fundus first through an anterior colpotomy. This technique provides greater visibility of the uterine vessels and a more effective vaginal suspension. LAVH is the procedure of choice when a minimally invasive procedure is desired, when salpingo-oophorectomy may be necessary, and when the uterus is only moderately enlarged.

ABDOMINAL PROCEDURES

The open abdominal approach may be used for a fixed or enlarged uterus, exploration, inflammatory disease, and most malignant lesions of the uterus, fallopian tubes, and ovaries. This approach permits inspection of pelvic and abdominal organs, as well as lymph glands for biopsy or treatment. Open laparotomy or minimally invasive endoscopic procedures are performed as appropriate to achieve desired outcomes.

Abdominal Hysterectomy

Medical, psychosocial, and sexual ramifications must be considered when contemplating hysterectomy (removal of the uterus). Medically the procedure may be lifesaving in patients with a malignant lesion or severe hemorrhage. However, the gynecologist has an obligation to consider the individual patient's attitudes when another mode of therapy is available as an alternative to hysterectomy. Signaling as it does the end of the patient's reproductive potential, a hysterectomy may cause psychologic stress and a sense of incompleteness, even though sexual responsiveness is not dependent on the uterus. Patients whose families are complete, however, may welcome reproductive sterilization.

The uterus is removed through an abdominal incision and opening of the peritoneal cavity. The most frequent indication for abdominal hysterectomy is leiomyofibroma, commonly known as benign fibroids or myomas. Fibroids are composed of muscle and fibrous connective tissue. They may be single or multiple and most often are present in the wall of the uterus. Some may be attached by a pedicle or protrude into and distort the uterine cavity. Fibroids, which are usually slow growing, are treated conservatively if they are small and present no problems. The tumor ceases to grow at menopause. If symptoms such as menometrorrhagia, bladder or bowel pressure, pelvic discomfort, or rapid tumor growth develop, surgical treatment is essential. Differential diagnosis includes dysfunctional uterine bleeding caused by disturbed endocrine function, tubal or ovarian masses, and pelvic cancer. In addition to these indications, hysterectomy is performed for uterine prolapse, extensive endometriosis, and cervical or uterine cancer. Various types of hysterectomy are performed.

Total Abdominal Hysterectomy

The entire uterus, including the cervix, is resected. Normal ovaries are preserved for hormone production whenever possible in women under 45 years of age. Studies have shown that after hysterectomy, women have a 20% increased risk for ovarian cysts within 5 years of the surgical procedure. Bilateral oophorectomy followed by hormone replacement therapy has eliminated the need for subsequent surgery for ovarian pathologic conditions.

The abdominal peritoneal cavity is entered through a vertical midline or a transverse Pfannenstiel incision. Vertical incision facilitates exploration. The patient is placed in a deep Trendelenburg position. Incision through the uterine peritoneum is carried out laterally. The abdominal organs are retracted and protected with laparotomy packs moistened with warm sterile normal saline solution. The fallopian tubes and round and broad ligaments are clamped, cut, and ligated. The ovaries, when not removed, are suspended to avoid adherence to the vaginal vault. With the uterus forward, posterior sheets of the broad ligaments are incised, the ureters are identified, and the uterine vessels and uterosacral ligaments are clamped, divided, and sutured. All uterine-supporting ligaments must be divided and ligated. The bladder is mobilized from the cervix and vagina, the vaginal vault is incised, and the cervix is dissected from the vagina. After the uterus is removed, the connective tissue ligaments are anchored to the vagina. The vaginal mucosa and muscular wall are approximated by absorbable sutures or staples, and the bladder, vault, and rectum (i.e., pelvic floor) are reperitonealized (i.e.,

covered with peritoneum). Abdominal layers are closed as for laparotomy. The following considerations apply:

1. When the surgeon is closing the vaginal vault following removal of the uterus, the needle, suture, needle-holder, or stapler and all instruments used on the cervix and vagina are considered contaminated. Separate instruments may be used for abdominal closure.
2. Complications of hysterectomy include injury to the ureters, with possible fistula formation or renal failure, injury to the bladder or bowel with fistula formation, or massive hemorrhage from damage to major vessels.

Radical Hysterectomy with Pelvic Lymph Node Dissection (Radical Wertheim's Procedure)
A radical Wertheim's procedure may be performed for early stages of invasive cervical cancer and sometimes for endometrial cancer. It involves wide en bloc removal of paracervical and uterosacral tissues (uterus, tubes, ovaries, ligaments) and at least the upper third of the vaginal canal. Bilateral pelvic lymph nodes and channels surrounding the external iliac artery and vein, the hypogastric artery and vein, and the obturator fossae are also dissected and removed.

Some surgeons perform a modified Wertheim's procedure for microinvasive carcinoma. This is somewhat less extensive than the radical procedure and may omit lymphadenectomy.

Because radical hysterectomy involves excision of paracervical and paravaginal tissue, bladder innervation is disrupted. This results in bladder dysfunction postoperatively, sometimes for as long as 6 months. Bladder complications are related to the extent of dissection.

Hysterosalpingo-oophorectomy
Fallopian tubes and ovaries are removed along with the uterus. This procedure may be done for endometrial, tubal, or ovarian cancer; excessive vaginal bleeding; or large fibroids. In postmenopausal women when total hysterectomy is indicated, bilateral salpingo-oophorectomy is often performed to avoid future ovarian pathologic conditions.

Myomectomy

In myomectomy single or multiple fibroid tumors are removed from the uterine wall in premenopausal women who may still desire pregnancy. The procedure is especially adaptable to pedunculated tumors, which may become necrotic from interference with the blood supply. Removal of large submucous fibroids may require opening the uterus.

Pelvic Exenteration

An ultraradical procedure for invasive, persistent carcinoma, exenteration is not performed for palliation but only when a possibility of cure exists. The extent of the disease determines the amount of exenteration. In anterior exenteration the reproductive organs and the distal part of the ureters, bladder, and vagina are removed. This modification is performed for cancer of the cervix, vagina, or vulva with extension to the bladder. The ureters are diverted to an ileal conduit, whereas the bowel remains intact. Posterior exenteration removes the reproductive organs, sigmoid colon, and rectum. It is done for cervical carcinoma involving the rectum or advanced rectal carcinoma involving the uterus and posterior vaginal wall. The urinary system remains intact; fecal diversion is by colostomy. Total or complete exenteration, rarely performed, involves en bloc dissection of the bladder, reproductive organs, perineum, rectum, and pelvic lymph nodes. Two setups are needed: abdominal and perineal. These procedures affect structure, function, body image, and sex life and should be preceded by intensive physical and psychologic preoperative preparation.

Numerous complications may occur involving any major system. Anesthesia and procedural times are long. Blood replacement and extensive monitoring are essential. Multiple stomas and gross pelvic defect with much dead space predispose the woman to infection; therefore wound drainage is used. Vascularized omental and myocutaneous flaps are used to fill pelvic defects.

Fallopian Tubes

The fallopian tubes are also referred to as the uterine tubes, oviducts, and salpinges.

Tubal Ligation

Tubal ligation should be considered a permanent method of reproductive sterilization because reversal cannot be guaranteed. Thorough preoperative counseling of the patient and her husband or partner should preface this procedure. A number of surgical techniques are used for tubal ligation. They are essentially similar, involving removal of a portion of the middle part of the fallopian tube on each side for pathologic confirmation and ligation of both the distal and proximal ends to prevent the cut ends from growing together. Frequently performed by laparoscopy, tubal ligation by open abdominal approach may be done alone, in conjunction with other abdominal surgery, immediately postpartum, or for patients in whom laparoscopic technique is contraindicated. Ligation may be performed through a small transverse incision in the pubic hairline area. An infraumbilical incision is used for postpartum patients. This is referred to as minilaparotomy. Tubal ligations are often performed immediately following cesarean delivery and closure of the uterine wall. No additional instruments are required other than those used for the cesarean section.

The Pomeroy technique of ligation is the most reliable, provides a surgical specimen of each tube, and causes minimal tubal destruction. The tube is tied with suture material, and a section is removed. The tube eventually pulls apart, destroying the passage between the ovary and uterus.

Sterilization may also be performed following vaginal delivery on the first to third postpartum day through an infraumbilical incision. In the cauterization technique the bipolar electrosurgical electrode transects and seals the ends of the fallopian tube or excises a section of the tube and seals the ends. Application of a stretchable Silastic band (Falloperring) or a ligating spring-loaded (Hulka) clip may also produce occlusion. In some patients, however, the Pomeroy and other occlusion techniques may be reversible by a subsequent reparative procedure. An estimated 1% of sterilized women will seek reversal because of sterilization at an early age, remarriage, or death of a child.

Tuboplasty

Removal of an obstruction may restore tubal patency to reverse infertility caused by diseased, damaged, or occluded tubes. Microsurgical techniques with fine suture materials and lasers have vastly improved results of tubal reconstructive procedures. Success depends on the extent of abnormal tissue or tubal destruction and/or the site of obstruction. The location of the previous ligation and normality of tissues at the severed ends of the tubes will influence the reversibility of a tubal ligation. Although tubal patency may be restored, abnormal function may persist in tubes damaged by pelvic inflammatory disease (PID). The chance of successful uterine pregnancy may remain limited. The risk of a tubal pregnancy can increase following tuboplasty. Preoperative assessment may include a hysterosalpingogram to determine the length and patency of tubal segments and/or laparoscopy with tubal dye perfusion or ultrasound imaging with installation of sterile normal saline solution to demonstrate patency. Contraindications for tuboplasty include active infection or disease and a tube that is less than 3 cm long.

Tuboplasties are microsurgical procedures performed through an abdominal incision. They include the options described in the following sections.

Salpingolysis Adhesions caused by an inflammatory process, such as a ruptured appendix or ovarian cyst, may surround the fallopian tubes. The tubes may function normally following lysis of adhesions.

Salpingostomy Tubal mucosa and/or fimbria may become occluded secondary to PID or other infectious process. A salpingostomy creates an opening in a distally obstructed tube. A CO_2 laser may be used through the microscope to open fimbriated ends and to divide adhesions in blocked tubes. An incision in a tube also may be performed to evacuate an early small tubal pregnancy.

Tubal Anastomosis A proximal obstruction in the tube is resected. The remaining patent segment is then reimplanted into the uterus and anastomosed at the cornu. Salpingitis usually occludes the tube near the cornu, which may need to be shaved to reach healthy tissue. A previous sterilization procedure usually occludes the mid-isthmus. This anastomosis will be midtubal in the ampulla.

Salpingectomy, Salpingo-oophorectomy

Salpingectomy (removal of a fallopian tube) is often performed in association with salpingo-oophorectomy (partial or total removal of the corresponding ovary). Procedures may be unilateral or bilateral. Indications are extensive damage from PID or endometriosis, cysts, primary adenocarcinoma of the tube, and ectopic pregnancy. Total abdominal hysterectomy and bilateral salpingo-oophorectomy may be performed for bilateral disease. Removal of a large tubo-ovarian abscess is essential to prevent rupture and dissemination of pus in the abdominal cavity.

Ovaries

Ovarian pain usually is referred to the lower abdomen just above either groin, making differential diagnosis from abdominal disease pertinent. Pelvic endoscopy, ultrasonography, and computed tomography (CT) scans assist diagnosis. An ovarian mass requires exploration for evaluation. The mass may be a cyst or a tumor. Ovarian tumors may be benign or malignant, cystic or solid. Epithelial ovarian cancer begins as a cystic intraovarian growth. It usually is asymptomatic until malignant cells have spread into the peritoneal cavity. Disease is usually confined to the peritoneal cavity and retroperitoneal lymph nodes, but advanced ovarian carcinoma can obstruct the urinary and intestinal tracts. Ovarian cancer is the leading cause of gynecologic cancer deaths in the United States.

Benign cysts, more common than tumors, may arise from the graafian follicle, corpus luteum, or epithelium (dermoid). As they grow in size, ovarian cysts can cause menstrual disturbances, pain, and abnormal uterine bleeding. They may leak contents into the peritoneal cavity, causing irritation, or they may rupture, causing massive bleeding that necessitates immediate laparotomy.

Cysts or solid tumors, even if asymptomatic, should be removed as a precaution because they may degenerate into a malignant lesion, increase in size, or lead to twisting of the pedicle. The type of procedure depends on the type of cyst or tumor, the age of the patient, and the importance of childbearing potential.

Incision or Biopsy

The surgeon incises an ovary to obtain tissue for frozen section. If a cyst or tumor is found in one ovary, the gynecologist transects the other ovary to rule out a neoplasm. Biopsy specimens may also be taken from paraaortic and pelvic lymph nodes.

Removal of an Ovarian Cyst

A procedure to remove an ovarian cyst may be scheduled as an oophorocystectomy, cystoophorectomy, or ovarian cystectomy. Many benign ovarian cysts and tumors are treated by local excision with preservation of the ovary. A large cyst may be aspirated before removal. Immediately after removal, the surgeon incises the cyst for examination to determine its character because gross appearance, as well as frozen section, are important. If there is reasonable assurance that the lesion is benign, removal of only the cyst or resection of a diseased portion (e.g., endometrioma) is justified, with preservation of normal tissue.

Oophorectomy

The most frequent indications for oophorectomy (removal of an ovary) are benign ovarian tumors. Many gynecologists believe that cystadenomas and all solid benign ovarian tumors should be treated by unilateral salpingo-oophorectomy because of the difficulty of clean dissection and the questionable assurance of their benign nature. In postmenopausal women, both ovaries, tubes, and uterus are removed to avoid future cancer.

If there is a strong probability or proof of malignancy in any ovarian cyst or mass, total hysterectomy and bilateral salpingo-oophorectomy are usually performed, regardless of age. Partial or complete omentectomy may be included because the rich blood supply of omentum contributes to rapid metastases. The extent of the surgical procedure is determined by the lesion. In malignant tumors a differentiation is made between primary and metastatic ovarian cancer, which influences treatment. As much tumor is removed as possible, a procedure referred to as debulking, for management of advanced ovarian cancer. An ultrasonic aspirator may be used for debulking. The procedure may require resecting parts of small and large intestines and the urinary tract. Following debulking, most patients receive chemotherapy. This often is followed by a "second-look laparotomy" to reassess the peritoneal cavity for further palliative or therapeutic therapy.

Muscles and Ligaments
Urinary Stress Incontinence Procedures

Urinary stress incontinence is the sudden, involuntary, and intermittent release of urine as a result of muscular changes around the proximal urethra, bladder neck, and bladder base. Differential diagnosis from fistulas, bladder neuropathies, and primary lesions is established by urethroscopy, a cystometrogram, and urodynamics. Surgical correction attempts to restore support. Three basic approaches are used. Anterior colporrhaphy with plication (i.e., reducing the size of the bladder neck) often is satisfactory. In a urethral sling procedure, a musculofascial sling is placed beneath the bladder neck and urethra; usually this is a combined vaginal and abdominal procedure. Urethral suspension procedures reposition the urethra and bladder neck retropubically by suspending the urethra in a plane with the symphysis pubis through a transverse abdominal incision. Sometimes a combined abdominoperineal approach is necessary for urethral suspension. Variations of these procedures have been devised, including an endoscopic suspension of the bladder neck.

Marshall-Marchetti Krantz Vesicourethral Suspension After mobilization through an extraperitoneal abdominal approach into the prevesicle space, the urethra and bladder neck are suspended to the posterior border of the symphysis pubis. Sutures are placed through the anterior vaginal wall on each side of the urethra and brought through the periosteum on the posterior surface of the symphysis pubis. Sutures may also be placed adjacent to the bladder neck and through the rectus muscle fascia to suspend the bladder neck. This procedure may be performed in conjunction with other pelvic surgery. It is 85% effective in the treatment of stress incontinence in women. A suprapubic catheter may be used for bladder drainage for 48 to 72 hours postoperatively. Urinary retention is a common complication for up to 7 days.

PERIOPERATIVE OBSTETRICS

Diagnostic techniques such as ultrasonography, specialization in fertility problems, and techniques of fetal monitoring and management have brought significant changes in the field of reproductive biology. Perioperative personnel become involved in the care of obstetric patients, both in elective and emergency procedures, for both obstetric and nonobstetric procedures. The pregnant woman experiencing trauma or an acute surgical disease, such as appendicitis, presents challenges to the perioperative team. The well-being of the fetus depends on maternal physiologic factors. Anesthesia and positioning are especially critical concerns. The anatomic changes of pregnancy alter the appearance and location of commonly identified surgical landmarks. Laboratory values are altered as a result of the growing fetus within the mother's uterus (Table 35-2).

Planning care for the surgical obstetric patient includes determination of the expected date of confinement. The size of the uterus, competency of the placenta, and condition of the growing fetus are prime considerations.

Considerations for the Care of the Pregnant Patient

Oxygen consumption increases about 20% during pregnancy and as much as 100% above normal during labor in response to the increased metabolic demand. Hypoxia and hypercapnia

develop rapidly. Fetal oxygenation varies in direct relation to that of the mother in normal and abnormal situations. In treating fetal distress, continuous 100% oxygen is administered to the mother until delivery or relief of the distress. Hypoventilation and hyperventilation are potentially harmful because they induce hypoxemia and hypercapnia in both the mother and the fetus. Maternal hypotension and hypovolemia diminish uterine blood flow and fetal perfusion. Hypoxia and acidosis threaten fetal well-being. The mother is safeguarded by appropriate anesthetic technique and selection of drugs. The fetus is protected by adequate uteroplacental perfusion and fetal monitoring by trained personnel. The patient should not be left alone in the holding area or OR. The fetal heart rate and uterine contractions are monitored continually. The procedure involves the care of two patients.

Position

Uterine displacement to the left during transport and until after delivery is necessary to shift the uterus away from the large abdominal vessels. The positional effect on cardiac output is of major importance in avoiding maternal hypotension and maintaining fetal well-being. In the supine position the enlarged uterus compresses the inferior vena cava and aorta, resulting in diminished venous return to the heart, stroke volume, and cardiac output. The patient is positioned supine with the right side slightly elevated by a wedge or small roll to tilt the uterus to the left (Figure 35-4). The operating bed may be tilted 30 degrees to the left. A slight Trendelenburg position assists venous return.

Anesthesia

Anesthesia is selected on an individual basis. Regional anesthesia, such as spinal or epidural, is preferred because it has a lesser impact on the physiology of the mother and her fetus. It is advantageous in patients with diabetes because of re-

| TABLE 35-2 | Altered Laboratory Values of Pregnancy |

Test	Nonpregnant Female	Change in Pregnant Female	Gestational Timing
Hemoglobin (Hgb)	12-16 g/dl	↓4%-7%	Drops to lowest point between 30th and 34th week, then stable.
Hematocrit (Hct)	37%-47%	↓1.5-2 g/dl	Drops to lowest point between 30th and 34th week, then stable.
White blood cells (WBCs)	5000-10,000/cm³	↑3.5 × 10³	Gradual increase throughout pregnancy.
Platelets	150,000-400,000/mm³	↓Slightly	Gradual decrease throughout pregnancy.
Fibrinogen	200-400 mg/dl	↑50%	Gradual increase throughout pregnancy.
Calcium (Ca)	9.0-10.5 mg/dl	↓10%	Gradual decrease throughout pregnancy.
Sodium (Na)	136-145 mEq/L	↓2-4 mEq/L	Decreases before 20th week, then stable.
Chloride (Cl)	90-110 mEq/L	↑Slightly	Gradual rise, almost negligible.
Potassium (K)	3.5-5.0 mEq/L	↓0.2-0.3 mEq/L	Decreases before 20th week, then stable.
Creatinine clearance	95-125 ml/min	↑40%	Rises through 20th week, then stable.
Blood urea nitrogen (BUN)	5-20 mg/dl	↓50%	Drops during first trimester, then stable.
Glucose (fasting)	70-115 mg/dl	↓10%	Gradual decrease throughout pregnancy.
Uric acid	2.0-6.6 mg/dl	↓33%	Decreases during first trimester, then stable.
Albumin	3.2-4.5 g/dl	↓1 g/dl	Rapid drop before 20th week, then stable.

duced metabolic expenditure, low incidence of vomiting, and earlier return to oral intake. General anesthesia is administered when the mother or fetus is in jeopardy and delivery is crucial, as in the presence of hemorrhage or severe fetal distress. The choice also depends on the reason for the surgical procedure, degree of urgency, and the patient's condition and wish. A cesarean section can be done with local anesthesia in an extreme emergency when an anesthesia provider is not immediately available. The anesthesia provider chooses the method safest for the mother and fetus. Gastric motility and emptying are inhibited by fear, pain, labor, and narcotic administration. Patients requiring emergency surgery may have eaten recently. A pregnant patient should always be regarded as having a full stomach.

Spinal or epidural anesthesia allows the mother to see her newborn in the OR. It also reduces neonatal depression and risk of maternal aspiration. Hypotension is treated with IV infusion and/or ephedrine given IV. Ephedrine, mephentermine (Wyamine), and metaraminol (Aramine) do not cause undesired uterine vasoconstriction. Other vasopressors can cause fetal hypoxia. Placentally transmitted drugs depressant to the fetus are avoided. A single injection of morphine may be given through the epidural catheter at the conclusion of the surgical procedure. With injection into the pain path, the drug significantly reduces postoperative pain for 24 to 36 hours with minimal side effects.

General anesthesia provides more rapid induction, less hypotension, greater cardiovascular stability, and better control of the airway and ventilation. Preoxygenation precedes induction. Rapid-sequence induction and intubation are used. Cricoid pressure during intubation occludes the esophagus to prevent regurgitation. Induction-to-delivery time is directly related to fetal hypoxia. Intervals greater than 3 minutes may lead to a lower pH of blood (metabolic acidosis) and respiratory depression of the infant from altered uteroplacental perfusion. All efforts are made to deliver the newborn as rapidly as possible, consistent with safety, to minimize anesthesia and surgical time and to protect the fetus. With general anesthesia, all preparations, such as patient skin preparation, insertion of an indwelling Foley catheter, draping, gowning, and gloving, are done before induction of anesthesia.

Threatened Loss of Pregnancy
Cerclage

Patients with painless dilation and effacement of the cervix during the second trimester may be at risk for preterm delivery caused by cervical incompetence. The pregnant patient at risk should be assessed for a history of previous preterm rupture of membranes or spontaneous abortion. The initial primipara cervical incompetence is rarely evident before 16 weeks' gestation. Diagnosis is commonly made between 18 and 26 weeks' gestation. Gestational ages appropriate for elective treatment of known cervical incompetence range between 12 and 16 weeks' gestation, before the cervix has dilated beyond 2 to 3 cm. Some patients may be suitable for this procedure up to 20 weeks' gestation. Cerclage is not usually performed after 26 weeks' gestation because the cervix is often too short to support suturing. Most cerclage is performed as an ambulatory procedure.

Occasionally cerclage may be performed as an emergency procedure when the cervix is dilating and membranes are bulging, as long as the membranes have not ruptured or premature labor has not begun. The patient is placed in a deep Trendelenburg position to take the uterine pressure off the cervix. No vaginal preparation is performed, to prevent accidental rupture of the membranes. It may be necessary to simultaneously perform transabdominal amniocentesis to decompress the membranes for the cerclage procedure. General anesthesia is commonly used to provide relaxation of the uterine muscle. Cerclage is contraindicated in active infection, ruptured membranes, bleeding, or active labor.

Rarely, transabdominal cervicoisthmic cerclage (TCIC) may be performed as an open pelvic procedure for patients who have had severe cervical lacerations, congenital malformations of the cervix, or multiple failed cervical cerclage procedures. TCIC can be performed as early as 11 weeks' gestation after ultrasonographic documentation of a viable pregnancy. A 5-mm Mersilene tape is sutured around the cervical isthmus in an avascular plane.

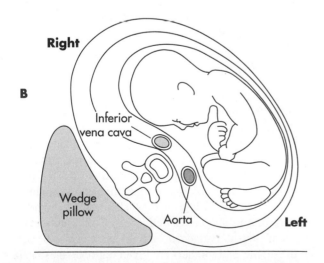

Figure 35-4 **A,** Pressure on aorta and vena cava caused by gravid uterus. **B,** Pressure is relieved by placing a wedge under right hip.

Shirodkar Procedure   A small incision is made in the anterior vaginal mucosa at the level of the bladder reflection and at the posterior cervix–cul-de-sac junction. A tunnel under the cervical mucosa is then made to join the anterior and posterior incisions. A polyester (Mersilene) tape is drawn around the internal os and tied. The knot is secured posteriorly to prevent erosion into the bladder. The suture tail is cut long so that it can be located and released at 37 to 38 weeks' gestation or if active labor begins (before delivery). Mucosal incisions are closed. A cesarean section may be necessary at term.

McDonald Procedure   The polyester suture tape is placed around the cervix with a circumferential running stitch without mucosal dissection. There is less cervical scarring, and the procedure is quicker to perform. The tape can be removed at term for vaginal delivery.

Aborted Pregnancy

Termination of pregnancy may be spontaneous or induced. The procedure will depend on the gestational age of the fetus. Ultrasonography may be used to determine the stage of intrauterine pregnancy.

Some patients are psychologically repulsed by the word *abortion*. They may associate the word with elective termination regardless of natural causes or therapeutic need. Religious or personal beliefs may influence decision making about a pregnancy that cannot continue to full term. In some circumstances the patient may accept and understand the word *miscarriage* and feel freer to select appropriate treatment options without fear of reprisal or rejection. Consideration for the support of psychologic coping mechanisms of the patient in crisis is more important than using absolute words such as *abortion*.

Suction Curettage

Intrauterine contents can be aspirated for voluntary pregnancy termination or for incomplete spontaneous abortion within the first 20 weeks of pregnancy.

Uterine Evacuation   A small flexible plastic tip or cannula is inserted into the uterus of women in the first 8 weeks of pregnancy. Suction created by drawing back on a large syringe attached to the cannula is sufficient to evacuate the contents of the uterus. Disposable equipment for suction curettage not requiring dilation or anesthesia is commercially available.

Dilation and Evacuation   For pregnancies of 8 to 16 weeks' duration, dilation and evacuation (D&E) must be performed. Cervical dilation is adjusted to the stage of pregnancy and the necessary cannula. A laminaria tent (i.e., a cone-shaped expansion plug) may be inserted preoperatively to gradually dilate the cervix, usually for 4 to 24 hours. Dilation with the laminaria, which is removed before the procedure, is gentler than instrument dilation, which can cause cervical tearing. Some instrument dilation may be necessary. A vacuum aspirator-cannula is inserted into the uterine cav-

ity and connected by tubing to an adjustable electric vacuum pump. With gentle suction the uterine contents are collected in a vacuum canister. Additional curettage with uterine curettes may be necessary to completely remove the uterine contents. The curetted contents are sent to the pathology department for gross examination.

Following an incomplete spontaneous or missed abortion, it is vital to remove all retained products of conception to prevent infection, especially from anaerobic bacteria, which may progress to septic shock. A D&C setup and suction curettage are used. The tissue is sent for culture and pathologic examination. Some patients may request baptism of an aborted fetus for religious reasons. Perioperative personnel may perform this function or request hospital clergy to assist. This has deep meaning for many patients.

Ectopic Pregnancy

A fertilized ovum may become implanted outside the uterine cavity. Referred to as an ectopic pregnancy, rarely does this fetus develop to term. This type of pregnancy usually involves the fallopian tube but can develop in the uterine cervix, on the ovary, or intraabdominally. Symptoms of ectopic pregnancy are irregular growth patterns of the uterus, abdominal pain, and vaginal bleeding. Diagnosis is made by ultrasonography, by laparoscopy, or by detection of blood in the cul-de-sac by aspiration. Hemorrhage results from extensive trauma to the tube and mesosalpinx. The patient often goes into severe shock. Immediate surgical intervention is necessary. Ruptured ectopic pregnancy is a true obstetric/gynecologic emergency. The affected tube is opened, and the products of conception are removed; hemostasis is attained; and the pelvic cavity is irrigated. The surgeon may attempt to repair the affected tube. Removal of the associated tube and possibly the ovary depends on the extent of damage from the rupture.

If an ectopic pregnancy is diagnosed by laparoscopy before rupture, conservative surgery may be able to restore fertility. Tubal pregnancy can be removed through a linear salpingostomy or by segmental resection, followed by tuboplasty. Laparoscopic techniques may be used. Some ectopic pregnancies can be managed through a vaginal colpotomy incision or abdominal minilaparotomy.

Cesarean Birth

Commonly referred to as C-section, a cesarean section is a method of delivery by abdominal and uterine incisions. Cesarean delivery may take place in the labor and delivery department or in the OR. Pregnancy and labor produce many physiologic alterations. Both the mother and the newborn have specific needs requiring comprehensive care. To promote a positive experience, the perioperative team should be cognizant of these physiologic and psychologic needs and of the reasons for transabdominal delivery. A C-section is a significant family event. Partners or support persons may be permitted in the OR, and mothers are given regional anesthesia and are usually awake.

The frequency of cesarean delivery is attributed mainly to diagnosis and management of uterine dystocia (ineffective labor), failure to progress, and fetal distress detected by fetal monitoring. A C-section is performed when safe vaginal delivery is questionable or immediate delivery is crucial because the well-being of the mother or fetus is threatened. Indications may include hemorrhage, placenta previa, abruptio placentae, toxemia, fetal malpresentation, cephalopelvic disproportion (CPD), chorioamnionitis, genital herpes in the mother within 6 weeks of delivery, fetal distress, or prolapsed umbilical cord. The multiparous pregnant patient who has had previous cesarean delivery may attempt vaginal delivery or may elect to schedule a planned cesarean birth.

Severe, unanticipated complications, such as bleeding or fetal distress during late pregnancy or labor, adversely affect the mother and/or fetus, creating an emergency. For these patients, preparations for immediate delivery are rapid. The patient easily senses a loss of control, especially if she participated in a childbirth education program for vaginal delivery. She needs special support. Most mothers fear more for the survival of the fetus than for themselves.

Admission procedures vary. Some hospitals admit an elective patient the morning of surgery. The patient is prepared by maternity personnel and taken to the delivery suite or to the OR. An emergency patient may go directly to the OR from the labor area. The trend is to perform C-sections in the obstetric suite. In any situation, the pediatrician and neonatal personnel from the nursery are notified before the procedure so that they will be available to resuscitate and care for the infant in the OR. Sterile pediatric equipment and supplies are made available.

Setup

Routine laparotomy skin preparation, draping, and setup are used for C-sections. Instruments are essentially those for a major gynecologic laparotomy with the addition of delivery forceps, a cord clamp, and a mucus aspiration bulb for infant suctioning on the field. A Foley catheter provides intraoperative bladder drainage. The patient is placed supine with the right side of the operating bed elevated or a small pillow under the right hip to displace the uterus from the inferior vena cava.

All preparations are made for the setup before the anesthetic is administered to the patient. If regional anesthesia is planned, the setup, counts, and preliminary routines can be performed simultaneously with the anesthesia procedures. The patient is prepped, catheterized, and draped after the anesthetic has taken effect. If general anesthesia is to be used, the setup, preparation, catheterization, and draping are performed before the anesthetic is administered to prevent prolonged depression of the fetus.

Incision and Delivery

A low transverse Pfannenstiel or low midline vertical incision is made in the skin and underlying tissue layers. The length varies with the size of the fetus. Dissection is expeditious. The uterine incision is made by one of the following methods:

1. *Low transverse (Kerr incision).* The bladder is dissected off the uterus and retracted gently downward. The lower uterine segment is entered through a low horizontal curvilinear incision. This approach causes less intraoperative blood loss and decreased chance of rupture with subsequent pregnancies. Some patients will be able to have vaginal deliveries in future pregnancies.

2. *Low vertical midline (Krohnig incision).* An 8-cm vertical incision is made in the lower uterine segment after the bladder is separated and retracted away. This incision is used when the fetus is small, preterm, and in the breech position. It is also used when cesarean hysterectomy may be performed following delivery.

3. *Classic uterine incision.* The uterus is incised vertically above the attachment of the bladder. The bladder is not dissected off the lower uterine segment. This approach is rarely used but may be necessary for a fetus in transverse presentation or for multiple fetuses. It may be indicated for a low anterior placenta, varicosities of the lower uterine segment, or cervical cancer. A major disadvantage is the high incidence of rupture with subsequent pregnancy.

As the uterus is incised, the amniotic sac will be opened. The amniotic fluid will escape rapidly, requiring suction. Retractors are removed, and the fetal head or the presenting part is gently delivered as pressure is applied to the fundus (Figure 35-5). Immediately on emergence of the head, the nares and mouth are aspirated with a bulb syringe to clear them of amniotic fluid. Newborns delivered by C-section have respiratory secretions. Delivery is completed, and the umbilical cord is double clamped and cut between the clamps with sterile scissors. The newborn is transferred via a sterile sheet to the neonatal resuscitation team. The circulator or neonatal team member who receives the newborn should wear protective eyewear, a gown, and gloves until all blood and amniotic fluid are wiped off the infant. The risk of exposure to blood and amniotic fluid warrants the same adherence to universal precautions as any other contact with blood and body fluids. The neonate is placed under a radiant warmer for resuscitation.

Low incision in uterus

Figure 35-5 Cesarean delivery after incising uterus and fetal membranes. As head is lifted through low uterine incision, pressure usually is applied to fundus of uterus through abdominal wall to help expel fetus.

IV oxytocin, 20 U, is administered to the mother to promote uterine contraction, minimize blood loss, and facilitate expulsion of the placenta and membranes. The placenta is delivered, visually inspected, and placed in a specimen basin. The uterine fundus is palpated for firmness and massaged as necessary to prevent hemorrhage from relaxation. Intrauterine injection of 10 U of oxytocin may be necessary to firm up an atonic uterus. The patient is returned to a horizontal supine position. The uterine incision is closed in layers with absorbable sutures, and hemostasis is ensured. Clots and excess intraperitoneal fluid are evacuated. After inspection of the pelvic organs and possible tubal ligation, the peritoneum and abdominal incision are closed.

Intraoperative assessment is the same as for any surgical patient. Sponges, tapes, and needles are counted before closure of the uterus and again before closure of the peritoneum, fascia, and skin.

Postpartum surveillance of the patient is essential. Lochia is observed. Abnormal bleeding, such as rapid saturation of the perineal pad, is immediately reported to the physician and recorded. Nurses' notes should include the mother's contact with the infant, the mother's emotional reaction to the surgical procedure, and persons in attendance, in addition to physical assessment data.

Neonate

Immediate postdelivery care is given in the OR by the neonatal team. The infant is taken to the nursery after careful examination by a pediatrician. The neonate traditionally has been evaluated by the Apgar score, acid-base status, and neurobehavioral examination. The Apgar score is an excellent screening tool for vital functions immediately (at 1- and 5- minute intervals) after birth, but the subtle effect of drugs may be overlooked. The Neurologic and Adaptive Capacity Score does not use noxious stimuli but emphasizes neonatal tone. Drugs that will produce significant neurobehavioral changes in the newborn must be avoided during labor and delivery.

In the newborn the apical pulse is the most accurate. Oxygenation is extremely important. Hypoxia (too little oxygen) can lead to intracranial hemorrhage, brain damage, or necrotizing enterocolitis. Hyperoxia (too much oxygen), administered at a rate in excess of 40% concentration, can cause bronchopulmonary dysplasia or retrolental fibroplasia.

Father or Support Person in the Delivery Room

Paternal or support-person participation in the birthing process is well established for vaginal delivery to provide support to the mother, a family-centered birth, and immediate bonding with the infant. However, the presence of the father or support person in the OR during cesarean delivery is not universal and requires the surgeon's consent. Hospitals adopting this policy report favorable experiences. This person is informed of the conditions permitting and excluding his or her presence. Those who have attended a structured childbirth education course have more understanding of pregnancy and birth. In compliance with hospital policy, donning of OR attire and supervised washing of hands with an antimicrobial soap before entrance to the OR are stressed. The father or support person sits by the mother's head. He or she may accompany the infant to the newborn examining area after delivery. If the condition of the newborn and mother permits it, the father or support person may rejoin the mother in the OR for bonding.

Prenatal Testing

Potentially useful for management of some congenital developmental disorders or genetic defects, prenatal diagnostic studies are performed during pregnancy in selected patients. Fetal anomalies are found in 2% of all women tested. Disorders in the fetus may be cause for induced abortion, elective cesarean delivery, or intrauterine fetal surgery.

Ultrasonography

Ultrasound is the standard tool for fetal imaging in utero. Ultrasonography, a noninvasive technique, permits accurate location of the placenta, determination of the gestational size of the fetus, assessment of fetal heart activity, and reliable diagnosis of structural defects (e.g., hydrocephalus or spina bifida). Other defects, such as missing limbs or conjoined twins, may be diagnosed.

Blood and Chorionic Villus Sampling

Ultrasound is also used for catheter or cannula guidance to obtain percutaneous umbilical blood samples or transcervical chorionic villus samples. Through direct fetal blood samples, anemia and some metabolic and chromosomal abnormalities can be diagnosed and treated in utero. Intravascular blood transfusions can be given to correct fetal anemia. Chorionic villi are a source of fetal genetic information. When obtained between the eighth and twelfth weeks of gestation, chorionic villi can aid in accurately diagnosing some enzymatic defects and in detecting the sex of the fetus.

Amniocentesis

Amniotic fluid is aspirated from the amniotic sac under ultrasound direction at 16 to 20 weeks' gestation for chromosomal analysis. This highly accurate test is indicated for known or suspected risk of chromosomal abnormality because of advanced maternal age, known parental translocation carrier, or a history of previous pregnancy with chromosomal defect in the fetus or infant. Maternal serum alpha-fetoprotein (AFP) measurement can predict neural tube disorders (e.g., myelomeningocele) or other defects in the fetus.

Fetoscopy

Fetoscopy permits direct visualization of the fetus. A fiberoptic needle scope (fetoscope) is inserted into the amniotic cavity to view fetal parts, to obtain a biopsy of skin, or to sample fetal blood. The fetoscope is 1.7 mm in diameter with a visual field of 70 degrees. To ensure an adequate volume of amniotic fluid, fetoscopy is done after 16 weeks of pregnancy. Because of the intent to view specific structures, the position of the fetus must first be determined and the procedure performed under sonographic-assisted visualization. Placental localization is important, especially in the area of umbilical cord insertion. Hemoglobinopathies and coagulation problems (e.g., hemophilia) may be rapidly diagnosed by aspiration of fetal blood from the placenta or umbilical cord. Congenital skin disorders and albinism may be detected by biopsy. Direct viewing of the fetus may reveal characteristic abnormalities of various congenital syndromes. The procedure is not without complications and should be performed only by trained physicians when genetic information is critical.

Intrauterine Fetal Surgery

Improvement and expansion in prenatal diagnosis have led to rapidly developing antenatal surgical intervention—intrauterine fetal surgery. Diagnostic screening by ultrasound, AFP, or some other method during gestation reveals abnormalities heretofore diagnosed after delivery. Some disorders can be treated in utero. Other conditions fall within the province of the surgeon. Prerequisites for fetal therapy include accurate diagnosis, known pathophysiology, workable treatment, and technical capability. Radiologists, perinatologists, pediatric surgeons, anesthesia providers, obstetric nurses, perioperative nurses, and surgical technologists comprise fetal surgery teams.

Most correctable malformations may be detected in utero but are best remedied by a surgical procedure after delivery at term. A full-term infant is a better surgical risk than is the fetus. Surgical treatment in utero is reserved for fetuses in whom continuing organ development could be normal if surgically treated (e.g., diaphragmatic hernia or hydronephrosis caused by urinary tract obstruction).

Minimally invasive procedures facilitate the placement of shunts and catheters. Highly invasive procedures require hysterotomy (opening of the uterine wall). Preoperative preparation includes the administration of tocolytic drugs (indomethacin suppository) to prevent the onset of labor caused by uterine manipulation. An irritable uterus requires cancellation of the procedure.

The procedure is performed in the late second trimester with the patient under general anesthesia using isoflurane because it is considered less hazardous to the fetus. The uterus is exposed through an abdominal incision, and a cannula is inserted through the uterine wall to decompress some of the amniotic fluid. The uterine anterior fundal incision is carefully extended down to the amnion. The sac is opened, and the edges are secured to the uterine edges with Raney clips. Meticulous hemostasis is necessary. ESU use is avoided. Small doses of fentanyl and pancuronium are administered to the fetus for anesthesia. A sterile pulse oximeter and electrocardiographic (ECG) leads are sutured to the fetus to monitor oxygenation and cardiac activity. Great care is taken to avoid manipulation of the placenta or cord. Warmed sterile saline irrigation is continuously perfused through the amniotic cavity during the procedure. After the repairs are complete, a small, wireless transducer is placed in the fetal chest for continued postoperative monitoring of the fetus in utero. This transducer is removed after birth. If fetal repairs require

thoracotomy and diaphragmatic patching, the pleural space is maintained with warmed Ringer's lactate solution to allow for continued lung growth.

On completion of the procedure, the amnion is sutured closed and fibrin glue is applied. The uterus is sutured, and the abdominal incision is stapled. The fetal wound healing is nearly scarless because of decreased inflammatory response and neotissue generation associated with continued fetal development. The pregnancy continues as long as possible after the open procedure, preferably a minimum of 32 to 36 weeks' gestation. Lung maturity is the key issue for success. Preterm labor usually precipitates cesarean birth. Vaginal delivery is contraindicated because a classic uterine incision of the fundus is used for open intrauterine fetal surgery.

ASSISTED REPRODUCTION

Infertility, the inability to conceive a child after a year or more of repeated attempts, can be emotionally devastating. Both partners undergo extensive testing to determine possible organic or functional causes. These may include a structural defect in either partner, past or present infections, genetic and/or immunologic abnormalities, or an endocrine imbalance or deficit. In the woman a hostile cervix, antibodies to sperm, endometriosis, or exposure to DES in utero may prevent conception. Tubal occlusion is the most frequent cause of infertility. A male partner may have an inadequate number, quality, or mobility of sperm or an absence of live spermatozoa in semen. When conventional infertility therapy has failed to produce a pregnancy, other options are available to assist in achieving pregnancy and birth of a mature, live infant.

In Vitro Fertilization

The term *in vitro* means *in glass.* Fertilization literally takes place in a culture dish or test tube. In vitro fertilization (IVF) refers to removal of ova from the prospective mother via endoscopy, fertilization with the husband's or a donor's sperm, and incubation in the laboratory with subsequent embryo transfer to the uterus. Ovulation may be stimulated by administration of hormones. Multiple follicles may mature, and several ova are procured. The first documented birth from IVF and embryo transfer, performed by Dr. Robert Edwards and Dr. Patrick Steptoe, took place in England in 1978 by cesarean section. The first IVF clinic in the United States using the Edwards-Steptoe method was established in Virginia in 1980.

IVF is most successful in woman younger than age 30 years. In women younger than 34 years the success rate is 30% to 40% for delivery per ovum retrieval. The success of this technology for pregnancy in woman over the age of 42 years is less than 10%. However, reports of a live birth by this method to a woman 60 years of age are found in the literature.

Patient Selection

IVF is accepted therapy for women with severely damaged or nonfunctioning fallopian tubes, for men with scarce or absent sperm, or for infertility of unknown cause. Contraindications include a uterine myoma, single uterine cornu, or a bicornate or septate uterus. The woman is evaluated preoperatively for a normal uterine cavity, an accessible ovary, and evidence of ovulation. These parameters are measured by pelvic ultrasonography and serum estrogen levels. A laparoscopy, endometrial biopsy, and hysterosalpingogram may be part of preoperative testing. Semen analysis is done to check the sperm condition and count of the male partner.

Some patients may be unable to provide an ovum, conceive, or carry a fetus to full term. In select situations, a surrogate mother will carry the developing fetus to term, surrendering the neonate at birth to the adoptive mother. Family members, such as a sister or other, may participate. Ethics and legal issues surround this event. Patient confidentiality is protected.

Induction of Ovulation

IVF is coordinated with timing of the ovulatory cycle. The medical protocol is prescribed for the individual couple. From day 2 or 3 of the menstrual cycle through day 6 or 7, the woman takes fertility drugs to stimulate growth and maturation of ovarian follicles. These drugs are a combination of clomiphene citrate (a synthetic hormone) and human luteinizing and follicle-stimulating hormones. Follicular growth is monitored daily, beginning about the eighth day, by ultrasonography and serum estrogen levels. The fluid-filled follicles on the surface of the ovaries contain ova (oocytes). When follicles reach a diameter of 15 to 20 mm, the woman is given human chorionic gonadotropin (HCG) intramuscularly to stimulate maturation of the ova.

Ovum Retrieval

The patient is scheduled for retrieval of mature ova about 35 hours after HCG injection. Ovum retrieval may be accomplished through ultrasound-assisted transvaginal, transvesicle, or transabdominal approaches. The procedure is performed with the patient under general anesthesia or IV sedation. Transvaginal ovum retrieval is the procedure of choice, but the approach depends on accessibility to the ovary. With the patient in the lithotomy position, the ultrasound probe with an aspiration needle guide attached is advanced through the cervix, uterus, and fallopian tube to the ovary. The needle guide is directed toward the follicle, as seen on a monitoring screen. The follicle is punctured with a 14-inch × 17-gauge needle. Follicular fluid is aspirated into a 5-ml syringe. Ova procured from the graafian follicle are placed in sterile solution designated by the treating gynecologist.

Extensive scarring in tubes may make ovaries inaccessible via the transvaginal approach. For a transvesicle approach, the ultrasound probe is inserted through the urethra and posterior bladder wall to the ovary. With the patient positioned supine, a retrieval probe can be inserted percutaneously through the abdominal wall to reach the ovary in the pelvic cavity.

Ova can be retrieved by laparoscopy. The surgeon visualizes the ovaries. The follicle is punctured with an 8-inch × 14-gauge needle and aspirated directly into a test tube through a catheter attached to the needle. All instruments and solutions used for retrieval are kept at a normal physiologic temperature of 98.6° F (37° C). After completion of aspiration, the syringe or test tube is carefully handed to the circulator using aseptic technique. To avoid contamination, fluid should not be exposed to the environment, including light. Dimmed room light also enhances the surgeon's view on the video monitor. The circulator labels the specimen and sends it immediately to the laboratory for confirmation of ovum retrieval while instrumentation is still in place. If the report is negative, the search for another ovum continues until the laboratory gives a positive response of retrieval. The procedure may be repeated on the contralateral ovary. Many surgeons prefer to retrieve at least three to five ova for fertilization. Other women can be suitable volunteer donors for ova for women who have been unable to provide a suitable ovum.

Fertilization

The aspirated ova are placed in a culture dish containing a nutrient mixture similar to tubal secretions at midcycle, which prepares the ova for fertilization. Fresh semen obtained an hour or so before the woman undergoes ovum retrieval, or previously collected frozen sperm from a partner or donor, is added. The culture dish is incubated for 40 to 48 hours for fertilization to take place. Cell division is detected by microscopic examination. When the embryo reaches the 4- to 8-cell stage of development, it is ready for transfer to the uterus. Multiple oocytes can be fertilized, and embryos can be stored frozen for a period of up to 3 years for later implantation if desired. Embryos frozen at the 2-, 4-, 8-, or 16-cell stage, after thawing, have a viability rate of 60% to 80%. The embryo is transferred during a natural ovulatory cycle for the best results.

Embryo Transfer

Approximately 48 hours after retrieval, the woman returns for embryo transfer. She is placed in the knee-chest position. Anesthesia is unnecessary. A catheter prepared in the laboratory, containing the embryo in culture medium, is inserted into the uterus. The patient remains in the knee-chest position for at least an hour to allow the embryo to gravitate to the upper uterine fundus. Immediately following embryo transfer, an injection of progesterone is given. Necessary for implantation, injections are given daily for the next 12 to 15 days. Implantation is necessary for progression of the cell mass to an embryo. The woman's own ovarian function sustains early gestation, as confirmed by ultrasonography.

Failure to implant may result from escape of the embryo from the uterus with removal of the catheter, excess uterine contractility, inadequate luteal phase affecting the endometrium, mechanical disturbance of the endometrium, or encapsulation of the embryo in blood or mucus.

Gamete Intrafallopian Transfer

The procedure for gamete intrafallopian transfer (GIFT), developed in 1984, is similar to IVF but is always done laparoscopically. The woman must have at least one patent, functional fallopian tube. Ovulation is induced as described for

IVF. Laparoscopy is scheduled 34 or 35 hours after injection of HCG. Fresh semen is obtained from the partner at least an hour before this procedure and is centrifuged and incubated at body temperature until use.

Ovum retrieval via laparoscope is accomplished as described for IVF. The follicular fluid is sent immediately to the laboratory, where an embryologist selects two or three ova. These and the sperm, along with the culture medium, are loaded into a catheter and sent back to the OR. The surgeon passes the catheter through the laparoscope and injects fluid into the ampulla of the fallopian tube. One or both tubes may receive an injection.

Other procedures, such as laser vaporization of endometriosis or lysis of adhesions, may be performed while the surgeon waits for the catheter. Additional ova may be inseminated and cryopreserved for IVF if GIFT is unsuccessful. Many implants may precede conception; it may never be successful.

Artificial Insemination

In vivo fertilization by artificial insemination of sperm may provide a reproductive option for a fertile woman. Homologous insemination deposits the partner's sperm into the upper vagina, cervical canal, or uterine cavity. Whole ejaculate is used when the man is unable to deposit sperm into the partner's vagina because of psychologic or physiologic factors. Washed sperm are used for intrauterine injection. Semen or sperm may be frozen and stored in a sperm bank for future use if reproductive capacity is threatened, such as by illness.

Artificial insemination is coordinated with the recipient's ovulation for conception to occur.

Donor insemination involves the same techniques, but sperm are obtained from a donor. Donors are screened for sexually transmitted diseases, including infection with human immunodeficiency virus (HIV) and hepatitis B virus (HBV). Genetic screening also may be required. Donor sperm may be sought when the partner has a genetically transmitted disease or defect. The couple may have concerns about donor selection.

NONOBSTETRIC SURGICAL PROCEDURES AND THE PREGNANT PATIENT

The pregnant surgical patient who is brought to the OR for reasons other than childbirth presents a unique challenge to the perioperative team. The plan of care includes consideration for two patients: the mother and her developing fetus. The effects of surgical intervention can be disastrous to a pregnancy, but in some situations it is necessary to save the mother and/or the fetus. These considerations apply to all pregnant patients.

The average gestation, or duration of pregnancy, is 38 to 40 weeks or 9 calendar months. This gestation period is divided into trimesters (3-month segments). Each trimester represents a specific developmental and viability concern (Box 35-1). Maternal anatomic and physiologic changes occur during each trimester of pregnancy (Table 35-3). Modifications to

---

Box 35-1	**Gestational Stages of Fetal Development and Viability Concerns**

First Trimester (1-3 Months, 1-12 Weeks)

Zygote implants in uterine wall by 14 days.

Communication of venous sinus and arterial supply of maternal circulation is completed at 17 days.

Teratogens can impair organogenesis until 14th week.

Primitive placental system with umbilical cord is established by 7th week.

Heart rate is detectable on ultrasound at 10-12 weeks.

Facial features and external genitalia are present by 12th week.

Crown-to-rump length is 6-7 cm by 12th week.

Second Trimester (4-7 Months, 13-27 Weeks)

Arms and trunk grow rapidly.

Little muscle tone.

Scalp hair, tiny nipples, and external ears develop by 20th week.

Meconium is present in intestine.

Body weight is 300 g.

Skeletal calcification is seen on x-ray film.

Sucks thumb and moves freely at will.

Fetal heart rate is audible with fetoscope at 120-160 beats/min at 20th week.

Fingertip pressure causes ballottement (fetal rebound) in amniotic sac during 16th-32nd week.

Teratogens may cause minor structural and functional abnormalities, especially endocrine, brain, and special senses, from 10th week to term.

Body is covered with vernix (gray-white cheeselike substance) and lanugo (soft, downy hair).

Eyebrows and eyelashes are present.

Body weight is 454-630 g (1-1.4 pounds) by 24th week.

May be viable.

Third Trimester (7-9 Months, 28-38 to 40 Weeks)

Subcutaneous fat begins to develop.

Crown-to-rump length is 25 cm.

Testes are descended in male.

Body weight is 1100 g (2½ pounds).

Surfactant is present in alveoli of lungs by 28th week.

Increased chance of survival.

Body weight is 1361-1814 g (3-4 pounds) by 32nd week.

Body is fuller and rounded.

Muscle tone is good.

Less vernix and absence of lanugo by 36th week.

Body weight is 3402-3629 g (7½-8 pounds) by 38-40 weeks.

Crown-to-rump length is 36 cm.

TABLE 35-3	Maternal Anatomic and Physiologic Changes of Pregnancy		
System	**First Trimester (1-3 Months' Gestation [1-12 Weeks])**	**Second Trimester (4-7 Months' Gestation [13-27 Weeks])**	**Third Trimester (7-9 Months' Gestation [28-38 to 40 Weeks])**
Cardiovascular	Cardiac output begins to increase at 6th week. Plasma volume begins to increase.	Cardiac output increases 30%-50% by 16th week. Plasma volume continues to increase. Hypervolemic and hemodiluted. Red blood cell (RBC) production increases 20%. WBC increases 30%-40%.	Cardiac output decreases slightly by 30th week. Plasma volume increase peaks 50% at 32-36 weeks. RBC increases, peaks at 33%.
	Breast veins dilate. Vasculature increases to vulva and vagina.	Capillary engorgement can cause epistaxis (nosebleeds) and epulis (bleeding gums). Heart rate increases 15-20 beats/min.	May develop hemorrhoids and varicosities in leg veins. Increased risk for venous thrombosis. Factors VII, IX, X increase causes hypercoagulative state. Plasma fibrinogen increases 40%-50%.
		Slight hypotension caused by decreased peripheral vascular resistance.	Normotensive by 26th week.
		Uterus presses on vena cava when supine. Physiologic anemia: hemoglobin, hematocrit, and platelets decrease.	Uterine circulation is 1 L/min by 38th-40th week.
Pulmonary Lung compliance and pulmonary diffusion remain constant throughout pregnancy.	Vital capacity and partial pressure of oxygen (PO_2) are unchanged.	Diaphragm is displaced upward by rising fundus; thoracic circumference increases by 6 cm. Tidal volume increases 30%-40%. Respiratory rate increases 15% to accommodate increasing metabolism. Mild dyspnea. Chronic state of compensated respiratory alkalosis. Nasal congestion caused by estrogen-induced edema.	Diaphragm is displaced 4 cm by risng fundus. Thoracic breathing replaces abdominal breathing. Venous stasis increases risk for thrombus formation and pulmonary emboli.
Gastrointestinal	Nausea and vomiting. Constipation. Salivation increases.	Nausea and vomiting diminish. Incidence of cholecystitis is increased. Progesterone causes decreased gastrointestinal motility. Esophageal sphincter tone is decreased; at risk for gastric reflux.	Gastric emptying time is decreased. Gallbladder sluggish, frequently develop gallstones.
Neurologic	May feel some slight Braxton Hicks contractions starting at 8th week.	Intraocular pressure decreases. Some temporary visual changes develop; vision returns to prepregnant state after delivery.	Braxton Hicks contractions increase and become regular.

TABLE 35-3	Maternal Anatomic and Physiologic Changes of Pregnancy—cont'd		
System	**First Trimester** **(1-3 Months' Gestation** **[1-12 Weeks])**	**Second Trimester** **(4-7 Months' Gestation** **[13-27 Weeks])**	**Third Trimester** **(7-9 Months' Gestation** **[28-38 to 40 Weeks])**
Endocrine	Human chorionic gonadotropin hormone secreted by corpus luteum of ovary is present in serum 9 days after conception. Progesterone production increases. Basal metabolic rate decreases. Blood glucose level decreases.	Protein binding causes increase in circulating hormones. Thyroid and adrenal hormone levels are elevated. Insulin production increases. Erythropoietin increases by 20th week. Metabolism increases.	Prolactin increases and peaks at delivery.
Genitourinary Ureters and renal pelves and calyces dilate, increasing risk of urinary tract infection. Dilation is present throughout pregnancy.	Urinary frequency caused by uterine pressure on bladder.	Bladder pressure decreases as fundus elevates. Bladder is displaced superior to pelvis. Glomerular filtration rate increases 30%-50%. Drugs are excreted faster.	Lateral position facilitates renal blood flow and increases urinary output. Increased frequency as presenting part enters pelvis.
Integumentary	No appreciable change.	Striae gravidarum (stretch marks) appear on breasts and abdomen.	Dark line (linea nigra) appears between umbilicus and pubis. Increased pigmentation of face (cholasma).
Musculoskeletal	Feels fatigue. Weight loss first few weeks caused by nausea and vomiting. Average weight gain 2.2 pounds (1 kg) by 10-12 weeks. Leg cramps.	Feels energetic. Weight gain 1 pound (0.45 kg) per week; desirable weight gain between 12th and 20th week is 8 pounds (3.62 kg). Gains ½-1 pound (0.24 kg-2.2 kg) per week between 20th and 38th week. Progressive lordosis to compensate for shifting center of gravity causes backache. Leg cramps increase by 24th week.	Energy declines. Ideal total weight gain 25-30 pounds (11-13.6 kg) total for entire pregnancy. Increased lordosis as uterus expands and protrudes forward. Pelvic joints relax and slight separation of symphysis pubis can be seen on x-ray film.
Reproductive	Menstruation ceases. Progesterone causes uterine lining to thicken. Estrogen causes uterine body to hypertrophy, anteflex, and become globular; by 3rd month fundus reaches pelvic brim. Cervix softens and vulva and vagina appear blue (caused by increasing vascularity). Vaginal discharge increases. Breast tissue enlarges and becomes sensitive.	Uterine fundus elevates halfway between symphysis pubis and umbilicus by 12th-16th week but rises above umbilicus by 24 weeks. Fetal movement is felt by 18th-20th week. Lower uterine segment elevates in pelvis. Areolae darken.	Uterine fundus elevates halfway between umbilicus and xyphoid process by 28th week and reaches xyphoid by 32nd week. Fundus decreases in height (caused by uterine weight) by 38th week. Uterine weight at term is 1100 g. Breasts feel full and tender. May secrete colostrum (precursor to milk).

the plan of care vary according to these changes. Risks associated with surgical intervention may be specific to the fetus. During the first trimester spontaneous abortion of the developing embryo (until the end of the eighth week) or fetus (from the eighth week) can occur. Preterm labor and/or delivery may be precipitated during the second and third trimesters. The surgeon and anesthesia provider should discuss the risks, benefits, and potential outcome with the patient and her family.

Nonobstetric surgical procedures on pregnant patients are usually performed for an urgent or emergent reason, such as cholecystitis, appendicitis, or trauma. Urgent surgical procedures are delayed until the second or third trimester if possible. Emergency procedures are performed immediately, regardless of gestational stage. If the maternal condition is critical, the primary concern is to save the mother. Elective surgical procedures should be deferred until after delivery of the neonate and the anatomic and physiologic changes of pregnancy have returned to normal.

Anesthesia Considerations in Pregnancy

The surgeon and anesthesia provider collaborate closely because the risks of anesthesia and surgical procedures are high for both the mother and the fetus. Perinatal morbidity and mortality are affected by maternal health, fetal viability, the type of anesthetic, and the surgical procedure. The incidence of preterm labor, low birth weight, and fetal death increases if general anesthesia must be administered. The objectives of anesthetic management in the pregnant surgical patient include, but are not limited to, the following:

1. *Maternal safety.* The pregnant patient should always be treated as if she has a full stomach. Nausea and vomiting are common and place the patient at risk for aspiration of regurgitated stomach contents during induction of anesthesia, intubation, and extubation. The condition of the mother directly affects the outcome of the pregnancy.
2. *Avoidance of teratogenic drugs.* Many anesthetic drugs cross the placenta and enter the fetus through the uteroplacental circulation. Some drugs that adversely affect the fetus during the first trimester include nitrous oxide, halogenated agents, sedatives, tranquilizers, antidepressants, and amphetamines. Halogenated agents and nitrous oxide have been given without teratogenicity in emergency situations during the second and third trimesters. Only short-acting drugs should be used. The fetal liver is immature and metabolizes tranquilizers and other narcotics slowly. Neonatal respiratory depression is common if these drugs have been used.

    Agents used in local and regional anesthesia have not shown teratogenicity in animal studies and may provide a safer anesthetic alternative than general anesthesia when a surgical procedure must be performed.
3. *Prevention of fetal asphyxia.* Maternal hypoxia rapidly affects the oxygenation of the fetus. The oxygenation capability depends on the hemoglobin content and arterial oxygen tension of maternal blood and uteroplacental perfusion. Maternal hypotension and decreased uterine blood flow cause fetal hypoxia.
4. *Prevention of preterm labor.* Studies have shown no association of any single anesthetic agent with an increase or decrease in preterm labor. Manipulation of the gravid uterus can cause preterm labor. The use of halogenated agents in advanced pregnancy decreases uterine tone and prevents uterine contractions. Vasopressors and drugs used to reverse muscle relaxants may stimulate the uterus to contract and initiate preterm labor.

Special Considerations
Intraoperative Care of the Pregnant Patient

Both the mother and the fetus should be monitored during the surgical procedure. The mother's physiologic and psychologic condition rapidly affects the well-being of her fetus. Changes in the fetal condition may be the first indicator of a physiologic change in the mother. Intraoperative care and monitoring of the pregnant surgical patient include special considerations regarding the following objectives:

1. Minimize the patient's time under anesthesia. Skin preparation and draping should be done before induction of general anesthesia. Devices for electronic fetal and uterine monitoring should be in position and in proper working order.
2. Monitor maternal oxygenation. Pulse oximetry is useful for noninvasive measurement of oxygenation in hemoglobin. Readings should remain above 94% to prevent fetal hypoxia. Continuous oxygen is usually administered.
3. Monitor the fetal heart rate. An electronic fetal heart monitor (EFM) should be used by appropriately trained personnel for continuous monitoring. Fetal tachycardia may be the first indicator of maternal hypoxia. EFM is most effective after 16 weeks' gestation. Personnel qualified in EFM should be assigned this role.
4. Monitor the uterine tone. The uterus should be palpated frequently during the surgical procedure to detect contractions. Uterine manipulation, bladder stimulation, and several anesthetic drugs may cause preterm labor.
5. Prevent aspiration. Assist the anesthesia provider during intubation by providing cricoid pressure (Sellick's maneuver) as directed.
6. Prevent maternal hypotension. If the uterus is enlarged to the level of the umbilicus or above (17 to 20 weeks' gestation), place a small pad or folded sheet under the right hip to laterally displace the uterus to the left. This redistributes the weight of the gravid uterus off the vena cava and abdominal aorta and facilitates a normotensive state. Renal perfusion is also improved.

7. Monitor urinary output. Minimum urinary output should be 25 ml/hr. Palpate the bladder every 30 minutes. Bladder distention can cause uterine irritability and preterm labor. The bladder is displaced above the pelvis during the second and third trimesters and is easily injured. An indwelling Foley catheter should be inserted if the surgical procedure is anticipated to exceed 1 hour.
8. Maintain a normothermic environment. Warm the room to 75° F (24° C) and maintain a consistent temperature during the surgical procedure. Maternal hypothermia causes decreased uteroplacental perfusion and can cause fetal bradycardia. Use prewarmed blankets and irrigating solutions. Keep the mother's head covered.
9. Prepare for emergency cesarean birth or preterm delivery. In the event of untimely rupture of the membranes, preterm labor, or fetal distress, it may be necessary to perform a cesarean section or precipitous delivery in an effort to save a viable fetus. A preterm fetus requiring immediate delivery after 24 weeks' gestation or 500 g (1 pound) weight may be considered viable. Fetal viability is individualized by measurement of lung maturity, body weight, and ability to sustain life after removal from the uterus.
10. Protect the fetus from hazards in the environment. The pregnant uterus at any stage of gestation should be shielded from ionizing radiation. During the first trimester, radiation may cause teratogenic damage. This may be unavoidable in trauma surgery.
11. Reassure the mother. Explain that she and her fetus will be monitored closely and that they will be carefully protected.

Intraoperative Risks

The enlarging uterus displaces abdominal organs and distorts anatomic landmarks, making diagnoses of trauma or a pathologic condition complex. A motor vehicle accident is a common cause of abdominal trauma. A seat belt (lap belt) without a shoulder restraint can cause compression injury to the enlarged uterus. Spontaneous laceration and/or rupture can occur. Peritoneal lavage, if used to assess for intraabdominal bleeding, should be done through an incision above the umbilicus to avoid injuring the uterus.

Surgical procedures for reasons other than trauma, such as pathologic causes, require careful differential diagnosis. Anatomic and physiologic changes of pregnancy must be considered. For example, the appendix is displaced to the upper right quadrant and may mimic cholecystitis. In advanced pregnancy, chest drainage tubes should be inserted one to two intercostal spaces higher, if needed. Diagnosis is complicated because laboratory tests are altered by the progressing pregnancy, and results vary according to the gestational stage.

Assessment of the patient's condition is difficult because compensatory mechanisms of pregnancy cause alterations in vital signs. The arterial blood pressure is lower than prepregnant values, and the pulse is elevated to accommodate an in-

crease in circulatory volume. Decreased peripheral vascular resistance prevents overt physiologic signs of shock, such as cool, clammy skin. Circulating blood volume can be reduced 30% to 35% before the patient shows any signs of hypovolemic shock, such as lowered blood pressure and increased pulse rate. In hypovolemic shock, blood is shunted away from the uteroplacental circulation at the expense of the fetus. The fetus becomes hypoxic. Fetal demise is 80% in maternal hypovolemic shock. An EFM can detect early signs of fetal hypoxia and uteroplacental insufficiency. Use of a fetal monitor is recommended during surgical procedures after 16 weeks' gestation. Personnel appropriately trained in fetal monitoring should perform this assessment throughout the perioperative period, including during the surgical procedure and postanesthesia recovery.

In the immediate postoperative period the pregnant patient must be assessed for uterine irritability, vaginal bleeding, and/or ruptured membranes. Any combination of these signs may signal impending labor and possible preterm delivery and must be reported to the physician immediately. Bladder distention can cause uterine irritability and stimulate preterm labor. The bladder should be palpated frequently. A distended bladder is felt as a bulge above the symphysis pubis that is cooler than the surrounding skin.

Psychologic Considerations

For most patients and their families, pregnancy is a time of joy and excitement. Their happiness is shattered when they are faced with the prospect of a surgical procedure and its inherent risks. In urgent and emergency situations there is little time for the family to adjust to the pending procedure. The outcome is uncertain, and the risks to the mother and her fetus are great. The patient and family are also facing the possibility of a preterm delivery. The perioperative team should take the special needs of the pregnant patient into consideration and provide as much reassurance as possible.

Bibliography

Bennett KL et al: Preventing intravasation in women undergoing hysteroscopic procedures, *AORN J* 64(5):792-799, 1996.

Berek JS, Hacker NF: *Practical gynecologic oncology,* ed 2, Philadelphia, 1994, Williams & Wilkins.

Bran DF et al: Outpatient vaginal hysterectomy as a new trend in gynecology, *AORN J* 62(5):810-814, 1995.

Brooten D et al: Early discharge and home care after unplanned cesarean birth: nursing care time, *J Obstet Gynecol Neonatal Nurs* 25(7):959-600, 1996.

Carlson KJ: Outcomes of hysterectomy, *Clin Obstet Gynecol* 40(4):939-946, 1997.

DeChurney AH, Pernoll ML: *Current obstetric and gynecologic diagnosis and treatment,* ed 8, Norwalk, Conn, 1994, Appleton & Lange.

Haspel-Siegel AS: Fallopian tube anastomosis procedures to restore fertility, *AORN J* 56(1):75-86, 1997.

Kendrick JM et al: Surveyed use of fetal and uterine monitoring during maternal surgery, *AORN J* 62(3):386-392, 1995.

Martyn P, Allan B: Long-term follow-up of endometrial ablation, *J Am Assoc Gynecol Laparosc* 5(2):115-118, 1998.

Murdoch JB et al: The outcome of pregnancy after CO₂ laser conization of the cervix, *Br J Obstet Gynecol* 101(3):277, 1994.

Raz S: *Atlas of transvaginal surgery,* Philadelphia, 1992, WB Saunders.

Reinhardt M: Emergency: ectopic pregnancy rupture, *Am J Nurs* 94(7):41, 1994.

Robinson BJ: The perioperative nurse's role in assisted-fertility procedures, *AORN J* 65(1):87-93, 1997.

Schneider D et al: Safety of midtrimester pregnancy termination by laminaria and evacuation in patients with previous cesarean section, *Am J Obstet Gynecol* 171(2):554-557, 1994.

Soderstrom RM: *Operative laparoscopy: the masters' techniques,* New York, 1993, Raven Press.

Steiert MJ: Clinical issues: male and female infertility; artificial insemination; in vitro fertilization; habitual abortions; patient care, *AORN J* 65(4): 810-812, 1997.

Ulmer BC: Cervical intraepithelial neoplasia: etiology, diagnosis, treatment, *AORN J* 59(4):851-860, 1994.

Weber AM et al: Uterine myomas and factors associated with hysterectomy in premenopausal women, *Am J Obstet Gynecol,* 176(6):1213-1217, 1997.

Wheeler SR: Psychosocial needs of women during miscarriage or ectopic pregnancy, *AORN J* 60(2):221-231, 1994.

Wiens AG: Preoperative anxiety in women, *AORN J* 68(1):74-88, 1998.

Chapter 36

Urologic Surgery

 Chapter Objectives

After studying this chapter, the learner will be able to:

- Identify the organs of the male genitourinary system.
- Compare the differences between male and female urinary systems.
- Describe the procedures performed for urinary incontinence.
- Describe the procedures performed for prostate cancer.

Urology is defined as that branch of medicine and surgery concerned with the study, diagnosis, and treatment of abnormalities and diseases of the urogenital tract of the male and the urinary tract of the female throughout the life span. Because of the shared responsibility in patient care with pediatricians, internists, nephrologists, endocrinologists, surgeons, and oncologists, close association with specialists in these disciplines is essential.*

HISTORICAL BACKGROUND

Writings from approximately 3000 BC tell of urinary diseases. The earliest known specimen of a bladder stone was found in an Egyptian grave that dates back to 4000 BC. People in India are known to have suffered from bladder stones around 2000 BC. Removal of a stone from the bladder through an incision is one of the earliest known surgical procedures. It was often performed by itinerant lithotomists, who flourished from the time of Hippocrates to the early eighteenth century. Hippocrates wrote that stone removal should be left to those trained for such work. For centuries this surgical procedure was not considered a part of medicine.

Although enlarged prostate glands were noted in the time of Hippocrates, attempts to remove part of them perineally or to tunnel through them with a sharp instrument were extremely dangerous.

Urethral sounds and bronze catheters have been found in the ruins of Pompeii, buried since 79 AD. Metal catheters were used until the advent of rubber ones in the late nineteenth century.

The first urologists were mainly venereologists and instrumenteurs of the urethra. Urology advanced as a science with the invention of the microscope in the seventeenth century. Attempts to visualize the interior of the bladder were not made until the early nineteenth century, and the instruments and source of light were inadequate. In 1877, Max Nitze (1848-1906), a German urologist, developed an electrically illuminated operating endoscope that is the basis of the modern cystoscope and urologic endoscopy. He systematically cauterized urinary tract tumors without using a fluid medium for bladder distention. He also authored an important monograph in 1889 that was dedicated to cystoscopy in patient care.

Urologists have contributed to the evolution of medicine in general. The use of antibacterial drugs by urologists freed all physicians from the time-consuming treatment of venereal disease. Urology has been and continues to be a supporting specialty within medicine and surgery and is interdependent with other specialties.

---

*American Board of Urology.

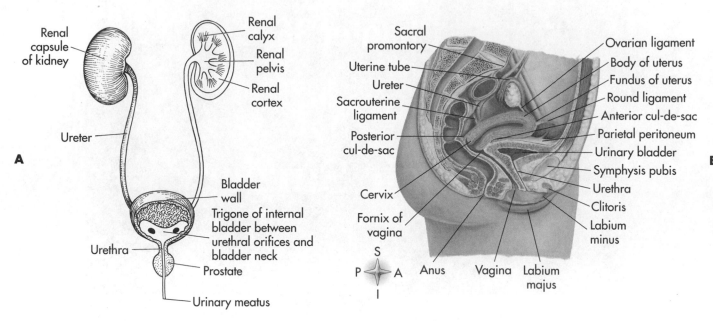

Figure 36-1 Anatomy of the urinary tract. **A,** Male urinary tract. **B,** Female reproductive organs and urinary system. (**B** from Thibodeau GA, Patton KT: *Anatomy and physiology,* ed 4, St Louis, 1999, Mosby.)

ANATOMY AND PHYSIOLOGY OF THE URINARY SYSTEM

The urinary system provides the vital life-sustaining functions of extracting waste products from the bloodstream and excreting them from the body. Organs of this system include bilateral kidneys and ureters, the bladder, and the urethra (Figure 36-1). An obstruction to blood flow in the renal arteries or in any part of the urinary system can cause renal damage, which ultimately results in uremia (a biochemical imbalance) or renal failure if left undiagnosed and untreated. Vascular hypertension, tumors, infection, trauma, and other systemic or neurogenic disorders are of major concern to the urologist.

Kidneys

The kidneys are large, bean-shaped, glandular organs located bilaterally in the retroperitoneal space of the thoracolumbar region behind the abdominal cavity. The arterial blood supply (renal artery) of the kidney originates from the aorta and enters the hilum on the medial aspect. Venous drainage flows through the renal vein and into the inferior vena cava. The lymphatics drain into the lumbar nodes.

Each kidney is enclosed in a thin, fibrous capsule. The renal parenchyma, the substance of the kidney within the capsule, is composed of an external cortex and internal medulla. The medulla consists of conical segments called renal pyramids. Each pyramid and its surrounding cortex form a lobe. Within these pyramids are the essential components of renal function: the nephrons (Figure 36-2). *Ren* is the Latin word for *kidney;* hence the adjective *renal* and combining forms of *ren-* and *reno-* in terms pertaining to the kidney as part of the renal system.

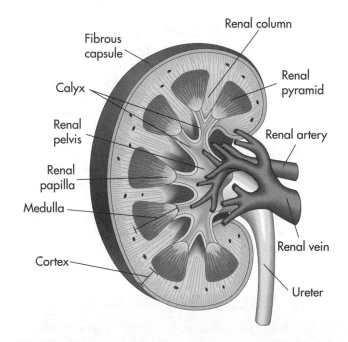

Figure 36-2 Cross section of the kidney. (From Thibodeau GA, Patton KT: *Anatomy and physiology,* ed 4, St Louis, 1999, Mosby.)

Each nephron consists of a glomerulus, glomerular capsule, and tubules. A glomerulus is an aggregation of capillaries formed by an afferent branch of the renal artery. These capillaries unite to form an efferent vessel. This capillary network is enclosed in a glomerular capsule (capsule of Bowman), which is the dilated beginning of the renal tubule. From the capsule, the tubule becomes tortuous and forms the proximal convoluted tubule. The distal portion forms the descending and

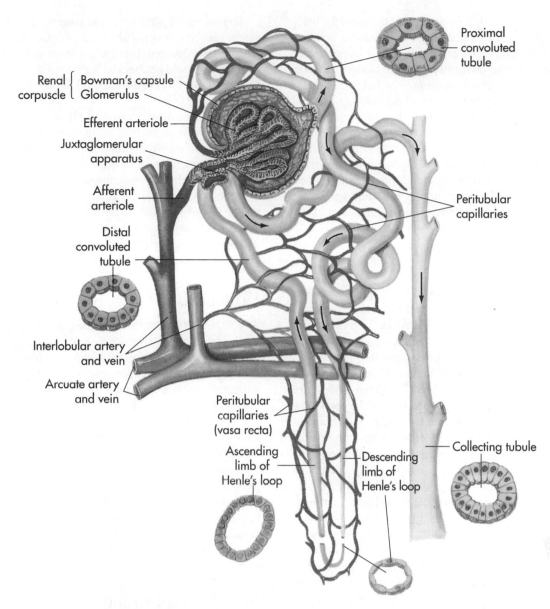

Renal { Bowman's capsule
corpuscle { Glomerulus

Efferent arteriole

Juxtaglomerular
apparatus

Afferent
arteriole

Distal
convoluted
tubule

Interlobular artery
and vein

Arcuate artery
and vein

Peritubular
capillaries
(vasa recta)

Ascending
limb of
Henle's loop

Descending
limb of
Henle's loop

Proximal
convoluted
tubule

Peritubular
capillaries

Collecting tubule

Figure 36-3 Cross section of the nephron. (From Thibodeau GA, Patton KT: *Anatomy and physiology,* ed 4, St Louis, 1999, Mosby.)

ascending limbs of the medullary loop (loop of Henle) (Figure 36-3). Nitrogenous wastes, salts, toxins, and water filtered from the capillary network form urine, which flows through the medullary loop and into the collecting tubule. The collecting tubules converge at the papilla (apex) of each renal pyramid. Urine flows continuously from each papilla into a calyx. Each kidney has between four and thirteen minor calyces that lead into two or three (rarely four) major calyces that form the renal pelvis. The renal pelvis forms the dilated proximal end of the ureter.

Ureters

The ureters are connecting tubes between the kidneys and bladder; they are 4 to 5 mm in diameter, have a 0.2 to 1.0 cm

lumen, and are approximately 12 inches (25 to 30 cm) long. They lie bilaterally beneath the parietal peritoneum and descend along the posterior abdominal wall to the pelvic brim. From there, they pass along the lateral wall of the pelvis and curve downward, forward, and inward along the pelvic floor to the bladder. The wall of each ureter is continuous with the renal pelvis and is composed of mucous membrane, longitudinal and circular muscles, and an outer layer of fibrous and elastic tissue. Slow, rhythmic, peristaltic contractions carry urine from the kidneys to the bladder.

Urinary Bladder

The bladder is a hollow muscular reservoir lined with mucous membrane; it is located extraperitoneally in the anterior pelvic cavity behind the symphysis pubis. The ureters enter the bladder wall obliquely on each side. The triangular area between the ureteral and urethral orifices is called the trigone. Valves formed by folds of mucous membrane in the bladder wall prevent the backflow of urine into the ureters. Urine collects in the bladder until an autonomic nerve stimulus from the sacral reflex centers causes micturition (urination) through the urethra. This stimulus opens the muscle fibers that form an internal sphincter at the bladder neck, the vesicourethral junction.

The arterial supply of the urinary bladder is derived from the hypogastric arteries, which branch from the internal iliac arteries. The venous drainage empties into the hypogastric veins. The lymphatics drain into the internal and common iliac nodes.

Urethra

The male urethra is approximately 25 to 30 cm long and has a diameter of 7 to 10 mm. It consists of two segments (proximal and distal) that are further subdivided into three segments referred to as the prostatic, the membranous, and the cavernous urethral segments. The proximal (posterior) prostatic urethra passes from the bladder orifice, through the prostate gland, and to the pelvic floor. The membranous urethra passes from the pelvic floor to the base of the penis. The distal (anterior) segment consists of parts of the membranous, bulbous, and anterior urethral segments that pass through the penis to the external urethral orifice. The membranous and anterior urethra also serve as a passageway for secretions from the male reproductive system (see Figure 36-1, *A*).

The female urethra is approximately 3.0 to 5.0 cm long and 6 to 8 mm in diameter. It is firmly embedded posterior to the clitoris and anterior to the vaginal opening. Females are predisposed to urinary tract infections because the urethra is anatomically located near the vagina and the anus, both of which have resident flora that can cause infection if introduced into the urethra. Mechanical injury during coitus and the use of a diaphragm for contraception may be contributing factors to urinary tract infection (see Figure 36-1, *B*).

SPECIAL FEATURES OF UROLOGIC SURGERY

Urologic Endoscopy

Cystoscopic diagnostic procedures and some conservative urologic procedures approached through the urethra are performed in an especially designed and equipped area that is often referred to as the cysto room or suite. This area may be located within the OR suite or in the urology clinic. X-ray control booths and developing units are located adjacent to or within the area. Because x-ray procedures are often performed, the walls and doors of the room should be lined with lead, and personnel remaining in the room with the patient during x-ray studies or fluoroscopy should wear lead aprons. Patients should be protected with gonadal and thyroid shields whenever feasible.

To protect the welfare of the patients and personnel, all safety regulations apply in the cysto room as they do elsewhere in the OR suite. All lighted instruments and electrical equipment should be checked for proper function before and after each use. Excess fluid should not be permitted to accumulate on the floor.

Proper OR attire is worn by all personnel entering the room. Personal protective equipment such as eyewear and masks should be worn if there is a possibility of splash or aerosolization. Many urologists don a water-repellent apron before scrubbing. It is recommended that the urologist wear a sterile gown and sterile gloves. Procedures performed in the cysto room should be performed as in a sterile field to prevent the introduction of microorganisms into the patient. Adherence to the principles of aseptic technique should be practiced to prevent nosocomial urinary tract infection.

Urologic Bed

A urologic bed differs from the standard operating bed in that it provides an x-ray–compatible base, a drainage system, and lithotomy knee supports with safety belts. Some urologic beds incorporate electrosurgical units (ESUs). Urologic radiographic studies use conventional x-ray studies, fluoroscopy and image intensification, and tomography. The imaging system is an integral part of the urologic bed. Some beds have a built-in automatic film handling system, others have a film cassette holder, and others adapt to a C-arm. The drainage system may have a drainage pan with tubing to drain port or single-use drainage bags. Under-knee/calf supports with gel pads and Velcro straps provide patient comfort in the lithotomy position. Urologic beds are equipped with hydraulic or electric controls to adjust height and tilt. Some have tray attachments for the light source and auxiliary ESU, as well as hooks for irrigating solution bags.

Patient Preparation for a Cystoscopic Examination

1. Unless the procedure will be performed with the patient under general or regional anesthesia, the patient may be encouraged to drink fluids before coming to the cysto room. Fluids ensure rapid collection of a urine specimen from the kidneys. Some tests require the ability to void for bladder strength studies or while contrast media passes through the urinary system. Electromyographic (EMG) data may be gathered during the process.
2. Intraurethral procedures are often performed with topical agents or local infiltration anesthetics. The patient should be reassured that the procedure usually can be performed with only mild discomfort. Respect the patient's modesty by providing appropriate drapes and keeping the cysto room door closed.
3. The patient is assisted into the lithotomy position with the knees resting in padded knee supports or stirrups. Gel pads behind the legs and knees help avoid undue pressure in popliteal spaces. Velcro straps are used to secure the

patient's legs. Some cystoscopic procedures are performed with the male patient in the supine position.

4. The drainage pan is pulled out of the lower break of the urologic bed after the patient's legs have been positioned on knee supports and the foot of the bed has been lowered.

5. The pubic region, external genitalia, and perineum are mechanically and chemically cleansed with an antiseptic agent according to routine skin preparation procedure. The solution should be warmed according to the manufacturer's recommendations before it is applied to an unanesthetized patient. To prevent burns, the temperature of the solution should not exceed 110° F (57° C). Scrub soaps can be diluted with warmed sterile saline or water.

6. Topical anesthetic agents are instilled into the urethra at the end of the prep procedure. A viscous liquid or jelly preparation of lidocaine hydrochloride, 1% or 2%, may be used. This medium remains in the urethra rather than flowing into the bladder.

   a. *For female:* The female urethra is most sensitive at the meatus. Thus a small, sterile, cotton applicator dipped into the anesthetic agent and placed in the meatus with a cotton tip is sufficient. The applicator is removed when the urologist is ready to introduce an instrument. Cone-shaped syringes are commercially available for intraurethral instillation of local jelly.

   b. *For male:* A disposable cylinder with an acorn tip can be used for intraurethral insertion. The agent is injected into the urethra, and the penis is compressed with a penile clamp for a few minutes to retain the drug.

7. A sterile stainless steel filter screen is placed over the drainage pan. The patient is draped as for other perineal procedures in the lithotomy position. The urologist may need to have access to the rectum. The perineal sheet has two fenestrations: one exposes the genitalia, and the other fits over the screen on the drainage pan. A gauze filter is incorporated into this latter fenestration to capture resected tissue.

The urologist may prefer to wear a sterile disposable plastic apron over his or her gown. The apron is attached to the bed, which provides a sterile field from the urologic bed to the urologist's shoulders. A receptor kit that attaches to the apron eliminates the need for the drainage pan. Tissue specimens are collected as irrigating fluid passes through a collecting basket.

Urologic Endoscopes

Urologic endoscopic instruments and catheters are available in sizes to suit infants, children, and adults. The sizes of these instruments and catheters are measured on the French scale: the diameter in millimeters multiplied by 3. The smallest ureteral catheter is 1 mm in diameter, or 3 French; the largest is 14 French.

Each type of procedure requires specific endoscopic equipment. All rigid urologic endoscopes have the same basic components, which are discussed in the following sections.

Sheath

The hollow sheath, through which the urologic endoscope passes, may be concave, convex, or straight in configuration at the distal end (the end inserted into the urethra). The other end has a stopcock attachment for irrigation. Sheath sizes range from 11 French for infants to 30 French for adults. Space is provided within the sheath to accommodate instruments for work in the bladder or urethra. Other instruments and catheters can be inserted through the sheath into the ureters and/or kidneys for diagnostic or therapeutic procedures.

Obturator

The stainless steel obturator, which is inserted into the sheath, occludes the opening of the sheath and facilitates introduction into the urethra without trauma to the mucosal lining.

Telescope

Telescopes are complex precision optical systems; they are costly, delicate instruments that are handled gently at all times. Each telescope contains multiple, finely ground optical lenses that relay the image from the distal end inside the bladder or urethra to the ocular (eyepiece) used by the urologist to view internal structures. Additional rod-shaped elements (i.e., field lenses) are located between each pair of relay lenses. Properly spaced throughout the length of the telescope, the lenses provide undistorted and clear vision at the desired angle and with some magnification. All telescopes are stainless steel and have a Bakelite ocular. Some telescopes have operating or working elements incorporated into them.

The optical systems provide several angles of vision (Figure 36-4):

- Direct forward or 0-degree vision is useful for viewing the urethra and for use with the optical urethrotome (an instrument for sharp resection of tissue in the urethra).

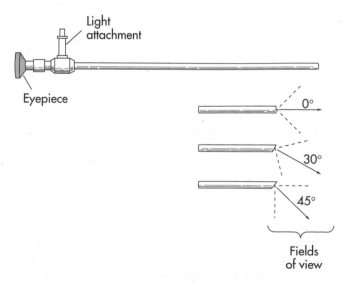

Figure 36-4 Viewing angles of telescopes.

- Right-angle or 30-degree vision is most suitable for viewing the entire bladder and for insertion of ureteral catheters.
- Lateral, which deviates 70 degrees but includes an additional visual field at a right angle in the line of vision, is used for wide-angle viewing within the bladder.
- Foroblique, which is a forward vision with an oblique view somewhat in front of a right angle, is used to examine the urethra and for transurethral surgical procedures.
- Retrospective, which provides an approximate 55-degree angle of retrograde vision, is used to inspect the bladder neck.

Light Source

The light source is a fiberoptic bundle and may be an integral part of the sheath or the telescope. A cable connects the instrument to a fiberoptic light source.

Types of Urologic Endoscopes

Many different types of urologic endoscopes and accessories are used, including nephroscopes introduced into the kidney and cystoscopes introduced through the urethra into the bladder. Before instrumentation is placed on the sterile instrument table, the preferred type and size of the endoscope for the examination and/or treatment should be verified with the urologist. The endoscopes and accessories most commonly used in the cysto room are described in the following sections.

Brown-Buerger Cystoscope

The stainless steel sheaths of the Brown-Buerger cystoscope range in size from 14 to 26 French. Size 21 French is used most often in adults with a right-angle examination telescope for routine inspection of the bladder. Size 24 or 26 French is used to accommodate larger instruments and catheters that cannot be used through size 21. The sheath contains the light carrier.

A Brown-Buerger cystoscope set usually consists of two sheaths—one concave and one convex, each with its own obturator—and two or three right-angle telescopes. Along with the basic examination telescope, the set may have a combination operating and double catheterizing telescope (i.e., a convertible telescope), or the operating and double catheterizing functions may be in separate telescopes. The convertible operating and catheterizing telescopes have a small deflectable lever on the distal end to aid in directing ureteral catheters or flexible stone baskets into the ureters. All corresponding parts of each set must be the same French size.

McCarthy Panendoscope

The stainless steel sheaths of the McCarthy panendoscope range in size from 14 to 30 French. These are used most often with the Foroblique telescope for viewing the urethra. Other telescopes are available for bladder visualization. The telescopes are interchangeable with all sizes of sheaths.

A bridge assembly is required to fit the telescope properly to the sheath. The light is supplied through the telescope.

Wappler Cystourethroscope

The Wappler cystourethroscope combines the functions of the Brown-Buerger cystoscope and the McCarthy panendoscope. The stainless steel sheaths range in size from 17 to 24 French. The Foroblique and lateral telescopes, which also supply the light, are interchangeable with all sheaths. A visual obturator may be used to permit visualization and irrigation during the introduction of the sheath into the urethra.

Resectoscope

The resectoscope uses electric current to excise tissue from the bladder, urethra, or prostate. Components of this instrument include the sheath, obturator, telescope, working element, and cutting electrode. The sheath, usually 24 to 28 French, is made of Bakelite or fiberglass to prevent a short circuit of the electric current. If the short beak post sheath is used with a wide-angle telescope, a Timberlake obturator is used to introduce the sheath into the urethra.

The working element of the resectoscope, which is inserted through the sheath, has a channel for the telescope and cutting electrode. The types of working elements differ by the method in which the cutting electrode moves:

- The Iglesias resectoscope uses a thumb control on a leaf spring–lock mechanism. The working element can be adapted for simultaneous irrigation and suction to control hydraulic pressure in the bladder.
- The Nesbit resectoscope uses a thumb control on a spring.
- The Baumrucker resectoscope uses finger control on a sliding mechanism.
- The Stern-McCarthy resectoscope uses a rack and pinion to move the loop forward and back. This requires two hands.

The cutting electrode is the most critical component of a resectoscope. Because it cuts and coagulates tissue, the electrode must be stabilized in the working element so it retracts properly into the sheath after each cut. The electrode has a cutting loop from which electric current is passed through tissue, an insulated fork, an insulated stem, and a contact that is inserted into the working element. Several loop sizes are available; the stem is usually color coded by size. Loop size corresponds to the French size of the sheath. The electrode is malleable and therefore is checked before use to be certain the insulation is intact and the loop is not broken. Electric current is applied only when the loop is engaged in tissue and is inactivated after a cut is completed. The sheath can be charred if electric current is maintained after the cutting loop has been retracted into it. Disposable loop electrodes are commercially available and are preferred for use by most urologists.

Conductive lubricants may provide a pathway for electric current and therefore should never be used on the sheath. Cleanliness of the sheath and all other components is essential to proper function.

Endoscopic Accessories

Ureteral catheters, bougies, filiforms and followers, stone baskets, and sounds are commonly used by urologist-endoscopists. Other accessories, such as retractable baskets and graspers, are used to remove tissue or calculi (stones).

Electrodes

In addition to the cutting loops used with the resectoscope, primarily for transurethral resections (TUR), other types of electrodes with tips of various shapes are used in the bladder. One type, referred to as a bugbee, is inserted through the operating telescope of the Brown-Buerger cystoscope or Wappler cystourethroscope. The bugbee is used mainly for fulguration of bladder tumors, coagulation of bladder vessels to control bleeding following biopsy, and ureteral meatotomy. More electric current is needed when working in solution (as in the bladder) than when working in air. A spark-gap generator is commonly used for transurethral resection and fulguration. A spark-gap ESU requires high-voltage arcing, which is described as spray coagulation. Spark-gap generator use requires the patient to be grounded with a grounding pad. The power control settings on the ESU should be as low as possible. Recommended practices as suggested by AORN, the Association of periOperative Registered Nurses, for the use and care of electrosurgical equipment (e.g., dispersive electrodes) apply also to urologic procedures.

Lasers

Argon, Nd:YAG, and Ho:YAG lasers can be adapted for use with urologic endoscopes. These are particularly useful for the ablation of hemangiomas and vascular tumors in the bladder and kidneys. The argon-pumped tunable dye laser is used for photodynamic therapy on solid bladder tumors. A flash lamp–pulsed dye laser will fragment a calculus in a ureter.

Lasers used through endoscopes require most of the same equipment as needed for standard urologic endoscopy. The fluid bladder expansion medium can be either saline or water because, unlike with the ESU and electrodes, no ionic charge is emitted from the laser.

Irrigating Equipment

Continuous irrigation of the bladder is necessary during cystoscopy to do the following:

- Distend bladder walls so the urologist can visualize them
- Wash out blood, bits of resected tissue, or stone fragments to permit continuous visibility and collection of specimens

A sterile, disposable, and closed irrigating system is used because it prevents airborne contamination of the solution. Two to four or more liters of sterile irrigating solution may be needed for a single examination. Disposable tandem sets may be used to connect several containers together. Tandem sets allow for a continuous flow and for replacement of containers without interruption of flow. Sterile disposable irrigating tubing is connected to the irrigating solution container before it is hung on a hook on the urologic bed, in the ceiling, or on a stand placed beside the bed. The solution container should be at a level 2½ feet (0.75 m) above the bed—a lower level decreases flow; a higher level increases hydraulic pressure with consequent fluid absorption by the tissues of the patient. Tubing should be filled with solution before being attached to the sheath of the cystoscope or resectoscope. The plastic tubing from the container to the instrument is for individual patient use only and is discarded after use.

Sterile isosmotic irrigating solutions that are nonhemolytic and nonelectrolytic are generally preferred by most urologists. Sterile distilled water may be used for visualization procedures and during resection or fulguration of bladder tumors with an ESU. Water may hemolyze red blood cells if a sufficient amount enters the circulation through open blood vessels. As much as 3 to 6 L of solution may be absorbed during a transurethral prostatectomy. Saline is contraindicated for use with an ESU, because the minerals in saline act as a conductor and disperse the current when the ESU is used.

Isosmotic solutions of 1.5% glycine (an amino acid) or sorbitol (an inert sugar) premixed in distilled water are commercially available in 1.5- and 3-L containers. Glycine solution is commonly used for transurethral resection with an ESU.

During the procedure, the flow of solution into the endoscope is controlled by the stopcock on the sheath where the tubing attaches. Rubber tips or sealing caps are used to seal other openings on the instrument to prevent solution from escaping during a procedure. The openings through which catheters or instruments are to be inserted are closed with rubber caps that have a central hole. The accessory can be inserted through this hole with the seal maintained. Silicone caps should be used instead of rubber caps if the patient or surgeon has a latex sensitivity.

When the urologist wishes, the irrigating solution flows away from the instrument and into the drainage pan through the filter screen. Solution drains from the pan, through the tubing, and into a collecting bucket that is emptied after each patient use. Some cysto rooms have floor drains, which are a source of environmental contamination unless cleaned thoroughly. If large quantities of solution are used, the level of drainage into the bucket should be observed to prevent overflow onto the floor or around the foot pedal of the ESU, which can be an electrocution hazard.

Evacuators

Evacuators may be attached to the endoscope to irrigate the bladder and to aspirate stone fragments, blood clots, or resected tissue. Stone or tissue fragments collected in the evacuator are retrieved and sent to the pathology laboratory. The two most commonly used types are the Ellik evacuator and the Toomey evacuator:

- *Ellik evacuator.* The Ellik evacuator is a double bowl–shaped glass or firm disposable plastic evacuator. It contains a trap for fragments so they cannot be washed back into the sheath of the endoscope during irrigation with pressure on the compression-bulb attachment.

- *Toomey evacuator.* The Toomey evacuator is a syringe-type evacuator with a wide opening into the barrel. It may be used with any endoscope sheath. A metal adapter permits its use with a catheter.

Care and Preventive Maintenance

1. Sterilization is preferred, although high-level disinfection with 2% glutaraldehyde is commonly used. Endoscopes and reusable accessories must be free of debris and residue for sterilization and/or high-level disinfection techniques to be effective.
   a. Disassemble all parts and open all outlets.
   b. Clean all parts in an appropriate liquid detergent solution. Clean the interior of sheaths and openings with a soft brush.
   c. Rinse in clean water, and dry thoroughly.
   d. Wipe lenses gently with a soft, dry cloth.
2. After cleaning, place endoscopes on a towel to drain. Air blow–dry the lumens. Moisture in the channels can dilute chemical sterilants and, if ethylene oxide is used, will form ethylene glycol, which is toxic to tissues.
3. Check the function of all moving parts, the clarity of vision through telescopes, and the patency of channels through instruments and catheters.
4. Keep sets of sounds, bougies, and filiforms and followers together so the urologist has a complete range of sizes readily accessible.
5. Wrap items for sterilization after cleaning. Flexible instruments should be protected by a rigid container.
6. Clean and dry stone baskets may be sterilized by low-temperature sterilization methods, such as plasma vapor, peracetic acid, or ethylene oxide. Retractable stone baskets are sterilized in the open position.
7. The principles and methods of sterilization apply to urologic endoscopy equipment.
8. Endoscopic processors and sterilizers, such as the Steris unit, are useful for sterilizing instrumentation between patient uses. The instrumentation is used immediately after processing and is not stored in the processing tray.
9. If sterilization between patient uses is not feasible, high-level disinfection may be the method of choice for processing urologic endoscopic instruments.

SURGICAL PROCEDURES OF THE GENITOURINARY SYSTEM

Most patients commonly seen by urologists are in the preadolescent or older age-groups. Congenital and common pediatric problems are discussed in Chapter 8. This discussion focuses on adult problems, most of which occur in men over 50 years of age who have prostatic disease.

An open surgical procedure is performed only after conservative treatment fails or examination of the genitourinary (GU) tract confirms a condition that does not yield to treatment. Fortunately, most urologic conditions can be diagnosed and treated conservatively through a urologic endoscope and its accessories. When a congenital or acquired condition does not respond to conservative therapy, the urologist performs open surgical procedures to repair, revise, reconstruct, or remove organs.

Obstructive and neuromuscular disorders are common problems in the urinary tract. Renal calculus disease and tumors in the urinary tract are most commonly diagnosed in middle age. These conditions may cause obstruction and subsequent infection in the kidneys, ureter, or bladder.

Kidney

Definitive renal surgical procedures are justified for the management of renal neoplasms, large cystic lesions that compromise renal function and/or produce obstruction, inflammatory diseases that necessitate drainage, or renal vascular disease. Chronic degenerative disease or severe traumatic injury can produce irreparable damage to renal cells. Computed tomography and magnetic resonance imaging identify the site, size, and extent of tumor involvement. Ultrasonography and intravenous urograms differentiate among solid tumors, stones, and cystic disease. A radionuclide scan may indicate renal function; arteriograms and venograms indicate the extent of renal vascular disease.

The kidney is usually approached posteriorly with the patient in a lateral position. (Figure 36-5). The kidney rest is raised, and the bed is flexed until the flank muscles become tense. After the patient is secured in position, the bed is tilted in the Trendelenburg position until the flank is horizontal to the floor. A flank incision is made parallel to and just below or over the eleventh or twelfth rib; the twelfth rib may be removed. The retroperitoneum is opened to expose the kidney.

The kidney can be approached anteriorly through a transverse, subcostal, or midline incision. A thoracoabdominal incision may be preferred in an obese patient or to reach a lesion in the upper pole of the kidney. These incisions, with the patient in the supine position, are often used for exposure of the aorta and vena cava for renovascular procedures. An anterior approach may be advantageous when prompt control of blood supply is important in renal trauma.

Nephrectomy

Removal of a lobe or the entire kidney is indicated when tumor, disease, or traumatic injury has resulted in the absence of renal function.

Figure 36-5   Surgical position for open kidney procedure.

The entire kidney can be removed through a laparoscope. The organ is dissected, fragmented, and aspirated; vascular pedicles are stapled. This alternative technique is used primarily for benign renal disease.

Partial Nephrectomy or Heminephrectomy
Partial excision of the kidney may be sufficient when a lobe has been destroyed by localized disease or injury but the remainder of the kidney remains functional. The vascular supply to the segment to be removed must be identified, ligated, and divided. The parenchyma of the lobe is resected from the capsule by blunt dissection. The renal pelvis and remaining capsule are closed.

Radical Nephrectomy
In a radical nephrectomy, the renal vessels are dissected free, ligated, and divided. Prerenal fat and fascia are dissected to remove the kidney. The ureter is ligated and divided close to the bladder. The renal pedicle is ligated and divided, and the kidney is removed. Massive hemorrhage from the renal artery and veins is a potential complication, as is injury to adjacent structures (i.e., inferior vena cava, aorta, and duodenum on the right side or spleen on the left side).

A nephrectomy is performed in the operating room (OR) on a living donor (unilateral) or on a cadaver donor (bilateral) to procure the kidney(s) for transplantation. Meticulous dissection is necessary to free the kidney, its blood vessels, and the ureter with minimal trauma. The ureter is dissected free and transected while the renal blood supply remains intact to ensure adequate urinary output. A living donor nephrectomy may last longer than the usual nephrectomy for kidney disease.

Bilateral Nephrectomy
Removal of both kidneys may be indicated before transplantation in a patient maintained on chronic dialysis who has severe hypertension. If rejection is uncontrollable following kidney transplantation, the patient may require a transplant nephrectomy and return to chronic hemodialysis. This is less likely following transplantation from a live donor than from a cadaver. Kidney transplantation is discussed in Chapter 45.

Nephrostomy or Pyelostomy

An incision through the renal parenchyma or into the renal pelvis may be necessary to establish temporary or permanent drainage when an obstruction prevents the flow of urine from the kidney. A tube placed in the kidney exits through the skin. A cutaneous nephrostomy tube may be used to drain a kidney postoperatively during healing following renal reconstruction or revascularization. Silastic tubes placed internally through a cystoscope via the ureter eliminate the need for an open surgical procedure for a temporary urinary diversion. More commonly, temporary urinary diversion is performed percutaneously under fluoroscopic or ultrasound guidance by a radiologist and/or urologist. A plastic disk is applied to the skin to secure the catheter, which is attached to a drainage bag in a manner to prevent tension. The tubing may be connected to a leg bag to avoid tension on the catheter during ambulation.

Pyeloplasty

Revision or reconstruction of the renal pelvis is performed to relieve an anatomic obstruction in the flow of urine by creating a larger outlet from the renal pelvis into the ureter. This may be performed to repair or excise damaged tissue so that kidney function will be restored without a partial or total nephrectomy.

Either a rigid or a flexible fiberoptic nephroscope may be used to visually inspect the renal collecting system. A laser fiber may be used to ablate some tumors.

Renal Revascularization

Stenotic lesions of renal arteries are surgically correctable causes of hypertension. Renovascular reconstructive procedures (renal angioplasty) are designed either to improve blood flow through the stenotic area to the kidney or to bypass the stenotic area. Revascularization procedures may have a dual purpose: to correct hypertension and to preserve renal function. The patient is placed in the supine position for these procedures because the renal arteries are approached through an abdominal incision.

In Situ Vascular Reconstructive Techniques
Obstruction of the renal artery most often occurs as a result of atherosclerotic stenosis at the origin of the artery or fibromuscular dysplasia (abnormal development) confined to the main renal artery. The obstruction is most often resected and replaced by an aortorenal-saphenous vein bypass graft. A reversed segment of proximal saphenous vein, gently distended and irrigated, is anastomosed first to the aorta and then to the renal artery. Prosthetic woven Dacron grafts may be used instead of an autogenous vein graft for renal artery bypass combined with distal aortic replacement. Segmental resection of diseased arterial segments with primary end-to-end anastomosis may be performed. Thromboendarterectomy is more often performed than is the latter procedure. All of these procedures may be performed bilaterally or as staged bilateral renal artery reconstructions. Percutaneous transluminal angioplasty may be preferred to these open procedures.

Ex Vivo Extracorporeal Kidney Surgery
When stenotic disease or another obstructive lesion extends into the branches of the renal artery, in situ reconstruction may be difficult, hazardous, or impossible. In these patients, a temporary nephrectomy with microvascular repair followed by autotransplantation of the kidney may be performed; this is referred to as workbench surgery. The kidney is completely mobilized from the retroperitoneal space. If one kidney is to be reconstructed, the ureter can remain intact and reconstruction is performed on a sterile bench (Mayo tray) placed over the patient's lower abdomen. For a bilateral reconstruction, one kidney is detached from its ureter to permit complete removal from the abdomen. A second team works on the contralateral kidney while the other kidney is reconstructed at an adjacent dissecting bench (table).

Extracorporeal perfusion is necessary for renal preservation during reconstruction. This may be accomplished either with perfusion of cold Ringer's lactate or other hyperosmolar solution by gravity flow or with a continuous hypothermic perfusion through a Belzer pump machine. A simple cold storage in saline slush may also be used for renal preservation.

A kidney may be autotransplanted into the patient's groin or pelvis for revascularization of the kidney, removal of renal tumors or calculi, or repair of ureteral injuries.

Traumatic Injury

Fatal or near-fatal hemorrhage may result if a kidney is ruptured or injured by blunt trauma, a bullet, or a stab wound. This requires an immediate surgical procedure. The surgeon makes every effort to save kidney tissue and the ureter. A Foley catheter is inserted to keep an output record and to check for the presence of hematuria preoperatively and postoperatively. Gross hematuria preoperatively usually indicates injury to the bladder or urethra. Kidney damage is diagnosed by the presence of blood seen microscopically.

Dialysis

End-stage renal disease and acute renal failure are potentially fatal conditions unless they can be controlled or reversed. Uremia and hypertension develop if renal failure is prolonged. Renal dialysis is the procedure of removing waste products and excess intravascular fluid from the body of a patient in acute or chronic renal failure by diffusion through a semipermeable membrane. This may be accomplished by either hemodialysis or peritoneal dialysis. The treatment modality alleviates the acute manifestations of uremia and controls many of the chronic long-term complications of end-stage renal disease. Grossly undernourished and anemic patients with severe electrolyte imbalances must be adequately stabilized by dialysis before kidney transplantation. Some patients require dialysis for the remainder of their lives. Patients undergoing chronic dialysis must have a means of arterial-venous access established for long-term maintenance.

Patients with chronic renal failure can tolerate extensive surgical procedures with minimal complications. Their management in the OR must include strict attention to maintaining a patent hemodialysis access shunt, fistula, or catheter; careful monitoring of fluid and electrolyte balance; and the avoidance of postoperative infections. Following kidney transplantation, the patient may require postoperative dialysis; thus access must remain patent during and after the surgical procedure.

Hemodialysis

In hemodialysis, waste products are removed from the blood through the semipermeable membrane of a dialyzer (artificial kidney machine). An arteriovenous (AV) shunt or fistula is created subcutaneously in either an arm or a leg to provide access to the patient's circulation. The Quinton-Scribner double-lumen shunt, developed in 1960, consists of two tips attached to tubing. One tip is placed in the artery and the other in a nearby vein. The tubing from each tip is exteriorized through a subcutaneous tunnel to form a loop. The arte-

rial and venous blood mix in this shunt. Variations and modifications of this basic external shunt are used to create an AV conduit; some have self-sealing devices to minimize the potential problems of clotting and infection.

An anastomosis, usually between the radial artery and the cephalic vein in the forearm, creates an arterialized peripheral vein that permits dialyzer connections to be made by venipuncture. Needles are placed in the venous limb of the AV fistula for blood outflow and return. The Brescia-Cimino radiocephalic AV fistula, first described in 1966, is easiest to construct and has the fewest complications. If creation of an AV fistula by direct anastomosis is not feasible, a biologic or synthetic graft may be interposed between the artery and the vein. Preserved human umbilical vein, saphenous or other autologous vein, bovine carotid artery heterograft, and polytetrafluoroethylene (PTFE) grafts are used.

Peritoneal Dialysis

For acute, intermittent, or continuous peritoneal dialysis, a Tenckhoff silicone catheter is placed into the peritoneal cavity. A paramedian incision is usually used to place a section of the catheter in subcutaneous tissue. The catheter has one or two synthetic fiber cuffs to anchor it in subcutaneous tissue and to block bacterial invasion along the catheter into the peritoneal cavity. Dialysate is instilled over time into the peritoneal cavity to draw solutes from body fluids into the dialyzing solution. This process selectively removes electrolytes, metabolites, toxins, and water normally excreted by the kidneys. Dialysate that has been warmed to body temperature is instilled, allowed to remain for a specified number of hours, and then withdrawn by a cycling machine or by gravity drainage. A Y-set disconnect system attached to the catheter allows separation of inflow and outflow. Peritonitis is always a potential complication. Infection is often treated by adding antibiotics to the dialysate. Heparin is added to prevent fibrin clots in the catheter. The patient may perform this routine at home several times per week, usually during the evening hours.

A patient being treated with peritoneal dialysis may come to the OR for an unrelated surgical procedure. Respiratory excursion may be impaired by pressure of retained dialysate under the diaphragm. A slight reverse Trendelenburg position may alleviate respiratory discomfort. Additional suction containers should be available if the abdomen must be evacuated while the patient is in the OR. Fluid removed from the peritoneal cavity is measured, and the appearance and volume are recorded on the intraoperative record.

Urolithiasis (Urinary Calculus)

A renal calculus (kidney stone) is a solid deposit or deposits of minerals and salts. These deposits are called calculi and accumulate in the renal collecting system. Calculi can be the result of cystinuria (amino acid metabolic disorder), hypercalcemia (immobility or hyperparathyroidism), oxalate (oxalic and glycolic acid in urine), and uric acid (dietary purines). Renal colic is an intense pain caused when a calculus or fragments of calculi partially or completely obstruct the calyces or renal pelvis. Renal calculi often dislodge and move from the renal pelvis into the ureter. A nidus (e.g., an infection or an exposed suture postoperatively) can be the focal point for the formation of a calculus in the ureter. If calculi are small enough, they pass into the bladder and are voided. Those that remain lodged, causing obstruction to outflow from any part of the urinary tract, must be removed.

Preservation of renal function is the primary objective of surgical procedures for urolithiasis. Lithotomy is removal of a calculus. Lithotripsy is fragmentation of a stone followed by removal. Chemolysis is dissolution with a chemical substance. Following removal from any location in the GU tract, urinary calculi should be placed in a dry container and sent to the pathology laboratory for chemical analysis.

Percutaneous Nephrostolithotomy or Nephrolithotripsy

With percutaneous nephrostolithotomy or nephrolithotripsy, a guidewire inside a transluminal angioplasty needle is introduced, under fluoroscopy, through the flank into the renal pelvis. The access point is carefully closed. This procedure may be performed in the radiology department with the patient under local anesthesia. In the OR, dilators are placed over the guidewire to enlarge a nephrostomy tract for introduction of a nephrostomy tube or nephroscope. The patient is placed in a modified prone position to elevate the surgical side slightly.

Renal calculi may be removed with stone forceps or baskets, or they may be fragmented with a lithotriptor. Lithotripsy is necessary for large calculi such as a staghorn calculus, which branches from the renal pelvis into the calyces and may extend into the ureter. Size, density, composition, and location influence the urologist's choice of lithotripsy.

Ultrasonic Lithotripsy With ultrasonic lithotripsy, ultrasonic waves are used to shatter the calculus into fragments. This procedure is usually performed with the patient under spinal or general anesthesia. Either a rigid or flexible fiberoptic nephroscope is inserted percutaneously; a hollow metal ultrasonic probe, which emits high-frequency sound waves, is inserted through the nephroscope. The probe is visually placed in contact with a calculus that is localized in the renal pelvis as identified on x-ray film or by fluoroscopy. The calculus fragments as the ultrasonic energy is absorbed, and the shattered particles are aspirated by suction through the probe. A nephrostomy tube may be placed in the renal pelvis for temporary drainage postoperatively; this tube is usually removed after 2 weeks.

Electrohydraulic Lithotripsy With electrohydraulic lithotripsy, an electrohydraulic lithotriptor is used to create an electrical discharge in fluid, and this discharge is transformed into a hydraulic shock wave. The calculus disintegrates when the probe is directed at it. Larger fragments may be removed with Randall stone forceps, and smaller

ones are flushed out with irrigation. A tube is left in the nephrostomy tract for continued irrigation for several days after lithotripsy. This procedure may be performed with a local anesthetic with intravenous sedatives and analgesics.

Nephrolithotomy or Pyelolithotomy

A large staghorn renal calculus that does not dislodge from the calyces or renal pelvis may need to be removed through an open incision. A nephroscope may be used during the surgical procedure for direct visual examination of the nephrons to locate and remove residual calculi. Ultrasound may also be used to identify retained fragments. Localized hypothermia provides the surgeon with a bloodless surgical field and extends the period of time in which the renal artery may be clamped safely without a loss of renal function during the search for and extraction of calculi.

Percutaneous Chemolysis

Hemiacidrin may be instilled through a small nephrostomy tube to alkalinize cysteine and uric acid calculi and to dissolve any debris that remains following other lithotomy procedures.

Extracorporeal Shock-Wave Lithotripsy

Many patients are scheduled for cystoscopy immediately before a noninvasive extracorporeal shock-wave lithotripsy (ESWL) procedure. A ureteral stent may be inserted to facilitate the passage of stone fragments. The ureteral stone may be manipulated back up into the renal pelvis. An x-ray film may be obtained to check the location of the calculus.

Waterbath Lithotripsy With a waterbath lithotripsy, the patient first receives a continuous epidural or general anesthetic and then is positioned in a gantry (a hoist) and hydraulically lifted into a tub filled with degassed, demineralized water. The calculus must be visualized by fluoroscopy to focus the shock waves. The shock waves are generated by rapid, high-voltage sparks that are discharged within an ellipsoid reflector at the bottom of the tub; they are focused and transmitted through water to enter the body. The impact of the waves against the calculus liberates high-energy mechanical stresses that cause fragmentation.

Up to 1500 shock waves are produced over a period of 45 to 60 minutes. After each series of 150 to 200 waves, the focus on the calculus is rechecked by fluoroscopy. Each shock wave is synchronized with the patient's respirations and resting phase of the heartbeat; an electrocardiogram (ECG) monitors the patient's R waves to avoid disrupting the cardiac rhythm. A loud report sounds in the room each time a spark is fired, and therefore both the patient and personnel must wear protective earplugs.

Tubless Lithotripsy For tubless lithotripsy, the patient is positioned on the bed over a shock-wave generator after receiving a local anesthetic or transcutaneous electrical nerve stimulation (TENS). Spark-induced shock waves may be transmitted through a water cushion that contains an electrode and curved reflector; the patient's back is in contact with this cushion. The shock-wave energy is generated electromagnetically and focused with an acoustic lens. Fragmentation of the calculus is verified with intermittent fluoroscopic images or x-ray films.

Shock waves also may be produced by piezoelectric transducers activated by an electronic generator. These transducers are mounted on a bowl-shaped spherical dish; a soft fluid membrane over this dish maintains contact with the patient's skin. Ultrasound images produced from an ultrasound localization system are used to position the stone at the focal point of the shock waves.

ESWL equipment may be located in the OR suite adjacent to or in the cysto room, in a separate unit, or in a mobile van. A mobile van may serve several hospitals within the region. Because this equipment is very expensive, patients are referred to regional centers. Perioperative nurses may be assigned to assist with ESWL.

Ureters

The ureters are the vital anatomic structures for the flow of urine from the kidneys to the bladder. An obstruction to urinary flow must be either corrected or diverted. The ureters may be approached either through an endoscope or through an open incision.

Ureteral Endoscopy

Both rigid and flexible, short and long, fiberoptic ureteroscopes allow direct visualization of the ureteral tumors, calculi, and strictures. These scopes are introduced percutaneously or cystoscopically. Tumors can be biopsied, and strictures can be corrected by balloon dilation. Ureteral calculi can be extracted with stone baskets or forceps or fragmented using ultrasound or lasers.

Percutaneous endoscopic techniques can be used in conjunction with cystoscopy. A complete cystoscopy implies that the procedure extends beyond the bladder into the ureters. This procedure may be performed for the following:

- Drainage of the renal pelvis for differential diagnosis or renal function
- Insertion of ureteral catheters to provide constant drainage for one or both kidneys or to outline the ureters for a difficult pelvic surgical procedure
- Insertion of a ureteral stent for internal drainage of an obstructed ureter
- Transluminal dilation of a ureteral stricture
- Manipulation and removal of a calculus
- Ureteral meatotomy to enlarge the opening of one or both ureteral orifices into the bladder

Ureteral Catheters   Made of flexible woven nylon or other plastic material, ureteral catheters range in caliber from size 3 to 14 French and are approximately 30 inches (76 cm) in length. Sterile, prepackaged disposable catheters

are available. Most are radiopaque so they can be visualized on x-ray film.

The urologist visualizes the ureteral orifice through the cystoscope. The catheter is inserted through the scope and introduced into the ureter. The catheter has graduated markings in centimeters so the urologist can judge the distance that the catheter has been inserted. The urologist will request a size and style of catheter tip best suited for the intended purpose. The most common tips are shown in Figure 36-6:

- *Whistle tips:* Used for drainage, as ureteral markers, or for the injection of a radiopaque contrast medium for retrograde pyelography. The largest sizes are used to dilate ureters to facilitate passage of a calculus.
- *Olive tips:* May be used for the same purposes as whistle tips.
- *Round tips:* May be preferred for drainage.
- *Flexible filiform tips:* May be used to bypass an obstruction for drainage.
- *Blassuchi curved tips:* May be used to bypass a ureteral stricture more easily than straight tips.
- *Braasch bulb with whistle tips:* Preferred to dilate the ureter or to inject contrast medium for a ureterogram.
- *Acorn or cone tips:* May be preferred for a ureterogram.
- *Garceau tapered tips:* Used to dilate ureters.

Ureteral catheters that are left indwelling to provide drainage must be attached to a sterile closed urinary drainage

Figure 36-6   Ureteral catheter tips. **A,** Whistle. **B,** Olive. **C,** Round. **D,** Flexible filiform. **E,** Blassuchi curved. **F,** Braasch bulb. **G,** Acorn/cone. **H,** Garceau tapered.

system. Because they are smaller in diameter than standard urinary drainage catheters, an adapter must be used. This adaptor may be a small rubber tip or nipple placed on one end of a straight connector or on both ends of a Y-connector. The catheters are put through the hole in the tip(s). The other end of the connector is attached to a constant drainage system with a piece of sterile tubing. A separate drainage system for each catheter may be desired by the urologist. Each drainage container must be labeled to identify the right and left ureteral catheters.

Ureteral Stent An indwelling ureteral stent is inserted for long-term drainage in a wide variety of benign and malignant diseases that cause ureteral obstruction. A stent also may be indicated for temporary drainage.

Several types of stents are used. They can be made of durable and biocompatible silicone, polyurethane, or another copolymer. The stent may have a collar, a double-J configuration, a pigtail, or a coil to minimize migration up into the renal pelvis or down into the bladder. The stent is passed through the cystoscope and over a guidewire into the ureter, and it remains fixed for internal urinary drainage. As described for ureteral catheters, some types of stents are used to identify ureters and provide external drainage intraoperatively.

Percutaneous Ureterolithotomy

As described for percutaneous nephrolithotomy and lithotripsy, a calculus lodged in the renal pelvis or upper tract of the ureter can be extracted or fragmented through a ureteropyeloscope.

Transurethral Ureteroscopic Lithotripsy or Lithotomy

A urologic endoscope can be introduced transurethrally for direct visualization and lithotripsy or for extraction of a calculus that is obstructing a ureter. Ultrasonic and electrohydraulic lithotripsy can be performed through a ureteroscope.

Laser Lithotripsy The use of laser technology has improved the minimally invasive treatment of calculi. A flash lamp–pulsed dye laser beam is directed through a flexible fiberoptic ureteroscope to a calculus in the lower tract. The fine tip of the laser fiber probe extends beyond the end of the scope and is placed in direct contact with the calculi to produce fragmentation without ureteral injury. This pulsed laser has a green wavelength and is attracted to the yellow color of a calculus. The energy generated through the intermittent laser pulses fragments the yellow calculus by mechanical action without increasing its temperature more than 50° F (10° C). This procedure may be performed with the patient under epidural or general anesthesia. Shattered calculi will pass with the patient's urine. An indwelling ureteral stent may be left in place for 48 hours and removed by the urologist in the office postoperatively.

Ureteral Stone Extraction A flexible-shaft, basket-type stone dislodger (stone basket) is inserted into the ureter through a cystoscope in the bladder for extraction of ureteral calculus. Several types of stone baskets are available, including the Dormia, Johnson, Levant, Pfister-Schwartz, and Lomac. These instruments have a fine wire or nylon basket that can be expanded through the shaft to ensnare a calculus located in the lower third of the ureter. Specialized stone baskets have a laser fiber port for calculi fragmentation. The basket is used to retrieve the central core after the exterior portion of the calculi is shattered.

Stone baskets must be cleaned promptly after use in a nonresidue, liquid-detergent solution to remove debris. Removable parts must be disassembled. Debris should be brushed away from the junction of the basket and shaft with a small, soft brush. Inspection of the basket wires is critical during cleaning. If the wires are cracked or broken at the end closest to the shaft, the basket may be passed into the ureter but cannot be withdrawn without trauma.

Ureterolithotomy

If a calculus fails to pass spontaneously through the ureter or cannot be removed with a stone basket, an open surgical procedure may be necessary. If the calculus is high in the ureter near the kidney, the patient is positioned for a lateral flank incision below the twelfth rib. An abdominal incision is used to reach a calculus in the lower segment near the bladder. The exposed ureter will be dilated proximal to the calculus and collapsed distal to it. The surgeon makes a small incision directly over the calculus and extracts it from the ureter with a stone forceps.

Cystolithotomy and Litholapaxy

Calculi usually can be removed from the bladder through the urethra. Crushing a urinary calculus in the bladder is referred to as litholapaxy or lithotrity. If a litholapaxy is unsuccessful or contraindicated, the removal of a calculus by incision into the bladder may be necessary; this surgical procedure is a cystolithotomy. For a litholapaxy, a lithotrite is introduced into the bladder through the urethra and is used to pulverize and remove calculi. The instrument used may be a lithotrite with hinged jaws, an ultrasound lithotriptor, or an electrohydraulic lithotrite. The electrohydraulic lithotrite generates energy shock waves at the tip of a flexible probe inserted through a cystoscope by direct vision. The stone fragments are then irrigated from the bladder.

Urinary Diversion Procedures

The ureters may be permanently or temporarily transplanted to maintain the excretion of urine from the body but to divert flow away from the bladder. Bilateral transplantation for permanent urinary diversion is performed when bladder function is impaired by neoplasm, chronic infection, congenital anomaly, trauma, or other cause. The procedure follows completion of a total cystectomy (removal of the bladder), a radical cystoprostatectomy in a male patient, or radical hysterectomy with salpingo-oophorectomy and cystectomy in a female patient, with or without pelvic lymphadenectomy. The ureters may be implanted into the intestinal wall, but more commonly they are transplanted to an isolated loop or segment of intestine that becomes a conduit for urinary flow. Ideally, a urinary reservoir collects and stores urine and expels it under voluntary control (i.e., functions as the lower urinary tract). The upper urinary tract should be protected from urine reflux, which can lead to kidney infection. Normal renal function and electrolyte balance must also be preserved. These objectives are not easily attained. Various procedures are used for urinary diversion.

Continent Reservoir   With a continent reservoir, an intestinal pouch is created with bilateral antirefluxing ureteroenteric anastomoses. This high-capacity (up to 800 ml), low-pressure pouch provides an intraabdominal reservoir (neobladder) for the storage of urine. A one-way outflow valve provides continence (i.e., the ability to control function). A cutaneous stoma also may be created to empty the reservoir (Figure 36-7). The procedure is performed through a low midline incision. Several techniques are used to create the reservoir from a segment of ileum. Anastomoses may be stapled or sutured to reestablish intestinal continuity.

Although creating a continent reservoir is a lengthy surgical procedure, the resultant quality of life for the patient makes this procedure, which prevents involuntary urinary leakage, the procedure of choice unless contraindicated by the patient's tolerance or pathologic condition.

Kock Pouch   With a Kock pouch, a U-shaped pouch is created from a segment (28 to 32 inches [70 to 80 cm]) of ileum. Nipple valves are created on two sides by intussusception (i.e., a portion of ileum is ensheathed in another portion). The afferent inflow valve prevents reflux. The ureters are anastomosed end-to-side distally near this inflow valve. The efferent outflow valve provides continence. Absorbable staples and/or mesh are used to help stabilize the valves. The reservoir will gradually increase in capacity to as much as 750 to 800 ml of urine. The patient does not wear a collection device but needs to use a catheter every 4 to 6 hours to empty the reservoir through the exteriorized cutaneous stoma.

Indiana Pouch   An Indiana pouch is constructed by mobilizing a segment (6 to 8 inches [15 to 20 cm]) of terminal ileum, cecum, and ascending colon. The ureters are anastomosed to the colonic segment, inferiorly on each side of the pouch, to prevent reflux. The terminal ileum is exteriorized to form a continent stoma for self-catheterization.

Camey Pouch   An ileocystoplasty can be performed on a male patient if a U-shaped segment (approximately 16 inches [40 cm]) of ileum reaches the urethra at the pelvic floor without tension. The ureters are anastomosed through small enterostomies to the distal ends of the mobilized and divided ileum. A urethroileal anastomosis in the midsection of the ileal reservoir allows the patient to void through the urethra. Continence is maintained by spontaneous contraction around the outflow valve at the site of anastomosis. Micturition occurs by relaxation of the perineal muscles and a Valsalva maneuver (i.e., a forced expiratory effort).

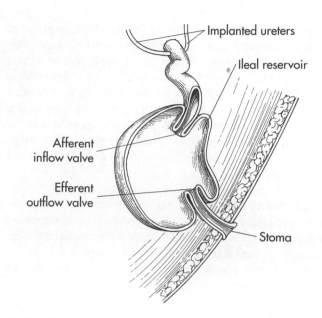

Figure 36-7   Ileal reservoir created from segment of ileum with ureters implanted distal to inflow valve. Exteriorized stoma allows self-catheterization through continent outflow valve. A continent reservoir includes implanted ureters, afferent inflow valve, ileal reservoir, efferent outflow valve, and stoma.

Mainz Pouch   With a Mainz pouch, a reservoir is formed by mobilizing a segment (4 to 6 inches [10 to 15 cm]) of cecum and ascending colon and detubularizing (opening out flat) two small segments of equal length of terminal ileum. The walls of the pouch are formed by anastomoses of the ascending colon and cecum with the ileal segments. The ureters are implanted into the ascending colon in an antirefluxive manner. To increase capacity, this pouch can be anastomosed to the urinary bladder remnant after partial cystectomy. Continent diversion can be achieved by inverting the appendix into the cecum and exteriorizing the intussuscepted appendiceal mucosa to form a continent stoma for self-catheterization. In the absence of a healthy appendix, an additional segment of ileum (3 to 5 inches [8 to 12 cm]) can be used to create a continent stoma.

Ileal Conduit   In the creation of an ileal conduit, a procedure popularized by Bricker in the 1950s, both ureters are anastomosed to an isolated segment of the terminal ileum near its proximal end. The distal end is everted and sutured to a predetermined stomal site on the skin, usually on the right side of the abdomen below the waist. A urinary collection appliance is secured over the stoma before the patient leaves the OR. An ileal conduit with an incontinent external stoma (Figure 36-8) creates the psychologic stress of an altered body image for the patient, but it may be the procedure of choice for the patient who will receive systemic chemotherapy following radical cystectomy. As a secondary procedure after chemotherapy, an incontinent ileal conduit may be converted to a continent ileal reservoir.

Ureterosigmoidostomy   With a ureterosigmoidostomy, the ureters may be anastomosed to a nonrefluxing seg-

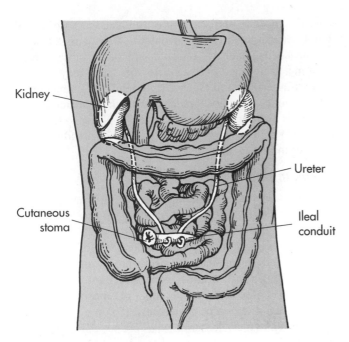

Figure 36-8 Ileal conduit created from isolated segment of ileum with ureters anastomosed to segment between closed end and external stoma. Urinary collection device must be placed over incontinent stoma. Incontinent urinary diversion carries urine from kidneys through implanted ureters and ileal conduit to stoma.

ment of sigmoid colon. Urine diverted into the colon may cause physiologic complications, making this alternative for permanent urinary diversion the least desirable therapeutically. However, the patient does retain an intact body image.

Cutaneous Ureterostomy To create a cutaneous ureterostomy, the end of the ureter closest to the bladder is brought through the abdominal wall to the skin. This procedure can be performed unilaterally or bilaterally with a single cutaneous stoma or double-loop stoma. The patient must be fitted postoperatively with an appliance for collecting urine directly from the ureter to the exterior of the body. This procedure may be performed as a temporary emergency measure following trauma to the bladder, such as a ruptured bladder.

Ureteroneocystostomy

Implantation of the ureters into the bladder wall can be performed to relocate the ureters into a different site for correction of ureterovesical reflux, to reestablish urinary flow following temporary diversion or ureteral injury, or to establish urinary flow from a kidney transplant following bilateral nephrectomy and ureterectomy.

Ureteroureterostomy

Anastomosis of two segments of one ureter is usually performed to reestablish ureteral continuity following traumatic injury. A ureteral catheter may be inserted as a stent and the ureter sutured over it. This procedure, a transureteroureterostomy anastomosis, may be indicated to bypass a ureteral stricture or to eliminate ureteral reflux that may be the result

of trauma. Injury to a ureter can occur as a complication of pelvic or abdominal surgical procedures, as well as from external penetrating wounds. Ideally, a transureteral anastomosis can be made 2 to 4 cm above the pelvic brim because the ureters are close at this point and the recipient ureter has a straight course into the bladder.

Vesicopsoas Hitch Procedure

The loss of a large segment of a middle or distal ureter can result from trauma or ureteral resection for tumor or stricture. A vesicopsoas hitch may be the procedure of choice when the length of the remaining ureter is insufficient for ureteroneocystostomy or ureteroureterostomy. The bladder is mobilized through an extraperitoneal approach into the retroperitoneal space. It is attached (i.e., hitched) to the psoas muscle to reposition the bladder cephalad. The segment of proximal ureter is brought through and sutured to the bladder wall. The kidney also may be mobilized and attached to the psoas muscle if too much tension will be placed on the ureterovesical anastomosis.

Urinary Bladder

The bladder may be opened through a suprapubic incision when a neoplasm, calculus, obstruction of the bladder neck, or traumatic injury is not amenable to treatment through the cystoscope. Diagnosis is usually established through urodynamics (the study of bladder function) and direct visualization via a cystoscope.

Cystometrogram

A cystometrogram measures voiding pressure within the bladder to determine muscle tone and to check nerve supply. A calibrated recording tidal irrigator cystometer is used for this measurement. The patient should feel a desire to void when 350 ml of solution is put into the bladder. Carbon dioxide gas is used with some electronic transducers or radio pressure gauges. The normal maximum capacity of the bladder is 450 to 550 ml. Normal bladder pressure is 40 to 50 ml of water. If the problem is neurogenic, the cystometric findings are not higher than normal. If the problem is a hypertonic bladder, these measurements are higher than normal.

Cystoscopy

Cystoscopy is a visual examination of the interior walls and contents of the bladder. This term is used broadly because various concurrent procedures may be carried out by using specially designed instruments through the cystoscope. Complete cystoscopy and litholapaxy have been described. A plain cystoscopy is a routine examination of the bladder. In conjunction with plain cystoscopy, the following procedures may also be performed within the bladder:

- Biopsy of a tumor with a flexible-shaft biopsy forceps to obtain specimens
- Cystogram for diagnostic x-ray studies after injection of a contrast medium into the bladder

- Fulguration of a tumor by use of an electrode to destroy tissue
- Resection of or incision into a bladder neck obstruction with a resectoscope
- Coagulation of a hemangioma with an argon laser, vaporization of a superficial tumor of the bladder wall with an Nd:YAG laser, or photodynamic therapy to a solid tumor with argon-pumped tunable dye laser
- Removal of a foreign body with a flexible-shaft, foreign body forceps
- Insertion of interstitial radionuclide seeds

Suprapubic Cystostomy

With a suprapubic cystostomy, urinary drainage from the bladder is established via a catheter inserted through a suprapubic incision or trocar puncture into the bladder. If the bladder or urethra is injured by trauma associated with bony and soft tissue injuries of the pelvis, the bladder may be drained with a catheter placed above the pubic arch. This method of drainage is also preferred following some ureteral, bladder, prostatic, and urethral surgical procedures to decrease tension on sutures, to ensure a patent route for urinary drainage, and to minimize urinary retention. A suprapubic catheter also can be used when the surgeon wants the patient to void some urine voluntarily via the urethra to maintain urethral function and tone, such as following bladder or vaginal repairs. Suprapubic catheters are connected to a sterile closed constant drainage system before the patient leaves the OR. The following are the most commonly used catheters for cystostomy drainage:

- Foley, 30-ml balloon, French sizes 20, 22, or 24.
- Foley, 5-ml balloon, French size 24, three-way irrigating catheter. The third lumen can be used for continuous irrigation.
- Bonanno suprapubic catheter.

Cutaneous Vesicostomy

In a cutaneous vesicostomy, urinary drainage is established directly from the bladder into a collecting device affixed on the abdomen rather than through a suprapubic catheter. The bladder is opened through a transverse suprapubic incision, and a flap is raised at the dome. A skin flap is raised in the midline of the abdomen below the umbilicus. The bladder flap is sutured to the defect created in the skin and then covered with the skin flap. A transparent adhering skin dressing and collection device form a seal around the resultant bladder stoma. A cutaneous vesicostomy may preserve renal function and/or improve upper urinary tract structure in patients with a neurogenic or atonic bladder, urinary incontinence, or bladder outlet obstruction.

Cystotomy, Cystoplasty

An incision into the urinary bladder through a suprapubic incision (cystotomy) may be performed to repair (cystoplasty) a bladder laceration or rupture as a result of trauma or a defect in the bladder wall. Various techniques are used to re-store the capacity and function of the bladder. Free fascial grafts, seromuscular grafts, myouterine flaps, and segments of stomach, ileum, or sigmoid colon are used to close defects. To stimulate regeneration of tissue, the defect may be covered with peritoneum, omentum, lyophilized human dura, gelatin sponge, or a biodegradable or synthetic material. The bladder is also incised to perform a Y-V-plasty to relieve a stricture or contracture of the bladder neck by broadening the outlet of the bladder into the urethra.

Cystectomy

In a cystectomy, the bladder is removed for invasive malignant disease. A radical total cystectomy with en bloc pelvic lymph node dissection is usually performed. The neurovascular bundle, which is required for penile erection, may be preserved in a male patient, or a penile prosthesis may be implanted during a subsequent surgical procedure. A salvage or partial cystectomy with intraoperative radiation therapy may be an alternative to a total cystectomy. If a urinary diversion procedure (previously described) has not been performed before removal of the bladder, transplantation of the ureters into the skin or into the intestinal tract for urinary drainage is required at the time of cystectomy. A gastrocystoplasty may be the procedure of choice following a partial cystectomy, especially in a patient with impaired renal function.

Urinary Incontinence

Involuntary, uncontrollable voiding may accompany congenital or acquired physiologic conditions, such as a loss of bladder control following spinal cord injury or neurogenic disease. Urinary incontinence may develop in males because of loss of sphincter control following prostatectomy and in females following obstetric injury, radiation therapy, or severe pelvic fractures. Surgical intervention is often necessary for stress incontinence—the intermittent leakage of urine as a result of a sudden increase in intraabdominal pressure (e.g., during coughing or sneezing) on weakened urethral sphincter muscles at the bladder neck. Various surgical procedures are performed as determined by urodynamics. Gynecologists perform some bladder suspension procedures (e.g., Marshall-Marchetti-Krantz suprapubic vesicourethral suspension, and urologists perform other procedures. Laparoscopic approaches have been developed for bladder neck suspension with the use of synthetic mesh and titanium staples. Surgical procedures that suspend, support, or reposition the bladder can correct urinary incontinence or improve urinary continence.

Stamey Procedure

In the Stamey procedure, sutures are placed on both sides of the urethrovesical junction from the anterior rectus fascia into the vagina. The patient is positioned in a modified lithotomy position so the legs extend laterally to flatten the lower abdomen. Short suprapubic incisions, right and left of midline, are extended to the anterior rectus fascia. The vagina is incised transversely and dissected from the urethra to expose the trigone of the bladder. The urethrovesical junction is located by palpating the balloon of the Foley catheter inserted into the bladder. A straight or angled Stamey needle is passed through the rectus fascia, along the internal vesicle neck, and out through the vaginal incision.

The cystoscopic equipment should be set up on a separate sterile table because contamination of the eyepiece is unavoidable. A cystoscope is inserted to ascertain correct needle placement without injury to the bladder. A heavy nylon suture threaded onto the needle is drawn from the vagina to the suprapubic incision; the needle is inserted again. The vaginal end of the suture is passed through a 1-cm length of polyester tubular graft before it is threaded onto the needle. When the suture is drawn to the abdominal wall, it establishes a suspending loop on one side of the bladder neck. The suture is tied over the anterior rectus fascia with enough tension to elevate the bladder neck by traction on the adjacent vaginal fascia. This procedure is repeated on the contralateral side.

Pereyra Procedure

In the Pereyra procedure, the bladder neck is elevated with sutures suspended from the anterior rectus fascia. The primary difference between this procedure and the Stamey procedure is that a Pereyra ligature carrier needle is passed blindly down through retropubic space and out into the vagina. Both procedures relocate the proximal urethra and bladder neck into the zone of intraabdominal pressure without necessitating open pelvic surgery. The Pereyra procedure is used for uncomplicated recurrent urinary stress incontinence and is 80% effective for long-term resolution of urinary leakage.

Artificial Urinary Sphincter

A prosthesis may be implanted to apply pressure to the urethra to maintain continence between periods of voiding. The pressure-regulating mechanism has a balloon, a cuff, and a pump constructed of silicone rubber. A balloon with a desired predetermined pressure is positioned intraabdominally beside the bladder. Depending on the preferred surgical approach, the cuff encircles either the bladder neck or the bulbous urethra. The pump is placed in the subcutaneous tissue of the scrotum (in males) or labium (in females). A control assembly lies subcutaneously adjacent to the external inguinal ring; tubing connects the components. A radiopaque isotonic solution is used to fill the prosthesis. When a patient squeezes the pump, solution is transferred from the cuff into the balloon, thus releasing pressure on the urethra and permitting urine to flow.

Periurethral Collagen Injection

Collagen may be injected into the tissues surrounding the urethra proximal to the external sphincter. The injection swells the tissue, narrowing the urethra sufficiently for sphincteric control. This procedure is performed in select patients with moderate to severe urinary incontinence, such as in a male following a transurethral resection or in a female in whom a suspension procedure has been unsuccessful. The injection is made transurethrally with a flexible syringe through a fiberoptic cystourethroscope. A suprapubic catheter is used for 3 to 5 days postoperatively to allow some voluntary passage of urine from the urethra. Postoperative complications include urinary retention, urethral fistulas, and infection.

Bladder Flap Urethroplasty

A bladder flap urethroplasty procedure is advisable when urodynamics show a resistance to urinary flow in a female with a neurogenic bladder. A lesion of the nervous system can cause bladder dysfunction.

Urethra

The urethra functions as the outlet for urine to pass from the bladder. Obstruction or dysfunction of the urethra may cause urinary retention or incontinence. Enlargement of the prostate may cause obstruction. Gonorrhea, other disease processes, or traumatic injury may cause a stricture.

Perineal Urethrostomy

When indwelling or intermittent urethral catheterization is contraindicated in a male patient with an obstructed or traumatized urethra, urinary drainage may be established through a perineal incision. An indwelling catheter is inserted into the bladder through an incision into the membranous urethra. Male patients may have a perineal urethrostomy after a total penectomy.

Urethral Dilation

Periodic dilation may be necessary for weeks to years following an infection or a trauma that has caused a urethral stricture. Either balloon dilators, woven filiforms and followers, bougies, or metal sounds are used. If the latter are preferred, curved metal sounds are used to dilate a male urethra; straight sounds are used for a female urethra. A short urethral stent may be inserted.

Urethral Stent   To prevent collapse of the lumen caused by stricture, a spring-loaded, stainless steel mesh stent can be placed into the male urethra via a cystoscope at a level proximal to the bulbar urethra and distal to the external urinary sphincter. The stricture is measured and dilated or incised by internal urethrotomy. To be effective, the stent selected should measure 1 cm greater than the length of the stricture. A special deployment applicator is used to place the stent in the urethra. The stent becomes a permanent urethral implant and is useful for males who suffer from benign prostatic hypertrophy. It is contraindicated in bleeding disorders or for males who are receiving anticoagulation therapy. After the procedure, antibiotics are administered as a prophylactic measure.

Urethrotomy

An Otis urethrotome may be used to cut into a urethral stricture. After the instrument is passed into the urethra, the blade is released to cut the stricture. If a specimen of the urethra is taken for biopsy, a rigid biopsy forceps is used through a cystourethroscope. This scope also is used with a laser to open a urethral stricture.

Urethroplasty

Reestablishment of continuity without stricture is the ultimate objective following a traumatic urethral injury and is usually associated with pelvic fractures in males. Scrotal-inlay urethroplasty or another method of urethral reconstruction is usually delayed until the extent of injury can be fully evaluated by urethrograms. A suprapubic cystostomy catheter inserted as an emergency measure can maintain urinary drainage for several weeks to months. Insertion of a urethral catheter into a ruptured urethra in the immediate posttraumatic period can produce periurethral infection, stricture, and other irreparable damage.

Perineum and Genital Surface Procedures
Ablation of Condylomata Accumulata

Condylomata are caused by a sexually transmitted human papillomavirus (HPV). Referred to as genital warts, this condition can affect the genitalia, perineum, perianal region, and mucus membranes of males and females. The incubation period is 1 to 2 months after exposure, but longer periods have been reported. HPV has been implicated in cervical cancer.

In the OR or office setting, and with the patient under local anesthesia, condylomata are surgically ablated with ar-

gon, CO_2, KTP, or Nd:YAG laser. Before the procedure, acetic acid 3% is applied to the area to make the lesions visible. As with all other laser procedures, laser precautions (e.g., appropriate eyewear for all persons in the room and proper instrumentation) are followed. Viral mutation in laser plume has been documented, and personal protective equipment is required. Appropriate laser eyewear and masks should be worn by the staff and the patient to prevent contamination of respiratory and ocular mucosa with virus-laden plume. The eyewear also protects from laser light.

MALE REPRODUCTIVE ORGANS

The primary functions of the male reproductive organs are procreation, sexual gratification, and hormone secretion. These organs are both internal and external (Figure 36-9).

Testes

The testes, or testicles, are both endocrine glands and male reproductive organs and are bilaterally suspended in the scrotum. They secrete hormones that influence growth and development, sexual activity, the production of spermatozoa, and the development of secondary sex characteristics. Disorders in or around one testis or both testes that inhibit sexual activity, reproductive capability, or cause discomfort in the scrotum may necessitate a surgical procedure. If both

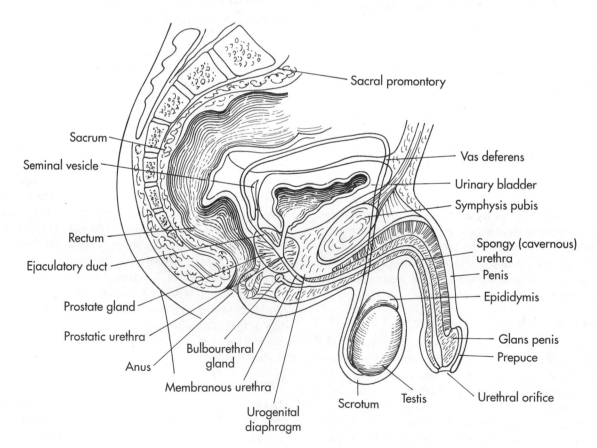

Figure 36-9   Male reproductive organs in sagittal section.

testes are excised (a bilateral orchiectomy), the patient becomes sterile and deficient in male hormones.

Male patients should be instructed to perform a monthly testicular self-examination (TSE), which should be performed when the scrotum is relaxed (after a warm bath or shower). When performing a TSE, each testis is gently rolled between the thumb and forefingers. The testis should feel smooth and oval, should be without lumps or hardened areas, and should move freely within the scrotal sac. Palpation should be pain free.

Orchiectomy

A bilateral orchiectomy may be performed in patients with prostatic cancer to alter the hormonal environment. Following this relatively simple procedure, control of the disease is attempted before the urologist considers other endocrine surgery, such as an adrenalectomy. Psychologic preparation is important to help the patient accept the sterilization and the other body changes, (e.g., breast enlargement) that may occur as a result of the alteration in the hormonal system.

In this procedure, bilateral oblique incisions in the inguinal canals extend into the upper anterior surface of the scrotum over the testes. The testes are removed from the scrotum following ligation of the spermatic cords at the external or internal inguinal rings. Silicone rubber prostheses may be implanted in the scrotal sac to improve aesthetic appearance, which helps with the psychologic rehabilitation of the patient.

The removal of one testis (unilateral orchiectomy) does not sterilize the patient. This procedure may be indicated following traumatic injury or infection, but it is more commonly performed to remove a tumor. Primary testicular tumors may be right- or left-sided; germ cell tumors may develop bilaterally. Accurate histologic findings and clinical evaluations of the type of tumor and stage of disease are mandatory for determining the appropriate therapy. Computed tomography and lymphangiography or lymphoscintigraphy are valuable diagnostic tools. Unilateral radical orchiectomy via an inguinal incision may be followed by radiation or chemotherapy and retroperitoneal lymph node dissection. The spermatic cord and vas deferens are ligated and divided separately at the internal ring so these structures can be identified if further dissection is needed for metastatic disease.

Retroperitoneal Lymphadenectomy A transabdominal midline incision is made for exposure of the lymph nodes and sympathetic nerve fibers in the paraaortic plane, usually along the anterolateral aspect of the aorta in the retroperitoneal space. A unilateral lymphadenectomy usually is performed on the ipsilateral (same) side as the tumor unless regional metastases have spread via lymphatic invasion, in which case a bilateral dissection is indicated. If possible, the neurovascular bundles extending from the hypogastric plexus to the corporeal tissues of the penis are preserved. These nerve fibers are identified and placed in vessel loops before lymphadenectomy is carried out, thus preserving ejaculatory function.

Scrotal-Testicular Trauma

An injury may require exploration of the scrotum to ligate bleeding vessels or to insert a Penrose drain. Infection is likely to develop following a penetrating wound; thus extraperitoneal spaces in the scrotum must be drained thoroughly.

Testicular Torsion

The testicle can become twisted on the spermatic cord, causing extreme pain. Immediate correction is necessary or the testicle will become ischemic and tissue death will follow. Manual detorsion may be tried, but surgical intervention is indicated if reduction is not successful within 1 hour of onset.

Hydrocelectomy

A hydrocele is an accumulation of fluid in the sac of the tunica vaginalis of the testis. Through an anterior incision into the scrotum, the hydrocele sac is dissected away from the testis and removed from the scrotum.

Spermatocelectomy

A small mass attached to the epididymis may be palpated in the scrotum superior to the testis. This painless cyst is a collection of testicular fluid and sperm cells. These cysts are repaired if they become annoying to the patient.

Varicocele Ligation

Dilation of the spermatic veins in the pampiniform plexus of the spermatic cord can cause a soft, elastic, often uncomfortable swelling in the scrotum. This condition, known as varicocele, occurs more often on the left side. It can cause a loss in testicular mass and a decrease of sperm density associated with male infertility caused by increased temperature. Ligation of the spermatic vein can improve sperm count if the testis has not atrophied.

The spermatic vein is ligated above the inguinal canal lateral to the inferior epigastric vessels or in the retroperitoneal space lateral to the iliac artery. In the latter approach, a transverse abdominal incision starts at the anterior superior iliac spine and extends toward the lateral aspect of the rectus abdominis muscle. The hemiscrotum must be manually emptied of all blood before the vein is ligated or the varicocele may persist postoperatively.

Laparoscopic approaches have been developed for spermatic vein ligation. In such a procedure, the internal inguinal ring is located laparoscopically and the spermatic cord and blood vessels are identified. The spermatic vein is dissected free, ligated with two endoscopic clips, and cut between the clips with endoscopic scissors. Most patients are able to return to work within 2 days of the procedure.

Vas Deferens

The vasa deferentia are the small fibromuscular excretory ducts that carry sperm upward through the spermatic cords from the epididymides (which lie along the upper portion of each testis) to the seminal vesicles, the pouchlike glands in front of the urinary bladder near the prostate gland. Interruption of or obstruction to a vas deferens inhibits normal spermatogenesis.

Vasectomy

Elective bilateral vasectomy is an established method of male sterilization and is usually performed as an ambulatory surgical procedure. In a vasectomy, a segment of each vas deferens is removed. Depending on the preference of the urologist, the cut ends are either ligated with suture or clips, or the endothelium of the lumen is coagulated with the ESU. Techniques vary, but all patients should be informed that spontaneous regeneration of a severed vas deferens does occur in a small percentage of patients. Follow-up care includes semen testing for sperm count; repeat testing should continue until no sperm is found in the seminal fluid. Patient teaching includes instructions to use alternative birth control methods until the seminal fluid contains no sperm.

Vasovasostomy

Recannulization of the vas deferens for the restoration of fertility requires a nonobstructed anastomosis. The vas deferens has a tough, 2-mm outer diameter and an inner diameter of 1 mm or less at the distal end, as well as dilation at the proximal end. This makes precise anastomosis under the operating microscope preferable to nonmicrosurgical techniques, in which it is difficult to see the lumen of the vas deferens on the distal side. One-layer microscopic anastomosis and splinting techniques for a vasectomy reversal often result in a stricture caused by scarring within the lumen of the vas deferens, which inhibits the passage of sperm.

After a scrotal incision is made to expose the vas deferens above and below the site of previous ligation, the two ends are cut to excise scar tissue and to open the lumen. Under magnification of the operating microscope, interrupted sutures are placed in the mucosal lining of the lumen to create a fluid-tight anastomosis. Muscularis is approximated separately. A carbon dioxide milliwatt laser may be used to weld tissue to overcome the scarring and stricture that may be associated with suturing. Sperm counts return to normal soon after the surgical procedure.

Male Infertility

Primary infertility is diagnosed after a failure to conceive during a period of 1 year of unprotected sexual intercourse. Causes of infertility include abnormality in the female and/or male reproductive systems. Male infertility can be the result of deficient sperm production, obstructed sperm passage, a mechanical inability to pass sperm, hormonal imbalance, testicular disease or injury, a low sperm count, and antibodies against sperm.

The history and physical should be concurrent with the female partner's gynecologic evaluation. Issues assessed should include sexual history, previous pregnancies, health history, the use of lubricants, drug use, radiation exposure, and timing or frequency of intercourse. Childhood illnesses such as high fevers and viral infections may be a factor. A

previous sexually transmitted disease can cause scarring that prevents the transport of sperm. Endocrine testing includes follicle-stimulating hormone, luteinizing hormone, testosterone, and prolactin levels. Urinalysis is performed to rule out infection and/or retrograde ejaculation.

The semen analysis includes determining ejaculate volume, sperm count and motility, morphology, and the presence or absence of white blood cells or red blood cells in the seminal fluid. The patient is advised to abstain from sexual intercourse for 2 to 3 days before the testing is performed.

Prostate Gland

The prostate gland, a musculoglandular organ in males, is encased in a fibrous capsule and surrounds the posterior urethra at the bladder neck. It is divided into five lobes. The normal function of this gland is to provide alkaline secretions to the seminal fluid for sperm mobility during ejaculation. The standard of care includes an annual digital prostate examination and prostate-specific antigen (PSA) testing after 40 years of age.

Although the prostate gland normally weighs 20 g, in most men it will enlarge to some degree by 50 years of age. Fifty percent of all men over 80 years of age will have prostatic cancer. Enlargement of the prostate gland can obstruct the urethra and interfere with voiding; this difficulty in voiding is what most often brings men with prostatic disease to a urologist. The urologist will examine the prostate and order a PSA blood test. If the tests indicate benign prostatic hypertrophy, surgery is not the first treatment method of choice. Conservative treatment for benign enlargement of the prostate includes administration of oral finasteride (Proscar). If the prostate does not respond to drug therapy by shrinking, balloon dilation or other surgical procedure may be indicated.

The entire prostate gland or one or more lobes can be resected from its capsule transurethrally. Prostatectomy can also be performed through a suprapubic or retropubic abdominal approach or a perineal incision. A radical prostatectomy, performed through a retropubic abdominal or perineal incision, includes extirpation of the prostate, periprostatic tissue, seminal vesicles, and vas ampullae en bloc. The approach and procedure depend on the urologist's preference for removing the type of pathologic condition.

Transrectal aspiration, core biopsies, or ultrasonography help establish the correct diagnosis. Prostatic carcinoma may be treated by surgical removal, interstitial and external beam radiation, chemotherapy, and/or hormonal therapy. Management depends on the stage of the disease and the age and condition of the patient. Carcinoma of the prostate is the second most common cause of cancer-related deaths in American men. Benign prostatic hypertrophy/hyperplasia (BPH) is a common indication for prostate intervention in men over 50 years of age if the prostate symptoms do not respond to drug therapy. Men younger than 50 years of age may not qualify for definitive treatment if prostate enlargement is caused by prostatitis. Conservative antibiotic therapy is the treatment of choice. More information about prostate health and patient teaching can be found at **www.prostate.org.**

Balloon Dilation of Prostatic Urethra

A balloon dilation probe can be inserted into the urethra and expanded to relieve obstruction caused by prostatic hypertrophy. This procedure is a temporary measure to relieve urinary retention.

Transurethral Microwave Thermotherapy

With transurethral microwave thermotherapy (TUMT), ultrasound guidance is used to insert a microwave probe into the urethra to the level of the prostate blockage. Microwaves are generated by a console and transmitted to the distal aspect of the probe. Heat generated by the microwave probe is absorbed by the urethral portion of the prostate for 1 hour. The probe is cooled with water circulation at 68° F (20° C) to protect nearby structures. A rectal probe is used to record rectal temperature. The heated tissue sloughs, which causes the urethral stricture to release. Most patients can void with ease, although a few patients require a Foley catheter for several days postoperatively.

Transurethral Needle Ablation

With transurethral needle ablation (TUNA), an ambulatory procedure, telescopic guidance is used to insert a probe into the urethra to the level of the prostate stricture. Two small needles are passed from the side of the telescopic probe into the prostatic tissue. Radiowaves are transmitted selectively into the tissue via the needles. Prostatic tissue in contact with the needles is ablated; nearby structures, such as nerves and vessels, are spared. Up to six select areas of stricture can be precisely ablated in the same procedure. Each application creates a defect in the prostate. The tissue reabsorbs over a period of 3 months, causing the stricture to release. The patient may complain of burning on urination for 24 to 96 hours after the procedure. The main side effect is the potential for retrograde ejaculation.

Transurethral Prostatectomy

Transurethral resection, also referred to as transurethral resection of the prostate (TURP), involves the removal of all or part of the glandular tissue within the prostatic capsule by electroresection. A resectoscope is introduced into the prostatic urethra. Using alternating currents from the ESU through the cutting loop electrode, the urologist resects tissue and coagulates bleeding vessels. The bladder must remain filled during resection. Nonconducting, isosmotic glycine irrigating solution is used; 10 to 12 L may be needed.

Resected tissue is collected in an Ellik or other evacuator. After the surgical procedure, tissue fragments must be sent to the pathology department for analysis and weighing. The urologist may insert a three-way 30- or 50-ml Foley catheter. The inflated balloon compresses against the bladder neck fossa to form a tamponade to help control bleeding. Some urologists place the Foley catheter under direct tension to increase the tamponade effect for hemostasis. The third lumen provides a means for continuous postoperative irrigation to prevent the formation of clots in the bladder.

Benign nodular hyperplasia of glands under 50 g in size is the usual indication for TURP. This approach has the potential complications of impotence and urinary incontinence. The technique is one of the most difficult for a urologist to master. Although electroresection is used most commonly, transurethral incision of small prostate glands (less than 25 g), balloon dilation of the prostate, laser surgery, and cryosurgery are other invasive techniques for treating BPH. TURP may be performed for the diagnosis or treatment of localized cancer.

Suprapubic Prostatectomy

The suprapubic approach for prostatectomy is limited almost exclusively to the removal of a large, benign, hypertrophied gland weighing more than 50 g. Through a midline vertical incision above the symphysis pubis, the superior bladder wall is opened to expose the prostatic urethra. The prostatic lobes are enucleated with a finger that is inserted through an incision into the mucosa of the urethra. This procedure may be termed *transvesicocapsular prostatectomy* because the prostatic capsule is approached through the bladder. Hemostatic agents are usually packed into the extremely vascular prostatic fossa to help control bleeding. Pressure from the Foley catheter balloon inserted after closure of the urethra also helps obtain hemostasis. A cystostomy tube is inserted to facilitate urinary drainage from the bladder during the healing process.

Retropubic Prostatectomy

In the retropubic approach, the prostate gland is exposed below the bladder neck through a vertical or transverse abdominal incision above the symphysis pubis. The gland is removed through an incision in the prostatic capsule; this procedure is called a transcapsular prostatectomy. The periprostatic tissue, seminal vesicles, and vas ampullae also may be excised.

Radical Retropubic Prostatectomy A limited pelvic lymph node dissection is performed for carcinoma with no evidence of spread beyond the prostatic capsule. This radical procedure may be carried out as initial curative therapy or following transurethral prostatectomy. After dissection of the lymph nodes, one of two approaches may be used to totally remove the prostate:

1. *Campbell technique.* An incision is made at the bladder neck, and the urethra is transected. The prostate and periprostatic tissue are widely dissected anterograde from the bladder. The bladder neck is reconstructed for the vesicourethral anastomosis. The patient will be impotent because the nerves responsible for erection are transected. A penile prosthesis may be implanted.
2. *Walsh technique.* The prostate is resected retrograde beginning at the urethra, working back to the bladder neck. Dissection is carried out close to the prostatic capsule to preserve the neurovascular bundle and thus maintain potency. The vesicourethral anastomosis is completed.

Perineal Prostatectomy

The perineum affords the most direct open surgical approach to the prostate through a relatively avascular field. With the patient in an extreme lithotomy position, the perineum is incised above the anal sphincter. The rectum may be dissected from the posterior surface of the prostate, or dissection may be carried out between the external anal sphincter and the rectum. The perineal approach may be used to enucleate the prostate gland from its capsule or for radical cystoprostatectomy. This latter procedure includes removal of the entire prostate gland, its capsule, the seminal vesicles, and a portion of the bladder. The classic radical perineal prostatectomy with pelvic lymph node dissection may be the surgical procedure of choice to reduce the morbidity of prostatic carcinoma.

Transperineal Prostatic Cryoablation

Transperineal prostatic cryoablation offers an alternative to radical prostatectomy in select patients with cancer of the prostate. This procedure is performed in the cysto room with the patient under general or spinal anesthesia. The entire prostate and periprostatic tissues are frozen. With the patient in the lithotomy position, an ultrasound probe is placed in the rectum for guidance in positioning five cryoprobes. Each cryoprobe is placed transperineally through a hollow sheath inserted in a small (18-gauge) needle puncture site. Liquid nitrogen is delivered to each probe from the cryosurgical device/console. Care must be taken to avoid freezing the rectum. Warm water is run through a urethral catheter to keep the urethra warm to prevent tissue sloughing, a potential complication of transurethral cryosurgery. Both the prostate gland and the tumor cells are destroyed. The side effects of this procedure include a high risk for impotence (80% to 90%) and urinary incontinence (30%).

Pelvic Lymphadenectomy

A pelvic lymphadenectomy involves either a low abdominal incision into the extraperitoneal space or a laparoscopic approach. The lymph nodes are dissected bilaterally from the iliac vessels, obturator spaces, and hypogastric vessels. These nodes may be examined by frozen section to detect early and subtle metastases from prostatic carcinoma. If several nodes are positive for cancer, the patient is unlikely to benefit from a radical prostatectomy. If the nodes are negative, the urologist may proceed with a radical retropubic prostatectomy. Pelvic lymphadenectomy also may be performed as a staged procedure before radical perineal prostatectomy. If feasible, at least one neurovascular bundle is preserved.

Penis

The penis is the cylindrical erectile male organ of copulation. Because it contains the urethra, a deviation or malformation in structure may affect normal urinary flow from the bladder. Circumcision or surgical procedures to repair congenital anomalies of the penis are usually performed during infancy and childhood. Penile anatomy consists of the glans at the distal section, the corpus spongiosum circumferentially the length of the urethra, and the corpus cavernosa bilaterally the length of the shaft (see Figure 36-9). The distal portion where the urethra exits is referred to as the glans. In its natural state, the glans is covered by redundant skin, which is referred to as foreskin. Some cultures electively remove this skin covering from males in infancy by circumcision.

The arterial supply of the penis arises from the inferior pudendal arteries. Venous drainage is from the venules in the periphery of the corpora and the superior and deep dorsal veins into the cavernosal and pudendal plexae. Innervation is from both sympathetic and parasympathetic origin combined with autonomic reflexes.

The erection and ejaculatory response is neurologically mediated by afferent and efferent pathways. Sacral efferent parasympathetic innervation causes both psychogenic and reflex erections. Destruction of these nerves during abdominal perineal resection and radical prostatectomy will result in impotency in 70% to 100% of patients. At the level of the penis, innervation is from adrenergic nerves in the arteriolar smooth muscle. Complete transsection of the spinal cord can result in impotence. Reflex erections may be found in patients with lesions of the upper cord. An exact loci of impulses in the brain has not been identified.

Impotence

The cause of erectile impotence can be classified as organic or psychogenic. Patients are thoroughly evaluated by a urologist and properly selected for surgical therapy. Organic causes are confirmed by angiography, neurologic testing, and papaverine injection–induced erection studies. A test dose of sildenafil (Viagra), a recently released drug for impotent males, appears to delineate vasculogenic causes.

Studies of penile activities include the measurement of erections during the rapid eye movement (REM) phases of sleep. A small band attached to a pressure-sensitive machine is placed around the penis. Erections, referred to as nocturnal penile tumescence, are recorded during sleep. This helps to rule out organic causes of impotence.

Psychogenic causes are suspected after organic causes have been ruled out. Some psychogenic causes may be attributed to a fear of sexual relations following a heart attack or surgical procedure. Antidepressants and psychologic counseling may be helpful.

Most procedures for the diagnosis and treatment of organic impotence are performed with the patient under regional anesthesia. Consideration for the patient's privacy should be included in the plan of care. More information can be found at **www.impotence.org.**

Dorsal Vein Ligation A failed erection can be caused by inadequate filling or inadequate storage of blood in the erectile tissue of the corpus cavernosa of the penis. Some patients are able to achieve erection but are unable to maintain it for more than a few minutes because of a cavernosal leak. The diagnosis is made by the dynamic infusion cavernosometry and cavernosography (DICC) procedure. In select patients with this condition, the urologist may elect to ligate the dorsal vein and several collateral vessels of the penis to delay the venous return from the erectile tissue and help sustain erection. This procedure is not always successful.

Penile Prosthesis Implantation of a penile prosthesis as treatment for organic impotence can enable some men to achieve a satisfactory return of sexual activity within 4 to 6 weeks postoperatively. Penile prosthetic implants are of three types: semirigid silicone, semiflexible silicone-braided silver, and an inflatable hydraulic device:

1. The Small-Carrion semirigid prosthesis consists of two foam-filled silicone rods that are inserted into the corpus cavernosum on each side of the penis, usually through a vertical incision in the perineum underneath the scrotum. The suitable-size prosthesis is selected from available lengths. This prosthesis maintains a permanent semierection.
2. The Finney Flexirod is similar to the Small-Carrion prosthesis except that it is hinged at the penoscrotal junction when implanted. This allows the penis to hang in a dependent position when an erection is not desired.
3. The Jonas prosthesis is constructed of malleable braided silver and silicone. It is semiflexible.
4. The Scott-Bradley inflatable hydraulic device is inserted through a midline incision that extends from the base of the penis to a point midway between the symphysis pubis and the umbilicus. Silicone cylinders are implanted into each corpus cavernosum. Tubing connected to these cylinders at the base of the penis is brought into the left inguinal canal, the prevesical space, and the right inguinal canal, where it is connected to tubing from the pump-release mechanism placed in the scrotum. A reservoir filled with a radiopaque solution is sutured into the abdominal fascia of the prevesical space; the tubing from this reservoir is also connected to the pump-release mechanism. To achieve an erection, the patient squeezes the pump in the scrotum (Figure 36-10).

Figure 36-10 Inflatable penile prosthesis.

Intraabdominal reservoir

Pump and release valve

Inflatable rods

Penectomy

The penis may be partially or completely resected because of neoplasm or trauma. A partial penectomy may allow the patient enough length for upright voiding. Cosmetic reconstruction may be possible in some patients. Invasive disease may necessitate a complete penectomy, including removal of the scrotum and testes. Reconstruction following a complete penectomy includes urethral diversion to the perineum. The plan of care should include consideration for psychologic counseling.

ENDOCRINE GLANDS

Two pairs of glands in the endocrine system are of primary interest to the urologist: the adrenal glands in both sexes and the testes in the male.

Adrenal Glands

The adrenal glands secrete substances that help regulate fluid and electrolyte balance, influence metabolism and the sexual organs, and assist the body in coping with stress. These glands are located in the retroperitoneal spaces immediately above the superior pole of each kidney. Total or partial excision of one or both adrenal glands is usually performed by the urologist. In some hospitals this surgical procedure has become the province of endocrinologic surgical specialists.

An adrenalectomy may be indicated to remove a benign, malignant, or metastatic tumor within the adrenal medulla or to eliminate adrenal hormonal secretions. The adrenal glands are a rich source of estrogens, and estrogens may stimulate a recurrence or metastasis from prostatic or breast cancer. A bilateral adrenalectomy may be performed as a supplemental treatment of advanced prostatic or breast cancer to reduce the hormonal environment within the body.

For a unilateral adrenalectomy, the adrenal gland is usually approached posteriorly through a lateral incision into the retroperitoneal space. The twelfth rib is usually resected on the right side because the adrenal gland lies above the kidney, behind the liver. The surgeon may also prefer a posterior approach for a bilateral adrenalectomy with the patient placed in a modified prone position for the bilateral incisions. Other surgeons prefer an anterior thoracoabdominal or transabdominal incision into the retroperitoneal space with the patient in the supine position. The circulator must verify with the surgeon the preferred position before the patient is positioned, prepped, and draped. Depending on the preoperative diagnosis, the thoracoabdominal incision may be preferred to extend the incision across the costal margin into the eighth or ninth intercostal space for exposure and exploration of the extraadrenal paraganglion system.

TRANSSEXUAL SURGERY (SEX REASSIGNMENT)

Transsexual surgery may be the only acceptable alternative for a patient who psychologically desires to become a member of the opposite sex—both physically and emotionally.

This type of surgery presents challenges to both the urologic and the gynecologic teams.

Sex transformation requires a stable personality, psychiatric counseling for feasibility, and careful preparation and support. The patient changes legal identity and social status.

Male to Female

Surgical techniques have been developed to eliminate the obvious external genitalia of a male by dissecting the penile structures, shortening the urethra, and removing the testes. The penile and scrotal skin are preserved for construction of a pseudofemale vaginal orifice. This surgical procedure is performed as the final stage following a change of secondary sexual characteristics by hormonal and/or surgical therapy to produce breast enlargement, suppression of beard and body hair, redistribution of adipose tissue, voice change, and removal of pronounced thyroid cartilage (Adam's apple). In this final stage of transsexual surgery, a vagina is created by inverting the hollow penis into the hypogastrium between the new urethral orifice and the rectum. Because the nerve endings from the penis are intact, the newly constructed vagina is capable of experiencing orgasm; the prostate and seminal vesicles are retained so that orgasm with emission is possible. The scrotal skin forms the labia.

Female to Male

Female to male transsexual surgery is also possible in satisfactory candidates. Management of this change is complex. A treatment schedule of hormonal substitution (i.e., androgens [male hormones] in the female patient) is begun well in advance of the procedure.

In a one-stage procedure, a bilateral subcutaneous mastectomy, total abdominal hysterectomy, and bilateral salpingo-oophorectomy are performed. Three additional stages are necessary to complete the transformation:

1. Urethral reconstruction, to the tip of the enlarged clitoris
2. Transfer of the labia for penile lengthening and scrotal construction
3. Prosthetic testicular implantation

An understanding, nonjudgmental, unembarrassed attitude on the part of health care personnel can help the patient adjust psychologically, as well as recover physically, after the radical change. Consideration should be given to the patient's family and significant others because they, too, must adjust. The patient may have married and produced children while in the role of his or her birth sex. In addition to confusion about parental roles, the patient may experience rejection or revulsion from offspring and other family members. Referral for family and individual counseling should be included in the plan of care.

POSTOPERATIVE COMPLICATIONS OF UROLOGIC SURGERY

Oliguria, the diminished capacity to form urine, is often seen after urologic surgery. Water and sodium are conserved by antidiuretic hormone, aldosterone, epinephrine, and norepinephrine secreted during stress; this decreases urinary output. Dehydration, shock, cardiac failure, renal failure, or third-space loss (e.g., edema or ascites) may contribute to oliguria. Because prolonged oliguria may result in renal failure, a urinary output of less than 30 ml an hour should be reported to the surgeon. Treatment depends on the cause.

The patient should be watched for infection following all urinary tract procedures because of the introduction of the catheter and instruments. Cloudy urine, dysuria, frequency, urgency, and pain or burning on urination are symptoms of urinary tract infections. Damage to bladder sphincters from instrumentation or urethral infection may lead to incontinence. Sharp abdominal pain following cystoscopy or the manipulation of a ureter to remove calculi may suggest peritonitis from bladder or ureteral perforation. Susceptibility to infection accompanies urinary diversion.

Bibliography

Aboseif S et al: The effect of cryosurgical ablation of the prostate on erectile function, *Br J Urol* 80(6):918-922, 1997.

Adams DH, Abernathy BB: Laser ureterolithotripsy for cystine calculi, *AORN J* 64(6):924-930, 1996.

Ang LP et al: Endoscopic injection of collagen for the treatment of female urinary stress incontinence, *Int J Urol* 4(3):254-258, 1997.

Bartholomew B, Grimaldi T: Collagen injection therapy for type III stress urinary incontinence, *AORN J* 64(1):75-86, 1996.

Carr HA: Prevention through care and technology, *Infect Control Today* 2(8):26, 28-29, 1998.

Choong S et al: A prospective, randomized, double blind study comparing lignocaine gel and plain lubricating gel in relieving pain during flexible cystoscopy, *Br J Urol* 80(1):69-71, 1997.

Cohen JK, Miller RJ: Thermal protection of urethra during cryosurgery of prostate, *Cryobiology* 31(3):313-316, 1994.

Eldh J et al: Long-term follow up after sex reassignment, *Scand J Plast Reconstr Surg Hand Surg* 31(1):39-45, 1997.

Emmert GK et al: Primary neoplasms of the penile shaft, *South Med J* 87(8):848-850, 1994.

Fisch M et al: The Mainz pouch II, *Eur Urol* 25(1):7-25, 1994.

Frank E et al: Postoperative epidural analgesia following radical retropubic prostatectomy: outcome assessment, *J Surg Oncol* 67(2):117-120, 1998.

Garber BB: Outpatient inflatable penile prosthesis insertion, *Urology* 49(4):600-603, 1997.

Gardner TA, Theodorescu D: Diagnosis and treatment of prostate cancer, *Surg Services Manag* 3(12):20-25, 27-28, 1997.

Gavaghan M: Surgical treatment of pheochromocytomas, *AORN J* 65(6):1041-1068, 1997.

Holschneider CH et al: The modified Pereyra procedure in recurrent stress incontinence: a 15-year review, *Obstet Gynecol* 83(4):573-578, 1994.

Johnson VY: Bladder neck suspension nursing care: preop, postop, and beyond, *Perspectives* 1(1):2-4, 1998.

Jordan GH et al: Penile prosthesis implantation in total phalloplasty, *J Urol* 152(2):410-414, 1994.

Keetch DW et al: Cryosurgical ablation of the prostate, *AORN J* 61(5):807-813, 1995.

Kim ED, Lipshultz LI: Advances in the treatment of organic erectile dysfunction, *Hosp Pract* 32(4):101-104, 107-108, 1997.

Koeneman KS et al: Sexual health for the man at midlife: in-office workup, *Geriatrics* 52(9):76-78, 84-86, 1997.

Mathias JM: New technology: cryoablation for prostate cancer, *OR Manager* 11(2):8-9, 1995.

Nagle GM: *Genitourinary surgery,* St Louis, 1997, Mosby.

Newton M et al: Prostate cancer: staging through laparoscopic lymphadenectomy, *AORN J* 59(4):823-836, 1994.

Ronk LL, Kavitz JM: Perioperative nursing implications of radical perineal prostatectomy, *AORN J* 60(3):438-446, 1994.

Rubin SO: Sex-reassignment surgery male to female, *Scand J Urol Nephrol* 154(3):1-28, 1993.

Salomon CG et al: Prostate carcinoma: transrectal US after cryosurgical ablation, *Radiology* 206(2):533-538, 1998.

Schivai RC et al: Erectile function and penile blood pressure in diabetes mellitus, *J Sex Marital Therapy* 20(2):119-124, 1994.

Schlatterer K et al: Multistep treatment concept of transsexual patients, *Exp Clin Endocrinol Diabetes* 104(6):413-419, 1996.

Serour F et al: Efficacy of EMLA cream prior to dorsal penile nerve block for circumcision in children, *Acta Anesthesiol Scand* 42(2):260-263, 1998.

Shandera KC, Thompson IM: Urologic prostheses, *Emerg Med Clin North Am* 12(3):729-748, 1994.

Stein P: Perioperative considerations of vascular access for dialysis, *AORN J* 60(6):947-958, 1994.

Strangio L: Interventional uroradiologic procedures, *AORN J* 66(2):286-294, 1997.

Swanson JM: Men's health: issues in prevention, *Surg Services Manag* 3(12):14-19, 1997.

Wallace MA: Anatomy and physiology of the kidney, *AORN J* 68(5):800-820, 1998.

Wespes E et al: Objective criteria in the long-term evaluation of penile venous surgery, *J Urol* 152(3):888-890, 1994.

Williamson ML: Circumcision anesthesia: a study of nursing implications for dorsal penile block, *Pediatr Nurs* 23(1):59-63, 1997.

Witt MA et al: The post-vasectomy length of the testicular vasal remnant: a predictor of the surgical outcome in microscopic vasectomy reversal, *J Urol* 151(4):892-894, 1994.

Chapter 37

Orthopaedic Surgery

 Chapter Objectives

After studying this chapter, the learner will be able to:

- Identify the pertinent anatomy and physiology of the musculoskeletal system.
- Discuss several types of fractures and the stabilization of each.
- Discuss bone healing.
- Describe the care of a patient undergoing orthopaedic surgery.

The word *orthopaedics* is derived from two Greek words: *orthos* (ορδοs), meaning *straight*, and *paithee* (παιδι), meaning *child*. As the name implies, orthopaedics began with the treatment of crippled children by means of rest, braces, and exercise. Degenerative diseases and disabilities affecting the musculoskeletal system cause loss of function and impair activity of the aged. Consequently, orthopaedic surgeons treat a large number of geriatric and pediatric patients in comparison with other surgical populations.

Orthopaedic patient care is individualized. As a branch of medicine and a contemporary surgical specialty, orthopaedics is "concerned with the diagnosis, care, and treatment of musculoskeletal disorders—that is, injury to or disease of the body's system of bones, joints, ligaments, muscles, and tendons."* Conservative, noninvasive medical and physical methods are used, if possible, to restore form and function.

Orthopaedics depends on many disciplines to help evaluate and treat patients. Diagnostic imaging, bioengineering, electrobiology, genetics, microbiology, oncology, and transplantation are but a few of these. Professional registered nurses who specialize in orthopaedic patient care are eligi-

ble for certification by examination through the Orthopaedic Nurses Certification Board. Eligibility includes current unrestricted licensure in the United States or Canada and a minimum of 2 years' experience as a registered nurse with a minimum of 1000 hours of nursing practice in orthopaedic patient care in the preceding 3 years. The certification period is 5 years and can be renewed through 100 contact hours of continuing education or by successful passage of the certification examination. More information about certification and the National Association of Orthopaedic Nurses (NAON) is available at **naon.inurse.com.**

HISTORICAL BACKGROUND

Records tell of the treatment of fractures in Egypt 4500 years ago. Mummies have been found with splints still in place made from the bark of trees; others were strips of linen impregnated with a gluelike substance. Egyptian mummies and murals show evidence of crippling diseases. One Egyptian tomb drawing, from 2830 BC, shows a man using a crutch.

Hippocrates (460-370 BC) described scoliosis, congenital dislocation of the hip, and clubfoot. Many of the treatment methods he advocated date back before his time, demonstrating an ongoing, organized manner of medical study. Almost

---

*American Academy of Orthopaedic Surgeons.

all of the principles of treating fractures currently followed are included in his book on fractures. Hippocrates discussed the use of traction, countertraction, bandages, splints, and treatment of compound fractures. He used mixtures of gelatinous substances and clay to coat bandages. He recognized the necessity of immobilizing a joint above and below a fracture. He described the proper position of fixing joints for the best possible future function. He wrote that exercise strengthens a part, but inactivity wastes it. He advocated mobilization of fractures as much as possible to prevent atrophy. For centuries, much of the wisdom in the books of Hippocrates was ignored or forgotten, then rediscovered.

Galen (129-199 BC) is often referred to as the father of sports medicine. He was surgeon to the gladiators. Galen described nervous system control of muscles and their function as a motor system. He named and treated the spinal deformities known as lordosis, scoliosis, and kyphosis. His description of osteomyelitis, sequestration, and regeneration of bone was very accurate for his time.

Of the orthopaedic surgeons in the late nineteenth century, no one contributed more to the development of the specialty than Charles Fayette Taylor (1827-1899). His investigations in kinesiatrics (movement therapy) and surgical mechanics contributed to the undertaking of exercise and rest in the treatment of musculoskeletal disorders.

The discovery of x-ray technology by German physicist Wilhelm Konrad Röntgen (1845-1923) in 1895 promoted orthopaedics as a specialty. American surgeon Austin Moore (1889-1963) performed the first metallic hip replacement in 1942. In 1959 John Charnley (1911-1982) suggested in England that methyl methacrylate, used in dentistry, might be used to hold prosthetic components in place. Charnley introduced the low-friction torque prosthesis for total hip replacement in 1962. Modified versions of the Austin Moore and Charnley hip are still in use today. The principles of biomechanics have revolutionized orthopaedic surgery.

ANATOMY AND PHYSIOLOGY OF THE MUSCULOSKELETAL SYSTEM

Structures that make up the musculoskeletal system provide bony shape, support, and stability; protect vital organs; and enable parts and the body as a whole to move. The musculoskeletal system includes bones, cartilage, joints, ligaments, muscles, and tendons. Orthopaedic surgery is concerned primarily with these structures in the upper and lower extremities, including the shoulder and hip joints, and the vertebral column.

Bones

The human skeleton (Figure 37-1) has 206 separate bones. The bony framework of the human body is divided into the axial skeleton, which consists of 80 bones that make up the skull, vertebrae, and rib cage, and the appendicular skeleton, which consists of 126 bones that make up the limbs. Each upper extremity is composed of 32 bones, and each lower extremity is composed of 31 bones. Bones are classified according to shape as long, short, flat, and irregular. The humerus in the upper arm, radius and ulna in the forearm, femur in the thigh, and tibia and fibula in the lower leg are long bones. The end of a long bone is referred to as the epiphysis, and the shaft is referred to as the diaphysis. Thin plates of cartilage are found in the ends of long bones. In immature bone this is the area of growth and elongation. In mature bone these plates are ossified and do not grow (Figure 37-2). The bones in the hand and foot are short bones. The scapula and patella are examples of flat bones. The vertebrae are irregular bones.

The cortex (outer layer) of bone is compact, hard connective tissue. This cortical osseous tissue surrounds porous, spongy, cancellous tissue. The innermost substance is bone marrow and is classified as either red or yellow according to its location and function (see Figure 37-2). The red marrow is found in the ends of long bones, in porosities of cancellous bone, and in flatter bones, such as the skull, sternum, and pelvic bones. This type of marrow is responsible for erythropoiesis, which is the formation of red blood cells and certain white blood cells. Yellow marrow is found in the medullary canals, or shafts of long bones, and has a higher adipose content.

Periosteum, a strong fibrous membrane, covers bone, except at joints. The blood supply and innervation penetrates through periosteum and enters the bone through structures known as Volkmann's canals. Lengthwise lamellar structures, referred to as Haversian canals, provide weight-bearing strength and passage for additional blood supply (Figure 37-3). The inner aspect of bone is lined with endosteum, which is tissue similar to periosteum. In small children this layer contains osteoclasts that destroy bone to enlarge the marrow cavity for circumferential growth.

Bone Healing

Broken bones heal by a process referred to as union. Union of bones takes place in a series of steps:

1. *Hematoma formation.* Blood accumulates in the area of break or injury. The inflammatory process ensues, and extravascular blood converts from liquid to a semisolid clot. Active phagocytosis removes necrotic tissue and debris.
2. *Callus formation.* Fibrin cells form a network around the injured area. The damaged periosteum is stimulated to generate osteoblasts, forming new bony substance referred to as osteoid. Minerals begin to accumulate in the network, forming a collagen callus. A callus is visible on x-ray examination within 1 to 2 weeks of injury.
3. *Calcification process.* Calcification begins and establishes support of the injury. Connective tissue proliferates across the site and is usually completely calcified within 6 weeks.

Bones   **Muscles and Tendons**   **Bones**

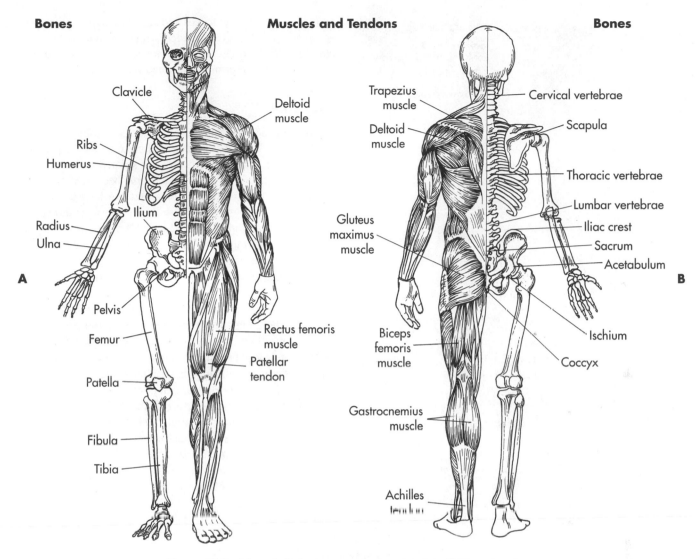

Figure 37-1   Musculoskeletal system. **A,** Anterior view. **B,** Posterior view.

4. *Remodeling phase.* Excess cellular material is resorbed, and the bone resumes its preinjury strength and configuration. This remodeling phase is enhanced by stress and exercise. Depending on the site and severity of the injury, complete remodeling can take 6 months to 1 year to complete.

Cartilage

Cartilage, a smooth, relatively firm, compressible connective tissue, cushions most articular surfaces at the ends of bones. It does not have a direct blood supply and is devoid of lymphatics and nerves. Cartilage derives its nutrition from synovial fluid and maintains a high water content except in pathologic states.

Joints

Bones give stability, but the body must bend and flex for locomotion. The ends of bones come together at joints. The ar-

ticular cartilage and construction of the joint prevent bones from scraping against each other. Tough, fibrous connective tissue forms the outside capsule of the joint, and a finer membranous lining secretes synovium, which is similar to egg albumin. The synovial fluid contains macrophages and white blood cells that keep the joint free of debris and bacteria that could interfere with mobility.

Joints are classified by variations in structure that permit movement (Figure 37-4). The hip and shoulder are ball-and-socket joints; the knee, ankle, elbow, and phalangeal joints of the fingers are hinged; the wrist is a condyloid joint; and the thumb is a saddle joint. The proximal and distal bone ends are held securely in place by the joint capsule attached to both bone shafts and by ligaments.

Ligaments

Ligaments are bands of flexible, tough fibrous tissue that join the articular surfaces of bones and cartilage. They become strong when the parallel configuration of their collagen fiber

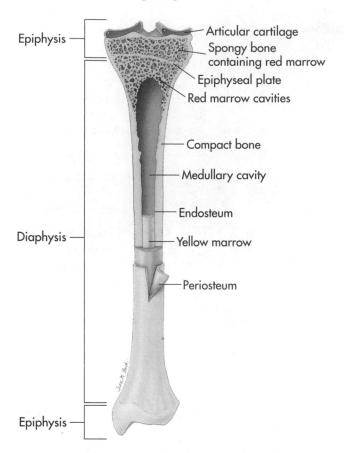

Epiphysis
— Articular cartilage
— Spongy bone containing red marrow
— Epiphyseal plate
— Red marrow cavities
— Compact bone
— Medullary cavity
Diaphysis
— Endosteum
— Yellow marrow
— Periosteum
Epiphysis

Figure 37-2 Long bone structure seen in longitudinal section. (From Thibodeau GA, Patton KT: *Anatomy and physiology,* ed 4, St Louis, 1999, Mosby.)

is oriented against the forces applied to them (e.g., the cruciate ligaments stabilize the knee joint). Ligaments are avascular and heal slowly. They do not readily reattach to bone when torn and are prone to subsequent reinjury.

Muscles

The human body has hundreds of muscles. Muscles are all the contractile tissues of the body and are classified as smooth (involuntary), branching (cardiac), or striated skeletal (voluntary). Muscles have a rich arterial supply because they require oxygen to perform many functions, and they have a multilevel venous drainage system because they perform as the venous pumps for resaturation by the lungs. They contract when an electrochemical impulse from the brain crosses the myoneural junction, causing fibers to shorten. Groups of muscles work together (i.e., contract simultaneously to bring about body movement).

Skeletal muscle is the largest category of muscle tissue. There are more than 600 skeletal muscles in the human body. Skeletal muscle constitutes approximately 23% of small female body weight and 40% of larger male body weight. Each muscle fiber is a single cell that ranges in length from 0.04 to 3 inches (1 to 80 mm). The fibers are bound together into fascia-covered bundles referred to as fasciculi. Several fascia-bound fasciculi constitute a skeletal muscle and contract in response to signals mediated by the nervous system and neurotransmitters, such as acetylcholine.

The peripheral attachment is referred to as the origin. The distal attachment is referred to as the insertion.

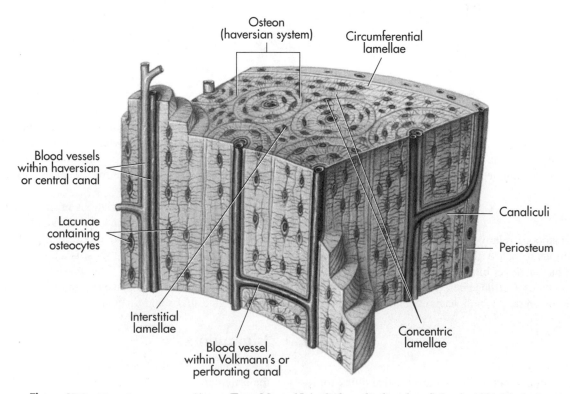

Osteon (haversian system)
Circumferential lamellae
Blood vessels within haversian or central canal
Canaliculi
Periosteum
Lacunae containing osteocytes
Interstitial lamellae
Concentric lamellae
Blood vessel within Volkmann's or perforating canal

Figure 37-3 Vascular structure of bone. (From Mourad LA: *Orthopedic disorders,* St Louis, 1991, Mosby.)

Tendons

Tendons are bands of extremely strong, flexible fibrous tissue that attach muscle bundles to the periosteum of bones (see Figure 37-1). They are encased in the synovial membrane sheath of movable joints.

SPECIAL FEATURES OF ORTHOPAEDIC SURGERY

The orthopaedic surgeon, also referred to as an orthopaedist or orthopod, attempts to restore function of the musculoskeletal system lost as a result of injury or disease. Surgical procedures may be performed to repair traumatic injuries, such as fractures, dislocations, torn ligaments, or severed tendons. Other procedures reconstruct joints, eradicate a benign or malignant disease process, or correct postural disabilities.

In addition to conventional x-ray films, computed tomography (CT), magnetic resonance imaging (MRI), and bone densitometers allow evaluation of conditions amenable to surgical correction. Arthroscopy enhances diagnosis and treatment of joint disorders, especially those caused by sports injuries. Highly sophisticated implants and instrumentation make many orthopaedic procedures possible. A large percentage of orthopaedic surgical procedures involve contaminated traumatic wounds or tissues highly susceptible to infection.

Osteomyelitis (infection in bone) typically occurs after bone is injured in an accident or is involved in a surgical repair. Microorganisms may harbor in a hematoma or in soft tissues and spread directly to bone. Acute osteomyelitis may

cause nonunion of fractures. Chronic infection may remain for life; it may cause loss of an extremity. Posttraumatic, postoperative, and nosocomial wound infections are leading causes of amputation. Chronic osteomyelitis is often associated with peripheral vascular disease. Meticulous attention to sterile technique is critical in all orthopaedic procedures to prevent or at least minimize the devastating effects of infection. Sterility of implants and fixation devices is absolutely essential.

Precautions also must ensure protection for the orthopaedic surgeon and team, especially when caring for a trauma victim. Manipulation of sharp bony fragments and instrumentation can be hazardous. Transmission of blood-borne pathogens is readily possible because of aerosolization of bone and debris during drilling and sawing, powered irrigation units, and the use of heavy instrumentation. In addition to standard precautions recommended by the Centers for Disease Control and Prevention (CDC), the American Academy of Orthopaedic Surgeons recommends the following:

1. Wearing of protective attire
   a. Wear knee-high, waterproof shoe covers or boots. Blood and body fluids frequently splash to the floor and lower legs. Shoe covers should be removed and changed if they become contaminated.
   b. Wear a fluid-impervious gown and/or a waterproof apron under the gown. Copious irrigation frequently is used.
   c. Double glove at all times and/or have additional protection for fingers. Cloth gloves or glove liners

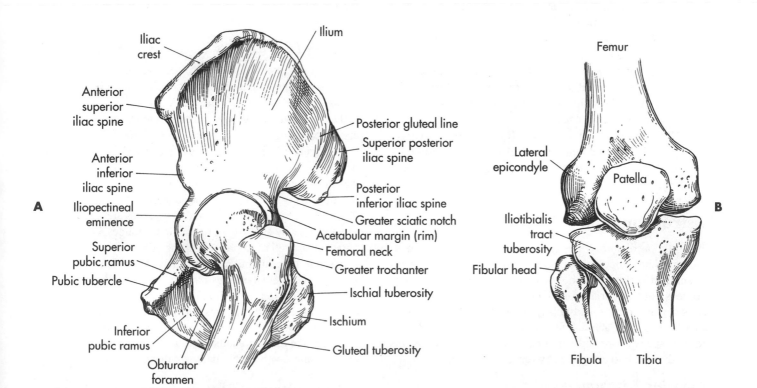

Figure 37-4   Joints. **A,** Ball-and-socket hip joint. **B,** Hinged knee joint.

Figure 37-5 Exposing instruments. **A,** Periosteal elevators. **B,** Bennett retractor.

of woven Kevlar may be worn between latex gloves in cases of trauma and major reconstructive procedures when sharp instruments and mechanical devices are used.

    d. Wear protective eyewear at all times. A full face shield should be considered when splatter is anticipated. Powered bone instruments can produce a fine mist. A space suit–type helmet should be considered when powered bone instruments are used.

2. Avoidance of inadvertent penetration of the skin of personnel during the surgical procedure

    a. Use instrument ties and other nontouch suturing and sharp instrument techniques whenever possible.

    b. Pass sharp instruments on a tray or magnetic mat, not hand to hand.

    c. Announce when instruments are being passed.

    d. Cover exposed internal wires and pins that extend through the skin with appropriate tubing, cork stoppers, or plastic caps.

3. Clean gowning and gloving (i.e., the scrub person should change contaminated gloves before gowning and gloving another team member during the surgical procedure)

Instrumentation

Each orthopaedic procedure must have the correct instrumentation for that particular bone, joint, tendon, or other structures the surgeon will encounter. An instrument used on a hip procedure is not appropriate for a hand. Orthopaedic instruments are heavy, often large and bulky, resembling carpentry tools, but also delicate. Each instrument has a specific purpose and requires special care and handling. Orthopaedic instruments can be divided into categories by functional design.

Exposing Instruments

To expose a bone or joint, special retractors and elevators are used (Figure 37-5). Retractors are contoured to fit around the

bone or joint without cutting or tearing muscles. Periosteal elevators are semisharp instruments used to strip periosteum from bone without destroying its ability to regenerate new bone.

Grasping Instruments

Grasping instruments are required to hold, manipulate, or retract bone. Bone-holding forceps should be selected appropriately for the size of the bone in the surgical field. Bone hooks are used for retraction and leverage (Figure 37-6). Heavy clamps are needed to hold smaller bones or to grasp a joint capsule, such as a meniscus clamp for fibrocartilage in the knee.

Cutting Instruments

Cutting instruments are used to remove soft tissue around bone; to cut into, cut apart, or cut out portions of bone; and to smooth jagged edges of bone. The surgeon's armamentarium includes osteotomes, gouges, chisels, curettes, rongeurs, reamers, bone-cutting forceps, meniscotomes, rasps, files, drills, and saws (Figure 37-7). These have sharp edges. Extra care should be taken not to nick or damage cutting edges; they should always be protected on the instrument table and during cleaning, sterilizing, and storing. Fitted sterilizable racks (Figure 37-7, *E*), trays, foam towels, or canvas cases are used to keep sets together by sizes (e.g., osteotomes, gouges, chisels, and curettes), as well as to protect cutting edges.

    Cutting instruments must be sharp. Osteotomes, chisels, gouges, and meniscotomes can be sharpened by operating room (OR) personnel with handheld hones or a honing machine designed for this purpose. Most manufacturers provide a service for sharpening and repairing instruments. Curettes, rongeurs, and reamers should be returned for sharpening. Small drill bits and saw blades usually are disposable (Figure 37-8).

Power-Driven Cutting Instruments   Instruments powered by electricity or compressed air or nitrogen offer precision in drilling, cutting, shaping, and beveling

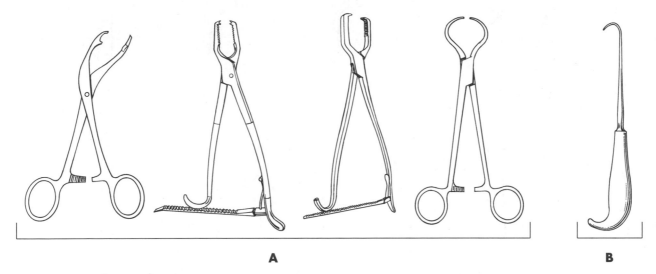

Figure 37-6 Grasping instruments. **A,** Bone-holding forceps. **B,** Bone hook.

bone. The instrument may have rotary, reciprocating, or oscillating action. Rotary movement is used to drill holes or to insert screws, wires, or pins. Reciprocating movement, a cutting action from front to back, and oscillating cutting action from side to side are used to cut or remove bone. Some instruments have a combination of movements and can be changed from one to another with hand controls. In some the change may be made by adjusting the chuck forward or backward and locking it into the desired position. Powered instruments increase speed and decrease the fatigue of manually driven drills, saws, and reamers. They also reduce blood loss from bone by packing tiny particles into cut surfaces.

Measuring Devices

Rulers, calipers, depth gauges, and flexible devices for measuring angles are important for the appropriate sizing of implants and selective bone cutting. Measurements of bone diameter are performed when selecting a joint prosthesis (Figure 37-9).

Implant-Related Instruments

Drivers, clamps, and retractors are used for inserting, securing, or removing fixation and prosthetic implants. Each type of implant requires its own instrumentation. Instruments used for insertion or extraction of metallic implants must be of the same metal as the implant to prevent galvanic reaction.

Items Used Frequently

The items to be discussed are handled frequently, although they are not used in every orthopaedic procedure.

Bone Grafts

When necessary to provide structural support, a piece of bone from one part of the skeletal system may be obtained from the patient to reinforce another part of the skeletal system. Autogenous cancellous and cortical bone is obtained from the crest of the ilium, and cortical bone is obtained from the

fibula. Free vascularized fibular grafts may be preferred to replace avascular (dead) bone or large segments of long bones following trauma or tumor resection. Autogenous bone may not have adequate shape or strength or may not be available in sufficient quantity, or the surgeon may deem it undesirable to subject the patient to a secondary incision or added operating time. Allograft bone, coraline hydroxyapatite, or a bone graft substitute of tricalcium may be used. Donors, both living and cadaver, should be tested for human immunodeficiency virus (HIV) antibody before a graft is transplanted. Living donors should be retested 90 days after procurement if possible. Persons who are HIV positive, have any immune disorder or active infection, and have a history of hepatitis are excluded as donors. The probability of transmission of HIV in frozen or freeze-dried bone is remote. Secondary sterilization by ethylene oxide or ionizing radiation may increase the margin of safety but will reduce the biologic effectiveness of the graft.

Soft Tissue Allografts

Cartilage, ligaments, and tendons obtained from cadavers may be frozen or freeze-dried for use to augment soft tissue repairs.

Fixation Devices

External and internal fixation devices are used to stabilize or immobilize bone, usually following skeletal injury. External devices provide temporary support during healing. Many types of screws, plates, and nails are used for temporary or permanent internal fixation of fractures or bone segments following a reconstructive procedure. Devices are also used to stabilize the vertebral column.

Prosthetic Implants

Prosthetic implants are used to permanently replace bone, joints, or tendons. They are made of nonmagnetic and electrolytically inert metals such as stainless steel, cobalt, and titanium alloys or of polymers such as silicone and polyethylene.

Figure 37-7 Cutting instruments. **A,** Osteotome, curved or straight tapered blade. **B,** Gouge, curved, straight, or angled tip. **C,** Chisel, straight blade. **D,** Curette with assortment of sizes of cutting loops. **E,** Sterilizing case for set of osteotomes, gouges, chisels, or curettes. **F,** Rongeur. **G,** Bone cutter, straight or angled blade.

Oscillating saw blades

Drill bits

Reciprocating saw blades

Sagittal saw blades

Figure 37-8 Saw blades and drill bits. (From Gregory B: *Orthopaedic surgery,* St Louis, 1994, Mosby.)

Berndt hip ruler

Townley femur calipor

Screw depth gauge

Protractor

Bone screw ruler gauge

Figure 37-9 Measuring devices used in orthopaedics. (From Gregory B: *Orthopaedic surgery,* St Louis, 1994, Mosby.)

Some modular implants are made of several materials. Others have a polymeric or porous coating for tissue ingrowth over a portion of the implant. Methyl methacrylate (bone cement) may be used to reinforce fixation or to increase the strength of the implant. An orthopaedic implant must withstand stresses within the internal environment. Fatigue strength, corrosion resistance, biocompatibility, and biomechanics are critical factors in selecting an implant.

Because of the high cost of prosthetic and fixation implants, the inventory is kept as low as possible, yet large enough to ensure availability when needed. These expensive implants are usually patient-charge items; they cannot be reused even if they are temporary. After measurements are taken, an implant of the correct size, shape, and design is selected from the sets available. Only the one to be used is handled, without the others being touched.

An infection around a fixation or prosthetic implant may require its removal, often resulting in permanent deformity or disability. Sterility at the time of implantation is imperative. Most implants are supplied sterile by the manufacturer. Others must be packaged and sterilized. Manufacturers may provide instructions for the recommended method of sterilization. Aeration time may be recommended following ethylene oxide sterilization. Reprocessing is appropriate only if an implant has not been implanted or contaminated by blood or body fluids and if guidelines are provided by the manufacturer. Implants should not be flash sterilized. Only standard cycles with appropriate biologic monitoring should be used. Some implants cannot withstand the heat of steam sterilization; ethylene oxide or some other appropriate method is used. The manufacturer's recommendations should be followed. Each sterilization cycle containing an implant(s) should be biologically tested and the implant(s) not used until a negative test result is known.

Implants made of or coated with polymers should be wrapped in an appropriate plastic or combination paper-and-plastic wrapper to prevent contamination with lint or other debris. A metal implant should not be removed from a package with an instrument. The surface could be scratched. An implant with a scratched or dented surface cannot be used because an electrolytic reaction will occur in the body. Powder-free gloves should be worn by team members who handle prosthetic implants.

Specifics about the device or prosthesis implanted must be recorded in the patient's intraoperative record. This includes the type, size, and other identifying information, such as the manufacturer's lot number. Lot numbers are recorded in the departmental lot number log as appropriate in case of recall.

Lasers

Although not used as commonly as in other surgical specialties, lasers are used in some orthopaedic procedures. They are useful in confined areas (e.g., through an arthroscope) to minimize bleeding.

Carbon Dioxide Laser Methyl methacrylate can be vaporized with a CO_2 laser to remove a cemented joint implant during a revision arthroplasty. Care is taken to use a smoke evacuator during the procedure. The CO_2 laser cannot be used in a fluid environment. A joint must be insufflated with gas; the distention medium is carbon dioxide. The vaporization of cellular water destroys soft tissue. The CO_2 laser is useful in arthroscopic surgery for sculpturing articular cartilage and for synovectomy. The joint is irrigated to remove charred tissue.

Holmium:YAG Laser Used primarily in the knee, ankle, shoulder, and elbow, the Ho:YAG laser is approved for all joints except the spine. The 2.1-μm wavelength with low penetration depth combined with pulsed high energy is delivered through a fine fiberoptic fiber. The Ho:YAG laser acts on water in cells without charring or damaging tissue extensively. It can ablate dense cartilage, bone, and soft tissue. It is used through an arthroscope to cut, shape, smooth, and sculpt cartilage and tissues in joints.

Neodymium:YAG Laser The Nd:YAG laser is used primarily in arthroscopy of the knee and shoulder joints on articular cartilage. It vaporizes protein and bonds collagen. It can be used for percutaneous disc procedures. Delivered fiberoptically, the Nd:YAG laser may have a reusable sapphire tip or a disposable, single-use ceramic contact tip. The Nd:YAG beam may be passed through a potassium titanyl phosphate (KTP) crystal, which has good cutting properties, to vaporize protein.

Bone Wax

Used for hemostasis in bone, bone wax is placed on the instrument table and opened as requested. The surgeon's preference card should be checked before the packet is opened.

Nerve Stimulator

A nerve stimulator is used occasionally to verify neural tissue during a partial nerve resection to control spastic muscles. When the popliteal nerve, for example, is given a slight shock with the nerve stimulator, the foot jerks. Both direct electric current and disposable battery-operated stimulators are available.

Sutures

Ligaments, tendons, periosteum, and joint capsules are fibrous tissues. They are primarily tough, stringy collagen and contain few cells or blood vessels. As a result, they heal more slowly than do vascular tissues. Nonabsorbable materials are generally used to suture ligaments, tendons, and muscles involved in movement of the bony skeleton. Absorbable suture is generally preferred to suture periosteum. The surgeon's preference card should be checked before the packet is opened.

Casts and Braces

A cast or brace is a means of obtaining external fixation of a fracture or a part following tendon repair, arthrodesis, or other surgical procedures. It is the means of putting a part at rest or attempting to correct an injury or abnormality. Cast application in the OR is discussed in detail later in this chapter.

Cast Room Casts are applied in the cast room, sometimes referred to as the plaster room. Many closed, noninvasive procedures are performed in the cast room, particularly those requiring general or regional anesthesia, when it is located within the OR suite. This frees the OR for open, invasive surgical procedures. It also keeps plaster dust from the perioperative environment, an important aspect of aseptic environmental control. Following an open surgical procedure the patient can be wheeled on the operating bed into the cast room for application of a cast, if the patient is hemodynamically stable.

Ultraclean Air System

Special care must be used to carry out strict asepsis. Infection is the most serious, dreaded, and costly complication of orthopaedic surgery. Therefore many surgeons prefer to operate within an ultraclean air system, especially for total joint replacement procedures. Orthopaedic surgeons use laminar airflow more frequently than other surgical specialists.

A surgical isolation bubble system or patient isolation drape may be used to isolate the sterile field from personnel and equipment. Surgical helmets are available that isolate airborne contaminants from each team member. Hoses exhaust exhaled air. This system can be used independently or in conjunction with a laminar airflow system.

Isolation suits are fully contained gowns with acrylic plastic face shields and a battery-powered air filtration system. Because the suits retain heat, the OR may be kept at 70° F (21° C) for the comfort of team members. The patient should be maintained in a normothermic state with forced-air warming or protected by some other warming method.

Orthopaedic Table

An orthopaedic table, often referred to as the fracture table, is used for many surgical procedures requiring traction, image intensification or conventional x-ray control, and/or cast application. The patient is anesthetized before he or she is positioned. The many available attachments make possible any desired position and traction on any part of the body. The table can be raised, tilted laterally, or put into a Trendelenburg or reverse Trendelenburg position. Attachments are designed not only for stabilizing the patient in the desired position, but also for exerting traction to help reduce a fracture, and for providing a means of evaluating the diagnosis or therapy by radiologic control. Bakelite or some other material that does not interfere with radiographic studies is used for attachments that might otherwise obscure the findings.

Essential standard component attachments on all models of orthopaedic tables include three-section patient body supports, a lateral body brace, a sacral rest, and traction apparatus. Optional accessories are available to accommodate the types of procedures performed and the model of the table. When the orthopaedic table is used, the following procedure is followed:

1. Consult the surgeon's preference card, procedure book, and manufacturer's manual for attachments needed for each desired position.
2. Check the patient's height and weight.
3. Assemble the necessary attachments. Pad all parts of the table and attachments to prevent pressure on joints, the sacrum, and the perineum.
4. Attach the standard components and accessories to the table frame so that all is in readiness for positioning the patient when the surgeon arrives.

X-Ray Control

Conventional x-ray equipment and fluoroscopy frequently are used during orthopaedic procedures. Considerations for patient safety and personnel protection described in Chapter 13 apply to the use of radiologic control for invasive or noninvasive orthopaedic procedures performed in the OR suite. Special positioning and draping techniques may be necessary, especially when C-arm fluoroscopy is used.

Often both anteroposterior (AP) and lateral views are necessary to assess the alignment of a bone or to determine the position of a fixation device or prosthetic implant. X-ray films or recorded fluoroscopic images document the work of the surgeon.

Special Considerations in Orthopaedic Surgery

1. Unit beds are used to transport patients in traction apparatus. Beds, frames, and stretchers can be decontaminated in the vestibular/exchange area.
2. A cast should be removed preoperatively in the cast room. If the OR suite does not have a cast room, a cast may be bivalved in the patient's room and then removed in the OR.
3. Positioning of the patient intraoperatively and postoperatively should be directed by the surgeon. Immobilization and good body alignment contribute to patient comfort and prevention of neurovascular injury. Pillows or other supports should not cause pain, impair function of unaffected muscles and joints, or compromise circulation.
4. Transcutaneous electrical nerve stimulation (TENS) may be used for postoperative analgesia. The electrode pads are affixed to the skin along the sides of the incision when a dressing is applied. Before application, the skin should be cleansed with water. (Saline is a conductor, so it cannot be used for cleansing.) The wires are connected to the stimulator in the postanesthesia care unit (PACU) or after recovery from anesthesia. The patient can be taught preoperatively how to use TENS for relief of pain postoperatively.
5. Electrostimulation promotes cellular responses in bone and ligaments. Mechanically stressed bone generates electrical potentials related to patterns of bone regeneration. If stimulated, healing may accelerate. Both internal direct-current stimulators and external pulsating electromagnetic field or electrical capacitor devices are used to stimulate bone and neural regeneration, revascularization, epiphyseal growth, and ligamental maturation.

EXTREMITY PROCEDURES

Although instrumentation varies by procedure and the size of structures involved, basic techniques apply to handling both upper and lower extremities.

General Considerations

1. A sterile irrigating pan is placed under an extremity to catch solution if an open wound is to be cleansed, irrigated, and debrided, as for a compound fracture.

2. A pneumatic tourniquet is usually used for a surgical procedure on or below the elbow or knee to provide a blood-free field. The tourniquet cuff is applied before the extremity is prepped. It is not inflated until draping is completed. Always check the pressure setting with the surgeon before inflating a tourniquet. Ischemia time is a critical factor in patient safety. Notify the surgeon of the time lapse after the first hour and every 15 minutes thereafter throughout tourniquet inflation. Document the tourniquet location, time, pressure, and unit number.

    An Esmarch's bandage may be applied to the elevated extremity before the pneumatic tourniquet is inflated to exsanguinate the limb.

3. An extremity is always held up for skin preparation. See that the area under it is dry before draping. Prevent prep solution from running under the tourniquet cuff.

4. A self-adhering incise drape may be used as the first drape applied. It may be impossible to drape adequately with self-adhering plastic drapes or fenestrated sheets. If the extremity must be manipulated during the surgical procedure, the entire circumference must be draped. A limb or split sheet may be used. A sterile glove can be placed over the foot to protect the sterile field during lower limb surgery.

5. Stockinette may be used over a self-adhering plastic drape or to cover skin. This is cut with dressing scissors over the line of the incision. The cut edges may be secured over skin edges with skin clips if a plastic drape is not used. A medicine cup is a handy receptacle for these clips after removal. The scrub person holds this at the field to receive clips as the surgeon removes them. They should be accounted for to prevent patient injury.

    A self-adhering incise drape eliminates the need for either stockinette and metallic skin clips or towels and towel clips that might interfere with the interpretation of x-ray films or image intensification.

6. A fluid-control drape collects blood and irrigating fluids in a pouch to prevent strike-through of and runoff from drapes. Fluids can be drained or suctioned for disposal. Blood may be suctioned for autotransfusion if blood loss is more than 400 ml, as in some hip procedures.

7. After a surgical procedure on a knee joint, a pressure dressing is usually applied to prevent serum accumulation. This may be a Robert Jones dressing, which includes a soft cotton batting roll, sheet wadding, and cotton elastic bandage. A cotton roll or other bulky material may be placed on each side of the knee and held in place with sheet wadding. A four-ply, crinkled-gauze bandage or cotton elastic bandage over this provides even, gentle pressure. Depending on the surgical procedure, a plaster splint or some other type of knee immobilizer may be preferred.

8. After a surgical procedure on a shoulder, the arm may be bound against the side of the chest for immobilization. An absorbent pad or a large piece of cotton or sheet wadding is placed under the arm to keep skin surfaces from touching, because they may macerate. The arm is held in a shoulder immobilizer that supports the humerus and wrist, or it may be bound firmly to the side of the chest with a cotton elastic bandage.

9. An extremity is elevated on a pillow placed lengthwise. This facilitates venous return, decreases swelling, and minimizes pressure on nerves. The hand should be elevated above the level of the heart; the toes must be higher than the nose.

Indications for Orthopaedic Surgery

Preoperative assessment of an acute or a chronic disability affecting the musculoskeletal system of an extremity includes evaluation of the extent of bony or soft tissue involvement with or without concomitant neurovascular compromise. Assessment for signs and symptoms of neurovascular impairment in an extremity includes the 6 *P*'s: *P*allor, *P*ulses, *P*ain, *P*arasthesia, *P*uffiness, and *P*aralysis. The six *P*'s are assessed postoperatively and monitored until support devices, such as castor splints, are removed from the surgical site.

Because they are the essence of adult orthopaedic surgery and are caused either by trauma or by a degenerative disease process, procedures on the following major anatomic classifications of structures are discussed:

- Fracture of bones
- Reconstruction of joints
- Repair of tendons and ligaments

FRACTURES

Intact bones are essential to the stability and mobility of upper and lower extremities. A comminuted (splintered) or fractured (broken) bone can cause malfunction and pain. Fractures vary by cause, location, type of fracture line, and extent of injury. They are either traumatic or pathologic:

1. *Traumatic fracture.* The impact, forced twisting, or bending of an accidental injury can break one or more bones in the body. Traumatic fractures can occur when bone has become fatigued from overwork or has inadequate muscle support during exertion; a stress fracture may result (e.g., in the tibia or fibula of an athlete). Traumatic fractures are either closed or open.
    a. *Closed fracture.* Sometimes referred to as a simple fracture, broken fragments do not protrude through adjacent tissue to puncture the skin (Figure 37-10, *A*).
    b. *Open fracture.* Also referred to as a compound fracture, either the proximal or distal end of bone, or both, protrudes from the fracture site through adjacent tissues and skin (Figure 37-10, *B*). Because of the risk of infection developing in the exposed bone, an open fracture is a surgical emergency.
2. *Pathologic fracture.* Demineralization of bone (e.g., from osteoporosis or the aging process) and primary or metastatic malignant bone disease can spontaneously fracture a bone without undue stress. Although they are technically simple fractures, pathologic fractures may

Figure 37-10 Fractures of a long bone. **A,** Simple closed fractures: *1,* transverse break runs across bone; *2,* oblique break runs in slanting direction across bone; *3,* spiral break coils around bone. **B,** Compound open fracture protrudes through skin.

require more than simple fixation of bone fragments. Bone allografts or alloplastic grafts may be needed. Methyl methacrylate bone cement may be used to increase the strength of a fixation implant or as an adjunct to fill a bone defect (e.g., following removal of a tumor around a pathologic fracture). A compound made from collagen protein mixed with ceramic material may serve to stimulate creation of cartilage and osteoblasts (bone-forming cells).

Mechanical means are used to reduce a fracture and immobilize the parts, maintaining the fragments in proper alignment. Fractures must be handled gently with support above and below the site to prevent further trauma. A physician should assume responsibility for supporting the fracture site during transfer of the patient to or from a stretcher, bed, or table. Other personnel must be instructed regarding the special care needed to move a patient. The surgeon removes or directs removal of temporary splints, traction, or a pneumatic counterpressure device. Adequate personnel must be available so that the patient can be lifted gently. All lifters should be on the affected side because this helps support the fracture during transfer.

In treating a fracture, the surgeon seeks to accomplish a solid union of bone in perfect alignment, to return joints and muscles to normal position, to prevent or repair vascular trauma, and to rehabilitate the patient as early as possible. Treatment of fractures usually includes three distinct phases: reduction, immobilization, and rehabilitation. The methods of treating fractures include the following:

• Closed reduction with immobilization
• Skeletal traction
• External fixation
• Internal fixation
• Electrostimulation

Closed Reduction

A fracture may be manipulated (set) to replace the bone in its proper alignment without opening the skin. This technique is referred to as a closed reduction. Many fractures of the lower leg or arm can be treated by closed reduction. When both leg bones are fractured, fibula fractures are generally disregarded and attention is directed to the tibia.

Often performed in the emergency department, closed reduction with the patient under anesthesia and application of a device for immobilization may be done in the cast room of the OR suite. A plaster, fiberglass, or other lightweight synthetic cast, cast-brace, or molded plastic fracture-brace may be used to hold the reduced fracture site in alignment during union.

Skeletal Traction

Traction is the pulling force exerted to maintain proper alignment or position. In skeletal traction the force is applied directly on the bone following insertion of pins, wires, or tongs placed through or into the bone. A small sterile setup is required. Traction is applied by means of pulleys and weights. Weights provide a constant force; pulleys help establish and maintain constant direction until the fractured bone reunites.

Forearm or Lower Leg

A Kirschner wire, either plain or threaded, or a Steinmann pin is drilled through the bone (preferably cortical) distal to the fracture site. For forearm fractures the wire or pin must be strong enough to prevent side-to-side, angular, and rotary motion while the fracture is healing. A traction bow is attached to the protruding ends of the wire or pin. The pulleys are fastened to this bow. The ends of the wire or pin are covered with corks or plastic tips to protect the patient and personnel from the sharp ends.

Finger

A fine Kirschner wire may be drilled through the distal phalanx. The ends may be attached to a banjo splint. Or a cast may be applied to the forearm with a loop of heavy wire incorporated in it that fans out beyond the fingers. The Kirschner wire is fastened to this loop by a rubber band.

External Fixation

External fixation devices are used for the treatment of selected types of skeletal injuries, especially to the pelvis and extremities, with marked soft tissue loss and instability. Skeletal pins and connecting bars permit rigid fixation, but with access to devitalized skin and soft tissue for wound management, especially for open injuries of the tibia. Fixation devices used for unstable pelvic fractures allow early ambulation.

Femur and Tibia

External fixation applies tension and compression forces to bone. Tension stimulates bone growth. Compression helps control infection and promotes union in fractures without bone loss. External fixators can also be used for correcting bone deformities and for lengthening the femur and tibia following osteotomy for limb length discrepancy. Several types of devices, used on the lower extremities, allow the patient to ambulate.

Stabilization Bar Two or more pins or screws, parallel to each other, are inserted into the cortex of each fragmented section of bone. These may be connected to a metal bar, such as the dynamic axial fixator, that runs parallel to the bone on one side of the leg, or the pins may protrude through the leg and be clamped onto bars on both sides, such as with the Hoffman external fixation system.

Ilizarov Technique Particularly useful for salvaging infected and nonunion fractures, the Ilizarov external fixator frame consists of a series of stainless steel rings connected by rods, nuts, and bolts. It can be assembled in various configurations and lengths. Wires are inserted percutaneously through the bone and connected under tension on both sides of the rings. Usually two wires are attached to each ring, at the proximal and distal levels, to stabilize bone fragments. The placement of wires is checked under C-arm fluoroscopy. Threaded rods are placed parallel to each other and in line with the longitudinal axis of the bone to connect and stabilize rings. The system has more than 120 interchangeable components, including wrenches, pliers, and wire cutters. Wire insertion is a sterile procedure. The frame is assembled on the sterile field. It weighs about 8 pounds (3.6 kg) when assembled.

Internal Fixation

Internal fixation is necessary for fractures that are not amenable to closed reduction and stabilization with cast or brace immobilization, skeletal traction, or external fixation

methods. The fracture must be reduced to align fragments. Open reduction exposes the fracture site for realignment under direct visualization; closed reduction sometimes precedes the insertion of an internal fixation device. If vascular structures have been traumatized, internal fixation followed by vascular repair may be necessary to restore arterial tissue perfusion and adequate venous drainage. The procedure may be performed with the patient under regional block anesthesia, especially in patients in poor physical condition, such as a geriatric patient or a patient who has suffered multiple trauma. Intravenous (IV) sedation may be given to dull the patient's awareness of the sound of drills and mallets.

Excellent results can be obtained with internal fixation of a fracture soon after it occurs. This method provides firm immobilization and close approximation of the fragments so that the gap between the ends is not too great for the callus to bridge. It reduces to a minimum, space between fragments and movement at the fracture site. Healing seems to take place faster. The patient starts non–weight-bearing exercises and progresses to ambulation early, which reduces joint stiffness and muscle atrophy and prevents a long period of rehabilitation.

Screws, Plates, and Nails

Many types of rigid fixation implants are available. The surgeon chooses the type best suited to serve its purpose. The implant may remain permanently, or it may be removed after the fracture has healed, especially in a young person. For example, a plate can cause a stress fracture from the shielding forces exerted over time along its rigid edges on the less rigid underlying bone. If osteomyelitis develops, an implant must be removed.

Screws, plates, nails, rods, and pins are made of stainless steel 316L, titanium, or cobalt alloys. These metals are nonmagnetic and electrolytically inert. Only one kind of metal is used in a patient. The instrumentation used to implant it must be of the same metal. Semirigid carbon fiber–reinforced plastic plates are also used in some situations. Biodegradable screws and rods provide stability during osteogenesis. A plate may be affixed to cortex of the bone, or an intramedullary rod can be inserted into the bone. The type and size of implant(s) must be documented in the patient's record and logged according to institutional policy and procedure.

Screws Screws alone may be used for fixation of an oblique or spiral fracture of a long bone. Screws must be long enough to penetrate both cortices. Hard cortical bone gives the best fixation, and two cortices generally hold better than one. Screws are available in various lengths and diameters. Not all screws have the same type of head (e.g., heads may be single slot, cross slot, concave cross slot, hexagon, or Phillips head [Figure 37-11]). The correct screwdriver must be used with each type of screw.

Compression Plates and Screws Many fractures requiring open reduction are rigidly fixed through the compression method. Compression plates are heavy and strong. They are held in place by specially designed cortical

Figure 37-11 Fixation plates and screws.

Figure 37-12 Compression hip screw for fixation of fracture of femoral neck.

lag screws. The threads of these screws are deeper than those on other types of screws and are farther apart, which allows a larger amount of bone between the threads. This construction gives maximum holding power and rigid fixation. A compression instrument may be used. It is connected to the end of the plate and then fastened to the bone with a short screw. When the nut on the compression instrument is tightened, the bone fragments are brought tightly together. The remaining screws are put into the plate, and the fracture is fixed. Screws alone are used only in selected situations. A cast may or may not be applied.

Following open reduction of an acetabular fracture, a compression plate may be bent to conform to the contour of the acetabulum and secured with long cortical and cancellous lag screws.

Eggers Plate and Screws The plate is slotted, which permits the muscle tone of the extremity to keep the ends of the fragments pressed closely together. The pressure stimulates osteogenesis.

Sherman Plate and Screws The appropriate-size plate is fitted to the contour of the bone, by bending it slightly if necessary, before the screws are applied. With a drill guide, holes for the screws are drilled with an electric or air-powered drill in the center of the screw hole and perpendicularly to the plate. The drill bit should be slightly smaller than the screws. The screws should pass through both cortices of the bone.

Nails An intertrochanteric or subtrochanteric fracture of the neck of the femur may be treated by inserting a nail, compression screw, or multiple pins through the neck into the head of the femur (Figure 37-12). Many different types of nails are used. They are usually inserted over or alongside a guidewire. The nail may form a continuous angulated unit with a plate that fits on the outer lateral cortex of the femur, or the plate may be attached and the nail, screws, or pins inserted separately. Screws secure the plate to the shaft of the femur before or after the nail is inserted, depending on the design of the implant.

The patient is usually positioned on the orthopaedic table. The surgeon and assistants assume responsibility for moving and positioning the patient. Figure 37-13 shows the position for nailing the left hip. If portable x-ray machines are used, one is on the unaffected side for an AP view, and one is at the foot of the table for a lateral view. The film for an AP view is placed on the cassette holder from the unaffected side. The procedure may be performed with C-arm fluoroscopic image intensification rather than conventional x-ray machines. All sterile tables are positioned on the affected side. The surgeon may sit to operate.

Intramedullary Nailing

An intramedullary nail, rod, or pin is driven into the medullary canal through the site of the fracture (Figure 37-14). This brings the ends together for union, splints the fracture, and eases pain. It permits early return of function so that the patient can be ambulatory. Intramedullary implants also provide a method of holding fragments in alignment in comminuted fractures. Rigid implants are usually used for pathologic fractures or impending fracture of diseased bone. Flexible intramedullary rods may be preferred for some traumatic fractures, particularly femoral fractures. The length, size, and shape of the nail or pin depend on the bone to be splinted.

The patient with a femoral or tibial fracture is positioned on the orthopaedic table. This permits traction as needed to maintain reduction. Figure 37-15 shows the position of the patient for intramedullary nailing of the left tibia. C-arm fluoroscopy is used for fluoroscopic control. The fracture may

Figure 37-13   Position on orthopaedic table for nailing left hip. Note arm on affected side suspended from screen to remove it from surgical field. Note traction on affected leg and support under knee. Elevated right leg permits x-ray tube to be adjusted under it for lateral view.

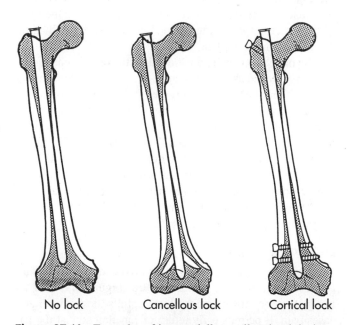

No lock   Cancellous lock   Cortical lock

Figure 37-14   Examples of intermedullary nail and rod devices. (From Gustilo RB, Kyle RF, Templeman DC: *Fractures and dislocations,* vol 1, St Louis, 1993, Mosby.)

Figure 37-15   Position on orthopaedic table for intramedullary nailing of left tibia. Note left foot anchored to foot holder and knee resting on elevated curved knee rest. Right foot is anchored, and knee rest is adjusted for support of leg.

be reduced with visual exposure of the fracture site or by closed reduction. In some situations the medullary canal must be reshaped or enlarged before an implant is inserted. The implant may be removed after union at the fracture site has taken place, especially if it causes pain. If nonunion occurs, the implant may need to be removed.

Interlocking Nail Fixation   After closed reduction of the fracture, an intramedullary rod or nail is inserted the length of the shaft of a long bone without exposing the fracture site. This technique is called closed intramedullary nailing and may be used for transverse or short oblique fractures of the midshaft of the femur or tibia. An incision is made to expose the femoral trochanter or tibial tuberosity. To stabilize more oblique, comminuted fractures and those beyond the midshaft region, transfixion screws are also used with locking nails. These screws pass through the cortices of the bone and holes in the intramedullary nail. This method of closed interlocking nail fixation may be static or dynamic, depending on the location and configuration of the fracture. In the static method, screws are inserted in both the proximal and distal fragments; in the dynamic method they are proximal or distal. Several types of interlocking nail systems are available, such as the Grosse-Kempf, Brooker-Wills, and Russell-Taylor systems. All systems prevent gliding and rotation of fragments, as well as shortening of the limb from bone loss.

JOINT PROCEDURES

Joint function depends on the quality of its structures. Articular cartilage covers the two ends of bone where they meet to form the joint. Bones are held securely in place at their articulation by ligaments and the joint capsule attached to both bone shafts. The synovial membrane lining the joint capsule secretes synovial fluid to lubricate the joint. When the joint is injured or altered by arthritis or some other degenerative disease, normal joint motion is impaired and/or painful.

Dislocations

Dislocation of one or more bones at a joint may occur with or without an associated fracture. Tendons, ligaments, and muscles are deranged. The articular surface of the bone is displaced from the joint capsule. The force of displacement damages the capsule and tears ligaments and surrounding tissues. Blood vessel and nerve damage can occur, impeding circulation and causing changes in sensation and muscle strength. Closed reduction, with or without skeletal traction, may be necessary at the time of an acute injury. If closed reduction fails to stabilize the joint and prevent recurrence, open reduction and internal fixation may be necessary. Surgical procedures to stabilize chronic recurrent dislocations are most frequently performed on the shoulder.

Arthrodesis

Fusion of a joint may be achieved by removing the articular surfaces and securing bony union or by inserting a fixation implant that inhibits motion. Arthrodesis may be performed following resection of a recurrent benign, potentially malignant, or malignant lesion that involves the ends of the bones and joint. After resection of the diseased portion of the bones, the joint may be stabilized with a bone graft or an intramedullary fixation implant. This procedure is performed most frequently for lesions in the distal femur and proximal tibia around or including the knee joint. Arthrodesis may also be performed to relieve osteoarthritic pain or to stabilize a joint that does not respond to other methods of treatment following injury, such as instability of the thumb. Because

Figure 37-16 Austin-Moore prosthesis to replace femoral head and neck in hemiarthroplasty. Shaft is driven into medullary canal of femur.

arthrodesis limits motion, other joint reconstructive procedures are usually attempted first.

Triple arthrodesis of the ankle is performed to correct deformity or muscle imbalance of the foot. The subtalar, calcaneocuboid, and talonavicular tarsal joints are fused. Staples are sometimes used to hold bones together.

Arthroplasty

Arthroplasty (reconstruction of a joint) may be necessary to restore or improve range of motion and stability or to relieve pain. This may be done by resurfacing, reshaping, or replacing the articular surfaces of the bones.

Femoral and Humeral Head Replacement

A metal prosthetic implant can replace the femoral or humeral head and neck (Figure 37-16). These prostheses have a shaft that is driven into the medullary canal of the bone. The head of the bone is removed. The neck is shaped or removed as necessary for accurate placement of the prosthesis. A reamer may be used to enlarge the canal for insertion of the prosthesis. These prostheses are used for the following purposes:

- To mobilize the joint in arthritic patients
- To replace a comminuted fractured head when soft tissue attachments are destroyed
- To replace the head if avascular necrosis or nonunion occurs following reduction of fractures

A free vascularized fibular graft may be preferred to decompress the femoral head, provide structural stability, and vascularize bone in an area of avascular necrosis. This procedure preserves the femoral head rather than replacing it with a prosthesis after removal of dead bone. The peroneal artery and vein are preserved with the graft. Under the operating microscope, these vessels are anastomosed to branches of the femoral circumflex vessels. Restoration of vascularization prevents progression of necrosis and stimulates osteogenesis (new bone formation).

Femoral Head Surface Replacement

As an alternative to femoral head replacement, a concentric metal shell is cemented over the femoral head. A high-density polyethylene shell is cemented into the acetabulum. Surface replacement to relieve severe hip pain and disability is reserved for young adults with good femoral and acetabular bone stock. Patients with sclerotic, well-vascularized subchondral bone of hypertrophic osteoarthritis, for example, may be candidates for this procedure. Resurfacing induces healing and reduces stress on the hip joint.

Total Joint Replacement

The surgeon's goal in total joint arthroplasty is to alleviate pain and to create functional mobility and stability. The prosthesis must maintain normal anatomic relationships and biologic fixation to bone. Correct alignment and fit of component parts are crucial aspects of their function. Although prosthetic implants for some joints have not been as well developed as those for others, total joint replacement is an accepted therapeutic modality, especially for the hip, knee, and elbow joints. Usually performed to improve mobility and relieve the pain of severe arthritic joints, total joint replacement may be indicated when other therapeutic measures have failed to correct a congenital defect, traumatic injury, or degenerative disease. A functional design for a prosthesis must consider a combination of load bearing, strain-stress, and kinetics in association with the pathologic condition. Positioning of the prosthesis influences the distribution of stress and rate of wear.

The bones on both sides of the joints are replaced or resurfaced. Both component parts must be solidly anchored to avoid movement of the prosthesis and wear on surrounding tissue. All movement must be between the smooth articulating surfaces of the prosthesis. Various alloys, ceramics, and high-density polyethylene or silicone are used; component parts of many prostheses are made of more than one material. Metal-to-plastic joints are self-lubricating. Natural synovial fluids help lubricate other types. The rate of wear on parts must be low so that the prosthesis will remain functional over a period of many years (the exact number is undetermined). The major complication of total joint arthroplasty is loosening of the prosthetic components over time, particularly in weight-bearing joints of obese and/or active patients. Configuration, surface features, and the method of fixation of component parts influence the mechanical stability of an "artificial" joint. The orthopaedic surgeon must consider the following:

1. *Biomechanics.* Ideally, a prosthesis provides full range of motion. The support provided by cartilage, ligaments, and the articular capsule surrounding the prosthesis influences its stability. Prostheses may be constrained or nonconstrained.
   a. A constrained prosthesis provides a stable joint but restricts motion to a single plane or limits motion in all planes.
   b. A nonconstrained prosthesis allows gliding and shifting motions resembling normal range of motion, but it is inherently unstable.
2. *Biophysical components.* A total joint prosthesis has at least two components, one for each side of the articulation. To determine the size and shape of components to fit the patient, measurements of bones that form the joint may be obtained preoperatively by developing templates (i.e., patterns on grids) from the patient's x-ray films. If templates have not been obtained, x-ray films and measurements are taken at the surgical field. The surgeon also takes trial measurements at the site to verify the correct selection of the implant.
   a. Solid components have a predetermined configuration. The surgeon must select the most appropriate size from those available. Bone may need to be reshaped to accommodate the prosthesis.
   b. Modular systems have interchangeable components so that the surgeon can customize the prosthesis at the operating bed. For example, the width, depth, or length can be adjusted to the patient's anatomy. A quick-setting Silastic mold may be formed for precise matching in three dimensions. The mold is sent to a laboratory, where the prosthesis is customized with the use of a laser scanner and a computer-guided milling machine.
3. *Fixation.* The bone into which the component part is implanted and the surface of the prosthesis will determine the method of fixation.
   a. Press-fit fixation relies on direct bone-to-prosthesis contact. This can be achieved by a variety of methods, including reshaping the bone to the size and/ or configuration of the implant and/or securing threads, pegs, or screws on the prosthesis into bone.
   b. Biofixation refers to a surface on the implant that allows tissue ingrowth for stability. Ingrowth is defined as the development of bony tissue in an empty hole. A portion of the implant has a porous or rough surface. Bone grows into pores or interstices. Many types of coatings are used, such as tricalcium phosphate or coraline hydroxyapatite sprayed on the surface. Others have a porous material, such as polysulfone bonded to metal. Surfaces that are porous enough for bone ingrowth without greatly expanding the surface area or weakening the implant are most desirable. These cementless prostheses require a precise fit in bones. They are particularly suited for young, active patients.
   c. Methyl methacrylate fixation uses self-curing thermoplastic acrylic cement to provide long-term fixation. Several different preparations of polymethyl methacrylate (PMMA), commonly referred to as bone cement, are available. The powder and liquid components are mixed at the instrument table immediately before insertion into the intramedullary canal of a long bone or socket of a joint.

PMMA hardens in response to an exothermic reaction that reaches 140° F (60° C) and destroys surrounding cells.

The liquid portion is highly flammable and should not be placed in close proximity to the pencil cautery. Use of appropriate venting devices during mixing provides an extra measure of safety for the team.

Bone cement is injected in a state of low viscosity under pressure to fill the interstices of bone. When the implant is placed, the cement fills the space around it for a secure fit. This is the method of choice for most patients over 65 years of age because it allows early ambulation. Cement can crack or break and cause loosening of the prosthesis over time.

Physiologic responses to bone cement are varied. Some patients experience hypotension and can suffer an embolus or cardiac arrest during the cementing process. Close collaboration with the anesthesia provider during the use of bone cement affords the patient an additional measure of safety.

d. Hybrid fixation refers to a combination of fixation methods. Some components are cemented; some are press fitted or held by screws or some other noncemented technique.

e. Bone grafts may be needed to replace bone loss around the joint. Either autologous or fresh frozen homologous bone may be used.

Total Hip Replacement

Total hip prostheses have greatly reduced the number of arthroplasty procedures previously described, especially in patients older than 50 years of age with degenerative hip disease. Several types and sizes of prostheses are available. Each has its own advantages and disadvantages. The surgeon must select the appropriate one for each patient's particular condition.

With the patient supine on the radiographic operating bed, an incision about 10 inches (25 cm) long is made along the lateral aspect of the thigh to remove the greater trochanter. Removal of the greater trochanter facilitates exposure to prepare sites for insertion of the prosthesis. However, its removal can cause abductor muscle weakness, instability, and other complications. Therefore some surgeons prefer an anterior approach to the hip joint with the patient supine; others prefer a posterior approach with the patient in the lateral decubitus position. With all approaches the femur is dislocated from the acetabulum. The femoral head is removed at the neck and replaced with a prosthesis. This may be a metal, usually titanium, head on a metallic stem that is seated into the medullary canal of the femur. Before the femoral prosthesis is inserted, the acetabulum is reamed to the configuration of the cup-shaped acetabular component (Figure 37-17). This may be high-density polyethylene or metal with a smooth, rough, or porous outer surface. The inner surface is smooth polyethylene to articulate with the smooth finish on the head of the femoral prosthesis. The acetabular component is fixed in the socket. Then the femoral prosthesis is po-

Figure 37-17 Components of total hip replacement prosthesis. **A,** Metallic stem with femoral head. **B,** Acetabular cup.

sitioned. This sequence is reversed if a Silastic mold is made for a customized femoral component.

A computer-assisted surgical robot may be used to help the surgeon plan the surgical procedure, select the most appropriate type and size of hip prosthesis, and prepare the surface of the bone. A drill in the end of the robotic arm precisely drills the cavity in the femur to hold the implant stem.

Total Knee Replacement

Insertion of a total knee prosthesis may be indicated to provide for mechanical deficiencies in the function of the knee. The patient, usually older than 60 years of age, may have significant chronic pain and joint destruction as a result of arthritis, an inflammatory condition, or an autoimmune disorder. One or both knees may be affected. Bilateral total knee replacement can be performed safely in a patient who has the ability to actively participate in postoperative rehabilitation. Selection of the appropriate prosthesis from among the types available depends on the deformity of the femorotibial articulation, patellofemoral articulation, and the structure of the cruciate and collateral ligaments. The prosthesis consists of a multiradius femoral component, a modular tibial component, and a patellar component. The tibial and patellar components of high-density polyethylene articulate with the polished metallic surface of the femoral component.

With the patient supine on the operating bed, the knee is maintained in a flexed position. Numerous commercial devices are available for this purpose. The pneumatic tourniquet cuff is placed on the thigh before prepping and draping. A vertical midline incision is made over the front of the knee. After the distal femur and the proximal tibia are cut, a trial prosthesis is inserted. The knee is taken through a range of motion to assess alignment, ligament balance, and patellar positioning before the components are fixed in place. To achieve stability, permanent bone ingrowth into a porous coated or rough-surface implant is desirable. Prostheses of this construction may not require bone cement for fixation. Hybrid fixation is used for others.

Total Ankle Replacement

Rheumatoid arthritis and posttraumatic osteoarthritis are the most common causes of ankle degeneration. Ankle joint replacement may be indicated as an alternative to arthrodesis in selected patients, usually older than 60 years of age, to relieve pain and secondarily to increase motion and provide stability in the tibiotalar joint. With the patient positioned supine, an anterior incision may be made from the base of the second metatarsal to the crest of the tibia. A posterior approach, with the patient positioned prone, may be preferred for wider exposure of anatomic structures. Procedures vary depending on the type of prosthesis to be implanted. The nonconstrained type allows normal dorsiflexion, plantar flexion, and rotation of the foot but is inherently unstable; the constrained type restricts motion to a single plane but is inherently more stable. The tibial components of both types are high-density polyethylene, and the talar components are metal. They are cemented in place.

Total Metatarsophalangeal Joint Replacement
Hallux rigidus and hallux abductus valgus deformities can lead to pain and altered gait. Through joint replacement the deformity can be realigned with stability and motion. Several types of implants are available. The Silastic hinge toe, a double-stemmed silicone prosthesis with a hinge, is popular to restore motion of the great toe and lesser metatarsophalangeal joints.

Total Shoulder Replacement
Shoulder replacement may be indicated for severe destruction by disease or posttraumatic degeneration of the humeral articular surface with resultant loss of motion, instability, and pain. The prosthesis replaces the humeral head and resurfaces the glenoid cavity, the articular surface of the scapula. Preferred if ligamentous or capsular support is sufficient, a nonconstrained prosthesis has a plastic component for the glenoid socket and a metal humeral head. Only the articular surfaces are replaced with these gliding metal-to-plastic components. A stable fixed-fulcrum, constrained prosthesis with interlocking components may be required to prevent dislocation. The patient is placed in a semi-Fowler's position with the affected shoulder slightly off the edge of the operating bed for these surgical procedures.

Total Elbow Replacement
Prosthetic replacement may be indicated to correct intraarticular problems within the elbow joint, especially one with severe surface damage. Surface replacement with a nonarticulating, constrained prosthesis provides internal stability. A hinged or articulated, nonconstrained capitellocondylar prosthesis improves the functional range of motion in the humeroulnar articulation. Both the metallic humerus and ulnar components are cemented in place following shaping of the bones. High-density polyethylene bushings facilitate articulation of the hinge assembly connecting the humoral and ulnar components.

Total Wrist Replacement
Silicone rubber implants are used to replace the radiocarpal joint in the wrist, primarily to improve function. A resection arthroplasty is done, usually from an anterior approach. The proximal row of carpal bones (i.e., scaphoid and lunate) and the trapezium are resected. Stems of the flexible, hinged implant are inserted into the intramedullary canals of the radius proximally and capitate carpal bone distally. A silicone cap is placed over the distal end of the ulna. Flexion and extension of the wrist are possible through free sliding of stems within the medullary canals. Some other types of prostheses have fixed stems.

Trapeziometacarpal Joint Replacement
A metal ball-to-plastic socket prosthesis restores function of the thumb. This prosthesis is cemented in place.

Metacarpophalangeal Joint Replacement
Known as implant replacement arthroplasty for small joints in the hands, the head of the affected metacarpal or proximal phalanx is removed. The silicone rubber implant bridges the excised joint. One stem fits into the medullary canal of the proximal metacarpal, and the other fits into the distal phalanx. The hinged body of the implant keeps the bones separated and mobile.

Patient Care Considerations in Arthroplasty

Patients of all ages have debilitating and painful arthritis; many are over 65 years of age. Attention must be paid to support all joints during moving and positioning of these patients. Other unique aspects of joint replacement should be kept in mind:

1. The prosthesis must be handled carefully.
   a. Use only instruments specifically designed for implantation of the prosthesis.
   b. Avoid causing dents and scratches.
   c. Avoid glove powder and lint. Silicone implants should not be placed on fabrics; place the implant in a metal basin or transfer it directly to the surgeon.
   d. Open sterile packages just before use, after the surgeon determines the size and style.
2. Bone cement, if needed, must be mixed by the scrub person immediately before use.
   a. Follow the manufacturer's instructions for handling this material. The scrub person should know by feel and appearance when the cement is of the correct consistency. A practice session is helpful before mixing for the first time during an actual surgical procedure.
   b. Avoid excessive exposure to vapors. In addition to causing irritation to the eyes, vapors may damage soft contact lenses if worn. A scavenging system should be used. A fume evacuator, if used, may need to be recharged before and after use.
   c. Avoid getting lipid solvent on gloves. It can diffuse through the latex to cause allergic dermatitis.
   d. Cement is poured into a syringe for injection into the intramedullary canal for joints such as hip or shoulder joints. Cement may be shaped manually for hinged joints.
   e. Room temperature can affect the time necessary for cement to set.

3. A Silastic mold, if used to customize the prosthesis, must be prepared at the sterile field. The scrub person mixes the catalyst and silicone quickly and thoroughly and then pours the mixture into the injector tube immediately before it is inserted into the bone. The customized prosthesis must be steam sterilized when it arrives from the laboratory. A standard sterilization cycle, not flash sterilization, is used.

4. Air-powered drills, saws, and reamers must be properly connected with adequate pressure. Check the pressure in tanks of compressed air or nitrogen before the surgical procedure begins. It must be more than 500 pounds.

5. Suction tubing must be kept open and collection containers changed as necessary to maintain suction for irrigation during the surgical procedure.

6. Blood loss should be appropriately monitored. It can be extensive during total hip arthroplasty. Blood may be salvaged from the sterile field and processed (e.g., through a cell saver) for autotransfusion.

7. Closed wound suction drainage usually is used, especially following hip, knee, and shoulder arthroplasty.

8. The exhaust system for personnel must be functioning properly if the surgical procedure is performed within an ultraclean air system.

9. Traffic through the OR should be restricted to minimize air turbulence. Infection is a major potential hazard of all bone and joint surgery. It can be both disabling and expensive.

10. The type of prosthesis used must be documented, including the manufacturer's identifying information. The label of a sterile implant can be affixed to the patient's record.

Arthroscopy

Arthroscopy, the visualization of the interior of a joint through an arthroscope, allows diagnosis and conservative treatment of some cartilaginous, ligamentous, synovial, and bony surface defects. Most frequently used for definitive treatment of meniscal, articular cartilage, and ligamentous defects in the knee, an arthroscope may also be used in the shoulder, ankle, elbow, wrist, and hip. Fiberoptic arthroscopes have diameters ranging from 1.7 to 6 mm to accommodate the size of the joint. Angles of the viewing lenses also vary from 0 to 90 degrees.

Sterile irrigating solution, either Ringer's lactate or normal saline solution, at room temperature is necessary to distend the joint, although some arthroscopists prefer air or carbon dioxide. The solution is injected initially via a needle and syringe. Then through a small stab wound, a cannula is inserted into the medial aspect of the knee, for example, for inflow of irrigation. Outflow tubing is connected to the metal sheath of the arthroscope. It can be attached to suction or placed in a drainage bucket and allowed to drain by gravity.

The sheath (sleeve) over a sharp trocar is inserted through a stab wound in the skin at the selected site of entry for the arthroscope. When the trocar penetrates the capsule, the capsule and synovium form a tight seal around the sheath. The sharp trocar is replaced with a blunt obturator to advance the sheath into the joint. The obturator is removed, and the arthroscope inserted through the sheath. The inflow and outflow irrigating tubes are connected to the stopcocks on the sheath.

An operating arthroscope may have a channel for passage of long, thin, manually operated instruments such as probes, hooks, scissors, knives, punches, and grasping forceps. Or these instruments may be manipulated through separate puncture sites (portals) into the joint under visualization through the scope. Power-driven shavers are also used to smooth rough articular cartilage or bony surfaces. A pulsed-energy Nd:YAG, Ho:YAG, or CO_2 laser may be adapted to some arthroscopes for use in a confined area and to minimize bleeding. A video camera attached to the eyepiece allows projection of the view to a closed-circuit television monitor so that the surgeon can manipulate instruments more comfortably than by squinting through the eyepiece. Some cameras attach to the side of a beam splitter on the scope. Daylight film should be used with fiberoptic lighting.

Patient Care Considerations in Arthroscopy

1. All metal components are steam sterilized. Some optical systems and fiberoptic cords can be steam sterilized; others require Steris, Sterrad, or EO gas sterilization. Protective sterilizing cases are recommended to protect the optics when the components are batch processed. Follow the manufacturer's recommendations for sterilization of the arthroscope and its component attachments.

2. The scrub person checks all sterile equipment and instruments while setting up.
   a. Check the arthroscope for clean lenses and unbroken optics.
   b. Check the patency of the inflow and outflow irrigation stopcocks and ports.
   c. All component parts must be the correct size; the optics, trocar, and obturator must fit securely into the sheath. Surgical instruments must pass through the channel. Fiberoptic cord must fit the arthroscope and projection lamp.
   d. Inspect the edges of cutting instruments, such as blades, burrs, knives, and scissors, under magnification. Blades must be sharp, set properly, and glide smoothly.
   e. Assemble power equipment. Rings must fit tightly. Forward and reverse rotating actions must function smoothly. Blades must be locked properly. The power source should be checked.

3. The circulator checks all nonsterile equipment (i.e., fiberoptic projection lamp, video equipment, and laser).

4. The video camera and cable must be enclosed in a sterile cover unless the camera has been sterilized. The scrub person and circulator coordinate draping.

5. The extremity must be firmly supported in a leg or arm holder that allows flexion of the joint. A tourniquet is

applied for arthroscopy of the knee, ankle, elbow, or wrist. Care is taken not to allow prep solution to run under the tourniquet cuff.

6. The patient is prepped and draped as for any sterile procedure on the extremity, with extra precautions to provide a waterproof barrier against contamination by irrigating solutions.

7. The circulator hangs bags of sterile normal saline or Ringer's lactate irrigating solution on an IV pole at least 3 feet (1 m) above the joint to ensure adequate hydrostatic pressure to keep the joint distended and to maintain the flow of the irrigating solution. Some facilities use irrigation pumps. Two to four 3000-ml bags may be needed. The solution is maintained at room temperature to avoid hyperemia from warm solution, which may appear as inflammation of synovium, or blanching, which produces an avascular appearance from cold solution. Used solution should be disposed of per biologic waste protocol.

8. Equipment must be appropriately attached after the patient is draped.

   a. The scrub person secures drainage tubes, fiberoptic cord, suction, air-power cables, and the like, to drapes in a location that will not impede movement of the extremity.

   b. The circulator attaches tubing to irrigating and suction systems, cords to power sources, and so on.

Arthrotomy

Arthrotomy (i.e., incision into a joint) may be necessary to remove bone or cartilage fragments or to repair a defect in the synovium or joint capsule. Synovectomy may be the procedure of choice for relief of pain and control of inflammation in a rheumatoid arthritic joint. If a joint is ankylosed (fused), fibrosed, or deranged, open arthrotomy rather than arthroscopy may be necessary. Occasionally during arthroscopy, an injury or disease process that cannot be adequately treated requires arthrotomy while the patient is anesthetized, or it may be performed at a later time. In the knee, for example, potential neurovascular complications may preclude arthroscopic repair.

Bunionectomy

Hallux valgus, a lateral deviation in position of the great toe, increases the prominence of the adjoining metatarsal head. Pressure at the base of the first metatarsophalangeal joint causes inflammation that creates formation of an exostosis or bunion beneath the bursa and joint capsule. A bunionectomy is done to remove a painful exostosis and to functionally or cosmetically correct the deformity (Figure 37-18). A capsulotomy must be performed to enter the first metatarsophalangeal joint. The procedure may be done with the patient under local infiltration anesthesia and IV sedation. A pneumatic tourniquet around the ankle provides hemostasis, unless contraindicated in a patient with a circulatory problem in the foot. One of several procedures may be selected:

1. *Keller arthroplasty.* The proximal third of the proximal phalanx of the great toe is resected. A silicone im-

Figure 37-18   Bunionectomy.

plant may be placed in the intramedullary canal to stabilize the metatarsophalangeal joint.

2. *Metatarsal osteotomy.* The metatarsal alignment is corrected by moving the metatarsal head laterally.

3. *McBride operation.* The abductor tendon is fixed to the lateral portion of the metatarsal neck, and the sesamoid bone is excised.

4. *Silver bunionectomy.* The medial aspect of the exostosis is removed from the first metatarsal head.

Bunionectomies are only one of many procedures performed by podiatrists, as well as orthopaedic surgeons, in the treatment of foot-related disorders, including degenerative diseases and injuries of the foot and ankle.

Neurolysis

Neuropathy caused by entrapment of a nerve produces tingling, numbness, and a burning sensation with radiating pain and compromise of function. Known as a tunnel syndrome, this most frequently occurs in the wrist from entrapment of the median nerve (i.e., carpal tunnel syndrome). It may originate from compression of the radial nerve in the lower arm (i.e., radial tunnel syndrome) or from the posterior tibial nerve in the foot (i.e., tarsal tunnel syndrome). The cause of formation of scar tissue or adhesions around the nerve may be related to repetitive stress, trauma, or inflammatory disease. Neurolysis, freeing of the nerve from the surrounding structures, relieves pain and restores sensation and function. For example, in the wrist, the transverse carpal ligament overriding the median nerve is incised. A segment may be excised, and a synovectomy may be performed to relieve the symptoms of carpal tunnel syndrome. Release of the median nerve may also be accomplished endoscopically.

REPAIR OF TENDONS AND LIGAMENTS

Tendons and ligaments may be severed, torn, or ruptured. These injuries are frequently seen in athletes. Total or partial avulsion of the major ligaments and tendons torn from their attachments in or around an extremity joint requires repair to stabilize the joint.

Tendons can be lengthened, shortened, or transferred. When a surgical procedure is indicated, tendon repair is a meticulous but tedious procedure. Tenorrhaphy (close apposition of the cut ends of tendons, particularly extensor tendons) is imperative to successfully restore function. Tendons heal slowly. Nonabsorbable or slow-absorbing suture is widely used in tendon repair because of its durability and lack of elasticity. A tendon may be wrapped in a silicone membrane to prevent adhesions after repair. Artificial tendons are made of a polyester center covered with silicone rubber. A double-velour polyester prosthesis is used for ligament repair of a shoulder separation.

Hand Surgery

Hand reconstruction has become a subspecialty of both orthopaedics and plastic surgery. Tendon surgery is within the realm of orthopaedic surgeons; however, many plastic surgeons also perform tendon repair and transfer for hand reconstruction. Restoration of function is the goal of the hand surgeon. The surgeon often manages surgical correction of fractures and rotational deformities of the fingers. Tenosynovectomy (excision of the tendon sheath) may be performed to release arthritic contractures.

Sports Medicine

Sports medicine deals with the anatomic, biochemical, physiologic, and psychologic effects of motion, strength, and coordination on physical activity. Public awareness of and surgeons' concerns about athletic injuries have led to the development of sports medicine centers that emphasize physical conditioning, injury prevention, and rehabilitation of athletes. Sports medicine is a rapidly growing area of orthopaedics, primarily as a result of interest in exercise among the general population. The intensity of a sports activity places physical demands on the musculoskeletal system that can result in injury. Most injuries involve ligaments, tendons, and muscles rather than broken bones. Most injuries, such as a strained muscle or tendon, do not require surgical intervention. MRI is a reliable method of assessing intraarticular injuries, either acute or chronic. The knee, shoulder, and ankle are most prone to athletic injuries of ligaments and dislocations of joints. Arthroscopy is useful in the diagnosis and treatment of some injuries. Others require open surgical reconstruction to regain joint stability. For example, a complete ligament tear usually requires surgical repair. Some procedures combine arthroscopy and arthrotomy. Postoperative rehabilitation aims to restore range of motion, to minimize muscle atrophy, and to reestablish muscle endurance and joint position. The patient should commit to a long-term conditioning program to prevent reinjury.

Knee Injuries

The knee is the joint that is most vulnerable to both contact and noncontact sports injuries. Hyperextension, for example, can result from a noncontact activity. Contact sports can result in a combination of injuries to the cruciate and collateral ligaments, meniscus, and posterior capsule.

Anterior Cruciate Ligament Knee stability is influenced by the dynamics of the anterior and posterior cruciate ligaments. Injuries to these ligaments are the most common and most serious types of knee injuries. The anterior cruciate ligament (ACL) can be partially or completely torn, ruptured, or avulsed. The extent of the injury determines the method of reconstruction. Arthroscopically, the ACL may be transferred into the posterior aspect of the lateral femoral condyle and secured with sutures, staples, or screws.

After an autograft is harvested through an open incision, the knee may be reconstructed through the arthroscope. One technique places a bone–patellar tendon–bone autograft and fixes it with cancellous or interference bone screws into tibial and femoral tunnels. In another method a composite of autogenous semitendinosus muscle with a polypropylene ligament augmentation device sutured to it extends from the tibial attachment across the joint and is stapled to the distal femur. In the open Insall procedure a bone-block graft with an iliotibial band of fascia lata is secured to the tibial tubercle.

Artificial ligamentous substitutes may be preferred for ACL reconstruction. These materials are also used to stabilize torn or ruptured ligaments in the ankle. Expanded polytetrafluoroethylene can be secured with screws. Allograft ligaments also are used. Woven bovine collagen, bovine and carbon fiber material, or a partially absorbable matrix of polylactic acid polymer and filamentous carbon may be used as a scaffold for new collagenous tissue ingrowth for disrupted ligaments. Concomitant partial meniscectomy or meniscal repair may be performed with ACL reconstruction.

Meniscus Partial meniscectomy or repair of a meniscal tear may be done by open arthrotomy or closed arthroscopy. Neurovascular injury is a potential complication of these procedures. Patients selected for arthroscopy usually have a single vertical longitudinal tear that can be debrided. Localized synovium can be abraded. Sutures must be placed to reduce displacement and stabilize the meniscus.

Ankle Injuries

Ankle sprains are commonly caused by inversion injury. Ankle fractures are usually eversion injuries. Rupture of the Achilles tendon can occur spontaneously during a physical activity, such as basketball or racquet sports, usually from indirect trauma. A gap is palpable at the back of the ankle. Severed ends of the tendon may be brought together through an open or percutaneous repair with heavy (size No. 2) nonabsorbable suture.

Ankle arthroscopy may be the procedure of choice for placing internal fixation devices or for removing osteophytes (bony outgrowths) in the joint after healing of an ankle fracture.

Shoulder Injuries

Many anterior glenoid labrum and minor rotator cuff tears, the most common acute injuries, can be repaired arthroscopically. Some recurrent dislocations also can be stabilized with sutures, staples, or screws. For a major rotator cuff tear, an open Bankart repair usually is necessary to suture the labrum and reattach the glenohumeral ligament. An open Putti-Platt correction for recurrent dislocation will limit external rotation of the shoulder.

VERTEBRAL SURGERY

Because of the proximity of the vertebral column to the spinal cord, both surgeons and neurosurgeons perform surgical procedures in this area. Orthopaedic procedures on the back are usually performed to excise vertebral lesions, to relieve pressure on the spinal cord, to stabilize the vertebral column, or to correct gross deformities. Primary neoplasms such as a giant cell bone tumor, bone cyst, hemangioma or osteoid osteoma, and metastatic tumors can occur in vertebrae. Osteomyelitis, spondylolisthesis (a condition in which one lumbar vertebra slips onto another), and degenerative diseases such as arthritis and osteoporosis may cause severe low back pain unresponsive to nonsurgical treatment. Fracture, with or without dislocation of one vertebra or more, may be reduced by traction, internal fixation, or excision of bony fragments. Scoliosis, a progressive curvature of the spine, may be stabilized. Further discussion of spinal surgery is found in Chapter 41.

CAST APPLICATION

For closed reduction of fractures, traction, and postoperative applications, many orthopaedic appliances must be available and at hand when needed. An orthopaedic cart can provide the necessary items for these situations (Box 37-1). The items may vary somewhat at different hospitals, but many are universally used. The cart can be taken wherever needed in the OR suite. One shelf should be kept for sterile items.

Casting supplies are commonly found on the orthopaedic cart. A cast is a rigid form of dressing used to encase a part of the body. It supports and immobilizes the part in optimum position until healing takes place. A cast usually includes the joints above and below the affected area. It may suffice as a

---

Box 37-1	**Contents of an Orthopaedic Cart**

Suture removal supplies
Webril and soft roll
Assorted gauze dressings and bandages
Sterile and nonsterile gloves
Skin antiseptic agents
Disposable razors

Nonsterile Items on Another Shelf
Pulleys and attachments for bed traction
Ropes, weights, and carriers
Felt padding and foam rubber
Arm and shoulder immobilizers
Pelvic slings and rods
Assorted sizes of gauze bandages and stockinette
Stapler
Safety pins
Cold cream and talcum powder
Disposable plaster pail or bucket with plastic liner bag
Plastic bag for trash
Assorted sizes of plaster and/or fiberglass rolls and splints
Cast cutters, knives, scissors, spreaders, and bender

---

conservative mode of treatment (e.g., for fractures). It can be fitted to any body contour or position and can be worn for months. The following are requirements of a cast:

1. It must fulfill its intended function of maintaining position of the desired parts.
2. It must not be too tight and must have no pressure areas. Postapplication pain is an important symptom and must be promptly investigated. Circulation may be impaired.
3. It must not be too loose. It must be as light as possible, yet strong enough to withstand usage.
4. It must be comfortable, with no binding or chafing.

Fiberglass Casts

A woven fiberglass tape impregnated with a water-activated polyurethane resin can be used for casting or bracing. Polypropylene stockinette is applied over the patient's skin. Polypropylene web wrap may be used for extra padding over bony prominences and pressure points. The person applying the cast must wear gloves or coat his or her hands with a silicone hand cream to facilitate smoothing and blending the layers of the fiberglass tape and to prevent resin pickup on the hands. The resin is activated by warm water. The tape is applied in the same manner as plaster.

The cast is lighter and thinner, yet stronger, than a plaster cast and is more porous, providing better ventilation. The outside may get wet without deterioration. X-rays penetrate synthetic materials better than they do plaster to evaluate the healing process. A combination of plaster and synthetic resin on a gauze backing produces a thinner, more waterproof cast that weighs less and is as strong as a plaster cast. Because of these advantages, casting tapes are preferred by many orthopaedic surgeons for extremity casts.

Plaster Casts

Plaster is gypsum or anhydrous calcium sulfate. It is finely ground to break up the crystals and is then heated to drive out the water. When water is added again, recrystallization takes place and the plaster sets. It was first used as a method of splinting fractures in the nineteenth century.

Plaster bandages and splints are made of crinoline or some other fabric, with the plaster powder entrapped in the mesh. These are available in rolls or strips 2 to 8 inches (5 to 20 cm) wide. Plaster splints are either supplied precut or made from rolls as the need arises. Usually six or eight thicknesses of the desired length are used. To provide added strength, splints are applied over areas that may weaken from extra strain. Plaster bandages and splints are available with three types of plaster:

1. Slow-setting plaster requires up to 18 minutes to set. It is used in large casts requiring more time to apply and mold. It permits blending of the layers.
2. Medium-setting plaster requires up to 8 minutes to set. This type is used in average-size casts.
3. Fast-setting plaster requires 4 to 5 minutes to set. It is advantageous for small casts on children who are difficult to keep in position. Many surgeons prefer using the fast-setting type in all kinds of casts; it is the most universally used type of plaster.

Application of Plaster

1. Spread a disposable plastic or nonwoven fabric sheet on the floor around the operating bed to catch drips.
2. Protect the table. If the orthopaedic table is used, spread a sheet over table parts after the patient is suspended.
3. Protect the patient's hair with a cap.
4. Use a disposable plaster pail or a plastic liner bag in a plaster bucket.
5. Fill the bucket with water at room temperature. Water warmer than 70° to 75° F (21° to 24° C) will speed up the setting time and may cause excessive loss of plaster from the fabric. More important, plaster will get even hotter than its normal exothermic reaction if it is dipped in hot water. The patient could get burned.
6. Don nonsterile disposable gloves to protect the hands from irritation by lime content.
7. Remove the outer wrapping. Start soaking the plaster only when the surgeon is ready to apply it. Keep just ahead in soaking it. Have the next roll ready when needed but do not prepare several rolls ahead of time. They may harden and, if used, can produce an ineffective laminated cast. Avoid waste.
8. Hold the bandage under water in a vertical position to allow air bubbles to escape from the rolled end. When air bubbles stop rising, the bandage is soaked through.

Compress the ends between the fingers and palm of each hand to remove excess water. This procedure prevents telescoping during use.

9. Open the end about 1 inch (2.5 cm) and hand the roll to the surgeon.
10. Fan fold a strip once toward the center, before soaking, leaving the ends free to grasp. When soaking, grasp an end in each hand, press the hands together, and submerge the strip in water for a few seconds; remove it and pull the strip taut by the ends. It may seem drippy, but the layers blend together well when quite wet.
11. Ask the surgeon if another roll will be needed before soaking it when the cast appears near completion.
12. Handle the cast with flat, open hands, never fingers, and support the patient in such a way that he or she cannot attempt to bend an incorporated joint. Wet plaster has only one third to one half its ultimate strength when dry. The person who supports an extremity while a cast is being applied takes care not to make finger pressure areas in the plaster that will damage the tissue under it.
13. Elevate an extremity on a pillow until the cast hardens. If it is laid on a hard surface, flat pressure areas may be pressed onto it.
14. Clean up as much as possible while the cast is being applied. Wipe plaster off equipment, as well as off the patient, before it dries. Plaster is easy to remove when still damp; after it dries, it must be scraped off. A cast dryer, if used, hastens drying.
15. Avoid splashing plaster on the furniture, walls, and floor.
16. Clean the equipment and table thoroughly. If the sink has a plaster trap, all plaster drip can be washed down the sink and the contents of the bucket poured into the sink. If there is no plaster trap, leave the bucket until the plaster in the bottom hardens; then empty the water and throw the plaster pail or plastic liner bag into the trash. Clean a reusable bucket as soon as you are finished with it.

Padding Under Casts

Padding is usually placed under casts and serves several functions:

1. It absorbs inevitable ooze from the wound following an open surgical procedure. Sterile padding is put on over the dressing before applying the cast.
2. It protects the wound and the patient's skin.
3. It protects bony prominences.

Materials used for padding include the following:

- *Stockinette.* A seamless tubing of knitted cotton 1 to 12 inches (2.5 to 30.4 cm) wide, stockinette stretches to fit any contour snugly.
- *Sheet wadding.* A glazed cotton bandage 2 to 8 inches (5 to 20 cm) wide is available as a sheeting. It is used over stockinette or in place of it.

- *Soft roll.* A soft roll of thin cotton batting has some stretch for smooth contour.
- *Felt.* Available in sheeting made of wool or blends of wool, cotton, or rayon in thicknesses ranging from ⅛ to ½ inch (3 to 13 mm), felt is cut into desired sizes to fit bony prominences. Felt pads are applied over sheet wadding. The plaster adheres to pads and prevents them from slipping.
- *Foam rubber.* Available in sheets ¼ to 1 inch (6.4 to 25 mm) in thickness, foam rubber may be used in place of felt.
- *Webril.* Webril is a soft, lint-free cotton bandage. The surface is smooth but not glazed, so that each layer clings to the preceding one and the padding lies smoothly in place.

Common Cast Configurations

1. *Cylinder.* A circular cast, made by wrapping the plaster bandages around an extremity, is used after closed or open reductions of fractures, after some surgical procedures for immobilization, or for the purpose of resting a part of an extremity.
2. *Walking cast.* A rubber walking heel or polyurethane sole is applied to the sole of a cylinder cast for ambulation. Use of a lower extremity helps to maintain strength and muscle tone and to prevent atrophy.
3. *Hanging cast.* A cylinder is applied to the arm with the elbow flexed. It extends from the shoulder over the hand, leaving the thumb and fingers free. A wire loop is incorporated at the wrist. A strap through this loop and around the neck suspends the arm. The weight of the cast provides needed traction on the humerus.
4. *Shoulder spica.* Applied to the trunk, arm, and hand, leaving the fingers and thumb free, a spica cast is used after some surgical procedures on the shoulder or humerus or for a fracture of the humerus. The orthopaedic table may be used for its application, or the patient may sit on a stool with the surgeon supporting the arm in the desired position.
5. *Hip spica.* A hip spica cast is applied to the trunk and one or both legs following some hip procedures and fractures of the femur. The orthopaedic table is used. The sacrum rests on a sacral rest. The perineal post provides countertraction. Attachments may be used to support the legs of an adult.
6. *Minerva jacket.* A Minerva jacket is applied from the hips to the head. If the head is to be completely immobilized, it is included in the jacket. The plaster is molded to fit around the face and lower jaw. A part of the plaster at the back of the head is cut out. It is used for fractures of the cervical or upper thoracic vertebrae. The orthopaedic table is necessary.
7. *Body jacket.* A body jacket extends from the axillae to the hips to immobilize vertebrae. Application of this cast usually requires the orthopaedic or Risser table with the necessary attachments, although sometimes the patient may stand on the floor. Traction may be applied by an overhead sling. If an open surgical procedure is to be performed with the patient in a body cast, a cast cutter must be at hand in case of respiratory difficulty. However, a body cast is usually bivalved before a patient is given an anesthetic.

   An opening is always made over the abdomen of a Minerva or body jacket to allow space for lung expansion and decompression of abdominal distention that normally occurs with ingestion of food. A folded towel may be placed over the abdomen before the stockinette is pulled over the body. This is removed when the opening is made in the cast to allow more space between the body and cast.
8. *Plaster shell.* A body jacket is cut along each side, into anterior and posterior parts. The parts may be fastened together by heavy straps with buckles, or the patient may rest in one while the other is removed temporarily.
9. *Wedge cast.* A wedge-shaped portion is cut from the cast. The edges are brought together and held with plaster reinforcement. This cast is used to overcome angulation in a fracture.
10. *Plaster splint.* Six or more thicknesses of plaster of the desired width and length may be applied to the posterior part of an extremity and secured with gauze or a cotton elastic bandage. Excess water is pressed from the plaster splint after it is immersed in water. A splint may be used for immobilization of a fracture of the ulna or fibula. Inflatable air splints are commercially available.
11. *Hairpin or sugar tong splint.* A splint twice as long as the lower arm and hand is used for a fracture of the ulna or radius. After the plaster is soaked, it may be covered with stockinette. Starting with one end on the back of the hand, the splint is placed around the flexed elbow. The palm of the hand and fingers rest on the other end of it. It is secured with a bandage.
12. *Abduction hip splint.* An abduction hip splint keeps hips in constant abduction. If desired for postoperative management, it is applied immediately after a hip procedure.
13. *Plaster rope.* Plaster rope may support the arm in a shoulder spica or join legs in a bilateral hip spica. It is made by twisting a wet roll of plaster bandage into a rope as it is unwound, fanfolding to the desired length and drawing it through a cupped hand to blend the strands. A wooden splint may be incorporated into the rope for reinforcement.
14. *Molds.* Molds are made as plaster patterns for removable metal or leather braces for the body, neck, or extremities.

Trimming, Removing, and Changing Casts

Rough edges of plaster are trimmed off, and the edges of a cast are covered with stockinette or adhesive tape to protect the patient's skin. Instruments specifically designed for cutting through plaster must be used for trimming or removing casts. These include the following:

- Plaster knives, which have short, slightly curved blades.
- Plaster scissors, which are heavy bandage scissors.

- Electric cast cutter, which is an oscillating saw. It cuts the cast but not the stockinette or other padding under it because the padding moves with the oscillations. The patient's skin also moves somewhat and is not injured if touched lightly, although care should always be taken not to touch the skin. One model has a vacuum attached to pick up the plaster dust created by the saw. A carbide steel blade is recommended for cutting a fiberglass cast. (A regular blade dulls quickly and can result in an inadvertent burn to the patient.)
- Cast spreader, which is a long-handled instrument that has thin, serrated jaws that can be inserted in the cutting line to pry open the cast.
- Cast bender, which is a heavy forceps-type instrument used to bend a small portion of the edge of a cast away from an area, such as a portion of a jacket away from the mouth and chin, to give freer movement.

Sharp plaster knives or scissors are usually used to trim casts. For large casts the electric cast cutter may be used, for example, to cut an opening over the abdomen of a body jacket. In a hip spica, adequate space is provided for use of the bedpan without soiling. If it is necessary to cut a "window" (i.e., a small opening in a cast to remove sutures or to inspect an area), it is put back in place and secured with a few turns of the plaster bandage. An opening in a cast encourages swelling of the tissues under it, known as window edema.

When the edema in a wound under a cast recedes, the cast does not furnish as much immobilization as may be desired. The cast is usually changed at this stage. A cast may be changed periodically during long-term immobilization because muscles atrophy with disuse. The cast becomes loose as muscle size decreases.

Skin sutures are removed at the time of a cast change if the cast was applied following a surgical procedure. A sterile suture removal tray should be ready for use when requested. Sterile sheet wadding may be needed to cover the wound after sutures are removed and before another cast is applied.

If the patient has been in a cast for some time, the skin is apt to be oily, somewhat soiled, and rough. If the surgeon wishes the skin cleansed before applying another cast, only superficial dirt can be removed. Scrubbing off oily scales may cause irritation. Usually skin is not washed but rubbed with cold cream or powdered with talc before sheet wadding and a new cast is applied.

A large, plastic-lined trash container is used for disposal of the wrappings, trimmings, and removed cast during cast application and removal. The knives, scissors, cutter, spreader, and bender are washed promptly after use. Before instruments are put away, oil is applied to all instrument joints to prevent rust and corrosion.

COMPLICATIONS FOLLOWING ORTHOPAEDIC SURGERY

Thromboembolism is the most common postoperative complication of orthopaedic surgery, particularly if the patient must be immobilized for an extended period. Pneumonia can be fatal for older persons. Urinary tract infection and skin breakdown also are potential problems, particularly in geriatric patients. As previously emphasized, wound infection can be devastating.

Embolus

Fat embolism is possible following fracture of a long bone or crush injury. The yellow bone marrow at the point of the fracture of the long bone releases adipose cells into the circulation. The fat emboli enter the pulmonary circulation and cause the release of fatty acids. The alveoli are damaged, and the lung surfactant is rendered ineffective.

Thromboemboli can result from deep vein thrombosis. Any vessel wall injury can cause this event. Pulmonary emboli prevent the gas exchange in the lung. Air can enter the lung, but ventilation cannot take place because of vascular obstruction at the level of the pulmonary artery. Waste gasses cannot be exchanged. A vena cava filter may be indicated.

Bibliography

AAOS Task Force on AIDS and Orthopaedic Surgery: *Recommendations for the prevention of human immunodeficiency virus (HIV) transmission in the practice of orthopaedic surgery,* Park Ridge, Ill, 1989, American Academy of Orthopaedic Surgeons.
Baehser-Griffith P et al: Arthroscopic repairs of triangular fibrocartilage complex tears, *AORN J* 66(1):101-111, 1997.
Brown C et al: Surgical treatment of patients with open tibial fractures, *AORN J* 63(5):875-896, 1996.
Clasby L, Young MA: Management of sports-related anterior cruciate ligament injuries, *AORN J* 66(4):609-630, 1997.
Farrell LA: Arthroscopic rotator cuff repairs using suture anchors, *AORN J* 62(5):739-750, 1995.
Gregory B: *Orthopaedic surgery,* St Louis, 1994, Mosby.
Klinger DL: Acetabular fractures, *AORN J* 61(1):157-178, 1995.
Lenke LG et al: Lumbar disc herniation, *AORN J* 59(6):1230-1248, 1994.
Meeker MH, Rothrock JC: *Alexander's care of the patient in surgery,* ed 11, St Louis, 1999, Mosby.
Owens RA: Total shoulder arthroplasty, *AORN J* 65(5):927-932, 1997.
Pellins TA: How to manage hip fractures, *Am J Nurs* 94(4):46-50, 1994.
Roth M: Metacarpophalangeal joint implant arthroplasty, *AORN J* 60(6):929-942, 1994.
Schramm CA et al: Triple arthrodesis, *AORN J* 64(1):31-52, 1996.

Chapter 38

Ophthalmic Surgery

 Chapter Objectives

After studying this chapter, the learner will be able to:

- Identify the pertinent anatomy of the eye and surrounding structures.
- Describe the procedures performed on the eye for glaucoma.
- Discuss the advantages and disadvantages of intraocular lens implantation.
- Describe the actions of mydriatic and miotic drugs.

The main causes of blindness are retinal disorders, glaucoma, and cataracts. Although a substitute system for vision in the eye, one of the most intricate organs in the body, does not exist, modern ophthalmic techniques can cure or greatly improve many types of impaired vision. Ocular disorders may be the initial manifestations of a systemic disease, such as diabetes. Early detection and referral on the part of an alert ophthalmologist can be both lifesaving and sight-preserving.

HISTORICAL BACKGROUND

Disorders of the eye have been well documented throughout history. The word *cataract,* an opacification of the crystalline lens of the eye, is originally derived from the Greek word *kataraxtos* (was translated in Arabic to mean *mist of a waterfall*). The cataract has been called by various names throughout history (e.g., *pearl of the eye*).

Cataract awareness probably extends back at least 3000 years. This belief is supported by the finding of Bronze Age (2000-1000 BC) instruments, such as those used for an ancient couching or reclination treatment. Couching consisted of striking a blow to the front of the eye with a sharp instrument to spontaneously dislocate the opacified lens and push it back into the vitreous cavity. Light then entered the pupil. Couching was performed by the Hindus, Greeks, Romans, and Arabs.

In the early Christian era, Celsus differentiated between incipient (beginning) and mature cataracts. Galen thought the white opacity to be partly in the lens and partly in the aqueous humor in the form of a membrane floating between the lens and the iris. That belief was held, and couching was practiced sporadically until 1748, when Jacques Daviel (1693-1762), a French surgeon, performed the first deliberate lens extraction. During the first half of the twentieth century, extracapsular cataract extraction was the accepted technique until an intracapsular technique became popular in the mid-1940s.

The first corneal transplant in which a scarred cornea was replaced with a clear donor cornea was performed around 1817. It failed because animal tissue (xenograft) was used instead of human tissue (allograft). The first reported full-thickness graft of full corneal depth to remain clear occurred in 1905. Although attempted in the interval, corneal transplantation did not become an established technique until after World War II. Since then, the technique has been refined to produce a high rate of favorable outcomes.

In the early eighteenth century, attempts to implant lenses were unsuccessful. The modern era of plastic intraocular lens implantation evolved from an incidental observation. Surgeons in England noted a lack of reactivity to plastic fragments from shattered plane canopies that penetrated the eyes of fighter pilots during World War II. Posterior chamber lenses placed in the 1950s produced disappointing long-term results, mainly because of dislocation. These lenses had to be removed because of inadequate fixation. The first series of anterior chamber lenses, which were placed in front of the iris, sometimes produced delayed corneal damage. The iris-supported lenses were designed to avoid this complication but are seldom used because of mechanical problems such as dislocation and corneal irritation. Modifications in the design of anterior chamber lenses have reduced complications. Since the 1960s the posterior chamber lens has attained the greatest popularity.

The development of fluorescein angiography, visualization of the entire retinal vascular tree by the injection of a fluorescing dye, has expanded the knowledge of retinal and choroidal physiology and disease. This increased knowledge has resulted in improved therapy.

The advent of ophthalmic lasers that provide ablation of pathologic conditions with light energy was a great step forward. In many patients, laser therapy obviates the need for some surgical procedures. Initially used primarily for vascular diseases such as diabetic retinopathy, laser use has expanded to include corneal reshaping and the treatment of glaucoma and secondary membranes. Ophthalmologists pioneered the use of medical lasers and operating microscopes.

ANATOMY AND PHYSIOLOGY OF THE EYE

A thorough understanding of the anatomic structure and physiology of the eye is fundamental to a comprehension of the surgical procedures.

The eyeballs are framed bilaterally by the bony orbits. Each orbit is comprised of seven separate bones: the maxilla, palatine, frontal, sphenoid, zygoma, ethmoid, and lacrimal bones. Foramina, fissures, and grooves provide stability and access for vessels, nerves, and attachments. Adjacent anatomic structures include the lacrimal apparatus medially, the extraocular muscles and their attachments, and the sinuses.

The globe, or eyeball, is situated within the bony orbit and is surrounded by a padding of fatty tissue. Its position is maintained by extraocular muscles and fascial attachments. The sclera, the white outer tissue layer of the globe, is contiguous with the transparent avascular cornea anteriorly. The conjunctiva is the mucous membrane that lines the inner side of the upper and lower eyelids and the exposed portion of the sclera, except for the cornea (Figure 38-1).

The eyeball is divided into two segments: anterior and posterior. The anterior segment of the eye includes the cornea, the anterior chamber filled with aqueous fluid (humor), the circular pigmented iris, and the lens. The lens consists of a

Figure 38-1   Front view of eye.

Figure 38-2   Anatomy of the eye. **A,** Anterior segment: *1,* cornea; *2,* anterior chamber; *3,* pupil; *4,* iris; *5,* lens; *6,* ciliary body; *7,* zonule. **B,** Posterior segment: *8,* vitreous body; *9,* retina; *10,* choroid; *11,* sclera; *12,* optic nerve; *13,* central retinal artery.

clear, transparent gelatinous protein encased in a capsule. It is supported by a series of suspensory ligaments called zonules. The posterior segment, the portion of the eye behind the lens, contains the vitreous fluid (which must be clear for vision), the retina, and the choroid linings, which are the vascular nourishing layers (Figure 38-2).

Innervation of vision and sensory transmission is derived from the second cranial nerve (optic nerve) (Figure 38-3). Motor innervation extends from the third cranial nerve (oculomotor nerve) to the rectus muscles. The superior oblique muscles are innervated by the fourth cranial nerve (trochlear nerve). The lateral rectus muscle is innervated by the sixth cranial nerve (abducens nerve).

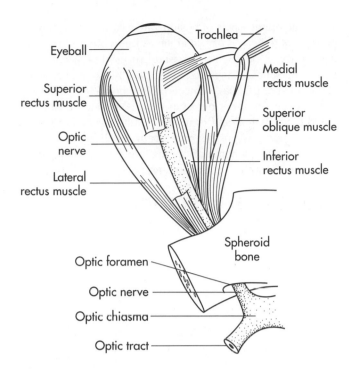

Eyeball
Trochlea
Superior rectus muscle
Medial rectus muscle
Optic nerve
Superior oblique muscle
Lateral rectus muscle
Inferior rectus muscle
Optic foramen
Spheroid bone
Optic nerve
Optic chiasma
Optic tract

Figure 38-3 Location of optic nerve in relation to eye muscles.

The arterial supply of the eyeball, muscles, and eyelids comes from the ophthalmic artery, which is a branch of the internal carotid artery. The retina has a separate blood supply that is derived from the central retinal artery and vein.

The physiology of vision requires the following:

- Functioning visual apparatus
- Source of light
- Intact neurovascular communication with the brain
- Interpretation by the brain of what is seen

The eye resembles a camera with a compound lens system. Light rays emanating from an object in the field of vision are transmitted to the eye, where they traverse the optical system to reach the retina. The retina corresponds to the film of the camera. The area of highest sensitivity for details is called the macula, which is located approximately in the center of the retina at the posterior pole. The intensity of light is automatically determined by the size of the pupil, which is controlled by the iris muscles. The iris functions like the shutter of a camera.

The optical system is comprised of the transparent cornea, or window of the eye; the aqueous fluid behind the cornea; the pupil, or opening in the colored iris; and the lens. The naturally flexible lens focuses light rays by bending them to form an image on the retina, the innermost layer of the eye that contains the visual sensory nerve endings. These cells are connected to nerve fibers that converge toward the brain to become the optic nerve. The sensory cells translate patterns of light into nervous impulses, which are transmitted to the brain via the optic nerve. The occipital portion of the brain interprets the images of light rays registered on the retina.

OPHTHALMIC SURGICAL PATIENT CARE

Impaired vision may produce prolonged severe stress and alter the patient's self-image. Most patients with impaired vision are older adults. When caring for these patients, the health care provider should reassure them, exercise patience, give directions clearly, anticipate needs, and check their comfort level. Specific patient care considerations include, but are not limited to, the following:

1. Urinary urgency can be a problem in geriatric patients or in patients receiving diuretic medication. Although the patient should void before coming to the operating room (OR), offer the patient the use of a bedpan before he or she transfers to the operating bed. Severe urinary urgency can cause increased intraocular pressure (IOP) during the procedure. Strain and gross movement are dangerous and are to be avoided.
2. The surgeon and circulator verify the intended surgical site with the patient and with the office records. After confirmation and to avoid error, some surgeons place an indelible mark on the side of the patient's neck that corresponds to the affected eye. A small, removable sticker can be used for the same purpose.
3. The patient is placed in the supine position on the operating bed so the head and body are aligned. The top of the head is in line with the edge of the operating bed for accessibility. The head should not be turned greatly in either direction; the head is stabilized in a ring-shaped pillow (donut). The patient's gown is untied at the neck to prevent pressure. Any obstruction to venous circulation can cause undue increased IOP, which can produce a loss of vitreous humor when the eye is opened. To assist venous return from the head, the operating bed is tilted so the patient's head is elevated by 5 to 10 degrees. For long procedures, an egg crate or gel pad mattress may be placed on the bed.
4. Skin preparation and draping procedures are performed according to routine. Sterile plastic drapes are often placed over woven textile drapes to contain lint, especially before lens implantation. A patient with a drape over the face is often apprehensive and afraid of suffocating. To help eliminate the feeling of claustrophobia, the drape can be placed over a Mayo stand or clipped to an IV pole to create a tentlike space above the patient's nose and mouth. Oxygen is delivered via nasal prongs or insufflated to the facial area beneath the drape at 6 to 8 L/min.
5. A quiet, stimulant-free environment is provided for the awake patient who is receiving a local anesthetic.
6. Because the patient has no defensive blink reflex to protect the retina from light exposure, some surgeons use a sterile, opaque pupillary shield to protect the patient's retina from phototoxic damage caused by prolonged exposure to illumination of the microscope. Some scopes have a sensor near the eyepiece that dims the light

source when the surgeon is not looking directly into the scope. The light reverts back to the desired intensity when the surgeon is positioned at the eyepiece.

7. The team should prepare for emergencies by anticipating problems. Fast action can make the difference between a seeing eye or nonseeing eye postoperatively. The following are potential complications:
   a. A systemic reaction to medications or local anesthetic drugs and cardiac arrest.
   b. A loss of vitreous, which requires the removal of vitreous from the anterior chamber with a vitreotome to prevent prolapse of the wound, severe inflammation, or an updrawn pupil.
   c. An expulsive hemorrhage or an expulsion of ocular contents, which requires a sharp knife (e.g., Beaver blade or Wheeler knife) for fast cutdown into the pars plana area and an 18-gauge needle or cannula attached to a syringe to aspirate blood and reduce pressure in an effort to save the eye and vision.
   d. Instrument failure. Hand aspiration devices should be available for immediate use.

8. A wide variety of fine-sized absorbable and nonabsorbable sutures are used. The scrub person follows the manufacturer's recommendations for handling these delicate materials and needles with the appropriate needleholders. Special techniques are used in microsurgery.

9. Sponges consist of precut compressed cellulose on sticks.

10. No foreign material should be introduced into the surgical wound. In intraocular procedures, no portion of any instrument or item intended to enter the eye should be touched by a gloved hand. To remove any debris or impurity, intraocular lenses (IOLs) are soaked and rinsed in balanced salt solution (BSS) and sometimes lubricated with sodium hyaluronate (Healon) before insertion.

11. Inflammation should be kept as minimal as possible because even slight inflammation may result in total functional loss. Steroids are often administered locally, subconjunctivally and, sometimes, systemically. The eye may respond violently to the slightest amount of trauma.

12. Antibiotic drops are often instilled topically for 24 hours preoperatively and postoperatively.

13. A sterile eye pad is applied at the conclusion of the surgical procedure. A protective shield is secured over the eye pad to guard against mechanical injury. Absorbable corneal shields may be used.

14. The patient should not be permitted to participate in the move from the operating bed following intraocular procedures; this prevents a sudden rise in IOP and/or dislocation of the IOL implant.

15. Arm restraints are essential for infants and young children. Restraints are applied to adults only under extreme circumstances, such as disorientation. The use of side rails is standard procedure for all patients undergoing ophthalmic surgery.

An important aspect of postoperative care is informing the patient not to get out of bed alone. A fall or injury to the eye can nullify an otherwise successful surgical procedure. The patient must not do anything to increase IOP (e.g., bend over at the waist or lift heavy objects). Deep breathing postoperatively is encouraged, but coughing is avoided because it could increase IOP and rupture the suture line. The patient should report any postoperative pain, swelling, redness, or discharge. The outcome of ophthalmic procedures includes a cosmetic as well as a functional aspect.

SPECIAL FEATURES OF OPHTHALMIC SURGERY

The patient undergoing ophthalmic surgery faces impairment or loss of vision if the outcome of the surgical intervention is unfavorable. Special features of ophthalmic surgery aim to prevent such a loss. Surgical procedures on the eye are extremely delicate and require precision instrumentation, a steady hand, and quiet surroundings. The operating microscope, all accessory equipment, and microinstruments should be set up and checked before the surgical procedure. The outcome of the procedure depends on the condition of the instruments. The tips of these expensive, fragile microinstruments should be protected and handled with extreme care before, during, and after use.

Operating Microscope

Most ophthalmic surgeons use the operating microscope for intraocular procedures. When the operating microscope is used, the operating bed should be mechanically secure and the patient's head should be stabilized. Inadvertent movement is not tolerated because of the minute surgical field. The headrest should be narrow so it does not obstruct the surgeon's approach to the surgical site from the sides of the vertical column of the microscope. The patient is instructed about the importance of remaining still during the surgical procedure. Otherwise, the patient could easily move out of the field of vision under the microscope or precipitate a complication.

The assistant observes the surgical procedure through an assistant's ocular and irrigates the cornea with BSS to prevent drying. The assistant should bring to the surgeon's attention any potentially unsatisfactory situation that the surgeon cannot observe from his or her position. Some scrub persons are trained to first assist. The caffeine intake of the surgeon and the assistants should be limited before the procedure to promote a steady hand when using microinstrumentation under the microscope.

Ophthalmic Drugs

Many drugs are critical to the preparation of the eye for the surgical procedure. Orders for patient preparation often contain common abbreviations that identify the eye(s) to receive drops: OD (right eye), OS (left eye), and OU (both eyes). Before skin preparation, a registered nurse instills the medications and anesthetic drops as ordered. The following procedures should be observed when instilling eye drops:

1. Wash your hands.
2. Identify the correct medication, eye, and patient.
3. Explain the procedure to the patient.
4. Tilt back the patient's head and tell the patient to look up. While gently pulling down on the lower lid, instill the medication in the middle third of the inner aspect of the lower lid. Release the lid while the patient slowly closes the eye to retain the drop; let the patient close the eye between repeated drops. In a struggling child, have the patient tilt the head back and close both eyes. Instill the medication at the inner canthus. The drop will roll into the eye as child reopens it.

   Some medications, such as atropine, may have a systemic effect. To prevent drainage into the tear duct, nose, and stomach, gently blot excess fluid. In small infants or young children, systemic absorption is avoided by applying finger pressure over the lacrimal sac region (inner canthus) of both eyes simultaneously for 1 minute.
5. Administer only the specified number of drops.
6. Read the label on the vial before each instillation.
7. Each patient should receive a fresh, single-use, disposable vial of medication, which is discarded after use.

Mydriatic or Miotic Drugs

Medications may be given to alter the size of the pupil:

- *Mydriatic drops:* 2.5% or 10% phenylephrine hydrochloride (Neo-Synephrine) to dilate the pupil.
- *Mydriatic-cycloplegic drops:* 1% cyclopentolate hydrochloride (Cyclogyl), 1% atropine, and 0.25% scopolamine hydrobromide (Isopto-Hyoscine) to dilate the pupil, paralyze the ciliary body, diminish the reaction to trauma, and prevent anterior synechiae (e.g., adherence of iris to the lens). These drugs are longer acting than phenylephrine.
- *Miotic drops:* 2% pilocarpine hydrochloride to constrict the pupil.

Local and Topical Anesthesia

Except in children and select patients, local and topical anesthetics are commonly used for ophthalmic surgical procedures. Most surgical procedures are scheduled as monitored anesthesia care (MAC) or attended local. An anesthesia provider is present to monitor the patient and to administer oxygen and/or supplement the local anesthetic if necessary. Intravenous (IV) midazolam (Versed) and/or fentanyl (Sublimaze) or propofol (Diprivan) are often given to relax the patient. The sedative effects of these agents increase the patient's tolerance to procedures. If a general anesthetic is used, the usual general anesthesia routines are followed.

Local anesthesia consists of the following:

1. Topical instillation of anesthetic drops. The drug used may be 0.5% proparacaine hydrochloride (Ophthaine), 0.5% tetracaine hydrochloride (Pontocaine), or 2% lidocaine hydrochloride (Xylocaine MPF [methylparaben free]).
2. Local infiltration by injection of the lids and tissue around the eyes with anesthetic medication.
3. Retrobulbar block. An absolutely quiet eye is necessary, especially at high magnifications of the microscope. When general anesthesia is used, some surgeons administer a retrobulbar block for immobility and to lower IOP. A popular solution for this block consists of a mixture of equal parts of 2% or 4% lidocaine hydrochloride and 0.75% bupivacaine hydrochloride with or without hyaluronidase (Wydase), 3.75 units/ml for penetration. A 25-gauge × 1½ inches (3.8 cm) needle with a sharp, rounded point (e.g., Atkinson needle) and a 5-ml syringe are used. The surgeon inserts the needle behind the eyeball to obtain anesthesia of the globe and paralysis of the muscles. The patient is asked to look up and away from the injection site and is told that a slight burning sensation may accompany the injection. Up to 5 ml of solution may be slowly and carefully injected.

   Retrobulbar block may be followed by intermittent massage of the eye to soften it, lower IOP, and facilitate surgical manipulation during cataract extraction, especially when insertion of an IOL is being contemplated. Massage is continued until the IOP is lowered to a satisfactory level (e.g., 10 to 12 scale reading on sterile Schiötz tonometer). Some surgeons apply the Honan balloon pressure device to soften the eyeball after a retrobulbar block. In using this device, a small inflatable balloon is placed directly over the closed eyelid and is secured with a strap around the head. The balloon is inflated to 30 to 40 mm Hg for 5 to 10 minutes to lower intravitreal pressure.
4. Peribulbar anesthesia. This is an alternative to retrobulbar injection. With this method, injections are made in the soft tissue superior and inferior to the globe rather than behind it. A greater amount of the same anesthetic solution used for retrobulbar injection is used for peribulbar anesthesia. With this procedure, adequate anesthesia is obtained without the risk of retrobulbar hemorrhage.

Ophthalmic Solutions

Extreme and constant care must be used with ophthalmic solutions. Nearly all of these solutions are colorless and may be stored in similar receptacles. These solutions are immediately and individually labeled by the scrub person; the solution is discarded if the identification is missing. Solutions for intraocular use must be separated from all other solutions. Ideally, these solutions should be filtered with micropore filters before injection.

Epinephrine or other sympathomimetics may have side effects when used with some anesthetic agents. Therefore the surgeon should check with the anesthesia provider before using medications intraoperatively. Medications that may induce vomiting are also avoided. Any straining or gross movement may cause intraocular hemorrhage, a sudden rise in IOP that results in a loss of vitreous, or the expulsion of ocular contents through the wound; all of these conditions can cause blindness.

OCULAR SURGICAL PROCEDURES

For convenience, surgical treatment of the eye can be divided into two main classifications:

1. *Extraocular:* conditions affecting the exterior surface of the eye or the orbit
2. *Intraocular:* conditions pertaining to the interior contents of the eye

Extraocular Procedures

Eyelid

Excision of Neoplasm of the Eyelid   Tissue may be excised with a knife, an electrosurgical unit (ESU), diathermy, or cryosurgery. An extremely common but benign tumor of the lid is the chalazion, a cystic alteration of one of the oil-secreting meibomian glands in the lid. The resulting accumulation of oil forms a hard tumor of the lid and requires excision. The excision is usually an office or ambulatory surgical procedure.

Following removal of a malignant lesion of the lid, plastic procedures such as Z-plasty, sliding flaps from adjacent areas, or full- or partial-thickness flaps from the opposing lid are used to close the defect.

Correction of Ptosis   Ptosis, a drooping of the upper lid, may be acquired in adulthood but is more commonly congenital. For the levator aponeurosis procedure, an incision is made on the front surface of the lid to expose the tarsus and the aponeurosis. The tarsus is sutured to the aponeurosis, and the skin incision is closed. For the frontalis suspension procedure, the anterior surface of the upper lid is incised at the crease, and two smaller incisions are made above the eyebrow. A graft of fascia or synthetic material is attached to the tarsus and passed through the deep lid tissue and brought out through the eyebrow incisions. The graft material is secured and the skin incisions are closed.

Repair of Acquired Malformation of the Eyelid   Conditions such as senile ectropion or entropion most commonly affect the lower lid. Ectropion is a condition in which either lid is everted (turned out) so as to expose the conjunctival surface. Entropion is the opposite condition, in which the lid margin is inverted (turned in). As a result, the eyelashes often abrade the cornea. Various procedures may be used to correct both conditions.

Blepharoplasty   A common result of aging is the stretching of the eyelid skin and the bulging of orbital fat from between the muscle fibers of the lids. Both conditions cause cosmetic disfigurement or baggy lids and, in extreme cases, may obstruct vision. In blepharoplasty, redundant fold(s) of skin and herniated pockets of fat are removed, and defects in the muscle layer are repaired. Transconjunctival blepharoplasty is performed by making a small incision into the conjunctiva of the lower lid and removing fat pads. Small bleeders are cauterized with a disposable electrosurgical pencil.

Lacrimal Apparatus

Lacrimal Duct Dilation   Lacrimal duct dilation is performed for excessive tearing. A series of probes, graduated in size, is introduced one by one into the duct system to permit freer drainage of tears.

Dacryocystectomy   Extirpation or removal of the lacrimal sac is performed for chronic dacryocystitis. This procedure does not reestablish the tear drainage system.

Dacryocystorhinostomy   Construction of a new opening into the nasal cavity from the lacrimal sac is performed to correct congenital malformation of or trauma to the nasolacrimal duct. A new tear drainage system is constructed.

Extraocular Muscle

Procedures on the oculomotor muscles, which control eye movement, are performed to correct misalignment that interferes with the ability of the two eyes to remain in simultaneous focus on a viewed object. The surgical procedures correct muscle imbalance by strengthening a weak muscle or by weakening an overactive one. Although commonly performed on children, these muscle procedures may be required in adult patients for the following:

- Untreated childhood strabismus (squint)
- Unsatisfactory result from a childhood surgical procedure
- Trauma to the brainstem or to the orbit with resultant muscle injury or paralysis
- Systemic disease (e.g., thyroid exophthalmos) and muscle paralysis
- Cerebrovascular accident (CVA) with resultant muscle paralysis

Orbit

Decompression   Decompression is the treatment for severe exophthalmos, or a protrusion of the eyeball(s), that does not respond to medical treatment.

Orbital Tumors   Depending on the location of the orbital tumor, exploration may be approached through a lateral wall or the roof of the orbit. This procedure may involve a multidisciplinary team of surgeons.

Surgical Removal of the Eye

Following removal of an eyeball, the patient is fitted with an artificial eye to restore cosmetic appearance. A spherical implant, such as silicone, plastic, tantalum, or hydroxyapatite, may be used to line the orbit and provide support for a prosthetic eye. The eye muscles are sutured to the implant, thereby providing natural movement, allowing the growth of surrounding tissue, and preventing the lower lid from sagging. The type of prosthesis that can be used depends on the procedure used to remove the eyeball.

Enucleation Enucleation is the complete removal of the eyeball and the severing of its muscular attachments. The muscle stumps are preserved, with the space between the stumps forming a pocket for the spherical plastic artificial eye. Overlying fasciae and conjunctivae are closed to hold the prosthesis in the socket. The contraction of eye muscles causes the prosthesis to move in the socket, simulating normal eye movements.

Evisceration Evisceration removes the contents of the eyeball only; the outer sclera and muscles are left intact for attachment to a prosthesis. This procedure reduces the danger of transmitting an intraocular infection to the orbit and brain. Predisposing factors for evisceration include destruction of the eyeball by injury or disease and absolute glaucoma (hard blind eye).

Exenteration Exenteration is the removal of the entire eye and orbital contents, including tendon, fatty, and fibrous tissues. This procedure is performed for a malignant tumor of the lids or eyeball that has extended into the orbit. Extensive plastic reconstruction is necessary before an artificial eye can be fitted.

Intraocular Procedures

Many ophthalmic surgeons subspecialize in anterior segment surgery on the cornea, iris, and lens or in posterior segment surgery on the vitreous body, retina, and sclera. Both types of surgery require specialized instrumentation. Most surgeons use the operating microscope for intraocular procedures.

Cornea

Although it consists of resilient tissue, the continually exposed cornea is especially susceptible to injury and infection.

Cauterization Cauterization with chemicals or heat is sometimes used for a corneal ulceration that does not respond to antibiotics. This is sometimes performed for herpes simplex virus infections of the corneal epithelium. Cauterization may be used in conjunction with topical antiviral agents.

Pterygium Pterygium is a benign growth of conjunctival tissue over the corneal surface. Although usually slow growing, pterygia can become fairly aggressive, especially in southern climates. A significant decrease in visual acuity secondary to induced astigmatism and corneal scarring can result from the abnormal growth. A popular surgical technique devised for the eradication of pterygia is the bare sclera method. This method involves excision of the entire pterygium, leaving an area of bare sclera. Beta radiation may be used as an adjunct to surgical treatment.

Corneal Transplantation (Keratoplasty)

With keratoplasty, a damaged cornea is removed and replaced with a healthy cornea from a human donor (Figure 38-4). The cornea must be clear to permit light to enter and focus on the retina. Thus this procedure is indicated when scars or opacities on the cornea reduce or destroy vision by preventing the transmission of a clear image. Corneal opacity may result from degenerative changes, scars from chemical burns, perforated corneal ulcers, trauma, or edema following a cataract surgical procedure. In addition, ocular surgery such as phacoemulsification, vitrectomy, and IOL implantation has the potential to damage the corneal endothelium.

Because the cornea is avascular, keratoplasty is the most successful transplantation procedure and has considerably less rejection phenomena than all other tissues except bone. The greatest advance in technique to reduce the rate of rejection and the restriction of activity during convalescence

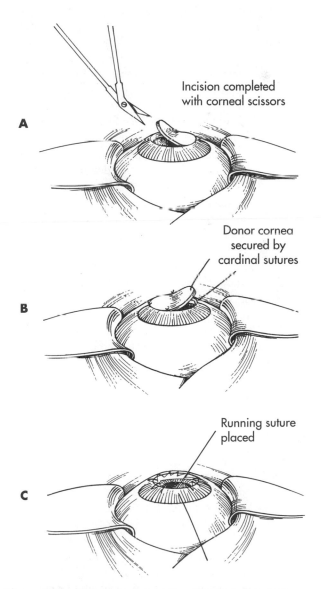

Incision completed
with corneal scissors

A

Donor cornea
secured by
cardinal sutures

B

Running suture
placed

C

Figure 38-4 Corneal transplantation (keratoplasty). **A,** Damaged cornea is excised with corneal scissors. **B,** Donor cornea is secured by cardinal sutures. **C,** Continuous suture remains in situ.

has been the use of the operating microscope and microsutures. Continuous 10-0 or 11-0 nylon sutures are left in situ with minimal tissue reaction. Two types of grafts are used:

1. *Full-thickness grafts:* The common type. The entire thickness of the cornea, usually 6.5 to 8 mm in diameter, is replaced (penetrating keratoplasty).
2. *Partial-thickness or lamellar grafts:* Less popular. Only the top layer of the cornea, not its entire depth, is replaced (lamellar keratoplasty).

An opaque cornea is an optically nonfunctioning one. The goal is to provide recipients with the highest quality corneal tissue. A fresh, healthy cornea cut from the promptly enucleated eye of a relatively young donor within 4 to 6 hours of death is considered the best for transplantation. The cornea should be inserted in the recipient eye, which has a healthy retina and optic nerve, as soon as possible to preserve viability and to prevent opacity. The acceptable times for collection of tissue after death and transplantation may vary among eye banks.

Donor tissue criteria include the following:

1. The consent for enucleation must conform with state laws. Responsibility for obtaining legal consent may rest with the person who will perform the enucleation. A certified eye bank technician may enucleate the eyes.
2. Medical information about the potential donor is evaluated. Some conditions that preclude the use of donor tissue are an unknown cause of death, previous intraocular surgery, Reye's syndrome, lymphosarcoma, rabies, and transmissible diseases such as hepatitis, human immunodeficiency virus (HIV), and Creutzfeldt-Jakob disease (CJD). Donor information must be documented on the donor screening form that accompanies the tissue. A copy should be filed at the eye bank.
3. The endothelium, the very sensitive inner single layer of corneal cells, must be kept intact for eventual transparency of the graft. Either the entire donor globe is removed, or the cornea with scleral rim is excised for transplantation. Important factors to optimize the success of the transplant include sterile technique, the removal of as much conjunctiva as possible from the donor globe, the avoidance of damage to or contamination of the removed eyes, and the use of appropriate transport containers and preservation methods.
4. The donor's eyes are cooled as soon as possible to prevent deleterious effects. The placement of ice bags over the eyes promptly after death slows the metabolism of corneal cells. In general, the sooner the enucleated eyes are refrigerated or the corneas are removed from the globe, the better the quality of the donor tissue. Enucleated eyes are placed in a controlled environment at the eye bank and should be used within 5 hours of procurement.
5. The donor's cornea is carefully evaluated for epithelial defects, clarity, the presence of any foreign body, or any evidence of jaundice or infection. Endothelial cell count is a determining factor in estimating the prognosis of the transplant. The higher the count and the more regular the cellular pattern, the better the tissue. Age is not a deterrent if tissue is acceptable for transplantation, but donors younger than 70 years of age are preferred. The evaluation form must be completed and must accompany the tissue. The transplant surgeon also may receive specular microscopic photographs of the endothelium.

Donor tissue preservation methods include the following:

- *Preservative medium.* Favored by many eye banks, Optisol GS sterile buffered tissue culture contains the antibiotics gentamicin and streptomycin and allows storage for 3 to 7 days. In the OR, the surgeon should inspect the container before using the cornea. If the cornea is used, the remaining corneoscleral rim should be placed in a culture medium and sent to the laboratory for culture. The incidence of positive cultures is low. The cornea should not be used and the eye bank should be notified if the medium is turbid or contaminated, such as by a crack in the container.
- *Cryopreservation.* Both cryopreserved corneal and scleral tissue can be used for transplantation or for patching purposes. In general, their use is limited to emergency procedures when fresh tissue is not available. Usually this tissue is used less than 6 months after cryopreservation. Precise freezing and defrosting methods are of crucial importance in preventing injury to the endothelium. Corneal metabolism resumes with defrosting; therefore when the solution is thawed, the team should work rapidly because of the extreme time limitation. The tissue should be placed immediately within its natural anatomic environment to enhance the potential for successful grafting.

Regardless of the storage method, tissue is preferably used as soon as practical after donation. In the OR, adequate preparation, teamwork, and standardized transplantation procedures are imperative. The recipient eye is trephined to receive the donor cornea. A separate sterile donor table is set for the surgeon to use in preparing the donor tissue to the exact measurement needed for the recipient eye.

Following a surgical procedure, a tissue recipient information form is completed to indicate how the tissue was used. This form is mailed to the eye bank, where it is kept on file. If the tissue is contaminated, the donor number and source can easily be traced. Information on the forms includes recipient medical information; previous keratoplasties; the date, type, and details of the current surgical procedure; and the estimate of success.

Available corneal tissue is in limited supply, which places restraints on transplantation. Numerous eye banks in the United States constitute the Eye Bank Association of America, which is tangentially associated with the International Eye Bank. These groups are central clearinghouses for the distribution of accessible tissue. They follow a stringent code of ethics in their functions to inform the public of the need for eye donations, to procure donated eyes, to assist in the optimal use of donor corneas locally, or to arrange for transportation to an area of greater need. Tissue procurement is facilitated by the following:

- Distribution of donor forms from eye banks and organ donation organizations.
- Organ donation consent forms affixed to driver licenses. Family consent is still required before procurement.
- Education of medical and health care personnel to alert them to ask families of deceased patients for donations. Some state laws require a donation request.

Phototherapeutic Keratectomy

In phototherapeutic keratectomy (PTK), scar tissue is removed from the cornea with an excimer laser. This procedure restores vision that has been blocked by scars from an infection, injury, or inherited condition. PTK may obviate the need for a corneal transplant. More information about excimer lasers can be found at **www.excimernet.com.**

Refractive Keratoplasty (Corneal Reshaping)

Refractive keratoplasty includes a group of surgical procedures designed to alter the shape and refractive power (i.e., focusing power) of the cornea to minimize the optical problems of myopia, aphakia, keratoconus, hyperopia, and astigmatism:

1. Radial keratotomy reduces myopia (nearsightedness) by making multiple small radial incisions in the cornea to approximately 90% of its depth (Figure 38-5). These incisions allow stretching and flattening of the anterior corneal surface, which corrects the refractive error by reducing corneal curvature and bringing light to a focus closer to, or on, the retina (Figure 38-6).

   Radial keratotomy is performed on patients who have occupational requirements for a visual acuity level without the use of glasses or contact lenses, such as certain airline, police, and firefighter positions. The procedure also may be performed for cosmetic reasons. Potential complications include perforations of the cornea, permanent corneal scarring, glaring or variable vision, injury to the lens (causing cataract), and infection. Long-term results are somewhat unpredictable but are improved with microsurgical techniques. This procedure should be limited to patients with healthy eyes. Only low amounts of nearsightedness can be corrected with this procedure.

2. Keratomileusis and keratophakia procedures modify corneal refractivity by using a computerized technique to insert a lathed button of corneal tissue into the cornea. If the patient is the donor (keratomileusis), the anterior lamellae of the cornea are removed, reshaped by cryolathing, and then sutured in place. For keratophakia, the tissue is obtained from another donor and may be preserved. The lenticule is cryolathed during the surgical

Figure 38-5 Corneal incisions for visual improvement of myopia. **A,** Radial keratotomy (RK). **B,** Astigmatic keratotomy (AK).

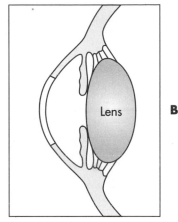

Figure 38-6 Side view of incised corneas. **A,** Radial keratotomy (RK). **B,** Astigmatic keratotomy (AK).

procedure, inserted intralamellarly into the recipient cornea, and sutured in place.

Keratomileusis and keratophakia require a highly specialized experienced team and costly equipment—the computer and the cryolathe for shaping the corneal button. With keratophakia, research is ongoing to develop other materials that may be used in place of human donor tissue. Plastic with a very high water content (similar to continuous-wear contact lens material) has been used.

3. Epikeratophakia is performed to correct extreme refractive errors such as aphakia (absence of lens, which induces extreme hyperopia), myopia, or keratoconus (cone-shaped cornea, which causes extreme astigmatism). The recipient corneal epithelium is removed, and a previously cryolathed and preserved donor button of corneal tissue is sutured onto the corneal surface of the recipient.

4. Corneal sculpting (photorefractive keratectomy) (PRK) is performed to reshape the corneal surface or to remove scars or other surface irregularities. The excimer laser is used to reshape the front corneal contour to correct nearsightedness, farsightedness, and astigmatism. The laser beam removes minute amounts of corneal tissue with each pulse wave without burning through or heating the tissue.

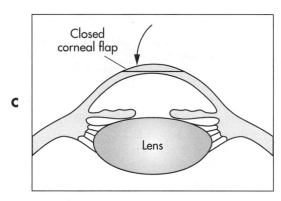

Figure 38-7 Laser in situ keratomileusis (LASIK). **A,** Top layer of cornea is opened like a flap with keratome. **B,** Excimer laser removes thin layers of exposed corneal surface. **C,** Cornea is replaced.

5. Laser in situ keratomileusis (LASIK) is performed to correct myopia (nearsightedness). A combination of excimer laser and keratome is used to remove layers of the cornea. A small flap is raised in the center of the corneal dome. The laser is used to remove micro layers of tissue. The flap of corneal tissue is replaced without the need for suturing (Figure 38-7).
6. Intrastromal corneal rings can be placed to elevate the border of the cornea, causing the central portion to recede. This implantable device was approved for use in 1998 and consists of two arc-shaped segments that are implanted in the circumferential stroma of the cornea. It can be removed surgically if vision correction is not satisfactory (Figure 38-8).

Figure 38-8 Intrastromal corneal rings are used to form a depression in the center of the cornea for correction of myopia. **A,** Intrastromal corneal ring in place. The center of the cornea flattens. **B,** Two arcs form a circle under the edges of the cornea.

Iris

Excision of Iris Prolapse Prolapse may follow an eye laceration or a surgical procedure on the anterior segment. Fresh prolapses may be reduced mechanically during the surgical procedure or pharmacologically with drugs. Older prolapses should be excised to avoid an intraocular infection.

Glaucoma Glaucoma is a disease characterized by abnormally increased intraocular fluid pressure; it often involves the iris. If uncontrolled, glaucoma progresses to atrophy of the optic nerve, hardening of the eyeball, and blindness. The incidence of glaucoma in persons over 40 years of age increases with each decade. There is a familial predisposition to the disease.

IOP is estimated in one of three ways:

1. A Schiötz tonometer records the depth of indentation of the cornea by a plunger of known weight. The degree of indentation is calibrated on the tonometer to correspond to the IOP. The normal numerical value is 10 to 22 mm Hg. The tonometer can be sterilized for use in the OR for preoperative pressure measurement.
2. An applanation tonometer attached to a biomicroscope (slit lamp) records the force required to flatten a specified area of cornea. This method is considered to be the most accurate. The normal value is 10 to 21 mm Hg.
3. An air puff device measures the force of a reflected amount of air blown against the cornea.

Persons suspected of having glaucoma undergo additional testing. Tonography continuously measures the rate of aqueous outflow with an electric tonometer. Visual fields detect diminished peripheral vision. Gonioscopy determines the structure of the angle between the iris and the cornea. Two basic types of glaucoma are classified anatomically by the size of this angle: (1) narrow-angle or angle-closure glaucoma, and (2) wide-angle or open-angle glaucoma.

If the angle is narrow, the iris may mechanically obstruct the outflow of aqueous. This will cause the pressure within the eye to rise and will precipitate an attack of acute glaucoma, an emergency situation that is very painful. Surgical intervention, usually a laser iridotomy, affords relief. It is always necessary to widen the angle for this condition and reduce pressure to avoid damage to the optic nerve. Surgical iridectomy occasionally is necessary.

Wide-angle or open-angle glaucoma is the most common type of glaucoma. It is a chronic type, is often of insidious onset, and may cause permanent visual loss before being detected. The obstruction is not mechanical but is a physiologic lack of ability to filter aqueous. Surgical procedures for this type of disease are performed only if medical and laser therapies are unsuccessful. Laser therapy to the trabecular meshwork (trabeculoplasty) offers an alternative to conventional surgical procedures for some glaucoma patients. One of the following surgical procedures may be preferred:

1. Iridectomy (excising a sector of iris) or iridotomy (cutting a small opening in the iris) is performed to deflate the mechanical obstruction, thus increasing drainage by permitting the normal outflow of aqueous from the posterior to the anterior chamber. Another use of iridectomy is to create a new optical pupillary opening to improve visual acuity for patients with corneal or lens opacity caused by injury or cataract not associated with glaucoma.
2. Filtering-type procedures, of which there are many variations such as trephining and trabeculectomy, create an artificial fistula between the angle of the anterior chamber and the subconjunctival space to bypass the usual blocked outflow channels. Iridectomy is usually performed as part of the procedure to eliminate blockage of the fistula by the underlying iris. The Nd:YAG laser may be used to reopen filtering sites that have scarred closed following previous surgery for glaucoma. The Ho:YAG laser may be used to create an opening in the sclera (sclerostomy) to promote filtration.
3. Cyclodialysis, cyclodiathermy, and cyclocryotherapy are performed to diminish aqueous secretion by the ciliary body. Cyclodialysis involves severing the blood supply of the ciliary body. Cyclodiathermy and cyclocryothermy use the application of heat or cold, respectively, for the same purpose.

Secondary glaucoma is often a complication of an inflammation such as iritis, which usually responds best to medical treatment. On the other hand, neoplasm, vascular obstruction, trauma or hemorrhage, and other causes of obstruction to aqueous drainage may require surgical intervention. Treatment is directed to the primary cause.

Congenital glaucoma, from an inherent defect in the trabecular meshwork or a systemic disorder, manifests soon after birth.

Cataract

A cataract is an opacification of the crystalline lens, its capsule, or both. The more or less opaque lens does not transmit clear images to the retina. Symptoms are related to the location and configuration of the opacity. The cause may be a known metabolic or systemic disease, toxic material, radia-

tion, trauma, or genetic factors, or the etiologic factors may be unknown. Persons are more prone to develop degenerative cataracts with advancing age. Although cataracts often develop in both eyes, each cataract tends to mature at a different rate, and only one is removed at a time. Most ophthalmologists perform cataract surgery as an ambulatory surgical procedure.

Cataracts may be classified as one of the following:

- Congenital
- Senile or primary
- Secondary, resulting from local or systemic disease or eye injury

Surgical removal, followed by appropriate optical rehabilitation, is the only treatment. The surgical procedure to be performed is determined by the patient's age and type of cataract. The procedure is selected according to visual requirements, general health, and the potential for rehabilitation. Cataract extraction is the most frequently performed surgical procedure in adults, and the advent of microsurgery has revolutionized this procedure.

Extracapsular Extraction With extracapsular extraction (ECCE), the lens is delivered through a small incision in the region of the limbus (the junction of the cornea and sclera). The anterior capsule is incised with a cystotome (a miniature hook-shaped knife) or with a capsulorhexis forceps. The nucleus is delivered by manual expression, or it may be aspirated by phacoemulsification (see the discussion of phacoemulsification later in this chapter). The remaining cortex is extracted by irrigation-aspiration, sparing the posterior capsule, which is left in place. Automated mechanical irrigation-aspiration devices are usually used. Some surgeons prefer a manual technique using a two-way cannula and syringe. The wound is closed with a few sutures.

ECCE with preservation of the posterior capsule has revolutionized the practice of artificial lens implantation. The implant can be placed at the time of cataract extraction. It resides in the posterior chamber behind the iris and rests on the posterior capsule. The implant is therefore positioned in almost the identical location of the lens it replaces.

The physiologic advantage of ECCE, with or without phacoemulsification and/or lens implant, is protection of the vitreous and retina by the clear posterior lens capsule, which then serves as an anatomic barrier between the posterior and anterior segments of the eye. Occasionally the posterior capsule remains opaque. Nd:YAG laser capsulotomy is performed at a later date to provide an optically clear opening.

The following innovations have enhanced the advantages of ECCE:

1. An operating microscope with coaxial illumination to clearly view the posterior capsule during aspiration.
2. A phacoemulsifier to remove the nucleus through a tiny (3- to 3.5-mm) incision. The smaller wound facilitates healing and causes less distortion of corneal curvatures.

3. An automated irrigation-aspiration system with an electronic sensor to remove all cortex remnants. This minimizes local foreign protein reaction.
4. A Nd:YAG laser to atomize posterior capsule opacity. The laser achieves a better result than discission/needling, which requires a second surgical intervention. The laser can be used immediately postoperatively, or the procedure can be delayed. The laser can be used under a drop of local anesthetic without requiring an incision and without causing blood loss.
5. An intraocular foldable lens designed to achieve insertion into the posterior chamber through a small incision.

Intracapsular Extraction

Intracapsular extraction (ICCE) is not commonly used unless the natural lens is displaced. Advance planning is necessary on the rare occasions in which it is performed. The entire lens, intact within its capsule, is delivered through a moderately sized incision made in the region of the limbus. Before delivery, an iridectomy or multiple iridotomies are performed, chiefly to prevent iris prolapse and to preserve communication between the anterior and posterior chambers. Depending on the surgeon's preference, the lens is grasped by a forceps, suction device, or cryoextractor.

A miniaturized, sterile disposable cryoextractor facilitates the removal of fragile or dislocated cataracts. The cryoprobe freezes onto the surface of the cataract, thus obtaining secure adherence. The freezing technique greatly reduces the inadvertent rupture of the capsule during extraction. The scrub person should have a BSS irrigator available for use in case it is necessary to unfreeze an unintentional attachment of the cryoextractor to the iris or cornea. The wound is closed watertight with multiple sutures, commonly 10-0 nylon.

With ICCE, the visual axis is free of remnants that might proliferate or opacify to obstruct vision. The success rate for regaining vision is high, but the popularity of this procedure has waned. Fluorescein angiography has identified a number of patients who developed cystoid macular edema postoperatively, resulting in marked loss of visual acuity. ICCE may also be followed by retinal detachment, which is discussed later in this chapter.

Linear Extraction

Linear extraction is performed in young adults. In this procedure, a small incision is made through the limbus. The anterior capsule is incised, and the major portion of it is excised with a cystotome. The soft cataractous material is irrigated from the anterior chamber.

Phacoemulsification

Although the aspiration technique is commonly used in young persons, it was not successful in older adults with senile cataracts until the late 1960s. At that time a sophisticated machine, the phacoemulsifier, was developed to break up (fragment) and remove firm, insoluble lens nuclei. This machine, with components for ultrasonic vibration and irrigation-aspiration, permits extracapsular extraction through a very small incision in the limbus. All functions are controlled by foot pedal.

The handpiece of the phacoemulsifier consists of a disposable hollow titanium alloy needle surrounded by a silicone sleeve. The needle is inserted into the anterior chamber following removal of the anterior capsule with a cystotome. The activated needle breaks up the lens with ultrasonic vibrations; the linear motion of the ultrasonic vibrations is created by electrical impulses. This process generates heat. A cooling pump circulates coolant, either fluid or air, through the power cord. While the lens is thus emulsified, a constant flow of BSS irrigating solution through the sleeve prevents heat buildup. The irrigation-aspiration flow is automatically regulated to maintain anterior chamber depth. The aspirator removes the fragments. After the cortex (material surrounding the lens nucleus) is removed by irrigation-aspiration, the posterior capsule may be polished with an instrument to remove any residual cortex. The posterior capsule is left intact unless an opacity remains, in which case it may be incised during the initial surgical procedure or at a future time. The limbal incision is closed with one stitch.

Appropriate checks should be made before use of the handpiece, and the integrity of the vacuum and irrigating systems must be confirmed. The handpiece should be disassembled for cleaning and sterilization and then reassembled on the sterile field before use. The handpiece can be steam sterilized as a single unit.

In the newer computerized machines, the phacoemulsification and aspiration settings are preset. To avoid error, the scrub person and circulator work closely with the surgeon to monitor the various functions of the machine in use. They should also observe the transparent tubes for the flow of aspirate. Aspirated fluid is contaminated and is discarded postoperatively in the same manner as all blood or body fluid.

Phacoemulsification has certain advantages:

1. It dramatically shortens convalescence time. The patient usually returns to full activity in 1 or 2 days.
2. It uses a small incision and minimal sutures, which promotes healing.
3. It retains the posterior capsule of the lens to preserve a more physiologically normal condition. The occurrence of post–lens extraction edema and retinal detachment is thereby diminished.
4. The posterior capsule supports an implanted IOL. Postoperative astigmatism is minimized.

Phacoemulsification also has disadvantages:

1. It is not suitable for all patients. Contraindications are corneal disease, a dislocated lens, a shallow anterior chamber, difficult-to-dilate pupils, and completely hard, stonelike cataracts.
2. It requires special techniques which, if not thoroughly mastered, may precipitate surgical complications such as temporary or permanent corneal damage (opacification), prolapse of the lens into the vitreous, and vitreous loss.
3. It may injure the cells because of the necessary substantial amount of anterior chamber irrigation. Corneal cells are very sensitive to manipulation and can respond by loss of function.

4. It requires meticulous technical monitoring of the machine. The usual precautions for the use of electrical equipment are also observed.

Clear Corneal Cataract Procedure Foldable IOLs and topical anesthetic techniques have been integral with the use of "no stitch" corneal incisions. Patient selection includes the ability to fixate vision on a focal point and cooperate with commands from the surgeon. Tetracaine intraocular drops are used preoperatively and intraoperatively. Additional intraoperative anesthetics include injectable lidocaine without preservatives for infusion into the anterior chamber.

Rehabilitation Following Cataract Extraction Rehabilitation following cataract extraction consists of substitution for the missing part, the lens, so the optical system can function to focus incoming light on the retina. Patients with no optical substitute see only blurred objects of large size with no detail. Rehabilitation may be accomplished by spectacles (glasses), contact lenses, or IOL implantation.

Spectacle correction of aphakia, the absence of the lens, provides focusing of light. The spectacle lens is approximately 2 cm in front of the original lens and magnifies images so they are approximately 35% larger than those the patient saw before development and extraction of the cataract. This magnification requires considerable readjustment to judge distances. In addition, peripheral areas are distorted. The spectacle type of replacement is intolerable in patients who have good vision in the unaffected eye, because an attempt to fuse the dissimilar images of the two eyes causes double vision.

A contact lens is often used to replace the optical deficiency caused by cataract extraction. This lens rests on the cornea only 2 to 3 mm from the original lens and thus causes only 7% magnification and provides a full, undistorted field of vision. It is difficult for some elderly persons to handle and care for contact lenses because of a lack of manual dexterity, arthritic hand and finger joints, or visual defects in the opposite eye. For these patients, an implanted IOL is a feasible and popular alternative.

Implantation of Intraocular Lens

IOL implantation is a microsurgical procedure in which an IOL is implanted in almost the identical position of the original lens and therefore does not change the size of the retinal image. Spatial displacement as seen by the aphakic eye and narrowing and distortion of the visual field are eliminated, thereby producing early visual rehabilitation. With spatial displacement, orientation in space is changed—objects are not where they appear to be.

An IOL is intended to remain in situ permanently. The implant is usually inserted through the same incision used to remove the defective, natural lens; this is called primary insertion. Some surgeons prefer to implant the lens at a later time; this is referred to as secondary insertion. The type of IOL used is contingent on the type of cataract extraction the surgeon chooses. Anterior chamber lenses are inserted in conjunction with ICCE or as secondary implants. Posterior chamber lenses are used after ECCE.

The prescription of the implanted lens (refractive power) involves complex preoperative calculations based on the patient's corneal curvature as determined by keratometer readings, anterior chamber depth, and eyeball axial length. Ultrasonography is helpful in making these determinations preoperatively. The information obtained is fed into a computer that automatically calculates the appropriate refractive power of the IOL.

Numerous IOLs of different shapes and sizes are available. The optical portion of a hard lens is made of an inert plastic, polymethyl methacrylate (with or without an ultraviolet blocker) that has been polished to a microscopic smoothness. Flexible and foldable lenses are made of silicone elastomer and acrylic resin.

The fixation portion has springlike supports or loops, called haptics, that are made of plastic (usually polypropylene). Some lenses are secured with polypropylene sutures. Lenses differ in design and method of fixation, and they can be classified according to placement or method of fixation.

Anterior Chamber (Angle Fixation) An anterior chamber lens consists of a band of plastic long enough to traverse the anterior chamber from one angle to the other. The optical portion is centrally located in the anterior chamber, in front of the pupil and iris. The pupil remains mobile because iris adhesions are not required for fixation. Although anterior chamber lenses are sometimes inserted primarily, they are popular lenses for secondary insertion.

Posterior Chamber (Capsular or Ciliary Body Fixation) Posterior chamber lenses are placed behind the iris and pupil, where the patient's own lens used to be. Placement of the IOL in the most normal physiologic position results in stabilization of the iris; less irritation of the uveal tract; a reduced tendency to iritis, secondary glaucoma, and cystoid macular edema; and stabilization of the optics. Posterior lenses permit safe dilation of the pupil if necessary to examine or treat posterior structures of the eye, such as the retina.

With capsular fixation, the lower loop of the haptic is inserted into a pocket of capsule created during extraction of the cataract. The lens does not touch the iris, and the pupil is free to move. With ciliary fixation, the haptics are placed between the iris and the posterior capsule. They rest on the corona (inner rim) of the ciliary body.

Pros and Cons of Intraocular Lens Implantation The final decision to implant an artificial lens rests with the surgeon, who should exercise good judgment to avoid serious complication.

Indications for implantation are the following:

1. Geriatric patients with disabling bilateral cataracts and others who cannot adapt to contact lenses
2. Patients with occupations having specific visual requirements (e.g., airplane pilots) or a difficult working environment (e.g., ranchers in a dusty area)
3. Children with a traumatic cataract, thus preventing amblyopia

Contraindications for implantation are the following:

1. Impossibility for follow-up to observe patient for late complications
2. Ocular conditions such as poorly controlled glaucoma or previous retinal detachment
3. Diabetic proliferative retinopathy
4. Poor result in previous implant
5. Patient anxiety in regard to the procedure
6. Young patients with congenital cataracts
7. Endothelial corneal dystrophy
8. Cataracts associated with recurrent iritis

Advantages to IOL implantation are the following:

1. Superior spatial orientation and binocular vision
2. Permanency of device unless complications develop
3. Additional option for postcataract refractive correction
4. Unrestricted pupillary dilation if necessary

Complications with IOL implantation are the following:

1. Corneal damage or latent edema
2. Prolonged inflammation such as iritis or vitritis
3. Cystoid macular edema
4. Secondary cataract (i.e., opacification of the anterior vitreous) from recurrent iritis
5. Corneal opacity (rare with posterior implants)
6. Dislocation or malposition of the lens, which can damage the cornea (fortunately rare)

The type of approach used to repair a dislocation depends on the amount of dislocation. With the anterior approach, an anterior vitrectomy is performed to remove the vitreous in front of the lens, followed by removal or repositioning of the lens. With the posterior approach, the vitrector is used to remove the lens and/or vitreous through the pars plana. The IOL can be repositioned or removed.

Retina

Defects in the continuity of the retina can occur following accidental or surgical trauma or as a result of certain degenerative diseases. The dense network of capillary vessels in the retina makes the eyes vulnerable to microvascular disease. Retinopathy is a noninflammatory degenerative disease of the retina. Retinal changes can occur in patients with diabetes (i.e., diabetic retinopathy). Diabetes can affect every part of the eye, causing lens changes (cataract), palsied extraocular muscles, glaucoma, or corneal problems. A person who has had diabetes for more than 15 years has a significant likelihood of having some form of retinopathy, which generally occurs bilaterally. The severity of retinopathy may differ from one eye to the other. Retinopathy is classified as one of the following:

- *Background or nonproliferative.* With this type of retinopathy, disease is confined to the retinal surface. Bulges or microaneurysms form in retinal capillary walls, eventually permitting leakage and the deposition of exudates. Intraretinal hemorrhages occur and are reabsorbed. Progressive changes in capillary membranes lead to the blockage of capillaries, resulting in retinal ischemia. Deterioration then progresses to the proliferative stage.

- *Proliferative.* In the proliferative stage, new blood vessels emerge from the retina and form in the surrounding tissues in an effort to relieve retinal anoxia (i.e., neovascularization). These fragile vessels may rupture spontaneously, producing hemorrhage into the retina and/or vitreous humor. The eventual result may be partial or complete blindness. Panretinal photocoagulation (PRP) is one method of eliminating abnormal vascularization. PRP consists of the application of hundreds of laser burns to the peripheral retinal tissue to partially destroy it, thereby reducing the retinal metabolic need for oxygen. After neovascularization has occurred, laser therapy is less effective in delaying or stopping the destructive process. Therefore early diagnosis and treatment are crucial. In an effort to prevent the formation of new vessels, lasers are used to cauterize minute hypoxic areas of tissue before damage occurs.

Laser light is used for cauterizing bleeding vessels, for diabetic retinopathy, and for other retinopathies such as central serous retinopathy with swelling of the macula, angiomas and hemangiomas, aneurysms, and small tumors. Laser light is absorbed selectively by three pigments in the retina: macular xanthophyll, hemoglobin in the retinal and subretinal blood vessels, and melanin in the retinal pigment epithelium. Laser therapy is not effective in correcting severe retinal damage or detachment.

Repair of Detached Retina The retina can become separated from its surrounding nourishing layer, the choroid (Figure 38-9). This detachment may occur in any region of the retina. Primary retinal detachment is characterized

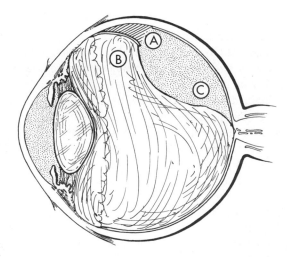

Figure 38-9 Detached retina. **A,** Retinal break. **B,** Vitreous. **C,** Fluid or blood behind the retina. (From Glaser BM: Surgical retina. In Ryan SJ, editor: *Retina,* ed 2, vol 3, St Louis, 1994, Mosby.)

by a hole in the retina. Secondary detachment may result when blood, fluid, or a tumor gets behind and displaces the retina; this type of detachment is not necessarily accompanied by a hole. The seepage of vitreous fluid into the potential space between the retina and the choroid causes the retina to become detached, and a serious visual disturbance results. Enucleation is usually indicated for tumor-caused detachment.

Reattachment is effected only by surgical intervention. The retinal defect is sealed off, and often the subretinal fluid is drained. The specific procedure used to achieve retinal reattachment is determined by the type and location of the detachment. All or some of the following procedures may be used in combination:

1. *Diathermy.* The traditional procedure involves diathermy coagulation to the area of the sclera overlying the region of the retinal defect. The resultant localized inflammation acts to seal off the break. Coagulation is delivered by a specialized short-wave diathermy unit.
2. *Cryosurgery.* Some surgeons prefer cryosurgery because of the type of adhesion obtained. The therapeutic applications of cryosurgery are basically similar to those of diathermy, and the tissue reactions superficially resemble each other. Cryosurgery is often used for anterior tears.
3. *Scleral buckling.* Internal elevation of the sclera may be increased by the scleral buckling procedure. This technique involves implantation of a wedge of silicone episclerally or intrasclerally. An encircling band of silicone may be used to keep constant external pressure on the buckle. Figure 38-10 depicts the result of this procedure.

4. *Intraocular gas tamponade.* Injection of room air or absorbable inert gas into the vitreous cavity can be used to create an intraocular tamponade. Room air absorbs after 5 days. Inert gases such as short-acting sulfahexafluoride (SF_6), intermediate-acting perfluoroethane (C_2F_6), or long-acting perfluorooctane (C_3F_8) are sometimes used to approximate the retina to the choroid (i.e., flatten the retina against the choroid). With pneumoretinopexy, the patient remains in a seated position for a superior tear or prone for a tear near the macula. This position is maintained for several weeks postoperatively so the gas bubble can successfully rise to close the retinal hole. The position and length of time in that position is determined by the ophthalmologist according to each patient's need. Pneumoretinopexy is less invasive than scleral buckling for securing a retinal detachment (Figure 38-11).
5. *Intraocular fluid tamponade.* Silicone oil has been approved by the Food and Drug Administration (FDA) for use as a vitreous substitute in securing a retinal detachment that cannot be corrected through conventional surgical intervention. Silicone oil is used for long-term intraocular tamponade. It is removed by the ophthalmologist several months postoperatively.
6. *Laser therapy.* Laser therapy can be used to secure the retina, except in severe detachment. A laser is often used to secure small posterior tears. (See the following discussion of laser therapy.)

Glaucoma and infection are potential postoperative complications of retinal reattachment. Glaucoma may be caused by congestion of the uvea by the buckle, increased IOP, or movement of injected gas from the desired site, causing blockage of outflow channels of aqueous humor. Infection is evident by swelling, purulent drainage, and a loss of optical clarity.

Laser Therapy   The laser delivery system uses the binocular microscope of the slit lamp, thus providing stereopsis and greater magnification. The nature of the laser beam permits extremely rapid delivery of radiant energy to produce a sharply defined burn. The small lesion it produces can be placed close to the macula. Exposure can be as brief as one hundredth of a second and the treated area as small as 50 μm (less than 2/1000 inch) in diameter. Because of this short exposure time, immobilization of eye is unnecessary unless the treated area is close to the macula, the central region of the retina with the clearest visual acuity. Accidental injury of the macula may result in a loss of central vision. Pupillary dilation is essential to avoid macular burn.

The argon laser is effective in treating retinal holes or tears and diabetic retinopathy. The krypton laser can be used to treat lesions closer to the macula and to treat retinal bleeding because of its poor absorption of the yellow pigment of the retina. The krypton spectrum is poorly absorbed by the red pigment of hemoglobin. Therefore it may be used effectively to treat retinal bleeding in the presence of blood in the vitreous humor. Under these circumstances the argon blue laser is ineffective because of absorption by even a small amount of blood.

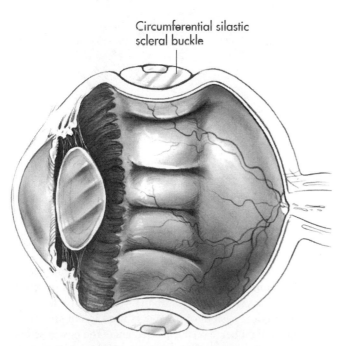

Circumferential silastic scleral buckle

Figure 38-10   Compressive effects of scleral buckle. (From Glaser BM: Surgical retina. In Ryan SJ, editor: *Retina,* ed 2, vol 3, St Louis, 1994, Mosby.)

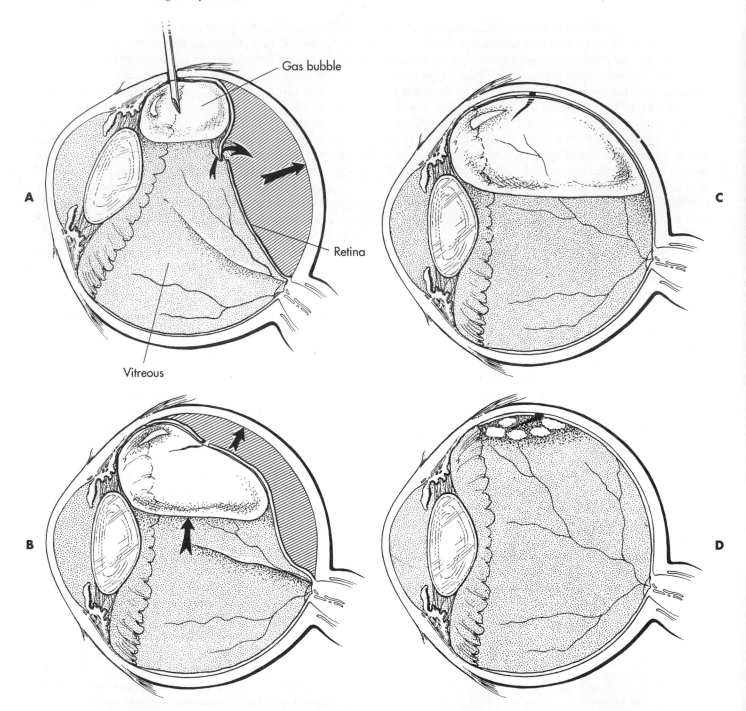

Figure 38-11   Pneumoretinopexy. **A,** Introduction of gas bubble. **B,** Gas bubble compresses retina. **C,** Tamponade formed by gas bubble. **D,** Gas bubble eventually absorbs. (From Glaser BM: Surgical retina. In Ryan SJ, editor: *Retina,* ed 2, vol 3, St Louis, 1994, Mosby.)

Photocoagulation   A retinal hole not surrounded by any detachment may be prophylactically sealed by xenon or laser photocoagulation. These therapeutic modalities, which are usually performed in an ophthalmic treatment area rather than the OR, were the outgrowth of traumatic retinal burns caused by watching an eclipse of the sun.

The xenon arc photocoagulator uses an intense source of multiwavelength light furnished by a xenon tube. The light is optically focused and concentrated into a delivering device

that is basically an indirect ophthalmoscope. The latter can be used both to view the area to be treated and to aim the light beam. The light may be directed to any of the pigmented (light-absorbing) layers of the eye, such as the iris or retina. These darker layers readily absorb the white light of the xenon tube. The optical system of the eye is used in the process of focusing the light beam on the desired area. The power setting and exposure time are completely controlled by the operating ophthalmologist. The pupil of the eye under therapy is dilated to give maximum visibility to the surgeon. The eye is immobilized by local anesthesia to prevent undesired movement, which could result in a burn to an area other than the one desired. Anesthesia also prevents pain from the intensity of the heat. Vitreous shrinkage that possibly leads to an inoperable detachment can be a complication.

Vitrectomy

Vitrectomy is the deliberate removal of a portion of the vitreous humor, also called vitreous body, that fills the space between the lens and the retina. Therapeutically it is performed for vitreal opacities, vitreal hemorrhage, and certain types of retinal damage or detachment. In addition to other causes, endophthalmitis (i.e., inflammation of the internal tissues of the eyeball) and the presence of an intraocular foreign body may result in vitreal opacity. In general, the candidates for vitrectomy have substantially impaired vision and complicated conditions preoperatively.

Whereas aqueous fluid is a clear liquid, vitreous is normally a transparent, gelatinous, viscid material containing fibrils. The vitreous helps give shape to the eyeball and serves a refractive function. It permits light rays to pass through it to the retina after the rays have traversed the lens. Diagnostically, the removal of a small amount of vitreous provides a sample for microbiologic study in suspected endophthalmitis. The procedure also provides tissue for biopsy to establish the diagnosis of intraocular tumors.

Alterations in the vitreous can have serious consequences. The loss of vitreous during surgical procedures is a dreaded complication, particularly of cataract extraction. Subsequent to retinal hemorrhage, which is common in patients with diabetes, bands of scar tissue may opacify the vitreous as well as adhere to the retina near the original bleeding vessel. Traction on the retina by these bands or further cicatrization (scarring) can lead to retinal tears or detachment. A persistent hemorrhage, lasting more than 1 year, is permanent. It will not absorb spontaneously.

For years the vitreous was considered an inaccessible, inoperable area. Research and the advent of microsurgery has changed this belief. A loss of vitreous from the posterior segment during a cataract procedure is relatively innocuous if the anterior segment is cleared of vitreous. Thus no residual strands are present to cause traction effects or to block visual function. In addition, the eye tolerates subtotal vitreal excision in the posterior segment if the vitreous body is proportionately replaced with BSS.

Vitrectomy is a microsurgical procedure that lasts 2 to 3 hours and requires a skilled retinal surgeon. It is performed with a vitreotome (vitrector) such as the Microvit. These devices, which incorporate a micromotor, terminate in a needle-like tube that contains a cutting mechanism for severing abnormal adhesions and cutting obstructive tissue into small pieces. In addition, the vitreotome has auxiliary connections for the aspiration of vitreous, debris, or blood from the posterior segment. Vitreous is replaced with BSS via a separate infusion cannula to maintain adequate IOP. A fiberoptic light source or pic is inserted into the vitreous to illuminate the

posterior portion of the globe. Various vitrectomy systems are available, but all have cutting, suction, and illumination systems. The machine may have an automatic or hydraulic pole for rapidly regulating the height of the BSS bottle.

The scrub person and circulator should assemble and check equipment before the surgical procedure begins. The vitreotome handpiece is attached to sterile tubing, which is connected to a power console. One person activates the various switches while the other tests the suction vacuum and cutting function. Suction is tested at maximum pressure. The tip is placed in sterile saline and activated until fluid reaches the collection bottle. The pressure is then lowered to the surgeon's preference. To assess cutting, the switch is activated and the tip is checked visibly and audibly for movement. The infusion catheter is primed with a solution of the surgeon's choice to remove air bubbles that could disturb the view in the posterior segment. The manufacturer's manual should be consulted.

A local anesthetic is administered unless the patient's condition necessitates a general anesthetic. There are two approaches to the vitreous body:

1. Through the posterior segment via the pars plana (i.e., the anterior attachment of the retina). Because the pars plana has no visual function, entry here is relatively atraumatic and poses minimal risk for retinal detachment. The anterior segment remains intact, and IOP is maintained. This approach is used to incise opacified vitreous, old hemorrhage, or bands of scar tissue, thereby giving a clear view of the retina and restoring visual function.
2. Through the anterior segment via incision at the limbus (i.e., junction of the cornea and sclera). A small opening is made and the tip of the vitrector is introduced. The vitreous is exposed through the pupillary opening. This approach is used to remove vitreous inadvertently displaced into the anterior chamber during cataract removal to avoid postoperative complications. The vitreous volume is replaced with BSS. Anterior vitrectomy also is used to correct retinal traction in retinopathy in premature infants (retrolental fibroplasia).

Vitrectomy is intricate and requires special equipment. The surgeon may request a bipolar cautery with a Charles clip attachment for actively bleeding intraocular vessels. A bipolar pencil or "eraser" may be used intraocularly. A handheld or "sew-on" contact lens placed onto the cornea enhances the view of the posterior chamber. A metal ring is sewn in place at two points around the limbus, encircling the cornea. Viscous material is placed on the cornea, and the lens of choice is placed down in the ring. Occasionally, a lensectomy is performed during vitrectomy to facilitate the view of the posterior segment.

After the removal of vitreous, before wound closure, and with the retina in clear view, the retina is inspected for defects such as holes or vascular abnormalities. If these are found, treatment is applied by means of endocryotherapy, a freezing application delivered by intraocular probe or by a laser delivered by an intraocular device. These maneuvers may be accompanied by the injection of air or inert gas to push the retina into physiologic position.

Postoperatively, patients may experience considerable pain that requires medication, ice packs, and steroid eye drops for treatment of inflammation. After vitrectomy, patients will experience aphakia if the lens was removed for visualization of the posterior segment, and they will eventually need optical correction such as that needed after cataract extraction. Vitrectomy can significantly improve vision.

Complications of vitrectomy include iatrogenic retinal damage, vitreous hemorrhage, or cataract formation from damage to the lens. A secondary surgical procedure may be required to repair the retina (e.g., a scleral buckling procedure or intraocular tamponade). No present treatment for retinopathy is free of danger. To save vision, some tissue is destroyed or sacrificed.

EYE INJURIES

Various forms and degrees of trauma may occur as a result of injury. All types of injury require immediate appraisal by an ophthalmologist. A delay in treating even minor injuries may result in a temporary or permanent loss of vision. Complications include hemorrhage, infection, iritis or tears of the iris, retinal tears or detachment, macular edema, and secondary cataract. Treatment may be immediate or secondary if a delay is necessary because of life-threatening injuries. Improved surgical management, such as vitrectomy and microsurgery, have reduced the loss of vision in severely injured eyes. An optimum result is especially crucial in patients with bilateral eye injuries. If possible, patients with eye injuries should be kept in the supine position until seen by an ophthalmologist.

Evaluation of the injury may necessitate sedating or anesthetizing the patient to prevent further damage at examination. Pressure to the eye must be avoided because bone fragments may be displaced or the globe contents emptied.

Injuries may be simple and involve only the external layers, or they may be compound and include the inner structures. They may be nonpenetrating (usually caused by a blunt object) or penetrating (caused by a sharp object). The more structures involved, the more difficult it is to salvage the eye.

Treatment is determined by the type or combination of injuries and aims to do the following:

- Promote healing and prevent anatomic distortion by reparative techniques
- Preserve and/or restore maximum vision
- Control pain by medication
- Prevent infection and inflammation through the administration of antibiotics and steroids

Nonpenetrating Injuries
Burns

Burns may be caused by ultraviolet radiation, such as sunlamps or sunlight, or by an electric flash. These types of burns are basically self-limited and are rarely surgical. A chemical burn constitutes an emergency. The initial treatment consists of flooding the cornea with water. Alkali burns may be further neutralized by prompt irrigation of the epithelium-denuded cornea with ethylenediaminetetraacetic acid (EDTA). This is especially important if discrete particles of alkali are superficially embedded within tissue. EDTA deactivates an enzyme (collagenase) and neutralizes soluble alkali such as sodium hydroxide (lye). Severe burns may be treated with specific amino acids, EDTA, or acetylcysteine (Mucomyst) to inhibit the continued destruction of the cornea by collagenase; however, these burns often progress to corneal opacity and blindness.

Contusions of the Globe

Contusions of the globe may or may not require surgical treatment. If hemorrhage is present, treatment consists of bed rest and antiglaucoma therapy to control IOP. It is not unusual for a secondary hemorrhage to occur on the third or fourth day after injury. If IOP remains high, blood staining of the cornea and damage to the optic nerve may result. It is then sometimes necessary to perform a paracentesis, in which an incision is made into the anterior chamber to drain the blood. If an organized clot is found, judicious irrigation may supplement the incision.

Penetrating Injuries

Lacerations of the globe may occur with or without a retained foreign body and with or without prolapse of the ocular contents. In injuries to the globe, an ophthalmic surgeon should repair both the eye wound and the tissues adjacent to the eye.

With a penetrating injury there is the possibility of an eventual sympathetic ophthalmia, an inflammation of the uninjured eye. Antitetanus therapy should be included in the treatment of these injuries.

Vitrectomy and lensectomy have rendered salvageable some massive injuries that formerly were inoperable. Such injuries include extensive lacerations with cataract formation, vitreous hemorrhage, and retinal damage.

Without a Foreign Body
Eyelid Laceration Lacerations are repaired according to anatomic principles. Plastic repair involves approximation of the anatomic layers. Penetrating wounds, such as animal bites, are debrided. If the laceration includes the lacrimal canaliculus (duct for the passage of tears), special probes are used to identify the proximal portions for rejoining. Lacerations of the lacrimal canaliculus may be repaired by suturing over one of two types of stents. The Quickert-Dryden tubing consists of a length of flexible silicone with a malleable metal lacrimal probe swaged onto each end. One end of the probe is inserted through the upper lid canaliculus, and the other end is inserted into the lower lid canaliculus. Both ends exit via the tear sac and nasolacrimal canal into the nose. The lacerated canaliculus is then sutured over the tubing, which is removed after healing takes place. Some surgeons prefer the rigid Veirs stainless steel rod, which is inserted into the lacerated canaliculus. A suture swaged to one end permits withdrawal of the rod after healing.

Conjunctival Laceration Conjunctival laceration is usually debrided and, unless large, is permitted to heal without suturing. If the laceration is large and there is a loss of conjunctival tissue, sutures or rotating flaps of conjunctiva may be necessary for repair.

Corneal and Scleral Lacerations A small corneal laceration may be covered with a protective soft contact lens to seal it and hold the edges together. A larger wound requires accurate appositional sutures that are best placed under the operating microscope. The microscope is especially useful for irregular, complicated, or multiple tears.

Some irregular corneal lacerations not easily closed by direct suturing may be closed and the leak stopped by the application of cyanoacrylate glue. A soft contact lens is usually placed as a bandage over the freshly glued cornea. A conjunctival flap can be placed to achieve a similar seal, but it is used less frequently. A large laceration may require a penetrating keratoplasty as an emergency procedure to ensure the integrity of the eye.

Adequate exploration, particularly of a scleral wound, is necessary both to determine the extent of injury and to ensure uncovering of the entire wound for repair. In instances of vitreous fluid presentation or loss, it is preferable to remove the fluid from the wound and the anterior chamber with the vitreotome before proceeding with repair. This is performed to prevent undesirable vitreous adhesions from developing postoperatively.

Posterior Rupture of the Globe Rupture of the globe usually involves the herniation of retinal and uveal tissue into the orbit. Although such injuries are self-healing, the eye is irreparably damaged. This injury usually results in enucleation. Avulsion (tearing) of the optic nerve produces permanent blindness even though the rest of the globe may be intact.

With a Foreign Body

Extraocular injuries are usually not extensive. An intraocular foreign object is removed very gently under sterile conditions to avoid secondary infection and further trauma. A corneal foreign body is removed with a sharp probe (spud), and the surrounding rust ring is removed with a rotating burr. The type, size, and position of other intraocular foreign bodies should be determined accurately before removal. Localization is accomplished by the following:

- Direct vision with an ophthalmoscope
- Computed tomography (CT) scan
- Berman locator, a small but extremely sensitive version of a metal detector, which may indicate the exact location of a ferrous metallic foreign body
- X-ray study, using a contact lens containing radiopaque landmarks (Sweet's localizer)

Fragments of ferrous metals often can be retrieved by using the attraction of a strong electromagnet. In some cases these foreign bodies can be withdrawn along the path of entry. Nonmagnetic foreign objects present a more serious

problem. Often they are secured only by passing a delicate forceps into the globe. Such instrumentation is combined with a partial vitrectomy, thus obtaining satisfactory results.

In summary, traumatic injuries may introduce infection or produce a severe inflammatory reaction to a greater degree than do elective surgical procedures. Proper early treatment is indicated to save vision. Early reintervention, before scar formation, may be necessary in some patients.

OPHTHALMIC LASERS

The use of an ophthalmic laser is often a safe alternative to conventional surgery for ablation of a pathologic condition. The color and wavelength of each laser determine which part of the eye it can best treat. Specific wavelengths destroy disease in tissues whose pigments are capable of discriminating absorption of that wavelength. Conversely, the selected wavelength should be only minimally absorbed by the vital adjacent tissues to be preserved. The ophthalmologist controls the power, intensity, and direction of the laser beam. The beam precisely cauterizes tissue and blood vessels, preventing bleeding. Each laser has selective uses:

- *Blue-green argon:* For a retinal detachment, tear, or hole; diabetic retinopathy; macular neovascular lesions; laser trabeculoplasty, to lower IOP and facilitate aqueous outflow in select patients with open-angle glaucoma; iridotomy, in place of iridectomy by incision; and to create a small opening in the iris that allows aqueous to enter the anterior chamber (angle-closure glaucoma). The use of this laser may reduce the threat of endophthalmitis, a serious postoperative complication. Adherence of the iris to laser treatment sites (synechiae) is a complication of laser trabeculoplasty. A portable laser is available for intraoperative use. It permits surgeons to work inside rather than through the eye while the patient is under general anesthesia.
- *Red-yellow krypton:* For blood vessel aberrations of the choroid (common to senile macular disease) in which abnormal vessels damage adjacent nerve tissue; for lesions in the perimacular region (the laser beam passes through cloudy vitreous hemorrhage); and for retinal vascular diseases, such as proliferative diabetic retinopathy and retinal detachment.
- *Invisible pulsed neodymium (Nd:YAG):* For preoperative anterior capsulotomy before extracapsular cataract extraction; posterior capsulotomy (discission) after extracapsular cataract extraction to make an opening in an opaque capsule and thus permit light to reach the retina; and lysis or severing of strands of vitreous and/or fibrous bands in the posterior segment that cause cystoid macular edema. Cloudy areas of tissue interfering with vision are painlessly pushed aside, resulting in immediate improvement in sight. Rather than producing the effect by absorption, energy is released almost entirely at the point of focus. Problems in both anterior and posterior parts of the eye are treatable (e.g., with optical iridectomy and photocoagulation of retinal disorders). Unlike with the

visible light lasers, the Nd:YAG laser does not require the target tissue to be pigmented for effectiveness.

- *Visible excimer:* Argon-fluoride in the ultraviolet range. Used for shaping the cornea, as in lamellar keratectomy, to correct refractive disorders.
- *Invisible holmium:YAG (Ho:YAG):* For sclerostomy to create an opening in the sclera that promotes filtration for glaucoma. It can also be used for corneal sculpting.

The following are advantages of laser therapy:

1. There is a minimal possibility of infection. Treatment is noninvasive and sterile, which is an advantage to diabetic and susceptible patients.
2. There is minimal pain. Only a topical anesthetic is required unless many retinal areas are treated with a high-energy laser.
3. It is performed as an ambulatory procedure.
4. The appropriate amount of energy is concentrated in very small area.
5. The light is highly flexible, which seems to do little damage to the clear media it traverses.
6. The laser light is selectively absorbed. Ideally, only desired tissue is affected.
7. It is useful in a poor-risk surgical patient or one who has had a previous unsuccessful surgical procedure.

Bibliography

Caramella F: Silicone oil as a vitreous substitute in vitreoretinal surgery, *J Ophthalmic Nurs Technol* 13(5):241-242, 1994.

Cataract Management Guideline Panel: *Cataract in adults: management of functional impairment (clinical practice guideline, no 4),* Rockville, Md, February 1993, pp 40-43, US Department of Health and Human Services, Public Health Service, Agency for Health Care Policy and Research, AHCPR pub no 93-0542.

Charpentier DY et al: Radial thermokeratoplasty is inadequate for overcorrection following radial keratotomy, *J Refract Corneal Surg* 10(1):34-35, 1994.

Evangelisto M: Phacoemulsification needle enhances cataract surgery, *Todays Surg Nurs* 18(6):19-22, 1996.

Garbee DD: Phacoemulsification procedures performed with topical anesthesia, *AORN J* 66(2):253-265, 1997.

Gill KS et al: Phototherapeutic keratectomy, *AORN J* 66(2):242-251, 1997.

Irvine AR, Lahey JM: Pneumatic retinopexy for giant retinal tears, *Ophthalmology* 101(3):524-528, 1994.

Koch PS: Managing the torn posterior capsule and vitreous loss, *Int Ophthalmol Clin* 34(2):113-130, 1994.

Kowalski CK: Cataracts at any age, *Home Healthc Nurse* 12(2):43-46, 1994.

MacKenzie M, Waterman M: Utilization of a clinical pathway in the care of the ambulatory cataract surgical patient, *Insight* 20(2):6-11, 1995.

Maclean H et al: Patient comfort during cataract surgery with modified topical and peribulbar anesthesia, *J Cataract Refract Surg* 23(2):277-283, 1997.

Maguen E et al: Results of excimer laser photorefractive keratectomy for the correction of myopia, *Ophthalmology* 101(9):1548-1556, 1994.

McEwen DR: Surgical treatment of dacryocystitis, *AORN J* 66(2):268-280, 1997.

Sandler RL: Clinical snapshot: glaucoma, *Am J Nurs* 95(3):34-35, 1995.

Schein OD et al: Variation in cataract surgery practice and clinical outcomes, *Ophthalmology* 101(6):1142-1152, 1994.

Schepens CL: Management of retinal detachment, *Ophthalmic Surg* 25(7): 427-431, 1994.

Szerenyi K et al: Keratitis as a complication of bilateral, simultaneous radial keratotomy, *Am J Ophthalmol* 117(4):426-467, 1994.

Updegraff SA et al: Pupillary block during cataract surgery, *Am J Ophthalmol* 117(3):328-332, 1994.

Wiedemann P et al: Reconstruction of the anterior and posterior segment of the eye after massive injury, *Ger J Ophthalmol* 3(2):84-89, 1994.

Yang KJ et al: Mitomycin-C–supplemented trabeculectomy, phacoemulsification, and foldable lens implantation, *J Cataract Refract Surg* 23(4):565-569, 1997.

Chapter 39

Plastic and Reconstructive Surgery

Chapter Objectives

After studying this chapter, the learner will be able to:

- Identify pertinent anatomy of the integumentary system.
- List four primary reasons for plastic surgery.
- Describe the techniques of skin and tissue grafting.
- Discuss the importance of fluid balance in the burn patient.

Plastic surgery has been called the "surgery of millimeters" because of the critical margin between good and poor cosmetic results. Each millimeter lack or excess of tissue can have a psychologic impact on the patient. If the patient thinks his or her appearance has improved, the patient's personality and self-image may improve and others may respond more positively to him or her. The term *plastic* means *to mold or fashion* and is derived from the Greek word *plastikos* (πλαστικος).

Plastic surgeons practice their art on virtually any part of the body. They attempt to restore both form (aesthetic appearance) and function. Some plastic surgeons limit their practice to specific areas, such as the head and neck, hand, or breast. The surgeon specifically trained in the art of plastic surgery frequently is a member of a multidisciplinary team to assist with the repair of defects and/or restoration of function. The results depend not only on the skill of the plastic surgeon and the team, but also on the age, health status, skin texture, bone structure, extent of the defect, and healing capacity of the patient. Many plastic and reconstructive surgical procedures are performed on an ambulatory basis;

many are performed with the patient under local anesthesia with sedation. The surgeon performs the simplest and safest procedure that will provide a realistic outcome.

HISTORICAL BACKGROUND

Plastic surgery was probably the first form of surgery. Egyptian papyrus scrolls tell of skin grafts and pedicle flaps to replace deficiencies as early as 3500 years ago. Egyptian mummies have been found with artificial ears and noses. In India more than 2000 years ago, the Hindus became skilled in transferring tissue to form noses for those who had lost them as a punishment. Ancient records verify other attempts to improve appearance.

During the fourteenth and sixteenth centuries, restorative procedures for the nose, lips, and ears were performed by Italian surgeons. Gasparo Tagliacozzi (1546-1599), an Italian surgeon, described the creation of a tube graft from the arm to the nose for reconstructive rhinoplasty. Further development of the art of reconstruction did not occur in

Europe until the nineteenth and twentieth centuries. The German surgeon Edward Zeis first used the term *plastic surgery* in his book published in 1863.

During World Wars I and II the development of military plastic and reconstructive surgery centers led to rapid progress in the rehabilitation of casualties with maxillofacial and hand injuries. Plastic surgeons worked closely with other specialists in treating many types of war injuries. They found that by replacing lost skin with grafts, fractures under these areas healed better and more quickly and parts returned to normal function sooner.

SPECIAL FEATURES OF PLASTIC AND RECONSTRUCTIVE SURGERY

Scars are inevitable whenever skin is incised or excised. The incision is made along natural skin lines whenever possible. The plastic surgeon attempts to minimize scar formation by meticulous realignment and approximation of underlying tissues and wound edges. Many plastic procedures involve only the subcuticular tissues and skin. Reconstructive procedures may include manipulation of underlying cartilage, bone, muscles, tendons, nerves, and blood vessels.

Preoperative instruction to patients includes instructions to avoid aspirin and not to smoke for at least 2 weeks before an elective surgical procedure. Aspirin and other substances have an anticoagulant action that can affect bleeding, causing hematoma formation. Box 39-1 lists medications and substances that may promote postoperative bleeding. Smoking causes vasoconstrictive ischemia that can affect wound healing, causing tissue necrosis. Photographs are commonly taken preoperatively, intraoperatively, and postoperatively for planning, documentation, and teaching purposes.

General Considerations

1. Pressure points are protected during prolonged procedures. Microvascular plastic and reconstructive surgical procedures may take several hours to complete. The patient should be positioned on a gel pad mattress. Bony prominences should be well padded to prevent tissue necrosis.
2. Sterile dye, such as methylene blue, gentian violet, Bonney's blue, or brilliant green, is often used to outline areas for incision. This can be done with a sterile marking pen or stylus after the skin is prepped.
3. Exposure of both sides for comparison is usually required for surgical procedures on the face, ears, and neck.
4. Draping often exposes much skin surface, which is unavoidable. A fenestrated sheet frequently cannot be used. The opening does not give adequate exposure, especially for skin grafting. Use towels, self-adhering plastic sheeting, and minor and medium sheets under and around the areas, according to need, to drape as much of the patient as possible. Drapes can be secured with nonpiercing towel clips, skin staples, or sutures.

Box 39-1	**Medications and Substances That May Promote Postoperative Bleeding**

Products Containing Aspirin (Examples)

Aleve
Aspergum
Bufferin
Congespirin
Darvon
Ecotrin
Empirin
Excedrin

Analgesics That Have an Aspirin-Like Effect on Bleeding (Examples)

Dolobid
Norgesic
Oxycodone
Pepto-Bismol
Percodan
Soma
Talwin
Voltaren

Medications Containing Ibuprofen (Examples)

Advil
Midol
Naprosyn
Nuprin
Postel
Sine-Aid
Toradol

Anticoagulants (Examples)

Coumadin
Dicumarol
Heparin
Panwarfin
Periactin

Other Substances That May Have an Anticoagulant Effect

Some fish oils
Vitamin E
Ginko Biloba

---

5. Local anesthesia is used for many surgical procedures on adults. Epinephrine may be added to help localize the agent, prolong the anesthetic action, and provide hemostasis. Care is taken not to use epinephrine in digits, ears, or other areas of terminal blood supply. Short 26- or 30-gauge needles are used for injection.
6. No. 15 and 11 scalpel blades are routinely used to cut small structures.
7. An electrosurgical unit (ESU) pencil may be used to cut or coagulate during incision. Small handheld, battery-operated units are useful for tiny bleeders. Overuse of the ESU can cause devitalization of tissue.

8. Instruments must be small for handling delicate tissues. Iris scissors, mosquito hemostats, fine-tipped tissue forceps, and other small-scale cutting, holding, clamping, and exposing instruments are part of the routine plastic surgery setup. Microinstruments are needed for microsurgical techniques.

9. Nerve stimulation may be used to help identify nerves, especially in craniofacial, neck, and hand reconstruction procedures.

10. Bone, cartilage, or skin grafts may be needed. Allografts may be obtained from the tissue bank rather than the patient's own tissues.

11. Prosthetic implants may be used in plastic surgery to reconstruct soft tissue and cartilage defects. They cannot be used unless there is adequate soft tissue coverage. They cannot be used in an infected area.

12. Suture sizes range from 2-0 through 7-0, depending on the location and tissue, with sizes 8-0 through 11-0 sutures for microsurgery. The material used varies according to the personal preference of the surgeon. Synthetic nonabsorbable and absorbable polymers are used more commonly than natural materials because they cause less tissue reaction.

13. Atraumatic swaged-on needles of small diameter with sharp cutting edges minimize trauma to superficial tissues. A needleholder with an appropriately fine tip is used with these delicate, curved needles.

14. Skin staples may be used to close skin or to secure skin grafts.

15. Wound closure strips may be used as skin dressings with sutures or to supplement closure with skin staples.

16. Closed wound suction drainage is frequently used to drain flaps to prevent seroma and hematoma formation.

17. Fine-mesh gauze may be used for the contact dressing. This may be impregnated with petrolatum or an oil emulsion, with or without medication, to cover denuded areas. Several types of sterile nonadherent dressings are commercially available. Dry gauze is not used on a denuded area because it adheres and acts as a foreign body, causing granulomas.

18. Pressure dressings may be used following extensive surgical procedures to splint soft tissues and prevent contractures. The mild, even pressure keeps fluid formation in tissues or under a skin graft to a minimum. Commercial compression garments or dressings for various body areas are preferred by some plastic surgeons. Some dressings may be sutured into place.

19. Stent fixation is a method of obtaining pressure when it is impossible to bandage an area snugly, such as the face or neck. A form-fitting mold may be taped over the nose. Long suture ends can be tied crisscrossed over a dressing to immobilize it and exert gentle pressure.

Tissue may be approximated, supplemented, excised, transferred, or transplanted. Many procedures are done in stages before complete reconstruction and restoration of function are achieved. Tissue flaps and grafts, prosthetic implants, and external prosthetic appliances may be required for functional and cosmetic restoration as a result of ablative surgery or trauma.

Psychologic Support for Patients Undergoing Plastic and Reconstructive Surgery

Physical appearance affects self-image and self-esteem. Patients can develop inferiority complexes and introverted personalities because of congenital or acquired alteration in body structure. The defect may not affect physiologic function but may predispose the person to psychologic crippling if it is not corrected to the individual's satisfaction.

Adults who are dissatisfied with their body image may believe that a change in personal appearance will solve their social, marital, sexual, or business problems. The plastic surgeon assesses the patient's psychologic status, motivations, and expectations before scheduling a surgical procedure. Realistic, attainable outcomes are identified. The patient should be emotionally stable and aware of the potential outcomes. The surgeon should carefully obtain informed consent. Psychologic assessment and preparation are advisable preoperatively and are essential before surgical procedures that may result in disfigurement.

Extensive reconstruction for severe congenital deformities is done in stages, often over a period of months or years. These patients require prolonged psychologic support and encouragement.

Plastic and reconstructive surgery, either therapeutic or cosmetic, evokes emotional responses from the patient, family or significant other, and the entire perioperative team. Anticipation of the final outcome, which can be seen by the patient and others, often creates temporary psychosocial reactions such as depression and isolation. Positive reassurance of progress in improvement of physical appearance and during emotional crises is essential throughout the perioperative period. Perhaps the surgeon-nurse-patient-family relationship is closer when a person undergoes alteration of physical appearance than with other types of surgery. The patient may be physically healthy but may suffer alterations in self-esteem related to his or her perception of a defect in appearance. Care must be given in a manner that protects the self-esteem of the patient and respects the dignity of the family. This requires communication, understanding, and empathy. Preoperative teaching and discharge planning prepare the patient and his or her family for postoperative rehabilitation.

Categories of Plastic and Reconstructive Surgery

Four main categories of problems are treated by plastic surgeons:

1. Congenital anomalies, especially in the structure of the face and hands.

2. Aesthetic appearance, especially of the face and breasts.
3. Benign and malignant neoplasms, especially those leaving large soft tissue defects. Resection of extensive tumors other than those involving the skin or head and neck are not usually within the province of the plastic surgeon initially, but the patient may be referred for reconstructive surgery and rehabilitation. Frequently, reconstructive procedures are done in conjunction with another specialty surgeon at the time of tumor resection.
4. Traumatically acquired disfigurements, especially facial lacerations, hand injuries, and burns. The objective of the plastic surgeon is to restore function, as well as body image.

GRAFTING TECHNIQUES

Denuded areas of the body are resurfaced by transplanting or transferring segments of skin and other tissues from an uninjured area (donor site) to the injured area (recipient site). The plastic surgeon prefers to transfer tissues of compatible color, texture, thickness, and hair-bearing characteristics. Soft tissue autografts are used whenever possible. They are classified as follows according to the source of their vascular supply (which is essential for viability):

- *Free graft.* Tissue is detached from the donor site and transplanted into the recipient site. It derives its vascular supply from the capillary ingrowth from the recipient site.
- *Pedicle flap.* Tissue remains attached at one or both ends of the donor site during transfer to the recipient site. The vascular supply is maintained from the vessels preserved in the pedicle of the donor site.
- *Free flap.* Tissue, including its vascular bundle, is detached from the donor site and transferred to the recipient site. Microvascular anastomoses between arteries and veins in the flap or autograft and recipient site establish the vascularity necessary for viability.

Deformities caused by loss of soft tissue substance, such as trauma from accidental injury, tumor resection, or radiation therapy, may require a graft to fill in deficiencies and restore contours or to cover tendons and bones. Free grafts, pedicle flaps, and free flaps may be taken from various areas of the body to reconstruct soft tissue defects.

Free Skin Grafts

The epidermis, including the basal layer of the dermis that generates new skin, is transplanted from a donor site to a recipient site in which it becomes a part of living tissue in that area. Adherence to healthy underlying tissue and adequate vascularity are necessary for graft survival. A fibrin layer forms to bind the graft to the recipient site and to provide nourishment until vascularization is established in the graft. The depth of the graft (Figure 39-1) will vary according to its purpose:

- *Split-thickness graft.* The epidermis and half of the dermis to a depth of 0.010 to 0.035 inch (0.3 to 1 mm) are

removed. The donor site heals uneventfully unless it becomes infected. Split-thickness grafts are widely used to cover large denuded areas on the back, trunk, and legs.
- *Full-thickness graft.* The epidermis, dermis, and occasionally subcutaneous fat at a depth greater than 0.035 inch (1 mm) are removed or elevated. Full-thickness grafts inhibit wound contraction better than split-thickness grafts and generally are preferred on the face, neck, hands, elbows, axillae, knees, and feet.

The desired thickness of a free skin graft is predetermined by the plastic surgeon before the skin is incised. The appropriate cutting instrument is selected to obtain the graft.

Dermatomes

A dermatome is a cutting instrument designed to excise split-thickness skin grafts. The thickness of the graft can be calibrated by adjusting the depth gauge. The width of the graft is determined by the width of the cutting blade. Blades are detachable and disposable, which always ensures a sharp new blade for every patient. The length of the graft may be limited by the type of dermatome used.

Oscillating Blade Type Dermatomes may be electric or air powered with compressed nitrogen or air. The length of the graft is limited only by the donor site. The surgeon checks the adjustable-depth gauge before cutting the graft (Figure 39-2, *A*). The oscillating blade, free of vibrations, takes an accurate graft from donor sites that overlie firm structures, such as bone. The oscillating blade–type dermatome is not usually used on the abdominal wall, where underlying support is not firm.

Care is used in handling these precision dermatomes. If the dermatome is electric, the circulator should remove the foot pedal as soon as the graft is taken. If the dermatome is air powered, the scrub person and surgeon should place a thumb under the lever on the handle while preparing the instrument for use. These dermatomes cannot be immersed in water or put in a washer-sterilizer or ultrasonic cleaner. The manufacturer's instructions should be followed for use, care, and sterilization.

Drum Type Padgett and Reese dermatomes consist of one half of a metal drum, which is one half of a circle (Figure 39-2, *B*). A metal handle through the center of the drum has an arm on each end. These arms hold the bar that carries the blade. The bar swings around the drum to cut the graft. The size of the graft is limited by the width and length of the drum. An adhesive is placed on both the skin surface and the drum to keep the skin in contact with the drum. The knife blade is moved from side to side as slight tension is exerted on the skin by rotating the drum. The drum-type dermatome is used on flat, open areas because it is bulky. Its use is limited by the body contour and the amount of suitable skin on the donor site.

ANATOMIC LAYERS

Epidermis

Dermis

Subcutaneous
tissue

Muscle

SKIN GRAFTS

0.01 inch
Thin

0.02 inch
Moderate

0.035 inch
Thick

Split
or
partial
thickness

Free flap

0.04 inch
Pedicle
flap

Full
thickness

BURNS

First
degree

Superficial

Second
degree

Deep

Third
degree

Fourth
degree
↓

Figure 39-1   Cross section of skin and subcutaneous tissue, relative thickness of skin grafts, and categorization of burn injury.

A

B

Figure 39-2   Dermatomes. **A,** Powered oscillating blade–type dermatome with depth gauges on each side of blade. **B,** Drum-type dermatome to manually cut skin graft.

Dermatome tape is used with the Reese dermatome. Packaged sterile, the tape has an adhesive coating on each side covered with a paper backing. The backing is removed on one side and applied to the drum, taking care to line up the edges of the tape and the drum. After the backing paper is removed from the other side of the tape, the drum is placed on the skin, which adheres to it.

When a drum-type dermatome is being handled, the blade carrier is always grasped to prevent its swinging around the drum and seriously injuring the hands. The dermatome is left in the rack when not in use or until the blade is removed.

Types of Free Skin Grafts

Split-Thickness Thiersch Graft   Removed with a free-hand skin graft knife or dermatome, Thiersch grafts are used to cover superficial defects. The surgeon may use sutures or skin staples along the edges of the graft to hold it to underlying subcutaneous tissue. An even-pressure dressing is secured over the top of the graft. This prevents movement and helps obliterate dead space in the recipient site. The skin of the donor site regenerates rapidly, and the same area can be used again in 2 or 3 weeks if necessary. If a thin graft is taken and the site remains infection free, that donor site may be used again sooner.

Split-Thickness Mesh Graft   A mesh graft makes it possible to obtain a greater area of coverage from a split-thickness skin graft. After removal with a dermatome, the graft is placed on a plastic derma carrier, cut side down. This is a rigid base to keep the graft spread out flat while it is put through a mesh dermatome. This instrument cuts small parallel slits in the graft. When expanded, the slits become diamond-shaped openings (Figure 39-3). This permits expansion of the graft to cover an area three times as large as

Figure 39-3   Split-thickness skin graft being passed through mesh dermatome. Mesh graft expands to obtain greater coverage of recipient graft area.

the original graft obtained from the donor site. The mesh graft can be placed over the recipient site with slight tension. The increased edge exposures are conducive to rapid epithelialization. The mesh allows serum to escape through the openings. If a mesh dermatome is not available or is not feasible to use, slits can be made with a knife blade in the donor graft to accomplish the same purposes.

Full-Thickness Wolfe Graft   Wolfe graft is cut exactly to the size and shape of the recipient site with a skin graft knife. It is sutured into place under normal skin tension. Full-thickness grafts are used on the face, neck, or hands to fill in superficial denuded areas and over joints to prevent contractures. This graft does not become viable readily on granulated surfaces, and the amount that can be transferred is much more limited than with Thiersch graft.

To ensure viability, the donor graft must be held in apposition to healthy tissue in the underlying recipient site. The surgeon tacks the edges of the graft with sutures or staples. The middle portion may be "quilted" (i.e., affixed) with sutures or staples. The graft is covered with an even-pressure dressing.

Free Composite Grafts

A composite graft usually includes skin, subcutaneous tissue and cartilage, bone, or other tissues. The viability of the graft depends on ingrowth of the vascular system from the recipient site.

Free Omental Grafts

A free graft of omentum can be used to provide contour in a soft tissue defect in the face or neck, to resurface an area such as the scalp, to provide vascular support for bone and skin grafts around prosthetic materials, and to control wound infection, such as in the chest wall. Omentum will localize inflammation and wall off infection. It will not resorb when grafted. Omentum resected from the peritoneal cavity can be transplanted to an avascular area if sufficient blood vessels are available for microvascular anastomoses to the gastroepiploic artery and vein in the graft. Split-thickness skin grafts cover the omental graft.

Pedicle Flaps

Creation of a pedicle flap may be the procedure of choice to reconstruct deformities of soft tissue loss that will create, or that have created, an obvious aesthetic or functional disability for the patient. The pedicle, which is the attachment of elevated tissue to the donor site, must contain a vascular bundle to maintain blood supply to the tissue. Pedicle flaps are constructed from several types of tissues and sources of vascular bundles. Flap survival seems to depend on a reduction in vascular resistance or an increase in arterial perfusion pressure, or both. Several techniques are used to monitor circulation in the flap intraoperatively and postoperatively.

Arterialized Tissue Flap

A full-thickness skin graft contains a vascular bundle within subcutaneous tissue and skin. Arterialized flaps may contain the following:

- Axial vasculature from axial vessels that supply a fairly definite area of skin and subcutaneous tissue. A direct cutaneous artery flows through the length of the flap.
- Random or local vasculature from a subdermal plexus. Random flaps do not have a specific blood vessel within the flap. These are usually small flaps created around the head or neck.
- Both axial and random vasculature. A deltopectoral flap, for example, has axial vessels from the sternal region and random vessels in the deltoid area.

Depending on the proximity of the recipient site to the donor site, the pedicle flap will be one of the following types.

Rotational Flap One end of flap is rotated and sutured to the recipient site to cover a denuded area. The flap tissue is obtained from an area near the recipient site. Arterialized skin pedicle flaps with axial vasculature are rotated in a one-stage procedure. Random rotational pedicle flaps can be used in the face because vascularity is sufficient in the head and neck.

Cross-Finger Flap Tissue at the donor site is undermined and rotated to cover a small defect in an adjacent digit.

Tissue Expansion Flap The surface of the dermal-epidermal layer can be increased by implanting a tissue expansion device subcutaneously, close to the defect. Available in many sizes and shapes, the device has a soft, pliable silicone pouch connected by tubing to a self-sealing inflation reservoir. After insertion under a designated area for the skin flap, the pouch is filled with saline by injecting small amounts into the reservoir. Rapid expansion may be achieved immediately in the head or neck area or gradually over a period of weeks to months in other areas. Natural physiologic skin expansion occurs. The dermis stretches and thins while the epidermis duplicates itself without changing thickness. Tissue will increase to about 1½ times the width of the device. The vascular network that develops produces more viable tissue than that of other pedicle flaps. The tissue has similar color, texture, and thickness as the recipient site. The expanded tissue is advanced or transferred to cover the defect, helping to minimize scarring and donor site deformity. Tissue expansion flaps are used for scalp and facial defects, breast reconstruction, and other soft tissue defects. They can be used for closure of large donor site defects.

Myocutaneous Flap

Pedicle myocutaneous flaps allow safe and rapid transfer of tissue over long distances to cover large defects and vital structures. They are used, for example, to close soft tissue defects in the lower extremities, to cover pressure sores on

paraplegics, and to reconstruct contour following head and neck resection and mastectomy.

A myocutaneous flap incorporates the muscle with its overlying fascia, subcutaneous tissue, and skin. It receives a vigorous blood supply from the vascular pedicle that supplies the underlying muscle (Figure 39-4). It may include a neurovascular bundle with nerve fibers to innervate the muscle in the flap. Usually done as a one-stage procedure, myocutaneous flaps can be created from the following and other muscles:

- Trapezius
- Sternocleidomastoid
- Platysma
- Latissimus dorsi
- Pectoralis major
- Rectus abdominis
- Gracilis
- Gluteus maximus
- Tensor fascia lata
- Biceps or quadriceps femoris

Fasciocutaneous Flap

Mobilized fascia, subcutaneous tissue, and skin are transferred as pedicle flaps similarly to the way myocutaneous flaps are transferred. The donor site may need to be covered with a split-thickness graft.

Muscle Flap

A divided section of a muscle with its proximal blood supply intact can be rotated over a soft tissue defect, such as an ulcer on the leg or buttock. A vascularized muscle flap may be covered with a split-thickness skin graft.

Neurosensory Flap

Sensory nerves may remain intact in a flap with other tissues or be restored by microneural anastomosis or by nerve grafting. Preservation of nerves in a vascularized flap becomes important when sensation is critical to function, as in the hand or foot.

Omental Flap

Omentum is mobilized from the peritoneal cavity, without compromise of the vascular pedicle, to cover an infected

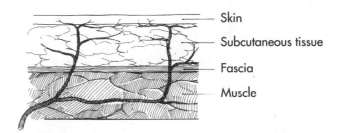

Figure 39-4 Myocutaneous flap. (From Ruberg RL, Smith DJ Jr: *Plastic surgery: a core curriculum*, St Louis, 1994, Mosby.)

mediastinal wound or a defect in the chest wall, such as following resection for irradiation necrosis or a neoplasm. The vascularity of donor omentum revascularizes the reconstructed chest wall recipient site. Split-thickness skin grafts, which may be mesh grafts, cover the omental flap. If additional rigidity is needed to restore the chest wall, polypropylene mesh may be sutured inside the rib cage to supplement the strength of the omental flap.

Microsurgical Free Flap Transfer

Composite free flaps or grafts of tissue are resected and transplanted from one area of the body to another to cover a denuded area, to restore function, or to restore body contour. Microsurgical techniques allow one-stage transfer of tissues. The main artery and vein supplying donor tissues must be anastomosed to vessels in the recipient site under the operating microscope. Often two teams work simultaneously at donor and recipient sites. These are lengthy, tedious procedures, often taking many hours to complete.

Fasciocutaneous Graft

Free grafts of fascia with overlying skin, with or without underlying muscle, may be transferred. For example, temporalis fascia may be transplanted into another area in the face.

Free Muscle Graft

Free island grafts of functional muscle can be resected and transplanted to replace motor function in another area. Although a small percentage of the graft survives, significant regeneration of muscle occurs. Free muscle, transferred by microvascular techniques and covered with a split-thickness skin graft, promotes healing of infected wounds.

Vascularized Muscle Pedicle Free Flap

In a multistaged procedure a myocutaneous flap is raised at the donor site and allowed to develop a new, isolated vascular system before free transfer to a recipient site. The vascular system in the muscle underlying the skin flap branches out to supply the skin. At the final stage the newly vascularized muscle pedicle is dissected free from the donor site. The donor site may need to be covered with a split-thickness graft. Under the operating microscope, arteries and veins in the flap are anastomosed to vessels at the recipient site. Two teams may complete the final stage: one to prepare and close the recipient site and the other to free the flap and close the donor site. The advantage of this type of flap is that the surgeon can select donor skin that will best provide color, texture, bulk, and contour at the recipient site, such as on the face.

Neurovascular Free Flap

Fascicles of nerves must be anastomosed to restore sensation; in addition, microvascular anastomoses of arteries and veins are needed to maintain viability of the donor tissue. A neurovascular free flap, also known as a sensate flap, may be taken from the scapular region. Many surgeons use the scapular flap because it is easy to dissect, has a long vascular pedicle, and creates a minimal donor site deformity. Other donor sites include the medial and lateral thigh and the lateral aspect of the upper arm.

Free Autologous Bone Graft

Vascularized autografts of bone are superior in strength and are less prone to deossification and structural weakness than conventional bone grafts. Anastomosis of the vascular bundle with a free rib, for example, may increase the chance of survival of the donor bone graft in a poorly vascularized recipient site (Figure 39-5).

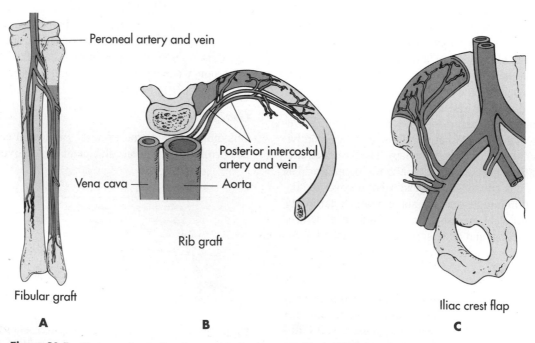

Figure 39-5 Common donor sites for vascularized bone grafts. **A,** Fibular graft. **B,** Rib graft. **C,** Iliac crest graft. (From Fortunato NM, McCullough SM: *Plastic and reconstructive surgery,* St Louis, 1998, Mosby.)

Composite Myoosteocutaneous Free Flap

A composite flap of skin, muscle, and bone provides soft tissue bulk, internal structural support, and external coverage in one-stage reconstruction of compound defects following head and neck resection. The skin and iliac crest on a vascular pedicle from the deep circumflex artery may be preferred. The scapula and tissue from the upper arm provide an alternative donor site. Or the skin, soft tissue, and latissimus dorsi muscle along with a portion of an underlying rib may be dissected free, preserving the thoracodorsal vessels for anastomosis at the recipient site. Other donor sites include the radial forearm and the fibula with the dorsalis pedis muscle.

Digital Transfer

Microneurovascular techniques are used for replantation of traumatically amputated digits. Less common is the toe-to-thumb transfer, called the free wraparound neurovascular flap, performed when an amputated thumb cannot be salvaged. Skin from the dorsum of the foot, the great toe (including tendons and bone), and the second toe web space are transferred as a sensate flap to the hand. After bone fixation and tendon anastomoses, arterial and venous circulation is established under the microscope. Digital nerves are anastomosed to reinnervate sensation and function. Other toes can be similarly transferred for finger reconstruction.

Replantation of Amputated Parts

Replantation may be attempted to salvage a traumatically amputated digit, hand, or entire upper extremity. A severed foot or lower extremity presents more formidable problems because of the functional necessity for weight bearing. The victim of amputation of the scalp, nose, external ear, or penis also is a candidate for replantation. Using microsurgical techniques, replanted parts can survive with varying degrees of effectiveness. Functional recovery, up to 80% of normal in some patients, may take up to a year or longer because it takes time for nerves to regenerate (approximately 2 inches [5 cm] per month). A team of specialists in hand surgery or of plastic and orthopaedic surgeons with microvascular skill is vital to success in these arduous procedures.

Correct care and preservation of the severed part for transport with the patient is also vital to success. The amputated part should be placed dry into a plastic bag, which is then sealed and immersed in crushed ice inside an insulated container (e.g., Styrofoam) to retard melting of the ice during travel. The part should not be warmed, frozen, or packed in dry ice. Rapid transport and cooling with ice will buy time.

Initial treatment involves assessment of the total patient. The patient and family should be supported emotionally but not given definitive promises in regard to outcome. The surgeon considers numerous factors when planning for replantation: the need for the part, associated disease and injuries, economic and psychologic factors, and age. Two criteria are of special significance:

1. The replanted part should have potential for being useful.
2. There should be no undue risk to the general safety of the patient if the procedure is performed.

Replantation is more successful in young patients than in older patients. Also, incomplete amputations are more successful because they have intact subcutaneous venous circulation in the skin bridges. Restoration is much more difficult in crush injuries than in sharp, clean amputations. Contraindications to replantation include the following:

- Prolonged warm ischemia
- Severe bruising or crushing injury
- Multiple fractures or injury at different levels in the same digit
- Associated injuries that preclude the effort

Supportive therapy following injury includes tetanus toxoid, intravenous (IV) antibiotics, fluid replacement therapy, blood products, and judicious administration of anticoagulants.

Preoperative patient preparation is in anticipation of a long procedure. The surgical procedure may take from 4 to 16 hours. The patient is placed on a gel-filled mattress. The head, scapulae, sacrum, and heels are padded. A footboard may be used, and antiembolic stockings or sequential compression devices applied. An indwelling Foley catheter is inserted. Most replantations of the hand are done with the patient under IV conscious sedation and an axillary or supraclavicular block with a long-acting agent, such as bupivacaine hydrochloride (Marcaine) without epinephrine. General anesthesia is used for children and may be needed for adults for a long procedure.

These surgical procedures usually involve a two-team approach; one team prepares the recipient site and the other prepares the severed or distal part. In the operating room (OR) the amputated part is cleansed with Ringer's lactate or normal saline. Debridement of crushed tissue is carried out. Vessels are isolated for repair, and vessel patency is ensured. The basic steps of replantation of digits or extremities include the following:

1. Identify proximal and distal tendons, nerves, and vessels.
2. Shorten bone within an acceptable limit necessary for tension-free repair of blood vessels, nerves, and soft tissues.
3. Stabilize the skeletal structure, such as with internal wire fixation techniques, to maintain joint continuity and fusion in functional position. Small plates and screws may be used.
4. Suture tendons and ligaments, both extensors and flexors, appropriately to lessen the junctional scar process that can inhibit motion.
5. Anastomose veins. A general rule is that more veins are anastomosed than are arteries to provide sufficient venous return and thereby minimize edema. Swelling

creates pressure that impedes circulation, leading to necrosis. Leech therapy may be indicated to lessen the effects of diminished venous drainage and swelling.

6. Anastomose arteries. The vessels may be flushed with heparin solution, and systemic anticoagulants may be given. Antispasmodic agents may be needed.

7. Repair nerves and soft tissues.

8. Perform a skin graft or tissue flap or transfer if necessary.

Microsurgical techniques are necessary for nerve, artery, and vein repairs of structures that have an external diameter of 1 mm or less.

To avoid constriction, a circumferential bandage is not applied. Instead, a foam bandage is used. The dressing is padded to prevent pressure sores and nerve damage. The original dressing is not changed for 10 days unless indicated.

Postoperative care is extremely important. Dressings must be checked carefully because even slight manipulation can cause great damage. Checking only the tip of the digit for circulation is not adequate. Circulation is verified by cautiously looking into the dressing to check the capillary refill, color, temperature, and drainage. A Doppler and a temperature probe may be used to evaluate arterial circulation. Patients are not permitted to smoke because nicotine is a vasoconstrictor. Constriction of vessels may reduce circulation.

The many hours expended by the OR team initially to achieve a successful repair of all structures can relieve the patient of subsequent procedures. The objective is to obtain maximal return of function by minimizing permanent disability. Physical and occupational therapies are important in rehabilitation.

General Considerations for All Tissue Autografts

1. Hypothermia is avoided. Room temperature should be increased to 75° to 80° F (24° to 27° C).

2. For long procedures, the patient should be positioned on a gel pad mattress.

3. Skin may be prepped with a colorless antiseptic agent so that the plastic surgeon can see the true skin color and assess the vascularity of the donor graft.

4. Donor and recipient sites are prepped and draped separately but concurrently. Care is taken that cross-contamination does not occur from one site to the other.

5. The recipient site is covered with a sterile drape until the surgeon is ready to apply a free graft or pedicle flap if preparation of the donor site will be the first procedure. If the recipient site must be prepared to receive the donor graft or flap, the donor site is covered.

6. A separate sterile instrument table is prepared for the donor site. This includes appropriate instruments for obtaining the graft or flap and dressings for the donor site. Two surgical teams may work simultaneously.

   Place the dermatome on a separate, small sterile table, never on the recipient instrument table. Handle dermatomes carefully so that the depth gauge is not disturbed.

7. Grafts are kept moist by covering them with a sponge wet with normal saline. A free flap should be kept in iced saline slush until the recipient site is prepared.

8. The operating microscope and appropriate microinstruments must be in readiness for microvascular and neuro anastomoses.

9. Tissue viability must be ensured. A sterile device may be needed during the surgical procedure to identify major blood vessels underlying a graft. Assessment of the patency of vessels and perfusion of the flap is possible through several types of monitoring.

   a. *Doppler probe.* A Doppler probe is placed on the recipient site preoperatively to obtain baseline measurements for comparison with postoperative measurements. The microcomputer machine has a digital readout. Ultrasonic Doppler probes also may be used for monitoring.

   b. *Photoplethysmographic disk.* A disk applied to the flap surface measures reflected light from pulsatile blood flow changes in tissue. A change in blood volume in tissue produces a corresponding change in the amount of light reflected. These changes are amplified and displayed on an oscilloscope.

   c. *Fluorometer.* A fluorescing dye is injected IV, and fluorescence is measured with a fluorometer for perfusion of the flap. Fluorescein and an ultraviolet Wood's lamp are used to check patency and perfusion. The room is darkened to see fluorescence. A photomultiplier may be used to amplify skin fluorescent emission.

   d. *Thermocouple probe.* The patency of a microvascular anastomosis can be assessed by the temperature in surrounding tissues.

10. Hemostasis is obtained during the surgical procedure with the use of warm saline packs, pressure, or thrombin.

11. An ESU is used very sparingly to prevent the devitalization of tissues.

12. Dressings over grafts vary by surgeon preference. Stent fixation to obtain pressure on the grafted area may be preferred. Some plastic surgeons omit pressure dressings and use an exposure technique on grafts so that they can watch the graft and incise a hematoma if necessary. The graft is kept covered with sterile, moist saline gauze dressings to keep the skin moist until revascularization occurs. Synthetic adhesive dressings that are moisture and vapor permeable are impermeable to liquid and bacteria. Healing under these occlusive dressings may be more rapid and less painful than at donor sites covered with fine-mesh gauze. A cast may be applied to immobilize extremities for pedicle flaps.

HEAD AND NECK PLASTIC AND RECONSTRUCTIVE PROCEDURES

Some plastic surgeons specialize in head and neck oncology or reconstruction, or both. Others limit their practice to aesthetic, or cosmetic, surgery.

Soft Tissue Reconstruction

Defects in soft tissues of the face or scalp, usually as a result of trauma, may be reconstructed by advancement of tissue expanded from an adjacent area. This technique ensures consistent skin color, texture, and hair-bearing characteristics. Other types of grafts or flaps may be necessary or preferred.

Craniofacial Surgical Procedures

The plastic surgeon usually heads the multidisciplinary team that performs the complex craniofacial procedures discussed in Chapter 40. Many of the concepts developed for these procedures are applied in less complicated surgical procedures. A variety of extracranial osteotomies, with or without bone grafts, reshape the bony framework of the face and skull. The desired aesthetic and functional results can be obtained only by painstakingly careful planning, dissection, and repositioning.

Maxillofacial and Oral Surgical Procedures

Plastic surgeons reconstruct soft tissue defects around and in the mouth that are caused by trauma or surgical resection. Those maxillofacial procedures involving bony structures that may also be performed by plastic surgeons are discussed in Chapter 40. Congenital deformities are discussed in Chapter 8.

Facial Nerve Grafting

Restoration of the quality of facial expressions in a patient with severe facial nerve paralysis can be accomplished by transfacial nerve grafting. Segments of nerve grafts are brought through tunnels across the lips from the normal side of the face to the paralyzed side. These are anastomosed to the distal facial nerve on the normal side and then to the proximal branches of the injured nerve on the paralyzed side. The overpull of the mouth and lower face toward the normal side is balanced when the nerve graft is anastomosed between fascicles of the intact facial nerve innervating the facial muscles to the same fascicles on the denervated side. If the facial muscle has been paralyzed for a prolonged period, the serratus muscle from the chest wall may be transplanted and innervated by the facial nerve.

Repair of Lacerations of the Lip or Mouth

Wound edges of the lip(s) and/or mucosa in the mouth are carefully sutured to repair lacerations. The borders of the vermilion line are carefully realigned.

Excision of Leukoplakia

Chronic irritation can result in an abnormal whitening of the mucous membrane of the lip and tongue (leukoplakia), a lesion primarily seen in heavy smokers. Sharp dissection or a CO_2 laser is used to resect a precancerous lesion.

Excision of a Lip Tumor

Excision of a lip tumor may be minor, with V-wedge excision, or extensive, depending on the stage of malignancy. Extensive lesions require a flap procedure for reconstruction.

Lip Reconstruction

Lips can be adequately reconstructed by a variety of techniques to restore sensation and motor function following trauma or surgical resection. Lip cancer is the most common type of cancer in the upper respiratory and digestive tracts. Surgical procedures to reconstruct lips may be classified as follows:

- Repair by primary closure of the remaining lip segments.
- Full-thickness cross-lip flaps from the opposite lip.
- Arterialized or myocutaneous flaps from adjacent cheek or nasolabial tissue.
- Distant flaps. Arterialized and innervated myocutaneous flaps from the forehead or deltopectoral region may be used. These require staged procedures. Free microvascular composite grafts are done in one stage.

The ideal repair yields a lip that is not tight and that has a good vermilion border, an adequate sulcus (philtrum), good sensation, and good muscle tone.

Aesthetic Procedures

Procedures are not always performed for aesthetic purposes alone. They may restore function as well as correct a facial deformity or defect.

Blepharoplasty

Redundant skin and/or protruding orbital fat is excised to correct deformities of the upper or lower eyelids of one or both eyes. Blepharochalasis (loss of elasticity of the skin of the eyelids) can occur at any age and usually is of unknown cause. Dermatochalasis primarily involves hypertrophy of the skin of the upper lids. Resection of the excessive redundant skin removes the mechanical visual obstruction caused by these two conditions. Protrusion of intraorbital fat into the lids is the most common eyelid deformity. It is often familial and is sometimes seen in patients as young as 20 years of age. This fat is removed from the compartments in the upper and/or lower lids to correct the deformity. This may be associated with dermatochalasis. A free graft of cartilage and mucosa from the nasal septum may be necessary to reconstruct lower eyelid defects following excision for tumor. Hypertrophy of the orbicularis muscle appears as a horizontal bulge below the lower lid margin. A skin-muscle flap resection may be performed. A surgical procedure for lifting the eyebrows will secondarily correct a hooding deformity of the upper lids caused by ptosis of the eyebrows.

These procedures are usually performed with the patient under local anesthesia. An upper lid incision is made in a natural skin fold; an incision in the lower lid is just under the eyelash line (Figure 39-6). The patient should wear dentures to the OR because facial contour is distorted without them. The surgeon could remove too much or too little redundant skin.

Because of the proximity to the eyes, protrusion of periorbital fat may impair vision. Oculoplastic procedures may be performed by an ophthalmologist. Through a conjunctival incision, subconjunctival fat may be removed with a CO_2

Figure 39-6 Incisions for blepharoplasty. **A,** Upper eyelid. **B,** Lower eyelid. (From Ruberg RL, Smith DJ Jr: *Plastic surgery: a core curriculum,* St Louis, 1994, Mosby.)

laser. An eyelid procedure also may be necessary to protect the eye in a patient with facial nerve paralysis caused by trauma or tumor resection. A gold weight, between 0.05 and 1.2 g, or a spring can be inserted in the upper eyelid with the patient under local anesthesia. This protects the eye by allowing the eyelid to blink.

Otoplasty

Deformities of one or both external ears of an adult are usually the result of burns or traumatic avulsion. A segment of external ear that is partially or completely amputated often can be reattached to the remaining segment and buried beneath a flap of postauricular skin. The area over a completely severed auricular cartilage, which cannot be sutured back in place, is covered with a split-thickness skin graft initially. Later reconstruction may include insertion of cartilage taken from the patient's rib cage, a cartilage allograft, or a porous polyethylene or silicone prosthetic implant. The porous implant allows vascular and soft tissue ingrowth that reduces the risk of infection and extrusion—potential complications with a silicone implant. The graft or implant is buried beneath a segment of turned-down temporoparietal fascia. Then the area is covered with a split-thickness skin graft from the scalp or a full-thickness graft from the opposite postauricular area.

Rhinoplasty

Reshaping of the nose, although usually performed for cosmetic alteration desired by the patient, may be necessary to correct defects caused by trauma or surgical resection of neoplasms. Subtle changes with limited nasal reduction or aug-

mentation of the nasal tip with the patient's own nasal cartilage can result in an aesthetically attractive and physiologically normal nose in most patients. Through an intranasal incision, the nose can be shortened or narrowed by rearranging, reshaping, and/or removing bone and cartilage. This may be done to relieve breathing problems. Nasal packing and a nasal splint support the structures postoperatively.

A free composite graft or pedicle flap may be necessary to close a large tissue defect. Bone or cartilage grafts may be needed for skeletal support. Prosthetic reconstruction for partial or total loss of the nose may be the procedure of choice.

Mentoplasty

The shape and size of the chin can be altered for aesthetics and/or functional bite disorders. The mandible can be repositioned forward or backward to change alignment in relation to the maxilla. Sections are removed to reduce size, or osteotomies are made to reshape the chin. An abnormally small jaw (micrognathia) is augmented with bone or cartilage grafts or a silicone implant, or by advancing the mandible. Lip incompetence (inability to bring the lips together without tension) may be corrected during the same surgical procedure.

Rhytidoplasty

Commonly referred to as a face lift, rhytidoplasty involves extensive dissection from above the ear, both in front of and behind the pinna, downward along the jaw line and upper neck (Figure 39-7, *A*). The skin is freed from underlying fascia. Wrinkles and folds caused by the normal aging process smooth out as the skin is lifted up and sutured in place. Dissection beneath the platysma muscle, referred to as the submuscular aponeurotic system (SMAS) procedure, minimizes the amount of skin undermined. The platysma is sutured back to the mastoid (Figure 39-7, *B* and *C*). Redundant skin is trimmed away. Frequently other procedures, such as blepharoplasty or rhinoplasty, accompany this surgical procedure. Meticulous hemostasis is essential to prevent hematoma formation, the foremost complication of rhytidoplasty. Hypotensive anesthesia may be used to help reduce this incidence. Closed wound suction drainage is frequently used with or without a pressure dressing applied after the surgical procedure.

Soft Tissue Augmentation

Fat transplantation may be done by mini-liposuction and injection of the patient's own tissue. Fat cells are withdrawn from the lower abdomen, hips, or thighs into a syringe through a hypodermic needle. The fat then is injected into areas around the lips or eyes to smooth wrinkles or into hollow spaces in the cheeks or other facial defects. This procedure may be done in conjunction with a rhytidoplasty. The correction is not permanent because some of the fat cells will die.

A purified form of bovine dermal collagen can be injected for the same purposes. A series of injections of small amounts of the collagen are deposited to fill small soft tissue defects or to smooth out wrinkles.

Figure 39-7 Rhytidoplasty (face lift). **A,** Incision from above ear and in front of and behind pinna. **B,** Dissection beneath and elevation of platysma flap (SMAS procedure). **C,** Platysma muscle is sutured back to mastoid. (From Ruberg RL, Smith DJ Jr: *Plastic surgery: a core curriculum,* St Louis, 1994, Mosby.)

Hair Replacement

Hair follicles can be transplanted from the posterior aspect of the scalp to bald or balding areas. Hundreds of micrografts (4 mm) and minigrafts (4.5 mm) are randomly scattered over the entire bald area to change the hairline. A new hairline can be initially established with rotational flaps from other parts of the scalp. This may necessitate tissue expansion. If hair loss is not complete, hair follicle grafts complement and thicken the

existing hair. Several transplantation sessions may be necessary to achieve the final result the patient is seeking.

Neck Dissection

Dissections for tumors originating in the head, neck, or tongue region are discussed in Chapter 40. Following primary resection by a laryngologist, head and neck oncologist, or oral surgeon, the plastic surgeon may be called on to reconstruct the resultant defect. The plastic surgeon may be the primary surgeon who resects a tumor or lesion approached through the oral cavity or neck, followed by an immediate reconstruction.

PLASTIC AND RECONSTRUCTIVE PROCEDURES OF OTHER BODY AREAS

Adipose Tissue

Lipectomy is an excision of excessive fat and redundant skin from the upper arms, abdomen, buttocks, thighs, or other body areas.

Liposuction

Localized areas of fat deposits are removed by suction-assisted lipectomy, known as liposuction, to alter body contours. Most surgeons prefer to inject target tissue with 1% lidocaine with 1:100,000 epinephrine in saline to create a tumescent effect. This solution also reduces blood loss during the surgical procedure. A blunt, hollow, curved or straight metal cannula (Mercedes cannula) measuring 1.5 to 6 mm with multiple openings in the distal shaft connected to a suction machine is inserted through small skin incisions (Figure 39-8). The cannula is moved back and forth along the axial plane, parallel to the skin surface, to bluntly dissect and aspirate cores of fat in a honeycomb pattern. This pattern allows for uniform tissue contouring. A laser beam may be used through the cannula to vaporize fat rather than suction it out. The laser diminishes bleeding by coagulating vessels. The patient's hematocrit level decreases by 1% for each 150 cc of fat removed by conventional liposuction.

Suction-assisted lipectomy may be used in conjunction with conventional abdominoplasty. It is also used to remove fat from the neck and chin, upper arms, breasts, flanks, buttocks, thighs, knees, and ankles. It can be used to defat transfer flaps and to treat some forms of lymphedema and lipomas. The amount of fat removed should not exceed the ability of the overlying skin to contract and may be between 1500 and 2000 cc. If tumescence is used, 2500 to 3000 cc may be removed without complications. Large fluid volume shifts follow lipectomy. The incisions are sutured and reinforced with wound closure strips, and compression garments are worn for 10 days to 2 weeks postoperatively to control edema.

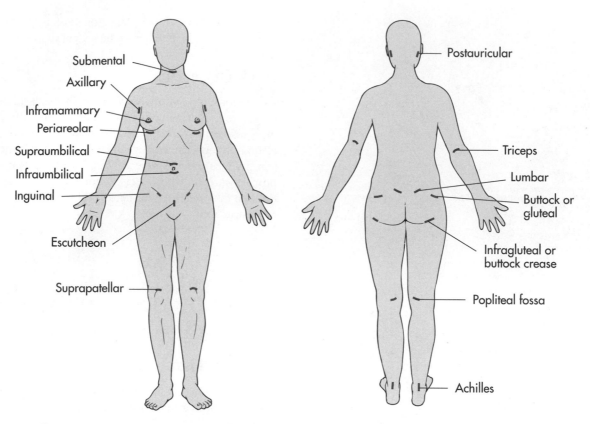

Figure 39-8 Incision areas for suction-assisted lipectomy. (From Fortunato NM, McCullough SM: *Plastic and reconstructive surgery,* St Louis, 1998, Mosby.)

Abdominoplasty

Abdominoplasty includes excising excess, lax abdominal wall skin and adipose tissue and tightening abdominal wall musculature. This is usually a cosmetic procedure referred to as a "tummy tuck." Physical discomfort or the inability to perform personal hygiene because of a large panniculus that hangs like an apron over the lower abdomen and genital region may be a functional indication for the procedure. Its purpose is not to make an obese person thin. The most suitable patient is of ideal weight and in good health. Causes of the abdominal wall laxity include pregnancy, marked weight loss, and the aging process.

Preoperatively the primary incision line is marked along a natural skin fold using a marking pen with the patient in a standing position. After the administration of anesthesia, the head and foot of the operating bed are elevated 15 to 20 degrees to anteflex the patient's torso and decrease abdominal tension. The surgeon chooses either a low transverse incision from one anterior superior iliac spine to the other or a combination transverse–secondary vertical incision (Figure 39-9). The typical area of dissection extends subcutaneously to the costal margins and xiphoid process superiorly and to the mid to lateral axillary lines laterally. The umbilicus is preserved on a vascularized stalk and repositioned in the abdominal wall after the rectus muscle is tightened (plicated) and excess skin, subcutaneous tissue, and fat are resected. When wound closure is completed, the abdominal wall should be flat and

smooth. Closed suction drainage, a bulky pressure dressing, and an abdominal binder are used to prevent hematoma formation and eliminate dead space.

Postoperatively the patient is restricted to complete bed rest with the head and foot of the bed flexed for 24 hours and then may ambulate progressively.

Breast

Breasts can be enlarged, reduced, or reconstructed. Unilateral augmentation or reduction is sometimes performed to correct asymmetry of the breasts.

Augmentation Mammoplasty

A bilateral mammoplasty usually is performed for aesthetics on a woman who desires larger breasts. Inflatable implants are inserted under either breast tissue or the underlying pectoralis muscles and then filled with sterile saline solution through self-sealing valves.

The breast implant can be inserted through a periareolar, transaxillary, inframammary, or supraumbilical endoscopic approach. The periareolar incision, made around the outside border of the lower half of the areola, is the most difficult for insertion of the implant, but it leaves the most inconspicuous scar. The transaxillary incision in the axilla does not scar the breast. The inframammary incision, the most common, is made transversely along the submammary fold. The implant

Figure 39-9 Abdominoplasty incisions. **A,** Medial to iliac crest for patient who desires high "French cut" swimsuit. **B,** In natural abdominal skin crease fold below iliac crest. (From Ruberg RL, Smith DJ Jr: *Plastic surgery: a core curriculum,* St Louis, 1994, Mosby.)

is inserted into a pocket formed between the mammary gland and pectoralis muscle or under the muscle.

An implant can also be inserted through a supraumbilical endoscopic approach. This technique eliminates an incision into the breast. A single incision is made in the superior border of the inner aspect of the umbilicus. An endoscope is inserted between the fascia and subcutaneous tissue up to the breast. The endoscope permits visual placement of a deflated expander between the breast tissue and the pectoralis muscle. The expander is filled with sterile saline solution, through a fill tube, to create a pocket for the implant. After insertion through the endoscope into the pocket, the deflated implant is inflated with sterile saline solution and the fill tube is removed.

Most implants are supplied sterile by the manufacturer. The manufacturer's instructions for sterilization of nonsterile implants must be followed. Sterile packages should not be opened by the circulator until the surgeon selects the appropriate-size implants. Silastic sizers are frequently used to make this determination. The implant identification card should be put in the patient's chart, and each implant's catalog and lot number recorded.

The woman with breast implants is not excluded from routine screening mammography programs. Additional radiologic images may be taken to visualize all of the breast tissue. Ultrasonography may be performed at the same time to confirm the integrity of the implant. Studies have shown that the risk of rupturing the implant is not increased by compression during mammography if performed according to the American College of Radiology standards.

Capsular contraction, hematoma, infection, and skin necrosis are potential complications following prosthetic implantation for breast augmentation performed either unilat-

erally or bilaterally. Because of reported incidences of rupture and leakage, with the possibility of the development of autoimmune disease, implants containing silicone gel are not used for breast augmentation or reconstruction unless women are enrolled in a controlled clinical study.

Removing a ruptured or leaking silicone implant frequently is complicated by intracapsular adhesions. Control of bleeding points is critical, to prevent silicone emboli in open blood vessels. This necessitates meticulous capsular dissection and hemostasis during removal of the implant shell, as well as irrigation with copious amounts of sterile saline solution to remove viscous silicone from the wound.

Reconstructive Mammoplasty

Breast reconstruction following mastectomy psychologically helps the patient cope with an altered body image. The type and timing of reconstruction are influenced by the patient's psychologic response to the mastectomy, the type of mastectomy, and the patient's diagnosis and prognosis. Technical maneuvers of the general surgeon at the time of mastectomy will influence the possibility of an aesthetically acceptable result following breast reconstruction by the plastic surgeon.

To reconstruct breast contour, an implant may be inserted beneath the muscle layers at the time of subcutaneous mastectomy. Following modified radical or radical mastectomy, the wound should be well healed, the scar mature, and the skin well vascularized before implantation. A prosthesis can be implanted only when reliable skin is available to cover it. Skin flaps should be cut as thickly as is consistent with a curative mastectomy. If sufficient skin flaps are not available, the plastic surgeon may use a tissue expander or transfer a pedicle skin flap from the abdomen or back to the chest wall.

Immediate breast reconstruction, or a delay of only a few days, after a modified radical mastectomy can be psychologically advantageous in women who have small lesions and no metastases. A latissimus dorsi myocutaneous flap may be used with an inflatable implant. A vertical or transverse rectus abdominis myocutaneous (TRAM) island flap with the vascular bundle from the superior epigastric vessels can be used without an implant. These flaps can also be used weeks to months after mastectomy for reconstruction. Aesthetically, the end result is a semblance of a breast in weight and consistency. An areola and nipple complex may be constructed in a second-stage surgical procedure. Dermapigmentation (a form of tattooing) may be used to create natural color and shading resembling the nipple-areola complex.

The techniques described may be contraindicated in markedly obese patients and in some patients because a sufficient amount of autogenous tissue is not present for breast reconstruction. Another option is to place a tissue expander under the pectoralis muscle. When the desired expansion is achieved, usually slightly larger than the other breast, the expander can be replaced with a permanent prosthesis. One type of expander/mammary prosthesis has a detachable reservoir and tubing to convert the expander into a permanent prosthesis. If this technique is not an option and the patient does not have adequate tissue in the lower abdomen or back, transfer of a microvascular free flap may be the procedure of choice. The vascular pedicle from a transverse abdominis rectus, superior gluteal, or inferior gluteal myocutaneous free flap may be anastomosed to the axillary or thoracodorsal vessels.

Reduction Mammoplasty

Hyperplasia of the breasts is reduced by resection of skin and glandular tissue. Reduction mammoplasty is usually sought by women for comfort, as well as aesthetic improvement of body image. The nipple-areola complexes are mobilized and transferred intact with the underlying breast tissue, maintaining the blood and nerve supply. The excess skin and glandular tissue may be excised with a scalpel, dermatome blade, or laser. Because breast tissue is very vascular, attention to hemostasis is important. The CO_2 laser offers the advantage of coagulating small blood vessels and sealing lymphatics as tissue is incised. A hemostatic scalpel can be used for the same purposes.

Scars

Scar formation, the body's mechanism for healing wounds, is inevitable whenever skin is incised or injured. The plastic surgeon attempts to make a scar a fine line and as level and smooth as possible at the time of primary wound closure or as a secondary scar revision.

Scar Revision

The plastic surgeon can excise an aesthetically displeasing scar, realign wound edges, and resuture or close them with anticipation of a better cosmetic result. The direction of a scar can be changed to be less conspicuous in the natural skin lines. Scars are frequently revised following extensive reconstructive procedures or following a laceration with or without soft tissue trauma, particularly a facial scar. Z-plasty, W-plasty, M-plasty, lazy-S, Y-V–plasty, and other techniques are used to improve the appearance of a hypertrophied or prominent scar.

Keloid formation, an abnormal deposition of collagen in healing skin wounds, presents a particularly difficult problem for the plastic surgeon and a psychologic problem for the patient. Keloids may require excision and grafting. The administration of a lathryrogenic agent and colchicine to inhibit cross-linking of newly synthesized collagen following grafting may prevent the development of recurrent keloid formation. The argon laser also is used in treatment of keloid scars to reduce the blood supply to the scar and to alter the balance of collagen synthesis and lysis.

Dermabrasion

Dirt and cinders can become embedded in the dermis from a brush-burn injury. The plastic surgeon may use a wire brush or sandpaper to scrub out dirt and irrigate it from the area with warm saline solution. Sandpapering is also done to improve acne scars. This procedure is not always satisfactory if many pitted scars are too deep to reach or there are changes in the pigment of scars. Some plastic surgeons prefer to use chemical preparations, such as phenol, trichloroacetic acid, or alpha-hydroxy acid, to produce dermal peeling for a skin-smoothing effect in selected patients with facial scars or fine wrinkles. The patient is advised to avoid direct sun exposure for at least 6 months. Patients with fair complexions and thin skin have more favorable results than patients with dark, oily complexions because the chemicals used decrease melanin in the skin and cause discoloration.

A high-speed dermabrader with rotating tips covered with diamond dust can be used on moderately damaged or tattooed skin. The rotating speed is controlled by regulation of pressure from the compressed nitrogen gas power source. Older dermabraders have narrow bands of waterproof, steam-sterilizable sandpaper mounted on an electric, air-powered, or battery-operated drill.

Facial resurfacing also can be accomplished with the CO_2 laser. The depth of beam penetration is controlled by the focus of the beam. Full-face laser resurfacing promotes continuity of skin color and texture rather than spot removal of facial scars (Table 39-1).

Skin Cancer

Because overexposure to sunlight is the primary cause of skin cancer, most skin cancers occur on areas of the face, neck, and ears. Basal cell carcinoma, squamous cell carcinoma, and malignant melanoma are the three types of skin cancer. Certain types of nevi are skin lesions that may be precancerous and therefore should be removed. Skin lesions may be removed by the following methods:

- Excision and closure with sutures, grafts, or flaps
- Punch biopsy with closure by second intention

TABLE 39-1	Examples of Lasers Used for Skin Surface Modifications	
Type of Laser	**Spectrum of Light**	**Notes**
Argon	Blue-green	Used for treatment of superficial vascular lesions, pigmented areas and some inflammatory lesions; absorbed by hemoglobin
CO_2	Infrared	Has a red aiming beam to make the invisible infrared laser visible; absorbed by water
Tunable dye (Candela)	Yellow	Used to treat port-wine stains and vascular ectasis; very selective vascular destruction; absorbed by pigmented tissues
KTP:YAG	Green	Used to treat tattoos, vascular lesions, and pigmented lesions; good for removal of black, yellow, or blue colors; works well for dark-skinned patients; articulated arm
Alexandrite	Red	Used to treat tattoos, particularly blue, black, and green; not good for orange or yellow; fiberoptic: flexible arm

From Fortunato NM, McCullough SM: *Plastic and reconstructive surgery,* St Louis, 1998, Mosby.
KTP:YAG, Potassium titanyl phosphate:yttrium-aluminum-garnet.

- Cold knife excision for frozen section
- Electrosurgical curettage and electrodesiccation
- Cryosurgery
- Laser surgery
- Radiation therapy

Mohs' micrographic surgery is a technique used to excise advanced, recurrent, or poorly defined basal cell or squamous cell carcinomas of the skin with minimal excision of normal tissue. The bulk of the clinically evident tumor is excised initially. Then the lesion is resected by serial tangential excision (i.e., underlying tissue layers are removed with 1- to 3-mm borders). Each layer is numbered and charted for size and location. A map of the corresponding margins of each layer is drawn. The tissue is frozen, cut into sections, and examined microscopically. The patient may be allowed to leave the OR and wait in a waiting room for the results. The surgeon removes additional layers of tissue or extends dissection until microscopic examination determines that all cancer cells have been removed. A map of the excisional area is created. Then the wound is closed. Small wounds may be left open to heal by second intention. Others may be sutured or covered with a rotational myocutaneous flap from an adjacent area. Large denuded areas may require a split- or full-

thickness skin graft. If a cartilage graft is needed, cartilage may be transferred from the auricle (pinna) of the ear to the transplant site.

Mohs' surgery is not used for excision of malignant melanomas. Primary melanomas are treated according to their anatomic site and level of cutaneous penetration. A wide margin of normal tissue is excised around the melanoma. Skin grafts often are required. Regional lymph node dissection may be indicated to control metastatic disease.

BURNS

Skin and underlying tissues can be destroyed by thermal, chemical, or electrical injury. Burns are open wounds. As in other injuries, initial treatment is aimed at saving the patient's life. Then the treatment is directed toward preserving or restoring to normal, or as near normal as possible, the patient's bodily functions and appearance as rapidly as possible. Depending on the depth, extent, and location of the burn, reconstruction may extend over long periods of time, from months to years. The patient must be helped to accept the disfigurement; thus rehabilitation from a psychologic standpoint is important. Psychotherapy, as well as surgery and physiotherapy, may be necessary to promote as early a return to normalcy and usefulness as possible.

Classification of Burns

The severity of the injury is determined by the location and the cause of the burn. The Abbreviated Burn Severity Index (ABSI) is a five-variable scale used to evaluate burn injury severity and the probability of survival. The five variables are sex, age, presence of inhalation injury, presence of full-thickness burn, and percentage of total body surface burned. An ABSI score of 2 to 18 is calculated by the summation of coded values for each variable. Burns are classified by depth and extent as soon after injury as possible. The depth of a burn is classified by the degree of tissue involvement:

- *First-degree superficial burn.* Only the outer layer of the epidermis is involved in a first-degree burn. Superficial erythema, redness of the skin, and tissue destruction occur, but healing takes place rapidly.
- *Second-degree partial-thickness burn.* All epidermis and varying depths of the dermis are destroyed in a second-degree burn. This is usually characterized by blister formation, pain, and a moist, mottled red or pink appearance. Hair follicles and sebaceous glands may be destroyed. Reepithelialization can occur provided that the deepest layer of the epithelium is viable. Superimposed infection can interfere with healing. Thickened scars form following healing of deep second-degree burns.
- *Third-degree full-thickness burn.* The skin, with all of its epithelial structures and subcutaneous tissue, is destroyed in a third-degree burn. This is characterized by a dry, pearly white or charred-appearing surface void

Relative percentage of areas
affected by growth

	Age in Years					
	0	1	5	10	15	Adult
A—½ of head	9½	8½	6½	5½	4½	3½
B—½ of one thigh	2¾	3¼	4	4¼	4½	4¾
C—½ of one leg	2½	2½	2¾	3	3¼	3½
Total percent burned			2° +		3° =	

Figure 39-10   Lund-Browder chart to determine relative percentage of areas of burns on child's body.

of sensation. The destroyed skin forms a parchmentlike eschar over the burned area. If removed or left to slough off, eschar leaves a denuded surface that can extend to the fascia. Third-degree burns require skin grafts for healing to occur unless the area is small enough for closure by reepithelialization.

- *Fourth-degree burn.* Sometimes referred to as char burns, fourth-degree burns may damage bones, tendons, muscles, blood vessels, and peripheral nerves. An electrical burn, for example, causes damage much deeper than is apparent on the skin surface. Often, necrotic muscle and bone must be excised.

Estimation of Burn Damage

Two methods are used to estimate the total percentage of body surface burned and the percentage of each degree of burn.

Lund-Browder Chart

The percentage sizes of the head and lower extremities differ in infancy, childhood, and adulthood. According to the guide-

lines of the Lund-Browder chart (Figure 39-10), the percentage of burn is estimated on the basis of age in addition to the anatomic location of the burn.

Rule of Nines

The body surface of an adult can be divided into areas equal to multiples of 9% of the total body surface (Figure 39-11).

Initial Care of the Burn Patient

Patients admitted to the emergency department with obvious burns may have multiple injuries and/or a pretrauma medical history that will complicate treatment. Initial care must include the following measures:

1. Stop the burning process. All clothing, jewelry, metal, and synthetic objects in contact with the patient's skin are removed.
2. Ensure a patent airway. The respiratory system may be damaged from inhalation of superheated air or toxic gases. Immediate nasotracheal intubation with assisted

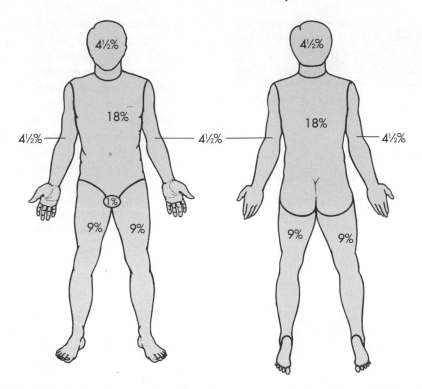

Figure 39-11 Rule-of-nines chart to estimate burn injury to an adult. (From Fortunato NM, McCullough SM: *Plastic and reconstructive surgery*, St Louis, 1998, Mosby.)

mechanical ventilation may be necessary. Soft endotracheal tubes are preferred for prolonged intubation. Tracheotomy may be required several days later for prolonged respiratory assistance if the patient cannot be weaned from the ventilator. Bronchoscopy is performed routinely to evaluate the extent of tracheobronchial damage.

3. Establish IV fluid therapy. Blood samples are drawn for laboratory analysis and type and crossmatching when a venipuncture or cutdown is performed to establish an IV route for fluid and nutritional administration. Fluid and electrolyte balance must be restored as quickly as possible. Fluid, electrolytes, and protein are lost through changes in capillary permeability, causing intravascular volume shifts to interstitial tissues. Fluid shifts are directly proportional to the depth and extent of the burn. Several formulas for determining fluid replacement have been developed to maintain plasma volume during the first 24 hours (Table 39-2). The calculated fluid replacement time begins at the time of injury, not when the patient arrives in the emergency department. A crystalloid solution of Ringer's lactate is infused initially because its hypertonic state decreases fluid loss from the intravascular space. Colloid-containing fluid, fresh frozen plasma, and other nutrients may be infused after the first 24 hours.

4. Insert an indwelling Foley catheter. Urine specimens are sent for analysis. Urine is checked for pH and specific gravity at frequent intervals. The hourly output is recorded. Adequate fluid replacement should maintain an output of at least 30 ml/hr.

5. Cleanse the wound. All burns are treated aseptically. A mild cleansing agent, such as povidone-iodine, and warm water or saline solution are used to gently remove debris and loose, devitalized tissue. Copious amounts of water, along with appropriate neutralizing agents, are used to cleanse and irrigate chemical burns. After cleansing, wet sheets under and around the patient must be removed and dry, sterile ones applied. Nonwoven sheets specifically designed for burn care are commercially available.

6. Estimate the percentage and depth of the burn. Definitive treatment may be completed in the emergency department, or the patient may be transported to an immersion tank for further cleansing and debridement or to the OR for initiation of further therapy as indicated by assessment of the burn. The burned area is covered with sterile or clean linen for transfer of the patient from the emergency department.

7. Assess the patient's preexisting medical history and other injuries. The patient may have a chronic illness, such as diabetes or heart disease, that must be stabilized as part of the treatment regimen. Withdrawal from alcohol or drugs may cause physiologic disturbances. The patient may have suffered other injuries in the accident causing the burn. Abuse may be suspected, particularly in a child or older person. Appropriate interventions must be taken. The burn may not be the first priority if, for example, the patient has a head injury, ruptured internal organs, or fractures.

8. Prepare the patient for transport. The patient may go from the emergency department directly to a burn unit, the OR, or some other care area. The attending physician may

TABLE 39-2	Fluid Replacement Formulas* for Burn Patients Developed at Major Burn Centers	
First 24 Hours	**Second 24 Hours**	

First 24 Hours	Second 24 Hours
Parkland Hospital	
Crystalloid	
4 ml Ringer's lactate/% burn/kg	Dextrose 5% in water
One half during first 8 hours	maintenance
One half during next 16 hours	
Colloid	
None	0.5 ml/% burn/kg
Brooke Army Hospital	
Crystalloid	
2 ml Ringer's lactate/% burn/kg	Dextrose 5% in water
One half during first 8 hours	maintenance
One half during next 16 hours	
Colloid	
None	0.5 ml/% burn/kg
Massachusetts General Hospital	
Crystalloid	
1.5 ml Ringer's lactate/% burn/kg	None specified
One half during first 8 hours	
One half during next 16 hours	
Colloid	
0.5 ml/% burn/kg	None specified
None during first 4 hours	
One half during second 4 hours	
One half during next 16 hours	

*Formula is calculated as percent of total body surface (% TBSB) × each kilogram (kg) of body weight × milliliters (ml) of fluid.

initiate therapy before referral to a plastic surgeon. If available, hyperbaric oxygen (HBO) therapy may be used. HBO produces marked vasoconstriction, decreasing the loss of serum through the burn surface. This may reduce the need for fluid replacement. Oxygen in cells around the burn may positively affect burn tissue to regenerate and begin healing. Partial-thickness burns may be prevented from progressing to full-thickness burns.

Methods of Surgical Treatment

Prevention of infection and promotion of healing are of utmost concern in the treatment of burn patients. The probability of infection developing increases in proportion to the percentage of body surface burned. Colonization may begin as early as 24 hours after the burn.

Excisional Debridement

Primary excision of necrotic tissue from deep second-degree and all full-thickness third-degree burned areas, followed immediately by skin grafting, is performed as soon as possible after the injury. Debridement can be accomplished with a

scalpel, scissors, or other specialized instrument. The surgeon selects the most appropriate instrument for the particular burned area to be excised. Layers of burned tissue are removed sequentially until capillary bleeding indicates that tissue is viable. Hypotensive anesthesia may help control massive blood loss during extensive excisions.

Mesh grafts are frequently used to expand available autografts. Micro–skin grafting is another alternative for maximizing a split-thickness autograft. The donor skin is cut with scissors into tiny particles. These are placed on the dermal side of an allograft. This dermal surface is placed on the recipient burn site. The skin particles grow together to resurface the area; then the allograft is rejected.

An allograft or xenograft may be applied to temporarily cover an area until regeneration proceeds or sufficient autografts can be harvested. Skin substitutes also are available to temporarily cover wounds, both recipient and donor sites. A composite silicone-nylon membrane with a chemically bonded polypeptide of collagen (Biobrane) will adhere to the wound surface to inhibit infection and control fluid loss. Another artificial material incorporates a layer of bovine hide collagen onto a layer of silicone. These biologic dressings and skin substitutes must be changed periodically.

Tangential Excision Burned tissue is excised until normal dermal tissue is reached below the depth of the wound. Tangential excision is usually the procedure of choice for deep partial-thickness burns of the dorsum of the hands or on the arms or legs. It is advantageous to minimize contractures. The wound base, containing some viable dermal structures necessary for regeneration, is covered with a split-thickness autograft. Early tangential excision and grafting in one procedure for body surface burns can reduce mortality and septic complications and shorten hospitalization.

Escharectomy Full-thickness eschar is excised down to the fascia when viable tissues in more superficial layers are not evident, except on the hands, neck, or face. All denuded areas created by excision are covered with a biologic dressing for 3 to 5 days. They are then grafted with full-thickness autografts. Frequently, split-thickness mesh grafts must be used to spread over large areas and allow seepage of serous fluids. These are not placed on the face and neck or over joints. If sufficient skin is not available for autografting, allografts or xenografts continue to be used as biologic dressings for short periods. They are changed every 3 to 5 days.

Other Surgical Procedures

During the course of hospitalization a burn patient may come to the OR for one or many procedures.

Escharotomy Shrinkage of eschar may occur and cause a tourniquet effect in circumferential burns of the extremities or thorax. Bilateral incisions through the eschar, not including the fascia, are made to improve circulation to a lower extremity. Multiple incisions on the chest wall relieve respiratory distress. Sites of incisions avoid major peripheral nerves to prevent irreversible neurologic complications.

Fasciotomy If adequate decompression does not occur following escharotomy, the incision may be extended into underlying fascia. Fascia may need to be incised in the arm if compromised circulation is evident.

Amputation of Digits Amputation may be necessary to control infection in the extremity and prevent septicemia if escharotomy is unsuccessful.

Debridement Debridement of underlying tissues helps prevent extension of tissue loss. Nonviable tendons, cartilage, or bone may be excised, such as from the hand, ear, or skull.

Full-Thickness Skin Grafts With or without tarsorrhaphy, full-thickness skin grafts are used to prevent contracture of the eyelids. The cornea must be protected from exposure.

Split-Thickness Skin Grafts Autografts are applied to debrided areas as rapidly as possible. The hands and face are the first priority to restore function; joints and flexion creases are second to prevent contractures; and the extremities and trunk are the lowest priority. Skin from donor sites is cut thin if the site will be used again. Mesh grafts are frequently used to cover very large surfaces or irregular areas such as the perineum. Grafts are held in place with staples or sutures and dressings to achieve apposition and immobilization.

Tissue Expansion If sufficient normal skin is available, a tissue expander may be placed beneath subcutaneous tissue to broaden the width for future use as a local flap to cover an adjacent burned area following excision of scar tissue or for better closure of the donor site.

Myocutaneous Flaps Myocutaneous flaps, either on a pedicle or by free microvascular transfer, may be used in the reconstruction of burn wounds.

Biologic Dressing Changes Instead of leaving a biologic dressing in place until rejection, with attendant inflammatory reaction, a biologic dressing is usually replaced every few days until the area is ready for an autograft or skin for an autograft is available. Biologic dressings may be allografts of human skin from a living or cadaver donor, placental or amniotic membranes, or a xenograft of porcine skin. Porcine dressings frequently are applied initially on second-degree burns as a temporary dressing or used in conjunction with extensive excisional therapy. Synthetic skin substitutes may be preferred. A biologic dressing is used for several reasons:

1. It helps to control infection by covering denuded areas.
2. It prevents loss of serum.
3. It decreases pain.

4. It seems to stimulate the formation of epithelium in dermis under it.
5. It promotes growth of granulation tissue.

Dressing Changes Occlusive dressings, if used, must be changed frequently to control infection harboring under them. An antimicrobial or chemotherapeutic agent may be applied as an integral part of the dressing. The following considerations apply:

1. Silver sulfadiazine (Silvadene) cream applied directly onto the burned area makes removal of a dressing less painful and does not disturb the healing process as it is removed. It is an effective topical antimicrobial and produces no metabolic side effects; some patients have developed neutropenia and delayed wound healing after its use. Fresh cream is applied after cleansing and debridement. A layer of fine-mesh gauze is laid over it (unless the open-exposure method will be used for further healing). Then soft, absorbent material, such as fluffed gauze, and a preformed splint may be used. These are held in place by a cotton elastic bandage. An occlusive dressing may be used to hold a hand, foot, or joint in functional position. This product is not used if the patient has a sulfa allergy.
2. Mafenide acetate (Sulfamylon) cream penetrates intact eschar rapidly and is quite successful in reducing bacterial counts to optimal levels for skin grafting. Application directly on the burned area is painful for the patient after cleansing and debridement. It may cause maceration under the dressing. Absorption may result in metabolic acidosis; thus the acid-base balance must be closely monitored. Prolonged use may lead to renal or pulmonary complications.
3. Silver nitrate solution is used infrequently. After cleansing and debridement, multiple-thickness dressings are applied to the area. These are kept saturated with 0.5% silver nitrate solution and changed every 12 hours. For debridement, sterile distilled water is used for irrigation because saline may cause the precipitation of silver salts. It is ineffective in treating established wound infection because it does not penetrate intact eschar. Care is taken to avoid splashing silver nitrate solution onto walls and floors because staining can occur. If disposable drapes and gowns are not used, stained linen must be laundered separately from other linen.

Serial Biopsy Cultures Through two linear incisions, a biopsy of tissue, including subcutaneous fat, is excised for culturing. This is done every 2 or 3 days, until the eschar begins to separate, to monitor the colonization of microorganisms in the wound. The results of serial biopsy culture enable the surgeon to make decisions specific to the therapeutic needs of the patient. An antimicrobial or chemotherapeutic topical agent is selected or changed according to these results.

Treatment of Curling's Ulcer   Gastrointestinal complications may occur anytime from the early postinjury period through rehabilitation. Complaints must be carefully evaluated. The patient who develops massive bleeding from a stress ulcer in the stomach and duodenum (Curling's ulcer) must be operated on. Vagotomy with antrectomy is most frequently performed by a general surgeon.

Treatment of Marjolin's Ulcer   An ulceration caused by malignant changes (Marjolin's ulcer) can develop in the surface area of a burn scar. As long as 20 years after the burn, a prolonged ulceration can lead to squamous cell carcinoma of the skin. The ulcer should be excised.

Environmental Considerations for Burn Patients

1. Environmental control is perhaps the essence of burn therapy. The environment must protect the wound from further injury and microbial invasion. A burn wound is always potentially contaminated until epithelialization occurs. Open exposure of the wound to room air may be the choice of the plastic surgeon for selected patients. Regardless of the method of treatment, the following adjuncts are used—if the equipment is available—in the care of burn patients, in addition to strict adherence to all of the principles of aseptic technique.
   a. Reverse isolation technique may be practiced to protect the patient, whose resistance is low, from infection from personnel. Caps, masks, shoe covers, sterile gowns, and sterile gloves are worn by all personnel attending the patient. This may be referred to as protective isolation.
   b. Laminar, or downward unidirectional, airflow away from the wound helps minimize airborne contamination.
   c. A plastic isolator protects the patient. Personnel do not directly enter this isolation unit. Patient care is given through clear plastic access walls. The environment around the patient inside the isolator is controlled at 90° F (32° C) and 94% relative humidity to conserve heat loss by evaporation.
2. Patients with extensive burns may be placed on a Stryker frame or a Circolectric bed specially designed to facilitate handling and turning. They are transported to the OR on these frames or beds. Patients must be turned slowly and gently because they are often hypovolemic after the injury.
3. Hypothermia must be prevented. The patient's thermoregulatory mechanism is altered by the destruction of skin that normally acts as an insulator. Heat loss is the greatest single problem the burn patient faces in the OR.
   a. The room temperature should be increased to between 80° and 90° F (27° and 32° C) with low relative humidity of about 30% to 40%.
   b. The OR must be ready to receive the patient directly from the burn unit. The patient should not wait in a cool holding area or corridor. Concern is for the patient's thermoregulation and potential for infection.
   c. A warm hyperthermia blanket should cover the operating bed. The patient should be exposed as little as possible. Cover with warm blankets.
   d. The patient's temperature should be monitored with a rectal or esophageal probe.
   e. Solutions should be warmed before irrigation or infusion.
   f. Operating during nighttime hours is advantageous for the patient because the normal schedule for oral intake is not interrupted.
4. Hypnosis and biofeedback techniques can reduce potential postanesthetic complications when many surgical procedures are necessary to achieve acceptable functional and aesthetic results after a burn. The OR environment must be quiet to be conducive to hypnotic suggestions given to the patient.

After the initial assessment of a severely burned patient, a prolonged period of treatment begins. A multidisciplinary team must coordinate the treatment plan to achieve the best possible clinical outcome for the patient. As with all plastic surgery patients, both physiologic and psychosocial support is essential to successful rehabilitation.

Bibliography

Clamon J, Netscher DT: General principles of flap reconstruction: goals for aesthetic and functional outcome, *Plast Surg Nurs* 14(1):9-14, 1994.

Dinman S, Giovanne MK: The care and feeding of microvascular grafts: how nurses can help prevent flap loss, *Plast Surg Nurs* 14(3):154-164, 1994.

Fortunato NM, McCullough SM: *Plastic and reconstructive surgery,* St Louis, 1998, Mosby.

Golden MA et al: Leech therapy in digital replantation, *AORN J* 62(3):364-375, 1995.

Goodman T: *Core curriculum for plastic and reconstructive surgical nursing,* ed 3, Pitman, NJ, 1998, American Society of Plastic and Reconstructive Surgical Nurses.

Hom DM: The wound healing response in grafted tissues, *Otolaryngol Clin North Am* 27(1):13-24, 1994.

Jones CE, Wellisz T: External ear reconstruction, *AORN J* 59(2):411-422, 1994.

Lutz DA, Hallock GG: Microsurgical transfer of vascularized tissue to close problem wounds, *AORN J* 62(2):234-243, 1995.

Rivera ML, Gross JE: Scalp replantation after traumatic injury, *AORN J* 62(2):175-184, 1995.

Ruberg RL, Smith DJ Jr: *Plastic surgery: a core curriculum,* St Louis, 1994, Mosby.

Simler AG: Endoscopic augmentation mammoplasty: the umbilical approach, *Plast Surg Nurs* 14(3):149-153, 1994.

Chapter 40

Otorhinolaryngologic and Head and Neck Surgery

Chapter Objectives

After studying this chapter, the learner will be able to:

- Identify the pertinent anatomy of the ear, nose, and throat.
- Describe the care of the patient having an otorhinolaryngologic procedure.
- List the main types of hearing loss and the treatments.
- Discuss the psychologic effects of head and neck surgery.
- List the precautions of caring for the patient with a tracheostomy.

Surgical procedures of the structures of the head and neck region are not within the province of any one surgical specialty. Subspecialists from many disciplines, most notably general surgeons, plastic surgeons, otolaryngologists, and dentists, limit their surgical practice to specific types of problems involving areas of the head and/or neck. Training in these subspecialties is included in specialty postgraduate programs.

Otorhinolaryngology has traditionally been concerned with research and surgical treatment of diseases of the ear *(oto),* nose *(rhino),* and throat *(laryngo).* Advances in scientific knowledge, diagnostic capabilities, and technology have broadened the scope of this field, which has led to subspecialization. General otorhinolaryngologists, commonly called ear, nose, and throat (ENT) surgeons, practice within the total scope of this specialty. Other surgeons confine their practice to one of the subspecialties: otology, facial surgery, or head and neck oncology. The certifying body for this specialty is the American Board of Otolaryngology, Head and Neck Surgery.

Dental and skeletal deformities of alignment and function coexist with aesthetic appearance. These deformities may be congenital, or they may be caused by trauma or disease. They may interfere with breathing, eating, swallowing, speaking, seeing, or hearing. A multidisciplinary team of surgical specialists is often required to reconstruct complex deformities. This team may be all-inclusive with a plastic surgeon, neurosurgeon, oral surgeon, orthodontist or prosthodontist, otolaryngologist, ophthalmologist, and general surgeon; or it may be limited to two or three specialists. The team may also include a radiologist, anesthesia provider, psychiatrist, speech pathologist, and social worker, plus, of course, the patient care staff. A team includes all of the specialties needed for complete preoperative assessment, intraoperative care, and postoperative rehabilitation of the individual patient.

HISTORICAL BACKGROUND

Recognition of abnormal conditions of the ear, nose, and throat began in early times. Some of the first permanent records are attributed to the Egyptians. Breathing was thought to occur through the ears via the eustachian tubes. Therefore attempts were made to remedy deafness and ear discharges. The study of anatomy of the ear, nose, and throat antedated the Christian era, leading to the practice of primitive procedures in India.

Hippocrates realized that irregular teeth could cause various mouth and ear disorders. He also recognized otitis media, as well as the fact that congenital deafness was incurable.

GENERAL CONSIDERATIONS IN EAR, NOSE, AND THROAT PROCEDURES

1. Preoperative explanations and postoperative instructions are vital to the outcome. For example, following ear or nasal procedures the patient must avoid blowing the nose, which would force air up the eustachian tube, potentially causing infection; force air through the incision; or dislodge a graft. To sneeze, both the nose and mouth should be open.

2. Communication is a major problem for patients with loss of hearing or voice. Touch is an effective means of conveying concern and letting the patient know he or she is not abandoned. Pencil and paper or a Magic Slate can be useful for the patient to communicate.

3. Care with antiseptic solutions is necessary because they are very painful and irritating if they are allowed to touch a perforated eardrum or get into the eyes. Some solutions, such as chlorhexidine or hexachlorophene, can cause permanent damage. Consult the manufacturer's recommendations before use.

4. The patient may experience anxiety with drapes over the head. Air and oxygen (6 to 8 L/min) administered during the otologic procedure afford relief.

5. Although a surgical area, such as the oral cavity, is often contaminated, sterile equipment and sterile technique are preferred to avoid introducing blood-borne exogenous microorganisms.

6. Anesthesia is mainly local. Use of local anesthesia minimizes bleeding and postoperative discomfort in addition to affording the surgeon observation of patient response. It allows patient cooperation. The presence of an endotracheal tube during general anesthesia can distort features during the surgical procedure.

   a. A qualified perioperative nurse monitors vital signs and the electrocardiogram (ECG) in the absence of an anesthesia provider. The nurse records the amount of local anesthesia administered and documents the patient's intraoperative responses.

   b. Patients undergoing local anesthesia may wear pajama-type bottoms or underpants to the operating room (OR) in some facilities.

7. Microsurgical otologic and laryngeal procedures, endoscopies, and laser procedures commonly require general anesthesia.

   a. The patient is intubated to maintain the airway and prevent aspiration of blood.

   b. The anesthesia machine may be positioned near the patient's side or feet. The endotracheal tube is taped; all connections must be tight, and tubes must be unkinked. The anesthesia provider usually sits alongside the operating bed.

   c. Eyelid edema caused by facial trauma may expose the conjunctiva. Lubricate with ophthalmic ointment or artificial tears to minimize corneal damage.

8. Various solutions and medications are on the table. Each container should be accurately and clearly labeled for foolproof distinction between, for example, cocaine, lidocaine, and epinephrine.

9. Illumination is provided by the overhead spotlight, the operating microscope, the endoscope, or the surgeon's fiberoptic headlight. Some want the room darkened.

10. Instrumentation is varied to suit the area. It includes very delicate, small endoscopic and microsurgical implements in addition to bone instruments because of the extensive involvement of cartilage and bone in the facial structures and skull. These areas have relatively little soft tissue. Many instruments are angulated to permit insertion without obscuring visualization.

11. Special care with electric appliances is indicated. Electrocoagulation is used to control oozing. Compressed air or nitrogen drills with a foot-pedal control are used on bone, such as the mastoid area. A number of drills for extremely fine work, such as stapes sculpturing, are powered by small electric motors fitted into a handpiece.

12. Various types of fiberoptic endoscopes with appropriate accessories are used. The diameter of aspirating tubes and forceps is small enough to pass through, and the length is long enough to extend beyond the end of the scope. The lighting mechanism and all accessories should be checked for working order before the patient is brought to the room.

13. Cryosurgery may be used to destroy tissue in accessible areas, especially those that bleed profusely if incised.

14. CO_2 lasers are used to vaporize tissue. Argon lasers coagulate tissue by heat generation. KTP lasers coagulate to shrink or debulk tissues. Nd:YAG lasers cut and coagulate to minimize bleeding. Appropriate instrumentation and attachments must be available for each type of laser. Laser surgery is usually done in conjunction with the operating microscope or endoscope. All safety precautions are taken to avoid ignition and injury when a laser is used. Laser safety is described in detail in Chapter 20.

15. Microsurgical techniques are used because they facilitate distinction between normal and diseased tissue and allow more accurate dissection.

16. Sponges and compressed patties are relatively small and are a distinct hazard when blood soaked because they can occlude an airway. All items used in the OR are counted or accounted for in their entirety at the end of the procedure.

17. One or two drops of blood can obscure a microsurgical field. Hemostatic aids should be ready at all times. Gelfoam pledgets soaked in 1:1000 epinephrine are used

frequently. Handle tissue grafts and gelatin sponges with forceps, not the hands. Gelfilm, which is brittle, may be cut while in the primary wrap.

18. Irrigation equipment and solution at body temperature should be available to remove bone dust, clean burrs, and rinse suction apparatus. Cannulas with very fine suction should be irrigated constantly to avoid blockage.

19. Suction should be available at all times and should include several patent cannulas. The degree of suction should be variable. Suction-irrigators are used with sinus endoscopes.

20. Tissue grafts must be kept from drying out before use. A convenient method is to place the graft on a moist cellulose sponge in a sterile, covered Petri dish. Some surgeons intentionally dry a temporalis fascia graft to facilitate handling. This type of graft may also be flattened and thinned in a small press.

21. Many procedures are done with the patient in a slight reverse Trendelenburg position or with a roll under the shoulders. This helps anatomic positioning and controls bleeding.

EAR

Anatomy of the Ear

The structures of the ear (Figure 40-1) are concerned with two functions:

1. Hearing (i.e., receiving sound, amplifying it, and transmitting it to the brain for interpretation)
2. Maintaining body equilibrium

Anatomically, the ear is divided into three parts: the external, middle, and inner ear.

External Ear

The outer ear consists of the auricle, or pinna, composed of cartilage except for the lobe; skin; and the external auditory canal. The meatus of the auricle leads via the ear canal to the tympanic membrane or eardrum. This membrane separates the external and middle ear. A color change of the translucent eardrum, visible through a speculum, may be indicative of middle ear disease. The outermost lining of the tympanic membrane is derived from tissue of the ear canal. The inner lining is continuous with the middle ear mucosa. The eardrum protects the middle ear but may be perforated by injury or pressure built up in the middle ear by infection.

Middle Ear

The middle ear consists of the tympanic cavity, a closed chamber that lies between the tympanic membrane and the inner ear. Within this cavity are the three smallest bones in the body: an ossicular chain comprising the malleus, incus, and stapes. They resemble a hammer, anvil, and stirrups, respectively. The malleus, which is attached to the eardrum, joins the incus, the extremity of which articulates with the stapes, the innermost bone. The footplate of the stapes fits in the oval (vestibular) window, an opening in the wall of the inner ear. The bones of the ossicular chain must be able to move mechanically to conduct sound from the eardrum to the inner ear. The round (cochlear) window, also between the middle and the inner ear, equalizes pressure that enters through the oval window.

The middle ear opens into the nasopharynx by way of the eustachian tube. Normally closed during swallowing or yawning, the eustachian tube aerates the middle ear cavity. This mechanism is essential for adequate hearing.

Posteriorly the middle ear exits to the mastoid process. This inferior projection of the temporal bone is a honeycomb

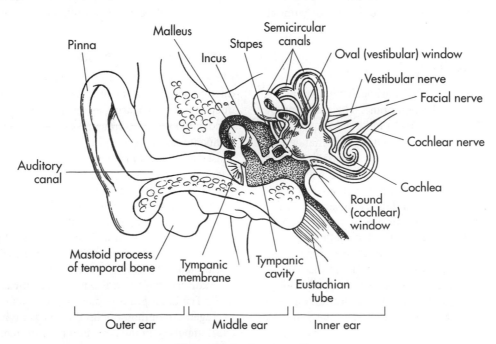

Figure 40-1　Anatomy of ear.

of air cells lined with mucous membrane. Because the antrum of the mastoid process connects with it, middle ear infection may produce mastoiditis. The middle ear is situated in the tympanic portion of the temporal bone; the inner ear is situated in the petrous portion, which integrates with the base of the skull. The tympanic portion also forms part of the ear canal.

Inner Ear

The end organs of hearing and equilibrium are situated in the inner ear. The two main sections—cochlear and vestibular—have distinct, although coordinated, functions. The cochlea, a bony spiral, relates to hearing. The vestibular labyrinth, which is composed of three semicircular canals, relates to equilibrium. These structures house two separate fluids—endolymph and perilymph—which nourish and protect the hearing receptors. Neuroepithelium of the organ of Corti, the end organ of hearing, holds thousands of minute hair cells, which respond to sound waves that enter the cochlea via the oval window. Neuroepithelium of the vestibular portion also contains hair cells. Rapid head motion produces current in the endolymph that may result in nausea or vertigo. The eighth cranial (vestibulocochlear) nerve governs reflexes to muscles to maintain equilibrium and controls hearing.

Proximal Structures

The middle and the inner ear are adjacent to many important structures. The seventh cranial (facial) nerve is enclosed in a bony canal running through the tympanic cavity and mastoid bone. The meninges of the temporal lobe of the brain are also near the middle ear and the mastoid. Facial paralysis, meningitis, and intracranial infection, such as brain abscess, are potential complications of ear infection.

The major blood vessels are the internal carotid artery and internal jugular vein, as well as the lateral sinus. Thrombosis and infection of the lateral sinus of the dura mater are potentially lethal complications of otitis media, with or without mastoiditis.

Physiology of Hearing

Sound or pressure waves enter the auricle. They pass along the ear canal to the tympanic membrane. The vibration of the waves is transmitted across the middle ear sequentially by the ossicles. Amplification of sound is enhanced to some extent by mechanical action of the ossicles but mainly by aerial ratio. A large volume of sound wave pressure from the tympanic membrane funnels to a small reactive area, the stapedial footplate, intensifying sound. At the footplate of the stapes, sound pressure is transferred to the inner ear via the oval window. The hair cells of the organ of Corti are set in motion by disturbance of the inner ear fluids as sound wave pressure moves from the oval to the round window. Mechanical energy is converted to electrical potential, which is delivered to the brain along the eighth cranial nerve. The brain interprets the impulse (sound) as hearing.

Pathology of Hearing

Hearing affects the quality and quantity of interpersonal interactions. It is a major sense for communicating within one's environment. Loss of hearing therefore affects social relationships. The type of deafness or hearing loss in varying degrees may result from the following:

1. Disease, such as otosclerosis, in which changes in the bony capsule of the labyrinth occur. Otosclerotic bone invades the stapedial footplate, resulting in its fixation and ultimate inability to vibrate in the oval window. Hearing loss is gradual but progressive. This type of deficiency can be surgically corrected when auditory nerve endings are not destroyed.
2. Trauma, such as a perforated eardrum, requiring repair to restore function and aerial ratio.
3. Infection, usually controlled by antibiotics. Although it is more common in children, infection may also occur in adults. It may cause accumulation of fluid in the middle ear. Mastoiditis results from extension of otitis media.
   a. Serous otitis media may result from obstruction of the pharyngeal orifice of the eustachian tube. If blocked, for example, by hypertrophied adenoid tissue, infection, or allergic swelling, the eustachian tube is unable to equalize pressure because air cannot enter the middle ear from the pharynx. The vacuum or negative pressure thus created causes serum to be drawn into the tympanic cavity from blood vessels in the middle ear mucosa. Recurrent otitis media may require drainage of purulent exudate if conservative treatment fails.
   b. Acute otitis media may require drainage of purulent exudate if conservative treatment fails.
   c. Chronic otitis media with or without mastoiditis may follow recurrent otitis media with tympanic membrane perforation. It can produce a chronically draining ear.

Differential Diagnosis

Measurements that compare bone conduction with air conduction are important in differential diagnosis. Bone conduction refers to hearing as transmitted through the skull; air conduction refers to transmission of sound waves from the tympanic membrane to the inner ear via air. Hearing loss caused by a defect in the external or middle ear, referred to as conductive loss, is a mechanical obstruction of air conduction that usually can be helped by surgical intervention. When the decrement is in the inner ear, referred to as perceptive or sensorineural loss, damage to nerve tissue and/or sensory paths to the brain is not benefited by a surgical procedure. Cochlear nerve endings are the main component of sensorineural hearing (Figure 40-2).

Auditory acuity and function are measured by various tests. The audiogram is one measurement tool. Computer-averaged tomography is used to measure and analyze electrical impulses, known as auditory brainstem responses, from

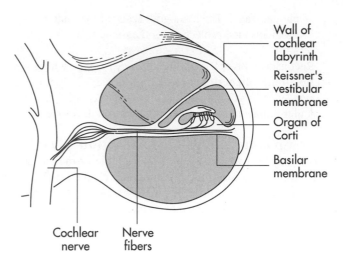

Wall of
cochlear
labyrinth

Reissner's
vestibular
membrane

Organ of
Corti

Basilar
membrane

Cochlear
nerve

Nerve
fibers

Figure 40-2 Cross section of cochlear labyrinth with sensory neural mechanism.

the brain and cortical auditory pathway. An acoustic reflex latency test of the stapedius reflex provides information about hearing sensitivity. Auditory brainstem evoked potentials assess the patient's hearing threshold.

Surgical Procedures of the Ear

Current techniques, instrumentation, lasers, and the operating microscope have enhanced the capability of otologists.

General Considerations

1. Local anesthesia may be used for a minor procedure on the external ear, but general anesthesia is usually used to avoid patient movement while the surgeon is manipulating delicate structures in the middle or inner ear.
   a. Inhalation anesthesia may be given by face mask for a short procedure, with the anesthesia provider seated at the head of the operating bed.
   b. The anesthesia provider sits alongside the operating bed with the patient facing him or her when the patient is intubated for a major procedure.
   c. Hypotensive anesthesia may be employed to create a bloodless field, especially during microsurgery.
   d. Nitrous oxide diffuses into cavities, causing expansion of the middle ear. This can present a hazard in a grafting procedure, for example; nitrous oxide is discontinued before placement of a graft in the middle ear.
   e. General anesthesia may be supplemented with a local agent in some procedures, often with epinephrine to control bleeding.
2. The patient's head is turned with the affected side up and stabilized in a donut. The dependent pinna should be protected from pressure.
3. Lint-free drapes are preferred. It is mandatory that gloves be free of powder and lint. The formation of a granuloma in the oval window can cause irreversible sensorineural hearing loss.

4. The operating microscope is used for many otologic procedures.
   a. The surgeon sits at the head of the operating bed to use the microscope.
   b. Microinstruments should be carefully handled before, during, and after use.
5. Compressed absorbent patties (cottonoids) moistened with normal saline solution, rather than gauze sponges, are frequently used. They must be counted.
6. Hemostasis may be achieved with epinephrine, absorbable hemostatic sponges, or oxidized cellulose, laser, and bone wax.
7. Prosthetic devices should be available in an assortment of types and sizes. Tissue homografts may be used.
8. A nerve stimulator may be used to identify facial, acoustic, cochlear, and/or vestibular nerve branches. Evoked potential audiometry also may be used to monitor the seventh and eighth cranial nerves.
9. Bone instruments, including powered drills, are used for opening the temporal bone.
10. CO_2, Nd:YAG, argon, and KTP lasers are used during otologic procedures to control bleeding, divide nerves, and/or vaporize tissues.
11. Pressure dressings are usually applied.

External Ear Procedures

Removal of a Foreign Body Removing a foreign body from the outer canal is performed most frequently in children. The object is washed out or removed to prevent purulent infection. A plant seed or vegetable foreign body, such as a pea, is not irrigated because it may swell in the ear and increase the difficulty of removal. General anesthesia sometimes may be required. Trauma should be minimal during removal of a foreign body to prevent stenosis of the canal or perforation through the eardrum.

Drainage of a Hematoma Usually a result of injury, a hematoma is drained to avoid infection with subsequent chondritis and deformity of the auricle.

Excision of a Tumor The extent of the surgical procedure to excise a tumor, either benign or malignant, depends on the size and type of tumor. The skin of the pinna is vulnerable to actinic (chemical) changes caused by radiant energy during exposure to the sun. Basal cell lesions do not metastasize, but squamous cell carcinoma often does. Primary cancer may be excised by a wide or wedge excision with primary closure or a wide excision with a skin graft. If the lesion is extensive, partial or total pinnectomy may be necessary. The area can be skin grafted and reconstructed cosmetically with a prosthesis. Radical temporal bone resection is indicated if the bone (canal) is involved. Neck dissection may be indicated if nodal metastases are present.

Middle Ear Procedures

Mastoidectomy Mastoidectomy, the eradication of mastoid air cells, may be indicated to relieve complications of acute or chronic mastoiditis. Mastoidectomy is more commonly performed in conjunction with a reconstructive procedure (see Tympanomastoid Reconstruction).

SIMPLE MASTOIDECTOMY   The mastoid process is opened behind the ear. Air cells are removed by drilling through bone with small burrs, without involving the middle ear or external canal.

MODIFIED RADICAL MASTOIDECTOMY   Simple mastoidectomy and removal of the posterior wall of the ear canal provide drainage from the mastoid into the canal. The tympanic membrane and middle ear ossicles are preserved.

RADICAL MASTOIDECTOMY   A radical mastoidectomy is performed for chronic mastoiditis. The middle ear cavity and mastoid antrum are combined into a single cavity for inspection and cleaning. Mastoid air cells are removed. The ossicles and tympanic membrane are partially removed. The stapes and facial nerve are preserved.

Tympanoplasty

Tympanoplasty, as a general term, refers to any procedure performed to repair defects in the eardrum and/or middle ear structures for the purpose of reconstructing sound conduction paths. The degree of hearing improvement following tympanoplasty is related to the degree of damage. Preferably, the ear should be uninfected at the time of the surgical procedure. If not, infected tissue is debrided. As microsurgical procedures, tympanoplasties are classified into five types:

1. Type I (myringoplasty) is closure of a perforation in the tympanic membrane caused by infection or trauma. The ossicular chain is normal. Autogenous fascia or a vein is used to repair the perforation. A vein graft is taken from the patient's forearm or hand. Fascia, more commonly used as a patch over a perforation, is obtained from the temporalis muscle.
2. Type II is closure of a perforated tympanic membrane with erosion of the malleus. The graft is placed against the incus or remains of the malleus.
3. Type III replaces the tympanic membrane to provide protection for the stapes and round window. The tympanic membrane, malleus, and incus have been destroyed by disease. The stapes is intact and mobile. A homograft of tympanic membrane with attached malleus and incus is placed in contact with the normal stapes, permitting transmission of sound.
4. Type IV is similar to type III except that the head, neck, and crura of the stapes are missing. The mobile footplate may be left exposed with the graft placed around it. The air pocket between the graft and the round window provides sound protection for the round window. To conserve the middle ear hearing mechanism, homograft transplantation of tympanic membrane and ossicles may be used to rebuild the chain.
5. Type V is similar to type IV except that the stapedial footplate is fixed because of otosclerosis (osteospongiosis). A fenestra (small opening) is made in the horizontal semicircular canal. The homograft seals off the middle ear to provide sound protection for the round window.

Reconstruction of the middle ear may be done with a synthetic bioinert material such as high-density polyethylene sponge (Plastipore). Fibrin glue also is used. Partial and total ossicular replacement prostheses have been developed.

Tympanomastoid Reconstruction

Tympanoplasty may be combined with either simple or radical mastoidectomy. The mastoid is drained and cleaned before reconstruction of the eardrum or middle ear ossicles. Following incision behind the auricle, the tympanic membrane and tympanic cavity are inspected. The mastoid antrum is entered by drilling through mastoid bone.

Sometimes in chronic otitis media, the mucous membrane of the tympanic cavity is replaced by epithelium from the ear canal as it grows through a perforation in the eardrum. Desquamated skin cells that cannot escape form a ball or cyst, known as a cholesteatoma. If present in the middle ear or mastoid, a cholesteatoma is removed during mastoidectomy and/or tympanoplasty. If left intact, a cholesteatoma can cause permanent hearing loss, balance disturbance, infection, and facial nerve paralysis.

Stapedectomy/Stapedotomy

Conductive hearing loss can result from fixation of the stapes, most often caused by otosclerosis. The surgeon aims to restore vibration from the incus to the mobile oval window membrane to transmit sound. A stapedectomy involves partial or total removal of the stapes. A partial stapedectomy removes only the fixed footplate (Figure 40-3); a total stapedectomy removes the entire stapes, including the footplate. A stapedotomy (small opening into the footplate) may be the preferred procedure. The opening is made with a handheld perforator, microsurgical power drill, or laser. An argon, CO_2, or KTP laser may be used for this purpose. A low-wattage lasing beam avoids thermal damage to the perilymph and inner ear structures. Following partial or total stapedectomy or stapedotomy, the remaining superstructure is used to reconstruct the sound-conducting mechanism.

An incision is made deep in the canal near but not in the eardrum. The eardrum is folded over, giving access to the middle ear. The stapes is disconnected from the incus, fractured by fine microinstruments, and removed. The oval window is sealed by a graft of vein, perichondrium, fascia, fat, or an absorbable hemostatic sponge over the oval window. A prosthesis is inserted and connected to the incus and to the graft, thus restoring sound conduction. Prostheses are made of various inert materials such as polyethylene, stainless steel, or tantalum.

By performing the microsurgical procedure with the patient under local anesthesia, the surgeon can reposition the eardrum and use his or her voice to test whether the patient's hearing is improved. Otosclerosis usually involves both ears, but stapedectomy is performed on only one ear at a time.

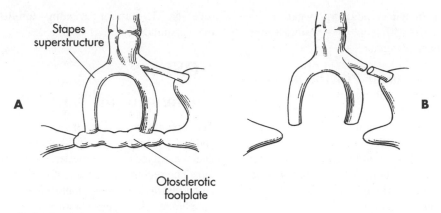

Figure 40-3 Partial stapedectomy. **A,** Stapes superstructure attached to fixed otosclerotic footplate. **B,** Footplate removed; superstructure remains.

Stapes Mobilization The stapes is manipulated at the footplate to restore normal function. A break through an otosclerotic lesion is achieved by means of transcrural pressure or direct application of chisels and picks to the footplate. A mobile, unaffected portion of a functioning stapes remains. Various techniques are used, with or without the use of prosthetic devices. The advantage of the procedure is that the preserved stapedial footplate provides natural protection for the inner ear. The disadvantage is that frequently a continuing otosclerotic process causes the footplate to become refixed. Therefore stapedectomy is more popular because it produces long-lasting results.

Stapes procedures are performed under direct vision with the operating microscope. The procedures do not disturb the integrity or position of the eardrum.

Removal of Middle Ear Vascular Tumors The argon laser is absorbed by red pigment. Therefore it is suited for removal of small vascular tumors in the middle ear, such as glomus tympanicum tumors. The argon laser acts by photocoagulation.

Inner Ear Procedures

Endolymphatic Sac Shunt The endolymphatic sac is an appendage of the membranous inner ear located in the posterior fossa, anterior to the lateral sinus and posterior to the semicircular canals. An excessive accumulation of endolymph in this sac causes the episodic vertigo (dizziness), tinnitus (ear ringing), and sensorineural hearing loss of Ménière's disease. Through a simple mastoidectomy approach, the sac is opened and the inner ear is drained into either the subarachnoid space or the mastoid. A shunt tube is inserted to maintain drainage.

Labyrinthectomy In labyrinthectomy the vestibular labyrinth is removed from the inner ear to correct incapacitating vertigo. This results in loss of vestibular function and hearing.

Vestibular Neurectomy A middle fossa approach to the internal auditory canal for vestibular neurectomy combines otologic and neurosurgical procedures. Through a temporal bone craniotomy incision, dura of the floor of the middle fossa is elevated to expose structures in the superior portion of the internal auditory canal. The superior and inferior vestibular nerves, which control equilibrium, are sectioned to control intractable vertigo. The cochlear nerve, the hearing portion of the eighth cranial nerve, is not damaged, thus preserving hearing. A graft of temporalis muscle is placed over the exposed internal auditory canal to prevent leakage of cerebrospinal fluid.

Removal of an Acoustic Neuroma Acoustic neuroma resection may be performed by an otologist and/or a neurosurgeon, depending on its location and the extent of neurologic involvement. An acoustic neuroma is a slow-growing encapsulated benign tumor of the eighth cranial (acoustic) nerve. It originates in the neural sheath in the internal auditory canal but grows to involve nerve fibers in the posterior fossa. Initially the patient experiences unilateral hearing loss and disturbances, especially tinnitus, and equilibrium problems such as mild vertigo. The syndrome may resemble Ménière's disease or an expanding intracranial tumor. Early differential diagnosis is enhanced by brainstem evoked response audiometry, vertebral angiography, and small-volume air-contrast computed tomography (CT).

A small neuroma, confined to the internal auditory canal, may be resected by the otologist using microsurgical technique through a middle fossa approach to preserve hearing. If a translabyrinthine approach is used to gain access to the internal auditory canal posterior to the inner ear structures, the patient will have total hearing loss after the surgical procedure. Acoustic neuromas extending into the cranial cavity are resected by the neurosurgeon. The CO_2 laser may be used to excise acoustic neuromas through a transmastoid or craniotomy approach. Cerebrospinal fluid leak and meningitis are complications of the craniotomy approach.

For selected patients, stereotactic radiosurgery can be performed on an outpatient basis with local anesthesia. Hearing is preserved in 50% of these patients.

Implantation of a Cochlear Prosthesis Cochlear implants have been used for adults since the 1980s, but it was not until the 1990s that they were used for children. A cochlear implant can restore perception of sound to patients who have profound sensorineural deafness not responsive to external amplification of a hearing aid. They are indicated for use in patients who have intact eighth cranial nerve function and are over 2 years of age. The implant is an electronic device that converts sound waves into electrical signals to stimulate cochlear nerve fibers in the absence of functioning hair cells. Several devices are available. All of them have external and internal components. The external part, which is attached behind the ear, has a microphone/ transmitter and a speech processor/receiver. The internal part has a receiver/ stimulator and electrode/ channel(s) that is threaded through the cochlea.

The internal electrode attaches to wires permanently implanted in the cochlea. Through a postauricular incision, a simple mastoidectomy is performed. Under the operating microscope, the facial recess between the posterior canal and the facial nerve is enlarged to expose the chorda tympani nerve and the middle ear. The electrode is securely seated in the mastoid cavity and placed through a recess into the middle ear. It is directed through an opening made in the round window into the scala tympani until it meets resistance. Placement is critical. A plug of fascia from the temporalis muscle is placed around the electrode at the round window to prevent perilymph leakage.

The internal electrode stimulates the auditory nerve to interpret sound. The single-channel model stimulates the nerve randomly so that the patient can discern environmental sounds but not speech. A multichannel electrode enables the patient to distinguish environmental sounds and some speech by differentiating the frequency, volume, and pitch of sound waves. With a single-channel electrode, a ground wire is placed under the temporalis muscle in the mastoid or middle ear. A multichannel electrode does not have a ground wire. The internal receiver is sutured in position over the temporal bone behind the ear. Electromagnetic components and/or a titanium enclosure for the receiver may act as an electrical ground device. Only a bipolar active electrode should be used if electrosurgery is necessary after placement of the receiver.

The external microphone/transmitter component of the implant activates the internal receiver/stimulator. Transmission may be percutaneous or transcutaneous. In the percutaneous model a direct wire to a receiver implanted behind the ear connects the transmitter. In the transcutaneous model the transmitter converts electrical energy into magnetic currents that pass through intact skin to the receiver. In both models sound enters the microphone and is transmitted to a speech processor, worn outside the body, where it is encoded into electrical signals or energy and amplified. The coded signals return to the transmitter and are passed to the internal

receiver. The patient can adjust amplification of environmental sounds.

NOSE

Anatomy of the Nose

The supporting structures of the nose consist of two nasal bones and the nasal processes of the maxillary bones superiorly, the lateral cartilages and connective tissue inferiorly, and the septum. The septum, composed of bone posteriorly and cartilage anteriorly, divides the nose into two chambers lined by mucous membrane. The anterior portion or vestibule holds the nasal hairs. The external anterior orifices are called nares.

The internal portion of the nose, the nasal cavity (Figure 40-4) extends to the nasopharynx, the space behind the choanae or funnel-like posterior nasal orifices. The nose communicates with the ear via the eustachian tube. The hard and soft palates divide the nasal and oral cavities. The ethmoid bone separates the nasal and cranial cavities.

The paranasal sinuses are the frontal, maxillary, ethmoid, and sphenoid sinuses. Ostia (openings from the sinuses and nasolacrimal ducts) are located in the nasal lateral walls. The ostia provide a drainage system for the sinuses, as well as aerate them. Three turbinate bones (superior, middle, and inferior) are also situated in the lateral walls. These bones are covered with a vascular mucosa. Beneath each turbinate is a corresponding meatus. Tears drain into the nose through the nasolacrimal duct that enters the inferior meatus. Drainage from the paranasal sinuses is passed to the nose through the middle and superior meatuses.

External and internal carotid arteries and their branches supply blood to the nasal region. Because of the extensive vascularity, lymphatic supply, and proximity to the brain, infections on or about the face are potentially very dangerous. Microorganisms may readily be carried to or thrombi may form in the cavernous sinus. The sense of smell is derived from the first cranial (olfactory) nerve. The sensory nerve supply of the nasal area is associated with the trigeminal or fifth cranial nerve.

Physiology of the Nose

1. It provides filtered air to the respiratory system. Fine cilia in the mucous membrane propel mucus toward the nasopharynx. Air is warmed and moistened as it passes to the trachea and lower respiratory tract.
2. It contains the end organs for smell in the olfactory epithelium, which differs from other nasal epithelium. When nasal obstruction blocks off the olfactory epithelium, loss of smell (anosmia) results. The senses of smell and taste are closely related.

Surgical Procedures of the Nose

Nasal procedures are concerned with two factors: adequate ventilation to accessory spaces and adequate drainage from

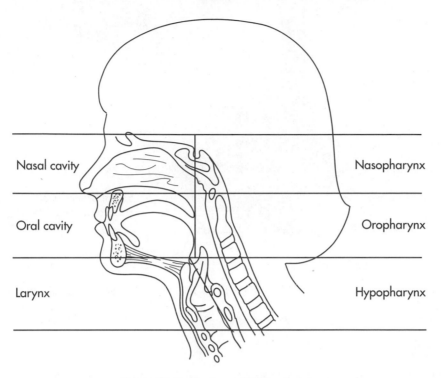

Figure 40-4 Regions of head and neck.

them. Abnormalities in structure, congenital or traumatic, and disease processes hinder function. Corrective procedures are done to relieve obstruction, to ensure drainage, to resect tumors, or to control bleeding (epistaxis).

General Considerations

1. CT and rhinoscopy are often performed preoperatively to diagnose the nature and extent of pathologic conditions, especially in the paranasal sinuses.
2. Many nasal procedures are performed with the patient under local anesthesia with or without intravenous (IV) sedation.
   a. Topical 4% cocaine may be sprayed on the nasal mucosa or applied with soaked compressed absorbent patties (cottonoids) or sponges put in the nostrils. Cocaine produces vasoconstriction, as well as anesthesia. The patties should be accounted for at the end of the procedure.
   b. A local agent, often lidocaine hydrochloride, 1% or 2%, is injected into the middle meatus. Epinephrine usually is used for vasoconstriction to control bleeding.
   c. When general anesthesia is indicated, a pack is placed in the pharynx to prevent aspiration of blood after the patient is intubated.
3. Paranasal sinuses and tissues underlying the mucosa are considered sterile. Therefore instrumentation should be sterile although the nasal cavity is considered a contaminated area because they are entering a vascular bed. Venous drainage could easily carry microorganisms to the cavernous sinus, causing an intracranial infection.
4. CO_2, Nd:YAG, and KTP lasers may be used. Endoscopes also are used. All equipment and accessories should be checked for working order.

5. Nasal packing is inserted at the end of most procedures except endoscopic sinus and laser procedures.

Nasal Cavity Procedures

The supporting structures surrounding nasal air passages can be injured or displaced. Acute or chronic disease processes can cause dysfunction or obstruction.

Epistaxis Most nosebleeds are caused by trauma, usually at Kisselbach's plexus of arteries and veins (also known as Little's area) in the anterior part of the nasal septum (Figure 40-5). Dehumidified air may cause changes in the mucosa and splitting of tiny vessels. Bleeding may be spontaneous, as in patients with arteriosclerosis, hypertension, or blood dyscrasia. Epistaxis is usually anterior and unilateral. In persons with systemic disease, such as leukemia, or with severe fracture, the bleeding is frequently posterior and more severe. Management involves locating the precise bleeding site and promptly instituting appropriate therapy. Severe hemorrhage places the patient in a precarious condition. Hypovolemia should be corrected preoperatively.

ANTERIOR PACK Local vasoconstriction and pressure on the side of the nose will control most nosebleeds. Electrocoagulation or silver nitrate is used to provide hemostasis at the bleeding point as needed. When bleeding is from the anterior ethmoid artery, inaccessible to cautery, packing is applied to the area of depression between the septum and the middle turbinate.

POSTERIOR PACK A posterior pack may be necessary for constant pressure when bleeding is severe in the posterior part of the nose. The pack consists of rolled gauze securely

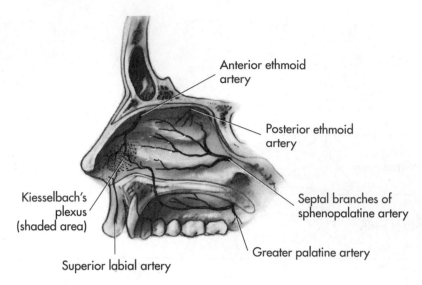

Figure 40-5 Blood supply to nasal cavity. (From Davis JH, Foster RS, Gamelli RL: *Essentials of clinical surgery,* St Louis, 1991, Mosby.)

tied to the middle of a length of narrow tape or strong string; commercial packs are available. To control infection and odor, gauze is lubricated with antibiotic ointment before insertion. After a catheter is passed into the mouth via the nose, one end of the tape is tied to the oral end of the catheter. The catheter and attached tape are then drawn back through the mouth and out one nostril, thereby pulling the pack up into the nasopharynx. Thus one end of the tape comes out the nose, the other end out the mouth. These ends are secured to the patient's cheek with adhesive tape. The nasal end is taped to prevent the pack from slipping into the throat; the oral end facilitates removal of the pack. Some oozing may persist in spite of packing. The pack is left in place until bleeding is arrested, usually for at least 48 hours, but prolonged use can lead to otitis media or paranasal sinusitis.

Patients with postnasal packs are often apprehensive and uncomfortable. They must breathe through the mouth. Posterior packs tend to reduce arterial oxygen tension. All patients, especially geriatric patients or those with marginal pulmonary function, should be observed carefully for respiratory problems that may result from the pack dropping into the hypopharynx.

ARTERY LIGATION A microsurgical procedure is performed to control persistent nasal hemorrhage by reducing the blood supply to the posterior portion of the nose. Some surgeons prefer artery ligation to packing, or it may be performed with a pack in place. Through an incision in the oral mucosa, removal of the posterior wall exposes the maxillary sinus for transantral ligation. Terminal branches of the internal maxillary artery, a branch of the external carotid artery, are exposed, identified, and ligated with metallic clips. Electrocoagulation is employed to control intraoperative bleeding, but if it is excessive, creation of a nasoantral window establishes drainage. The replaced posterior mucosal flap is covered with absorbable gelatin sponge, and the incision is closed.

Through an incision along the left side of the nose, ligation of the anterior and posterior ethmoidal arteries is helpful in controlling bleeding in the superior aspect of the nose.

The argon or KTP laser may be used to control severe epistaxis. If a laser is used to control bleeding, nasal packing usually is unnecessary.

Turbinectomy Chronic engorgement of the middle and/or inferior turbinate causes nasal congestion and rhinorrhea. Rhinitis is frequently an allergic reaction. A KTP laser shrinks turbinates without removing normal mucosa. A CO_2 or Nd:YAG contact laser vaporizes the superficial layer of mucosa without injuring the turbinate or ablating the turbinate. The KTP or CO_2 laser fiber handpiece is directed through a nasal endoscope. Because bleeding is minimal, nasal packing is unnecessary. Electrocoagulation and cryosurgery also have been used to treat soft tissue obstruction and refractory allergic rhinitis.

Nasal Obstruction Surgical intervention can provide relief for certain types of nasal obstruction. For example, after the mucosa is shrunk with a vasoconstrictor and secretions are suctioned, a foreign body is removed with a forceps. An abscess or hematoma may need to be drained to relieve pressure. Accumulation of pus or blood separates the perichondrium, the connective tissue, from underlying cartilage. This may cause necrosis of cartilage with resultant deformity. Infection must be eradicated to avoid extension to the brain.

POLYPECTOMY Polyps (soft edematous masses) projecting from the nasal or sinus mucosa can obstruct the posterior choanae. Polyps usually are bilateral, but they may be unilateral, single or multiple, and they frequently are infected. In addition to obstructing ventilation, they may obstruct the sense of smell if the olfactory epithelium is blocked. Some polyps may be excised with a wire-loop snare through a nasal speculum or with forceps through an endoscope. Packing is inserted to control bleeding. The KTP laser coagulates the base to debulk large, multiple polyps. The laser fiber can be directed through a straight or angled handpiece. A CO_2 laser can vaporize polyps. The laser is less invasive than other techniques.

Nasal Deformity   Surgical intervention can restore contour and/or improve function after an injury. A deformity in nasal structure also may be corrected to improve cosmetic appearance.

REDUCTION OF A NASAL FRACTURE   Fracture of the septum or nasal bones often accompanies other trauma to the head. Intranasal manipulation is required to elevate depressed bone or cartilage that may be pushed into the paranasal sinuses. This should be performed as soon as possible to bring the parts in apposition. A delay of 7 to 10 days to permit edema to subside will not affect the outcome. Bleeding from a laceration must be immediately controlled and drained. Intranasal structure compatible with air passage must be preserved.

SEPTOPLASTY, SEPTAL RECONSTRUCTION, AND SUBMUCOUS RESECTION   The terms *septoplasty, septal reconstruction,* and *submucous resection* are used interchangeably to describe correction of a deviated nasal septum. Often the result of injury, the condition interferes with breathing and drainage. With the patient under local anesthesia, one side of the septum is incised its entire length. Membranous coverings are detached from cartilage and bone. The deformed part of the septum is removed or straightened and replaced. Bilateral nasal packing is inserted to hold tissues in place and to prevent bleeding. The procedure creates a patent airway and straight septal line, thereby reducing sinus disease and polyp formation.

RHINOPLASTY   Rhinoplasty, a procedure to correct deformity of the nose, may be performed by a rhinologist or a plastic surgeon. It is a major procedure involving reconstruction and molding of the bones and cartilages. Septoplasty and rhinoplasty may be performed together; septorhinoplasty restores both function and cosmetic appearance. Local anesthesia is usually used. The skin is taped postoperatively to maintain the nasal structures in alignment. A rigid shield is applied for protection. This is not removed without a specific order from the surgeon. Temporary ecchymosis from surgical trauma surrounds the eyes postoperatively.

REPAIR OF A PERFORATED SEPTUM   Perforations occur most often in the anterior cartilage. If bleeding and crusting are severe, the perforation may be covered by rotated mucoperichondrial flaps. Or the mucosa of adjacent intact septum may be denuded and a skin graft applied to cover the perforation. Nasal packing is inserted.

Paranasal Sinus Procedures

The paranasal sinuses are air-filled spaces in the skull. Because the sinus mucous membrane lining is continuous with the mucous membrane lining of the nose, nasal infection may readily spread to the sinuses. Various procedures provide drainage for patients with chronic sinusitis that may result from allergies or repeated nasopharyngeal infection. Swelling of the nasal mucosa can trap microorganisms within a sinus cavity. Ostial occlusion and abnormalities in the walls of the nasal cavity interfere with breathing, drainage, and smell. Sinus procedures are executed through an external or an intranasal approach or through an endoscope.

Maxillary Sinus Procedure   The maxillary sinuses are located bilaterally between the upper teeth and the eyes.

CALDWELL-LUC PROCEDURE (ANTROSTOMY)   The maxillary sinus contents are approached through an incision of the oral mucous membrane above the canine teeth. The flap is retracted. A section of maxillary bone is cut out to create a large nasoantral window for aeration and permanent drainage by gravity into the nasal fossa under the inferior turbinate. Polyps and diseased tissue are removed, along with eradication of mucosa. At the completion of the surgical procedure, the sinus is packed with gauze impregnated with antibiotic ointment. One end of the gauze is brought through the window and into the nose. The incision under the upper lip is sutured. The packing is eventually removed through the nose. Antrostomy is usually limited to adults because of unerupted teeth in children. A Caldwell-Luc incision is also used for removal of a tumor in the maxillary sinus.

Ethmoid Sinus Procedures   The ethmoid sinus cells lie bilaterally between the nose and the orbits. The maxillary sinuses are below the ethmoid bones, and the frontal sinuses are above them.

ETHMOIDECTOMY   Diseased tissue is removed from the ethmoid labyrinth, middle turbinate, and meatus. A large cavity is formed to facilitate aeration and drainage. Severe ethmoiditis can cause orbital abscess requiring drainage through an intranasal or external (Lynch) incision that extends from the inner half of the eyebrow down alongside the nose.

TURBINECTOMY   Removal of portions of the inferior and middle turbinates increases aeration and drainage. The cavity is packed at completion of the surgical procedure.

Frontal Sinus Procedures   The frontal sinuses are situated above the eyes. They are usually approached through the external incision described for ethmoidectomy, or a coronal incision may be made for exposure across the scalp from ear to ear.

OSTEOPLASTIC FLAP PROCEDURE   The bone covering the frontal sinus is exposed and incised. The contents of the sinus, such as a mucocele (a cyst lined with mucus-secreting glands), are extracted. The lining of the mucocele sac is removed and the cavity packed with fat (from the abdominal wall) to obliterate the sinus with fibrous tissue that fills in the cavity. The incised bone flap is then repositioned, and the incision is sutured.

KILLIAN PROCEDURE   A frontal sinus cavity is reached by removal of the floor or anterior wall of the sinus through an external incision above the eye. A large communication and drainage channel into the nose is formed.

Sphenoid Sinus Procedure
The sphenoid sinus is deep, almost in the center of the skull. It may be approached intranasally or via the external ethmoidectomy incision through the eyebrow.

SPHENOIDOTOMY   Sphenoidotomy involves the creation of an opening into the sphenoid sinus for drainage.

Endoscopic Sinus Surgery
Sinuscopes permit direct visualization of the paranasal sinuses and the anatomy of lateral nasal walls. The site of diseased mucosa or obstructive tissue, such as polyps, can be localized for removal, with preservation of some mucosa and restoration of drainage. The mucosa of each sinus has cilia that move air in waveforms. With an endoscopic approach, some ciliary motion may be retained for aeration. The basic principle of endoscopic sinus surgery is that most sinus mucosal disease will resolve if aeration and drainage are reestablished. The extent of the procedure depends on the location of diseased mucosa and the resection necessary to establish drainage. Septal deformities or inferior turbinates causing nasal obstruction may be concurrently corrected (i.e., septoplasty and turbinoplasty). Minor procedures limited to removal of disease from maxillary or ethmoid sinuses usually can be done with topical and local anesthesia. IV sedation or general anesthesia is needed for more extensive procedures, such as ethmoidectomy or sphenoethmoidectomy.

The telescopes of sinuscopes are 2.7 and 4 mm in diameter with 0-, 25- or 30-, 70-, and 120-degree viewing angles. The quartz rod telescope has a solid quartz optical cone in the light post that attaches to a halogen light source. This system provides optimal light transmission through the fiberoptics of the miniaturized scope. An attached suction/irrigation device permits unobstructed viewing. The telescope is inserted intranasally and advanced into the frontal, ethmoid, or sphenoid sinus. It is inserted through a cannula in the canine fossa to reach the maxillary sinus. Many accessory grasping and cutting instruments, including the KTP laser, are used to remove mucosa, lamina, osteum, and cells. Hemostasis is controlled with epinephrine and cautery or laser. Nasal packing usually is not required.

FUNCTIONAL PROCEDURE   Known as the Messerklinger technique, the surgeon begins at the ethmoid and works anteriorly to the frontal and maxillary sinuses to clear ethmoidal compartments of disease. If a minimal opening of the narrow osteomeatal tract at the anterior ethmoidal sinus will not achieve adequate drainage from other paranasal sinuses, a posterior ethmoidectomy and sphenoidotomy are included in the procedure.

EXENTERATION   Known as the Wigand procedure, total sphenoethmoidectomy and partial middle turbinate resection are performed, beginning with a sphenoidotomy and working anteriorly to the frontal sinus. This creates a broad opening of the sphenoidal, ethmoidal, frontal, and maxillary sinuses. To avoid the optic nerve, dissection does not extend beyond the lateral wall of the sphenoid. Visual evoked potentials monitor optic nerve function; the eyes are uncovered. The endoscopic procedure may be done bilaterally.

Resection of Tumors   Osteoma, a benign tumor, can arise from bones around the paranasal sinuses. Although rare, primary carcinoma and sarcoma do occur in the frontal, ethmoid, sphenoid, and maxillary sinuses. Most originate in the maxillary sinus. The incidence increases with age. The sinuses are proximal to the orbits, oral cavity, and base of the skull. A tumor in the maxillary sinus may be associated with oral or nasal symptoms, such as loosening of the upper teeth, bleeding from the nose, or asymmetry of the face. A malignant lesion in the ethmoid sinus may be accompanied by displacement of the eye, disturbance of smell, and nasal obstruction. Chronic sinusitis is thought to play an etiologic role because of an associated replacement of respiratory epithelium by stratified squamous cells. Most sinus tumors are squamous cell carcinomas. Often the bony walls are invaded and destroyed by the time symptoms appear because the tumor tends to extend in all directions. Exploratory surgery by a Caldwell-Luc incision provides the best chance of early diagnosis. Radical craniofacial resection may be indicated.

ORAL CAVITY AND THROAT

Anatomy and Physiology of the Oral Cavity and Throat

The oral cavity is lined with thick mucous membrane. This squamous mucosa connects with the nasopharynx superiorly and the hypopharynx below. The hard palate, part of the maxillary bone, forms the floor of the nasal cavity and the anterior part of the roof of the mouth. The soft palate, a musculomembranous structure posterior to the hard palate, occludes the nasal cavity during speech and swallowing. These functions are aided by the uvula, a small conical appendage (tonguelike structure) that projects from the posterior free margin of the soft palate. It contains the uvular muscle covered by mucous membrane. The tongue, occupying much of the oral cavity, joins the soft palate and pharynx posteriorly by folds of mucous membrane.

The throat refers to space surrounded by the soft palate, the palatoglossal and palatopharyngeal arches, the base of the tongue, and the pharynx. The funnel-shaped pharynx is subdivided into the nasopharynx (above), oropharynx (middle), and hypopharynx (below). The nasopharynx communicates with the nasal cavity through the posterior choanae. The oropharynx includes the base of the tongue anteriorly, the tonsillar fossae laterally, and the oropharyngeal walls of the throat posteriorly. The hypopharynx leads from the oropharynx to the larynx, trachea, and esophagus. The pharynx, posterior to the larynx and the nasal and oral cavities, consists of constrictor muscles essential to swallowing. The proximity of food and air passages and the joint function of the pharynx in their passage contribute to the hazard of aspiration.

The nasopharynx and oropharynx contain masses of lymphoid tissue. The adenoids (pharyngeal tonsils) hang from the nasopharyngeal roof; the lingual tonsils are in mucosal crypts. The palatine tonsils lie on either side of the oropharynx. These, referred to as the tonsils, are supported in the tonsillar fossae by anterior and posterior pillars. A fibrous capsule adheres to each laterally.

The salivary glands are located in the soft tissue walls of the oral cavity. The six major paired glands are the submandibular, sublingual, and parotid glands. The parotid glands are the largest. The ducts of these major glands, in addition to lesser glands, secrete saliva into the mouth. Saliva functions to moisten and lubricate food to aid in swallowing, to dissolve some substances and enzymatically digest starches, and to facilitate tasting.

Surgical Procedures of the Oral Cavity and Throat

Pathologic conditions may affect the lips, tongue, floor of the mouth, palates, salivary glands, or pharynx. The oral region is one of the most vascular areas of the body. Hemostasis may be achieved with an electrosurgical unit, hemostatic scalpel, argon beam coagulator, or laser. Lasers are used to vaporize both benign and malignant superficial and subepithelial lesions.

Abnormalities result from congenital malformation, improper occlusion or jaggedness of teeth, and infection, but most commonly they result from trauma and neoplasms. Adequate reconstruction restores the lining, internal structural support, soft tissue, and external coverage. Many of the craniofacial, maxillofacial, and dentofacial procedures previously described in this chapter are performed through intraoral incisions. Plastic surgeons, oral surgeons, laryngologists, or a multidisciplinary team may perform the following procedures through intraoral or extraoral incisions.

Excision of Salivary Gland Tumors

Benign mixed tumors of the salivary glands are more common than are malignant tumors and most frequently are located in a parotid gland. Most tumors can be removed by dissection, and some can be removed by cryosurgery. The incision is of adequate size to expose the entire gland and the facial nerve. A nerve stimulator is used to identify the nerve and its branches. Injury to the nerve results in postoperative facial paralysis.

Parotidectomy Parotidectomy, excision of a parotid gland, is performed through an incision in the neck below the angle of the mandible and extending upward to one or both sides of the ear. A swelling beneath the skin in the area in front of or below the ear is almost invariably within the substance of the parotid gland. This may be a benign, mixed, or malignant tumor. Benign lesions localized superficially may be excised by superficial subtotal parotidectomy. Lesions

deep within the gland, extending under the mandible, frequently displace the soft palate in the oral cavity. Radical neck dissection or hemimandibulectomy may be indicated to remove a highly invasive malignant tumor. For most parotid tumors the facial nerve can be isolated and preserved during total parotidectomy, unless the nerve is inextricably involved by the tumor. If the facial nerve is to be sacrificed, the nerve may be primarily grafted, with the great auricular nerve as a graft, to prevent total facial nerve paralysis.

Excision of Oral Carcinoma

Primary malignant lesions may occur in the lower lip, tongue, or floor of the mouth. Because of the proximity of cervical lymph nodes, metastasis occurs early. A painful, bleeding ulcer is considered a suspicious symptom. Oral cancer in its earliest stages may be asymptomatic and painless. Small tumors may be treated with only irradiation, local excision with primary closure, or vaporization with a laser beam. Larger lesions compel more extensive procedures.

Subtotal Glossectomy or Hemiglossectomy In subtotal glossectomy or hemiglossectomy, part *(subtotal)* or half *(hemi-)* of the tongue is removed *(glossectomy)*. The extent of the resection will determine the type of reconstruction to resurface the oral cavity. Innervated free flaps may be used to maintain bulk and tone.

Total Glossectomy All of the tongue and often the floor of the mouth are resected. A pectoralis major myocutaneous island flap is more advantageous than are the cervical, pectoral, or forehead flaps also used to restore the intraoral lining. Respiratory embarrassment and chronic aspiration are significant problems after glossectomy. Cricopharyngeal myotomy may be performed to facilitate swallowing and reduce aspiration. The tip of the epiglottis is often sutured to the pharyngeal wall (epiglottopexy) to decrease aspiration. Unless it is involved directly with tumor, the larynx is preserved. Laryngeal suspension, achieved by placing a heavy suture around the mandibular ramus, holds the larynx laterally. Extension into the larynx and cervical metastases are indications for unilateral or bilateral neck dissection, usually with laryngectomy. A tracheotomy is always performed with a total glossectomy to maintain an airway. For postoperative alimentation a nasogastric tube is inserted before closing the pharynx.

Procedures of the Nasopharynx

Uvulopalatopharyngoplasty Increasing the air space in the oropharynx corrects obstructive sleep apnea (OSA) caused by anatomic relationships in some patients. OSA can cause oxygen desaturation during apneic episodes that occur during sleep. This can lead to life-threatening pulmonary and systemic hypertension, cardiac dysrhythmias, and neurologic dysfunction if untreated. Upper airway obstruction may be caused by nasal obstruction, a deviated nasal septum, hypertrophied adenoids and/or tonsils, or mandibular retrognathism (overbite), which may be surgically corrected. To diagnose OSA in patients who do not have obvious abnormalities, airway obstruction can be viewed during sleep with fiberoptic nasopharyngoscopy and fluoroscopy. Obstruction of air passage for more than 10 seconds is diagnostic. Oxygen saturation of the blood is 85% in moderate cases and less than 60% in severe obstructive cases. Some of the oropharyngeal muscles may become atonic and collapse inward, and the soft palate may drop down. Patients who have a large, drooping soft palate and at least moderately redundant lateral pharyngeal walls or large tonsils are good candidates for uvulopalatopharyngoplasty. These patients have moderate apnea but do not have severe cardiac dysrhythmias.

The patient is continuously monitored during induction of anesthesia. The surgeon is present and an emergency tracheotomy tray is available in case the patient's airway becomes obstructed.

The full thickness of mucosa is resected from the posterior margin of the soft palate, including the uvula, and most of the anterior tonsillar pillar. The lesser palatine artery is ligated. The tonsils or mucosa of the tonsillar fossae are resected. The remaining posterior tonsillar pillar is sutured to the resected anterior pillar. The palate is closed laterally. The extent of tissue removal varies according to the width and depth of the patient's oropharyngeal space.

Adenoidectomy   Adenoidectomy, the removal of hypertrophied adenoid tissue from the nasopharynx and behind the posterior choanae, may be performed in adults to relieve upper airway obstruction. This is more commonly performed in children, often to prevent recurrent otitis media. Adenoid tissue usually atrophies after adolescence.

The patient is supine. General anesthesia is administered, and the patient is intubated. Adenoids can be resected with an adenotome and curette or vaporized with a CO_2 laser. Bleeding is more easily controlled with the laser. An electrocautery and/or gauze sponges soaked in epinephrine may be used following sharp dissection. Occasionally a posterior nasal pack is needed.

Procedures of the Oropharynx

Tonsillectomy   Chronically infected or hypertrophied tonsils are most frequently removed in childhood. Even slightly enlarged tonsils can obstruct airflow to the lungs during sleep in an adult. Tonsillectomy may significantly improve symptoms of sleep apnea, with or without uvulopalatopharyngoplasty.

A CO_2, Nd:YAG, argon, or KTP laser may be used to excise tonsils from the tonsillar fossae. The patient is supine. General anesthesia is administered. The endotracheal tube and cuff must be protected, and other laser precautions must be taken around the oral cavity. A smoke evacuator should be available with a CO_2 laser. A handheld laser may be used, or a beam may be directed through the microscope.

Local anesthesia is frequently used for adult tonsillectomy. The patient is in semi-Fowler's or a sitting position on the operating bed or sits in a specially designed chair. The throat is anesthetized with a topical agent and local infiltration. With sharp and blunt dissection, each tonsil is separated from the pillars and capsule and removed from the fossa with

a tonsil snare. Attention is given to hemostasis to prevent aspiration; suture ligatures, free ties, and/or absorbable ligating clips may be used. Bleeding can be difficult to control and can occur postoperatively with this technique. Less intraoperative bleeding occurs with laser tonsillectomy.

Incision and Drainage of a Peritonsillar Abscess   Less common since the advent of antibiotics, incision into the anterior tonsillar pillar may be necessary to drain purulent material posterior to the tonsillar capsule following acute tonsillitis.

Resection of a Tonsillar Tumor   A localized squamous cell carcinoma of the tonsil may be resected by dissection or with cryosurgery. An en bloc resection includes the primary tumor and nodes. Metastatic nodes are common. Superior progression of the tumor may reach the supratonsillar fossa, soft and hard palates, and uvula. Inferiorly the tumor may spread to the posterior and lateral walls of the larynx, base of the tongue, and pyriform sinus. Neck dissection may be indicated for regional disease. Surgery may be combined with preoperative or postoperative radiation therapy. The most common complications are fistula formation and delayed healing.

Pharyngeal Diverticulectomy   Diverticulectomy, or removal of sacs or outpocketings of lower pharyngeal mucous membrane in which food collects, may be performed in extreme cases in which regurgitation presents a hazard of aspiration. The neck of the sac is dissected from the posterior pharyngeal wall and ligated. The stump of the excised sac is inverted into the pharyngeal wall. Diverticuli may be removed endoscopically.

Dental Procedures

Just as the scope of many medical-surgical specialties, such as otolaryngology–head and neck surgery, has broadened, so has dentistry. Likewise, subspecialization within dentistry, through extensive specialized postgraduate education, has given OR practice privileges to dentists who perform surgical procedures in and around the oral cavity. Among these are the following:

- *Oral surgeon.* Oral surgery may be limited to exodontia (extraction of teeth) and minor surgery in the oral cavity. It may also include correction of dentofacial deformities (i.e., oral and maxillofacial surgery). A qualified oral surgeon is competent to complete a history and physical examination and thus determine the patient's ability to undergo the proposed surgical procedure.
- *Orthodontist.* Orthodontics focuses on irregularities of the teeth, malocclusion, and associated facial problems.
- *Prosthodontist.* Prosthodontics is concerned with artificial restoration of intraoral and external facial structures.
- *Periodontist.* Periodontics is the treatment and prevention of disease in the gingiva (gum), underlying soft tissues, and alveoli surrounding the teeth.

Patients with medical problems admitted to the hospital by oral surgeons and all patients admitted for dental care have an admission history, physical examination, and evaluation of their overall medical risk by a physician preoperatively. This physician is responsible for the care of a preexisting condition and any medical problem that arises during hospitalization.

Just as physicians from various specialties function as members of a multidisciplinary team, so do oral surgeons and dentists, each contributing to the dental health of the patient. Frequently they also function as collegial members of the teams involved in craniofacial or maxillofacial surgery. They assist with reconstruction of the face, correction of jaw deformities, and establishment of optimal dental occlusion. For example, the orthodontist may move teeth before a maxillofacial or oral surgeon repositions the jaws to correct malocclusion. Many patients undergo both preoperative and postoperative orthodontia. Prosthodontics may be necessary to replace missing teeth. Prosthodontists also may fit an artificial nose postoperatively following rhinectomy for a tumor or trauma.

Patients seeking dentofacial treatment usually have functional problems. These may include difficulty with mastication (chewing) and deglutition (swallowing), speech problems, abnormal tongue posture, or lip incompetence. A dental surgical procedure is defined as any manipulation, cutting, or removal of oral or perioral tissues and tooth structures where bleeding occurs. Oral surgeons and periodontists perform these procedures.

Periodontics

Diseases that affect the gingiva, bone, and supporting structures such as periodontal ligaments can occur at any age. Periodontal disease is the primary cause of tooth loss in adults over 35 years of age. Treatment usually takes place in the periodontist's office. Patients who have medical problems, such as hemophilia or some other blood dyscrasia, severe diabetes, or heart disease, are admitted to the hospital. Periodontal plastic surgery encompasses resective, regenerative, and reconstructive techniques.

Gingivectomy   Portions of the gingiva, mucous membrane, and underlying soft tissue that covers the alveolar process and surrounds the teeth are excised to remove deep pockets of plaque, calculus, and inflamed soft tissue. The CO_2 laser may be used for this procedure.

Mucogingivoplasty   Plastic surgery around the teeth and gums is done primarily to reduce inflammation, prevent accumulation of bacteria, and stop sensitivity. Another indication is to rebuild bone and soft tissue destroyed by disease or trauma. Excessive gum tissue is excised to contour or reshape the gingiva for improved physiologic form or aesthetics. The alveoli may be reconstructed to change their shape and height. Gingival margins may be reshaped for the site of a false tooth or fixed bridge. Gingival grafting or augmentation done before or during orthodontic treatment may reduce the risk of recession of gum tissue from around the roots of teeth. Autogenous mucogingival free grafts from the hard palate or pedicle flaps from adjacent tissues may be used to cover receded alveolar mucosa or an exposed tooth root. Flaps or grafts are used to augment inadequate zones of masticatory gingiva. Gingival onlay grafts are also used to enhance ridges where trauma or extraction has resulted in a reduced ridge, thus correcting an aesthetic defect.

Alveolar Ridge Reconstruction

The alveolar ridge is the bony remains of the alveolar process of the maxilla or mandible that formerly contained the teeth. Some edentulous patients have atrophic maxillae and/or mandibles or bony defects caused by trauma or tumor resection that will not support artificial dentures. The alveolar ridges can be augmented or reconstructed.

Inlay Bone Grafts   Bone grafts are used for augmentation of the maxillae and/or mandible. A prevascularized autogenous rib graft may be transplanted into a maxillary defect; microvascular anastomoses revascularize the graft. Composite grafts of freeze-dried cadaver rib with autogenous particulate cancellous bone and marrow may be preferred in the maxilla. Iliac bone is used to augment the mandible (see Mandibular Reconstruction). Calvaria may be harvested from the frontal, parietal, or occipital cranial bones for maxillofacial bone grafts. Calvarial bone undergoes less resorption than rib and iliac bone because of its dense blood supply; graft tissue revascularizes rapidly. Titanium osseointegration fixtures may be used to secure calvarial bone grafts in place.

Dental Implant   Fixtures are implanted into the gingiva and attached to bone to replace or augment lost dentition. Dental implants may replace a single tooth or missing teeth. They are made of biocompatible metals, most commonly titanium, and may be coated with ceramic, carbon, or sapphire. Several types are used, as follows:

1. *Endosteal implant.* A threaded screw, cylinder, or flat blade is implanted in an alveolus in the maxilla or mandible. The number of implants placed depends on availability of bone and the number of teeth to be replaced. The fixture is covered with soft tissue. By the process of osseointegration, a perimucosal seal and bond develop between the gingiva and the surface of the implant. Some implants have small holes that allow bone to grow through them to secure the implant. After a minimum of 3 (for the mandible) to 6 (for the maxilla) months, a second-stage procedure is performed to connect a solid post to the implanted fixture. This extends slightly above the gingiva. The artificial tooth is attached to this post with tiny screws. Osseointegration provides firm, immobile support and distributes the stress of chewing evenly within the jaw.
2. *Subperiosteal implant.* The implant is placed beneath the periosteum directly onto the alveolar bone. This type of implant is used when bone is insufficient to support an endosteal implant.

3. *Transosteal implant.* A bone plate with retaining posts, similar to the mandibular staple (see below) is used when the patient has severe mandibular alveolar ridge atrophy.

Mandibular Staple The staple fastener prosthesis is implanted as an alternative to bone grafting to restore the ability of the mandible to support a denture. The titanium alloy (Tivanium) device has two transosteal pins with a set of fasteners and lock nuts between them on the curved cross-arch connecting plate. The staple is inserted with a drill guide and twist drills specifically designed for it. The staple is evenly seated in the holes drilled in the mandible to the point of contact with the inferior border.

A scratch or bend may weaken the staple and may result in a fracture of the device. A deformed staple will not fit into the drill holes properly. The prosthesis is carefully protected and handled very little before implantation.

NECK

Anatomy and Physiology of the Neck

The neck connects the head and trunk of the body. It is supported by the cervical vertebrae posteriorly and muscles anteriorly and laterally. The larynx, leading to the trachea, and the proximal end of the esophagus pass within the muscular structure. The vascular, nervous, and lymphatic systems leading to and from the head also pass through the neck. The thyroid and parathyroid glands lie along the trachea on the anterior aspect at the base of the neck.

Larynx

The larynx, situated anteriorly between the hypopharynx superiorly and the trachea inferiorly, consists of three major cartilages supported by ligaments and muscles: the thyroid cartilage, which protects the soft inner structures; the cricoid cartilage directly beneath it; and the paired arytenoid cartilages posterior to the thyroid and joined to the cricoid. The thyroid cartilage is incomplete posteriorly, but the cricoid is a complete ring. The cricothyroid space lies between the thyroid and cricoid cartilages.

The larynx functions as an organ for speech and for closure of the glottis during swallowing to protect the respiratory passage and prevent aspiration. The epiglottis, an elastic cartilage covered with mucous membrane at the root of the tongue in the hypopharynx, covers the superior opening of the larynx during swallowing.

Extrinsic muscles open and close the glottis, the space between the true vocal cords. Intrinsic muscles regulate vocal cord tension. Movement of the paired arytenoid cartilages opens and closes the glottis. Folds of mucous membrane covering muscle line the larynx. The two upper folds are the false cords; the two lower folds are the true vocal cords. The true vocal cords attach to the arytenoid cartilages posteriorly and to the thyroid cartilage anteriorly. The cords are an integral part of phonation. They vibrate to produce sounds by rhythmically moving air particles. Production of vocal sound involves coordination of the musculature of the lips, tongue, soft palate, pharynx, and larynx. The mouth and pharynx are the resonating cavities.

The tenth cranial (vagus) nerve innervates the larynx. Its major branch to the larynx is the recurrent laryngeal nerve. Trauma to the nerve can result in laryngeal paralysis, which is devastating if both nerves are paralyzed.

Trachea

The trachea is a 10- to 11-cm tube composed of rings of cartilage anteriorly and membrane posteriorly. This membrane also forms the anterior wall of the esophagus (the musculomembranous canal between the pharynx and the stomach). The trachea extends from the lower larynx to the carina in the chest, where it bifurcates to form the right and left main bronchi, leading to the lungs.

Surgical Procedures of the Larynx

Trauma or disease involving laryngeal cartilages, mucous membrane, or the vocal cords can obstruct respiration and/or speech. Surgical procedures are directed toward diagnosis of the cause and elimination of obstruction to maintain the larynx's dual functions in respiration and phonation.

Laryngoscopy

Laryngoscopy is a visual examination of the mucous membrane lining of the larynx and vocal cords with a lighted instrument, with or without the adjunct magnification of the operating microscope. Laryngoscopy is performed for diagnosis, biopsy, and/or treatment of laryngeal lesions, including the following:

- Foreign body, such as a coin, watch battery, or small toy.
- Papilloma of the vocal cords, which prevents accurate cord approximation and a normal voice.
- Laryngeal polyps, with stripping of polypoid mucosa to alleviate recurrence.
- Juvenile papilloma (multiple growths on the larynx, epiglottis, vocal cords, and trachea). These may be treated by cryosurgery or a laser beam in lieu of excision.
- Leukoplakia (a white thickening on the vocal cords, causing hoarseness). The lesion is examined histologically for differentiation from carcinoma.
- Laryngeal web (adherence of the anterior aspects of the vocal cords as a result of removal of mucous membrane or following inflammation). After excision, a metal or plastic plate may be placed between the cords until normal mucous membrane regenerates. The plate is then removed.

Preoperative preparation and endoscopic technique are similar for laryngoscopy, esophagoscopy, and bronchoscopy. General anesthesia is usually used, but local topical anesthesia may be preferred for some patients. The patient is supine with the neck hyperextended and head supported. As following any anesthetization of the throat, postoperative orders include nothing by mouth for a specific number of hours until throat reflexes have returned, to prevent aspiration.

Indirect Laryngoscopy   In indirect laryngoscopy a laryngeal mirror is inserted through the mouth to the base of the tongue. With the patient in a sitting position, light is reflected to the area by the surgeon's headlamp. During this simple diagnostic procedure, a biopsy or polypectomy can be performed.

Direct Laryngoscopy   In direct laryngoscopy a rigid, hollow tubular laryngoscope is inserted into the larynx for direct visualization. Suction tubes and grasping forceps are maneuvered through the handheld laryngoscope. Fiberoptic light carriers are connected to a light source. Endoscopic principles as discussed in Chapter 20 are applicable.

Suspension Microlaryngoscopy   For microlaryngoscopy the laryngoscope becomes self-retaining by suspension in a special appliance placed over the patient's chest. This gives the surgeon bimanual freedom in use of the operating microscope. The microscope provides binocular vision and magnification in critical inaccessible areas or areas difficult to visualize by direct laryngoscopy. A standard operating microscope with a 400-mm lens is used. Microlaryngeal instruments are added to the basic setup for direct laryngoscopy. Suspension microlaryngoscopy is used for most intralaryngeal procedures.

Laser Microlaryngoscopy   The CO_2 laser was introduced in laryngology by Jako and Strong in 1971. It was initially used for removal of recurrent laryngeal papillomas. Now CO_2 and other lasers are used to remove a variety of benign and malignant lesions in the respiratory tract, particularly in the larynx. For example, the argon laser may be used for treatment of hereditary hemorrhagic telangiectasia (dilated groups of capillaries) in the larynx.

A micromanipulator, used to direct the laser beam, is coupled to the operating microscope. The microscope lens focuses the beam. Reflecting mirrors defocus the beam to reach into otherwise inaccessible areas. Microlaryngeal instruments are used in addition to specific laser instruments. For example, anterior commissure vocal cord retractors with suction attachments are used to clear the smoke of tissue vaporization for visibility.

LASER SAFETY   The laser is a safe instrument when used around the oral cavity and neck only when safety precautions are taken as follows:

1. The patient's eyes should be taped shut and covered with moistened sponges to prevent injury from inadvertent reflection of the laser beam from a metal surface.
2. The patient's face should be covered with a moist towel so that only the oral cavity is exposed.
3. The patient's teeth should be protected from the pressure of the laryngoscope and from the laser beam.

4. Only noncombustible anesthetic gases are used. Anesthetic gases potentially can be ignited by the laser. Nitrous oxide should not be used. Oxygen concentration may be decreased to between 21% and 30% during the lasing phase of the procedure.
5. A stainless steel or laminated aluminum and silicone endotracheal tube or a ventilating bronchoscope avoids the danger of ignition. Polyvinyl chloride and latex endotracheal tubes cannot be used because they are heat labile. Red rubber and silicone tubes may be wrapped with reflecting aluminum tape, but the tip is not always sufficiently protected if exposed to the laser beam. Ignition of endotracheal tubes has occurred. Moist gauze or compressed patties, attached to strings, are placed through the suspended laryngoscope to protect the balloon in the cuff of the tube from rupture by stray or reflected laser beams. The balloon should be filled with sterile normal saline solution, which may be tinted with methylene blue dye, so that the balloon will not ignite if ruptured. If a cuff does rupture, immediate replacement of the tube is necessary. A tracheotomy tray should be available for emergency use.
6. Combustible materials, such as sponges and drapes, are kept moist. Water effectively inhibits penetration of laser energy into surrounding tissue and materials.
7. Division of a blood vessel larger than 0.5 mm requires ligation or electrocoagulation.
8. All other precautions for laser surgery are taken.

Laryngeal Injuries

Patients with abnormal laryngeal conditions bear close watching for respiratory distress. The anterior, unprotected location of the larynx predisposes it to trauma, such as a crushing injury. Treatment is concerned primarily with maintenance of the airway, which may be occluded by edema, hematoma, torn mucosa, or cartilaginous fragments.

Cricothyrotomy (emergency incision into the larynx) and/or tracheotomy (incision into the trachea) may be necessary to open the airway or to prevent asphyxia. An intraluminal stent inserted into the larynx superiorly to the tracheostomy tube and fixed to it for stabilization may be worn for several months until the laryngeal laceration heals and an intralaryngeal airway re-forms. The stent is used to mold the tissues.

Preservation of the voice is also a major concern. Severe laryngeal injury may result in permanent voice impairment. In unilateral vocal cord paralysis, because of muscle atrophy and muscle imbalance, a weak, hoarse ("air-spilling") voice is present. Inadequate glottic closure can be treated by injection of Teflon (Polytef) paste into the affected cord to augment its size and thus help to bring the two cords into apposition. The injected material becomes firm and retains its shape. A functioning cord and marked improvement in voice quality result. This modality is used commonly when the recurrent laryngeal nerve is affected. It is not indicated for acute glottic incompetence. A suspension of Gelfoam powder in saline can be used for temporary augmentation until compensation or the need for permanent augmentation occurs.

Procedures for Carcinoma of the Larynx

Procedures vary depending on the size and location of the lesion, extent of invasion, and presence of regional or distant metastasis, as well as the patient's age, general condition, and rehabilitative capacity. Classification of malignant lesions by location includes glottic (true cords), supraglottic (above true cords), and infraglottic (below true cords) lesions. In the early stages, cancer of the larynx is one of the most curable of all malignant tumors because of the sparse lymphatic supply in the region of the vocal cords. Radiologic study of the lesion by various methods, such as contrast laryngography, is a valuable adjunct in selecting an appropriate therapeutic modality. Laryngograms can identify mucosal irregularity, vocal cord thickening, or a tumor and outline the lesion, as well as portray functional alteration of laryngeal structures.

Symptoms vary as well. Hoarseness for more than 2 weeks' duration often is a result of cord fixation by a malignant glottic lesion. Dysphagia is suggestive of a tumor at the esophageal opening. Dyspnea from airway obstruction is a late manifestation.

Whenever possible, the surgeon will perform a conservative laryngectomy to retain some natural voice. These procedures yield the same rate of cure of selected cancers as a radical procedure—total laryngectomy—without sacrificing phonation, deglutition, or respiratory function. A neck stoma is usually necessary for breathing.

Laryngofissure with Partial Laryngectomy

Laryngofissure (division of or opening into the larynx) may be necessary to remove a foreign body or tumor. Laryngofissure with partial laryngectomy through an incision in the thyroid cartilage is performed to remove a large tumor confined to one vocal cord. A tracheotomy is performed to maintain the airway. Postoperative hoarseness may diminish as scar tissue forms to replace excised vocal cord.

Supraglottic Laryngectomy

The epiglottis, false cords, and hyoid bone are removed in a supraglottic laryngectomy when a tumor is located in the epiglottis (i.e., is supraglottic). A horizontal incision is made above the true vocal cords, thus preserving voice and a normal airway. Neck dissection may be done simultaneously. A temporary tracheotomy is always part of the procedure because of the danger of aspiration and postoperative edema. With the epiglottis removed, liquids in particular can easily spill into the trachea. A cuffed tracheostomy tube is a necessary precaution postoperatively.

Vertical Hemilaryngectomy

In hemilaryngectomy through a vertical incision, one true cord, false cord, arytenoid, and half of the thyroid cartilage are removed. The epiglottis, cricoid, and opposing cords are preserved. Following healing, scar tissue fills in the surgical defect, almost approximating the remaining vocal cord. Thus the patient has a usable although hoarse voice and satisfactory airway and can eat normally. Sometimes a muscle flap is used for glottic reconstruction to improve voice quality. A prophylactic tracheotomy usually is done to protect the airway. Subcutaneous emphysema (i.e., infiltration of air under the skin) is a potential complication.

Total Laryngectomy

A radical procedure, total laryngectomy is performed for advanced lesions involving the larynx and/or hypopharyngeal area, with or without neck dissection. The entire larynx, hyoid bone, cricoid cartilage, two or three tracheal rings, and strap muscles are removed. This resection destroys the connection between the pharynx and the trachea. Pharyngeal walls and the lower trachea are preserved. The pharyngeal opening to the trachea is closed, thus leaving the pharynx open only to the esophagus. The patient breathes and expels bronchial secretions through a permanent stoma at the base of the anterior neck. This is created by suturing the tracheal stump to the skin (tracheostomy). The size of the stoma should be recorded on the patient's record in the event of emergency need for a tube at a later time. In patients with a permanent stoma, resuscitation is always via the stoma.

The nose no longer humidifies the air to the lungs. The sense of smell is also lost because the nasal olfactory epithelium is not stimulated by inhalation. Acclimatization to air intake through the neck constitutes a major adjustment for the patient.

A nasogastric tube is inserted during the surgical procedure for temporary feeding. Although the patient no longer has a normal voice, normal eating is resumed after healing takes place.

The formation of a salivary fistula is one complication of laryngectomy. Swallowed saliva leaks out through a weakness in the pharyngeal suture line and through the skin. Rupture of the carotid artery, especially in preirradiated patients, is another complication. This may occur if radical neck dissection was performed also, which places the artery in the surgical area.

Rehabilitation should begin preoperatively at the time of diagnosis and include the family. It incorporates input from many professional disciplines because major disability results from the surgical procedure. In working with a speech pathologist, some patients learn to develop esophageal speech. By intake of a bolus of air into the esophagus and vibration by cricopharyngeal muscles, sound is produced to articulate speech. Persons unable to perfect the technique may use an artificial larynx, an electronic device that includes pitch and volume.

Many patients are unable to acquire usable esophageal speech, with or without the artificial larynx. Some of these patients have undergone surgical procedures to rebuild a functioning glottis or to create a permanent tracheoesophageal fistula to shunt pulmonary airflow to the pharynx for phonation. Aspiration pneumonia caused by leakage of saliva and food is a major problem following these procedures. Also, pharyngeal constrictor muscle spasms or stenosis may inhibit speech rehabilitation. Voice restoration for these aphonic patients may be enhanced by a valved prosthesis. This is inserted through a tracheoesophageal fistula to allow free flow of air into the esophagus for phonation, to prevent aspiration, and to maintain patency of the fistula. Three types of one-way valve voice prostheses are used:

1. The Blom-Singer duckbill prosthesis, so named from the shape of the slit valve, is a silicone tube with retention flanges (collarlike projections). The fistula for the prosthesis is created through an esophagoscope inserted into the cervical esophagus. A needle is introduced to puncture the posterior tracheal wall and anterior esophagus at the superior aspect of the laryngectomy stoma. A rubber catheter stent is inserted through the puncture to maintain patency during healing. When the prosthesis is fitted, the flanges are taped to the peristomal skin. The patient occludes the stoma to produce a voice.
2. The Blom-Singer tracheostoma valve and low-pressure prosthesis has a diaphragm that opens during normal respiration and closes in response to expiratory airflow for speech. The circular valve is recessed slightly into the tracheostoma, with the housing fixed to the peristomal skin with a hypoallergenic adhesive. The patient does not manually occlude the stoma during speech.
3. The Panje voice prosthesis, commonly known as the voice button, is a biflanged silicone valve inserted into a simple tracheoesophageal stab wound. An insertion guide is used to place the prosthesis through the tracheostoma into the created fistula. The patient occludes the stoma to speak.

Practical help and moral support are offered to the newly laryngectomized patient by others who are members of support groups, such as the International Association of Laryngectomees and the Lost Chord Club. The American Cancer Society is also a resource for assistance.

Laryngeal Transplant

In January of 1998 Marshall Strome of the Cleveland Clinic Foundation transplanted a larynx and a portion of a trachea into a 40-year-old man whose larynx was crushed in a motor vehicle accident 19 years previously. He was able to speak a few words within 12 hours of the procedure. The full extent of recovery will not be known for several years. The only other documented attempt to transplant a larynx was in 1969 in Belgium.

Surgical Procedures of the Esophagus

Esophageal disorders may be acquired or congenital. Abnormalities result from trauma, inflammation, or a neoplasm. A gastroenterologist and/or laryngologist may study them.

Esophagoscopy

Endoscopic direct visualization of the interior of the esophagus is performed to remove foreign bodies; to obtain biopsy, brush cytologic, or secretion specimens for diagnosis; and to examine the esophagus and esophageal orifice of the stomach for organic disease. Inspection is made for diverticula, varices, strictures, lesions, or a hiatal hernia, which may manifest as symptoms of obstruction, regurgitation, or bleeding.

Esophagoscopes are either rigid, hollow metal tubes or the flexible fiberoptic type of scope that reduces discomfort and trauma. Accessory instruments, such as aspiration tubes and biopsy forceps, are similar for all endoscopes. Removal of an obstructing mass, such as a steak bolus in the esophagus, is better accomplished with the rigid metal scope. Various sizes of scopes are available to suit the individual patient's situation.

The patient is positioned with the shoulders even with, or a little over, the edge of the body section of the operating bed. The head section is lowered. An assistant holds the patient's head. The patient is encouraged to relax by breathing deeply if the procedure is done with local topical anesthesia. The head is raised or lowered slowly, at the direction of the endoscopist as the esophagoscope is passed, until the neck is hyperextended. The esophagoscope is passed through the mouth and cricopharyngeal lumen to the cardiac sphincter at the esophagogastric junction. The entire area is carefully scrutinized. The esophagus may be distended by insufflation of air to assist in viewing in the presence of stenosis, or a lumen finder may be necessary. The scrub person introduces tips of aspirating tubes, grasping forceps, bougies, and other long accessories into a rigid esophagoscope for the endoscopist.

Removal of Foreign Bodies

Removal of foreign bodies from the pharynx and/or esophagus is relatively common. Persons who wear upper dentures are especially prone to swallowing sharp bones that cannot be felt against the covered palate. Pieces of meat or dental bridgework may lodge or become impacted in the food passage, occluding the airway by pressure. This is an emergency situation necessitating provision of a patent airway by endotracheal intubation or tracheotomy and endoscopic removal of the bolus or foreign object. Acute esophageal obstruction increases salivation, creating the danger of tracheopulmonary aspiration.

Children frequently swallow objects, such as watch batteries, coins, buttons, parts of toys, or safety pins, that may remain in the throat. Metallic objects are visible on roentgenograms, but many others are not.

It is dangerous to attempt to push an object toward the stomach because esophageal perforation can result. Esophagoscopy is the method of choice for removal, although the procedure is often difficult and painstaking. All effort is made to prevent trauma, with resultant mediastinitis.

Dilation of a Stricture

The esophageal lumen can narrow because of the formation of scar tissue resulting from inflammation or a burn at any level. Treatment consists of regular dilation with bougies of graduated sizes. Steroid administration is adjunctive therapy.

When an individual suffers a severe burn, such as from swallowing a caustic material, gastrostomy may be indicated to bypass the esophagus until it heals. Dilation of such strictures uses retrograde fusiform bougies with spindle-shaped shafts that are linked together. They are carried through the gastrostomy, up the esophagus, and out the mouth. The treatment is continued for an extended period.

Dilation of a stricture at the cardioesophageal junction may be necessary in patients with cardiospasm (achalasia). Gross dilation above the stricture, often a result of muscular atrophy, leads to regurgitation. Diagnosis is made by roentgenography, esophagoscopy, or gastroscopy. If dilation is unsuccessful, a myotomy at the esophagogastric junction (Heller procedure) is performed to enlarge the opening into the stomach. Severe, unyielding strictures may necessitate stent placement, resection, or esophageal replacement.

Neoplasms of the Esophagus

Most often malignant, neoplasms of the esophagus are treated by resection, photodynamic therapy, or irradiation. Dysphagia or obstruction demands immediate investigation. Surgical procedures fall under the classification of gastrointestinal surgery.

Cervical Esophageal Reconstruction Restoration of continuity of the alimentary tract is a major challenge following ablative surgery of the neck, particularly after cervical esophagectomy or circumferential pharyngectomy. The location of the primary tumor and its extension and the extent of resection are contributing factors in determining the most satisfactory reconstruction. A pectoralis major myocutaneous flap or a free revascularized intestinal autograft will satisfactorily restore continuity in some situations.

Transposition of the mobilized stomach, jejunum, or colon into the neck may be performed when the entire esophagus is resected. Two teams working simultaneously perform this pull-up procedure. The team of general surgeons performs the abdominal dissection to mobilize the stomach or intestine while the other team resects the primary tumor in the neck. The tumor may arise from the hypopharynx, cervical esophagus, or thyroid gland. Radical neck dissection is carried out for extension into the cervical lymph nodes. Anastomosis of the stomach or intestine to an esophageal remnant may be accomplished with a circular intraluminal stapler if the primary esophageal tumor is above the level of the thoracic inlet. Primary pharyngogastric anastomosis may be required for high transection of the pharynx.

Surgical Procedures of the Trachea

Upper respiratory tract obstruction and ventilatory failure may require surgical intervention when the need for intubation or positive pressure ventilation would be long term or of indefinite duration or when severe laryngeal obstruction is present. The obstruction is bypassed or resected.

Tracheotomy/Tracheostomy

Tracheotomy is an incision into the trachea below the larynx. Tracheostomy is the formation of an opening into the trachea into which a tube is inserted through which the patient

breathes. Performed in any age-group to improve or maintain patency of the airway or relieve obstruction, the opening in the trachea provides easy accessibility for suctioning secretions from the tracheobronchial tree or administering anesthesia to patients with facial trauma or burns. A tracheotomy is commonly a controlled prophylactic procedure but can be an acute emergency. An endotracheal tube may provide temporary airway relief before and during the tracheotomy. Indications for tracheotomy include severe trauma to the hypopharynx or larynx, acute laryngotracheal bronchitis or epiglottitis in infants and children, laryngeal edema, prolonged intubation, or any other condition that obstructs respiration.

Tracheotomy is often done with the patient under local anesthesia. The patient is supine with support under the shoulders to hyperextend the neck. A transverse incision is made, producing a better cosmetic result, or a midline vertical incision is made between the cricoid cartilage and the suprasternal notch. The overlying isthmus of the thyroid gland is retracted or divided, and the exposed third and fourth tracheal rings are incised through a midline vertical incision (Figure 40-6). Use of the electrosurgical unit is avoided near the open trachea, because the oxygen-rich environment supports combustion.

After tracheal aspiration to remove blood and secretions, a tracheostomy tube is inserted with the obturator in place. Immediately after insertion of the tube, the obturator is re-

Figure 40-6 Tracheotomy incisions. Midline vertical incision *(a)* is made between cricoid cartilage and suprasternal notch. Transverse incision *(b)* is used for emergency tracheotomy and cricothyrotomy.

moved to open the airway. (This remains with the patient constantly in case of future need.) The outer cannula is suctioned, and the inner cannula is fixed in place. The wound is closed with a few sutures, or the superficial edges of the area above the tube may be sutured and the area below left with natural tissue approximation to facilitate drainage. A smooth-edged dressing split around the tube protects the skin. Commercial tracheostomy dressings are available. Tapes tied to the ends of the outer cannula are secured around the neck. Proper tension allows insertion of one finger between the tape and skin. If the tapes are tied too tightly, they may compress the jugular vein; if the tapes are tied too loosely, the tube can obtrude with coughing. The tube should not be removed during the first 24 to 48 hours by any person unable to perform a tracheotomy because the tract to the trachea may occlude and not be immediately located.

A sterile tube identical to the one inserted and a tracheotomy set accompany the patient from the OR and constantly remain with him or her until otherwise indicated by the surgeon's order.

A tracheotomy is the creation of an open wound. Although rigid asepsis is not possible, every effort is made to keep contamination to a minimum. Only sterile equipment, with minimal handling, is used to prevent infection. Suctioning through a tracheostomy tube is done as a sterile procedure with a sterile catheter and gloves. Careful suctioning prevents trauma. The catheter is inserted without application of suction, which could injure the tracheal walls and suction out oxygen in the patient with borderline oxygen saturation levels. Suction is applied as the catheter is withdrawn. Sterile solution is run through the catheter after use to clean it and maintain patency. Disposable catheters are recommended; they are used once and discarded.

Some patients who have undergone tracheotomy come to the OR for a change of the tube or other procedure. These patients may require suctioning while waiting in the holding area. Knowledge of and preparation for each patient is a prime responsibility of the circulator. These patients require humidified air, which can be delivered by various devices, to keep secretions liquefied and to prevent drying of tissues. Other needs are constant observation and special communication (e.g., pencil and paper, Magic Slate, or picture board).

Tracheostomy Tubes Although an endotracheal tube may provide ventilation for short-term therapy, a tracheostomy tube is easier to suction and immobilize for extended use. It also reduces the possibility of laryngeal injury and tracheomalacia.

Most tubes have three parts—the outer cannula, inner cannula, and obturator (Figure 40-7). The inner cannula is periodically removed and cleaned to prevent blockage by crusting of secretions. It is replaced immediately within the outer cannula so that the latter remains free of crusting. The obturator provides a smooth tip during tube insertion to prevent trauma to the tracheal wall. Some plastic tubes do not require an inner cannula because they remain relatively free of crust. If crusts do form, the tube is changed.

Some tubes have a built-in soft cuff that is inflated to eliminate any free space between the tube and the tracheal wall, thus preventing aspiration of drainage down the trachea. Cuffed tubes also facilitate function of any ventilatory apparatus. A pilot balloon in the inflation line, attached to the outer cannula, indicates cuff inflation or deflation. Proper cuff inflation-deflation is very important. Irritation and pressure of the cuff against the tracheal wall can cause damage such as ulceration and necrosis of the mucosa, which can lead to infection, tracheobronchial fistula, erosion into the innominate artery, or stenosis from scarring. Precautionary measures include deflation at regular intervals, by the physician's written order, to increase blood flow to the cuff site; use of a low-pressure or controlled-pressure cuff; constant monitoring of intracuff pressure; and minimum inflation to ensure a leak-free system. Overinflation can reduce the tube diameter, as well as cause the cuff to extend over the tip of the tube, thus obstructing ventilation. Or the tracheal wall may herniate over the tube end. Underinflation may cause subcutaneous emphysema. Cuffs also should inflate symmetrically. The amount of air needed for inflation varies with the size of the trachea and the tube. Understandably, less air is needed for larger tubes. Usually 2 to 5 ml of air provides a closed system.

Specific tubes have special variations, such as an opening in the wall opposite the bevel to permit ventilation in case of bevel occlusion. Others have a radiopaque tip that allows radiologic visualization of the tube position. Many have connectors, some of which are a built-in swivel type, permitting lightweight, flexible, easy connection to a ventilating system. These connectors reduce the hazard of accidental disconnection. Still others have a fenestration in the outer cannula, permitting air to flow through the larynx. These tubes are used to allow assessment of spontaneous breathing and coughing in preparation for decannulation in patients no longer requiring mechanical ventilation. With air passing through the larynx, the patient can speak with the proximal end of the cannula plugged. A so-called speaking tube permits introduction of

Figure 40-7 Tracheostomy tube. **A,** Outer cuffed cannula. **B,** Inner cannula. **C,** Obturator. **D,** Pilot balloon in inflation line.

humidified air and oxygen through a special line, and with upward flow of the gas through the larynx, the patient can speak.

Tracheal Resection

Tracheal obstruction can result from trauma or a tumor, thus occluding the patient's airway. Localized erosion and scarring, causing narrowing of the trachea, can develop from prolonged endotracheal intubation or a tracheotomy. An obstructive or stenotic lesion can be resected and the trachea reconstructed by end-to-end anastomosis. Through a cervical, low-collar skin incision, the upper trachea and subglottis are mobilized. A right posterolateral thoracotomy incision is used for lesions in the distal trachea near the carina, where the trachea bifurcates into the right and left bronchi. A longitudinal incision is made in the stenotic area, and an anode tube (a flexible wire-reinforced endotracheal tube) is inserted into the distal trachea to maintain respiration. The trachea is transected circumferentially above and below the obstructed segment. The laryngeal attachments to the trachea are released, and the suprahyoid muscle is transected. Up to 5 to 6 cm of trachea can be resected and closed by primary anastomosis. The neck is flexed so that the edges of the trachea can be approximated without tension. The neck may be kept flexed during postoperative healing by a heavy suture from the chin to the chest. The patient remains intubated, with the end of the tube located beyond the anastomosis, as a stent, for 1 or 2 days.

Surgical Procedures of the Anterior Neck

Many laryngologists and plastic surgeons, as well as some oral and general surgeons, perform neck dissection when cervical lymph nodes are involved in cancer of the head and neck. A multidisciplinary team, including a thoracic and/or general surgeon, may perform some complex resections and reconstructive procedures.

The patient may be positioned with the neck extended, usually over a thyroid elevator. The arms are secured at the sides of the body and not on armboards, thus preventing distortion of the body contour in the neck region. The operating bed may be tilted into a reverse Trendelenburg position.

Thyroid Procedures

The thyroid gland, located in the anterior aspect of the neck, is composed of two vascular lobes that lie on either side of the trachea and are united by a narrow band, the isthmus (Figure 40-8). The thyroid hormone controls the rate of body metabolism and may influence physical and mental growth.

Hyperthyroidism (Graves' disease), hypothyroidism, and an enlarged gland (goiter) are the main disorders of the thyroid gland. Drugs, radioactive iodine, and/or surgical resection are used to treat hyperthyroidism. This disease, which is rare in geriatric patients or the very young, affects women more frequently than it does men. Replacement of the thyroid hormone with drug therapy is the specific treatment for

Figure 40-8   Anterior view of thyroid gland.

hypothyroidism. Oral administration of thyroid extract or iodine may reduce the size of the gland, but surgical excision is frequently necessary to remove benign or malignant tumors.

Thyroid Biopsy   A needle biopsy or an excisional biopsy may be performed to aid in establishing a diagnosis of thyroiditis or differentiating between nodular goiter and carcinoma.

Thyroidectomy   During all thyroidectomy procedures, care is exercised not to damage the laryngeal nerves and parathyroid glands. A transverse collar incision is made in a natural skin crease about 1 inch (2 cm) above the clavicle. The cervical fascia is incised vertically in the midline. Throughout the surgical procedure, meticulous hemostasis is maintained. Blood supply arises from the external carotid arteries to the upper poles of the thyroid gland and from the subclavian arteries to the lower poles. The superior laryngeal nerves, which innervate the cricothyroid muscles, and recurrent laryngeal nerves, which innervate the vocal cords, are identified. Trauma to these nerves can result in temporary or permanent laryngeal paralysis. Voice disturbances with hoarseness occur with paralysis of one vocal cord.

Postoperative complications of thyroidectomy include hematoma, edema of the glottis, injury to a recurrent laryngeal nerve, muscle rigidity and spasm (tetany), and acute thyrotoxicosis. A tracheotomy set should remain at the patient's bedside postoperatively for at least 24 hours in the event of respiratory obstruction.

A general surgeon usually performs thyroidectomy. Depending on the pathologic diagnosis, the surgeon chooses the most appropriate procedure for removal of a part of or the entire thyroid gland.

THYROID LOBECTOMY   An entire lobe is removed, especially for toxic diffuse goiter, which is usually benign. In case of malignant growth, the lobe and lymph nodes in the neck that drain into the involved area may be dissected.

SUBTOTAL THYROIDECTOMY The usual procedure for hyperthyroidism is removal of approximately five sixths of the thyroid gland. This procedure generally relieves symptoms permanently because the remaining thyroid tissue secretes sufficient hormone for normal function.

TOTAL THYROIDECTOMY Excision of both lobes plus the isthmus may be the procedure of choice for palpable disease in both lobes.

SUBSTERNAL INTRATHORACIC THYROIDECTOMY Invasion of the gland into substernal and intrathoracic regions can cause tracheal obstruction. The sternum may have to be split to remove a large, adherent intrathoracic goiter.

Parathyroid Gland Procedures

The parathyroid glands are small endocrine glands that regulate metabolism of calcium and phosphorus. Four or more glands are located within or are attached to substance of the thyroid gland (two on each side), or they may migrate into the neck or mediastinum. Primary hyperparathyroidism is associated with hypercalcemia, which may be secondary to renal, skeletal, or gastrointestinal disease. A single or multiple glands may be diseased and surgically excised. The incision and exposure are the same as described for thyroidectomy.

Subtotal Parathyroidectomy

A single diseased gland, confirmed by frozen section, is excised. Up to three and a half glands may be removed if all glands appear to be involved, as in diffuse hyperplastic disease. Parathyroid glands are handled by their pedicles to avoid crushing, suturing, or violating the capsule. Inadvertently implanted parathyroid tissue may cause recurrence of disease or persistent or recurrent hypercalcemia. A remnant of normal tissue is left to prevent hypoparathyroidism, which may cause severe tetany. Removed normal tissue may be cryopreserved for autotransplantation in muscle, usually in the forearm, if hypoparathyroidism develops or reoperation is necessary for recurrent or persistent hyperparathyroidism.

Total Parathyroidectomy with Autotransplantation

All parathyroid tissue is removed when all glands are abnormal. First described by William Halsted in 1907, a portion of a gland is immediately transplanted into a vascularized muscle, usually the sternocleidomastoid, which is in the surgical field. Some surgeons prefer to put the transplant in a forearm muscle. This procedure may be done when embedded parathyroid glands are removed in conjunction with a total thyroidectomy. Postoperative supplemental calcium and vitamin D should be considered for treatment of hypoparathyroidism.

Thyroglossal Duct Cystectomy

During fetal development the thyroid gland descends through the thyroglossal duct from the foramen cecum near the base of the tongue to the neck below the larynx. In adulthood, remnants of this embryonic duct may form a cyst in the anterior midline of the neck. Excision requires removal of the entire cystic sac and a portion of hyoid bone that surrounds the duct.

Cervical and Scalene Lymph Node Biopsy

Biopsy specimens are taken of the cervical and/or scalene nodes for diagnosis of metastatic extension of cancer or tuberculosis into these lymphatic nodes. A thoracic surgeon may perform the procedure.

Neck Dissections

Tumors, benign and malignant, occur in the head and neck regions. Although the origin of many of these neoplasms is technically in the head, the cervical lymph nodes frequently are involved secondarily by metastases from a primary head or neck malignant tumor. Treatment is directed toward definitive management for eradication of the tumor and metastases, with consideration for rehabilitation. In an attempt to eradicate all cancer foci, neck dissection may be performed at a time later than removal of a primary lesion of, for example, the parotid gland or tongue or simultaneously as a one-stage procedure. This composite resection removes the primary tumor and metastatic lesions at the same time en masse. Sometimes metastasis occurs before a primary lesion is discovered.

Various reconstructive techniques provide immediate restoration to improve speech, reestablish oral function, or prevent airway obstruction. Others involve delayed reconstruction. The method of repair depends on the type of defect resulting from excision of the lesion. Preoperatively, the patient's emotional stability is analyzed if the surgical procedure will result in a cosmetic deformity. Reconstruction is planned so that local tissue can be used whenever feasible and normal function is preserved whenever possible. The aim of reconstruction is to restore function and appearance.

Radical Neck Dissection

Malignant tumors of the oral or pharyngeal cavities, cutaneous malignant melanoma, and skin cancer in the head and neck region often require wide resection of the primary lesion and excision of all of the cervical lymph nodes on one or both sides of the neck. This procedure gives the patient with cancer of the cervical lymphatic chain a chance for cure and arrest of spread. When metastasis is known to be present or is highly suspected because of the location or stage of the malignancy, the surgical procedure is predicated on the assumption that metastases are regional and not distant.

The head and neck surgeon plans the surgical procedure with reconstruction in mind, so that the incisions will allow good exposure but provide as much local flap tissue as possible for reconstruction. Incisions used for the tumor resection will necessarily vary according to the type of reconstruction planned. No single surgical procedure can be used to treat all lesions, but certain basic features remain common to all neck dissections.

All lymph-bearing tissue from the midline anteriorly to the trapezius muscle posteriorly and from the mandible superiorly to the clavicle inferiorly is removed. All tissue between the deep cervical fascia and the platysma muscle externally is removed except the carotid artery system; the vagus, phrenic, and hypoglossal nerves; and the brachial plexus.

The massive tissue resection (removal en bloc) includes the jugular vein, eleventh cranial (spinal accessory) nerve, sternocleidomastoid muscle, and submandibular salivary gland. Elimination of the motor nerve to the trapezius muscle contributes to muscular atrophy, subsequent shoulder drop on the affected side, and possibly decreased strength in raising the arm.

Various techniques are used to close the large defect in the anterior neck. When the occipital, posterior auricular, facial, and superior thyroid arteries can be preserved, arterialized skin flaps designed to incorporate branches from these vessels can be constructed with the length up to three or four times the width. Otherwise, the length of a flap should not exceed twice the width. A deltopectoral pedicle flap or a pectoralis major myocutaneous free flap may be needed (Figure 40-9). An exposed carotid artery is covered. Cervical flaps carrying their own blood supply may be used for this and to restore the oropharyngeal lining intraorally. A pedicle flap of sternocleidomastoid muscle from the clavicle may be an alternative.

The mandible is preserved unless it is involved by direct extension of the tumor into the bone. Access through a mandibular osteotomy or partial mandibulectomy is usually required for effective resection in the posterior oral cavity. Solid bony continuity and realignment of the dental arches are established for functional restoration of speech and chewing. A revascularized free fibular graft, a bone graft from the rib or iliac crest, cancellous bone chips, or a composite graft may be used to stabilize the mandible.

Effective drainage of the wound is important to healing. This is accomplished by use of closed wound suction drains inserted through stab wounds below the clavicle. Prevention of hematoma protects the viability of the thin skin flaps and facilitates approximation of wound surfaces.

A tracheotomy may be performed to protect the patient from respiratory distress in neck dissection alone. A tracheostomy is always done in a composite radical neck resection.

A feeding gastrostomy tube may be inserted for anticipated extended feeding. This permits suction to avoid aspiration and gastric distention in addition to providing a feeding route. The tube is usually inserted in the OR.

Potential complications of neck dissection are numerous, depending on the tumor itself, irradiation therapy, or necessary sacrifice of vital structures. Intraoperatively hemorrhage may occur from injury to a major vessel or the thoracic duct. Postoperatively invasion of overlying skin necrosis into a major vessel wall, such as the carotid artery, can cause an often fatal blowout of the vessel. Slight previous bleeding may be a forewarning. Balloon occlusion of the carotid artery may be used to prevent hemorrhage.

Although reconstruction begins at the time of primary neck dissection, the patient usually requires considerable postoperative rehabilitation psychologically and staged procedures before cosmetic and functional reconstruction is complete.

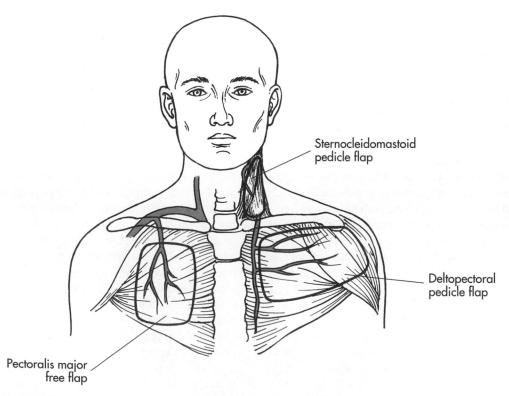

Figure 40-9 Myocutaneous flap to close defect following radical neck dissection may be deltopectoral pedicle flap, pectoralis major free flap, or sternocleidomastoid pedicle flap.

FACE

Anatomy and Physiology of the Face

The face is the anterior part of the head, including the forehead, cheeks, nose, lips, and chin, but not the ears. The eyes, situated in the bony orbits, contribute to the features of the face, although they are not technically a part of the face.

The skeletal structure of the face (Figure 40-10) includes the frontal bone of the forehead. It forms the upper part of the orbits. Divided by sutures (i.e., lines of union between bones), the frontal bone joins the sphenoid and ethmoid, and the paired nasal, lacrimal, maxilla, and zygomatic bones. The posterior orbits are formed by the sphenoid bone, which is shaped like a butterfly with extended wings, and the palatal bones. The medial walls are formed by the ethmoid, lacrimal, and nasal bones and maxilla. The lateral aspect is formed by the zygoma (malar bone), or the cheekbone. The irregularly shaped ethmoid bone also forms the roof and posterior lateral wall of each nasal cavity. The nasal bones form the bridge of the nose between the orbits.

The maxilla (the upper jaw that holds the palate) extends laterally to the zygoma and temporal bone, under the orbit, and along the anterior nasal cavity. The maxillary bones are paired and join in the midline between the nose and the oral cavity. The alveoli that hold the teeth are along the alveolar processes of the maxillae.

The ramus of the mandible (the arch-shaped bone of the lower jaw) articulates with temporal bones at the temporomandibular joints in front of the ears. The alveoli, the tooth-bearing bodies, meet at the alveolar process to form the chin (mental region).

The bony structure of the face is covered with muscles, superficial blood vessels and nerves, epidermis, and dermis. Other structures (i.e., ducts and sinuses [air spaces]) are also in the soft tissues or bony structure of the face.

Craniofacial Procedures

The term *craniofacial* refers to the cranium and face. Craniofacial surgery of increasing complexity has been performed since World War II. The approach developed by Paul Tessier has led to previously inaccessible anatomic areas. Exposure for dissection of soft tissues and bone to restore contour and symmetry in practically every type of facial deformity, whether congenital, neoplastic, or traumatic in origin, can be accomplished by a multidisciplinary team of surgeons. This team may include a plastic surgeon, neurosurgeon, anesthesia provider, ophthalmologist, oral surgeon, and otorhinolaryngologist. Some procedures require more than 100 separate maneuvers and may take as long as 14 to 16 hours to complete.

Many of the concepts developed for these very complex procedures are applied in the more common and less complicated procedures to reshape sections of the skull or reconstruct soft tissues. Craniofacial reconstruction should be performed as soon as indicated by the physiologic and psychologic impacts of the deformity on the patient, regardless of age. An early surgical procedure not only decreases psychologic trauma but also may prevent craniofacial distortion caused by brain and nerve damage of a disease process or traumatic injury.

Analysis of three-dimensional CT scans and cephalometric tracings accurately superimposed on transparent photographs

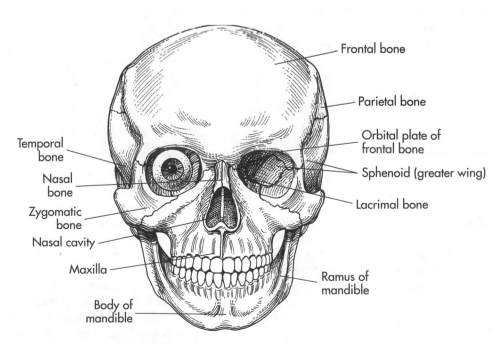

Figure 40-10 Anterior view of skull.

of the patient preoperatively are essential to determine the extent of the facial deformity and the plan for skeletal re-arrangement. The exact size of the defects that will need bone grafts can be determined.

Many procedures involve correction of malocclusion of the mandible at the same time that the orbitocranial skeleton is restructured. Dental models are cut and mounted on an articulator for reference.

Hypotensive anesthesia reduces blood loss during these extensive procedures. The patient is continuously monitored throughout the procedure to estimate blood loss. A preoperative tracheotomy may be necessary to maintain an adequate airway postoperatively.

Midface Advancement

The base of the anterior cranial fossae can be exposed through a bifrontal incision to elevate a frontal bone flap. While the neurosurgeon is raising the flap, the plastic surgeon may take donor bone from a rib and/or the iliac crest if autogenous bone grafts will be needed. Harvesting of bone from the calvarium (the upper, domelike portion of the skull) may be preferred.

The facial skeleton is separated from the cranial base. The plastic surgeon raises the periorbita, orbital contents, and soft tissue over the dorsum of the nose. The subperiosteum of the anterior maxillae is elevated. Osteotomies are cut in the supraorbital region to mobilize the lateral walls. An anterior maxillary osteotomy, through an infraorbital approach, extends across and below the frontal processes of the maxillae. Osteotomies of the anterior cranial fossae and the medial and lateral orbital walls and floors are completed. The mobilized bones can be functionally advanced in three dimensions as desired. They are then stabilized with a plating system or wired into position. To maintain stability, bone grafts also are wired into place in the resulting defects. Demineralized bone blocks, chips, or powder often are preferred to bone grafts to induce osteogenesis. The frontal bone flap is replaced, and the incision is closed.

Mandibular osteotomies may be done before closure to correct alignment of the jaws. Whether this is necessary or not, the mandible is stabilized after closure with intermaxillary wires and suspension wires to the zygomatic arch.

Depending on the deformity, variations of the intracranial and extracranial osteotomies are done to advance, align, or reposition the facial bones and reconstruct soft tissues. Many patients return to the OR for additional corrective procedures: eyelid ptosis and/or extraocular muscle surgery performed by the ophthalmologist; dacryocystorhinostomy and/or nasal reconstruction performed by the rhinologist; and bone augmentation or resection of the maxillae and/or mandible for repositioning by the plastic surgeon or oral surgeon. During all procedures the surgeons avoid injury to optic and facial nerves and to arteries and veins.

Procedures of the Orbit

An abnormally wide space between (hypertelorism) or malposition of (dystopia) the bony orbits is usually secondary to other craniofacial malformations. The medial orbital walls by themselves may be moved to correct minimal hypertelorism. Advancement of the superior and lateral walls, rather than total orbit advancement, may suffice to correct a dystopia. A combined intracranial and extracranial approach may be necessary to change the angle of the orbits and reposition the medial canthal ligaments of the eyes.

Resection of Nasal or Paranasal Sinus Tumors

Radical craniofacial resection may be indicated to remove gigantic benign nasal dermoid tumors and malignant tumors of the paranasal sinuses. In a one-stage procedure, all involved soft tissue is excised with simultaneous correction of the underlying skeletal structure.

Basal cell carcinoma is a common type of nasal tumor. The surgical procedure may be performed alone or as combined therapy. Immediate repair by skin graft or pedicle flap accompanies excision of well-defined lesions. Reconstruction is postponed in multicentric (many-centered) cancer or if there is doubt regarding extension of the tumor. More advanced lesions require replacement of the nose by a prosthesis or a tissue flap.

Erosion of a growth in one of the sinuses into an adjacent nasal wall can occlude the air passage. Resection may include partial or total maxillectomy and removal of surrounding tissues. The cavity usually is covered by a skin graft. Unilateral enucleation of the eye may be necessary. A radical surgical procedure for an ethmoid tumor also may involve removal of part of the base of the skull and excision of the maxillary antrum and the palate on the affected side.

In providing maxillofacial prostheses to replace facial structures following various procedures, the prosthodontist works closely with the surgeon and radiation therapist. Splints or stents hold tissue grafts in place, seal cavities from each other, or unite bony segments. A dental prosthesis to close the defect in the upper jaw and an eye prosthesis following enucleation contributes to the patient's rehabilitation following an extensive surgical procedure.

Resection of Craniofacial Tumors and Dysplasia

Malignant tumors can originate from soft tissues of the face and scalp, the oropharyngeal mucosa, the ear canal, or the lacrimal gland. They can invade the base of the skull. Fibrous dysplasia, a congenital metabolic disturbance that causes an abnormal proliferation of fibrous tissue, can result in asymmetric distortion and expansion of craniofacial bones. These conditions can collapse the paranasal sinuses; compress the optic nerve or chiasm, causing loss of vision; and cause other functional disabilities. An acute epistaxis (nosebleed) can be life threatening. A combined intracranial and extracranial approach may be used to completely remove the tumor or dysplastic bone. The remaining bony structures may be reshaped or repositioned. Bone grafts and/or prosthetic implants may be used for reconstruction of the forehead, orbits, nose, maxilla, and/or mandible.

Midfacial Fractures

The facial bones provide a shield for the brain. They also protect the senses of sight, smell, hearing, and taste. Although midfacial fractures and soft tissue injuries are seldom fatal, inadequate treatment can result in disfigurement and sensory impairment. For example, virtually all blindness secondary to trauma is permanent.

Facial fractures should be suspected when the patient complains of pain, malocclusion of the jaws, or diplopia (double vision). Swelling and asymmetry of the face may be obvious. Diagnosis is confirmed by x-ray film or a CT scan to identify the bone(s) involved. The LeFort classification of fractures, which is useful in determining the appropriate method of reduction and stabilization (Figure 40-11), is as follows:

1. LeFort I fracture is a transverse fracture of the maxilla, fragmenting the upper alveoli and palate.
2. LeFort II fracture is a pyramidal fracture of the frontal processes of the maxillae, the nasal bones, and the orbital floor. The maxillae are freely movable.
3. LeFort III fracture includes zygomas, maxillae, and nasal bones and the ethmoid, sphenoid, and other orbital bones. This creates a craniofacial dysjunction (separation).

Facial fractures are reduced, stabilized, and immobilized. Priorities of initial treatment following injury concern airway obstruction, possible cervical spine injury, and hemorrhage. Treatment of the fracture may be delayed. The surgeon follows the principles of approaching fractures from "inside out, downward up." This means that bony structures are repaired first, then the soft tissues; the mandible or most distal fracture is reduced first before working upward toward the cranium.

The method of bony repair is determined by the complexity of the fracture(s). Intermaxillary fixation combined with interdental wiring, external pin fixation, or rigid internal fixation effect stabilization. Minifacial and midfacial plates, microplates, and mandibular plates may be combined with arch bars or bone grafts.

Reduction of Orbital Fractures   If orbital contents are depressed into the maxillary sinus, surgical exploration through an orbital or a transspinal approach is indicated. The extent of the trauma should indicate the most appropriate surgical management. The injury may involve the rim or the floor of the orbit, or both:

1. Fractures of the orbital rim, frequently associated with fractures of the zygoma, are usually detected by the resulting deformity. The fracture is reduced by appropriate means. Fragments are wired into place as necessary.
2. A blowout fracture of the orbit may result from a direct blow to the eyeball, which is, in turn, transmitted to the very thin floor of the orbit. A typical fracture is in the medial third of the floor with dislocation of floor fragments into the maxillary sinus. The fracture occasionally may extend into the ethmoid plate. Consequently, orbital contents, which may include the inferior extraocular muscles, are usually herniated into the antrum. This produces limitation of upward gaze and some degree of enophthalmos (recession of the eyeball into the orbit). The herniated orbital contents are reduced from the antrum back into the orbit with special attention to freeing the entrapped muscles. Plastic or silicone sheeting may be used to close the defect in the floor. Or the fragments may be elevated by packing the antrum through a Caldwell-Luc (sinus) approach. The diagnosis may be overlooked unless a laminogram is taken.

Reduction of Nasal Fractures   Fracture of the nasal bones and septum often accompanies other trauma to the head, such as a blowout fracture of the orbit (see above). If the zygoma or maxilla is involved, reduction may be accomplished through a small incision anterior to the ear and superior to the zygomatic arch. Periosteal elevators are used to raise depressed bone and cartilage fragments. Nasal fractures are splinted with nasal packs and an external splint.

Reduction of Zygomatic Fractures   Dislocations of the zygoma are more common than fractures of the cheekbone (malar bone). Zygomatic fractures always involve the orbital bones. Those of the zygomatic arch are particularly unstable and require intraosseous or transosseous wire fixation following internal reduction with counterpressure from underneath the arch. Transantral Steinmann pinning may be necessary to maintain reduction of fragments in severely fragmented fractures.

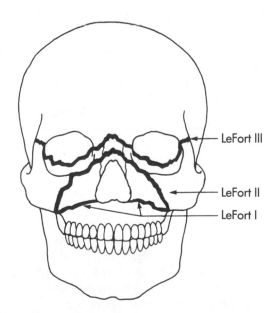

Figure 40-11   LeFort facial fractures. (From Neff JA, Kidd PS: *Trauma nursing: the art and science,* St Louis, 1993, Mosby.)

Maxillofacial and Mandibular Procedures

The term *maxillofacial* pertains to the part of face formed by the upper and lower jaws. Most maxillofacial procedures are designed to reconstruct defects in the lips, buccal sulcus, maxilla, alveolar ridge, floor of the mouth, mandible, and/or chin. These defects may be a result of trauma or resection of tumor. Whenever feasible, intraoral incisions are used to minimize facial scarring.

Intermaxillary Fixation of Fractures

Following closed or open reduction, fractures of the maxilla and mandible are usually immobilized by interdental wiring if the patient has upper and lower teeth. If the patient is edentulous (without teeth), open reduction and skeletal fixation by circumferential wiring over an intraoral splint or screws and connecting bars may be necessary.

Erich arch bars are shaped along the dental arches. Wires are passed between the teeth to anchor the splints on the upper and lower jaws. Each splint contains a series of small lugs. Tiny rubber bands, placed around opposing lugs, hold the teeth in occlusion. Splints frequently are not used for fixation of these fractures. The teeth may be held in occlusion by wires passed around opposing teeth. Following fixation of the mandible or maxilla, wire cutters accompany the patient from the OR and remain at the bedside as long as wires or rubber bands are in place. If the patient experiences respiratory difficulty or vomiting, the wires may have to be cut to prevent aspiration. Fluids may be difficult to swallow.

If microplates can be used for rigid fixation, the interdental wiring may be released after the fixation procedure is completed.

Mandibular Fractures

Some fractures of the mandible can be immobilized by transoral placement of noncompression miniplates. This technique obviates the necessity for interdental wiring. Vitallium, titanium, or stainless steel plates and screws are used for rigid fixation.

Mandibular Reconstruction

Skeletal defects creating loss of mandibular continuity are usually a result of trauma or benign disease. Bone replacement is the most common method of restoring function and contour. The patient's own ilium provides cancellous bone that can be shaped into the configuration of the jaw. A composite graft of a freeze-dried cadaver mandible packed with autogenous cancellous bone chips also can be used. These grafts fill a bony defect but do not provide soft tissue coverage. A vascularized iliac graft is preferable to reconstruct the mandible and a large intraoral defect.

Temporomandibular Joint Syndrome

Persistent pain and dysfunction of the temporomandibular joint (TMJ) can be associated with stress-related bruxism (tensing muscles and grinding teeth), the position of teeth, malocclusion, trauma, arthritis, and other degenerative changes in one or both joints. If TMJ syndrome is unresponsive to conservative treatment, surgical intervention may be indicated.

ARTHROSCOPY Arthroscopy, usually performed bilaterally, is used to diagnose problems such as scarring or adhesions that do not show up on a CT or magnetic resonance imaging (MRI) scan. Lysis of adhesions, mechanical debridement, and lavage of the TMJ may relieve symptoms. Repositioning or release of the fibrocartilaginous articular disc (meniscus) between the mandibular condyle and the glenoid fossa of the temporal bone may restore function. A 1.7- or 1.9-mm arthroscope with a fiberoptic camera attached is locked into a cannula sheath inserted through an inferolateral puncture wound into the joint capsule. Continuous inflow and outflow of fluid, usually iced Ringer's lactate solution, is necessary to keep the joint distended for visibility and lavage. Therapeutic synovectomy and partial or complete meniscectomy may recontour the joint. A rotary shaver and/or the Ho:YAG laser may be used. The laser rapidly resects and vaporizes cartilaginous tissue and coagulates bleeding vessels.

ARTHROPLASTY Open, direct visualization of the disc and condyle may be necessary to correct abnormal relationships. Either a preauricular or postauricular incision may be used to approach the TMJ. The condyle, fossa, and/or articular eminence may be reshaped or resurfaced. A damaged or displaced articular disc can be recontoured and repositioned. It is recontoured with a scalpel or by electrosurgical cutting and then repositioned and sutured in place. If the disc is torn or perforated, it is usually removed. A silicone elastomer implant or titanium alloy prosthesis may be used to reconstruct the joint. The jaw may be immobilized with interdental wiring to stabilize the TMJ during healing.

Orthognathic Surgery

The jaws can be reshaped or repositioned to correct functional bite disorders and/or for aesthetics. Occlusion (closure of teeth) depends on the anteroposterior relationship of the upper and lower jaws. The term *orthognathia,* derived from the Greek words *orthos* (ορθος), meaning *straight,* and *gnathos* (γναθος), meaning *jaw,* relates to treatment of conditions involving malposition of the maxilla or mandible, or both. Malocclusion occurs when teeth do not close together properly. It can cause difficulty in chewing and/or speaking, periodontal disease, and/or temporomandibular joint dysfunction. Psychologically debilitating facial deformity and bite disorders of genetic origin or as a result of growth disturbances or trauma include the following:

- *Prognathism.* One or both jaws project forward beyond the normal relationship with the cranial base. If the mandible (lower jaw) protrudes beyond the maxilla (upper jaw), it creates a prominence of chin, concave profile, and underbite. If the maxilla grows beyond the mandible, it creates an overbite.
- *Retrognathism.* One or both jaws are positioned posterior to the normal craniofacial relationship (i.e., behind the frontal plane of the forehead). In reference to the mandible, the condition is commonly known as a receding chin; this may create an overbite.
- *Apertognathia.* The front teeth do not close because the back teeth come together first, creating an open bite.

- *Micrognathia.* The dental arch, usually of the mandible, is too small to accommodate the teeth. Teeth are pushed out of alignment because they are crowded together.
- *Asymmetry.* A discrepancy in size, shape, or position of the jaws creates an imbalance between the right and left sides of the face.

Preoperative orthodontia may be required to align and level the teeth. The ultimate goal is to achieve functional stability of dentofacial structures with acceptable facial aesthetics. Surgical correction may include extraction of one or more teeth, maxillary and/or mandibular osteotomies with repositioning of bone segments, and/or repositioning of alveoli. Intraorally, bilateral maxillary osteotomies may be performed in conjunction with mandibular osteotomies, or either of these procedures can be done independently to change the shape of the facial contour.

LeFort Osteotomy For maxillary deformities, an incision is made in the mucosa of the upper lip. Osteotomies (i.e., bone cuts) are made in the medial and lateral maxillary sinus walls. The vomer is cut just above the floor of the nose. Pterygoid plates are sectioned from the maxilla. The maxilla is movable for reduction, augmentation, or repositioning. The maxilla can be detached from the base of the skull, maintaining vascular supply via the soft palate, and cut into segments to reconstruct the lower face as described for midface advancement. Usually miniplates anchored with screws bridge the osteotomy cuts.

Mandibular Osteotomy Sagittal split osteotomies through the ramus and vertical osteotomies through the molar region on each side allow backward or forward repositioning of the mandible. If moved posteriorly, bone on the anterior aspect is trimmed for good medullary bone contact. Rigid fixation may be obtained with miniplates or with screws placed percutaneously through stab wounds. The latter are stabilized with an external fixator. If plates and screws are used, intermaxillary fixation as described for fractures may not be necessary.

Postoperative orthodontia may be required to complete closure of spaces around the osteotomies and thus stabilize occlusal function.

Mandibulectomy Partial or total removal of the lower jaw is performed for extension of a tumor into the bone of the floor of the mouth. It may be performed with glossectomy and radical neck dissection for wide excision. Mandibular replacement combines bone graft and synthetic materials for restoration of speech and appearance. A compound osseocutaneous flap from the iliac crest, with microvascular anastomosis of the deep circumflex iliac artery vascular pedicle, may be transferred for reconstruction. If the patient is dentulous, the relationship of opposing teeth is maintained; if edentulous, the patient wears a denture. Whenever possible, mandible-sparing procedures are done for carcinoma of the tongue.

Bibliography

Bruno BJ, Gustafson PA: Cranial bone harvest, grafting: a choice for maxillofacial reconstruction, *AORN J* 59(1):242-251, 1994.

Colman JJ: Osseous reconstruction of the midface and orbits, *Clin Plast Surg* 21(1):113-124, 1994.

Fina DK: Is it only a tonsillectomy? *AORN J* 66(6):1073-1075, 1997.

Guyuron B, Friedman A: The role of preserved autogenous cartilage grafts in septorhinoplasty, *Ann Plast Surg* 32(3):255-260, 1994.

Haskins DR: Pediatric dental rehabilitation procedures in the OR, *AORN J* 64(4):573-579, 1996.

Hayes KM, Combs NL: Perioperative nursing care of patients with craniofacial injuries, *AORN J* 64(3):385-406, 1996.

Jones CE, Wellisz T: External ear reconstruction, *AORN J* 59(2):411-422, 1994.

Krouse HJ et al: Powered functional endoscopic sinus surgery, *AORN J* 66(3):405-414, 1997.

Loftus BC et al: Epistaxis, medical history, and the nasopulmonary reflex: what is clinically relevant? *Otolaryngology* 110(4):363-369, 1994.

McEwen DR, Sanchez MM: Complications associated with excision of a submandibular salivary gland tumor, *AORN J* 64(1):109-111, 1996.

McEwen DR, Sanchez MM: A guide to salivary gland disorders, *AORN J* 65(3):554-567, 1997.

McEwen DR et al: Dental restorations using titanium osseointegrated dental implants, *AORN J* 62(2):189-205, 1995.

McHenry A, Piotrowski JJ: Thyroidectomy in patients with marked thyroid enlargement: airway management, morbidity, and outcome, *Am Surg* 60(8):586-591, 1994.

Miller MA, Saltvoll B: Absorbable gelatin powder injection for transient vocal cord paralysis, *AORN J* 61(5):821-826, 1995.

Moore S, Haughey BH: Surgical treatment for thyroid cancer, *AORN J* 65(4):710-725, 1997.

Petroff PF: Computer-assisted endoscopic sinus surgery, *AORN J* 66(3):416-425, 1997.

Sanders RA et al: Dental surgery standards for perioperative nurses, *AORN J* 62(2):227-233, 1995.

Steur K: Pediatric fibromatosis requiring mandibular resection and reconstruction, *AORN J* 62(2):212-226, 1995.

Stinson A: Cochlear implantations in children, *AORN J* 64(4):561-571, 1996.

Stone CD, Heitmiller RF: Simplified, standardized technique for cervical esophagogastric anastomosis, *Ann Thorac Surg* 58(1):259-261, 1994.

Truelson JM, Pearce AN: Tongue reconstruction procedures for treatment of cancer, *AORN J* 65(3):528-551, 1997.

Waddington C et al: Treatment of conductive hearing loss with ossicular chain reconstruction procedures, *AORN J* 65(3):511-525, 1997.

Weilitz PB, Dettenmeier PA: Back to basics: test your knowledge of tracheostomy tubes, *Am J Nurs* 94(2):46-50, 1994.

Yantis MA: Decreasing surgical risks for patient with obstructive sleep apnea, *AORN J* 68(1):50-55, 1998.

Chapter 41

Neurosurgery

Chapter Objectives

After studying this chapter, the learner will be able to:

- Identify the pertinent anatomy of the brain and spinal cord.
- Describe the significance of neurologic monitoring.
- Discuss the risks associated with neurosurgery.

Neurosurgeons specialize in procedures associated with dysfunction, disease, or injury of the nervous system. The nervous system includes the brain and spinal cord, also known as the neuraxis (central nervous system [CNS]) and the cranial, spinal, and autonomic peripheral nerves (peripheral nervous system [PNS]). Neural tissues control motor and sensory functions throughout the body. Generalized cerebral function is manifested in overall behavior, level of consciousness, orientation, and intellectual performance. These functions may be altered by a metabolic disorder, a chromosomal defect, a disease process, or a traumatic injury. Assessment of neurologic deficits or changes in functional activity establishes the indications for neurosurgical intervention. The scope of neurosurgery is broad and includes removal of pathologic lesions; relief of pain, spasm, or other neurophysiologic conditions; and repair of nerve injuries and tissue defects.

HISTORICAL BACKGROUND

Prehistoric skulls have been discovered that have evidence of successful craniotomy. Studies of trephined skulls have shown that new bony tissue regenerated around the skull perforation, demonstrating that the early patients frequently survived the procedure. Hippocrates (460-379 BC) described the use of a trephine to treat headache and postulated that the brain was the seat of intelligence. Herophilus (335-280 BC) described the ventricles of the brain. He believed that they were the seat of intelligence.

Early anatomists and physicians, such as Egyptian physician Marinus (first century AD), who identified cranial nerve X, began to realize that nerve pathways in the periphery led to the brain and cord. During his lifetime seven pairs of cranial nerves were identified. English anatomist Thomas Willis (1621-1675) identified cranial nerve V and the communication of the cerebral vasculature known as the Circle of Willis. By the eighteenth century the remainder of the 12 pairs of cranial nerves had been identified by German anatomist Samuel Soemmering (1755-1830).

Cranial surgery progressed slowly and until the early 1880s was limited to palliative treatment of hematoma or infection. English surgeon Sir Rickman Goodlee is credited with the first surgical procedure for removal of a brain tumor in 1884. American surgeon William Keen (1837-1932) is credited with the first intracranial meningioma excision in the United States in 1888. He devised linear craniotomy, referred to as Keen's operation.

The recognized father of modern neurosurgery is Harvey W. Cushing (1869-1939). Among his many accomplishments,

809

Cushing described the relationship of intracranial pressure (ICP) to blood pressure in 1900, and in 1932 he described pituitary basophilism, commonly known as Cushing's disease. At Harvard he established the first school of neurosurgery, which led to the development of a discipline recognized throughout the world.

Application of increasing knowledge of neurophysiology and advances in diagnostic methods, such as those of American surgeon Walter E. Dandy (1886-1946), who performed ventriculography in 1918, and Portuguese neurologist Antonio Egas Moniz (1874-1955), who perfected cerebral arteriography, led to the success of intracranial and intraspinal procedures.

English anatomist Sir Charles Sherrington (1857-1952) was a pioneer in the study of the physiology of the spinal cord. He originated the term *synapse* to denote the gaps between nerve fibers, identified the stretch receptors, and demonstrated that the cerebellum is responsible for proprioception and balance.

English surgeon Sir Victor Horsley (1857-1916) developed a stereotropic brain stimulus–lesion locator in 1908. Stereotaxis led to the development of less destructive techniques to replace some extensive invasive procedures and to treatment of some otherwise inoperable lesions.

The sophistication of physiologic monitoring techniques was enhanced by the development of the electroencephalogram in 1924 by German neurologist Hans Berger (1873-1941). Further developments in monitoring included evoked potentials in 1933 by Ralph Gerard.

The use of lasers has further enhanced neurosurgery. The operating microscope opened up a new field of microneurosurgery that has created interest in cerebral revascularization techniques previously unattempted and offers advantages in surgical management of many other pathologic lesions. The sophistication of physiologic monitoring techniques has facilitated these therapeutic modalities.

ANATOMY AND PHYSIOLOGY OF THE BRAIN AND SPINAL CORD

An understanding of basic anatomy and physiology is essential for preparing for the approach used to reach intracranial and spinal cord structures.

Cranium

The brain is enclosed within the bony vault of the cranium. Eight bones form the cranium: the single frontal, sphenoid, and ethmoid bones anteriorly; the paired temporal and parietal bones forming the middle fossa; and the occipital bone posteriorly. Although these bones are fused together by nonmobile joints referred to as sutures, the cranium is described as being divided into three areas: the anterior, middle, and posterior fossae. Galea (tough fascia-like tissue over the cranium) connects muscles of the temples, forehead, and base of the skull. The scalp (skin) covers the muscles and extracranial vessels and nerves in subcutaneous tissue.

Meninges

The membranous covering of the CNS, referred to as meninges, lines the cranium and covers the brain. The three distinct layers are the dura mater (in direct contact with the cranium), arachnoid (a weblike space), and pia mater (in direct contact with the surface of the brain). Cranial dura mater, firmly attached to the inner aspect of the cranium, has two layers that separate in planes to form venous sinuses. The arachnoid, which lies under the dura mater, has weblike connections with the pia mater, which closely adheres to the gray matter of the brain. Cerebrospinal fluid (CSF) circulates through the arachnoid layer to bathe the brain. The pia mater follows the convolutions of the surface of the brain.

The dura is arranged in three large folds: the falx cerebri, which covers the hemispheres; the falx cerebelli, which separates the lobes of the cerebellum; and the tentorium cerebelli, which supports the temporal and occipital lobes. The tentorium is a surgical landmark denoting supratentorial structures and infratentorial structures, such as the brainstem and cerebellum.

Brain

The brain is divided into five main subdivisions composed of gray matter (neurons, cell bodies) and white matter (axons, dendrites, nerve fibers). The brain has three distinct anatomic units that consist of several subdivisions, as shown in Figure 41-1. The cranial nerves (Table 41-1) originate from several locations in the brain and its subdivisions (Figure 41-2).

The blood supply to the brain is derived from the carotid and vertebral arteries. The arterial component collectively joins at the circle of Willis (Figure 41-3).

Cerebrum

The right and left hemispheres of the cerebrum are connected centrally by the corpus callosum, a broad band of nerve fibers. The cerebrum, also known as the telencephalon, occupies most of the area within the cranium and is arranged into superficial folds (called gyri) and furrows (called sulci), which are surgical anatomic landmarks. The outer cerebral cortex is the gray matter; the inner tissue is the white matter. Cranial nerve I originates here. Each hemisphere of the brain is divided into four anatomic lobes:

1. The frontal lobe lies within the anterior fossa.
2. The parietal lobe lies in the superior and anterior portion of the middle fossa.

Figure 41-1   Left lateral view of cerebral hemisphere.

TABLE 41-1	Cranial Nerves

Number	Name	Origin	Action
I	Olfactory	Telencephalon	Smell
II	Optic	Diencephalon	Vision
III	Oculomotor	Mesencephalon	Somatic motor for eyeballs, iris, and ciliary body
IV	Trochlear	Mesencephalon	Somatic motor for eyeballs
V	Trigeminal	Metencephalon	Motor and sensory
VI	Abducens	Myelencephalon	Somatic motor
VII	Facial	Myelencephalon	Motor and sensory
VIII	Vestibulocochlear	Myelencephalon	Hearing and balance
IX	Glossopharyngeal	Myelencephalon	Visceral motor and sensory, general sensory
X	Vagus	Myelencephalon	Visceral motor and sensory, general sensory
XI	Spinal accessory	Myelencephalon	Visceral motor
XII	Hypoglossal	Myelencephalon	Somatic motor

3. The temporal lobe lies inferior to the frontal and parietal lobes within the middle fossa.
4. The occipital lobe lies posteriorly within the middle fossa.

The hypothalamus and thalamus, referred to as the diencephalon, also lie within the cerebrum to form the floor and lateral walls of the third ventricle. All afferent impulses except smell pass through here to the cerebrum. The optic chiasma forms the anterior border. The diencephalon controls body temperature, emotion, hunger, thirst, sleep, and some hormones. Although it lies in the sella turcica outside the cerebrum, the pituitary body attaches to the inferior aspect of the hypothalamus.

The cerebral pedicles and the corpora quadrigemina form the midbrain, which is also referred to as the mesencephalon. The cerebral aqueduct runs through the full length of the structure. Cranial nerves III and IV originate here.

Brainstem

The brainstem lies anteriorly within the posterior fossa. It extends from the cerebral hemisphere to the base of the skull, where it merges with the spinal cord.

Pons and Cerebellum

The pons and cerebellum form the metencephalon. The pons is a bridge between the cerebrum and the medulla. It

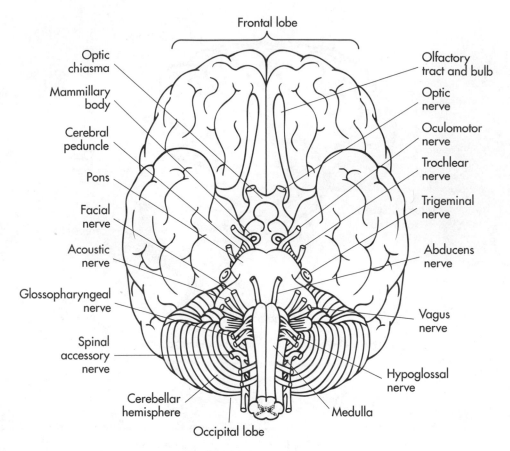

Figure 41-2   Cranial nerves.

lies anterior to the bilobed cerebellum and is the origin of cranial nerves V, VI, VII, and VIII. The cerebellum lies below the occipital lobes of the cerebrum, posterior to the brainstem, within the posterior fossa. It is about one fifth the size of the cerebrum. The cerebellum controls motion and equilibrium.

Medulla

The medulla oblongata forms the floor of the fourth ventricle and contains the origin of cranial nerves IX, X, XI, and XII. It contains the vital centers, such as cardiac, vasomotor, and respiratory function.

Ventricles

Four spaces within the brain are referred to as ventricles (Figure 41-4). The lateral ventricles, one lying in each hemisphere of the cerebrum, drain into the foramen of Monroe. It opens into a central cavity, the third ventricle, which is connected by the aqueduct of Sylvius with the fourth ventricle lying anterior to the cerebellum and posterior to the brainstem. CSF is a clear substance produced in the choroid plexuses, which are vascular extensions of the pia mater lining the ventricles. CSF is predominantly produced in the lateral ventricles and circulates through the subarachnoid space around the meninges covering the brain and spinal cord. The normal adult volume of circulating CSF is 125 to 150 ml. Obstruction of the CSF flow causes increased ICP.

Vertebral Column and Spinal Cord

The bony structure of the vertebral column extends from the foramen magnum at the base of the skull to the coccyx. The 33 vertebrae, which provide support for the body, vary in size and are classified according to location: the 7 cervical vertebrae are in the neck; the 12 thoracic vertebrae articulate posteriorly with the ribs; the 5 lumbar vertebrae are posterior to the retroperitoneal cavity; the 5 sacral vertebrae are fused to form the sacrum; and the 4 fused coccygeal vertebrae form the coccyx. The vertebral column measures about 28 inches (71 cm) in the average-sized adult.

Disc

An intervertebral disc is held between each cervical, thoracic, and lumbar vertebral body by the annulus fibrosus and posterior longitudinal ligament. The disc itself, a fibrocartilaginous substance known as nucleus pulposus, acts as a shock absorber or cushion between the vertebrae.

Anterior
cerebral
artery

Middle
cerebral
artery

Posterior
communicating
artery

Posterior
cerebral
artery

Vertebral
artery

Anterior
spinal
artery

Anterior
communicating
artery

Internal
carotid
artery

Superior
cerebellar
artery

Basilar
artery

Anterior
inferior
cerebellar
artery

Posterior
inferior
cerebellar
artery

A

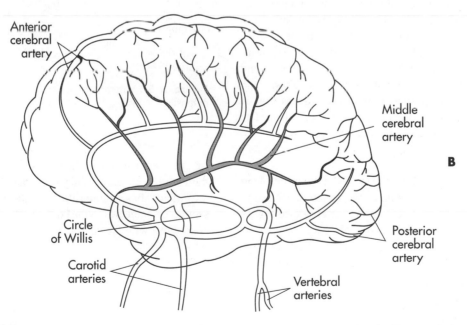

Anterior
cerebral
artery

Middle
cerebral
artery

Circle
of Willis

Carotid
arteries

Vertebral
arteries

Posterior
cerebral
artery

B

Figure 41-3   Cerebral vasculature. **A,** Circle of Willis and principal arteries of brain. **B,** Lateral view of cerebral circulation.

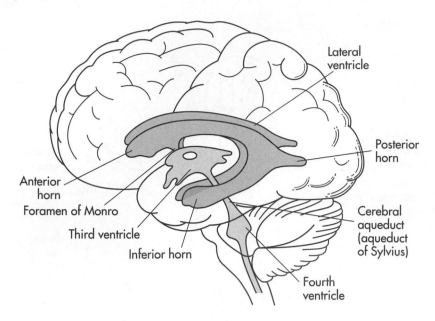

Figure 41-4   Ventricular system of brain.

Vertebrae

All vertebra have similar bony characteristics that form a circular canal to house the spinal cord (Figure 41-5). The structure of a vertebra includes the following:

1. A thick, cylindrical body that bears the weight of the torso.
2. Two posterolateral extensions that form the proximal bony vertebral (neural) arch. These extensions form thick pedicles that connect to flatter laminae posteriorly. The laminae connect at the spinous process, forming a circle. Each pedicle has a notch superiorly and inferiorly to seat the vertebrae above and below.
3. A transverse, wing-shaped spinous process that is formed by the connection of the posterior laminae. The central foramen shapes the spinal canal.

Spinal Cord

The spinal cord is between 17 and 20 inches (43 to 50 cm) long and passes through a central canal in the vertebral column to the level of the second or third lumbar vertebra (see Figure 41-5). Pairs of spinal nerve roots branch off to each side of the body from 31 segments of the spinal cord as it passes through the vertebrae (Figure 41-6). The spinal nerves are as follows:

- Eight pairs cervical
- Twelve pairs thoracic
- Five pairs lumbar
- Five pairs sacral
- One pair coccygeal

The spinal nerves carry sensory and motor impulses between the CNS and the PNS. The cord is composed of gray matter on the inside (cell bodies) and white matter (nerve fibers) on the outside.

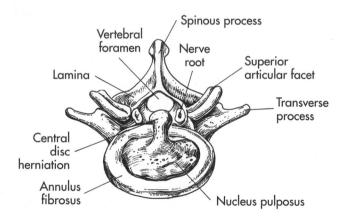

Figure 41-5   Vertebra. Superior view with herniation of nucleus pulposus.

The meninges cover the cord to the level of the second or third lumbar vertebrae. They terminate in a fibrous band (filum terminale) that extends through the lumbar vertebrae and sacrum and attaches to the coccyx. The dura is not attached or continuous with the central canal of the vertebral column.

SPECIAL CONSIDERATIONS IN NEUROSURGERY

Neurosurgical procedures are classified according to the anatomic location in the nervous system: brain and cranial nerves, spinal cord and nerve roots, or autonomic and somatic peripheral nerves. Regardless of the location of the surgical site, neural tissue is handled gently to minimize functional disability from surgical trauma. Hemostasis is a critical factor to sustain the vital functions of circulation and respiration. The visibility of structures in the surgical site also should be ensured.

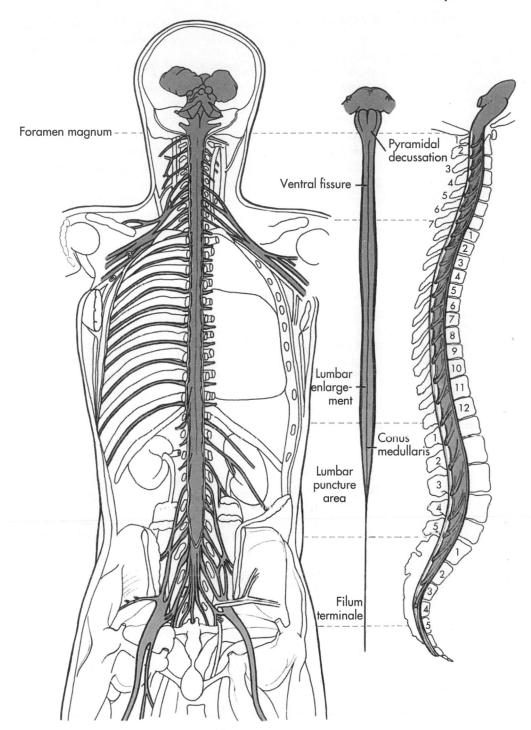

Figure 41-6 Spinal nerves. (Modified from Mettler FA: *Neuroanatomy,* ed 2, St Louis, 1948, Mosby.)

Hemostatic Agents

The hemostatic agents commonly used by the neurosurgeon for most procedures include the following.

Scalp Clips

The scalp is highly vascular. Bleeding is controlled by Leroy or Raney clips placed over the edges of the wound with a special clip applier as the primary incision is made.

These disposable clips are used as temporary wound pressure for hemostasis and are removed during closure of the wound.

Bone Wax

Bone wax is used on cranial and vertebral bones. The sterile wax is rolled into small 4- to 5-mm balls and placed on a smooth surface within reach of the neurosurgeon.

Compressed Absorbent Patties (Cottonoids)

Compressed absorbent patties, made of rayon, cotton, or polyester, rather than gauze sponges are used on fragile, delicate neural tissues to absorb blood and fluids. They are also used for protection of wound edges and for hemostasis. Assorted sizes are moistened with normal saline or Ringer's lactate solution and pressed out flat on a smooth surface that is easily accessible to the neurosurgeon. Although they have no loose fibers, they could pick up lint if placed on a towel.

The standard for sponge counts includes counting these patties. They are retrieved before the surgical site is closed. Some neurosurgeons use only patties with a radiopaque thread securely attached to each one. This reminds the surgeon that they are in the wound and facilitates their removal. They are x-ray detectable.

Chemical Agents

Chemical hemostatic agents may be used following resection to control bleeding from large vessels, sinuses, or the surface of a tumor bed. The scrub person moistens a gelatin sponge with normal saline or topical thrombin before handing it to the neurosurgeon. Microfibrillar collagen, supplied in fibers or knitted sheet form, is applied dry. The tips of tissue forceps should be dry to prevent this substance from adhering to them. Oxidized cellulose also is applied dry but is removed after hemostasis has been attained, because it can interfere with wound healing.

Ligating Clips

Clips are applied on larger vessels where electrocoagulation would be insufficient or its thermal effect would be hazardous. Some permanent clips, such as intracranial aneurysm clips, are specifically designed only for neurosurgical use. Titanium is preferred because it causes less interference with diagnostic cranial studies such as computed tomography (CT) or magnetic resonance imaging (MRI). Each type and size of clip requires a specific applier.

Electrosurgery

Monopolar current is used to cut and coagulate tissue and small vessels of dermis and epidermis. Current is conducted through hemostatic forceps, fine smooth-tipped tissue forceps, or a metal suction tip to bleeding vessels. A combination suction-fulguration tip also may be used. Bipolar current is frequently used for more precision in coagulation of tiny vessels without damage to surrounding tissue.

Lasers

Argon, CO_2, KTP, Nd:YAG, and tunable dye lasers are selectively used in neurosurgery in conjunction with the operating microscope, endoscopes, and stereotaxis. Each type has benefits, but all have definite limitations. Depending on the type of laser and the location and type of tumor or vascular lesion, the laser may vaporize, shrink, or coagulate tissue. Precise hemostasis, minimal damage to contiguous structures, and visualization of effects are definite advantages of laser surgery for removal of brain and spinal cord tumors. Lasers are also used to assist in microvascular anastomoses.

Ultrasonic Aspiration

Although not technically a method of hemostasis, ultrasonic emulsification and aspiration devices fragment and remove tissue with minimal bleeding. The emulsification process assists in hemostasis of small vessels. The technique can be used to debulk or remove benign tumors in relatively inaccessible areas of the brain and intramedullary spinal cord. The high-frequency sound waves of the ultrasonic probe fragment the tumor while sparing adjacent structures, such as nerves and blood vessels. The tumor is emulsified and removed by suction. Various settings on the instrument allow the surgeon to adjust for removal of firm or calcified tumor or soft masses.

Interventional Neuroradiology

With fluoroscopy, a team consisting of a neurosurgeon and a neuroradiologist may insert a percutaneous transfemoral catheter into a strategic point in the intracranial circulation feeding an arteriovenous malformation, an aneurysm, or a vascular occlusion. A substance such as silicone or isobutyl 2-cyanoacrylate or a detachable microballoon is injected to effectively embolize the lesion or its major deep-feeding arteries. This facilitates surgical resection of the lesion by minimizing potential hemorrhage. The intravascular procedure may be done preoperatively or intraoperatively.

Adjuncts to Visibility

Neural tissues should be as clean, dry, and visible as possible without damaging them. Visibility is enhanced by the following procedures.

Irrigation

Most wounds are irrigated frequently with normal saline or Ringer's lactate solution. The scrub person should keep a bulb syringe filled and ready for use. The solution should be maintained at 105° to 110° F (40.5° to 57° C). A sterile thermometer in the basin of the solution helps provide a safety check.

Suction

Suction is necessary to evacuate blood, CSF, and irrigating fluid from the surgical site so that the neurosurgeon can identify structures. Necrotic tissue, pus, or cystic matter also may be aspirated. Usually a Frazier tip is used. Caution is taken to avoid applying vacuum directly on normal neural tissue, especially brain tissue. This tissue is protected by compressed absorbent patties. Suction should be available for all neurosurgical procedures.

Retractors

A variety of self-retaining retractors, such as Leyla or Greenberg, are used to retract scalp or skin and muscles. Dura mater is usually retracted with traction sutures. Blunt, malleable, flat and spoon-shaped spatulas are used to retract brain tissue. Because visibility of structures is critical, retractors with a fiberoptic lighting system incorporated into them may be used, especially for intracranial procedures.

Headlight

A fiberoptic headlight is used by some neurosurgeons for supplemental lighting in the surgical site.

Endoscope

A side-viewing fiberoptic endoscope may be used to enhance visibility at obscure angles in otherwise visually inaccessible areas. This endoscope is particularly useful to identify lesions in the sella turcica, cerebral aneurysms, and intervertebral discs, for example. An endoscope may be used for placement of electrodes for stimulators or a catheter for radioisotopes. The argon laser can be used through a ventriculoscope for intraventricular obliteration of the choroid plexuses and for intravascular treatment of lesions and neoplasms. The Nd:YAG laser can be used through a flexible or rigid neuroscope to vaporize a cyst. A straightforward, rigid 0-degree scope may be used for electrocoagulation or laser obliteration of tissue and to obtain a CT-assisted stereotactic biopsy.

Neuroguide Intraoperative Viewing System

The Neuroguide intraoperative viewing system provides capabilities for viewing structures through a tiny opening in the brain for diagnostic and therapeutic procedures with minimal trauma to tissues.

Operating Microscope

The operating microscope provides an intense light, as well as magnification for visualization of intracranial structures. Microsurgery permits removal of tumors and vascular lesions that are otherwise inaccessible or inoperable. The CO_2 laser may be used through a micromanipulator. The microscope also is used for some spinal procedures and peripheral nerve repair. A fiberoptic camera attached to a microscope projects the surgical site onto a video monitor screen. This provides a clear view for the assistant and scrub person. In lieu of using the microscope, the surgeon may wear binocular loupes to magnify the surgical site.

Patient Care Considerations

The patient's fear of an inability to function independently as a result of intracranial surgery is paramount, either consciously or subconsciously. The brain is the core of one's being. Many neurosurgical patients are not premedicated, which allows neurologic assessment before induction of anesthesia or during a procedure performed with the patient under local anesthesia. The circulator should be sensitive to the patient's fears and offer reassurance. Psychologic support is especially significant for an awake patient. Explana-

tion of what to expect is critical. The following considerations apply:

1. Preparation of the patient in the OR usually begins with clipping hair with electric clippers. Hair on the head is considered the patient's personal property. When all of it is removed, it is saved. Hair removal is documented on the patient's chart.
2. The incision and the type of procedure determine the head holder that will be needed to position the patient. The basic unit of a neurosurgical headrest attaches in place of the headpiece on the standard operating bed. The head holder, either a headrest or a skull clamp, stabilizes and supports the head. The circulator should be familiar with the desired neurosurgical positions and the headrests, skull clamps, and attachments for each.
   a. For the supine position, the configuration of the headrest contours to the back of the head. The supine position is used most commonly for approaches to the frontal, parietal, and temporal lobes within the anterior and middle fossae. A lateral position may be preferred for some of these surgical procedures, such as a unilateral approach to the right or left temporal lobe.
   b. For the prone position, a padded circular or horseshoe-shaped headrest equalizes weight distribution around the face. The eyes are lubricated and taped closed for protection. The prone position is used to reach the occipital lobe. It may also be used for a suboccipital approach, but most neurosurgeons prefer a sitting position to approach the posterior fossa.
   c. For the sitting position, the headrest is attached at the head end of the operating bed to support the back of the head for a unilateral or nasal approach. For a posterior approach, a head holder supports the forehead. The frame of the head holder is attached to side rails of the back section of the operating bed (Figure 41-7) so that the patient's head can be lowered in the event of an air embolus. The sitting position allows greater torsion and flexion of the neck than either a lateral or the prone position and a more accessible approach to the cerebellopontine angle.
   d. For rigid fixation of the skull, a skull clamp provides stability that is necessary for microsurgical procedures and is desirable during lengthy procedures. This eliminates the risk of pressure-related complications around the face or eyes with the patient prone or in a lateral position and minimizes the risk of air embolism with the patient sitting. Three pins on the clamp partially penetrate the outer table of the skull. Pins on one side may be spring loaded, such as on the Mayfield skull clamp (Figure 41-8), to join the skull and the clamp into

Figure 41-7 Neurosurgical sitting position for posterior approach. Frame of head holder is attached to side rails of back section of operating bed. Note that legs are flexed at thighs and are approximately at level of heart. Feet are padded at right angles to legs. Subgluteal padding protects sciatic nerves.

Figure 41-8 Mayfield skull clamp stabilizes head for right frontotemporal craniotomy. Single pin on left and two spring-loaded pins on right penetrate outer table of skull.

one rigid mechanical unit. The skull clamp is attached to the operating bed with a frame that accommodates the desired position.

3. Infiltration of a local anesthetic agent with epinephrine beneath the scalp is desirable for many intracranial procedures. The scalp, extracranial arteries, and portions of the dura mater are the only structures covering the brain that are sensitive to pain. Epinephrine may be added to the agent to prolong its effectiveness

and to constrict superficial blood vessels. The anesthetic may be injected before the patient is prepped and draped.

4. Administration of general anesthetic agents via an endotracheal tube may be preferred for extensive intracranial procedures, although the skull and brain are insensitive to pain. The patient is positioned after he or she is anesthetized and before prepping and draping.

5. Anticipation of difficulty in achieving hemostasis by the methods previously discussed is not unusual in some procedures to remove vascular intracranial lesions. Controlled hypotension may be initiated by the anesthesia provider, with the concurrence of the neurosurgeon, to lower the blood pressure.

6. Prevention of cerebral edema during repair of cranial injuries may be accomplished with hypothermia. Hypothermia may also be used to decrease cerebral blood flow and venous pressure and to decrease brain volume and ICP. Patients are cooled to a core temperature between 57° and 68° F (14° to 20° C) by surface-induced hypothermia, bloodstream cooling, or a combination of both. Core body temperature can be monitored via a thermal probe placed in the esophagus or rectum or contained within the indwelling Foley catheter.

   Hypothermia with elective circulatory arrest and extracorporeal cardiopulmonary bypass is an alternative when conventional approaches to the control of blood loss would be unsatisfactory. The desired core temperature before beginning extracorporeal cardiopulmonary bypass is 64° F (18° C). The cooling process may take 1 hour. An 18 to 24 French arterial perfusion cannula is placed in the right femoral artery for oxygenated blood return, and a 28 or 32 French venous return cannula is placed in the left femoral vein for venous drainage. Normally the brain cannot tolerate ischemia for more than a few minutes. This time is extended with lowering of body temperature. The average circulatory arrest time is between 12 and 45 minutes at 64° F (18° C). Hypothermia decreases cellular metabolism and therefore decreases oxygen consumption of the brain and heart during interruption of circulation. Intermittent administration of cold crystalloid cerebroplegia solution also may help protect the brain during cardiopulmonary bypass and profound hypothermia.

   Blood viscosity increases as body temperature decreases. Two or three units of the patient's blood may be withdrawn and replaced with chilled normal saline solution. During rewarming, this blood is autotransfused. Crystalloid priming solution from the cardiopulmonary bypass machine also causes hemodilution.

7. Air embolism is a potential problem when a sitting position is used. The brain is higher than the heart in this position. Venous pressure may be lower than atmospheric and can allow for entry of air into the heart via an open venous channel. A pneumatic counter-

pressure device may be used. An antishock garment extends from the patient's rib margin to the ankles and is inflated if the patient becomes hypotensive. In lieu of an antishock garment, antiembolic stockings or sequential compression stockings are worn. If a Gardner-Wells frame with pin fixation is used, antibiotic ointment is applied around each fixation pin to form an airtight seal. This reduces the risk of air embolism and infection.

8. Reduction of ICP and brain volume may be accomplished by withdrawing spinal fluid. An intrathecal catheter or Tuohy needle is inserted, before prepping and draping, for the anesthesia provider to remove CSF during the surgical procedure as desired by the neurosurgeon.

9. Demarcation of the desired outline for the incision may be made on the scalp after the skin preparation and before draping. A sterile disposable skin marker is available.

10. Instrumentation is usually arranged on a Mayfield or Phalen table or on a double Mayo stand setup over the patient positioned supine or prone. The scrub person stands on a tiered platform to easily set up and reach the instruments as they are needed. The instrument table surface can be raised or lowered. The drapes over the head are attached to the table drapes. A one-piece sheet that provides a combined sterile table cover and the patient's cranial drape with a self-adhering incise area is available.

    If the patient will be in Fowler's or a sitting position, the instrument table is placed above and lateral to drapes over the patient. The drapes form a tent on the side of the anesthesia provider so that he or she can have access to the patient throughout the procedure.

11. Prevention of sudden movement around the surgeon and of bumping the operating bed or microscope is crucial. A slip of the surgeon's hand under the operating microscope or in the cranial cavity could be fatal for the patient.

12. Prevention of peripheral nerve and circulatory damage requires that the circulator check pressure points on the patient's body during prolonged procedures. Some microneurosurgical procedures take 10 hours or longer to complete. A foam mattress similar in configuration to an egg crate or gel pads should be used if the patient is supine or prone on the operating bed.

Physiologic Monitoring

Cerebral edema (brain swelling), cerebral arterial perfusion, and ICP can be safely controlled before, during, and after the surgical procedure. These parameters are continuously monitored. An intraarterial catheter is often inserted for continuous direct arterial blood pressure monitoring and for drawing samples for arterial blood gas analyses. A central venous pressure line may be established also. A pulmonary artery catheter may be inserted to measure fluid volume and to di-

agnose air embolism. Capnography is used routinely. Mass spectrometry is the most sensitive method of monitoring concentrations of inspired and expired gases. This sensitive device detects any type of gas, including nitrogen.

Doppler Ultrasound

A precordial Doppler ultrasound transducer is secured over the precordium (i.e., over the right side of heart to the right of the sternum between the third and sixth intercostal spaces). This is used primarily for continuous monitoring for gas entrapment or air embolism in the patient in a sitting position. An altered ultrasound response results if air is present in the right atrium. A catheter can be passed transarterially to evacuate air from the right atrium.

A sterile transcranial Doppler ultrasound transducer monitors changes in redistribution of cerebral blood flow, such as following obliteration of a large intracranial vascular malformation. This technique is also used to monitor cerebral vasospasm. Elevation of transcranial Doppler velocities precedes clinical signs of cerebral ischemia. The transducer can also be placed over the cerebral cortex to verify the location and depth of a tumor or cyst.

Evoked Potentials

Somatosensory evoked potentials guide the anesthesia provider in handling arterial blood pressure, ventilation, inspired oxygen concentration, or patient positioning. Changes in cortical evoked potentials can indicate cerebral ischemia and systemic hypoxia. Both cortical and subcortical sensory evoked potentials can record surgical invasion of the spinal cord, peripheral nerve, nerve plexus, brainstem, or midbrain. To avert permanent injury to the patient, the surgeon may adjust retractors, alter the approach to a tumor, or perform a subtotal tumor resection on the basis of changes in evoked potentials. The anesthesia provider may adjust the depth of anesthesia.

Auditory brainstem evoked potentials, with a stimulus to the ear, may be used to monitor the eighth cranial nerve and brainstem during surgical procedures in the posterior fossa, if performed with the patient under local anesthesia.

Visual evoked potentials may be used during the surgical procedure for pituitary tumors, optic nerve decompression, aneurysms, and some other types of lesions. A strobe light flash is used to elicit responses. The light-emitting diodes are placed over closed eyelids and secured before the patient is prepped and draped.

Intracranial Pressure

ICP rises with an increase in volume of the brain, CSF, and/or cerebral blood supply, or with decompensation (inability to compensate for pressure changes). In adults normal ICP ranges from 10 to 20 mm Hg (or 13 to 27 cm H_2O). When an abnormal elevation is sustained, ICP prevents adequate perfusion of the cerebral cortex. The brain is deprived of its blood supply. Pressure monitoring is the only exact method to determine a rise in ICP and impending neurologic crisis during cranial procedures or following head injury.

ICP monitoring is accomplished by implanting a ventricular catheter, subarachnoid screw, or epidural sensor.

A ventricular catheter is an invasive, but the most accurate, method of ICP monitoring. The cannula and reservoir are inserted into the ventricle through a burr hole or twist drill hole in the skull. Proper positioning of stopcocks is important because incorrect placement may result in excessive CSF drainage with a sudden drop in ICP and possible brain herniation. This method evaluates volume/pressure responses and permits drainage of large amounts of CSF and installation of contrast media and antibiotics. Catheter patency should be checked frequently. Postoperatively the patient is observed for signs of infection, such as meningitis or ventriculitis.

A hollow steel subarachnoid screw is placed in the subdural space via a twist drill hole in the skull and a small incision in the dura mater. Although this method measures ICP accurately and directly from CSF, it cannot be used to drain large amounts of fluid; it can provide access for CSF sampling. The screw may become occluded with blood or tissue. It should be checked frequently for patency.

A small epidural sensor is implanted in the epidural space of the brain through a small burr hole in the skull. The sensor is attached to a transducer, which converts CSF pressure to electrical impulses. The sensor cable is plugged into a monitor that produces a continuous readout. This is the least invasive method of ICP monitoring, but its accuracy is questionable.

Electroencephalogram

The function or organic activity of the brain may be monitored periodically throughout the surgical procedure by an electroencephalogram (EEG). Sterile subdermal needle electrodes may be used if surface scalp electrodes cannot be used.

SURGICAL PROCEDURES OF THE CRANIUM

Craniectomy

Craniectomy is removal (*-ectomy*) of a portion of the bones of the skull *(cranium)*. The bone is perforated or removed to approach the brain. This may be accomplished through one or more burr holes or twist drill holes. Each hole is drilled with an electrical or air-powered instrument or manually with a Hudson brace. Burr holes are approximately ½ inch (13 mm) in diameter. Some diagnostic and therapeutic procedures are performed through them. Additional bone may be removed with a rongeur to increase exposure of the brain for more extensive procedures, such as an approach to the cranial nerves or tumors in the posterior fossa or suboccipital region.

The bone may be cut between the burr holes with a flexible multifilament wire (Gigli saw) or air-powered craniotome. A dura guard attachment protects the dura mater. A large area of bone is raised for temporary or permanent removal. Attached to the muscle, which acts as a hinge, the bone may be turned back to expose the underlying dura. This is referred to as raising a bone flap.

Burr holes may be plugged with a soft, pliable silicone, disk-shaped cover, with or without a channel for introduction of a hypodermic needle. The cover may be used to eliminate a cosmetically undesirable indentation of the scalp into the created bone defect. Postoperative access to the cranial cavity through the hole or channel in the cover can be used for drainage of fluid or instillation of chemotherapeutic drugs. ICP monitoring devices also can be attached. Other types of implantable infusion pumps also are inserted through a craniectomy.

Brain Pacemaker

Electrode plates of a brain pacemaker or cerebellar stimulator are implanted through small occipital and suboccipital craniectomies. Silicone-coated polyester fiber mesh plates, each with four pairs of platinum disk electrodes, are applied to the anterior and posterior surfaces of the cerebellum. One or two receivers, implanted just below the clavicle, are attached to the electrodes on the cerebellum by subcutaneously placed leads. Stimulation of the pacemaker electrodes is controlled by an external transmitter through an antenna placed on the skin over the subdermal receiver. This device is used to control muscular hypertonia and seizures related to cerebral palsy, epilepsy, stroke, or brain injury.

Craniotomy

Scalp, bone, and dural flaps are raised to expose a large area of the cerebrum for exploration, definitive treatment, or excision of lesions within the brain. The three semicircular or U-shaped flaps are turned in opposite directions. Hemostatic forceps or compression clips designed to control bleeding from the scalp are applied to the galea and over the edge of the skin flap. The bone flap is turned as described for craniectomy. Moistened sponges protect both the scalp flap and the bone flap. The dural flap is protected with large compressed patties. For wound closure, the thin but tough fibrous dural flap is laid over the brain. Usually it is sutured with many interrupted stitches to provide a tight seal that prevents leakage of CSF. The bone flap may be anchored with stainless steel sutures, silicone burr hole buttons, or plates and screws. Absorbable screws can be used for aesthetic appearance. The galea is closed with interrupted sutures before the scalp is sutured or approximated with staples.

A silicone rubber suction drain may be placed in the subdural space to drain residual fluid from a subdural hematoma or the bed of a brain tumor, or to remove red blood cells in CSF after a craniotomy.

Intracranial tumors can originate from the neural tissues of the brain, the meninges, glandular tissue, choroid plexuses, cranial nerves, blood vessels, embryonal defects, or metastatic lesions (Table 41-2). A craniotomy may be performed to remove a circumscribed, encapsulated, slow-growing, benign brain tumor. Some of these tumors, such as a meningioma, are highly vascular. Primary or metastatic malignant tumors are broadly classified as gliomas. These have an unregulated cellular proliferation of rapidly growing cells,

TABLE 41-2 Intracranial Neoplasms

Cell of Origin	Site	Age and Sex	Degree of Malignancy
Astrocytoma—Grades I and II			
Astrocyte	Cerebum	Young adults Equal between genders	Low malignancy; slow-growing tumor; becomes cystic, well-differentiated cell structure; average survival is 6 years
Astrocytoma—Grades III and IV			
Astrocyte	Cerebrum and white matter	Middle age Males > females	Highly malignant, slow-growing tumor; poorly differentiated cell structure; 20% of all brain tumors are this type; average survival is 6 years
Ependyoma			
Cells lining ventricular system of brain; most common in fourth ventricle	Fourth ventricle and distal spinal cord	Children and young adults Equal between genders	Low malignancy; slow-growing tumor; variable differentiation of cell structure; may calcify; 10% of all brain tumors are this type; survival is measured in months according to location of tumor
Glioblastoma Multiforme			
Glial cells	Cerebral hemispheres and corpus callosum	Middle age Equal between genders	Highly malignant; infiltrative, rapidly growing; highly cellular with many necrotic foci; 50% of all brain tumors are this type; average survival is 1 year
Medulloblastoma			
Uncertain, primitive bipotential cells	Cerebellum, fourth ventricle, and subarachnoid space	Children Males > females	Moderate malignancy; rapidly growing tumor; moderate differentiation of cell structure; 10% of all brain tumors are this type; average survival is 15 months
Meningioma			
Arachnoid cell	Parasagittal and lateral convexities, sphenoidal ridge, and thoracic spinal cord	Middle age Females > males	Usually benign; encapsulated and easily separated from nervous tissue
Neurilemoma (Schwannoma)			
Schwann cells of cranial nerves and spinal nerve roots	Cranial nerve VIII in cerebellopontine angle and thoracic spinal cord	Middle age Equal between genders	Usually benign; pain and parasthesia are common
Oligodendroglioma			
Oligodendrocyte	Cerebrum, white matter	Middle age Equal between genders	Low malignancy; slow-growing tumor; moderate differentiation of cells; 5% of all brain tumors are this type; average survival is 5 years

which invade surrounding brain tissue. Glioblastoma multiforme, one of the most common brain tumors, is the most malignant type. Hemorrhagic and edematous effects of a rapidly growing tumor may be an indication for a lobectomy to give the brain an area for expansion and to impede mortality. The rigid characteristics of the skull prevent its expansion or contraction; however, the brain can expand or contract. Subdural decompression by craniectomy to reduce ICP and papilledema may be the palliative procedure of choice. By anatomic location, some benign tumors are considered malignant because they cannot be safely removed without severe neurologic deficits or a threat to life-sustaining functions. Microneurosurgery and stereotaxis provide access to tumors in some anatomic locations that are otherwise impossible to reach, such as in third-ventricle and pineal regions.

Cranioplasty

Traumatic or surgically created skull defects are corrected with autogenous bone grafts or a synthetic or titanium prosthesis. Large defects in the anterior or middle fossae are covered for protection of the brain and for cosmetic effect. The bone flap may be removed following an intracranial procedure to allow cerebral decompression postoperatively. It is stored under sterile conditions in the bone bank until it can be placed in the skull.

Bone removed because of an extensively comminuted fracture or bone disease may be replaced with sterile methyl methacrylate. This material contours better than preformed titanium plates. Under sterile conditions the sterile resin powder is mixed with the sterile liquid polymer to form a doughy mass. This is placed in a sterile plastic bag and rolled to the thickness of the skull with a roller. While still pliable, it is molded to the contour of the head and the size of the defect. When hardened, it can be trimmed with a rongeur and the edges smoothed with a special small emery wheel mounted on the electric bone saw. The prosthesis is wired to the skull in several places. The brain expands to meet it and leaves no dead space between it and the dura.

Dural defects can be closed with autogenous fascia graft, fibrin film, polyethylene film, synthetic absorbable mesh, or freeze-dried human cadaver dura mater grafts.

Intracranial Microneurosurgery

The magnification and lighting afforded by the operating microscope have refined intracranial microneurosurgical techniques and made possible approaches to many neurologic problems. A CO_2 laser may be adapted to the microscope for ablation of benign or malignant intracranial tumors. Some other microneurosurgical procedures include the following.

Excision of an Acoustic Neuroma

Middle fossa or translabyrinthine approaches may be used by otologists for removal of small acoustic neuromas confined in the internal auditory canal. A neurosurgeon resects an acoustic neuroma that more commonly extends into the posterior fossa of the cranial cavity. An acoustic neuroma can grow progressively into the trigeminal, facial, and abducens nerves and into the cerebellopontine angle (the area between the pons, medulla oblongata, and cerebellum). Potentially life threatening, these involvements manifest symptoms of facial weakness, paresthesia, and dysphagia.

The suboccipital retrolabyrinthine approach is preferred by most neurosurgeons. The patient is placed in a semi-Fowler's or a sitting position, with pin fixation in the Gardner-Wells frame. This position provides good exposure but has the potential risk of air embolism. The operating microscope offers the potential for preservation of functional hearing. Particular caution is taken to obtain meticulous hemostasis, to spare the auditory artery if hearing is to be preserved, and to avoid trauma to or resection of the facial nerve. It is impossible to salvage facial nerve function in a percentage of patients. If the facial nerve is sacrificed, the patient may return for a facial-hypoglossal or facial-accessory nerve anastomosis 4 to 6 weeks postoperatively.

A retromastoid, transtemporal approach with the patient in a lateral position or a subtemporal, transtentorial approach with the patient supine may be preferred. The surgeon's decision to preserve or sacrifice the facial nerve and/or hearing will influence the approach to an acoustic neuroma. The ultrasonic aspirator and/or CO_2 laser may be used to remove the tumor.

Decompression of Cranial Nerves

Microvascular decompression relieves the severe and disabling symptoms of some cranial nerve disorders, such as trigeminal neuralgia (tic douloureux), glossopharyngeal neuralgia, acoustic nerve dysfunction, and hemifacial spasm. Initial symptoms of hyperactivity in a cranial nerve can progress to loss of function. Some disorders are caused by mechanical cross-compression, usually vascular, of the nerve root at the brainstem. Symptoms depend on sensory and/or motor functions of the nerve.

With the patient in a sitting position, a retromastoid craniectomy is performed to explore the cerebellopontine angle. A supracerebellar exposure is used for the trigeminal nerve, and an infracerebellar exposure is used for the remainder of the cranial nerves. An artery or vein compressing the nerve root may be mobilized away from the nerve. A tiny piece of Silastic sponge may be placed between the vessel and nerve to relieve the pulsating pressure on the nerve. A tissue sling may be created to lift the vessel off the nerve. Tumors that were not diagnosed preoperatively are excised. If vascular decompression or another pathologic condition is not evident, the nerve may be sectioned to relieve pain.

Cerebral Revascularization

For cerebral revascularization an extracranial artery is anastomosed to an intracranial artery for bypass of stenotic or occlusive vascular disease distal to the bifurcation of the common carotid artery. This provides an additional and significant source of blood to the cerebral circulation. An artery in the scalp, such as the superficial temporal or occipital artery or another branch of the external carotid artery, is anastomosed to a branch of the middle cerebral artery or to a cortical branch of the cerebral artery. Vessels must be 1 mm in diameter or larger for the anastomosis to work. The procedure is primarily prophylactic to prevent development of a major brain attack (stroke) in patients who have had transient ischemic attacks or minor strokes with temporary disruption of brain function caused by blockage of the cerebrovascular system.

The patient is positioned supine with the head turned or laterally with the head stabilized flat on the operating bed for an approach through a temporal craniectomy. The anastomosis is made on the surface of the brain, either end-to-end, side-to-side, or end-to-side of the arteries.

In some patients plaque can be removed from the middle cerebral artery rather than bypassing the occlusion. Cerebral embolectomy with a detachable balloon or other intravascular technique may be done to obliterate a carotid-cavernous fistula or arteriovenous malformation in conjunction with an extracranial-intracranial arterial bypass. Cranial bypass is the procedure of choice for cerebral revascularization in a patient who has a vascular lesion that cannot be treated by carotid endarterectomy.

Excision of an Arteriovenous Malformation

An arteriovenous malformation (AVM) is an abnormal communication between the arterial and venous systems involving many dilated blood vessels. As the fistulous connections gradually enlarge under pressure, blood is diverted from surrounding brain tissue, causing scarring and compression as a result of poor perfusion. This process is accelerated by multiple small hemorrhages from the thin, engorged vessels. Progressive neurologic deficits can cause seizures and life-threatening subarachnoid, intraventricular, or intraparenchymal hemorrhage.

A large, diffuse AVM involving multiple vessels and high-flow shunts can be difficult to excise. The strategy of the neurosurgeon may be to perform a staged resection with intraoperative embolization initially to reduce the number of fistulous arteries and size of shunts. For embolization, small Silastic beads may be introduced into an AVM via a catheter placed into the internal carotid artery. This procedure usually is done a month before surgical resection.

Using the operating microscope, the surgeon carefully coagulates or clips the arteries as close to the AVM as possible. Normal arteries that perfuse the brain beyond the AVM are preserved. At least one vein must remain patent to drain the AVM until other vessels are occluded. Then this vein is occluded, and the AVM is removed.

Occlusion of Aneurysms

Aneurysms of the cerebral and vertebral arteries vary from the size of a pea to the size of an orange. Most intracranial aneurysms are located near the basilar surface of the skull and arise from the internal carotid or middle cerebral arteries. Cerebral artery (berry) aneurysms are usually located on the circle of Willis at the base of the brain between the hemispheres of the cerebrum. Most aneurysms are associated with a congenital defect of the media of the intracranial vessel wall. Hemodynamic forces of pulsatile pressure cause enlargement, outpouching, and thinning of the arterial wall, which eventually ruptures. This is the most common source of subarachnoid hemorrhage. Most aneurysms seal spontaneously, but a surgical procedure may be indicated to prevent rebleeding. If diagnosed, an unruptured asymptomatic aneurysm may be occluded before rupture.

With the patient in a sitting position for suboccipital or subfrontal craniectomy, the aneurysm is exposed for occlusion. The neck (base) is occluded with a low-pressure aneurysm clip or ligated if it can be isolated. If it cannot be isolated, the aneurysm and parent vessel may be wrapped in fine-mesh gauze and coated with methyl methacrylate, isobutyl 2-cyanoacrylate, or other epoxy resin to reinforce the wall. More commonly the aneurysm is coagulated with bipolar electrosurgery or a laser. Induced hypotension may be used to decrease blood flow in the artery feeding the aneurysm. This aids in dissection and occlusion. The operating microscope is used for delicate dissection of the arteries at the base of the brain.

Stereotaxis

Stereotaxis is the accurate location of a definite circumscribed area within the brain from external points or landmarks on the skull. It defines three-dimensional coordinates (planes) by

which to approach deep structures without damaging overlying structures. The technique is used to create or ablate a lesion in otherwise inaccessible parts of the brain. By determination of specific reference points on a CT, positron emission tomography (PET), or MRI scan, the exact area for the target site of the lesion is calculated by computer. The computer, especially designed for stereotactic surgery, provides measurements for correct alignment of instrumentation and calculation of the depth of target tissue within the brain.

A stereoencephalotome, a specially designed mechanical apparatus, is attached to the skull with the patient in a sitting position. After this is in place, computerized data show localizers of the apparatus in relation to intracranial structures. The ventricular system provides the internal landmarks. Of the many models available, three basic types of stereoencephalotomes are used:

1. *Semicircle arc system.* Steel screws are tapped through each of four burr holes for fixation of the head to a ring supported from a table attachment or a pedestal on the floor. The ring is secured to arc plates. The head is moved rather than the apparatus.
2. *Rectilinear system.* The apparatus can be moved back and forth and from side to side around the head to make adjustments.
3. *Single arc system.* An arc over the head allows angular adjustments.

The stereoencephalotome can obstruct the surgeon's access for an intracranial procedure. A frameless stereotaxic system enables the neurosurgeon to continually interact with CT scans and MRI displays via a computer linkage throughout an intracranial procedure. Known as an interactive image-guided stereotactic neurosurgery system, the system incorporates three-dimensional images from cameras mounted over the operating bed, position-sensing probes and forceps, and a computer system.

With a stereoencephalotome in place, stereotactic surgery can be performed through a burr hole, rigid or flexible endoscope, or open craniotomy. A lesion may be made or removed by laser, high-frequency or radiofrequency electrocoagulation, cryosurgery, ultrasound, radiation, hyperthermia, or mechanical curettage. Procedures are performed with the patient under local anesthesia when patient cooperation to test motor or sensory function may be needed during the surgical procedure. Various types of intracranial procedures are performed with computer-assisted stereotaxis. Operating room (OR) personnel must know how to sterilize and assemble the apparatus and must prepare necessary instrumentation.

Aspiration

A needle or cannula is placed into target tissue to aspirate a cyst, abscess, or hematoma. Tissue may be obtained for biopsy.

Functional Neurosurgery

For functional neurosurgery, lesions are created in the brain to reduce intractable pain or to control tremors or psychotic behavior.

Electrostimulation Intermittent electrostimulation of the brain by stereotactically implanted electrodes can control a variety of benign intractable pain problems. One electrode is placed in the somatosensory system to evaluate pain of central origin, and another is placed in the paraventricular gray matter to evaluate pain of peripheral origin. Following postoperative evaluation of the effectiveness of electric stimulation of each electrode, the patient returns to the OR to have a receiver placed under the skin on the anterior chest wall. A connecting wire is tunneled from the receiver to the electrode. An external transmitter and antenna placed over the receiver stimulate the electrode as desired by the patient.

Radiofrequency Retrogasserian Rhizotomy

Radiofrequency retrogasserian rhizotomy relieves the pain of trigeminal neuralgia, also known as tic douloureux. The fifth cranial (trigeminal) nerve carries sensory impulses for touch, pain, and external temperature from the face, scalp, and mucous membranes in the head. Trigeminal neuralgia is an intense paroxysmal pain in one side of the face. It can be controlled by damaging the gasserian (trigeminal) ganglion.

An insulated cannula with an uninsulated tip is placed through the cheek and foramen ovale and is advanced to the gasserian ganglion. The ganglion is coagulated when a radiofrequency generator activates the tip of the cannula. Several lesions can be made to achieve the desired extent of paresthesia.

Thalamotomy The forerunner of other stereotactic procedures, thalamotomy destroys a selected portion of the thalamus for relief of pain, epileptic seizures, involuntary tremor or rigidity of muscles (e.g., in Parkinson's disease), and occasionally for emotional disturbances. Functionally the thalamus, located in the midbrain, is the principal relay point in the cerebrum for sensory impulses passing from lower parts of the nervous system to the cerebral cortex.

Cingulotomy Bilateral symmetric radiofrequency electrolytic lesions are placed to disrupt pathways of cingulum. The cingulum is a bundle of connecting fibers in the medial aspect of each cerebral hemisphere between the frontal and temporal lobes. Cingulotomies are performed for severe chronic pain, addiction, or some intractable psychoses that have not responded to other methods of treatment.

Palidotomy Stereotactic palidotomy can be performed to decrease muscle rigidity associated with Parkinson's disease.

Psychosurgery

Intractable depression, obsessive-compulsive disorders, or chronic anxiety may be treated by cingulotomy as described or by frontal lobotomy. Under stereotaxic control, a probe is inserted into the white matter of the frontal lobe of the brain to create a lesion by cryosurgery or electrocoagulation. The lesion disrupts neural cortical/subcortical connections in the frontal lobe anterior to the lateral ventricles that control emotions. Some surgeons implant fine electrodes that remain indwelling for weeks to months. These can be used for chronic stimulation of surrounding tissue or to create additional electrocoagulative lesions. Complications include epilepsy, indecisiveness, and altered personality. Studies have shown that memory and intellect are not impaired. Psychosurgery is performed only if other treatments, such as medication or psychotherapy, have failed to provide relief.

Intracranial Vascular Lesions

Some cerebral aneurysms or AVMs can be electrocoagulated, coagulated with an argon laser, vaporized with a CO_2 laser, or clipped through stereotactic instrumentation. Thrombosis of an aneurysm or embolization of an AVM may be performed for lesions that are otherwise inoperable or before a microneurosurgical procedure to control bleeding.

Intracranial Neoplasms

Computer-assisted stereotaxis helps locate and reach the margin of a deep-seated intracranial tumor either by open craniotomy or through an endoscope. Then a CO_2 or KTP laser beam or other agent can be directed to destroy the tumor while preserving normal cerebral tissue.

Cryohypophysectomy Creation of cryogenic lesions may be the procedure of choice for treating growth hormone–producing pituitary adenomas with no suprasellar extension. The cryosurgical probe is introduced into the sella turcica through a frontal burr hole. During creation of the lesion, ocular movements and visual acuity are carefully monitored.

Interstitial Radiation Radioactive substances may be stereotactically implanted into malignant brain tumors. Multiple catheters can be placed throughout the target volume. The catheters are afterloaded with radioactive iridium-192 or iodine-125 seeds. The catheters are inserted percutaneously through twist drill holes. For photoradiation therapy a hematoporphyrin derivative may be injected preoperatively and activated by argon or a tunable dye laser to create a cytotoxic photochemical reaction in tumor cells.

Interstitial Hyperthermia Catheters and remote sensors are implanted into the tumor volume. Sufficient heat is conducted through sensors to raise the temperature within the tumor to a degree that destroys its cells. This is effective against radioresistant hypoxic cells and poorly vascularized and metabolically inactive tumors.

Stereotactic Radiosurgery Intense beams of high-energy gamma radiation or microwave-generated energy photons from a linear accelerator are directed to specific targets within the brain while sparing normal brain tissue. Gamma knife stereotactic radiosurgery does not actually use a knife and is technically not surgery as the name implies. This noninvasive procedure uses stereotaxis to identify the location of an intracranial tumor or AVM. A specially designed helmet fits over the patient's head and the stereoencephalotome frame. A single high dose of cobalt-generated gamma radiation is directed through holes in the helmet. The beams are collimated and focused on the lesion. The gamma unit is a specific installation for this procedure. The treatment takes 5 to 30 minutes. It does not remove the lesion, but it can stop its growth and reduce its size.

Control of Epilepsy

Epilepsy, caused by erratic electrical rhythms in the brain, manifests in a variety of intermittent disabling behaviors, most commonly convulsive seizures. Epilepsy may result from a congenital anomaly within the brain or can develop following trauma, meningitis, or acute febrile illness. Patients with intractable seizures uncontrolled with medication may be candidates for surgery to remove the focal point of the seizures.

EEG monitoring and CT, PET, and MRI scans help identify the specific location of abnormal brain tissue causing seizures. One of two invasive procedures may be necessary if these tests are inconclusive:

1. *Subdural grid implantation.* Via a frontotemporoparietal craniectomy, a Silastic grid with metal disks attached to stainless steel or platinum electrodes is placed on the cortex of the brain. The grid size varies depending on the area to be monitored. The grid is anchored to the dura mater. The electrodes are tunneled under the skin to an area outside the incision before the dura, bone, and skin flaps are closed. Subsequently, seizure activity coming from the surface of the brain is monitored for several days by an EEG monitor connected to the electrodes. The grid also maps the brain to locate areas of motor, sensory, visual, speech, and memory control. The patient returns to the OR for removal of the grid. Cortical resection also may be performed at this time.
2. *Stereotaxic depth electrode implantation.* By correlating CT, PET, and/or MRI images with reference points on the stereotactic frame, electrodes are implanted directly into the brain. These are connected to an EEG to determine the focus of seizures within specific areas of the brain. After weeks of monitoring, the patient returns to the OR for removal of the electrodes. The epileptic focus may be destroyed by creating a stereotactic lesion at this time.

After an epileptic focus is identified, a definitive surgical procedure can be performed to stop or reduce seizure activity. The objective is to maintain cerebral capabilities for language, speech, memory, vision, movement, and other sensory and motor neurologic functions.

Cortical Resection

Epileptogenic tissue is resected from the cerebral cortex where the epileptic focus is localized. An anterior temporal lobectomy is most commonly performed. Frontal and other extratemporal sites may be resected if the epileptic focus does not interfere with neurologic functions.

Corpus Callosotomy

The corpus callosum (a fibrous band of neurons) or the anterior commissure connecting the two hemispheres in the midline of the brain is severed. This prevents passage of neuronal discharges from a focal seizure between the hemispheres, thereby preventing secondary generalized seizures.

Hemispherectomy

A hemisphere severely damaged by widespread, persistent, multifocal seizures may be removed. This radical procedure is usually performed only on children with unilateral pathologic foci, including infantile hemiplegia (palsy), hemiparesis (paralysis), and hemianopia (loss of vision). The hemisphere (i.e., half of the brain) is resected with preservation of the basal ganglia. If an abnormal hemisphere is removed at an early age, the normal half of the brain can take over much of the missing function.

Extracranial Procedures

The cranial procedures previously discussed include access to the surgical site through the skull. A few cranial neurosurgical procedures do not require craniectomy or intracranial incision.

External Occlusion of the Carotid Artery

When an internal carotid or middle cerebral artery aneurysm cannot be reached or controlled by other surgical techniques, a carotid clamp can be applied extracranially in the neck. Progressive turns on the clamp over several days cause it to occlude the carotid artery gradually until complete occlusion of the blood supply to the aneurysm is accomplished.

Endovascular Procedures

A thin catheter with a very fine guidewire can be advanced into a cerebral vessel to fix a problem within the brain. For example, a thrombotic material may be injected to seal off a cerebral aneurysm. Cerebral angioplasty uses a tiny balloon catheter to reopen the clogged or narrow lumen of a cerebral blood vessel.

Transsphenoidal Procedures

As a palliative surgical procedure, hypophysectomy (enucleation of the pituitary gland) may be performed for pain relief and endocrine ablation in patients with disseminated metastatic carcinoma of the breast or prostate gland or to relieve intractable pain from other types of disseminated carcinoma. The microsurgical transsphenoidal approach also is used for removal of intrapituitary tumors or other lesions within the region of the sella turcica, a cavity of the sphenoid bone. Visual loss and endocrinopathy are the main symptoms of a pituitary tumor. Tumor tissue in the sella turcica is distinguished both by color and texture from the normal firm, yellowish anterior and red-gray posterior lobes of the pituitary.

The patient is placed in a semi-Fowler's position with the head slightly flexed and tilted so that the patient's body is out of the way when the neurosurgeon sits in front of the face to work in the midsagittal plane. The image intensifier is positioned lateral to the patient's head with the horizontal beam centered on the sella turcica. A television monitor is placed behind and just above the patient's head so that the surgeon can look at the screen in line with the binocular of the microscope. Televised radiofluoroscopy is used as an aid in placing instruments and resecting tissue. The image intensifier is switched on and off, as needed, to minimize exposure to radiation.

The floor of the sella turcica is exposed through the sphenoid sinus. A horizontal incision is made under the upper lip, at the junction of the gingiva, and carried deep to the maxilla. Soft tissues are elevated; bone and nasal cartilage are resected. The resected nasal cartilage is preserved on the instrument table for possible replacement. A specially designed nasal speculum is inserted in the oral incision to visualize the sphenoid sinus. This is opened wide until the floor of the sella turcica can be identified. The floor is opened with an air-powered drill. The microscope is brought into position for visualization of the pituitary and other structures and lesions inside and around the sella turcica.

Treatment of Head Injuries

A patient with severe head injury requires first a patent airway. A relaxed jaw and tongue should be raised; if necessary, suction should be applied through the mouth. An endotracheal tube may be inserted. Ultimately a tracheotomy may be necessary.

Vital signs, blood pressure, dilation of pupils, and level of consciousness are checked frequently. An intravenous (IV) osmotic dehydrating solution, such as mannitol, may be ordered to reduce cerebral edema if there is no evidence of intracranial hemorrhage. After these supportive measures have been carried out, definitive treatment is initiated:

1. Scalp lacerations are thoroughly cleansed, debrided, and sutured. Because the scalp is highly vascular, lacerations bleed profusely. Hypovolemic shock is rare but possible.
2. Simple linear or comminuted fractures usually require no treatment. A depressed skull fracture must be elevated when bone is pressed 5 mm or more into any part of the brain.
3. A compound fracture requires debridement. The extent of the surgical procedure depends on the specific extent of injury. Dura may need to be sutured. Some macerated brain tissue may have to be excised.
4. An intracranial hematoma may be present. Depending on the location, intracranial hemorrhage may require an immediate emergency surgical procedure.
   a. *Epidural hematoma.* Bleeding caused by rupture or tear of the middle meningeal artery (or its branches) forms a hematoma between the skull and the dura.

Usually associated with a skull fracture, symptoms of increased ICP caused by rapid compression of the brain may occur immediately or within a few hours. An arterial hemorrhage presents an extreme surgical emergency to evacuate the clot and clip or electrocoagulate the bleeding vessel through a burr hole or small craniectomy.
   b. *Subdural hematoma.* Bleeding between the dura mater and arachnoid is usually caused by laceration of veins that cross the subdural space. A large encapsulated collection of blood over one or both cerebral hemispheres produces increased ICP and other neurologic changes. The onset and extent of these changes depend on the cause, size, and rapidity of growth of the hematoma. Treatment may necessitate a burr hole. A bone flap may be raised if more extensive exploration is indicated. Subdural hematoma may be:
      (1) *Acute.* Usually caused by arterial bleeding, symptoms occur rapidly. The vessel is ligated with clips or electrocoagulated.
      (2) *Subacute.* Usually caused by venous bleeding, symptoms appear within 24 to 48 hours to 5 days after the injury.
      (3) *Chronic.* Symptoms do not appear until 6 or more months after the injury.
   c. *Intracerebral hematoma.* Tears in the brain substance at the point of greatest impact most commonly occur in the anterior temporal and frontal lobes. Although it is usually absorbed, a hematoma may require evacuation and debridement of necrotic tissue.

Complications of Cranial Surgery

All cranial procedures present risks of postoperative seizures and neurologic deficits. Paralysis, muscle weakness, gait disturbances, and ataxia may be temporary or permanent. Neurologic damage can follow hemorrhage, occlusion of cerebral circulation, and increased ICP. Any sudden, sustained rise in ICP raises blood pressure to maintain the cerebral blood flow and elevates pulmonary vascular pressure. This can lead to acute neurogenic pulmonary edema. This is also a complication of venous air embolism. Both venous and arterial air embolism can result in ventricular dysrhythmias and fibrillation. Infection is always a potential complication.

SURGICAL PROCEDURES OF THE SPINE

For diagnosis of spinal conditions, CT detects abnormal bone. CT and MRI evaluate spinal injuries. MRI and myelography outline soft tissue abnormalities, such as disc degeneration, protrusion, or rupture. Because it is noninvasive and seems as effective, MRI is replacing myelography.

Surgical procedures to relieve low back pain or to stabilize the spinal column are most commonly performed by orthopaedic surgeons. The use of intraoperative spinal cord monitoring with cortical and spinal somatosensory and motor evoked potentials increases the safety of these procedures. Dermatomal mapping and Stagnara "wake-up" tests also are reliable techniques for monitoring spinal cord function. In the latter test, the patient must be awake enough to respond to the surgeon's command to move the foot.

Because of the proximity of the vertebral column to the spinal cord, both neurosurgeons and orthopaedic surgeons perform surgical procedures in this area. They may work together as a multidisciplinary team. For example, the neurosurgeon may remove a herniated lumbar intervertebral disc, and the orthopaedist will do the spinal fusion or stabilization. The most common spinal surgical procedures are described here.

Ligamentum Flavotomy

The ligamentum flavum is the yellowish elastic tissue that connects laminae of adjoining vertebrae. It is incised and retracted laterally. The disc is removed. Then the ligamentum flavum is sutured back in place. Some surgeons prefer this simple, limited discectomy rather than laminectomy for selected patients.

Laminectomy

Removal of the spinous process(es) and lamina from one or more vertebrae is performed to expose an intervertebral or spinal cord lesion. A laminectomy is usually carried out through a vertical midline skin incision with the patient prone or in a lateral position. Some neurosurgeons prefer a transverse skin incision with the patient in a modified prone position. The patient may be positioned on a Hastings, Wilson, or Andrews frame to hyperextend the spine, to reduce epidural blood loss by lowering the blood pressure in the vena cava, and to relieve pressure on the abdomen.

The extent of the incision depends on the number of laminae to be removed. Fascia and muscles are retracted to expose the spinous processes and laminae. These are cut off with a rongeur, as necessary, for exposure of the spinal cord dura, spinal nerve roots, or an interlaminar lesion. An intervertebral disc, spinal cord tumor, bone fragments, and extradural or intradural foreign bodies may be removed after the laminectomy is completed.

Discectomy

Intervertebral disc injuries usually occur between the lumbar vertebrae; they are often caused by lifting heavy objects or by the stress of twisting the spine. The nucleus pulposus can herniate or rupture through a tear in the annulus fibrosus and posterior ligament. This protrusion, referred to as a herniated disc or ruptured or slipped disc, compresses the spinal nerve roots or spinal cord within the spinal canal against the vertebra. This causes pain from the lumbar or sacral region to the lower back. Pain may radiate down the sciatic nerve pathway to the leg. During the surgical procedure the herniated nucleus pulposus or ruptured portion of the annulus fibrosus is excised. Microdiscectomy or percutaneous discectomy may be used to remove a herniated lumbar nucleus pulposus with minimal surgical manipulation.

Microdiscectomy A unilateral, one-level discectomy is performed under the operating microscope. Microdiscectomy permits exposure of the herniated nucleus pulposus through a 1- or 2-inch (2.5- to 5-cm) incision without extensive manipulation of the paraspinal muscles or removal of a large section of lamina. The skin incision is shorter than required for a standard laminectomy; therefore recovery time is decreased.

Percutaneous Discectomy Percutaneous lumbar discectomy is an endoscopic procedure to remove a focal bulge-type herniated disc, usually at the level of L4-5. It is done with the patient under local anesthesia, usually with IV sedation, because the patient must be alert enough to assess radicular pain in the leg. The patient may be either prone or in a lateral decubitus position. A trocar is inserted through the skin and soft tissue into the disc capsule. Under fluoroscopic control, a cutting probe (Nucleotome) is inserted through the outer cannula. The herniated nucleus pulposus is excised and aspirated to relieve pressure on the spinal nerve root.

Excision of a Spinal Cord Tumor

Primary tumors of the spinal cord include ependymomas, lipomas, meningiomas, and neurofibromas. The posterior segment of the vertebral arch is removed to expose the dura over the involved section of the spinal cord. The dura is incised and retracted with sutures. The tumor is excised, and the dura is closed tightly to prevent leakage of CSF. Both intrinsic and extrinsic spinal cord tumors can be removed by laser with decreased tissue trauma. The laser is especially useful in areas difficult to reach by dissection, such as the foramen magnum or anterior spinal cord.

Rhizotomy

Anterior motor roots of spinal nerves can be divided to control the involuntary muscle contractions associated with torticollis and spastic paralysis. Cutting the roots of cervical spinal nerves controlling the neck muscles, for example, relieves the muscular imbalance that causes the head to rotate intermittently and tilt significantly in patients with torticollis.

Treatment of Spinal Injuries

Vertebral fractures, with or without dislocation, can cause spinal cord compression that denervates nerve tracts below the injury. Spinal cord injury may also be caused by penetrating or stretching trauma or by damage to blood vessels that supply the cord. Spinal cord injuries are classified as follows:

- *Complete.* The patient lacks sensation, proprioception (position sense), and voluntary motor function below the level of the spinal cord damage. Lesions above the fifth cervical vertebra (C5) will cause partial to complete diaphragmatic paralysis. Injury in the cervical region will result in quadriplegia (i.e., functional impairment from the neck down). Lumbar cord injuries lead to paraplegia (i.e., excluding paralysis of the upper extremities).

- *Incomplete.* Some sensory, proprioceptive, and motor impulses are present. Loss of function depends on the extent and location of the injury.

Spinal cord edema or hematoma can cause a cord lesion to ascend and worsen the neurologic deficit. Resultant paralysis may be relieved if the surgical procedure to remove bone fragments or to drain a hematoma compressing the spinal cord is done within a very short time after injury. Results are frequently discouraging. Damage to the cord may be too extensive for return of function, or at best, return may be incomplete. Care is taken in moving and positioning the patient to avoid further paralysis. The patient should be log rolled (i.e., turned or lifted without flexing the vertebral column).

A lumbar puncture with pressure readings may be done. If a block in the flow of spinal fluid is present, a laminectomy is done to decompress the spinal cord in a patient with complete paralysis or partial paralysis that is becoming progressively worse. A laminectomy may also be done to remove bone fragments. Internal fixation may be combined with decompression for thoracolumbar fractures.

Temperature control and monitoring of fluid and electrolyte balance are essential to the outcome for the patient with a spinal cord injury. The patient loses thermoregulatory ability after injury and tends to assume the temperature of the environment. Lack of vascular adaptation affects fluid balance. Pulmonary edema and left ventricular failure can occur. Pulmonary embolus also is a potential complication.

Spinal Stabilization

Immobilization of vertebrae in segments of the vertebral column may be necessary to treat chronic, degenerative diseases of the spine. Progressive instability, especially in the upper cervical spine, may lead to compression of the spinal cord with resultant neurologic deficit. After decompression of the spinal cord or excision of a bone tumor or following trauma, the vertebral column may need stabilization to protect the spinal cord or to relieve pain. Surgical alignment is indicated for scoliosis or other curvature when it progresses to a cosmetic deformity, when pain becomes a handicap, or when cardiopulmonary functions are decreased.

Spinal Fusion

Spinal fusion may be indicated following spinal injury or excision of bone to stabilize the vertebral column. Either a posterior or an anterior approach may be used to place the bone grafts. A combined anterior and posterior spinal fusion may be required for severe deformities. The anterior fusion is performed first. Unless the lesion or bone fragment to be removed is on the right side of the vertebral column, an anterior thoracolumbar approach is used through an incision with the patient in the right lateral position (left side up). A retroperitoneal incision is made for an anterior lumbar approach. These approaches are safer on the left side because the surgeon works near the aorta, which is more resistant to inadvertent injury than is the vena cava on the right.

Bone grafts are placed in the intervertebral spaces or along the spinous processes to bridge over or to stabilize the defect. The rib removed for an anterior thoracolumbar approach is used for grafting. Homogeneous cancellous bone from the bone bank may be needed to provide a larger quantity of bone than can be obtained from the rib or an autogenous graft from the crest of the patient's ilium. Cancellous bone rather than cortical bone is usually preferred for spinal fusion. Bone grafts may be used with or without internal fixation devices. The goals of spinal fusion are to achieve stability, rigidity, and correction of deformity. The combined use of internal fixation devices with bone grafts may facilitate postoperative care and early ambulation.

Internal Fixation

Complex procedures are performed for sublaminar wiring, pedicle screw fixation, and internal vertebral stabilization or fusion. Many spinal implant systems are available. All have the common goal of immobilizing spinal segments; each offers significant biomechanical advantages, but all have potential complications. The surgeon chooses the most appropriate device for the location, approach, and type of deformity and instability. For example, the posterior body and ligamentous structures in the cervical spine may be disrupted by a flexion-compression type of injury. Interspinous wiring and bone grafting provide posterior neck fusion for stability. In the thoracolumbar spine, pedicular screw and plating systems can be used in conjunction with spinal fusion in treatment of fractures, spondylolisthesis, and idiopathic scoliosis. Cotrel-Dubousset rods, hooks, and screws; the Texas Scottish Rite Hospital (TSRH) system of pedicle screw fixation with rods and cross-links; Luque rods and sublaminar wires; or Wisconsin spinous process wires may be used to provide decompression of spinal nerve roots and vertebral alignment following posterior thoracolumbar spinal fusion. Kaneda, Zielke, Dwyer, or Dunn devices are used when an anterior approach is preferred. Each device has its own set of instrumentation; these are not interchangeable.

Anterior Cervical and Thoracic Procedures

The anterior cervical spine can be exposed through a transverse skin incision in the neck and dissection through the cleavage plane between the carotid artery and the esophagus. The spinous processes and laminae remain intact. A ruptured intervertebral disc and/or a fracture-dislocation with bone fragments compressing the cervical spinal cord or nerve roots can be completely explored. Removal of the posterior margins of the vertebral bodies may be indicated to decompress the nerve root. The operating microscope is a valuable adjunct to anterior cervical intervertebral discectomy and for an anterior approach to other cervical spinal lesions. A bone graft may be placed between the vertebral bodies for interbody fusion, usually by an orthopaedic surgeon.

An anterior approach is also the procedure of choice for thoracic vertebral disc herniations, spinal cord tumors, or fractures. A thoracic surgeon assists with a transthoracic approach. Fractured bone fragments can be stabilized by anterior spinal fusion or placement of posterior rods by costotransversectomy in the thoracic region.

Cervical Traction

To stabilize the head and neck of a patient with a cervical spine injury, traction is applied by means of a Sayre sling as an emergency measure. A Sayre sling is a canvas or leather halter that buckles around the neck and chin. The patient lies with the head at the foot of the bed. Traction appliances are attached to the footboard. Countertraction is accomplished by the weight of the patient, who rests in bed in a semi-Fowler's position.

If the patient has a cervical fracture and/or dislocation, the Sayre sling may be replaced in the OR by an appliance, such as Gardner-Wells, Vinke, or Crutchfield tongs, for skeletal traction. A sterile table setup with a dissecting set of instruments and a drill is necessary. Through a small incision over the lateral parietal bones on each side of the head, holes are drilled in the skull for positioning the mechanical apparatus. Pins of Crutchfield tongs, when tightened, are controlled by a locking and positioning mechanism that forces points medially and upward away from the inner table of the skull. Traction is then transferred from the Sayre sling to the tongs, giving the patient free movement of the jaw. The amount of weight applied to the tongs depends on the extent of injury and the patient's weight. Halo traction allows the patient to be ambulatory.

Relief of Intractable Pain

Many patients suffer intractable pain in advanced stages of some illnesses, such as cancer, occlusive arterial disease, or demyelinating or degenerative diseases, or from some benign lesions. Intractable pain cannot be relieved satisfactorily by drugs without the hazard of narcotic addiction or incapacitating sedation. Implantation of a continuous infusion pump for intraspinal administration of low doses of morphine may be the procedure of choice for chronic pain of malignant tumor origin. Other surgical techniques may be indicated to interrupt the sensory fibers carrying pain sensations through the spinal cord to the brain.

Anterior Cervical Cordotomy

Cervical cordotomy is performed by exposing the cervical portion of the spinal cord through an anterior incision. A mi-

crosurgical technique may be used to sever sensory fibers at the base of the brainstem to relieve intractable pain of advanced carcinoma. This procedure provides good relief from severe pain for some patients.

Commissural Myelotomy

Commissural or sagittal midline myelotomy may be preferred to relieve intractable midline or bilateral pain in the lower half of the body. The sensory nerve fibers of the cervical or thoracic spinal cord are exposed and severed. The operating microscope is a valuable aid to the neurosurgeon in identifying the nerve tracts to be cut or resected.

Percutaneous Cervical Cordotomy

To avoid an open surgical procedure, a percutaneous approach to cervical cordotomy may be used to destroy sensory fibers. With the patient under local anesthesia, a spinal needle is introduced just below the ear into a cervical interspace. The neurosurgeon avoids the pyramidal tract that carries motor impulses. The position of the needle is checked on x-ray film or an image intensifier. An electrode wire, inserted through the needle, is connected to a radiofrequency lesion generator. The fibers are destroyed when the positive charge is activated through the electrode. The patient retains the sense of touch but not pain.

Electrostimulation

Chronic intractable pain of organic origin may be relieved by electrostimulation in some selected patients. Fibers of the peripheral nerves conduct pain impulses to the spinal cord. These pain impulses can be blocked by induced electrostimulation that modifies the impulses transmitted from peripheral nerve receptors through the spinal cord to the brain. Electrodes to transmit an electric current to the spinal cord or peripheral nerve are placed transcutaneously or percutaneously or are implanted.

Transcutaneous Electrical Nerve Stimulation Transcutaneous electrical nerve stimulation (TENS) is applied to the surface of the skin over the spinal cord or a peripheral nerve. These devices are used for many types of chronic pain problems.

Percutaneous Stimulation With the patient under local anesthesia, an electrode is inserted into the spinal canal or subcutaneous tissue adjacent to a peripheral nerve. This procedure is performed in the OR or radiology department with fluoroscopic control and sterile conditions. The patient is prepped and draped as for an invasive procedure. For spinal cord stimulation two platinum-tipped electrodes are threaded cephalad through needles placed in the epidural space. After the electrodes are connected to a percutaneous transmitter, they are manipulated until paresthesia is achieved in the desired area. When the electrodes are in the correct position, they are secured to the lumbodorsal fascia by Silastic patches. The distal ends are attached to a lead wire brought through the skin. This connects to an external transmitter for temporary stimulation. When conversion is to be made from temporary to permanent stimulation, the electrodes are attached to a receiver implanted in the lateral chest wall, usually on the left side midway between the axilla and the waistline. An antenna, placed on the skin over the implanted receiver, connects to the external transmitter.

Dorsal Column Stimulation The dorsal column stimulator operates on the same principle as the percutaneous stimulator. A laminectomy is performed to suture the electrode over the dorsal column of the spinal cord. For permanent peripheral nerve stimulation the electrode is attached to a major sensory nerve. The receivers for these stimulators are implanted in subcutaneous tissues.

PERIPHERAL NERVE SURGERY

The PNS includes the cranial nerves, spinal nerves, and autonomic nervous system located outside the CNS. Ganglions, a group of nerve cell bodies also located outside the CNS, can transmit either autonomic (involuntary) or somatic (both reflex and voluntary) impulses. Somatic nerves supply voluntary muscles, skin, tendons, joints, and other structures controlling the musculoskeletal system. Afferent nerve fibers carry sensory impulses from the organs and muscles to the CNS. Efferent fibers transmit motor impulses from the CNS back to them. Peripheral nerve procedures are performed on both the autonomic and somatic nervous systems. The neurosurgeon may identify nerves and test function with a nerve stimulator before or after dissection or repair.

Autonomic Nervous System

The autonomic nervous system is an aggregation of ganglions, nerves, and plexuses through which the viscera, heart, blood vessels, smooth muscles, and glands receive motor innervation to function involuntarily. This system is divided into the following:

1. *Sympathetic nervous system.* This thoracolumbar division, arising from the thoracic and first three lumbar segments of the spinal cord, includes the ganglionated trunk near the spinal cord, plexuses, and associated preganglionic and postganglionic nerve fibers. The efferent fibers transmit impulses that stimulate involuntary activity in the heart, blood vessels, smooth muscle of the viscera, and all of the glands in the body.
2. *Parasympathetic nervous system.* This craniosacral division includes the preganglionic fibers that leave the CNS with cranial nerves III (oculomotor), VII (facial), IX (glossopharyngeal), and X (vagus); the first three sacral nerves; outlying ganglions near the viscera; and postganglionic fibers. In general, this system innervates the same structures but has a regulatory function opposite that of the sympathetic nervous system. These efferent fibers act to restore stability for quieter activity.

Surgical procedures most frequently performed on the autonomic nervous system are discussed, but other surgeons perform some of them.

Sympathectomy

Resection or division of the sympathetic ganglions and nerve fibers of the autonomic nervous system is performed in an attempt to increase peripheral circulation or to decrease the pain of peripheral vascular disease or intractable pain of other organic origin. It may be an emergency procedure to relieve severe vasospasm following arterial embolism or freezing of an extremity. The paravertebral ganglionic chains and/or nerve fibers that innervate the affected area are resected or divided. The procedure may be termed sympathetic ganglionectomy or splanchnicectomy, but usually the surgical procedure is specified by the location of the ganglions and nerves. (General and vascular surgeons also perform some of the following surgical procedures.)

Upper Cervical Sympathectomy Upper cervical sympathectomy is done to increase the blood supply in the internal carotid arteries. Through an anterior cervical approach in the neck, the superior cervical ganglion is resected. Ptosis of the eyelid may occur postoperatively because this ganglion innervates eyelid retraction.

Cervicothoracic Sympathectomy Cervicothoracic sympathectomy may be performed to treat Raynaud's phenomenon of the upper extremities by relieving the chronic vasoconstrictive process or to relieve angina pectoris or causalgia. Through a transaxillary-transpleural incision, the stellate ganglion of the middle cervical ganglionic chain is hemisected and the lower half resected along with the second through fifth thoracic nerve ganglions. In selected patients video-assisted thoracoscopy is used to perform sympathectomy to treat Raynaud's phenomenon, thoracic outlet syndrome, reflex sympathetic dystrophy, and hyperhidrosis of the upper limbs.

Thoracic Sympathectomy Thoracic sympathectomy is usually done for relief of the chronic intractable pain of biliary and pancreatic disease. Through a posterior paravertebral incision over the transverse processes of the thoracic vertebrae, the ganglions of the sixth through twelfth thoracic nerves are resected and the splanchnic nerves divided.

Thoracolumbar Sympathectomy Thoracolumbar sympathectomy is performed for the treatment of essential hypertension. Usually done in two stages, bilateral resection is necessary to reduce blood pressure by altering the vascular tone and denervating the viscera. With the patient prone or in a lateral position, a paravertebral incision parallel to the vertebral column extends from the ninth rib downward and then curves anteriorly toward the iliac crest. The lower half of the thoracic and the first through third lumbar chains with the ganglions and splanchnic nerves are resected.

Lumbar Sympathectomy Lumbar sympathectomy may be of some value in the treatment of lower extremity vasospastic disease, such as Raynaud's phenomenon and Buerger's disease; ischemic ulcers as a result of vasospasm of the peripheral vessels; and some types of causalgia. Usually through a flank incision, the lumbar chain and ganglions located in the retroperitoneal space between the vertebral column and the psoas muscle are resected from above the second to below the third ganglions.

Presacral Neurectomy

The hypogastric nerve plexus may be resected for relief of idiopathic intractable dysmenorrhea and pelvic pain.

Vagotomy

Truncal vagotomy is total vagal denervation of all structures below the diaphragm. Selective vagotomy is performed more frequently to denervate a specific branch of the vagal nerve.

Somatic Nervous System

As cranial and spinal nerves extend out from the CNS into plexuses and peripheral nerve branches throughout the body, the somatic nervous system provides involuntary control over sensations and both voluntary and involuntary control over muscles. Loss of sensation and muscular control occurs distal to the site of severed or compressed nerve fibers. Sensation and function will be restored only if regeneration of nerve axons takes place distally from an unobstructed axis cylinder proximal to the site of disruption.

Nerve injuries in the lower extremity tend to be a result of a major impact, such as an automobile accident; upper extremity injuries are more often associated with industrial accidents. Nerve injuries usually are associated with multisystem trauma such as fractures and lacerations. An injury may occur at any point along a peripheral nerve (e.g., from penetrating trauma that severs the nerve or blunt trauma that produces contusions or traction to the nerve). Lower extremity nerves do not recover as rapidly as upper extremity nerves.

Most peripheral nerve surgery is performed to repair traumatic nerve injury in an extremity. Dissection is also done to remove tumors or relieve pain. Etiologic factors determine the location and length of the skin incision.

Neurorrhaphy

Neurorrhaphy (suturing of a divided nerve) must provide precise approximation of the nerve ends if function is to be restored. Primary repair may be accomplished by suturing the epineurium, or outer sheath. Under magnification of the operating microscope, accurate fascicular alignment and epineural end-to-end suturing of larger nerve bundles constitute the desired technique to enhance regeneration of function. For a successful result, nerves are not repaired under tension.

Primary repair soon after injury may be advantageous to align the fascicles.

A tumor, such as a neurofibroma or posttraumatic neuroma, is excised. If the nerve ends can be brought together without tension, they are anastomosed. Silastic membrane may be wrapped around the anastomosis to prevent adhesions with the surrounding tissue.

Neurolysis

Neurolysis (freeing of a nerve from adhesions) relieves pain and restores function. Release of the transverse carpal ligament overriding the median nerve in the wrist affords relief of carpal tunnel syndrome, for example.

Neurotomy, Neurectomy, and Neurexeresis

Neurotomy is division or dissection of nerve fibers. Neurectomy is excision of part of a nerve. Neurexeresis is extraction or avulsion of a nerve. These procedures may be performed to relieve localized peripheral pain.

Bibliography

Bernstein M, Parrent AG: Complications of CT-guided stereotactic biopsy intra-axial brain lesions, *J Neurosurg* 81(2):165-168, 1994.
Brady S et al: Stereotactic biopsy procedures for brain tumor diagnosis, *AORN J* 65(5):890-900, 1997.
Connelly CS, Manges PA: Video-assisted thorascopic discectomy and fusion, *AORN J* 67(5):940-952, 1998.
Dzwierzynski WW, Sanger JR: Reflex sympathetic dystrophy, *Hand Clin* 10(1):29-44, 1994.
Eller T, Dan D: Stereotactic pallidotomy for treatment of Parkinson's disease, *AORN J* 65(5):903-916, 1997.
Gerzeny M, Cohen A: Advances in endoscopic neurosurgery, *AORN J* 67(5):957-965, 1998.
Kawakami N et al: Intraoperative ultrasonographic evaluation of the spinal cord in cervical myelopathy, *Spine* 19(1):34-41, 1994.
Kubo Y et al: Microsurgical anatomy of the lower cervical spine and cord, *Neurosurgery* 34(5):890-895, 1994.
League D: Interactive, image-guided, stereotactic neurosurgery systems, *AORN J* 61(2):360-370, 1995.
McEwen DR: Transsphenoidal adenomyectomy, *AORN J* (61)2:321-337, 1995.
Pieper DR et al: Surgical management of patients with severe head injuries, *AORN J* 63(5):854-867, 1996.
Schott GD: Visceral afferents: their contribution to sympathetic dependent pain, *Brain* 117(4):397-413, 1994.
Schram J et al: Intraoperative SEP monitoring in aneurysm surgery, *Neurol Res* 16(1):20-22, 1994.
Tessman C: Exploring frameless stereotactic image-guided surgery, *AORN J* 69(3):498-512, 1999.
Walton PG, Broughton EL: Transoral resection of spinal cord tumors and posterior cervical spine stabilization, *AORN J* 65(1):48-68, 1997.
Wick J et al: Use of decompressive craniectomy after severe head trauma, *AORN J* 69(3):517-529, 1999.
Williams EM et al: Neuroendoscopic laser-assisted ventriculostomy of the third ventricle, *AORN J* 61(2):345-359, 1995.
Yamasaki T et al: Intraoperative use of the Doppler ultrasound and endoscopic monitoring in the stereotactic biopsy of malignant brain tumors, *J Neurosurg* 80(3):570-574, 1994.

Chapter 42

Thoracic Surgery

Chapter Objectives

After studying this chapter, the learner will be able to:

- Identify the pertinent anatomy of the thoracic cavity.
- Describe patient positioning for each type of thoracic incision.
- Discuss the setup of water-seal chest drainage.

Thoracic surgery concerns disorders of the lungs, mediastinum, thoracic esophagus, diaphragm, and chest wall. Surgical intervention is most frequently indicated for neoplasms, traumatic injuries, and vascular disease. Inclusion of vital organs of respiration and circulation within the thoracic cavity mandates special attention to sustaining an oxygenated blood supply to body tissues, especially the brain, during and after the surgical procedure.

HISTORICAL BACKGROUND

Interest in the thorax and lungs dates back to ancient times. The brutal practice of dissecting live criminals was documented by Aulus Cornelius Celsus, a Roman physician and author from the first century AD. He noted that when the diaphragm, or abdominal transverse septum, was cut, the thorax was widely opened and the person died. Flemish anatomist Andreas Vesalius (1514-1564) used animals to demonstrate to his students the transparent pleura and motion of the lungs beneath it. As exposure was widened and the pleural cavity entered, the lung was seen to collapse. Experimental animals were revived by tracheotomy with a reed pipe used as a tracheostomy tube. The invention of the stethoscope by French physician René Laënnec (1781-1826) facilitated the study of thoracic disease.

Learning safe access to the pleural cavity and lungs was a difficult step in the development of thoracic surgery. Thoracentesis with a needle and trocar for open drainage of acute empyema was performed in the United States in the mid-nineteenth century. Sporadic attempts at thoracic surgery (e.g., pulmonary resection) in the nineteenth century were accompanied by unacceptable mortality.

In 1913 American surgeon Franz Torek (1861-1938) successfully removed a carcinoma of the esophagus by resecting the ribs. Sucking wounds of the chest created by shell fragments during World War I drew new interest in thoracic problems. In 1920 American surgeon Evarts Ambrose Graham (1883-1957) brought attention to the relationship of the relaxation of vital capacity to the size of an opening in the thorax and in 1923 presented a staged procedure: cautery pneumonotomy and partial excision of the lung. The first successful pneumonectomy, using exposure by rib resection, took place in 1933.

The development of thoracic surgery paralleled advances in diagnostic and surgical endoscopy, endotracheal anesthesia, mechanical ventilation, closed chest drainage systems, and perioperative respiratory care techniques.

ANATOMY AND PHYSIOLOGY OF THE THORAX

An essential balance must be maintained between atmospheric pressure outside the chest and internal pressures within the thoracic cavity to sustain the vital function of respiration. Knowledge of the anatomy and physiology of the chest and thoracic cavity is necessary for an understanding of thoracic surgery.

Thoracic Cavity

The thorax, or chest, is the portion of the trunk between the neck and the abdomen. The thoracic cavity is divided into right and left pleural compartments separated by the mediastinum, which is a separate enclosed space located centrally. Alterations in pressure affecting one side of the thoracic cavity or the mediastinum cause a positional shift of the other compartments.

The bony framework of the thoracic cavity consists of the sternum and costal cartilage anteriorly, 12 pairs of ribs laterally, and 12 thoracic vertebrae posteriorly, all encased within soft tissue. The framework is bounded superiorly by structures of the lower part of the neck and inferiorly by the diaphragm. Eleven external and internal intercostal muscles, which lie between the ribs, have a corresponding artery, vein, and nerve, which require meticulous dissection to avoid inadvertent injury. The arterial blood supply is derived from the internal thoracic artery and the thoracic aorta. Venous drainage is through the mammary veins anteriorly and the azygos and hemiazygos veins posteriorly.

The first seven ribs articulate anteriorly in the midline with the sternum, which is composed of three parts: the manubrium (superiorly), the gladiolus (medially), and the xiphoid process (inferiorly). Ribs one and two articulate with the clavicle and the manubrium. Ribs three through seven articulate with the gladiolus via the costal cartilage. The eighth, ninth, and tenth ribs are joined anteriorly to the cartilage of the rib above each; the eleventh and twelfth ribs have no anterior fixation. The ribs articulate posteriorly with the tho-racic vertebrae. The esophagus, trachea, and great vessels leading to and from the neck and arms pass through the small space between the manubrium and the vertebrae. Any structure pushing into this narrow opening (e.g., a mediastinal tumor) may obstruct breathing, venous return from the neck and arms, and swallowing.

Lungs

The lungs lie in the right and left pleural cavities (Figure 42-1). The main function of these porous, spongy, conical organs is oxygenation of the blood with inspired air and expiration of carbon dioxide. The apex of each extends to the neck; the base rests on the diaphragm. The lungs are enveloped by serous membrane, referred to as pleura. The pleura has two layers. The external layer, the parietal pleura, lines the inner surface of the thorax. The inner layer covers the surface of the lung. Small amounts of serous secretion allow for smooth interaction of these layers without causing friction. Excess inflammation or fluid accumulation causes pain and impaired respiratory effort.

The trachea divides at the carina into two main branches—the bronchi—leading to the right and left lungs. The right lung, with three lobes, is wider and broader than the left lung, because the liver is positioned beneath the diaphragm directly below the base. The left lung has only two lobes and is thinner, longer, and narrower in shape. It shares space in the left side of the chest with the heart, which rests in an area of the left lung referred to as the cardiac notch.

The bronchopulmonary segments within each lung are wedges of tissue separated by veins and thin connective membrane. Although configuration of the segments differs and variations in the bronchi and blood vessels exist between the right and left lungs, it is generally accepted that both lungs normally have 10 bronchopulmonary segments. Al-

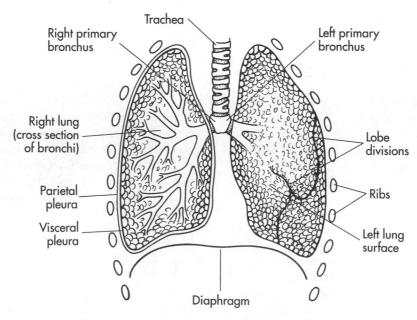

Figure 42-1 Respiratory system within thoracic cavity.

though not demarcated by surface fissures, these segments represent zones of distribution of the secondary bronchi and may be excised individually when the segment contains a small lesion, thus preserving the uninvolved portion. Each segmental bronchus subdivides into numerous, increasingly smaller branches that eventually end in terminal bronchioles. These fine tubules invested by smooth muscles can constrict to close off the air passage, as in asthma. The terminal bronchioles give rise to respiratory bronchioles from which arise the alveoli. The approximately 300,000,000 alveoli are the functional units wherein oxygenation takes place at the capillary level.

The hilus of the lung, on the mediastinal surface, is the point of entry for the primary bronchus, nerves, and blood vessels. The right primary bronchus is straighter and is a more direct continuation of the trachea. Arterial supply to the lung tissue is derived from the bronchial arteries. Venous drainage is through the bronchial veins, which empty into the azygos system. The pulmonary veins and arteries to and from the heart provide systemic pulmonary circulation. Innervation of the breathing mechanism is by the autonomic nervous system.

Mediastinum

The mediastinum has superior, anterior, middle, and posterior sections, each containing anatomic structures: the thymus lies in the anterior and superior sections, the thoracic aorta lies in the posterior section, the base of the heart and the great vessels lie in the middle, and the esophagus and trachea lie in the superior section. The organs are surrounded and suspended by the loose tissue diffused throughout the mediastinum.

Physiology

The size of the thorax varies with the bellows action of the thoracic wall and diaphragm, increasing with inspiration and decreasing with expiration. A partial vacuum between the parietal and visceral pleurae expands the lungs. A negative (subatmospheric) pressure normally within the thorax is essential to life. Alterations of intrapleural pressure are of major concern because an uncontrolled opening in the thoracic wall and pressure change can be fatal. Uncontrolled increased positive pressure in one side causes a collapse of the lung on the other side. Referred to as a mediastinal shift, this reaction occurs with entrance of either air or fluid into the pleural cavity, compressing the opposite lung and causing dyspnea. When the mediastinum has moved its limit, it can no longer accommodate a great pressure change; the lung on the affected side collapses. Air in the pleural space between the parietal and visceral pleurae constitutes pneumothorax. Blood in the pleural space constitutes hemothorax.

A mediastinal shift disturbs heart action and circulation. Changes in pressure balance within the thorax reduce vital capacity, the greatest amount of air that can be exchanged in one breath. Many diseases and conditions alter vital capacity (e.g., anesthesia, thoracic tumors, chest trauma).

SPECIAL FEATURES OF THORACIC SURGERY

Entry into the thoracic cavity can be accompanied by pulmonary distress. Team members especially skilled in meeting emergency situations are essential. Patients require close observation and monitoring because changes may occur rapidly. A pulmonary artery catheter is inserted to monitor pulmonary capillary wedge pressures and arterial blood gases. Equipment for bronchoscopy, esophagoscopy, and mediastinoscopy must be readily available. Other preparations are routinely completed for entry into the chest for intrathoracic procedures:

1. Endotracheal anesthesia permits the lungs to expand and function even when subjected to atmospheric pressure. Administration of anesthesia under controlled positive pressure prevents physiologic imbalance and lung collapse in the presence of controlled pneumothorax. Use of a double-lumen endotracheal tube permits expansion of the unaffected lung and collapse of the lung on the surgical side. At the conclusion of the surgical procedure, the affected lung is reexpanded by the anesthesia provider and negative pressure in the chest is restored. Portable chest x-ray films may be taken immediately to assess the status of the surgical area, pleural cavities, and lung reexpansion.

2. Instrumentation includes a basic laparotomy setup with the addition of thoracic instruments. These include bone instruments and a power saw (Figure 42-2 shows rib strippers/raspatories, shears, and an approximator/contractor), a large self-retaining chest retractor/rib spreader (Figure 42-3), bronchus clamps and lung forceps (Figure 42-4), and long instruments for work in a deep incision.

3. A variety of sutures may be used for soft tissues, vessels, and bone. The bronchus usually is closed with staples.

4. Sponges for hemostasis or blunt dissection are placed on long, ring-handled forceps. Periosteal bleeding may be controlled by electrocoagulation. Bone wax may be needed to control bone marrow oozing.

5. Blood for transfusion should be available at all times. Hemorrhage is a major threat intraoperatively and postoperatively. Blood may be salvaged for autotransfusion.

6. The surgical field is potentially contaminated by secretions and contact with open air passages when a bronchus is opened and sutured. Used items and instruments are isolated in a discard basin. Maintenance of a dry field is important to prevent aspiration of blood and fluid, which predisposes the patient to postoperative pneumonia.

7. An airtight pleural cavity must be restored and negative pressure maintained for maximum pulmonary function postoperatively. Except after a few specific procedures, a sterile closed water-seal drainage system is essential. Chest tubes are inserted through a stab wound and anchored to the chest wall with suture and tape. Two or three tubes are sometimes inserted

Figure 42-2   Rib instruments. **A,** Strippers/raspatories. **B,** Shears. **C,** Approximator/contractor.

Figure 42-3   Self-retaining chest retractor/rib spreader.

Figure 42-4   Thoracic tissue forceps. **A,** Bronchus clamps. **B,** Lung forceps.

into the pleural space and connected to separate drainage systems. The tube at the base of the pleural space is usually inserted at the seventh costal interspace, near the anterior axillary line, to evacuate fluid. An upper tube, if indicated, is inserted at the apex through the anterior chest wall at the third costal interspace to evacuate air leaking from the lung. Key points to remember include the following:

a. Connections must be physically tight and securely taped at the time of dressing application. The taped connections should not obscure the observation of drainage.

b. System components must be kept below the level of the patient's body to prevent reentry of air or fluid from the drainage collection system into the pleural cavity.

c. Tubes may be clamped before insertion and connection to the drainage system, depending on the surgeon's preference. Tubes are not routinely clamped at other times unless this is specifically requested by the surgeon.

Access to the Thorax

Surgeon preference and the procedure determine the method of entrance into the thorax. Access may be gained by anterior, lateral, or posterior approaches or a combination of these. Entrance through the rib cage may be intercostal between the ribs, through the periosteal bed of an unresected rib, or by rib resection. By incising near the top of a rib, the surgeon protects nerves and vessels that lie in the intercostal spaces. An intercostal approach may be used to drain an empyema pocket or mediastinal abscess or to obtain a biopsy specimen of lymph nodes or of a lung. To enter the thorax via the periosteal bed, the periosteum of the rib is incised and removed from the unresected rib, and an incision is made through the bed. For entrance via a rib resection, the periosteum is incised and removed superiorly and inferiorly with a periosteal elevator, and the rib is divided. Rib spreaders increase exposure, but if the exposure is still inadequate, the rib above or below the incision also may be resected.

Endoscopy

Elective surgery depends on accurate diagnosis by radiologic and physiologic pulmonary function studies and by biochemical, cytologic, and histologic determinations and evaluations. Frequently endoscopic procedures are performed to obtain secretions and tissue biopsy specimens. Some lesions can be treated endoscopically.

Bronchoscopy Disorders of the bronchus are most commonly infection, the presence of a foreign body, trauma, or neoplasms. Diagnosis is made by radiologic study and endoscopy. Bronchography (radiologic study of the tracheobronchial tree) is frequently done in conjunction with bronchoscopy. Bronchoscopy (direct visualization of the tracheo-

bronchial tree through a bronchoscope) is done for the following purposes:

- *Diagnosis:* securing an uncontaminated secretion for culture, obtaining a biopsy specimen, or finding the cause of a cough or hemoptysis
- *Treatment:* removing a foreign body, excising a small tumor, applying medication, aspirating the bronchi, or providing an airway during performance of a tracheotomy

Foreign bodies in the trachea and bronchi are very serious, requiring a careful history and immediate bronchoscopy with preparation for a potential tracheotomy. Maintaining a safe airway during extraction is a major risk. If the airway is not seriously obstructed, the aspirated foreign body may remain in the bronchus for months without producing symptoms until suppuration develops. Coughing and hemoptysis bring the patient to the physician.

Bronchoscopes are of two types: a rigid hollow metal tube or a flexible fiberoptic type. The rigid bronchoscope commonly uses a fiberoptic light carrier attached to a light source to allow visualization of the trachea and primary bronchi. It is the scope of choice for foreign body retrieval. It has a side channel incorporated into the length of the instrument and perforations along the sides of the tube to allow oxygenation of bronchi and administration of anesthetic gases if such gases are used. Aspirating tubes, foreign body or biopsy forceps, and CO_2 laser beams are manipulated through the rigid bronchoscope. Both rigid and flexible fiberoptic bronchoscopes are used for diagnostic and therapeutic procedures.

Flexible bronchoscopy is used frequently for the patient with decreased range of neck motion. Tiny forceps can be inserted through the working channel of the flexible fiberoptic bronchoscope to obtain a tissue biopsy specimen. Because the diameter is smaller, the flexible fiberoptic scope reaches into the bronchi of the upper, middle, and lower lobes for examination and/or biopsy. Diagnostic needle aspiration, forceps biopsy, and bronchial brushings and washings are performed in accessible areas. Mediastinal lymph nodes can be aspirated through the flexible bronchoscope. Various types and lengths of aspirating tubes, forceps, and brushes are used to remove tissue and secretions. The Nd:YAG or argon laser can be used with either a rigid or a flexible bronchoscope.

If the gag reflex can be controlled, bronchoscopy can be performed with the patient under local anesthesia and intravenous sedation. General anesthesia may be necessary. The bronchoscope is inserted over the tongue and through the vocal cords to the trachea. The patient's head is turned to the right to visualize the left bronchi with a rigid scope and to the left for the right bronchi. The bronchi may be examined to ascertain the patency of the tracheobronchial tree or to locate the source of an obstruction or bleeding. The person who assists the bronchoscopist introduces tips of instruments into the scope.

All persons involved with bronchoscopy should wear gowns, gloves, masks, and eye protection to protect themselves from bronchial secretions and blood.

Some pulmonary lesions are treated by laser. The CO_2 laser is used for stenosis, granulation tissue, or other obstructive lesions that are not highly vascular. Video-assisted flexible fiberoptic laser bronchoscopy is more commonly performed using the Nd:YAG laser. This laser is preferred for vascular lesions, such as neoplasms, to produce hemostasis as it cuts. The argon laser is used for photodynamic therapy to shrink or destroy bronchial tumors. Everyone in the room, including the patient, is required to wear appropriate eye protection of the correct optical density for the type of laser in use. All other precautions for the use of a laser also are observed as described in Chapter 20.

Airway obstruction can be relieved by insertion of silicone rubber stents. These may be either a T-tube or T-Y bifurcation prosthesis.

Ideally, a sterile bronchoscope should be used for each patient. When mucous membranes are intact, the bronchoscope is considered a semicritical item and may undergo high-level disinfection. Thorough cleaning of the bronchoscope and instrumentation is necessary immediately following the procedure. Terminal sterilization is recommended before storage.

Mediastinoscopy   Mediastinoscopy may immediately follow bronchoscopy. To prevent needless thoracotomy, mediastinoscopy is performed for assessment of resectability in patients with suspected bronchogenic carcinoma and for diagnosis of mediastinal lesions.

Mediastinoscopy uncovers mediastinal lymph nodes for direct visualization and biopsy. Subaortic nodes draining the left lobe of the lung may be out of reach for biopsy with this technique. With the scope, the mediastinoscopist can see down to the carina and about 4 cm distal to it along each bronchus. If more than one biopsy specimen is obtained, each specimen should be placed in a separate container and identified by location. The procedure gives a high percentage of accurate diagnoses and information in staging the extent of a lesion and determining its operability for curative resection. Sometimes a frozen section is done while the patient is in the OR, with resection performed immediately following a report from the pathologist.

General endotracheal anesthesia is used. The patient is supine with the neck hyperextended and the head turned slightly to the right. A small transverse incision is made in or about 2 cm above the suprasternal notch between the borders of the sternocleidomastoid muscle. Dissection is carried down to the pretracheal fascia. After blunt dissection the sterile mediastinoscope is passed behind the suprasternal notch and advanced behind the aortic arch into the superior mediastinum to the level of the carina. Care is exercised because of the proximity of the great vessels to the insertion point of the scope. Bleeding is controlled by coagulation with an insulated electrosurgical suction tip. Although mediastinoscopy usually is performed without complication, major bleeding may require immediate thoracotomy. A chest x-ray film frequently is obtained after mediastinoscopy.

Thoracoscopy   Thoracoscopy provides visualization of the pleural space, parietal and visceral pleura, mediastinum, pericardium, and thoracic wall. The need for evaluation of pleural effusion (i.e., the accumulation of fluid, pus, or blood in the pleural space) and the need for obtaining biopsy specimens of pleural or lung tumors are the most common reasons for thoracoscopy. Definitive treatment of spontaneous pneumothorax (e.g., in patients with cystic fibrosis or in pleural effusion using a sclerosing agent such as antibiotic powder or talc poudrage) may be performed under thoracoscopic guidance. A laser may be used to vaporize thickened tissues.

Recent advances in thoracoscopic techniques include video-assisted thoracic surgery for bullous emphysema, pneumonectomy, and debulking of thoracic tumors. Some procedures incorporate endoscopic and open techniques. An axillary approach to thoroscopy provides good access to the apex of the lung and satisfactory aesthetic incisional closure.

General anesthesia with endotracheal anesthesia is necessary. The patient is in a partial or full lateral position, depending on the insertion site that the surgeon selects. A small skin incision is made over and carried through the intercostal space of choice. The surgeon incises the parietal pleura to enter the pleural cavity. It may be necessary to resect a portion of a rib for access to the pleural space. After the anesthesia provider deflates the lung, the sterile thoracoscope is inserted into the pleural cavity. When the procedure is completed, the scope is removed, and a chest tube is inserted and connected to a sterile closed water-seal drainage system to remove residual air and fluid.

Complications of thoroscopy include bleeding; injury to thoracic nerves, ducts, or vessels; atelectasis; and respiratory failure. Contraindications to the procedure are a fused lung, inability to tolerate a unilateral deflated lung, and cardiac instability.

Thoracic Incisions

Factors influencing the location of the thoracic incision include the following:

- Adequate exposure into the thoracic cavity
- Physiologic intrapleural pressure changes and constant movement of the chest
- Maintenance of integrity of the chest wall and diaphragm
- The condition of the underlying pleura and lung
- The objective of a minimally invasive procedure if possible

Because of its continuity with the neck and abdominal structures, the thoracic cavity may be entered for neck and upper abdominal procedures, as well as for thoracic procedures. Examples include a thoracic aortic aneurysm and pathologic conditions of the esophagus.

Posterolateral Thoracotomy

With the patient in a lateral chest position, a posterolateral incision permits maximum exposure to the lung, esophagus, diaphragm, and descending aorta for exploration of the thoracic cavity. Beginning anteriorly in the submammary fold, about at nipple level, a curved incision is made, extending below the scapular tip, following the course of the underlying ribs. Then curving upward and posteriorly, it may be carried as high as the spine of the scapula. Subcutaneous tissue is incised; the latissimus dorsi, lower margin of the trapezius, rhomboideus, and serratus muscles are divided; and bleeders are ligated. In dividing the serratus muscle, special precaution is taken to avoid the neurovascular bundle on the surface.

In closure, the ribs are reapproximated with a rib approximator/contractor and sutures, the intercostal muscles are sutured, and the incision in the periosteal bed and pleura is closed. Muscles are reapproximated anatomically and sutured; subcutaneous tissue and skin are closed.

Posterolateral thoracotomy is used for pulmonary resections, for repair of a hiatal hernia, and for procedures on the thoracic esophagus or posterior mediastinum.

Anterolateral Thoracotomy

For an anterolateral incision the patient is supine. Supports are placed under the affected side to tilt the shoulder 20 to 45 degrees for extension of the incision posteriorly. A pad behind the buttocks may rotate the hips slightly. A submammary incision, immediately below the breast but above the costal margin, extends from the anterior midline to the midaxillary or posterior axillary line. To avoid the axillary apex and a painful scar, the posterior end of the incision is curved downward. Superiorly, access is desired at about the fourth interspace. Further anterior exposure can be gained, if desired, by transecting the sternum and continuing the incision to the contralateral interspace. The pectoralis muscles are divided, the serratus anterior fibers are separated, the intercostal muscles are divided, and the thorax is entered through an intercostal space. When an anterior incision extends to the sternal border, internal mammary arteries and veins are ligated and divided. If the incision is carried far laterally or posteriorly, injury to the long thoracic nerve must be avoided to prevent a winged scapula.

In closure, the sternum is reapproximated with heavy suture, the ribs are approximated with pericostal sutures, and the muscles, subcutaneous tissue, and skin are closed.

Anterolateral thoracotomy is used for resection of a pulmonary cyst or a local lesion or for open lung biopsy.

Thoracoabdominal Incision

With the patient in a lateral position, the thoracoabdominal incision extends from the posterior axillary line to the abdominal midline, paralleling the selected interspace (usually the seventh or eighth). Following insertion of a rib spreader, the incision in the intercostal muscles and pleura may be extended posteriorly from within for added exposure. The diaphragm may be divided peripherally. This incision exposes the upper abdomen, retroperitoneal area, and lower aspect of the chest (Figure 42-5).

In closure, the diaphragm is closed with interrupted sutures. The costal margin is secured by approximating the margins of the divided costal cartilages with suture. Tissue layers are closed in reverse order of incision.

A thoracoabdominal incision is used for repair of a hiatal hernia, for esophagectomy, and in general surgery for resection of retroperitoneal tumors and cardioesophageal lesions.

Figure 42-5 Left thoracoabdominal incision with patient in lateral position.

Median Sternotomy

The patient is supine for a median sternotomy. A vertical incision extends through the midline from the suprasternal notch to below the xiphoid process, which is removed. A power saw is used to split the sternum. In closure, heavy-gauge stainless steel sutures are used to close the sternum.

A median sternotomy incision is used for simultaneous bilateral pulmonary surgical procedures; for treatment of mediastinal neoplasms or trauma; for pulmonary embolectomy and cardiac and aortic procedures; and for access to the lower cervical and upper thoracic vertebrae. This incision may be preferred for resection of peripheral neoplasms in patients with impaired pulmonary function, particularly in the upper and middle lobes of the lungs.

Parasternotomy incisions are being used more frequently for minimally invasive cardiac procedures. An incision to the left or right of the sternum, without splitting the sternum, allows for visualization of the inner thorax.

Alternative Thoracotomy Incisions

Alternative incisions may be used, such as the following:

1. A transaxillary approach for lung biopsy or wedge resection, particularly in the lower lobe; for thoracic sympathectomy or exposure of the second to fifth thoracic ganglia; or for exposure for thoracic outlet syndrome. This vertical incision causes minimal injury to muscles of the chest wall and preserves muscles of the shoulder.
2. A supraclavicular (scalene) approach for phrenic nerve section, cervicothoracic sympathectomy, axillary vein thrombosis, or thoracic outlet syndrome. The incision is parallel to the clavicle. The first rib may be resected.

3. Cervical mediastinotomy for drainage high in the mediastinum, such as following esophageal perforation.
4. Anterior approach for upper dorsal sympathectomy, exposing upper thoracic ganglia.

Lung-Assist Devices
Extracorporeal Membranous Oxygenator

An extracorporeal membrane oxygenator (ECMO) is used as a resuscitative device for patients who have potentially reversible respiratory and/or cardiac failure. It also is commonly used to prolong extracorporeal circulation when the patient is in distress after removal from cardiopulmonary bypass. The ECMO also can be used for a short interim period (several days) to sustain the patient's life while waiting for an organ transplant or after major trauma. Potential complications include bleeding caused by the high-dose anticoagulants required to minimize clotting.

Two methods of extracorporeal membrane oxygenation include the following:

1. *Venoarterial bypass.* Cannulation points include the common carotid artery and the internal jugular vein, or the femoral artery and the femoral vein. Venoarterial bypass supports both the heart and lungs by removing deoxygenated venous blood via a vein, removing carbon dioxide, adding oxygen, and returning the oxygenated blood to the body via an artery. The device is used for patients of all ages. It is the method of choice for cardiopulmonary assistance in the preterm neonate because other appropriately sized assistive devices are unavailable.
2. *Venovenous bypass.* The right atrium and the femoral vein are common sites for cannulation. Venovenous bypass supports pulmonary function by oxygenating venous blood and decreasing the circulating venous carbon dioxide level. The advantages are lower mechanical flow rates and decreased risk of arterial emboli. The patient receives ventilatory assistance, which supplements the oxygenation process.

Intravascular Oxygenator

A lung-assist device such as an intravascular oxygenator (IVOX) may be used temporarily to assist the adult patient with acute respiratory failure or respiratory distress syndrome (ARDS). The IVOX allows the patient's damaged lungs to heal. The device is inserted into the common femoral vein and advanced into the vena cava. It has hundreds of thin-walled, hollow fibers made of polypropylene coated with gas-permeable membranes. The gas conduit that exits from the skin has two tubes: one delivers oxygen, and the other removes carbon dioxide. The oxygen inlet tube is connected to a pump to produce a flow of oxygen through the lumina of the fibers into venous blood. Carbon dioxide transfers through the outflow membrane, controlled by a vacuum pump. It can provide up to 50% of the patient's gas exchange requirements by bypassing the volume of oxygen to the lungs. By decreasing the airway pressure in the lungs, damaged tissue has a better chance to heal. The IVOX requires minimal anticoagulation and can remain in place for several weeks.

THORACIC SURGICAL PROCEDURES

Pulmonary resection often is the procedure of choice for malignant tumors and benign diseases such as bullous emphysema and tuberculosis. A bronchopleural fistula and pulmonary fibrosis are also among concerns of the thoracic surgeon.

Rib Resection

Rib resection for donor bone procurement requires much of the same instrumentation used for open thoracotomy. Reconstructive procedures of the ear, mandible, or facial structures commonly employ autologous rib grafts. Equipment and supplies should be immediately available for open thoracotomy or closed chest drainage if hemothorax or pneumothorax should occur.

Mediastinotomy

Anterior mediastinotomy may be indicated when x-ray studies show hilar or mediastinal nodal involvement inaccessible to mediastinoscopy. With the patient supine and under general anesthesia, an incision is made over the right or left third costal cartilage. The cartilage bed is incised. Extrapleural dissection is carried toward the hilus of the lung, and a biopsy specimen is obtained. If the desired nodes are deep, a mediastinoscope may be inserted through the incision to obtain the biopsy specimen. Alternatively, the pleural space may be entered for a lung biopsy. If this space is entered, closed water-seal chest drainage is required. If it is not entered, the incision is closed in layers without drainage. Mediastinotomy allows assessment of the extent of a lesion or a deformity.

Excision of Lesions

A median sternotomy (i.e., a vertical sternal splitting procedure) may be necessary to resect a cyst or a benign or malignant tumor in the upper anterior mediastinum. Through a posterolateral thoracotomy incision, a tumor may be resected or an abscess drained in the posterior mediastinum.

Correction of a Pectus Deformity

Congenital deformities of the chest wall are usually corrected in childhood. Pectus carinatum (pigeon chest) is forward projection of the sternum, resembling the keel of a boat. Pectus excavatum (funnel chest), which is more common, is caused by elongation of costal cartilages, which pushes the sternum back toward the spine.

Surgical correction of pectus excavatum, sometimes delayed until adolescence or adulthood, is performed to relieve respiratory distress or pressure on the heart from mechanical compression, or for cosmetic improvement. Various techniques may be employed. Usually, with the patient supine and the upper chest slightly hyperextended, costal cartilages are exposed by muscle splitting and/or division through an anterior midline or horizontal inframammary incision. Involved costal cartilages and deformed rib ends are freed from sternal attachments and resected or straightened. The sternum is mobilized and restored to normal position, and its corrected position is maintained by fixation. An alternative method corrects the contour deformity with a silicone prosthesis introduced through an inframammary incision. Dacron patches on the posterior surface stabilize the prosthesis.

Thoracotomy

An incision through the thoracic wall (i.e., thoracotomy) is indicated for drainage of pleural spaces, exploration of the thoracic cavity, or cardiac and pulmonary procedures. Thoracic surgical procedures, exclusive of cardiac procedures, include the following.

Thoracostomy

Closed thoracostomy is performed to establish continuous drainage of fluid from the chest (usually purulent from sepsis) or to aid in restoring negative pressure in the thoracic cavity. It involves insertion of a tube through an intercostal space via a trocar and cannula.

Poudrage   Sterile talc or some other substance, such as antibiotic powder, is instilled to cause pleural sclerosis in effusion caused by metastasis or other disease.

Exploratory Thoracotomy

Exploratory thoracotomy is performed as an open procedure to confirm the diagnosis and extent of involvement of bronchogenic carcinoma or other chest disease, such as a mediastinal lesion, when the pathologic process cannot be confirmed by endoscopy. A biopsy specimen is obtained, most often from the lower margin of the upper lobe, for disseminated lung disease. This may be done with the patient under local anesthesia through an anterior thoracotomy. Biopsy specimens are also usually obtained from the mediastinal lymph nodes. Through a posterolateral incision the lungs and hemithorax are exposed after the ribs are spread and the pleura is opened. Interstitial bleeding and chest trauma are other indications for exploration.

Open thoracotomy may be employed for spontaneous pneumothorax, for large air leaks that prevent reexpansion of the lung, or for persistent leaks and incomplete lung reexpansion. This type of pneumothorax usually occurs from rupture of a bleb on the lung surface. By posterolateral incision through the fourth interspace, an apical bleb may be ligated or the involved segmental area of the lung resected. Abrasion or cauterization of the parietal pleura effects adhesion to the visceral pleura, thereby eliminating future rupture of blebs. Open chest drainage also is used to eliminate an empyemic cavity, which accompanies chronic disease and lung adherence to the chest wall. With this procedure, portions of one or two ribs are removed to aid in the establishment of drainage.

Lung Resection

All or part of a diseased or traumatized lung may be resected. Generally, the indications are neoplasms; emphysematous blebs; and fungal infection, localized residual lung abscess, tuberculosis, and/or bronchiectasis resistant to nonsurgical treatment. Neoplasms are the predominant indication. An anterior intercostal incision with division of costal cartilages above and below the incision may be used for excision of pulmonary nodules or lung biopsy. A posterolateral incision is commonly employed for lobectomy and pneumonectomy. Endotracheal anesthesia is used. Special precautions in pulmonary resection include meticulous hemostasis and closure of the bronchus, as well as continual attention to cardiopulmonary function preoperatively, intraoperatively, and postoperatively. Particular hazards are hemorrhage, which is difficult to control because of the size and friability of major pulmonary vessels and the proximity of the lungs to the heart; cardiopulmonary insufficiency; and the risk of injury to other intrathoracic structures, such as the vagus, phrenic, and left recurrent nerves and the esophagus. Specific resections include the following.

Segmental Resection   Removal of individual bronchovascular segments of a lobe is preferred when wide excision is not necessary, such as for a pathologic process confined to a segment or for acute hemorrhage. The arteries, veins, and bronchus of the involved segment are ligated and divided. The segment is separated from surrounding lung tissue and removed. The proximal bronchial stump is closed with sutures or staples.

Wedge Resection   Wedge resection is a conservative procedure performed when a lesion is thought to be benign. Along with an adequate margin of normal lung tissue, the diseased peripheral portion of a lobe is removed, and the lung tissue is sutured. A stapler may expedite removal and closure. A frozen section is done. If a benign diagnosis is confirmed, the wound is closed in layers, and a chest tube is inserted for closed water-seal drainage. If the lesion proves to be malignant, lobectomy or another appropriate procedure may be done. The advantage of wedge resection is its simplicity with minimal blood loss and procedural time.

Lobectomy   One or more lobes of a lung are excised when disease or neoplasm is confined to the lobe. The remaining portion of the lung expands to fill the space formerly occupied by the removed lobe. Through a posterolateral incision, entrance to the chest may be intercostal or by rib resection. The pulmonary pleura is incised and freed from the hilus of the lobe. The arteries and veins to the pulmonary tissue being resected are ligated and divided. The bronchus of the lobe is identified by lung inflation while the bronchus to be resected is clamped. Suction of blood and secretions from the open bronchus may precede closure of the bronchus by sutures or staples. A suture line in the bronchus is covered with a flap of parietal pleura to prevent leakage. Dissection is completed, the specimen is removed, and the chest is closed.

Bronchoplastic Reconstruction   Extensive partial pulmonary resection may be followed by bronchoplastic reconstruction to ensure maximum preservation of residual pulmonary tissue. These techniques require successful bronchial anastomoses to retain a patent airway to the bronchioles.

Pneumonectomy   Major indications for excision of an entire lung are malignant neoplasms and extensive unilateral pulmonary disease. The chest wall is opened by a posterolateral incision, the pleura is incised, the lung is exposed, and the pleural cavity is examined. Following immobilization of the lung, the hilus is dissected free on all sides. The pulmonary artery and veins are ligated and divided. The bronchus is clamped, divided, and closed with sutures or staples. The bronchus is checked for air leaks by instillation of normal saline solution, and the bronchial stump is covered with surrounding pleura. After wound closure, intrathoracic pressure is measured and residual air aspirated from the hemithorax until the desired pressure is reached. Use of chest drainage is governed by surgeon preference, but usually no chest tube is inserted.

Sacrifice of one lung places the entire responsibility for respiratory and circulatory function on the remaining lung. Potential complications are respiratory insufficiency, cardiac dysrhythmia, and a predisposition for infection because of dead space. The empty hemithorax gradually fills with fluid and eventually consolidates, thus preventing a mediastinal shift. Dehiscence of the bronchial closure may produce a bronchopleural fistula.

Lung Reduction

Lung reduction can be performed for patients who have emphysematous lung disease. In emphysema the lungs have become enlarged because the air sacs are destroyed. By reducing the size of the lungs, efficiency is improved. Minimally invasive techniques have been employed with great success. Clinical trials are in process to validate the efficacy of the techniques.

Patient selection for the procedure is based on the patient's cardiac profile, pulmonary function, and exercise tolerance. Patients with severe disease of the heart or lungs and those who are over 70 years of age are usually poor surgical risks for the procedure and are not surgical candidates.

Thoracoplasty

Thoracoplasty is usually done extrapleurally. The chest wall is mobilized to obliterate the pleural cavity or reduce thoracic space by resection of one or more ribs. Indications are inadequate expansion of the lung to fill pleural space after resection, persistent shift of the mediastinum to the empty space after pneumonectomy, or chronic empyema. Tissue fibroses, contracts, and eventually obliterates the space. Thoracoplasty is reserved for patients in whom excessive space in the chest cannot be eliminated satisfactorily by other means to maintain the mediastinum in the midline.

Pulmonary Decortication

In patients with empyema a fibrinous thickening or peel on the visceral pleura may restrict pulmonary ventilation. Pulmonary decortication, a pleural procedure, removes the restrictive layer or membrane over the lung to reexpand the entrapped lung and fill space remaining after drainage of an empyemic cavity. Minimum damage to the rib cage by a thoracotomy incision is desired to permit motion of the chest wall that is as normal as possible. An intercostal incision is usually preferred, but in some patients resection of a rib may facilitate access to the intrapleural space. Adequate postoperative drainage via chest tube(s) is essential.

Transplantation of Thoracic Organs

Transplantation of either a single lung or both lungs may be an option for the patient with end-stage pulmonary fibrosis, obstructive lung disease, or cystic fibrosis.

Thymectomy

The thymus gland lies on the pericardium in the anterior mediastinum from its origin in the cervical region around the trachea. The lobes are separated from the arch of the aorta and great vessels by a layer of fascia. Thymectomy is usually performed through a median sternotomy, but the gland may be excised through a transcervical incision. The pericardium, the innominate vein, a portion of the superior vena cava, and a portion of the lung are removed en bloc to resect a thymoma. The phrenic nerve is spared to prevent diaphragmatic paralysis. Thymectomy without en bloc resection may be done to relieve symptoms of myasthenia gravis.

Thoracic Outlet Syndrome

The thoracic outlet is an area bordered by the manubrium anteriorly, the first rib anterolaterally, and the first thoracic vertebra posteriorly. The major blood vessels and nerves of the head and upper extremities pass through this space. Following a neck injury, changes can occur in the anterior and/or middle scalene muscles, causing pressure on these nerves and vessels. Symptoms include pain and paresthesia of the upper extremities extending into the fingertips. When conservative treatment fails to relieve pain, scalenectomy or scalenotomy is performed. A supraclavicular incision with resection of the first rib or a transaxillary incision is used. In extreme circumstances bilateral resection of the first rib may be necessary.

CHEST TRAUMA

Trauma to the chest varies in severity and may result in injury to the thoracic wall or intrathoracic organs such as the heart and lungs. If the trauma is severe, the patient is plunged into a critical condition. Rapid initial evaluation of the extent of injury is necessary to preserve life, with priority needs met first. These include resuscitation with relief of airway obstruction, treatment of shock and blood loss, and restoration of normal cardiorespiratory dynamics to the extent possible. Impairment of these dynamics may be caused by various factors such as disturbance of lung expansion or cardiac tamponade.

Trauma is categorized as blunt or penetrating. Blunt trauma usually results from a fall, blow, severe cough, blast, or deceleration injury. The patient may have little overt evidence of chest injury, even though he or she may be bleeding internally from pulmonary contusion. Penetrating wounds are usually caused by a low- or high-velocity missile, such as a knife stab or bullet. Surgical exploration may be required to control bleeding and/or air leak. Open thoracotomy may be performed in the emergency department and the patient brought to the operating room (OR) with the chest open for further exploration of the wound and for closure.

Blunt Trauma

Fractured Ribs

Rib fracture is the most common injury to the chest wall, the fourth to the eighth ribs being the ones mainly involved. Pain may be relieved by an intercostal nerve block. Surgical treatment is usually not required unless sharp edges or displaced bone fragments puncture the pleura or lung. Extensive pneumothorax requires immediate reexpansion of the lungs.

Multiple rib or sternal fractures often produce an unstable chest wall, resulting in flail chest. Normal respiration changes to paradoxic motion of the chest wall. The chest wall collapses on inspiration and expands on expiration. This results in ineffective respiration and coughing. As the chest wall expands, the free-floating sternum is sucked inward, thus impairing ventilation and producing hypoxia. The following measures are used to stabilize the chest wall:

1. Internal stabilization is achieved by controlled mechanical ventilation. An endotracheal tube or tracheostomy tube may be necessary to decrease pulmonary resistance and increase perfusion. Frequent suctioning maintains a clear airway; thus paradoxic motion and dead air space decrease.
2. Surgical stabilization is achieved by inserting pins or wiring fractures together. Fracture of the sternum, scapulae, and clavicles also may be involved in the injury.

Ruptured Organs

Blunt trauma can cause rupture of the diaphragm, aorta, or thoracic tracheobronchial tree, necessitating emergency thoracotomy. Contusions of the lung and pericardium may cause hemorrhage.

Penetrating Wounds

Anatomic visualization of the path of the projectile or instrument producing injury is important. A knife, for example, should not be removed except under the direction of a physician because it may be penetrating the heart or a major vessel.

An open chest wound must be converted to a closed chest wound. Air rushes into an open wound, building up atmospheric positive pressure inside the pleural space. Pneumothorax followed by a mediastinal shift ensues.

Thoracentesis

Air or blood in the pleural cavity may be detected and aspirated by a needle and syringe. A chest tube may be inserted into the pleural space percutaneously for closed thoracostomy drainage. If bleeding persists, the chest is opened and vessels are ligated or repaired.

Sucking Chest Wound

Pneumothorax is relieved and further air prevented from entering the chest during respiration by suturing the wound and inserting one or more chest tubes.

INTRATHORACIC ESOPHAGEAL PROCEDURES

Esophageal disorders may be congenital, or they may be acquired by trauma or disease. Thoracic surgeons may perform esophageal resections for a benign tumor (such as a leiomyoma) or for relief of obstruction in the thoracic esophagus (such as a stricture, stenosis, or achalasia). Esophageal myotomy with or without fundoplication may relieve obstruction in the lower segment. Resections are performed for malignant tumors. Early detection of esophageal carcinoma increases the rate of cure by surgical resection. Unfortunately, symptoms are not usually apparent in the early stages, so that carcinoma of the esophagus generally presents a poor prognosis. Most surgical procedures provide palliation rather than cure. Radical en bloc mediastinectomy may become the procedure of choice, but esophagectomy is more commonly performed.

Esophagectomy

For esophagectomy the patient is in a lateral position. A posterolateral thoracotomy or thoracoabdominal incision is extended across the chest wall to expose the affected segment of the esophagus (i.e., upper, middle, or lower third). The thoracic cavity is opened, and the mediastinal pleura is incised. The esophagus is dissected away from the aorta and transected above and below the lesion.

For combined thoracoabdominal exposure of a lesion in the lower third of the esophagus, the diaphragm is opened and the stomach mobilized for transection and intrathoracic esophagogastrostomy. In some patients resection and anastomosis may be performed without thoracotomy by means of a substernal resection to avoid morbidity associated with thoracoabdominal exposure.

High esophageal resection followed by hypopharyngeal reconstruction may be the procedure of choice for tumors in the upper third of the esophagus. Total esophagectomy for tumors in the middle third may be carried out through abdominal and cervical incisions, without thoracotomy. The stomach is mobilized for esophagogastric anastomosis in the neck.

Repair of a Hiatal Hernia

Repair of herniation of the stomach through the diaphragm may be performed by a general surgeon or by a thoracic surgeon using thoracic routines, such as chest tube insertion with closed water-seal drainage. The thoracic approach is preferred in the following situations:

- When exposure from an abdominal approach would be difficult, as with an obese patient
- When the hernia is incarcerated into the thoracic cavity and would be difficult to reduce through the diaphragm into the abdomen
- When the hernia is recurrent and direct visualization will facilitate the procedure
- When herniation is caused by blunt trauma or a penetrating abdominothoracic wound

COMPLICATIONS OF THORACIC SURGERY

Continuous movement of the chest causes postoperative pain. The patient is likely to breathe shallowly and not adequately raise secretions that accumulate as a result of inhaled anesthetics and sedation. Obstruction in the bronchi from retained secretions can lead to pneumonia and/or atelectasis. The plan of care should include preoperative teaching of breathing techniques to assist the patient in clearing airway secretions.

Development of one pulmonary complication frequently predisposes the patient to development of another. Other potential complications are pneumothorax from an air leak, hemothorax from hemorrhage, and pleural effusion. Empyema and persistent undrained fluid or air pockets can develop in intrathoracic spaces. A bronchopleural fistula may necessitate closure. Pulmonary shunting is also a major complication.

Chylothorax is a potential complication of thoracic surgery. Chylothorax is the leakage of chyle from the thoracic duct of the lymphatic system into the pleural space. This complication may occur in response to trauma or after a surgical procedure in the chest cavity. Surgical repair is performed.

ARDS, also known as progressive pulmonary insufficiency or shock lung, may develop in the first 24 to 48 hours following a traumatic injury such as pulmonary contusion or from diffuse or aspiration pneumonia. Beginning with dyspnea, grunting respirations, and tachycardia, signs progress to cyanosis, hypoxemia, and alveolar infiltration. Mortality is high. An IVOX/intravenacaval blood gas exchanger may be used as a temporary booster lung for a patient with ARDS or acute respiratory failure.

Bibliography

Boutin C, Astoul P: Diagnostic thoracoscopy, *Clin Chest Med* 19(2):295-309, 1998.

Caron EA, Hamblet-Berlandi JL: Extracorporeal membrane oxygenation, *Nurs Clin North Am* 32(1):125-140, 1997.

Cina C et al: Treatment of thoracic outlet syndrome with combined scalenectomy and transaxillary first rib resection, *Cardiovasc Surg* 2(4):514-518, 1994.

Cybulsky IJ, Bennett WF: Mediastinoscopy as routine outpatient procedure, *Ann Thorac Surg* 58(1):176-178, 1994.

Dickey DM: Bilateral lung volume reduction surgery for treatment of emphysema, *AORN J* 63(2):355-372, 1996.

Ellison DW, Wood VE: Trauma-related thoracic outlet syndrome, *J Hand Surg* 19(4):424-426, 1994.

Frank MW et al: Axillary thoracoscopy, *Ann Thorac Surg* 66(2):590-591, 1998.

Graling PR et al: Bilateral lung volume reduction surgery, *AORN J* 63(2):389-404, 1996.

Hayward RH et al: Access to the thorax by incision, *J Am Coll Surg* 179(2):202-208, 1994.

Ichiba S, Bartlett RH: Current status of extracorporeal membrane oxygenation for severe respiratory failure, *Artif Organs* 20(2):120-123, 1996.

Kaiser LR: Thymoma: the use of minimally invasive resection techniques, *Chest Surg Clin North Am* 4(1):185-194, 1994.

Lechin AE, Varon J: Adult respiratory distress syndrome (ARDS): the basics, *J Emerg Med* 12(1):63-68, 1994.

Lodenkemper R, Schoenfeld N: Role of endoscopy in the preoperative assessment of bronchial carcinoma, *Arch Chest Dis* 49(2):138-143, 1994.

Milanz JR et al: Intrapleural talc for the prevention of recurrent pneumothorax, *Chest* 106(4):1162-1165, 1994.

Nakanishi R et al: Combined thoracoscopy and mediastinoscopy for the evaluation of mediastinal lymph node metastasis in left upper lobe cancer, *J Cardiovasc Surg* 35(4):347-349, 1994.

Podbielski FJ et al: Thoracoscopic assisted pneumonectomy, *J Soc Laparoendosc Surg* 1(1):75-77, 1997.

Roviaro G et al: Videothoracoscopic excision of mediastinal masses: indications and techniques, *Ann Thorac Surg* 58(6):1679-1683, 1994.

Sarsam MA et al: Postpneumonectomy chylothorax, *Ann Thorac Surg* 57(3):689-690, 1994.

Sutedja G, Postmus PE: Bronchoscopic treatment of lung tumors, *Lung Cancer* 11(1-2):1-17, 1994.

Urschel JD, Horan TA: Mediastinoscopic treatment of mediastinal cysts, *Ann Thorac Surg* 58(6):1698-1700, 1994.

Wilson JM et al: ECMO in evolution: the impact of changing patient demographics and alternative therapies on ECMO, *J Pediatr Surg* 31(8):1116-1122, 1996.

Windsor PG et al: Sclerotherapy for malignant pleural effusions: alternatives to tetracycline, *South Med J* 87(7):709-714, 1994.

Chapter 43

Cardiac Surgery

 Chapter Objectives

After studying this chapter, the learner will be able to:

- Identify the pertinent anatomy of the heart and great vessels.
- List the types of conduits used for coronary artery bypass grafting.
- Describe the function of a cardiac pacemaker.

Cardiovascular surgery encompasses the spectrum of clinical pathologic processes associated with congenital anomalies and acquired diseases of the circulatory system. The often complex surgical procedures involving the heart, great vessels, and peripheral blood vessels mandate the need for experienced operating room (OR) teams with special education and training. The goal of cardiovascular surgeons is to restore or preserve adequate cardiac output and circulation of blood to the brain and tissues throughout the body. Technologic advancements in diagnosis, anesthesia, hemodynamic monitoring, extracorporeal circulation, myocardial preservation, prosthetic devices, and transplantation have made possible the correction of many defects and the treatment of cardiovascular diseases.

Cardiac surgery, more than any other surgical specialty, owes its successes to teams of experts in chemistry, biology, immunology, biomedical engineering, and electronics working cooperatively with courageous surgeons and cardiologists.

Congenital malformations corrected in infancy or early childhood are discussed in Chapter 8. This chapter focuses on surgical procedures performed for acquired heart diseases.

HISTORICAL BACKGROUND

Awareness of the heart transcends the ages. Ancient civilizations revered the heart and considered it the seat of loyalty,

bravery, and love. The physiologic properties, such as the heartbeat and its changes under the influence of emotion, gave rise to the importance of the symbolic heart. A warrior in a South American country would remove the beating heart from his enemy in a ritual ceremony and marvel at how it continued to beat. Some cultures performed this rite as part of religious celebration. The mystery associated with the heart and its electrical properties continued through the ages.

The circulation of blood was not understood until English physiologist William Harvey (1578-1657) demonstrated that blood makes a complete circuit in the body. Harvey derived knowledge of comparative anatomy from dissections and experiments on the heart chambers, arteries, and veins. Then in 1791 Italian anatomist Luigi Galvani (1737-1798) discovered the fundamentals of electrical stimulation of animal muscle and indirectly discovered how electrical impulses affect the heart.

Cardiopulmonary bypass (CPB) procedures were conceived of as early as 1812. A prototype of the CPB machine was built by Von Frey and Gruber in 1858 and was successful in perfusing a single organ. Development of the CPB machine, which permits safe direct vision for open heart procedures, is credited to John Gibbon, who conceptualized its use for cardiac surgery as early as 1938. In 1953 at Jefferson Medical College in Philadelphia, he performed intracardiac surgery using the first successful pump oxygenator. The procedure to repair an atrial septal defect in an 18-year-old woman was successful.

In 1998 the Cleveland Clinic developed vacuum-assisted venous drainage that decreases the amount of priming solution needed to promote blood flow through the bypass machine from 2.4 L to less than 1 L. This significantly minimizes the risk of postoperative complications such as bleeding, hemodilution, and hemolysis. Cannulas are smaller in diameter and work well in a minimally invasive environment.

Revascularization of an ischemic myocardium to increase blood supply has progressed from abrasion of the epicardium with talcum powder in the 1950s to internal mammary artery implantation and coronary bypass procedures developed in the 1960s. The Cleveland Clinic pioneered advances in coronary artery bypass procedures, starting with F. Mason Sones, who in 1957 developed and refined angiography methods to locate blocked coronary arteries. In 1964 H. Edward Garrett performed the first successful coronary bypass on a human as an emergency procedure in Texas. Rene Falvaloro performed the first successful planned coronary artery bypass in 1967 using an autologous interposition saphenous vein graft as a conduit.

The first successful heart transplant by Christian Barnard was performed in South Africa in 1967. The advent in 1981 of a combined heart-lung transplant and the implantation of a mechanical artificial heart in 1982 may provide hope in the future for patients with end-stage cardiopulmonary disease.

ANATOMY OF THE HEART AND GREAT VESSELS

Cardiac procedures involve the heart and associated great vessels. To understand diagnostic procedures, hemodynamic monitoring, myocardial preservation techniques, and CPB used in conjunction with cardiac surgery requires knowledge of the normal anatomy and physiology of the heart.

The cardiovascular system supplies oxygen and nutrients to body cells and carries waste away from cells by the flow of blood through the system. The heart, blood, and lymph vessels constitute this circulatory system. The heart—the hollow muscular organ located in the thorax—maintains the circulation of blood throughout the body.

Heart

The heart is located in the middle mediastinum slightly left of midline. The heart is a four-chambered muscular "pump" enveloped by a closed, double-layered, fibroserous sac—the pericardium. The outer parietal layer forms the sac that contains a small amount of clear serous fluid that lubricates the heart's moving surfaces. The base of the pericardium is attached to the diaphragm; the apex surrounds the great vessels arising from the base of the heart (Figures 43-1 and 43-2).

The layers of the heart are the epicardium (outer visceral pericardium), myocardium (muscle fibers), and endocardium (inner membrane lining). Divided into right and left halves by an oblique longitudinal septum, each half of the heart has two chambers: a thin-walled upper atrium and a thick-walled lower ventricle. The right side of the heart pumps the pulmonary circulation, and the left side of the heart pumps blood into the systemic circulation. The right atrium receives desaturated blood from the inferior and superior vena cava and the coronary veins. The left atrium receives oxygenated blood from the pulmonary veins. The left ventricle pumps blood into the aorta and the arteries. The heart's rounded apex, formed by the left ventricle, is behind the sixth rib slightly to the left of the sternum. The base is formed by the atria and great vessels.

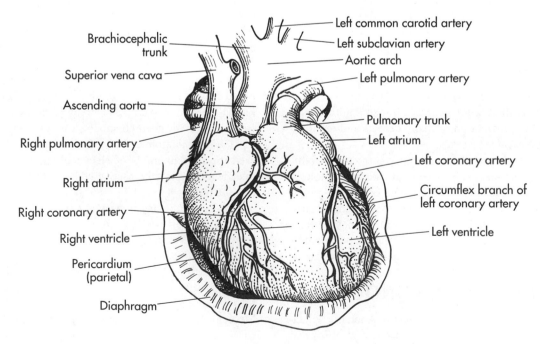

Figure 43-1   Anterior view of heart and great vessels.

Valves

Four heart valves promote unobstructed unidirectional blood flow through the chambers (Figure 43-3). These valves are of two types:

1. Atrioventricular (AV) valves. The bases of the cusps (the endocardial leaflets) of these valves attach to the fibrous ring that surrounds their opening between the atrium and ventricle on each side of the heart.
   a. The right tricuspid valve has three cusps.
   b. The left mitral valve has two cusps.
2. Semilunar valves. These valves open to allow blood to flow from the heart chambers into the great vessels.
   a. The pulmonary valve between the right ventricle and the pulmonary trunk has three cusps.
   b. The aortic valve between the left ventricle and the aorta has three cusps.

When the ventricle begins to contract, the AV cusps float up to close the opening, preventing a backflow of blood, as the semilunar valves open. Sequential heart sounds (S1 and S2) are heard by stethoscope as the valves open and close.

Coronary Circulation

Coronary circulation supplies oxygen directly to the heart muscle and is predominantly anatomically right or left. The coronary arteries arise from the aorta and, with their branches, supply oxygen and nutrients to the heart muscle. The left coronary artery divides shortly after its origin into two main trunks:

1. The anterior descending or interventricular branch courses toward the apex of the heart. Its branches distribute over the anterolateral wall of the left ventricle. Septal branches supply the anterior interventricular septum.

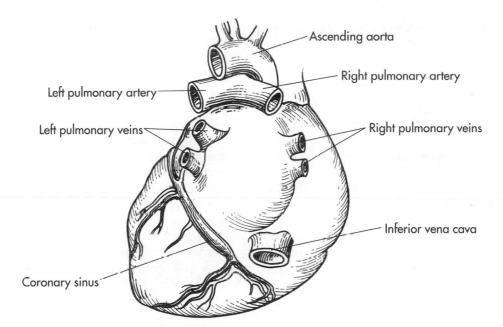

Figure 43-2   Posterior view of heart and great vessels.

Figure 43-3   Cardiac valves: superior view with atria removed.

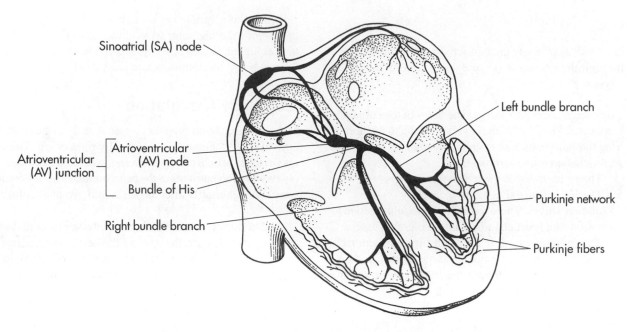

Figure 43-4　Conducting system within heart. Electrical system is composed of sinoatrial (SA) node, atrioventricular (AV) node, and bundle of His, at AV junction; left bundle branch; right bundle branch; Purkinje network of Purkinje fibers.

2. The circumflex branch passes posteriorly. Following the AV groove and passing under the left atrial appendage, it meets the right coronary artery at the base of the junction of both ventricles.

The right coronary artery is directed to the right, passing to the posterior aspect of the heart and eventually running between the two ventricles. Its branches supply the posterior interventricular septum. The desaturated coronary blood returns to the venous circulation through the coronary sinus.

The vagus nerve (parasympathetic nervous system) and cardiac branches of the cervical and upper thoracic ganglia (sympathetic nervous system) innervate the heart.

PHYSIOLOGY OF THE HEART

Electrical Conduction System

The conduction system of the heart (Figure 43-4) permits synchronous contraction of the atria followed by contraction of the ventricles. The right and left sides of the heart function simultaneously but independently. Muscular contractions of the atria and ventricles are controlled by an electrical impulse that originates in the sinoatrial (SA) node. This "pacemaker" is a dense network of specialized Purkinje fibers that begin at the junction of the right atrium and superior vena cava. These fibers become continuous with muscle fibers of the atrium at the node's periphery. The stimulus is passed to the smaller AV node beneath the endocardium in the interatrial septum. A mass of interwoven conductive tissue, this node's specialized fibers are continuous with atrial muscle fibers and the AV bundle of His. The bundle of His provides conduction relay between the atria and ventricles. Arising from the AV node, the band of conducting tissue passes on both sides of the interventricular septum, its branches dividing and subdividing to penetrate every area of ventricular muscle and to transmit contraction impulses to the ventricles. Thus expansions of conducting tissue, providing coordinated excitation of muscle areas, spread through both atria and ventricles. Each atrial contraction (depolarization) is followed by a period of recharging (repolarization) during which the ventricles contract. Ventricular contraction is followed by a period of recovery while the chambers fill with blood as the atria contract.

Cardiac Cycle

Myocardial contraction is referred to as systole; cardiac relaxation is referred to as diastole. Venous blood from the entire body enters the right atrium via the vena cava and passes through the tricuspid valve to the right ventricle, from which it is ejected through the pulmonary valve into the pulmonary arterial trunk (Figure 43-5). Right and left pulmonary arteries originating from the trunk carry the blood to the lungs, where it takes up oxygen and gives off carbon dioxide. Oxygenated blood is transported from the lungs to the left atrium by the pulmonary veins and enters the left ventricle through the mitral valve. Contraction of the left ventricle propels blood through the aortic valve into the aorta, from which it is carried to all parts of the body by arterial branches. The highest pressure reached during left ventricular systole is the systolic blood pressure. Following contraction the ventricle relaxes, during which time systemic intraarterial pressure falls to its lowest level—the diastolic blood pressure. Each contraction of the right ventricle forces blood through the pulmonary

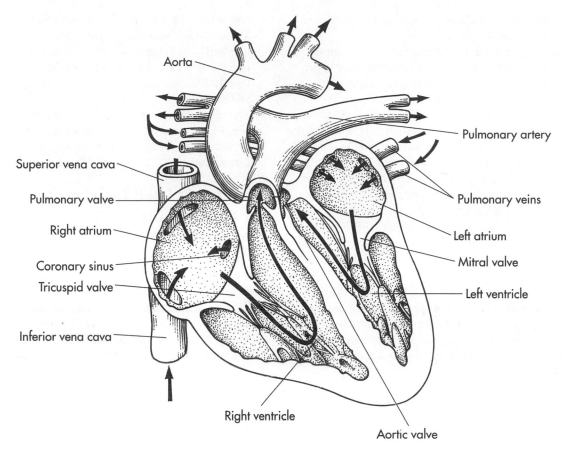

Figure 43-5 Circulation of blood through heart. Arrows indicate direction of flow from superior vena cava and inferior vena cava into right atrium, through tricuspid valve into right ventricle, and through pulmonary valve into pulmonary artery. Blood flows from pulmonary veins into left atrium, through mitral valve into left ventricle, and through aortic valve into aorta.

valve into the pulmonary arteries to the lungs. In summary, there are two circulations:

1. Pulmonary, from the right ventricle to the lungs and back to the left atrium
2. Systemic, from the left ventricle to the aorta, to body tissues and organs, and back to the right atrium

SPECIAL FEATURES OF CARDIAC SURGERY

The principles of general and thoracic surgery apply to cardiac surgery, but several factors require emphasis:

1. Extra minutes are not available; seconds save lives.
2. The team concept is of utmost importance. An experienced team working together can handle emergencies expeditiously.
3. Comprehensive physical and psychologic preparation of the patient precedes a surgical procedure. Postoperatively the patient is taken to an intensive care unit (ICU). The patient is continuously monitored intraoperatively and postoperatively, including during transport to the ICU.

General Considerations

1. The OR for cardiovascular surgery should be equipped with the following:
   a. Cardiac defibrillator, pacemaker, and intraaortic counterpulsation devices.
   b. Cardioplegia (to induce cardiac arrest) and inotropic (to modify cardiac muscle contractility) drugs, including, but not limited to, the following:
      (1) Calcium channel blockers
      (2) Dopamine hydrochloride (Intropin)
      (3) Dobutamine hydrochloride (Dobutrex)
      (4) Epinephrine hydrochloride (Adrenalin)
      (5) Intravenous nitroglycerin
   c. Laboratory facilities for blood gas and acid-base balance determinations. Modern analyzers have microprocessors to determine values.
2. The basic thoracic setup is used with the addition of cardiovascular instruments (i.e., various noncrushing vascular and anastomosis clamps, cardiotomy suction tips and sump tubes, and cardiovascular sutures).
3. Prosthetic devices are sterilized by the manufacturer. Care is taken to maintain sterility during placement in the patient. Many types of valves, patches, grafts, and catheters

are available. They should be biocompatible, nonthrombogenic, and nonbiodegradable.

4. Local and/or systemic hypothermia may be used intraoperatively to reduce the body's need for oxygen and to preserve myocardial function. Commercial preparations of sterile slush for local hypothermia are convenient.

5. Intraoperative autotransfusion is often used for blood volume replacement. Blood substitutes such as hetastarch, an albumin substitute for plasma expansion, may be administered. Properly crossmatched blood should be available for transfusion in the event of excessive blood loss. Platelets, stored at room temperature, may be given after CPB to enhance clotting. Often little or no blood is needed for transfusion in many procedures when CPB is used.

6. Closed water-seal drainage or suction drainage is used postoperatively to drain the mediastinum and/or pleural space(s).

7. Many devices are available for cardiac pacing, ventricular support, and treatment of cardiogenic shock. A portable cardiopulmonary support system, external pulsatile pump, and other devices are used. It is critical that these devices be properly sterilized and handled. Read package labels and inserts for the specific manufacturer's instructions. The circulator should affix labels and record serial numbers and identifying data in the patient's chart. In the event of a mechanical failure, this information becomes important. Lot numbers are logged according to facility policy and procedure.

8. The scrub person should set up a separate table for assembling devices. Check to be certain that all parts are available and functional. A missing component could be catastrophic.

Commonly Used Incisions for Cardiac Surgery
Median Sternotomy

For median sternotomy the patient is supine. A vertical incision extends through the midline from the suprasternal notch to approximately 2 inches below the xiphoid process (Figure 43-6). Retrosternal tissue is dissected. The sternum is split (divided) with a powered sternal saw. Caution is used to avoid injury to underlying mediastinal structures. The blade has a safety guard to prevent penetration into the mediastinum.

Figure 43-6   Median sternotomy. (From Waldenhausen JA, Pierce WS, Campbell DB: *Surgery of the chest,* ed 6, St Louis, 1996, Mosby.)

At closure, heavy-gauge stainless steel sutures are placed around or through the sternum, tightly pulled together, and twisted. The ends are buried in the sternum. Other nonabsorbable sutures may be used to provide firm fixation. The linea alba, subcutaneous tissue, and skin are sutured. Complications are brachial plexus injury, costochondral separation from too vigorous sternal retraction during the surgical procedure, and keloid formation. A median sternotomy incision is used for open heart procedures and pericardiectomy.

Paramedian Thoracotomy

An incision is made to either the immediate left or right of the sternum for minimally invasive cardiac procedures.

Transsternal Bilateral Thoracotomy

A bilateral submammary incision is made with the patient supine for transsternal bilateral thoracotomy. In the midline the incision curves superiorly to cross the sternum at the fourth intercostal space level. Lateral extension is to the midaxillary line. The pleural cavity is entered via the interspace after division of the pectoralis muscles. The internal mammary arteries and veins are ligated and divided. The sternum is divided horizontally.

At closure, the sternum is reapproximated securely, the ribs are approximated with pericostal sutures, and the remaining tissue layers are closed.

This incision is used for resection of a ventricular aneurysm, aortic arch grafts, and complicated pericardiectomies. This incision is less commonly used and causes more discomfort for the patient.

Anterolateral or Posterolateral Thoracotomy

Anterolateral or posterolateral incisions may be preferred for some cardiac procedures, such as valve procedures. For some procedures involving the posterior aspect of the heart, the thoracotomy incision is made on the right side (opposite side) of the chest.

Invasive Hemodynamic Monitoring

Although placement of invasive pressure monitoring lines is not their responsibility, perioperative nurses should be aware of the implications of data and the potential for complications, such as thrombus, embolus, cardiac arrest, and, postoperatively, infection. For assessment of tissue perfusion, invasive hemodynamic monitoring is used to determine blood pressures in major arteries, veins, and the heart chambers. Indwelling catheter lines are inserted to measure the following:

- Radial and femoral artery pressures.
- Central venous pressure (CVP).
- Pulmonary artery pressure. The Swan-Ganz catheter line also determines right atrial, right ventricular, and pulmonary capillary wedge pressures of left ventricular function.

Indwelling intravascular catheters are inserted preoperatively. During a surgical procedure they provide information relative to the effects of anesthetic agents, surgical manipulation of the heart, hypothermia, extracorporeal circulation, induced ischemia, and cardiac arrest. A registered nurse may draw blood samples from the pressure lines at intervals during CPB perfusion for blood gas analysis. Catheter patency is maintained with heparinized flush solutions.

In addition to arterial and CVP pressure lines, during the surgical procedure the surgeon may insert a small plastic catheter directly into the left atrium to assess left atrial pressure. Pulmonary artery pressures may be measured also. Postoperatively these catheters are connected to a transducer and monitor. The atrial transducer balancing port must be level with the right atrium. The catheter is flushed with heparinized 5% dextrose in water because inadvertent overload with this solution is less dangerous than is overload with normal saline. Also, an air filter is attached to the end of the pressure tubing as a precaution against fatal air embolism. Every part of the line and filter must be flushed and free of air, or the pressure bag could force a bubble into the left atrium, causing an embolus. In the absence of mitral valve disease, left atrial pressure at the end of atrial diastole, just before the mitral valve opens, indicates left ventricular end-diastolic pressure and therefore left ventricular filling pressure and function.

Postoperatively, hemodynamic monitoring detects dysrhythmias caused by impaired myocardial perfusion, transient reduction in cardiac output with subsequent hypotension, hypovolemia secondary to hemorrhage, and tamponade. Circulating blood volume, pulmonary volume overload leading to pulmonary edema, and reactions to titrated vasopressor drugs also can be identified.

Intraoperative Monitoring

Noninvasive technologies are used intraoperatively to evaluate the effectiveness of some repairs and/or tissue perfusion. These technologies include the following:

- *Transesophageal echocardiography (TEE).* A transesophageal ultrasound probe is used for assessment of graft patency, myocardial perfusion, adequacy of valve replacement, or ventricular function. A Doppler color flow probe also may be useful to quantitatively assess other repairs.
- *Electrophysiologic measurements.* A computerized mapping system is used to identify the focus of dysrhythmias.
- *Near-infrared reflectance spectroscopy.* A device equipped with a sensor is attached to the patient's head. Light transmitted through the skin and skull to the brain is reflected to light detectors in the sensor. Changes in oxygen levels in the brain change light absorption. These changes may alert the anesthesia provider and surgeon to a developing oxygen deficit.

Cardiopulmonary Bypass

CPB is the technique of oxygenating and perfusing blood by means of a mechanical pump-oxygenator system. This apparatus temporarily substitutes for the function of the patient's heart and lungs during cardiac surgery. CPB is used for most intracardiac (open heart) and coronary artery procedures. Venous blood is diverted from the body to the machine for oxygenation (extracorporeal circulation) and is pumped back to the patient (Figure 43-7).

In preparation for bypass, the patient is heparinized to prevent clot formation within the CPB circuit. Two-stage venous cannulas are inserted into the right atrial appendage. Bicaval cannulation is done by inserting venous cannulas into the inferior and superior vena cavae. A cannula for return of oxygenated blood to the systemic circulation is placed in the ascending aorta or femoral artery. Cannulas are connected to the machine by sterile tubing before institution of bypass. During bypass the lungs are kept deflated and immobilized.

Minimally invasive surgery has given rise to vacuum-assisted venous drainage (VAVD) for the attainment of a bloodless field. This method requires less priming medium for the machine and uses smaller cannulas. VAVD adds negative pressure of −25 to −40 mm Hg to the venous lines for faster decompression of the heart.

The perfusionist who operates the CPB machine must be familiar with its function, care, and operation. The perfusionist may be employed by the cardiac surgeon, a group practice, or the hospital.

Components of a Bypass System

Oxygenator   Oxygen is taken up and carbon dioxide is removed from the blood. The types of oxygenators include the following:

- *Bubble.* Bubbles of oxygen are supplied to the blood by direct blood/gas contact.
- *Membrane.* Oxygen and carbon dioxide diffuse through a permeable Teflon or polyethylene membrane that contains the blood. This method diminishes blood/gas interface. Several types of disposable membrane oxygenators are available.
- *Microporous membrane.* Blood film is separated from ventilating gas by a microporous polypropylene membrane folded like an accordion and operated like a bubble oxygenator. Blood pressure in this oxygenator exceeds gas pressure at all times, thus precluding gas bubbles passing through the microporous membrane.

Heat Exchanger   Incorporated in the circuit, a heat exchanger regulates blood temperature. Water at a thermostatically controlled temperature circulates through the exchanger, which can rapidly produce, control, or correct systemic hypothermia. Hypothermia is often used in conjunction with bypass to reduce oxygen demands of tissues and to protect the myocardium during arrest.

Figure 43-7   Cardiopulmonary bypass circuit. (From Waldenhausen JA, Pierce WS, Campbell DB: *Surgery of the chest,* ed 6, St Louis, 1996, Mosby.)

Pump Rollers turning over sterile plastic tubing propel reheated oxygenated blood in a relatively nonpulsatile flow through a blood filter and bubble trap to the arterial cannula for recirculation through the body. The rate of flow can be varied. It is calculated according to patient weight or body surface area. Reduced flow accompanies hypothermia.

Perfusion

Immediately before the surgical procedure the machine is primed (filled) with a combination of crystalloid and colloid solutions, a balanced electrolyte component, and a cardiopreservative solution including sodium bicarbonate and heparinized plasma volume expander. Some circuits are heparin coated by the manufacturer. For a hemodilution technique of priming, the system is filled with fluid that will replace blood diverted to the pump-oxygenator system and is recirculated through the circuit to remove air bubbles. The priming solution should be of sufficient volume and of a suitable hematocrit level so that when mixed with the patient's blood the resultant buffered plasma will be capable of achieving adequate perfusion and preventing myocardial acidosis. Blood is added as needed to maintain an adequate oxygen-carrying capacity and perfusion rate.

The bypass may be partial or total. In a partial bypass, only a portion of venous return is routed to the pump-oxygenator circuitry; the remaining portion follows the normal systemic circulation. In a total bypass, all venous return is diverted to the machine for total-body perfusion. Purse-string sutures in the vena cava are tightened around the caval cannulas inserted to drain all venous return to the machine. The heart is arrested.

During perfusion the patient is monitored intensely (i.e., arterial and venous pressures, body and blood temperatures, blood gases and electrolytes, and urinary output). General anesthesia may be maintained by an anesthetic vaporizer that adds vapor to the oxygenating mixture or by intravenous anesthesia.

At the conclusion of the defect repair, air is removed from the heart, the patient is rewarmed, the heartbeat is restored, oxygenation is reestablished by mechanical ventilation, and perfusion is gradually decreased to wean the patient from the CPB machine. After discontinuance of bypass, cannulas are removed and purse-string sutures around insertion sites are tied. Protamine sulfate is injected to reverse the effect of the heparin previously administered.

CPB may also be employed in conjunction with deep hypothermia during neurosurgical procedures, in major organ transplantation, and for pulmonary embolectomy. It is also used to assist in the event of ventricular failure, to treat some types of pulmonary dysfunction, and to perfuse an isolated segment of the body for cancer chemotherapy.

Myocardial Preservation

A bloodless, motionless field allows direct vision of the heart and its interior for repair of coronary circulation or intracardiac defects. CPB isolates the heart while the body is perfused with oxygenated blood. Cardiac arrest is purposely induced. During bypass, the perfusionist is in control of the patient's body temperature and preservation of the body and brain. The surgeon assumes responsibility for preservation of the heart. Bypass time is kept to a minimum because ischemia causes myocardial injury of time-related severity. Deliberate arrest may be effected by one or a combination of methods.

Aortic Cross-Clamping The aorta is occluded with a vascular clamp to block systemic circulation. Ischemic (anoxic) cardiac arrest occurs as the blocked systemic blood within the heart becomes deoxygenated and cardiac metabolic needs are depleted. This technique can be maintained for only a limited period, because myocardial damage and necrosis will occur when the oxygen supply and energy required to maintain the subcellular system are depleted. Cerebrospinal fluid pressure may increase.

Cardioplegia Modern, safe cardiac surgery is based on the use of cardioplegic solutions used alone or in combination with other techniques discussed. These are preparations of a small amount of potassium in crystalloid, blood, or other solution. Cardioplegia is delivered by two methods: either by direct antegrade infusion through the coronary ostium or retrograde through the right atrium into the coronary sinus.

When cardioplegic solution is injected into the coronary artery system, hyperkalemia immediately induces complete electromechanical cardiac arrest. The composition and temperature of the solution and infusion techniques can be determined for each patient's disease process. Some solutions have a calcium antagonist, such as verapamil or nifedipine, to help prevent myocardial ischemia. Some are infused warm; others are infused cold. Infusion may be continuous or intermittent. Coronary perfusion pressure during administration of the cardioplegic solution may influence regional delivery. When the solution is flushed out of the collateral circulation at the end of the surgical procedure, the heartbeat may resume spontaneously. If not, ventricular fibrillation is treated with countershock.

Hypothermia Hypothermia reduces systemic metabolic needs and oxygen requirements. It exerts a protective effect during CPB through a temperature-related decrease of intracellular metabolism, thus allowing tissues to tolerate a prolonged period of decreased perfusion. Hypothermia is an essential component to ischemic myocardial preservation, but because of its calcium-loading effect, cardioplegic arrest precedes initiation of hypothermia. Local hypothermia can be induced by topical application of iced saline slush around the heart or iced Ringer's lactate solution to the heart externally and/or internally. Cardiac arrest also can be induced by deliberately lowering systemic body temperature moderately to 78.8° to 89.6° F (26° to 32° C) or deeply to below 78.8° F (26° C). This is achieved by a cooling perfusate in the heart-lung machine.

Complications of Cardiopulmonary Bypass

Although excellent results are obtained with most procedures, significant derangements can occur following CPB. These are most obvious in infants or after prolonged surgical procedures in adults. Alterations in clotting may occur as a result of heparinization of blood, mechanical damage to platelets and clotting factors, and direct exposure of blood to oxygen. If trauma or transfusion reaction hemolyzes red blood cells, viscosity in renal tubules may cause tubular necrosis and renal failure.

Inadequate or extended perfusion and oxygenation may promote tissue anoxia and metabolic acidosis. Fluid and electrolyte balance merit close watching, particularly for hypervolemia. When nonblood fluids are used to prime the pump, they may diffuse into interstitial spaces. As this fluid returns to circulation postoperatively, hypervolemia may result. Furthermore, increased levels of aldosterone and antidiuretic hormone induced by the stress of surgery cause retention of sodium and water. Fluids are restricted for 24 hours postoperatively. Cerebral edema and brain damage at times ensue, for unknown reasons. These developments are generally temporary.

"Post-pump psychosis" consists of visual and auditory hallucinations and paranoid delusions. This often terminates when the patient is transferred from the ICU.

The most severe pulmonary complication of extracorporeal circulation is postperfusion lung syndrome. Its cause is unknown. It is often fatal because of the development of atelectasis, pulmonary edema, and hemorrhage. Metabolic acidosis during bypass may lead to low cardiac output syndrome postoperatively. This occurs most frequently in patients with long histories of cardiac disease. Finally, cardiac tamponade is another potential complication, reflected by a drop of more than 10 mm Hg in systolic blood pressure during the patient's inspiration (pulsus paradoxus).

Diagnostic Procedures

Interference in any part of the circulatory system can jeopardize survival. A surgical procedure is preceded by extensive cardiovascular assessment on the basis of noninvasive and invasive studies that dictate subsequent treatment.

Noninvasive Procedures

Routine examination and electrocardiography are augmented by determination of venous pressure, cardiac output, circulation time, and blood chemistry studies. Chest x-ray examination reveals the heart's size, position, and outline. Screening or functional capacity testing, such as stress testing, is informative. Pulmonary function tests may detect left ventricular failure. Echocardiography with ultrasonic waves reveals the heart structure and gives information pertinent to congenital heart disease and valvular disease. Radionuclide imaging may be used to detect regional reductions in myocardial blood flow and thus help to confirm or deny the diagnosis of myocardial infarction (necrosis of a portion of the myocardium caused by obstruction in a coronary artery).

Invasive Procedures

Radiographic visualization following injection of a nontoxic radiopaque substance permits study of the heart chambers, great vessels, and coronary circulation.

Angiography Angiocardiography, with intravascular injection of a radiopaque substance, permits radiographs of the heart chambers, thoracic vessels, and coronary arteries. Rapid serial radiographs or motion pictures on an enlarged fluoroscopic screen show the heart's outline and the passage of contrast materials in the great vessels. Selective angiocardiography or coronary angiography is done in association with cardiac catheterization to evaluate coronary artery disease and to determine the extent of obstructive disease in the coronary vessels. Aneurysms also may be diagnosed by angiography.

Cardiac Catheterization Under image intensification fluoroscopy, a sterile catheter is introduced through a cutdown into a brachial vessel in the arm or percutaneously into a femoral vessel in the groin and is passed into the heart or a coronary artery. The procedure permits the following:

- Evaluation of heart function
- Measurements of intracardiac pressure
- Visualization of the heart chambers

Catheterization is used to diagnose coronary artery disease, valvular heart disease, or congenital anomalies. It is the ultimate tool for diagnosis of ischemic heart disease.

For study of the coronary arteries, a single catheter is passed, and its tip is inserted into the ostia of the arteries for injection of dye and tracing of solution flow. Cinefluorograms record findings. After removal of the catheter, the incision is closed and pressure dressings are applied.

For right-sided heart catheterization a pulmonary artery catheter is inserted through the vein to obtain pressures in the right atrium and ventricle, pulmonary artery, and pulmonary artery wedge. Measurements of thermodilution, cardiac output, and oxygen saturation also may be obtained. The right internal jugular vein may be cannulated, and a bioptome (a specially designed biopsy forceps) may be advanced to obtain a right endomyocardial biopsy specimen. For left-sided heart catheterization a catheter is inserted into an artery and advanced through the aortic valve into the left ventricle.

Physiologic monitoring with a multichannel recorder is continuous during the procedure. Potential complications include dysrhythmias, air embolus, thrombosis, and vascular and/or cardiac perforation.

CARDIAC SURGICAL PROCEDURES

The purposes of heart surgery are to correct acquired or congenital anatomic abnormalities, repair or replace defective heart valves, revascularize ischemic myocardium, and improve or assist ventricular function. The hours immediately before the surgical procedure can be a highly stressful period for the patient. Mental stress can cause myocardial ischemia (inadequate blood supply to the heart) without symptoms of chest pain. Therefore the patient should be monitored from arrival in the OR suite, through induction of anesthesia, and throughout the surgical procedure. Administration of oxygen before induction of anesthesia may be indicated to help reduce stress. Procedures may be performed with or without CPB.

Valvular Heart Disease

Valvular heart disease may arise from a congenital abnormality or can be acquired. Abnormal vibrations or heart murmurs, referred to as S_3 or S_4, may be congenital or the end result of disease such as rheumatic fever or degenerative change. Valves can become thickened and calcified, resulting in loss of valve substance, narrowing of the orifice, and immobility. They then develop insufficiency, fail to close completely, and permit blood leakage or regurgitation. Failure to open completely is caused by stenosis, which impedes blood flow. A defective valve is reconstructed if possible. If the valve is not repairable or if symptoms return after repair, a prosthetic valve is implanted.

Incisional approaches for valve surgery include median sternotomy and other modifications of thoracotomy. CPB is used for all valve procedures to create and maintain a bloodless field.

Restorative Valve Procedures

Restorative and reparative valve surgery is the preferred procedure for most valve diseases. Reconstruction of the patient's own valve may restore normal valve function. Valvuloplasty and annuloplasty are valve-sparing procedures to maintain structural integrity and ventricular function. An annuloplasty ring, either flexible or nonflexible, may be used for support and to provide continuity and permanence of repair. Thromboembolism is less of a threat than it is following valve replacement; thus anticoagulant therapy is not indicated postoperatively.

Valve Replacement

A diseased mitral or aortic valve may be excised and replaced. Several types of prosthetic heart valves are available. They may be mechanical or biologic. One type of mechanical valve has disks resembling leaflets of human valves. The disks of some are tilted. The metal ring at the base of the cage may be covered with polyester fabric to facilitate suturing. It also encourages tissue ingrowth, an aid to long-term fixation. Biologic valves also have been developed from allograft or xenograft (porcine bioprosthesis or bovine pericardial xenograft) donor material. Cryopreserved fresh aortic valve allografts are carefully thawed before use. Glutaraldehyde storage solution is rinsed thoroughly from xenografts before use.

An effective prosthesis is nontoxic, nonthrombogenic, and nondeteriorating. The surgeon selects the most suitable type and size for the defect to be repaired. Contamination of a valve can cause a serious postoperative endocarditis. Sterility is maintained before and during insertion.

Mitral Valve Replacement Through a median sternotomy, right or left thoracotomy incision, the pericardium is incised and retracted. When bypass cannulas are placed, the left ventricle may be vented with a plastic tube to decompress the heart and prevent overdistention of the ventricle during unclamping of the aorta after anoxic arrest. The atrium is opened, depending on the approach. The mitral valve is exposed, inspected, and removed by circumferential excision and severance of muscular attachments to the ventricular wall. The surgeon usually prefers to leave the chordae tendineae and papillary muscles intact. The fibrous ring or annulus surrounding the valvular opening remains intact. A sterile prosthetic valve is inserted and sutured in place, and the atrium is sutured. Teflon felt pledgets are commonly used as a buttress under the sutures to prevent the annulus from tearing when the prosthetic valve is seated and the sutures are tied.

The probability of thromboembolic complications in a patient with chronic atrial fibrillation and an enlarged left atrium is sufficient to warrant postoperative anticoagulant therapy. Therefore a durable synthetic mechanical prosthetic device may be the valve of choice for this procedure.

Pacing wires are implanted in the wall of the right and left ventricles during the surgical procedure. Then the pericardium is closed. Air is removed from the heart, and blood flow is resumed. Partial CPB is resumed as the patient is being weaned from the machine. The incisions are closed, and closed water-seal chest drainage is used.

Aortic Valve Replacement The surgical procedure for aortic valve replacement is basically the same as that described for mitral valve replacement except that the aortic valve is exposed through a transverse incision in the aorta. Either a mechanical valve or bioprosthesis may be used. Biologic prostheses offer the advantage of a low embolic rate and obviate the need for prolonged anticoagulation therapy. Cryopreserved fresh aortic valve allograft, from either a donor bank or commercially available allograft, may be preferred. The aortic valve may be replaced with the patient's own pulmonary valve (i.e., an autograft).

Percutaneous Transluminal Balloon Valvuloplasty

An interventional cardiac catheterization procedure, balloon valvuloplasty may be an option to treat valvular stenosis in a high-risk patient who cannot tolerate valve replacement. A catheter with a deflated balloon is inserted under fluoroscopy across a stenosed aortic, pulmonary, tricuspid, or mitral valve. The balloon is repeatedly inflated until the valve is opened.

Coronary Artery Disease

Coronary arteries supplying the myocardium may become stenosed or obstructed, which is referred to as occlusive coronary artery disease or ischemic heart disease. Resultant myocardial ischemia may result in angina or myocardial infarction. Occlusive disease of the coronary arteries characteristically affects vessels in their proximal segments and at the origin of major branches. Significant obstructions occur most frequently in the right coronary, right posterior descending, left anterior descending, and circumflex arteries. More than one artery can be occluded. Revascularization to improve blood supply to the myocardium is possible by surgical intervention in selected patients.

Coronary Artery Bypass Graft

Single or multiple arterial bypasses are done, depending on the number of vessels affected and the degree of obstruction present. The internal mammary (thoracic) artery and segments of saphenous and cephalic veins are used to bypass coronary artery obstruction. The gastroepiploic, inferior epigastric, splenic, and radial arteries also may be used as free grafts. Cryopreserved saphenous vein and umbilical vein allografts also are used. Most cardiac surgeons wear loupes for magnification while constructing an anastomosis between the graft and the coronary artery.

The chest is opened by median sternotomy or some other thoracotomy incision for minimal access, and the pericardium is incised. CPB is established; techniques are influenced by the surgeon's preferred procedure and the extent of grafting. After the conduit or graft is anastomosed, CPB is discontinued; all incisions are closed and checked for leaks. The patient is hemodynamically stabilized. The wound is closed in the usual manner for sternotomy with closed water-seal chest drainage.

A patient with a heavily calcified aorta is at risk for embolization and/or dissection of the great vessels. In extreme circumstances bypass to the right coronary or left anterior descending artery can be performed without arresting the heart or using CPB. Bleeding is controlled with small clamps and occlusion with vessel loops. The heart is closely monitored for ischemia. CPB is instituted as an emergency measure if the heart tissue fails to perfuse adequately during the procedure.

Internal Mammary Artery Conduit Because of its long-term patency rate, at least one internal mammary artery is used as a conduit for myocardial revascularization. The left internal mammary artery is dissected up to its origin from the subclavian artery, freeing it from the retrosternal aspect of the chest wall (Figure 43-8). After mobilization the pericardium is notched to minimize the distance to the coronary artery. Side-to-side or end-to-side anastomosis is performed primarily between the internal mammary artery and the left anterior descending coronary artery, distal to the obstruction. The right internal mammary artery will reach vessels supplying all but the posterolateral wall of the left ventricle. To provide adequate drainage without tension on the arterial conduit, the pericardium is not sutured. Segments of either right, left, or both internal mammary arteries also are used as free grafts to bypass other diseased coronary arteries.

Saphenous Vein Graft The procedure for a saphenous vein bypass graft is expedited by two teams: one har-

Figure 43-8 Internal mammary artery procurement using mounted self-retaining retractor. (Courtesy Rultract, Inc., Cleveland, Ohio.)

vests the saphenous vein for the graft while the other opens the chest and prepares for CPB (Figure 43-9). Methods for saphenous procurement include the open method and the endoscopic approach (Figure 43-10). An adequate length of vein is removed to obtain sufficient graft material. The distal end of each vein segment is identified, and the graft is placed in heparinized normal saline solution after it has been harvested. It is handled gently to avoid trauma to the intima. The vein is reversed to permit a normal direction of blood flow through the venous valves into the aorta. The affected coronary artery is opened distal to the obstruction; the proximal end of the saphenous vein is anastomosed end-to-side to the artery, creating the distal anastomosis, thus bypassing the obstruction. Usually a fine 6-0 or 7-0 monofilament nonabsorbable suture is used. The proximal anastomosis is established by creating a small opening in the aorta with a punch and suturing the distal end of the vein to the aperture. Saphenous or other vein or artery bypass grafts are completed before the internal mammary artery is anastomosed to form a vascular conduit. Manipulation of the heart could stress the anastomosis.

Radial Artery Conduit An arterial conduit is preferred for patients who have had previous vein grafting or who may be at greater risk for clotting a new vein graft. Arterial grafts have a decreased incidence of clotting when used as a conduit. The radial artery arises 1 cm distal to the brachial

Figure 43-9   Open saphenous vein procurement. (From Waldenhausen JA, Pierce WS, Campbell DB: *Surgery of the chest,* ed 6, St Louis, 1996, Mosby.)

Figure 43-10   Endoscopic saphenous vein procurement.

artery and terminates at the distal aspect in the palmar artery. The harvested segment may measure between 12 and 25 cm. The end diameters measure between 3 and 5 mm. The procured segment is usually taken from the patient's nondominant hand.

Coronary Artery Angioplasty

Restoration of perfusion from the left coronary system is possible by direct enlargement of the left main coronary artery lumen in selected patients in whom clinical circumstances preclude bypass grafting. A curved incision is made in the lateral aortic wall. Either the posterior or anterior aspect of the left main coronary artery is incised across the stenosis. An autologous onlay pericardial or onlay saphenous vein patch is sutured between the artery and the aortic wall.

Endarterectomy (removal of an organized thrombus and attached endothelium or atherosclerotic fatty plaques from the arterial wall) may be performed in conjunction with left coronary angioplasty or right coronary bypass grafting. Small spatulas, wire loops, miniature abrasive drills, or ultrasonic devices may be used to remove plaque.

Laser angioplasty removes plaque in coronary arteries distal to the site for an anastomosis. A handheld excimer or a CO_2 laser may be used. The CO_2 laser may also be used for canalization of the myocardium. Tiny channels are created through the wall of the left ventricle into the myocardium. Blood seeps into sinusoids to revascularize the myocardium.

Coronary artery angioplasty procedures usually are performed in the cardiac catheterization laboratory or special interventional procedures room in the radiology department. A standby OR team should be available for emergency coronary artery bypass in the event that acute coronary artery obstruction or perforation occurs.

Percutaneous Transluminal Coronary Angioplasty
Percutaneous transluminal coronary angioplasty is performed under fluoroscopy with image intensification. Balloon dilation of the coronary arteries may be the procedure of choice for selected patients with significant atherosclerotic narrowing in a major coronary artery (Figure 43-11). The coronary arteries are approached by either percutaneous femoral artery entry or brachial artery cutdown. A balloon-tipped catheter is passed through a guiding catheter into the area of the coronary artery with atherosclerotic material (plaque). The balloon is inflated by a hydraulic pump to compress plaque against the arterial lining and dilate the arterial wall, thus enlarging the lumen. During the time the balloon is inflated, normal flow of oxygen supplied by the artery to the myocardium is interrupted. Oxygenation distal to the balloon may be maintained with oxygenated perfluorochemical emulsion (Fluosol) flowing through the catheter.

Catheters with ultrasonic devices or tiny drill heads may be used to pulverize atherosclerotic plaque before balloon dilation. Other procedures may be performed as an alternative to or in conjunction with balloon angioplasty.

Laser Angioplasty
An argon laser probe, an Nd:YAG optical fiber, or a pulsed excimer laser may be used for laser angioplasty. An integrated system combines direct laser energy and fiberoptics with a balloon angioplasty catheter. The catheter positions the laser fiber, which then vaporizes the plaque or thrombus obstructing the coronary vessels.

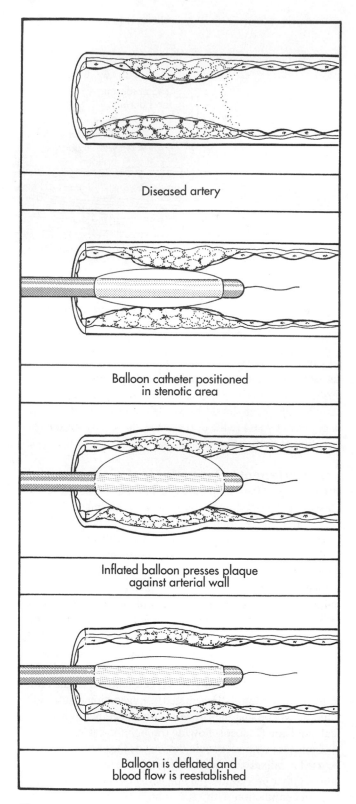

Diseased artery

Balloon catheter positioned
in stenotic area

Inflated balloon presses plaque
against arterial wall

Balloon is deflated and
blood flow is reestablished

Figure 43-11 Balloon angioplasty. (From Canobbio MM: *Cardiovascular disorders,* St Louis, 1990, Mosby.)

Intracoronary Stent A stent may be inserted to act as a buttress to keep an artery open. The coronary artery to be stented should be at least 3 mm in diameter. The stent, which is permanently implanted at the site of the stenosis, widens the arterial lumen by compressing atherosclerotic plaque against the arterial wall. The stainless steel mesh or spring-like coil stent is tightly wrapped around a balloon catheter. As the balloon is inflated, the stent expands. After the balloon is deflated and removed, the stent remains in place to provide structural support and keep the artery from collapsing.

Cardiac Dysrhythmias

Some cardiac rhythm disorders are unresponsive to drug therapy. Normally the electrical cardiac impulse begins at the SA node, thus controlling the rhythm of the heart rate. Fibers from the SA node conduct the impulse through the atria into the AV node and then transmit it along the bundle of His into the ventricles, ending in Purkinje fibers. Occasionally some other part of the heart develops a rhythmic discharge with a rate more rapid than the SA node. This causes tachycardia (a rapid heartbeat). The impulse also may repeatedly reenter the system, most often at the AV node–bundle of His junction (AV junction), causing overstimulation of the heart. With epicardial and endocardial mapping techniques, the surgeon is able to pinpoint electrical activity causing dysrhythmia. Preoperatively the mapping procedure is done under fluoroscopy. Electrical impulses from electrode catheters, placed in the heart via a femoral vein, activate sites in the heart to reproduce the abnormal rhythm and to obtain a direct electrocardiogram. Premature cycles, the origin of electrical signals, and accessory pathways can be pinpointed. Intraoperative mapping may be needed to correlate preoperative studies or to identify other sites or pathways masked by antiarrhythmic drugs. The origin and site of a dysrhythmia determine the surgical procedure.

Endocardial Resection

Severe ventricular dysrhythmias associated with ischemic heart disease and malignant ventricular tachydysrhythmias can be treated by ablating areas of endocardial damage (i.e., endocardial resection). The specific site or focus of the ventricular dysrhythmia is excised, or the reentry pathway is interrupted. Atrial incisions may be made to channel electrical impulses from the SA node to the AV node to treat atrial focal tachycardia.

Cryoablation

When the location of a ventricular tachycardia makes excision difficult, cryosurgery can be used to ablate the site. Cryoablation is also used to fuse the ends of fibers causing reentrant dysrhythmias from accessory pathways, as in Wolff-Parkinson-White syndrome. This syndrome is characterized by premature atrial beats that initiate supraventricular tachycardia or atrial fibrillation that can cause ventricular fibrillation. Many patients with this syndrome require cardioversion intraoperatively; thus external defibrillator pads are placed before the patient is draped. Partial CPB also is used as a precaution against hypotension and coronary damage from induced tachycardia during mapping and cardiac manipulation. Temporary pacing wires are sewn onto the heart (see Cardiac Pacemaker) before the chest is closed.

Balloon Electric Shock Ablation

For balloon electric shock ablation, CPB is established and a small incision is made in the left atrium. A deflated balloon is passed through this incision and across the mitral valve into the left ventricle. The balloon is inflated to make contact with the endocardium for mapping with the electrodes inside the balloon. Electric currents are passed through these electrodes to deliver electric shock to specific locations selected for ablation. Endocardial resection or cryoablation may be preferred when the focus of ventricular tachycardia is mapped intraoperatively using the balloon.

Ventricular Aneurysm

Atherosclerotic coronary disease predisposes an individual to myocardial infarction. Ventricular aneurysm (a segmental dilation of the ventricular wall) may develop any time from a few weeks to years after infarction. Predominantly occurring in the left ventricular wall, the aneurysm results from ventricular force on an area of nonfunctioning scar tissue. The thin-walled fibrous aneurysm often contains clots within it. A left ventricular aneurysm usually produces hemodynamic instability manifested by congestive heart failure and ventricular dysrhythmia. The surgeon can excise the aneurysm and reconstruct the ventricle.

The chest is opened by median sternotomy. CPB is established before the adhesion between the aneurysm and pericardium is detached. The ascending aorta is cross-clamped. The aneurysmal sac is opened with a vertical incision. Fibrotic myocardium is excised circumferentially, leaving a rim of fibrous tissue to hold the sutures used to close the ventricle. Before completion of closure, air is removed from the ventricle by suction. The heartbeat is restored, decannulation is performed, and all incisions are closed.

Aneurysmectomy may be done as a single procedure or in conjunction with cardiomyoplasty, valve replacement, coronary artery bypass, or endocardial resection.

Cardiomyoplasty

A skeletal muscle flap can be used to reinforce the damaged heart muscle (i.e., perform cardiomyoplasty) in patients who are not candidates for cardiac transplantation because of medical contraindications or other exclusionary problems. Structurally, skeletal muscle is different from myocardial muscle and is more easily fatigued. After conditioning by electrical stimulation for several weeks preoperatively, the skeletal muscle is less prone to fatigue and endures repeated contraction at a normal heart rate caused by an implanted stimulator.

The two-step cardiomyoplasty procedure can be performed in a single surgical procedure or in two stages for patients who are unable to withstand long periods under general anesthesia. In step 1, with the patient in the left thoracotomy position, a muscle flap of latissimus dorsi, rectus abdominis, pectoralis, psoas, or diaphragm is dissected free. A small segment of the second or third rib is resected to form a window through which the flap is rotated upward into the mediastinum. Intramuscular pacing wires are woven into the musculature of the flap. In step 2, with the patient supine, a sternotomy is performed. The flap is wrapped around the damaged portion of the myocardium and secured around the heart. The pericardium is not sutured closed. A small pocket is made in the skin of the upper abdomen, and a generator is implanted and attached subcutaneously to the ends of the pacing wires.

CPB is not routinely used during the procedure, but it is available on a standby basis if needed. Postoperatively some patients require ventricular counterpulsation with an intraaortic balloon pump until the muscle flap is fully functional. Postoperatively the stimuli for contraction is started at week 2 and gradually increased over a 4- to 6-week period so that the newly attached flap is not disrupted before proper healing has occurred. After 4 to 6 months the flap–myocardial contraction ratio can reach 1:1 or 1:2. Contraindications to cardiomyoplasty include a hypertrophic myocardium and end-stage cardiac disease because the muscle flap is unable to contract sufficiently over the thickened cardiac wall.

Cardiac Transplantation

Cardiac transplantation may be an acceptable option for the patient with limited life expectancy who is incapacitated by end-stage myocardial disease secondary to the following:

- Valvular disease with cardiomyopathy
- Coronary artery disease
- Postmyocardial aneurysm
- Idiopathic cardiomyopathy
- Congenital heart disease
- Cardiac tumor

Mechanical Assist Devices

Mechanical assist devices may be indicated for patients with cardiac dysfunction. These devices may be implanted in conjunction with other cardiac surgical procedures or to provide long-term assistance for life-sustaining cardiac function.

Cardiac Pacemaker

The conducting system of the heart may be altered or interrupted at any point by degenerative disease, drugs, or surgical trauma. This may cause syncope, diminished cardiac output, hypotension, dysrhythmias, partial or complete heart block, or sinus bradycardia (sick sinus syndrome). Patients with these conditions may be treated by artificial pacing (i.e., delivery of an electrical impulse by a pacemaker) to correct atrial and ventricular dysrhythmias and to interrupt chronic atrial fibrillation.

A pacemaker consists of a pulse generator, which produces electrical impulses, and leads to carry impulses to stimulating electrodes placed in contact with the heart (Figure 43-12). A pacing system includes electromyocardial conduction. Lithium batteries supply power for years to the microprocessor of the pulse generator. Platinum alloy or stainless steel electrodes, with leads encased in plastic, may be unipolar or bipolar. With bipolar systems, electric current flows between two electrodes during pacing; it flows between the electrode tip and the pulse generator in unipolar systems.

A pacemaker may be either a standby ventricular demand type or a physiologic type. Both types are intermittent and noncompetitive with the patient's own pacing system. They monitor the heart's normal activity. The impulse to stimulate the heart is not emitted unless the rate of the heartbeat falls below a preset level. Also known as the R wave–inhibited or QRS-inhibited pacemaker, electrodes of the ventricular demand pacemaker are placed in the ventricle. Stimulating electrodes are placed in the atrium or ventricle, or both, depending on the type of physiologic pacemaker to be used.

Effective external pacing for ventricular standstill led to the development of partially implanted electrode leads connected to an external stimulator for long-term pacing for other conditions. Fully implantable pacemaker systems for long-term use have been available since 1960. An implantable mi-croprocessor generator is hermetically sealed in a metallic container impermeable to body fluids. Selection of a system depends on the specific pacing requirements of the individual patient. Pacemakers may be temporary or permanent. Endocardial (transvenous) or epicardial (myocardial) electrode leads may be used. Most of these units are programmable to alter pacing function. Temporary pacing is often necessary before and during permanent-system implantation. Systemic complete heart block and sinus bradycardia are the most frequent indications for permanent-system implantation. A single-chamber ventricular pacemaker may be implanted. The dual-chamber pacemaker, most commonly in the DDD mode (Table 43-1), senses and synchronously paces both chambers and triggers or inhibits the response to vary the ventricular rate with the atrial rate. Permanent pacing may be initiated by the following devices.

Endocardial Pacemaker A transvenous electrode lead is placed in the endocardium and attached to a pulse generator. With the patient under local anesthesia, an incision is made just beneath the clavicle or in the deltopectoral groove, preferably on the side of the chest opposite the patient's dominant hand. The subcutaneous tissue is opened to underlying fascia to create a pocket for the pulse generator. The lead may be inserted through the cephalic, subclavian, or internal or external jugular vein. Under fluoroscopy the endocardial electrode catheter (lead) is advanced via the superior vena cava into the apex of the right ventricle, where it is wedged against the endocardium. Atrial leads are directed into the right atrial appendage. The lead is connected to the pulse generator, which in turn is placed into a previously prepared subcutaneous pocket. The incision is closed with or without suction drainage.

Epicardial Electrodes With the patient under general anesthesia, epicardial electrodes are placed via a transthoracic approach to the myocardium. For an extrapleural parasternal approach, the pericardium is entered by subperichondrial resection of the fifth costal cartilage. Two sew-on

Figure 43-12 Cardiac pacemaker. (From Waldenhausen JA, Pierce WS, Campbell DB: *Surgery of the chest,* ed 6, St Louis, 1996, Mosby.)

TABLE 43-1	**Identification Code for Cardiac Pacemakers***			
First Letter (Chamber Paced)	**Second Letter (Chamber Sensed)**	**Third Letter (Mode of Response to Sensing of Patient's Heart Rate)**	**Fourth Letter (Programmable Functions)**	**Fifth Letter (Tachyarrhythmia Function)**
A = Atrium	A = Atrium	I = Inhibited response	P = Programmable rate and output only	N = Normal rate
V = Ventricle	V = Ventricle	T = Triggered response	M = Multiprogrammable	B = Bursts
D = Dual/both chambers	D = Dual/both chambers	D = Dual function/ inhibited and triggered response	C = Communicating noninvasive program	S = Scanning
	O = No sensing	R = Reverse response	O = Nonprogrammable	E = External
		O = No response		

*Sequence of letters describes parameters and functions.

or screw-in–type electrodes are implanted 1 cm apart in the myocardium of the right or left ventricle and/or atrium. After the pacing thresholds are measured from an external source, electrode leads are tunneled under the costal margin to the pulse generator implanted in a subcutaneous pocket in the left upper quadrant of the abdominal wall. Water-seal chest drainage is necessary only if the pleura has been opened.

Precautions with Pacemakers
Use of an electrosurgical unit is usually avoided during placement of a pacemaker or when a surgical procedure is performed on a patient with a pacemaker. Electromagnetic interference may affect the pulse generator, depending on the type of pacemaker. If it is necessary to use the electrosurgical unit, it should be kept as far away from the pulse generator as possible. The dispersive electrode should be placed on the thigh area, not near the chest.

A pacing system analyzer measures the amount of energy in milliamperes (mA) needed to stimulate the heart. It is used to locate the area of the myocardium where the least amount of energy will be needed (generally 0.4 to 0.8 mA) and to test functioning of the electrode and pulse generator before placement. Telemetric communication capabilities of some pacemakers allow the surgeon to obtain direct evidence of battery output.

The patient with a pacemaker requires adequate follow-up care. He or she should carry identification containing the serial number, model, rate, manufacturer's name, and date of insertion. The circulator records this information in the patient's chart, along with the time of insertion. Patients with demand or radiofrequency units should be warned to avoid proximity to electromagnetic devices, such as microwave ovens, because electrical interference may stimulate heart activity. Newer models have metallic shielding to minimize this concern.

Battery depletion is the most common indication for replacement of the pulse generator. The old generator is removed from the subcutaneous pocket. A new one is connected to the electrode and inserted into the pocket. Occasionally, electrode problems and/or erosion of or infection around the generator require surgical intervention.

Cardioverter-Defibrillator

The automatic implantable cardioverter-defibrillator (ICD) has the capability of recognizing potential life-threatening episodes of ventricular tachycardia or fibrillation. The system has a pair of sensing electrodes to monitor changes in the heart rate, cycle length, and waveform (Figure 43-13). After the onset of ventricular tachycardia, two defibrillating electrodes deliver a synchronized shock to terminate it. The electrical conduction pattern of the heart is converted to a more normal pattern. Newer models are capable of pacing, as well as defibrillating. Supplied sterile, the pulse generator of the device is powered by lithium batteries hermetically sealed in a titanium case. The device may be implanted in addition to endocardial resection or other ablation, or instead of a surgical procedure for dysrhythmia. Placement of this

device is similar to procedures described for implantation of cardiac pacemakers.

The wavelength of the electrosurgical unit or magnetic field of magnetic resonance imaging (MRI) can deprogram the ICD and cause the device to discharge aberrant electric current into the myocardium. A specialized electromagnetic wand can be placed over the chest to deactivate the device for subsequent surgical procedures requiring the use of electrosurgery. The same electromagnetic wand can be used to reactivate and reprogram the ICD. ICDs are not affected by household appliances, such as microwave ovens, computer terminals, or television sets.

Intraaortic Balloon Pump

An intraaortic balloon pump (IABP) is a left ventricular supportive device used to assist a patient with prolonged myocardial ischemia, reversible left ventricular failure, or cardiogenic shock. It often is inserted in the OR in conjunction with an open heart procedure for circulatory support during weaning from CPB. An IABP reduces left ventricular workload and increases delivery of oxygen to the myocardium, thereby increasing cardiac output and systemic perfusion. An IABP cannot be effective without partial ventricular function.

The cylinder-shaped balloon is inserted into the descending thoracic aorta, just below the left subclavian artery, by way of a femoral artery (Figure 43-14). The balloon catheter may be inserted percutaneously or by direct vision, or it can be inserted via a prosthetic arterial graft anastomosed end-

Figure 43-13 Implantable defibrillator. (Courtesy Medtronic, Inc., Minneapolis, Minn.)

Left subclavian artery

Descending thoracic aorta

Renal artery

Figure 43-14 Intraaortic balloon catheter positioned in descending thoracic aorta, above renal artery and below left subclavian artery, via femoral artery.

to-side to the femoral artery. After insertion, the balloon catheter is connected to a pump console.

The IABP uses principles of counterpulsation. In contrast to systemic arteries, coronary arteries are constricted during systole and fill during diastole. Therefore inflating the balloon during diastole increases coronary perfusion, aiding contractility and oxygen transport. When the balloon is inflated, the blood volume displaced increases coronary artery pressure. When the balloon deflates during systole, the resistance against which the ventricle pumps is decreased. Balloons vary in size to provide 20, 30, or 40 ml of volume displacement, thus giving a maximum assist without total aortic occlusion. When the balloon is placed and the position is verified by chest x-ray film, the complete system is vented of air and filled with either helium or carbon dioxide for balloon inflation, depending on the type of counterpulsator. The ratio of ventricular assist is determined by the individual patient's hemodynamic status. The pump can be regulated automatically, triggered by an electrocardiogram signal, or operated manually. To prevent potential thrombi, pumping should be continuous. Intraaortic balloons are made of antithrombic

material. The manufacturer's instructions for use should be followed. Pumps are equipped with sensors (e.g., alarm and automatic shut-off) to minimize danger.

Weaning from the IABP is usually gradual, as tolerated by the patient. Lower extremity pulses are checked during and periodically after balloon catheter removal to assess circulation in the foot on the side of the catheter insertion and to check for the presence of clots. Complications associated with an IABP include distal extremity ischemia, thrombus or emboli, gas embolism, arterial or aortic perforation, bleeding, and infection.

Ventricular Assist Device

A powered ventricular assist device (VAD) can be used to wean patients from CPB when the IABP, drugs, and/or cardiac pacing are ineffective, to support circulation following postinfarction cardiogenic shock or traumatic myocardial contusion, and to provide a temporary bridge for support before transplantation. The mechanical device maintains systemic and myocardial perfusion while promoting metabolic and hemodynamic recovery of a reversibly damaged myocardium. The VAD does not depend on cardiac contractility or electrical conduction. It acts as an artificial ventricle. The VAD consists of a flexible polyurethane blood sac, a flexible diaphragm, and a pump assembly enclosed within a rigid polysulfone housing. Inlet and outlet valves maintain unidirectional blood flow. The VAD is attached to the patient via inflow and outflow cannulas. Support can be to the left, right, or both ventricles:

- *Left ventricular assistance (LVA).* Blood is withdrawn from the left atrium into a left ventricular assist device (LVAD) and returned to the ascending aorta. The polyurethane inflow cannula can be inserted into either the left atrium or the left ventricle. The outflow cannula has a segment of woven polyester that is anastomosed end-to-side to the thoracic aorta.
- *Right ventricular assistance (RVA).* Blood is withdrawn from the right atrium into the right ventricular assist device (RVAD) and is returned to the pulmonary artery. The inflow cannula is placed in the right atrium. The outflow cannula is anastomosed end-to-side to the main pulmonary artery.
- *Biventricular assistance (BVA).* Both an LVAD and an RVAD are used to support both ventricles simultaneously.

The cannulas exit the pericardial sac below the costal margin. They are connected to parts of the VAD after removal of all air. Depending on the intended duration of support, the housing is exteriorized or implanted:

1. Extracorporeal VAD, used for short-term ventricular assistance, is externally powered pneumatically with compressed air or electrically with centrifugal force. The housing rests on the patient's chest, with the inflow and outflow cannulas passing through the chest wall. The power source is attached to the air-inlet port

or pump head. The skin is approximated, or the chest is left open and covered with sterile material sutured to the wound edges. Then the chest is covered with a sterile occlusive dressing. The patient returns to the OR for removal of the device and chest closure or heart transplantation, usually within 10 days.

2. Implantable VAD, for long-term use, is an electrically activated pump implanted in the left upper quadrant of the abdomen. The internal battery pack and control unit in the housing are connected to an external battery pack. The cannulas pass through the diaphragm.

The rate of pumping and movement of the diaphragm inside the VAD are programmed by the power console. Another type of LVAD is mounted on a catheter connected to a pump and external motor. The catheter, inserted via the femoral artery or by transthoracic or retroperitoneal approach, draws blood out of the left ventricle and returns it to the descending aorta.

Extracorporeal Membrane Oxygenator

An extracorporeal membrane oxygenator (ECMO) is used as a resuscitative device for patients who have potentially reversible respiratory and/or cardiac failure. It is also commonly used to prolong extracorporeal circulation when the patient is in distress after removal from CPB.

Total Artificial Heart

Clinical trials are in process to test an artificial heart that can be permanently implanted to maintain circulation in the patient with irreparable myocardial damage or end-stage cardiac disease who does not meet the criteria for cardiac transplantation. A total artificial heart also could be used as temporary support while the patient is awaiting a transplant.

In 1982 William DeVries implanted the first total artificial heart. The Jarvik-7 was an air-driven, double-chambered device that replaced the ventricles. Connector cuffs were sutured to the atria, pulmonary artery, and aorta. These cuffs attached to rims of openings on the device. Power was supplied to the pumping chamber through percutaneous tubes to an external source of compressed air. The patient was essentially tethered to a machine. Many complications, such as emboli, hemorrhage, and infection, were associated with the device.

A newer, totally contained artificial heart is powered electrically with the addition of a hydraulic actuator that will increase cardiac output during exercise and decrease the potential for hematologic complications. A double-diaphragm type of pump is implanted in the chest to work in place of the ventricles. The power source is smaller and quieter than that of the Jarvik-7 and connects to the device via cables through the skin. The efficiency and compactness of the unit permit limited activity.

To date, there has not been a permanent total artificial heart. Complications include thromboembolism and infection. The VAD has been a significant bridge to transplantation and is useful for cardiac support until a suitable donor is available (Figure 43-15).

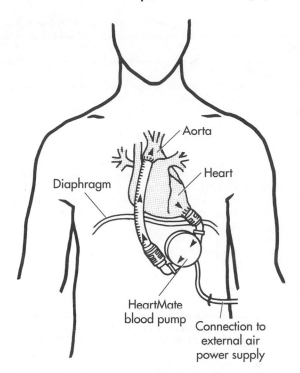

Figure 43-15 HeartMate ventricular assist device. (Courtesy Thermo Cardiosystems, Inc., Woburn, Mass.)

COMPLICATIONS OF CARDIAC SURGERY

Cardiogenic shock may be precipitated by coronary air embolism, pulmonary embolism, myocardial contusion, mechanical venous obstruction, or hypothermia. Precautions are taken intraoperatively to avoid postoperative cardiogenic and/or hemorrhagic shock. Excessive bleeding can result from stress to the clotting mechanism. Cardiac tamponade (the filling of the pericardial sac with blood, thus compressing the heart) is potentially fatal. Sinus bradycardia, supraventricular tachycardia, ventricular tachycardia, and other dysrhythmias are common in the immediate postoperative period following open heart surgery. Infections of the sternum and/or mediastinum may require additional surgical intervention, such as muscle grafting and debridement. Infection of the cardiac suture line can be a fatal complication. Infection of a prosthetic valve or implanted device can cause endocarditis, malfunction, hemodynamic abnormalities, or embolus. Attention to sterile technique and patient monitoring is especially critical during cardiac surgery.

Bibliography

Antonioli LC, Bennett HC: Vein harvesting for coronary bypass surgery: the RN first assistant's role, *AORN J* 59(5):969-982, 1994.

Bower JO: New therapy for ventricular arrhythmias: implantable cardioverter/defibrillators with pacing therapies, *AORN J* 59(5):985-996, 1994.

Bower JO: The Ross procedure for replacement of diseased aortic valves, *AORN J* 64(6):966, 969-972, 1996.

Brunet F et al: Extracorporeal carbon dioxide removal technique improves oxygenation without causing overinflation, *Am J Respir Crit Care Med* 149(6):1557-1562, 1994.

Chapek PE: A review of minimally invasive cardiac surgery, *Semin Periop Nurs* 6(3):165-169, 1997.

Collins MA: When your patient has an implantable cardioverter defibrillator, *Am J Nurs* 94(3):34-38, 1994.

Coulson AS et al: Mimimally invasive direct coronary artery bypass surgery, *AORN J* 66(6):1012-1037, 1997.

Coulson AS et al: Right thoracotomy approach to mitral valve surgical procedures, *AORN J* 65(2):347-364, 1997.

Donn SM: Alternatives to ECMO, *Arch Dis Child* 70(2):81-83, 1994.

Dougherty KG et al: Laser ablation of coronary arteries: preliminary findings, *AORN J* 54(2):244-261, 1991.

Ergin MA et al: Hypothermic circulatory arrest and other methods of cerebral protection during operations on the thoracic aorta, *J Cardiovasc Surg* 9(5):525-527, 1994.

Gallegos-Alvarez M, O'Brien M: Right gastroepiploic artery conduit use in myocardial revascularization, *AORN J* 60(5):763-777, 1994.

Gavaghan M: Cardiac anatomy and physiology: a review, *AORN J* 67(4): 802-822, 1998.

Hayashida N et al: The optimal cardioplegic temperature, *Ann Thorac Surg* 58(4):961-971, 1994.

Kurose M et al: Emergency and long-term extracorporeal life support following acute myocardial infarction: rescue from severe cardiogenic shock related to stunned myocardium, *Clin Cardiol* 17(10): 552-557, 1994.

Martella AT et al: Continuous normothermic retrograde cardioplegia for valve surgery, *J Heart Valve Dis* 3(4):404-409, 1994.

May D, Daley K: Percutaneous transluminal coronary angioplasty: study of open heart surgical standby: effective patient, OR management, *AORN J* 59(4):811-819, 1994.

McEwen DR: Postoperative complications related to coronary artery bypass grafting, *AORN J* 60(6):982-988, 1994.

McLean RF et al: Cardiopulmonary bypass, temperature, and central nervous system dysfunction, *Circulation* 90(5):250-255, 1994.

Phillips SJ: Resuscitation for cardiogenic shock with extracorporeal membrane oxygenation systems, *Semin Thorac Cardiovasc Surg* 6(3):131-135, 1994.

Plotkin JS et al: Extracorporeal membrane oxygenation in the successful treatment of traumatic adult respiratory distress syndrome: case report and review, *J Trauma* 37(1):127-130, 1994.

Quaal SJ: *Comprehensive intra-aortic balloon counterpulsation,* ed 2, St Louis, 1993, Mosby.

Schooler MP: A clinical pathway for patients undergoing minimally invasive direct artery bypass surgery, *AORN J* 67(1):237-241, 1998.

Seifert PC: *Cardiac surgery,* St Louis, 1994, Mosby.

Starling RC: Radical alternatives to transplantation, *Curr Opin Cardiol* 12(2):166-171, 1997.

Strimike CL: Caring for a patient with an intracoronary stent, *Am J Nurs* 95(1):40-45, 1995.

Wisniowski C, Stephen L: Minimally invasive treatment for coronary artery disease, *AORN J* 66(6):1002-1009, 1997.

Chapter 44

Peripheral Vascular Surgery

Chapter Objectives

After studying this chapter, the learner will be able to:

- Identify the pertinent anatomy of the peripheral vascular system.
- Describe the potential complications associated with peripheral vascular disease.
- Describe the care of the patient with peripheral vascular disease.

Circulation within the peripheral vascular system affects the brain, internal organs, and extremities. An expanding body of knowledge relating to vascular physiology and the development of the art of vascular surgery has improved the quality of life for many patients with peripheral vascular diseases. Circulatory problems may affect any part of the body, but this discussion focuses on the most common pathologic conditions amenable to vascular procedures performed by vascular surgeons and interventional radiologists. Current surgical trends include open procedures and endovascular techniques.

HISTORICAL BACKGROUND

For centuries human beings have been plagued with peripheral vascular disease and its complications, such as pain or the loss of an extremity or life. However, little was understood about vascular system disease that causes arterial stenosis or occlusion until the contributions of the Scottish brothers William and John Hunter. Their studies of aneurysm formation, pathology, and treatment provided the foundation for the concepts of modern vascular surgery. William Hunter (1718-1783) was the first to describe an arteriovenous fistula and aneurysm, and John Hunter (1728-1793)

performed a successful surgical procedure for a popliteal aneurysm. Others subsequently experimented with vascular anastomoses. Alexis Carrel (1873-1944) received the Nobel prize in 1912 for his work at the University of Chicago with blood vessel anastomoses, suturing techniques, and animal organ transplantation. The suturing of blood vessels was the vital link necessary for the development of successful vascular surgery.

An endarterectomy to remove a localized vascular occlusion was first performed in 1946. In 1948 the first bypass graft was implanted to treat diffuse vascular disease. In the following decades many surgical procedures have become feasible with the use of improved diagnostic techniques and instrumentation, sutures, synthetic grafts, and microvascular techniques.

In 1983 the American Board of Surgery began a certification program in general vascular surgery. To qualify, candidates must have specialized training and practice in peripheral vascular surgery and be a Diplomate of the American Board of Surgery or the American Board of Thoracic Surgery. The Society of Vascular Nursing was founded in 1982. Specialty certification for perioperative vascular nurses was established in 1996.

ANATOMY AND PHYSIOLOGY OF THE PERIPHERAL VASCULAR SYSTEM

Vessels in the thorax, abdomen, extremities, and extracranial cerebrovascular area constitute the circulatory system (Figure 44-1). The ascending aorta, which originates from the left ventricle, carries oxygenated blood from the heart to the arteries. The major arteries leading to the head and upper extremities—the brachiocephalic trunk, left common carotid, and subclavian arteries—branch off from the aortic arch in the middle mediastinum above the heart. The thoracic aorta then descends through the posterior mediastinum at the left side of the vertebral column. Passing through the diaphragm, the abdominal aorta descends to the level of the fourth lum-

bar vertebra, where it bifurcates (i.e., divides) to form the common iliac arteries that lead to the lower extremities. Arteries from the abdominal aorta carry blood to the kidneys and the abdominal and pelvic organs. The femoral artery, which originates from the iliac artery, is the main artery in each leg.

Oxygenated blood flows from the arterial system through the capillary network and returns deoxygenated to the heart via the venous system. The vena cavae enter the right atrium. The superior vena cava, formed by the union of the two brachiocephalic veins, returns deoxygenated venous blood from the head, neck, upper extremities, and chest. The inferior vena cava, which begins at the level of the fifth lumbar vertebra, returns blood from the lower extremities, pelvis, and abdominal organs. There are two exceptions to this oxygenation/deoxygenation pattern: (1) the pulmonary arteries

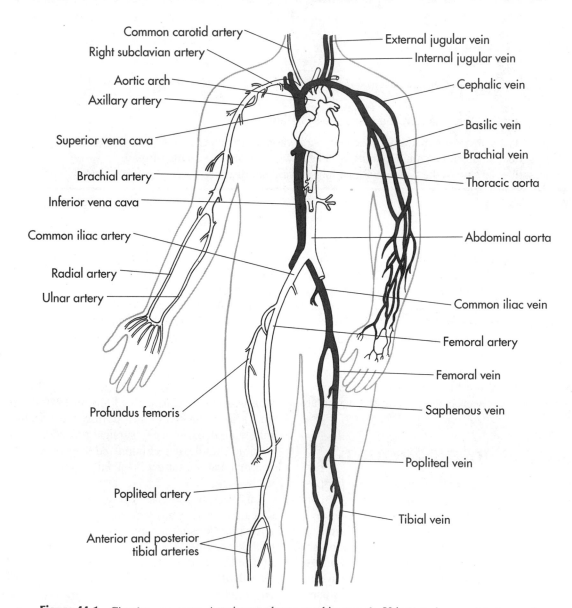

Figure 44-1   Circulatory system. Arteries are shown as white vessels. Veins are shown as black vessels.

carry deoxygenated blood to the lungs, and the pulmonary veins carry oxygenated blood to the heart; and (2) in fetal umbilical circulation, one vein carries oxygenated blood and two arteries carry mixed blood.

Innervation of the arteries and veins is controlled by the efferent vasomotor fibers of the autonomic nervous system. The nerve fibers enter the vessel adventitia (i.e., covering) along the same route as the blood supply. Stimulation of these nerves can cause vasoconstriction that shunts blood to larger organ groups such as the skin or gastrointestinal tract. Some medications cause vasodilation, which relaxes the vessels and slows heart rate to decrease intraluminal pressure.

The vessels are lined with endothelial cells, which when intact do not support platelet aggregation. This property is interrupted when a vessel is injured, and a clot is allowed to form. The endothelial lining also secretes factors that resist clotting, stimulate tissue repair, and synthesize clotting factors.

Arterial Anatomy

Arteries are elastic and constrict in response to hemorrhage. The arterial walls are made up of three layers that are separated by internal and external elastic membranes (Figure 44-2). The innermost layer is the intima (tunica intima)—a single layer of endothelial cells on a thin matrix of hyaluronic acid, collagen, and elastic fibers. The middle layer is the media (tunica media, or yellow fibrous). It is the thickest of the layers and is composed of a combination of smooth muscle fibers, yellow collagen, and some elastic fibers. The medial layer gives the arterial wall the flexibility and strength to withstand higher internal pressure. The outermost layer is the adventitia (tunica adventitia, or white fibrous). It is the thinnest layer but provides most of the external support for the arterial wall and resistance to overexpansion.

The tissues of the adventitia and the outer third of the media are nourished by a series of capillaries called the vasa vasorum. The rest of the medial layer and the intimal layer are nourished by diffusion from the luminal flow. Terminal arteries, referred to as arterioles, end at the level of the capillary beds in the tissues.

Venous Anatomy

Venous walls are structured in three layers. The innermost layer is the intima and is composed of endothelial cells that produce coagulation factors. The middle layer, or media, is much thinner in the deep venous system and may even be hard to identify microscopically. The superficial veins have a thicker medial layer mainly composed of smooth muscle fibers. This provides some resistance and response to intraluminal pressure changes. The external layer, or the venous adventitia, is composed of loose connective tissue (see Figure

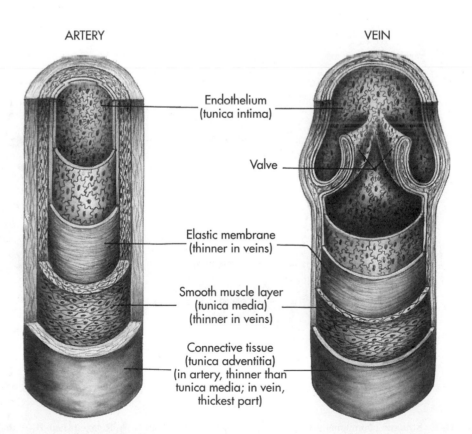

Figure 44-2 Cross section of an artery and a vein showing the three layers; tunica intima, tunica media, and tunica adventitia. (From Thompson JM et al: *Mosby's clinical nursing*, ed 4, St Louis, 1998, Mosby.)

44-2). Because of lower flow pressure, larger veins have internal semilunar valves to maintain the direction of the blood flow. The muscular component of the lower extremities provides force during contraction of large muscle groups, which facilitates venous return from the larger peripheral sinusoids. The cerebral veins are an exception; they have no valves. Veins are less elastic than arteries and tend to ooze instead of contracting in response to hemorrhage.

Venous anatomy has three structural components: superficial veins, deep veins, and perforators (also known as communicating veins) (Figure 44-3). The venous structure and flow of the lower extremities is an example of this system. At the tissue level, the origin of the venous system at the capillary bed are referred to as venules. The venous drainage of deoxygenated blood from the superficial veins returns through the perforators to the deep veins during muscular contraction. The deoxygenated blood then passes from the deep veins to the inferior vena cava.

Capillary Anatomy

Capillary beds are the vascular nutrition and waste exchange points of the arterial and venous systems. Capillaries are the diameter of a red blood cell and form a network throughout body tissues. Structurally they are a single epithelial cell layer thick, which facilitates the exchange of oxygen and carbon dioxide at the tissue level. They are semipermeable to water and crystalloids but are impermeable to larger molecules such as proteins. Oxygenated blood enters the capillary bed via the arterial system, and deoxygenated blood passively drains into the venous system. There are no fibrous or muscular layers of the vessels at this level. Lymphatic vessels passively exchange lipids, debris, fluids, proteins, antibodies, and other nutrients at this level in response to skeletal muscle contraction. This fluid is filtered by the lymphatics and is transported through the thoracic duct to the vena cava. The lymphatic vessels are structurally very pliable and have valves to maintain a unidirectional flow.

VASCULAR DISEASE

Vascular diseases that cause occlusion or stenosis are usually acquired diseases. Atherosclerosis is the most common arterial disease. It is a diffuse disease and begins as a disruption of the intima of a large artery. Cholesterol enters the media to stimulate muscle growth, and platelets accumulate around the disruption of the endothelial intima to form plaque or a thrombus. Often this process becomes localized around vessel orifices and branches (i.e., at bifurcations). The disease may produce stenosis (narrowing) and subsequent occlusion or ectasia (dilation) and aneurysm. Atherosclerosis is the principal factor in transient ischemic attacks (TIAs, or "mini strokes"), cerebrovascular accidents (strokes, or "brain attacks"), myocardial infarctions (heart attacks), and aortic stenosis. Risk factors include familial history, a high level of serum cholesterol, smoking, and hypertension (Box 44-1).

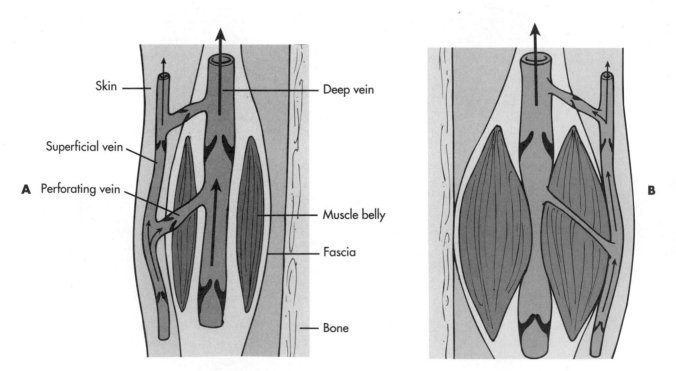

Figure 44-3 Structural components of venous anatomy in lower extremity. **A,** Relaxed state. **B,** With muscle contraction, the perforating veins are squeezed closed. (From MacVittie BA: *Vascular surgery,* St Louis, 1998, Mosby.)

Inadequate blood supply causes ischemia in tissues. If left untreated, this can lead to thrombus, embolus, ulceration, necrosis, or gangrene. Venous stasis disease or an obstruction of venous return can cause hemodynamic imbalances. Through vascular surgery, vessels are repaired, reconstructed, or replaced to improve peripheral (systemic) circulation. The most common procedures are performed to revascularize a lower extremity for limb salvage, to repair an aortoiliac aneurysm, and to improve cerebral blood flow through the carotid arteries.

Box 44-1	**Risk Factors for the Development of Peripheral Vascular Disease**

Advanced age
Diabetes
Familial predisposition
Habitual long periods of standing
High-fat diet causing high serum cholesterol
Hypertension
Obesity
Repeated pregnancies
Sedentary lifestyle
Smoking
Stress

DIAGNOSTIC PROCEDURES

Preoperative assessment of cardiac risk is critically important in planning the care of a patient who requires major vascular surgery. Peripheral arterial and venous diseases are then assessed. Table 44-1 compares the assessment factors of peripheral arterial and venous obstructive diseases in an extremity. Peripheral vascular laboratories, which are similar to cardiac catheterization laboratories, have been established in many health care facilities to perform noninvasive and invasive studies before and following surgical intervention.

Noninvasive Procedures

Computed axial tomography (CT scan) and magnetic resonance imaging (MRI) are noninvasive techniques of choice to confirm a diagnosis of aortic aneurysm, thrombus, or atherosclerotic plaque in arterial walls, especially in the abdominal and carotid circulation. CT scans are good tests to assess the sizes and stages of vessel occlusions. They can be performed with or without contrast and very quickly in emergency situations. CT scans are somewhat expensive and expose the patient to x-rays.

MRI is useful for evaluating a three-dimensional image of the vessel being studied. This method is contraindicated for patients with pacemakers, vena cava filters, or metal vessel clips, but many patients can benefit from its use. MRI is more expensive and slower to perform than CT scans.

TABLE 44-1	Comparison of Peripheral Arterial and Venous Obstructive Diseases in an Extremity	
Assessment of Extremity	**Arterial Obstructive Disease**	**Venous Obstructive Disease**
Color	Dusky, blue, gray, mottled, pallor distal to obstruction	Red, purple, brown hemosiderin spots, brawny
Temperature	Cool, cold	Warm, hot
Visual and palpable characteristics	Dry, shiny, flaking skin; vessels not obvious Lack of hair on affected part Thick nails	Moist, peeling skin Vessels may be tortuous and inflamed Thickened tissue Hair present on affected part Normal nails
Sensation	Numbness, tingling, pain during exercise (intermittent claudication) Pain at rest in severe disease Increased pain when exposed to cold Pain can be acute and severe	Aching, throbbing, tightness, feeling of heaviness; muscles feel fatigued Pain decreased by motion or elevation of legs Feels worse at end of day
Mobility	Painful range of motion; limited flexion and extension caused by avascular necrosis at the tissue level Diminished elasticity	Painful range of motion, limited flexion and extension caused by congestive edema in joints
Size	Not enlarged, average for body build	Swollen, edematous
Integrity of surface layer	Peeling, infarcted, painful, deep serous oozing ulcers with defined edges on or between toes	Stasis ulceration; open, draining, shallow ulcers with irregular borders
Pulses	Weak or absent	Present
Condition of digits	Mottled, blackened, fragile, painful; can become gangrenous	Edematous, reddened, painful; can become gangrenous

Carotid phonoangiography and oculoplethysmography (OPG) are techniques to obtain cerebral blood flow measurements to localize obstructions in the vessels of the head and neck. OPG is contraindicated in patients with intraocular lens implants.

Pulse volume recording (PVR) or photoplethysmography is used to measure systolic pressure in the extremities and digital arterial systems. This test is affected by artifacts and patient positioning. A diagnosis of deep vein thrombosis (DVT) may be made by phleborheography (PRG), a plethysmographic technique that records the rhythmic changes in venous volume in the legs; these changes are associated with respiration. PRG is not useful for small thrombi or for deep iliac or femoral veins, and the process is time consuming and expensive.

Ultrasonography is a major diagnostic tool for measuring segmental arterial pressures and venous patency in the extremities, and it may also be used for abdominal circulation. Doppler color-coded flow imaging and transcranial Doppler imaging are replacing carotid phonoangiography and OPG in the evaluation of carotid circulation. High-resolution, B-mode ultrasound provides real-time images of venous systems in the upper and lower extremities. Saphenous and cephalic vein mapping accurately measures vein diameter, location, and quality to determine preoperatively if the vein is suitable for use as an arterial conduit in arterial reconstruction. Ultrasound also detects venous thrombosis. With a pulse Doppler blood flow detector, longitudinal and/or transverse cross-sectional scans are obtained, and the images are recorded by oscilloscope. A computer-generated print of the image on the screen provides a permanent record of the arteriograph or venograph.

Intraoperative assessment of shunt performance or vessel patency or stenosis, as well as identification of an arteriovenous fistula (AVF), is easily performed with a sterile Doppler probe. An audible signal is transduced and is similar to the sounds transmitted by a Geiger counter (Figure 44-4).

Invasive Procedures

Selective angiography permits the radiographic study of a particular segment of the vascular system. Aortography visualizes the aorta (Figure 44-5). Arteriography shows the pa-

Figure 44-4 Doppler box and probe. (Courtesy Parks Medical Electronics, Aloha, Oregon.)

Hepatic artery

Splenic artery

Right renal artery

Left renal artery

Abdominal aorta

Right common iliac artery

Figure 44-5 Normal abdominal aortogram. (From Ballinger PW: *Merrill's atlas of radiographic positions and radiologic procedures,* ed 9, vol 3, St Louis, 1999, Mosby.)

tency of an artery or a branch of the aorta and its collateral circulation. Phlebography detects DVT, and a venogram visualizes the veins. An angiogram requires the injection of a nontoxic radiopaque substance. The pain associated with injection of intravascular contrast material can be so intense that the procedure may be performed under continuous epidural anesthesia or general anesthesia.

Angioscopy is an endoscopic technique used to visualize the interior of vessels. A small (1.5 to 3 mm) flexible fiberoptic angioscope is coupled to a camera, which allows the view from the angioscope to be seen on a monitor. The lining and structures within the blood vessels are visualized as the scope is advanced within each vessel. For many patients, angioscopy is an alternative preoperative diagnostic technique to angiography and may be used to evaluate the effectiveness of therapy intraoperatively. It can reveal retained atherosclerotic plaque or thrombi and suture lines.

Intravascular ultrasonic scanning uses a miniaturized ultrasonic probe at the end of a 5 to 9 French catheter. The probe is introduced into the vessel percutaneously. Images of the entire circumference are obtained to determine the thickness of the vessel wall and the distribution of plaque within the wall. This technique may be used both intraoperatively and percutaneously.

SPECIAL FEATURES OF PERIPHERAL VASCULAR SURGERY

Vascular injury can occur during invasive diagnostic, monitoring, or therapeutic procedures. Iatrogenic arterial injuries, those resulting from an unexpected outcome of a procedure, can cause loss of function or even death from ischemia, hemorrhage, or embolus. The patient must be carefully observed and monitored for signs of complications during and following vascular procedures. Infection is a devastating postoperative complication that must be avoided through strict adherence to aseptic and sterile techniques. Other considerations include the following:

- A thorough understanding of the principles of general surgery should be combined with special training in vascular surgical techniques. Speed and accuracy are imperative.
- Anesthesia considerations. Local or monitored anesthesia care (MAC) is usually preferred for most conservative interventional procedures. General anesthesia or regional block is used for longer or more extensive procedures.
- Temperature regulation may be a problem during long procedures or when multiple blood transfusions are given. Warmed fluids can be administered via rapid infusing pumps. Forced warm air blankets provide a normothermic temperature.
- Meticulous care is exercised during anastomosis of vessels to avoid the danger of postoperative thrombosis and stenosis:

To prevent undue trauma to vessels, an assortment of scissors, noncrushing vascular clamps, and forceps specifically designed for vascular surgery is included in the instrument setup. Umbilical tape or synthetic vessel loops are used for retraction and vessel control.

An operating microscope may be used for anastomosis of vessels. Appropriate instrumentation for microsurgery is made available.

Synthetic nonabsorbable suture materials are preferred because they are strong and pass through vessel walls and grafts easily with minimal trauma and tissue reaction. Swaged needles also minimize trauma. A larger swaged suture-to-needle ratio is advantageous to avoid leakage. Holes made in graft materials by the needle are occluded by the larger suture. Double-armed needle sutures are often used for vessel anastomosis.

- Anticoagulation. Heparinized solution is available for use as an anticoagulant. Preoperatively, heparin (5000 U) may be given subcutaneously for DVT prophylaxis. Intraoperatively, the optimal dose is 70 to 100 U/kg of body weight if given intravenously for immediate systemic effect. Thromboelastography may be used intraoperatively to monitor the effects of heparin administration. Sensitivity to bovine sources of heparin can result in heparin-induced thrombocytopenia (HIT), also know as "white clot" syndrome. Clots composed of fibrin and platelets form after 4 to 15 days of heparin therapy. A severe decrease in the platelet count predisposes the patient to thrombosis and acute arterial occlusion.

  Reversal of anticoagulation. Before closure at the end of the procedure, protamine sulfate, a heparin antagonist, is given to reverse the anticoagulant effect. One mg of protamine is given to counteract 100 U of heparin. Protamine is derived from fish semen and testicular tissue and may elicit a sensitivity reaction in patients who are allergic to fish. Insulin-dependent diabetics who take NPH insulin also may be predisposed to a sensitivity reaction to protamine. Some men who have had a vasectomy may exhibit allergic or hypersensitivity reactions.
- Hemostatic agents can be used independently or in combination (Box 44-2).
- A vasodilator such as papaverine hydrochloride is used to relax the smooth muscle of the vessel. This prevents endothelial damage during intraluminal irrigation. Vasopressors should be available.
- Blood replacement therapy. Blood is lost by the flushing of clots and debris. Blood loss should be calculated, and blood should be available for replacement if the hematocrit level falls below 26%. During procedures on the great vessels, blood may be salvaged from the thoracic or abdominal cavity for autotransfusion. An autologous blood salvage machine (cell-saver) may be used to collect the patient's own blood for autotransfusion. Care is taken not to aspirate hemostatic materials or other debris into the blood suction-salvage device.

Absorbable gelatin sponge (Gelfoam) can be used dry or dipped in saline. According to the manufacturer the patient may have an antigenic reaction when the sponge is soaked in thrombin. The sponge can be applied to the site and removed after 20 seconds or left in the wound; it is absorbed after 4 to 6 weeks. Because it may provide a favorable microbiologic growth medium, it is not used in the presence of infection. It is derived from porcine gelatin and has more of a mechanical than a chemical hemostatic property.

Absorbable collagen (Avitene, Hemopad, Helistat), either in powder, foam, woven, or nonwoven form, induces platelet adhesion and results in the formation of fibrin. It provides both a chemical and a mechanical hemostasis. Because it may provide a favorable microbiologic growth medium, it is not used in the presence of infection. The long-term effects of an in situ collagen hemostat are unknown, but animal studies indicate that it absorbs. It is of bovine origin and can be moistened, but it works better when dry.

Oxidized cellulose (Surgicel, Oxycel) is applied dry over a bleeding site for hemostasis. Although a single layer can be left in the wound and absorbed, it is preferred that a large wad be removed because it may interfere with healing or cause pressure. It chemically destroys thrombin and is not used concurrently with it. Because it may provide a favorable microbiologic growth medium, it is not used in the presence of infection. It has some bacteriocidal properties against gram-positive and gram-negative microorganisms. The mode of action is mechanical hemostasis when applied to an area of bleeding.

Fibrin glue is applied by simultaneously placing a combination of cryoprecipitate, bovine thrombin, and/or calcium chloride on the bleeding tissue surface to form a fibrin patch.

Topical thrombin should be available. Preparations from bovine origin are contraindicated in patients who are sensitive or allergic to these products.

Blood should be warmed before transfusion to help prevent inadvertent hypothermia. Consideration is given to the patient who does not want a blood transfusion. Patients undergoing nonemergent procedures should be given the option of donating autologous blood in advance of the procedure.

- DVT prophylaxis. Antiembolic stockings or sequential compression devices should be worn by the patient during and following the surgical procedure.
- Vascular monitoring. Doppler ultrasound, pulse volume recorder, and/or intravascular imaging techniques are used intraoperatively to monitor hemodynamic changes and to assess blood flow following peripheral vascular reconstruction. A pulmonary artery catheter (Swan-Ganz) is usually inserted to monitor pulmonary artery pressures during and following the procedure.

The most serious immediate postoperative complications are thrombus and hemorrhage. The patient may need to return to the operating room (OR) for immediate correction of these problems. Long-term complications include infection and graft failure by occlusion.

Vascular Grafts

Biologic or synthetic prosthetic vascular grafts are required to bypass a vascular obstruction or to reconstruct vessels. These substitute conduits for blood flow vary in length, diameter, and configuration to meet the requirements of each situation. A graft may be straight or bifurcated into a Y shape. Pieces of biologic or synthetic material may be cut to size for use as patch grafts.

The American National Standards Institute (ANSI) has established requirements for product characteristics and the labeling of textile and nontextile synthetic grafts, vascular homografts, and vascular heterografts. Grafts sterilized in see-through containers or packages permit the surgeon to select the appropriate size after exposure of the surgical site. Manufacturer's instructions for use and handling are strictly followed.

Biologic Vascular Grafts

Autografts, allografts, and xenografts have been used for arterial or venous conduits, but autologous grafts have a higher success rate. Allografts and xenografts have a higher failure rate.

Arterial Conduit   Autologous arteries are procured for coronary artery bypass grafting. The radial, gastroepiploic, or internal mammary arteries are commonly used.

Venous Conduit   An autologous vein is a suitable graft conduit because it is lined with endothelial cells, which inhibit clotting. These cells produce fibrinolytic substances and the plasminogen factor essential to maintain patency. The saphenous vein is commonly used for an autologous arterial bypass or vein graft. If the saphenous vein is not suitable, the basilic or cephalic veins of the arm are sometimes used. A vein graft is used as a conduit in one of three ways:

1. *In situ conduit/bypass.* To revascularize a lower extremity, the saphenous vein is exposed at the proximal and distal aspects but is left in place. The surgeon performs a venotomy at each end of the vein, inserts a valvulotome and/or a disposable valve cutter, and disrupts the internal valves. The occluded artery to be bypassed is ligated distally and proximally and then anastomosed proximally and distally to the saphenous vein. This technique reverses blood flow in the vein and reestablishes the flow of oxygenated blood beyond the level of arterial occlusion. Decreased manipulation and

not excising the length of vein minimizes endothelial trauma and preserves antithrombogenic properties. The vasovasorum and neurovascular components of the vessel remain intact.

2. *Nonreversed vein graft.* Renal and mesenteric revascularization also can be accomplished by grafting nonreversed segments of the saphenous vein.

3. *Reversed vein graft.* When a segment of saphenous vein is harvested for placement in the arterial system, the vein is reversed from its normal anatomic position so the valves will not obstruct arterial blood flow. Intact valves are used to keep the blood flow unidirectional after anastomosis. Endothelial integrity is maintained by gentle dissection and handling. The surgeon exposes the surgical site while the first assistant, resident, or another surgeon prepares the vein for grafting on a separate sterile table supplied with fine vascular instruments, ties, and vascular clips. Magnification loupes are worn to check for imperfections in the vein and to tie off leaking perforators. The valves may be cut, especially in small-diameter segments. The vein is flushed with sterile cold solution (commonly heparinized Plasma-Lyte with papaverine hydrochloride) and immersed in this solution until the recipient site is prepared.

Because the saphenous vein decreases in diameter as it courses distally, a size discrepancy may cause difficulty at the anastomosis attachment sites.

Synthetic Vascular Prostheses

Various forms of synthetic materials are used to construct arterial vascular prostheses. Certain materials are more suitable than others for specific applications. The surgeon selects the most appropriate graft for each patient. Rejection and tissue reaction are minimized if Dacron or Teflon are used.

Knitted Polyester   Knitted polyester (Dacron) grafts are porous enough to allow the ingrowth of fibrous tissue into the interstices. They also are porous enough to allow blood to seep through the material, and therefore they are preclotted before insertion. Preclotting causes the wall of the graft to become impervious to blood by filling the interstices with fibrin. For the preclotting process, the surgeon withdraws blood from the patient at the surgical site before anticoagulation therapy. The scrub person places the blood in a sterile basin containing the graft material. The blood saturates the lumen and all surfaces of the graft. The fabric-fibrin conduit later becomes firmly placed in tissue and provides a hypothrombogenic flow surface.

Filamentous Velour   Knitted velour construction of polyester grafts has uniform porosity for easy preclotting and ensures rapid tissue ingrowth. These types of grafts may be crimped or noncrimped, with velour inside and/or outside. One type, the exoskeleton (EXS) prosthesis, has a spiral polypropylene support fused to the outer surface of noncrimped velour. This graft was developed specifically for use across the knee joint. Another type, in which amikacin is bonded to knitted filamentous velour polyester with a bovine collagen matrix, provides an antibiotic in the prosthetic wall. This type of construction also renders the porous graft impervious to leaks, which eliminates the need for preclotting.

Bonded albumin also reduces porosity and potential thrombosis. Older style porous grafts required bonding. This was achieved by "baking on" autologous plasma. A porous graft was soaked in the patient's plasma or in allogenous albumin and was then steam sterilized. This thermal process altered the fibrin and protein elements in plasma.

Woven Polyester   The weave of woven polyester (Dacron) grafts is tight enough to be leakproof, and therefore these grafts do not require preclotting. However, the more inflexible construction limits their use to aortic replacement or for the bypass of large caliber arteries.

Polytetrafluoroethylene   The microporous wall of polytetrafluoroethylene (PTFE) serves as a lattice framework into which cells grow to become a microthin lining for contact with blood. These prostheses (Gore-Tex, Impra) do not require preclotting. Vascular grafts that are constructed of expanded and reinforced PTFE maintain dimensional stability. Configuration may be straight, tapered, or bifurcated. It may be supported by external rings to resist compression.

During the surgical procedure, the inside lumen of the graft may be seeded with the patient's own endothelial cells to sustain patency. The graft may be bonded with an antibiotic before implantation to prevent infection.

Composite Vein Grafts

A composite graft of autogenous vein and synthetic, usually PTFE, may be the surgeon's choice as a substitute for an insufficient length of saphenous vein. The prosthetic graft is anastomosed to a segment of reversed or in situ autogenous vein. The prosthetic graft is cut to match the diameter of the vein.

CONSERVATIVE INTERVENTIONAL TECHNIQUES

Peripheral vascular disease is often managed by a team of collaborating vascular surgeons, cardiologists, and radiologists. Multifaceted care encompasses invasive interventional procedures to treat occlusive disease conservatively. Endovascular procedures are considered minimally invasive conservative management. Vascular instruments and supplies for an open surgical procedure should be immediately available in the event that a vessel is perforated or injured during any of the conservative interventional techniques. A perforation may be closed with sutures; a patch graft, in situ conduit, or synthetic prosthesis may be necessary.

Percutaneous Transluminal Angioplasty

Severe ischemia or incapacitating claudication resulting from localized or segmental stenosis or occlusive disease can be conservatively treated by recanalization to restore the lumen in the obstructed vessel. Atherosclerosis in the iliac, femoral, and popliteal arteries is the most common indication for percutaneous transluminal angioplasty (PTA). Stenosis in the renal arteries also can be treated.

PTA is performed under local anesthesia and fluoroscopy, often in the interventional radiology department by a radiologist, in the angiography or cardiac catheterization laboratory by a cardiologist, or in the OR by a surgeon. In the Seldinger technique, the artery is punctured percutaneously with a large-bore needle, and a guidewire is introduced. A vessel dilator sheath is advanced over the guidewire into the vessel. The endovascular device is passed through the dilator sheath for the performance of several types of percutaneous procedures. Various techniques are used to dilate a stenotic lesion or to displace or ablate a plaque.

Balloon Angioplasty

A Gruentzig or other type of balloon dilation catheter is passed over the guidewire and positioned across the lesion. Catheters of several diameters with balloons of various widths and lengths are available. Determination of the appropriate balloon size and length is made on the basis of angiogram findings. When the balloon is inflated, atheromatous material is compressed against the arterial wall. It remolds and cracks, splitting the plaque and intima (inner lining) and stretching the media (middle layer) and adventitia (outer layer), thus dilating the lumen of a stenosis or recanalizing an occlusion. The balloon is repeatedly inflated and deflated until the lumen is dilated.

Intraluminal Stent A prosthetic stent may be placed along the vessel wall to maintain patency following dilation. The Palmaz stent, for example, is a stainless steel mesh tube mounted coaxially on a balloon angioplasty catheter. After the stent is positioned in the artery, the balloon is inflated to expand the stent. The stent remains in place when the balloon is deflated and removed. Stents made of titanium, polypropylene, or other materials either operate in a similar manner or are self-expanding, such as the Gianturco stent (Figure 44-6).

Aortic Intraluminal Stent A new procedure for the repair of abdominal aortic aneurysms is entering phase II clinical trials. Although this procedure is still in clinical trials, it shows great promise for treating aortic aneurysms with less invasive methods and at a reduced length of stay for and cost to the patient.

This procedure uses a balloon-mounted stent/graft. Delivery is under fluoroscopy and uses the same technology as the balloon angioplasty and intraluminal stents currently in use. The device, which combines the intraluminal stent and a Dacron graft material, is placed across the aneurysmal portion of the aorta through a percutaneous entry site in the femoral artery. Upon release the stent/graft is embedded in the aortic wall above and below the aneurysmal sac.

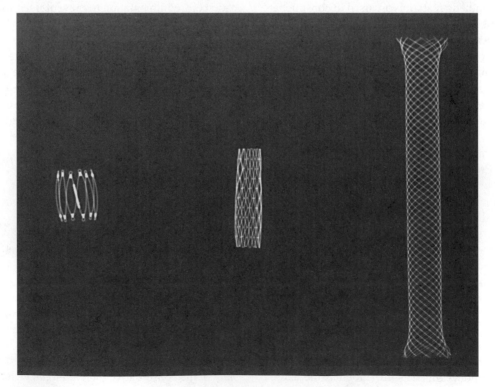

Figure 44-6 Examples of intraluminal vascular stents. (From Ballinger PW: *Merrill's atlas of radiographic positions and radiologic procedures,* ed 9, vol 3, St Louis, 1999, Mosby.)

Laser Angioplasty

With laser angioplasty, a laser fiber is introduced into an occluded artery to destroy plaque or thrombi. The laser usually is used to supplement balloon angioplasty. The procedure may be done percutaneously or as an open surgical procedure via an angioscope. Several different types of laser probes are available. The physician selects the most appropriate probe on the basis of the location and size of the artery and the determination of the degree of calcification in plaque or other cause of obstruction. The delivery system determines the mechanism of action:

- *Thermal laser.* A thermal laser uses argon or Nd:YAG laser energy to heat the tip of a metal probe at the end of a fiberoptic catheter to a temperature between 392° and 752° F (200° and 400° C). Plaque is vaporized as the tip is moved through the obstruction. This "hot-tip" technique may cause some damage to vessel walls. The laser fiber may be positioned within a balloon to destroy the thrombus selectively or to seal the arterial wall while the vessel is dilated. A temperature between 203° and 230° F (95° and 110° C) in the surrounding tissues dries and disintegrates the thrombus. The combination of pressure from the inflated balloon and diffuse laser energy adheres the loose flaps of arterial tissue back onto the arterial wall; this process is known as arterial welding.
- *Photothermal laser.* A photothermal laser uses contact Nd:YAG laser energy. A sapphire-tipped probe or catheter heats plaque by a photoptical effect at the point of contact for vaporization of plaque. This is followed by rapid cooling to prevent damage to the intima.
- *Photochemical laser.* A photochemical laser uses an excimer laser with pulsed energy or a tunable dye laser to destroy plaque with minimal generation of heat. With the athermal action of a "cold laser," the intima is not damaged. Heavily calcified plaque cannot be ablated by an excimer laser.

Intravascular Ultrasonic Energy

An ultrasonic probe on the tip of a catheter can be used to recanalize occluded or stenosed peripheral vessels.

Atherectomy

In an atherectomy, catheter-mounted instruments are used for transluminal removal of atherosclerotic plaque. A high-speed rotating cam, burr, and/or side cutter are positioned under fluoroscopic guidance. The plaque is pulverized and retrieved to restore the patency of the vessel. These instruments may be used intraoperatively.

Thrombectomy and Embolectomy

For a thrombectomy and embolectomy, a local anesthetic is infiltrated percutaneously. A Fogarty catheter is inserted proximally and advanced into a vessel distally beyond the obstruction. The balloon on the tip is then inflated. As the catheter is withdrawn, thrombotic or embolic material is removed to restore blood flow to an extremity. This procedure may be performed with fluoroscopy to selectively cannulate vessels. Different types of catheters may be used when the blockage is in a native vessel or an artificial graft.

Thrombolytic Therapy

In thrombolytic therapy, streptokinase, urokinase, or tissue-type plasminogen activator may be administered by local bolus infusion into the occluded vessel or directly injected into the thrombus. These drugs activate plasminogen and cause liquefaction of fibrin, thus dissolving the clot or loosening it for removal by balloon catheter. This therapy may be used in conjunction with angioplasty (thrombolysoangioplasty) or infused intraoperatively, especially in tibial vessels, for lower limb salvage.

Streptokinase

Treatment for DVT, pulmonary embolus, or another clotted vessel is facilitated by the use of streptokinase. Streptokinase is derived from a form of beta-hemolytic streptococci and has an indirect effect that breaks down fibrin. It may not be effective for patients who have antibodies against streptococcus infections. Clots more than 1 week old are not treated with this drug. The maximum effectiveness of this drug is evident within 10 minutes. Reversal of the anticoagulant effect can be accomplished by administering cryoprecipitate or fresh frozen plasma. Some patients will have a sensitivity reaction that can progress to anaphylaxis. Pretreatment with antihistamines and steroids may be indicated.

Urokinase

Urokinase is administered directly into the clot with a catheter in an interventional procedure room equipped with x-ray and fluoroscopy capabilities. Care is taken not to cause damage to the endothelial lining of the vessel. Urokinase causes fewer sensitivity reactions than streptokinase, but it is expensive to produce. It is derived from fetal kidney cells and urine, and it is reconstituted with sterile water without a bacteriostatic agent.

Tissue-Type Plasminogen Activator

More recent advances in thrombolytic therapy include tissue-type plasminogen activator (TPA), a chemical that occurs naturally as a secretion of the endothelial cell lining of vessels. There is a risk of bleeding when TPA is used.

PERIPHERAL VASCULAR SURGICAL PROCEDURES

If conservative therapy is unsuccessful or contraindicated, an open surgical procedure may be indicated.

Arterial Bypass

Occlusive disease or trauma may cause arterial blockage, or arterial injury may indirectly occur near the site of a fracture.

The vessel lumen above and below the lesion is usually normal. Vascular reconstruction is performed in an attempt to restore normal circulation. The surgeon selects an appropriate method to bypass the obstruction:

1. The involved segment may be excised and the ends anastomosed if they can be approximated without tension.
2. If direct anastomosis is impossible, the involved segment is excised, and an autograft or synthetic prosthetic graft is used as a replacement.
3. The lesion can be bypassed using the long saphenous vein from one thigh as a vein graft, or a synthetic prosthetic graft may be used. The ends of the graft are anastomosed to the artery proximal and distal to the lesion. The obstructed segment of the artery is not resected.
4. The lesion can be bypassed by interposing a prosthetic graft through the subcutaneous tissues between a patent artery and the artery distal to the lesion; this procedure is known as an extraanatomic bypass. For example, in a femoral-femoral bypass, the graft is placed from the femoral artery of the unaffected leg to the femoral artery of the ischemic leg. In an axillofemoral bypass, the graft is placed from the axillary artery to the femoral artery of the ischemic leg.

Femoropopliteal Bypass

The femoral artery is most prone to obstruction by occlusive vascular disease in a lower extremity. A femoropopliteal bypass, the most commonly performed bypass procedure in an extremity, may be the procedure of choice for severe ischemic disease and limb salvage. The patient is placed in the supine position on the operating bed with the thigh of the affected leg slightly abducted and the knee flexed and supported. The entire extremity is prepped and draped to allow adequate exposure. Incisions are made over the femoral and popliteal arteries to expose them and explore the area before bypassing the obstruction in the femoral artery. An autogenous in situ saphenous vein graft, PTFE or noncrimped velour graft, or composite graft may be used. Anastomoses may be visualized with an angioscope. During the surgical procedure, pulsations of the proximal and distal popliteal artery, as well as pulsations in the foot, are checked with a sterile Doppler pulse detector.

Endarterectomy

Atherosclerotic plaque may cause localized stenosis in the major peripheral arteries. An endarterectomy involves the excision of the diseased endothelial lining of the artery and the occluding atheromatous deposits; this leaves a smooth lining. Loosely attached plaque may be removed by dissection in the media with wire-loop strippers, spatulas, and/or catheters. A long-segment endarterectomy may be facilitated in the iliac, femoral, and popliteal arteries with a powered Hall oscillating endarterectomy valvulotome or other high-speed drill to pulverize plaque as described for atherectomy. A

saphenous vein or patch graft may be used to close the arteriotomy site. Plaque also can be vaporized from femoral and carotid arteries with a laser beam. Subsequent inflammation and fibrosis are minimal, and healing is rapid.

Carotid Endarterectomy

One of the most common vascular procedures, a carotid endarterectomy, is performed to prevent a brain attack (stroke) in a patient with severe carotid artery insufficiency. Atherosclerotic plaque at the bifurcation of the common carotid and/or in the internal and external carotid arteries causes localized stenosis or ulceration that impedes cerebral blood flow. Endarterectomy is indicated when this stenosis causes TIAs.

This procedure can be performed with the patient under superficial and deep regional cervical block, or a general anesthesia may be preferred to preserve metabolic demands. The patient may be continuously monitored by electroencephalogram (EEG) or computerized EEG topographic brain mapping (CETBM) to assess cerebral circulation and neurologic deficits.

The patient is placed in the supine position, with his or her head turned away from the affected side. Care must be taken not to place undue extension on the neck, because such pressure may occlude vertebral blood flow. The skin prep is performed without causing excessive pressure or massage over the carotid artery, which could dislodge the plaque and cause an embolic event in the brain.

In the neck, an oblique incision approximately 4 inches (10 cm) long is carried through subcutaneous tissue, platysma muscle, and the anterior border of the sternocleidomastoid muscle. Retraction of the sternocleidomastoid muscle and jugular vein allows exposure of the common carotid artery and its branches. After systemic heparinization, special vascular instruments are used to clamp above and below the occluded area. In certain instances an intraluminal shunt is inserted in the artery to maintain blood flow to the brain while the plaque is removed. Many surgeons use a shunt routinely; others use an alternative means of cerebral protection, such as deliberate production of mild to moderate hypertension or hypercapnia. Cerebral protection during carotid cross-clamping is a primary concern to prevent serious neurologic complications.

An arteriotomy (incision in an artery) is made in the common carotid artery below the plaque and is extended upward; in the internal and external carotid arteries it begins above the plaque and extends downward. The plaque is dissected free and is removed in its entirety. In addition, most of the underlying media layer is removed. A headlight and magnifying loupes are worn by the surgeon to enhance visibility during dissection and closure of the arteriotomy. To check blood flow, a Doppler pulse detector is used after the artery is closed. A PTFE or saphenous vein patch graft angioplasty or bypass grafting is occasionally necessary if an adequate lumen cannot be established. Bilateral endarterectomies may be indicated for severe bilateral occlusion, but the surgical procedures are performed at least a week apart.

Aneurysmectomy

An aneurysm is a localized abnormal dilation in an artery that results from the mechanical pressure of blood on a vessel wall that has been weakened by biochemical alterations. The loss of structural integrity is implicit because the aneurysm forms in the media. A fusiform aneurysm is a uniform circumferential dilation. Less common is a saccular aneurysm, a saclike outpouching in the media of the vessel wall (Figure 44-7). Cystic medial necrosis causes a dissecting aneurysm, usually in the thoracic aorta, in which the media separates from the intima.

Atherosclerosis is the most common cause of an aneurysm, but trauma may also be a factor. The abdominal aorta, thoracic aorta, aortic arch, and popliteal arteries are the vessels most often affected. Diagnostic evaluation combines a physical examination, laboratory findings, and the results of ultrasonography, CT scan, MRI, and aortography and/or angiography. The location and extent of the lesion determine the operability of the aneurysm and the type of reconstruction. For example, cross-clamping of the descending thoracic aorta to remove an aneurysm will impair blood supply to the spinal cord. Repair in the arch or ascending aorta can impair cerebral and coronary perfusion. Blood flow through the visceral, mesenteric, and renal arteries may be affected by abdominal aortic aneurysmectomy or aortoiliac reconstruction. Vital structures must be protected during aneurysmectomy.

A ruptured aneurysm is a surgical emergency and precludes further evaluation. A transbrachial or transfemoral occluding balloon catheter may be placed in the aorta to prevent an exsanguinating hemorrhage. The surgical procedure is performed immediately.

Resection of an Abdominal Aortic Aneurysm

An abdominal aortic aneurysm usually develops between the renal and iliac arteries. An abdominal aneurysmectomy may be a lifesaving procedure. Serious hazards, including massive hemorrhage, ischemic organs, and injury to ureters and other nearby structures, are associated with the procedure. Renal failure is a potential complication. Modern techniques have greatly reduced mortality. Survivors of the procedure enjoy the same life expectancy as do other patients with comparable atherosclerotic disease.

Constant monitoring of cardiac function with a Swan-Ganz pulmonary artery catheter is used in these high-risk patients. Patients whose condition is unstable may require frequent blood gas determinations. Central venous pressure monitoring is a guide for regulating fluid replacement. Blood must be available for transfusion. Autotransfusion may be used if massive hemorrhage is encountered, such as with a ruptured aortic aneurysm. An indwelling Foley catheter is inserted preoperatively, and urinary output is monitored. Mannitol can be infused before aortic cross-clamping to prevent ischemic renal failure. Blood flow in the extremities should be checked immediately preoperatively and postoperatively to detect embolic or occlusive problems. Marking the location of the pedal and dorsalis pedis pulses with a marking pen enables rapid location of the appropriate site when they need to be checked intraoperatively. An audible Doppler device is usually used.

With an abdominal aneurysmectomy, a long midline incision from the xiphoid process to the pubis usually is used. The abdomen is thoroughly explored, the small intestinal mesentery is mobilized, and the posterior peritoneum overlying the aorta is incised to expose the aneurysm. A self-retaining abdominal wall retractor helps provide needed exposure. The small intestine and ascending colon are delivered outside the abdomen to increase exposure and prevent injury. Warm moist tapes, plastic sheeting, or a Lahey (bowel) bag may be used to protect these structures.

Although the situation may be urgent or emergent, care is taken to account for plastic sheeting, towels, and other items used in the abdomen. If counts are aborted because of the patient's condition, documentation in the patient's permanent record should include that the count was not performed and the reason for not performing it. The count should not be listed as incorrect. An abdominal x-ray film should be obtained as the patient's condition permits.

An extended posterior retroperitoneal approach may be preferred, especially in a patient who is obese or has had previous abdominal surgery. The patient is placed in the right lateral position with the left side up. An oblique flank incision is extended along the superior margin of the twelfth rib, which may be resected. The entire abdominal aorta and left renal artery are exposed without needing to enter the pleural or peritoneal cavities. The kidney, ureter, and peritoneal sac are reflected anteromedially and packed with moist tapes. Exposure is maintained with self-retaining and handheld retractors. If access to the iliac or femoral arteries is required,

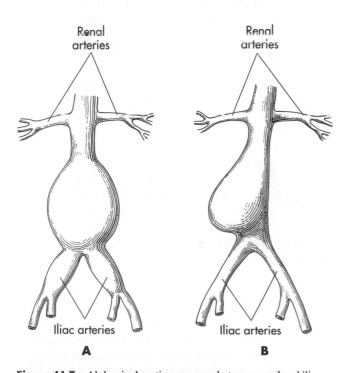

Figure 44-7 Abdominal aortic aneurysm between renal and iliac arteries. **A,** Fusiform (circumferential) type. **B,** Saccular (saclike) type.

the patient's hips are rotated to a prone position, and longitudinal incisions are made in the groin.

Before occlusion of the aorta, blood is withdrawn if needed for preclotting in the graft. Heparin is injected for anticoagulation. Aortic clamps are placed proximal to the aneurysm, and the iliac arteries are clamped distally. The distal aortic stump or iliac arteries may be closed with staples. If the aneurysmal wall is opened, clots and loose intraluminal debris are removed. A tube graft is used if the aneurysm is confined to the aorta (Figure 44-8, *A*). More commonly, a bifurcated graft is sutured in place above the aneurysm and to the common iliac or femoral arteries distally (Figure 44-8, *B*). Branches of other arteries are anastomosed to the graft as necessary, depending on the segment of aorta being replaced. The graft is commonly placed inside the aneurysm (open inclusion method), and the sac is closed over the graft. With the less commonly used closed exclusion method, the graft is placed beside the unopened aneurysm sac. Living tissue, either the aneurysm sac or the mesentery, must cover the prosthesis to prevent contact of the prosthesis with the intestines; otherwise a fistula can develop. After the aortic clamps are released, the anastomoses are checked for leakage. The incision is usually closed with nonabsorbable sutures; retention sutures are commonly used for a long abdominal incision.

Embolectomy

An embolus is a mass of undissolved matter carried by the bloodstream until it lodges in a blood vessel and occludes it. An embolus may be an air bubble, a fat globule, a clump of bacteria, a piece of tissue, or a foreign body. The occlusion of a blood vessel by an embolus causes various symptoms depending on the size and location of the occluded vessel. The occlusion of a vessel in the brain, lungs, or heart can cause rapid and sudden death.

Surgical intervention is the primary treatment for an embolus unless contraindicated. Select patients may be treated with heparin, vasodilators and, perhaps, sympathetic blocks. Renal or mesenteric emboli are usually treated by embolectomy or bypass grafting. With an embolectomy, the affected blood vessel is incised and the embolus is removed.

Pulmonary Embolus

The occlusion of a pulmonary artery or one of its branches usually occurs with emboli that originate from veins in the lower extremities or pelvis. Emboli pass up the inferior vena cava to the right side of the heart and are ejected from the right ventricle into the pulmonary artery. A pulmonary embolism may be diagnosed by lung scans, pulmonary angiograms, and phlebograms.

Pulmonary Embolectomy   A massive pulmonary embolism can cause irreversible cardiac arrest or profound refractory hypotension and hypoxemia. If portable cardiopulmonary bypass equipment is available, cannulae can be inserted at the patient's bedside or in the emergency department or intensive care unit. The patient is then trans-

Figure 44-8   Resected abdominal aneurysm replaced with tube graft (**A**) or bifurcated graft (**B**).

ported to the OR. A median sternotomy is performed to establish total cardiopulmonary bypass and to allow access to the pulmonary artery. Pulmonary emboli are removed by manual extraction; by the passage of forceps into both the right and left pulmonary arteries; by the passage of balloon catheters into pulmonary arterial segments; and by squeezing both lungs to force peripheral thrombi through a pulmonary arteriotomy. The incision can be extended for vena caval ligation to prevent recurrent embolization.

Pulmonary Thromboendarterectomy   Chronic pulmonary thromboembolic disease may develop from failure to resolve a massive pulmonary embolus, from repeated embolic episodes, or from a combination of both. The removal of obstructions in the main pulmonary arteries by thromboendarterectomy improves hemodynamics. The procedure is performed with the patient under induced hypothermia and cardiopulmonary bypass; thrombi are removed from the upper, middle, and lower branches of the right pulmonary artery and then from the left pulmonary artery.

Vena Caval Filter Devices   A surgical procedure may be indicated when anticoagulant therapy fails or is contraindicated to prevent the passage of emboli to the lungs from the deep veins in the lower extremities and pelvis. Blood flow within the vena cava may be partially interrupted with clips or filter devices (Figure 44-9). This allows blood to return to the right ventricle of the heart without passage of the emboli. Vena caval ligation or plication may be performed using an abdominal approach. A Moretz clip is placed on the vena cava using a retroperitoneal approach.

Figure 44-9 Vena cava filters. Left to right: Kimray-Greenfield, Titanium Greenfield, Simon-Nitinol, Gianturco-Bird's Nest, Vena Tech. **A,** Actual filter. **B,** Radiographic images. (From Ballinger PW: *Merrill's atlas of radiographic positions and radiologic procedures,* ed 9, vol 3, St Louis, 1999, Mosby.)

Under fluoroscopic control, the applicator of a Mobin-Uddin umbrella filter or Greenfield filter is inserted through a right internal jugular venotomy by using a guidewire. It is advanced through the right atrium into the inferior vena cava at the level of L 2-3. The cone-shaped titanium filter measures 4.6 cm from apex to base and is ejected and fixed in position below the renal veins and above the point of juncture of the iliac veins. Hooklike prongs anchor the device in the correct orientation to collect clots. A patient with an enlarged, dilated caval lumen >30 mm in diameter caused by right heart failure may require placement of a filter in each iliac artery. To avoid a second procedure, especially for a high-risk patient, a filter may be placed at the completion of a diagnostic angiogram. The titanium filter does not interfere with CT scans or MRI, but the radiologist should be informed of its presence before any imaging procedure is performed. Older stainless steel models cause distortion on imaging scans.

The Greenfield filter is a permanent implant that traps and hold clots of 3 mm or larger. If preferred, it can be placed

from a femoral vein route. Additional angiography may be performed during the placement procedure, and the appropriate contrast media should be readily available.

Natural body processes dissolve clots that become lodged in the device. Postoperatively, the patient usually begins to undergo anticoagulant therapy. Complications include lower extremity edema, which may indicate an obstruction in the filter that requires prompt medical attention. Other potential complications include premature deployment of the device or migration. If the device cannot be repositioned by endovascular methods, an open surgical procedure may be performed.

Venous Stasis Disease

When the valves of the veins fail to function normally, increased back pressure of blood causes the veins to become dilated, tortuous, or elongated. These are known as varicose veins. Pain and secondary complications, such as thrombophlebitis and venous stasis ulcers, may follow. It is believed there is a familial tendency toward varicosities caused by valve incompetency, which afflicts both males and females. Habitual long periods of standing, repeated pregnancies, and obesity are other predisposing factors.

A procedure may be performed to bypass a venous obstruction, such as iliac-venous occlusion or femoropopliteal occlusion. Venous valve repair (valvuloplasty) or venous valve transposition may be performed to correct femoral valvular incompetence and severe venous stasis and to salvage the saphenous vein. The perforator or superficial femoral veins may be ligated for severe venous stasis with marked fibrosis and ulcerations. Injection-compression sclerotherapy to treat varicose veins may be preferred to surgical treatment.

Ligation and Stripping of Varicose Veins

For ligation and stripping of varicose veins in a leg, the saphenous vein is excised in toto with the aid of a semiflexible stripping device; this procedure begins at the ankle. Additional incisions are made along the course of the vein to ligate perforator branches as the stripper is moved upward toward the groin. Perforators and branches are occluded with ligating clips and transected. At the groin, an incision is made over the palpated stripper, and the vein is ligated at the saphenofemoral junction.

Preoperatively, the surgeon may mark areas of varicosity for incision. During the skin prep, care is taken not to wash away the markings or to massage areas of potential thrombus accumulation. Following closure of the incisions and the application of dressings, the full length of the leg is wrapped in cotton elastic bandages for compression.

Fasciotomy

Decompression by fasciotomy is the treatment of choice for the prevention of compartment syndromes following acute ischemia in the upper or lower extremity. Vascular compromise can occur following a penetrating or crush injury. Release of the overlying fascia may be indicated for clinical evidence of increased pressure, such as pain, edema, pallor, and diminished sensation.

Epidural Spinal Electrical Stimulation

Epidural spinal electrical stimulation (ESES) may be used to improve nutritional blood flow in patients with severe lower limb ischemia. This can lead to the healing of ischemic ulcers. ESES uses a microscope connected to a television camera, television monitor, and video recorder. Intravital capillary microscopy is performed before and after ESES to measure red blood cell velocity in skin capillaries. With the patient in a sitting position, the dorsum of the foot is placed over the microscope. Fluorescein dye is injected intravenously, and the time for perfusion of the capillaries is measured. With the patient under local anesthesia and x-ray control, an epidural electrode is placed parallel to the spinal column. After stimulation of the electrode, perfusion in the foot is tested again.

Vascular Shunts

Normal circulation can be altered to increase or decrease blood flow to a specific organ, either temporarily or permanently. A vascular anastomosis or prosthetic device may be used to establish a route for the diversion of blood flow. For example, vascular isolation of the liver can be achieved with an atrial caval shunt. This shunt permits continuous venous return to the ventricle to sustain cardiac output during the repair of traumatized suprahepatic or retrohepatic vena cava and/or hepatic veins. A straight tube or inflatable balloon catheter may be inserted to establish the shunt.

Portosystemic Shunts

A shunt between the portal and systemic venous systems is definitive treatment for esophageal varices complicated by portal hypertension. This surgical procedure may be only palliative. Many patients have progressive liver disease that eventually leads to liver failure. Shunting does not repair an already damaged liver but can prevent further hemorrhage. Portal hypertension is an increase in portal venous pressure and is caused by the obstruction to intrahepatic blood flow as a result of cirrhosis, hepatitis, or thrombosis. The increased pressure thus produced results in venous dilation that causes varices. The patient also may have ascites. The purpose of the surgical procedure is to reduce portal hypertension and/or portal venous blood flow. The surgeon selects the most appropriate type of shunt to achieve the purpose.

Distal Splenorenal Shunts Known as the Warren shunt, this procedure involves anastomosis between the splenic vein and the left renal vein. The hilum of the spleen and the tail of the pancreas are exposed through a left subcostal incision. The splenic vein is completely dissected from the pancreas to its bifurcation at the splenic hilum. This technical maneuver preserves portal profusion but eliminates collateral circulation to control bleeding from gastric and esophageal varices by decompression. The splenoportal system must be patent, and there must be adequate distance between the splenic and renal veins for the anastomosis.

An autogenous jugular or external iliac vein graft may be interposed to ensure a tension-free splenorenal anastomosis. A splenectomy may be performed. Other modifications may be made to meet specific patient circumstances.

Mesocaval Shunt A mesocaval shunt is an option if a splenic vein is too small for a successful splenorenal shunt. A superior mesenteric inferior vena caval shunt is well tolerated by young patients. With a mesocaval shunt, the side of the superior mesenteric vein may be anastomosed to the proximal end of the divided inferior vena cava. An interposition autologous vein or synthetic H-graft may also be used to create a shunt between the inferior vena cava and the superior mesenteric vein.

Portacaval Shunt A portacaval shunt may be performed with end-to-side or side-to-side anastomosis between the portal vein and inferior vena cava or with an interposition H-graft inserted between the portal vein and inferior vena cava. A ringed PTFE graft may be used, or an autologous graft may be obtained from an internal jugular or saphenous vein. The shunt relieves hypertension by bypassing the obstruction and diverting the return flow of blood to the liver from the portal vein, thus decompressing esophageal varices.

Depending on the type of portosystemic shunt planned by the surgeon, either a subcostal or a transabdominal incision may be used. Two suction setups should be available to evacuate the copious amounts of ascitic fluid that can be anticipated when the peritoneum is opened. Both abdominal and vascular setups are prepared. Pressure within the portal vein is measured with a manometer, via a cannulated branch of the superior mesenteric vein, at the beginning and at the conclusion of the surgical procedure. Because of venous distention and the vascularity of the surgical area, hemorrhage is a major intraoperative hazard. Care is taken to avoid injury to adjacent structures, including the hepatic artery and the common bile duct.

Arteriovenous Shunts and Fistulas

With arteriovenous shunts and fistulas, blood flow from an artery to a vein is established directly and without going through the capillary network. Access to the vascular system through an arteriovenous shunt or fistula is necessary for a patient who is suffering from end-stage renal disease and who is being maintained on long-term chronic hemodialysis. With the patient under local anesthesia, the endogenous Cimino-Brescio arteriovenous fistula is established internally at the wrist by anastomosis between the radial artery and cephalic vein. If the vessels are inadequate, a synthetic PTFE graft may be interposed between the artery and vein. A loop fistula may be created with a graft from the brachial artery to the cephalic or basilic vein in the antecubital fossa or from the brachial artery to the axillary vein in the upper arm. Enzymatically treated bovine carotid artery heterografts are used occasionally to create arteriovenous shunts or fistulas. Thrombosis and infection are the most common complications. Using a Fogarty balloon catheter, a thrombectomy may reestablish patency. Total excision of the graft is necessary in the event of a generalized infection.

Vascular Anastomosis

The operating microscope is needed for microvascular anastomosis of small vessels to revascularize tissue. Patency of the anastomosis depends on factors related to blood flow, coagulation, and vessel spasm. The vessels must be approximated without trapping adventitia in the lumen. Collagen fibers, tissue thromboplastin, and other thrombogenic factors in the adventitia predispose the patient to rapid platelet aggregation that may cause thrombus formation. Interrupted sutures are placed through the full thickness of the vessel wall (i.e., adventitia, media, and intima). Veins are technically more difficult to anastomose than arteries because their walls are thinner and have less substantial mus-

cularis. Anastomoses may be end-to-end or side-to-side. An interpositional vein graft may be needed to add length or to bridge a gap between the ends of either an artery or a vein. A patent artery should pulsate distal to the anastomosis. Although this procedure is used most commonly for tissue transplantation (e.g., vascularized free flaps or replants such as severed digits), the peripheral vascular surgeon may be needed to assist with vascular problems that require microvascular techniques.

Laser-assisted vascular anastomosis, also referred to as vascular tissue welding, fuses medium-sized (6- to 8-mm) vessels together to form an anastomosis. The adventitial surface is less thrombogenic than it is following suturing and heals faster with less scar tissue. The argon laser is used for this technique. It may be used to create an arteriovenous shunt at the wrist for hemodialysis, to reattach severed limbs, and to repair damaged vessels.

Limb Salvage

Amputation of a lower extremity may be required for peripheral vascular disease or for lymphedema with lymphangitis. All efforts are made to salvage the limb; amputation is the last resort. Ischemia can cause debilitating pain, skin ulcers, and gangrene, often secondary to smoking or diabetes. Revascularization by the techniques described in this chapter may save the patient from the emotional trauma of amputation. This is a prime objective of the peripheral vascular surgeon.

Bibliography

Allen SL: Perioperative nursing interventions for intravascular stent placements, *AORN J* 61(4):689-698, 1995.

Belkin M et al: Abdominal aortic aneurysms, *Curr Opin Cardiol* 9(5):581-590, 1994.

Berengoltz-Zlochin SN et al: Subintimal versus intraluminal laser-assisted recanalization of occluded femoropopliteal arteries, *J Vasc Interv Radiol* 5(5):689-696, 1994.

Bunt TJ: Revascularization versus amputation for elderly patients, *AORN J* 62(3):433-435, 1995.

Chuter TA et al: Bifurcated stent-grafts for endovascular repair of abdominal aortic aneurysm, *Surg Endosc* 8(7):800-802, 1994.

Fahey VA: *Vascular nursing*, ed 2, Philadelphia, 1994, WB Saunders.

Fellows E: Abdominal aortic aneurysm: warning flags to watch for, *Am J Nurs* 95(5):26-32, 1995.

Gulli B, Templeman D: Compartment syndrome of the lower extremity, *Orthop Clin North Am* 25(4):677-684, 1994.

Henderson LJ, Kirkland JS: Angioplasty with stent placement in peripheral arterial occlusive disease, *AORN J* 61(4):671-685, 1995.

Kaufman JA et al: MR angiography in the preoperative evaluation of abdominal aortic aneurysms, *J Vasc Interv Radiol* 5(3):489-496, 1994.

Kupeli IA: Factors affecting outcome in patients undergoing peripheral vascular surgery, *Anesthesiology* 80(2):483-485, 1994.

Long J et al: Pulmonary thromboendarterectomy: clinical profile, surgical treatment, *AORN J* 59(4):801-810, 1994.

MacSweeny ST et al: Pathogenesis of abdominal aortic aneurysm, *Br J Surg* 81(7):935-941, 1994.

MacVittie BA: *Vascular surgery,* St Louis, 1998, Mosby.

McCance KL, Heuther SE: *Pathophysiology: the biological basis for disease in adults and children,* ed 3, St Louis, 1998, Mosby.

McEwen DR: Arteriovenous fistula: vascular access for long-term hemodialysis, *AORN J* 59(1):225-232, 1994.

Mills JL et al: The utility and durability of vein bypass grafts originating from the popliteal artery for limb salvage, *Am J Surg* 168(6):646-650, 1994.

Moody CA et al: Effects of intraoperative manual descending compressions on saphenous vein incision healing, *AORN J* 62(6):913-923, 1995.

Moore WS, Rutherford RB: Transfemoral endovascular repair of abdominal aortic aneurysm: results of the North American EVT phase 1 trial, *J Vasc Surg* 23(4):543-553, 1996.

Pace RM: Intraoperative preparation of autologous fibrin gel, *AORN J* 62(4):604-607, 1995.

Parodi JC: Endovascular repair for abdominal aortic aneurysms and other arterial lesions, *J Vasc Surg* 21(4):549-557, 1995.

Sales CM et al: *Handbook of vascular surgery,* St Louis, 1994, Quality Medical Publishing.

Sapienza P et al: Comparative long-term results of laser-assisted balloon angioplasty and atherectomy in the treatment of peripheral vascular disease, *Am J Surg* 168(6):640-644, 1994.

Soong CV et al: Bowel ischemia and organ impairment in elective abdominal aortic aneurysm repair, *Br J Surg* 81(7):965-968, 1994.

Stein P: Perioperative considerations of vascular access for dialysis, *AORN J* 60(6):947-958, 1994.

Volpicello C: Pulmonary embolism after repair of a traumatic Achilles tendon rupture, *AORN J* 64(4):599-601, 1996.

Yamamoto N et al: Monitoring for spinal cord ischemia by use of the evoked spinal cord potentials during aortic aneurysm surgery, *J Vasc Surg* 20(5):826-833, 1994.

Chapter 45

Organ Procurement and Transplantation

Chapter Objectives

After studying this chapter, the learner will be able to:

- List the criteria for validating brain death.
- Describe the testing performed on tissue before it is suitable for transplantation.
- Discuss the role of the host procurement facility.
- Discuss the psychologic impact of a transplant on the donor and recipient families.

Transplantation is the transfer of an organ or tissue from one person to another or from one body part to another. Concentrated efforts continue in search of compensation for or suitable replacements for deficient tissues and organs. The indication for organ transplantation is irreversible functional failure of the organ. The goals of transplantation include changing appearance, restoring function, and/or improving quality of life.

HISTORICAL BACKGROUND

The interest in transplantation is many centuries old. Celsus wrote that tissues could survive after grafting from one part of the body to another. Galen attempted to reconstruct facial defects. Centuries later it was observed that full-thickness autografts survived and allografts failed, although the reason for the difference was not understood.

Darwin's theory of evolution and Mendel's laws of heredity shed new light in the nineteenth century, spurring researchers to pursue the study of regenerative capacity in animals. In the early twentieth century, Alexis Carrel and Charles Guthrie performed blood vessel anastomoses, an essential component of organ transplantation. Performing het-

erotopic heart transplantations in animals, they demonstrated that a heart could be removed, transplanted, and resume beating.

In the 1930s the maintenance of organs in vitro opened the way to organ preservation. During the 1940s, expanded information concerning a patient's response to a surgical procedure marked advances in surgical therapy. Open heart surgery, as well as acquisition of the basic knowledge required for clinical transplantation, evolved in the 1950s. As pioneers in transplantation biology, Peter Medawar and Frank M. Burnet received the Nobel prize in 1960 for their work on immunologic tolerance of tissue transplantation in animals.

Many scientific disciplines contribute to and integrate information to aid the progress of clinical transplantation. Foremost among these areas are physiology, genetics, immunology, and pathology. The practical application of clinical transplantation became possible in the 1960s after investigative efforts led to the development of supportive techniques such as cardiopulmonary bypass and immunosuppressive drug therapy.

Kidney transplantation began in 1954 and preceded heart transplantation by more than a decade. The first successful

Types of Biologic Transplants

allografts   Tissue grafted between different or genetically dissimilar individuals of the same species.
autografts   Tissues grafted in the same person from one part of the body to another. The donor is also the recipient.
heterotopic transplant   Transplant to an anatomically abnormal location in the host. Heterotopic grafts may function normally in the unnatural site.
isografts   Tissues grafted between genetically identical donor and recipient, as between identical twins.
orthotopic transplant   Transplant to an anatomically natural recipient site.
xenografts   Tissues grafted between two dissimilar species; may be used when allograft material is unavailable or a temporary replacement is necessary.

Box
45-2

Donor Selection Criteria for Tissue Allografts

Negative for viral, bacterial, or fungal infection or disease
Negative for sexually transmitted disease
Negative for neurologic disease
Negative for autoimmune disease
Negative for metabolic bone disease
Negative for malignancy or suspected malignant neoplasm
Negative for disease of unknown origin
Negative for death of unknown origin
Negative for use of systemic medication
Negative for parenteral drug use
Negative for exposure to toxic substances
Not ventilator-dependent for more than 7 days before brain death
Not immobile or bedfast for more than 7 days before brain death
Normothermic 98.6° F (37° C) for more than 7 days before brain death

heart transplant, performed in 1967 by Christian Barnard in South Africa, expanded the era of clinical organ transplantation. Although survival rates vary, most body tissues and organs can be transplanted or grafted. The availability of donor organs remains a problem.

TYPES OF TRANSPLANTS

Certain tissues and whole organs can be transplanted and grafted to restore bodily function. The type of transplant selected depends on the purpose of the graft, anatomic function, and availability of the tissue or organ. The types of biologic transplants are listed in Box 45-1.

TISSUE TRANSPLANTATION

Some tissues can function normally even after being moved from one area of the body to another or after being obtained from a donor:

1. Skin grafts provide a protective surface covering, initially acquiring then eventually losing vascular connection with the host.
2. Corneal grafts replace nonfunctioning corneal tissue.
3. Bone grafts afford temporary structural supports and a pattern for regrowth of the host's bone; the grafts are then resorbed.
4. Ossicles and the tympanic membrane in the ear can be transplanted to restore bone-conduction hearing loss.
5. Cartilage restores contour in a defect of cartilaginous facial structures.
6. Blood vessel grafts bypass or replace diseased or obstructed segments of vessels.
7. Bone marrow restores hematologic and immunologic functions.
8. Heart valves replace stenosed or diseased valves.

Tissue transplants can be either autografts or allografts. Xenograft transplants are in the research phases. The American

Association of Tissue Banks sets standards for retrieving, processing, storing, and labeling tissues and for donor criteria for allografts (Box 45-2). Tissue for transplantation is procured from suitable cadaver (nonliving) donors, either heartbeating or nonheartbeating, or from a living donor. Table 45-1 details the procurement parameters for tissue allografts. Additional information is available from the National Institute of Transplantation at **www.transplantation.com** or the United Network for Organ Sharing at **www.unos.org.**

Potential donors are screened to avoid the transmission of infection or disease. Cultures are taken at the time of procurement for microbiologic and serologic testing. Tissue is not transplanted until negative test results are obtained; tissue is discarded if the test result is positive. Living bone donors are tested for human immunodeficiency virus (HIV) immediately after donation and again after 90 days because seroconversion can be delayed. Recipients also should be tested and should be negative for HIV and hepatitis B virus (HBV). A baseline is essential to establish that the patient was not infected by the act of grafting. Patients with HIV or HBV are not barred from receiving an allograft, but baseline data can help rule out causes for rejection or infection. Incidences of graft failure and superinfection are high in immunocompromised patients with HIV.

Banked tissues are labeled with the donor's name and/or identification number, pertinent medical history, the pathology report of the donor, final culture and serology reports of donors, type and site of donation, date and time of procurement, and method of procurement and preservation.

Bone Marrow Transplantation

Bone marrow transplantation is essentially a tissue transplant. However, because this type of transplantation is fraught with the hazards of rejection, bone marrow is procured and transplanted using a protocol similar to that of organ procurement

| TABLE 45-1 | Tissue Allograft Procurement Parameters | | | |

Age of Donor	Physiologic Status of Donor	Time Between Procurement and Grafting	Other Considerations
Cornea			
Both sexes: 3 months-80 years	Nonheartbeating cadaver donor	Procured 6-8 hours postmortem at room temperature	Corneas are not perfused tissue. Heartbeating status is unimportant. Tissue may be procured in morgue or setting other than OR, under sterile conditions.
		Procured 48 hours postmortem if donor has been refrigerated at 39.2° F (4° C)	
		Transplanted fresh 7-10 days after procurement	Corneas are usually used fresh rather than in cryopreserved state.
		Cryopreserved cornea may be stored for 1 year	Corneal tissue is not commonly cryopreserved.
Skin			
Both sexes: 14-75 years	Nonheartbeating cadaver donor	Procured 6-8 hours postmortem at room temperature	At least 75% of skin surface should be free of abrasions, scars, or deformities to qualify as donor.
		Procured within 24 hours postmortem if refrigerated at 39.2° F (4° C)	Skin is procured before bone and is taken only from below nipples to knees on ventral surface, and from scapulae to popliteal area on dorsal surface. Tissue is taken to the depth of dermal layer (split thickness). A 70-kg donor can provide 7-8 square feet of skin.
		Cryopreserved skin can be stored for 5 years at −238° F (150° C)	Newly procured skin is stored at 39.2° F (4° C) in preservation medium for a maximum of 24 hours.
			Cryopreserved skin is thawed at temperatures not to exceed 59° F (15° C) for use on recipient.
			Allograft skin is commonly used as a biologic dressing in combination with autograft skin. The recipient autograft is meshed 6:1 then covered by allograft that has been meshed 2:1. Allograft skin is temporary and is replaced on the recipient every 48-72 hours until natural reepithelialization at the autograft site begins.
Iliac Crest			
Female: 18-50 years Male: 18-70 years	Nonheartbeating cadaver donor	Procured within 12 hours postmortem at room temperature	Bone is procured after the recovery of any other internal organs and skin. Preferably, bone is procured under sterile conditions; however, it may be procured under clean conditions in a setting such as the morgue and secondarily sterilized by ethylene oxide followed by aeration. Sterile bone can be freeze-dried and stored at room temperature.
		Procured within 24 hours postmortem if refrigerated at 39.2° F (4° C)	
		Cryopreserved bone can be stored for 3 years at −112° F (−80° C)	

Continued

and transplantation. Bone marrow is transplanted only after conventional treatments have failed to replenish depleted bone marrow cells. The marrow given by infusion restores hematologic and immunologic functions. Indications for treatment are acute lymphoblastic leukemia, myelogenous leukemia, aplastic anemia, and certain other blood diseases. Bone marrow transplantation is the only cure for severe combined immunodeficiency disease, a genetic disorder in which a child lacks adequate immune defenses to fight infections.

Bone marrow transplants also are given to victims of severe radiation exposure. Contraindications to transplantation are renal or cardiac disease.

With bone marrow transplantation, blood type and human leukocyte antigen (HLA) compatibility are essential. A bone marrow transplant may be one of three types:

1. *Autologous.* The donor is the recipient. Stem cells are collected from the leukemic patient in remission,

TABLE 45-1	Tissue Allograft Procurement Parameters—cont'd			
Age of Donor	**Physiologic Status of Donor**	**Time Between Procurement and Grafting**	**Other Considerations**	
Joints and Long Bone				
Female: 18-50 years Male: 18-55 years	Nonheartbeating cadaver donor	Procured within 12 hours post-mortem at room temperature Procured within 24 hours post-mortem if refrigerated at 39.2° F (4° C) Cryopreserved bone can be stored for 3 years at −112° F (−80° C)	Bone is procured after the recovery of any other internal organs and skin. Preferably, bone is procured under sterile conditions; however, it may be procured under clean conditions in a setting such as the morgue and secondarily sterilized by ethylene oxide followed by aeration. Sterile bone can be freeze-dried and stored at room temperature. Joints are not used as joints per se but are cut into pieces to fit a defect.	
Both sexes: femoral head not age dependent; usually acceptable to age 75	Living nonrelated donor (femoral head or rib)		Living nonrelated donor femoral head can be salvaged during total joints arthroplasty procedure and processed for use as bone plug or ground bone grafting tissue.	
Heart Valves				
Female: 0-40 years Male: 0-35 years	Nonheartbeating cadaver donor	Cryopreserved valves can be used within 1-2 years	Size match is important.	

cryopreserved, and stored to be infused during a subsequent relapse.

2. *Allogeneic.* The donor is HLA-compatible with the recipient. Marrow is harvested for immediate infusion into the recipient.
   a. A syngeneic donor, an identical twin, is preferred.
   b. A genotypically compatible sibling or parent has identical tissue type.
   c. An unrelated allogeneic donor must be HLA-compatible. Graft-versus-host disease (GVHD) is unique to allogeneic bone marrow transplantation. With GVHD, donor T cells immunologically attach to recipient cells, causing tissue damage at the site of antigen localization.
3. *T cell–depleted marrow.* To prevent GVHD, mature T lymphocytes are removed from donor marrow before infusion into the recipient.

Before transplantation, the recipient is given a high-dose regimen of immunosuppressive chemotherapy to eradicate leukemic, lymphoid, and bone marrow cells, thereby inducing marrow depression. The recipient also receives total body irradiation (TBI) to penetrate the areas resistant to the drugs. During this period of pretransplant preparation, the patient is placed in reverse isolation, preferably in a laminar airflow clean or sterile (germ-free) environment. The patient is closely monitored for the side effects of immunosuppressive chemotherapy and TBI.

After pretransplant protocols have been completed, the donor is hospitalized before the scheduled transplantation. In the operating room (OR), with the patient under general or spinal anesthesia, 500 to 700 ml of bone marrow is aspirated at multiple sites from the iliac crests; the sternum may also be used. The marrow is filtered, heparinized, and placed in sterile containers for infusion. The donor is watched for bleeding and may need blood and fluid replacement.

Marrow is infused into the recipient intravenously or via a Hickman or Broviac catheter over several hours. During this time the patient is constantly attended and closely monitored for adverse reactions. By an unknown process, the marrow migrates into the marrow cavities of the bones. For 10 to 30 days after transplantation, the recipient may receive daily transfusions of lymphocytes, platelets, and granulocytes, preferably taken from the donor, to counteract the predictable side effects of pretransplant immunosuppressive therapy (mainly hemorrhage and infection). If the marrow is not from an identical twin, blood is irradiated before transfusion to destroy the lymphocytes. Mature blood cells and platelets are unaffected by the irradiation process. Daily marrow aspirations and complete blood counts are performed on the host. The success or failure of transplantation is usually decided after 10 to 20 days, when the new marrow begins to function.

ORGAN TRANSPLANTATION

Organ transplantation can be a lifesaving treatment for some end-stage diseases. Although tissue grafts are commonplace, transplantation of functional, whole, vital organs presents physiologic, philosophic, and ethical dilemmas. A biologically related donor (referred to as a "living related donor") makes a supreme sacrifice to become an organ donor; therefore cadavers are the primary source of organs for transplant. Organ donation is the ultimate gift of life and is given by the donor to the recipient. Transplantation can potentially restore the recipient to near-normal physiologic status.

Kidney transplantation was initially the most successful and principal clinical application of organ transplantation. If a kidney graft fails, the patient may survive by returning to hemodialysis indefinitely before receiving another transplant. This option does not exist for transplants of the heart, liver, pancreas, or the lungs. No practical prolonged artificial support exists for these organs in the event of an allograft failure.

Transplantation of each organ involves unique technical and physiologic problems, but the major barriers and causes of transplant failure are immunologic rejection and infection. Immunodeficiency depends on the amount of immunosuppression the patient receives to prevent rejection. Immunosuppressive agents cause the patient to be prone to opportunistic infection. Reverse protective isolation may be advisable if the patient develops leukopenia, a decrease in white blood cells. In other aspects of care, transplant recipients are similar to other critical surgical patients with severe chronic illnesses who require measures that minimize the risk of infection.

The American Society of Transplant Surgeons (**www.asts. org**) and the International Society of Transplantation meet regularly to exchange ideas and information among persons of different scientific backgrounds. The aim is to achieve the best possible patient survival rather than merely transplant survival.

The Organ Transplant Registry of the American College of Surgeons, in conjunction with the National Institutes of Health, collects data on transplantation procedures and approves and funds various registries. The Federal Organ Transplantation and Procurement Act of 1983 provided financial grants for the initial development of regional organ procurement centers and a transplant registry. A national task force has also been established to analyze medical, legal, ethical, economic, and social issues of concern in organ procurement and transplantation.

Organ banks collect organs and tissues from donors, exchange organs geographically, and register patients in need of a transplant. The register includes information about the patient's blood grouping and tissue typing. Computer lists of patients waiting for donor organs are maintained by the United Network for Organ Sharing and the North American Transplant Coordinator Organization 24-Hour Alert. Regional organ procurement organizations coordinate with these registries to match donated organs with compatible recipients nationwide. The position of the recipient on the waiting list is determined by the severity of the illness. Other countries have similar mechanisms. For example, the United Kingdom (UK) Transplant Register has membership in the Euro Transplant Register. Organs procured within the UK can be transported by air to another country in Europe, and vice versa, for a histocompatible recipient. The number of patients awaiting transplants exceeds the supply of available

donor organs. As a result, many patients die while waiting for a suitable organ to become available.

Many persons carry a signed *Uniform Donor Card* or other identification (e.g., the reverse side of a driver's license) that states that certain or all organs and tissues may be removed for transplantation in the event of death. Such cards or a living will constitutes legal written consent under the Uniform Anatomical Gift Act enacted by all 50 states. Written or telephone consent is still obtained from the family of a potential donor before procurement may commence. Federal and state laws mandate required-request or routine-inquiry. These laws require that the family of every medically suitable potential donor be asked to consider the donation of organs and tissues. As a result of these laws, organs and tissues are procured in many hospitals and are then transported to organ banks or transplantation centers. Procurement teams from these centers may go to the community hospital (host facility) to procure organs and tissues.

Time is paramount when critical organs are involved, because their value depends on preserving maximum functional viability. The time factor is less urgent with less critical tissue. When a potential donor has been identified, a transplantation coordinator contacts the regional registry and procurement team(s).

Organ Procurement

Immunologic rejection and the shortage of donor organs remain the principal deterrents to transplantation. The goal is selection of a donor-recipient match with adequate histocompatibility to permit an organ to function without complications. Organs and tissues come from two primary sources: cadaver (heartbeating and nonheartbeating) and living related donors (Table 45-2). Tissue donors may be between newborn age and 80 years of age. All donors of vital organs must be free of sepsis or malignant processes, between newborn age and 65 years of age, and have good function of the donor organ(s). Technical aspects of the procurement procedure must ensure the viability of organs throughout the entire period between procurement and transplantation.

Cadaver Donor

Death is confirmed by irreversible cessation of all functions of the brain and brainstem. The criteria for brain death are listed in Table 45-3. To be suitable for organ or tissue donation following death, cadaver donors are classified as either *heartbeating* or *nonheartbeating*.

Heartbeating donors are persons with confirmed brain death in whom the vital organs can be preserved in vivo. In these donors brain death usually has resulted from severe neurologic trauma, such as from head or spinal cord injury, hemorrhage, or anoxia. Death must occur in a location in which a cardiopulmonary support system is immediately available (i.e., in the emergency department, OR, or other critical care unit). To be a potential organ donor, an individual who is brain dead is maintained on mechanical ventilation and/or cardiopulmonary bypass to prevent ischemic

TABLE 45-2	Organ Procurement Parameters		

Age of Donor	Physiologic Status of Donor	Time Between Procurement and Transplantation	Other Considerations
Heart			
Female: 0-40 years Male: 0-35 years	Heartbeating cadaver donor	3-6 hours, fresh tissue	Heartbeating cadaver donor: total heart and segments of great vessels.
	Nonheartbeating cadaver donor	Cryopreserved valves can be used within 1-2 years	Nonheartbeating cadaver donor: heart valves only. Size match is important. Donor criteria include no cardiac disease and normal cardiac enzymes.
Lung			
Both sexes: 0-45 years	Heartbeating cadaver donor	1-4 hours	Heartbeating cadaver donor lung(s) may be given en bloc to one recipient. The lungs may be separated and/or divided into segments (lobes) for several recipients.
	Living related donor		One lobe from living related donor is transplanted into recipient. Size match is important. Donor criteria include no evidence of trauma, negative sputum culture, normal chest x-ray film.
Heart-Lung En Bloc			
Both sexes: 0-50 years Younger ages preferred	Heartbeating cadaver donor	1-4 hours	Heartbeating cadaver donor heart and lungs are transplanted en bloc into recipient. Size match is important. Donor criteria same as for individual heart or lung donation.
Liver			
Both sexes: 0-45 years	Heartbeating cadaver donor Living related donor	8-24 hours	Heartbeating cadaver donor liver may be divided into two segments for two separate recipient patients. Small segment of living related donor's liver is transplanted into recipient. Size match is important. Donor criteria include normal liver function, normal liver enzymes and bilirubin, no evidence of trauma.
Kidney			
Both sexes: 6 months- 60 years	Heartbeating cadaver donor	48-72 hours Ideally, should be transplanted within 12 hours	Heartbeating and nonheartbeating cadaver donor kidneys are given to two separate recipients.
	Nonheartbeating cadaver donor in highly selected circumstances	Procured within 45 minutes of cardiac arrest, with immediate in situ cooling	
	Living related donor		One kidney from living related donor is transplanted into recipient. Donor criteria include normal renal function, normal serum creatinine, no evidence of trauma.

damage to the vital organs. Maintenance of a heartbeating donor before and during organ procurement includes the following:

- Systolic blood pressure above 90 mm Hg
- Central venous pressure of 5 to 10 mm Hg
- Hydration with crystalloids and colloids
- Urine output minimum 100 ml/hr—ideally 200 to 300 ml/hr
- Ventilation with 100% oxygen
- Core body temperature of 98.6° F (37° C)

Nonheartbeating donors are not suitable for the procurement of parenchymal organs. With nonheartbeating donors,

TABLE 45-2 Organ Procurement Parameters—cont'd

Age of Donor	Physiologic Status of Donor	Time Between Procurement and Transplantation	Other Considerations
Pancreas			
Both sexes: 3 months-60 years	Heartbeating cadaver donor Living related donor	12-24 hours	Heartbeating cadaver donor pancreas is transplanted as a whole or partial organ for one recipient. Tail segment of pancreas from living related donor may be transplanted into recipient. Donor criteria include normal pancreatic function, normal blood glucose regulation, normal serum amylase, no evidence of diabetes mellitus, no evidence of trauma.
Kidney-Pancreas			
Both sexes: 3 months-60 years	Heartbeating cadaver donor	12-24 hours	Heartbeating cadaver donor kidneys and pancreas are simultaneously transplanted into recipient. Usually performed for diabetic nephropathy. Donor criteria is the same as for individual kidney or pancreas donation.

TABLE 45-3 Brain Death Criteria

Criteria	Clinical Assessment
Irreversible coma not caused by pharmacologic agent, hypothermia, or unknown cause	No response to external stimuli. No cerebral brain activity on EEG over a period of 10 minutes. EEG activity has no prognostic value for estimation of cerebellar and brainstem activity.
Absence of spontaneous movement, decerebrate posturing, and decorticate posturing	Spinal nerve reflexes may be unaffected because these reflexes do not require cortical (brain) activity.
Apnea with no spontaneous respiration not influenced by hypothermia or pharmacologic agent	Elevated carbon dioxide in the blood is not a stimulus for breathing. No spontaneous respiratory effort for 3 minutes when removed from ventilatory assist device. $Paco_2$ greater than 55.
No cranial nerve reflexes	Fixed and dilated pupils. Pupils are unreactive to light. No corneal reflex (no blinking when cornea is touched). No oculocephalic reflex (doll's eyes). No oculovestibular reflex (no response to ice water instilled in ear). No response to pain on face and head (pin prick, supraorbital pressure). No response to upper or lower airway stimulation (no gag or cough reflex when suctioned or stimulated by endotracheal tube).

cardiopulmonary or ventilatory support was not provided after brain death. As a result, the major organs have suffered thrombosed vascular structures and ischemia. Skin, bone, heart valves, blood vessels, and corneas may be acceptable for procurement from select nonheartbeating donors (see Table 45-1).

Multiple Organ Procurement The heartbeating donor is brought to the OR and treated with the same respect and care given to any other patient. Organs and tissues are removed under sterile conditions by a procurement team and are preserved and transported to the recipient(s). The procurement team includes two surgeons, two assistants, and a scrub person. A circulator and a scrub person from the host facility assist with the procedure. An anesthesia provider also is necessary to maintain vital functions until the aorta is cross-clamped and cardiopulmonary support is no longer needed. A procurement coordinator from an affiliated organ procurement agency or organ bank usually accompanies the team and assists wherever needed throughout the procurement process. The procurement team brings the necessary supplies for packaging the organ(s) and tissue(s) for transport.

The procurement process includes the following functions:

1. The procurement coordinator facilitates the procurement process by:
   a. Obtaining blood samples and arranging tissue typing to assist the organ bank with the potential placement of procured organs
   b. Documenting necessary information, making any needed phone calls, and coordinating the host facility personnel with the procurement team
   c. Assisting the physician with communications with the donor family
   d. Calling the procurement team
   e. Assisting the circulator and scrub person with the setup of the procurement room
2. The circulator and scrub person assist in the procurement process by:
   a. Gathering sterile supplies that include the following:
      (1) Laparotomy drape pack and extra medium drapes
      (2) Nonabsorbable sutures for ligating ties (usually 0, 2-0, 3-0, 4-0 silk) and for closure (usually a size 2 monofilament suture on a large cutting needle) as requested by the surgeon
      (3) Umbilical tapes at least 30 inches long
      (4) Suction tubings with tips
      (5) Electrosurgical handpieces with blades
      (6) Scalpel blades, No. 10
      (7) Bone wax
      (8) Bulb syringes
      (9) Laparotomy sponges
      (10) Cold normal saline solution for irrigation
   b. Setting up sterile instrumentation that includes the following:
      (1) Chest tray with sternal saw and self-retaining chest retractor
      (2) Major abdominal laparotomy tray and large self-retaining abdominal retractor
      (3) Vascular tray
      (4) Minor tray for organ preparation table (benching table)
      (5) Basin sets
   c. Providing nonsterile equipment that includes the following:
      (1) Electrosurgical units
      (2) Suction containers to accommodate at least 24 L of fluid
      (3) Power source for sternal saw
      (4) Extra intravenous (IV) poles
      (5) Hyperthermia/hypothermia blanket
      (6) Defibrillator
      (7) Skin preparation solution
      (8) Isopropyl alcohol (70%) to make slush or slush machine, if available
      (9) Crushed ice; dry ice is not used for organ preservation

Figure 45-1   Midline, sternal-splitting incision from suprasternal notch to pubis is made for procurement of thoracic and abdominal organs from heartbeating cadaver donor.

3. The anesthesia provider assists in the procurement process by:
   a. Ventilating the donor with 100% oxygen
   b. Monitoring electrocardiogram (ECG), blood pressure, urinary output, and fluid and electrolyte balance
   c. Administering drugs as necessary (e.g., dopamine or dobutamine for vasomotor regulation, muscle relaxants to neutralize spinal reflexes and relax the abdomen, osmotic diuretics for renal function, and heparin for anticoagulation)
   d. Monitoring and replacing blood as appropriate
   e. Monitoring and maintaining core body temperature and initiating cooling: cold fluids, usually Ringer's lactate or Collins' solution with 30,000 U of heparin, are infused intravascularly 10 minutes before the aorta and vena cava are cross-clamped for heart removal
4. Incisions are made by the procurement surgeon to provide maximum access to organs and tissues:
   a. A midline, sternal-splitting incision is made from the suprasternal notch to the pubis to remove vital thoracic and abdominal organs (Figure 45-1). It takes 2 to 3 hours to procure parenchymal organs.
   b. Eyeballs are enucleated to procure the corneas. Glass balls may be put in the sockets.
   c. Skin is taken with a dermatome from flat body surfaces, excluding the upper chest, neck, face, arms, lower legs, and feet (Figure 45-2). Skin procurement may take 1 to 1½ hours.
   d. Skin is excised and the muscles are separated. Long bones and iliac crests are removed in toto (Figure 45-3) and are replaced with wooden, fiberglass, or metal dowels to maintain structural integrity. Bone procurement may take 5 to 6 hours to complete.
   e. Multiple incisional closures may take 1 to 1½ hours.

Figure 45-2 For cadaveric allografts, skin is removed with dermatome from anterior and posterior flat surfaces between midchest and knees.

Figure 45-3 Long bones and iliac crests are procured for bone allografts. Humerus, tibia, and fibula are cut distally. Radius, ulna, and femur are disarticulated at both ends. Pelvis is cut at pubic and sacroiliac joints.

5. The sequence of organ removal is coordinated to maintain the viability of the organs. The kidneys and liver are mobilized and cannulated for in situ cooling. The aorta is cross-clamped, and the heart is removed first, followed by the liver and then the kidneys, pancreas, and intestines. A combined heart-lung procurement may be performed after the other organs have been removed. Enucleation of the eyes for corneal procurement usually follows retrieval of the parenchymal organs. Skin is then taken, followed by bone.
   a. A small, sterile table should be set up so that organ and tissue packaging for transport can be completed away from the main sterile field.
   b. Closure should be as aesthetic as possible for later viewing at funeral services, if desired.

Additional Considerations in Cadaver Organ Procurement The procurement coordinator remains at the host facility after the procurement team has departed. The coordinator's role extends into the aftercare given to the donor's body and the psychologic support and debriefing of the OR team. After the closure and dressing of all incisional wounds, the donor's body should be bathed, and all drainage tubes and IV access lines are removed. The body should be labeled with identification tags and placed on a clean transport cart. The head of the stretcher should be elevated 20 to 30 degrees. Ice packs should be placed over the eye sockets to decrease serous pooling. This will be of benefit to the mortician who prepares the body for viewing. The donor's body is prepared as aesthetically as possible for the benefit of the family and loved ones.

The OR team may experience a sense of sadness and loss. This is normal and to be expected. Death is not a common event in the OR. Although the patient is technically brain dead before arriving in the OR, he or she gives the outward appearance of being sustained on life support as in general anesthesia. After the aorta and vena cava are cross-clamped, ventilatory support is no longer needed, and the anesthesia provider turns off the ventilator. The sudden silence can feel overwhelming. The OR team may need the added support given by the procurement coordinator, who has experienced the same feelings and understands the psychologic impact of each stage of the procurement process. Personnel who specialize in procurement state that they feel the same sense of loss despite years of experience and exposure. An understanding of the outcome is important in the grieving process. Participation in the aftercare of the body helps to provide the OR team with a sense of closure and completion of patient care. Some of the same sadness may be shared by the critical care nursing staff members who helped monitor and maintain the donor's vital signs before transfer to the OR. Although the urge to be emotionally strong may exist, it is therapeutic to shed tears of sorrow.

The donor's family also needs support and communication from the procurement coordinator. The coordinator makes himself or herself known to the family and maintains communication with them for several months or longer as needed; he or she also provides referrals for follow-up counseling if the need arises. The coordinator informs the family of the progress of the recipients. In select situations, donor and recipient families may be brought together, thus forming lasting friendships.

The financial aspects of donor maintenance and subsequent organ procurement are paid by the procurement agency and are not the responsibility of the donor's family. Medical bills accumulated before the patient was identified as a potential donor are paid by the donor's family.

Living Related Donor

There are distinct advantages to procuring a kidney, lobe of the liver or lung, tail segment of the pancreas, or marrow from a living related donor. The results are better than are those with non–biologically related cadaver organs because donor-recipient matches are usually good (identical twin sources are ideal for compatibility). Waiting time is also reduced, and the procedure is planned and performed under controlled circumstances.

The use of living donors involves a special protocol:

1. Adult donors, who are preferred over adolescents or children, must be able to give informed consent voluntarily and without coercion. Children are used as donors only for a twin or for a patient with predictable results. If the donor is a minor, court (legal) and parental or guardian consents are required to avoid bias. The donor must fully comprehend the sacrifice; if the physician deems it advisable, a psychiatric examination is included along with intelligence testing.
2. The donor must be in excellent health. The donor's physician confers with him or her and performs the preoperative physical examination to facilitate informed consent. Before a nephrectomy, renal arteriograms are performed to confirm the presence of bilateral kidneys and to identify the renal vasculature.
3. The donor should have no psychiatric complications. Donor reactive depression may follow organ removal if adequate gratitude is not shown by all concerned.

Preservation of Organ Allografts

The successful use of donor tissue depends on rapid organ resection and cooling because the period of ischemia must be kept to a minimum. Long-term preservation of tissue remains a problem; current techniques use a variety of cryoprotective agents. Uncontrolled freezing may produce lethal cell injury. Therefore this technique is used for skin, bone, semen, and blood suspensions but not for whole organs. Hypothermia above freezing at 39.2° F (4° C), with or without the perfusion with cold solutions, reduces general metabolic demands and thereby provides a safety margin. Methods of hypothermia include the following:

- Simple flush techniques with cold electrolyte solutions and storage by immersion in an electrolyte or flush-out solution in a plastic container that is kept at a hypothermic temperature
- Hypothermic continuous pulsatile perfusion with an oxygenated electrolyte solution

In 1987, potassium-based organ-preservation solutions were developed at the University of Wisconsin by Dr. Folkert Belzer (1930-1995). These solutions are known as UW (ViaSpan) and Belzer MPS solutions, and they extend the preservation time of the liver to 24 hours and of the kidney and pancreas to 72 hours. A total organ perfusion system (TOPS) consists of a machine that pumps an artificial blood substitute through the donor organ during transport. Minicomputers and microsensors regulate pH levels, blood pressure, and nutrient levels. The potential for altering the immunogenicity of an organ and improving its regenerative processes are the focus of research in perfusion techniques. More information about organ preservation research at the University of Wisconsin is available at **sapphire.surgery. wisc.edu/home.htm/.**

The organ is placed in a sterile container filled with perfusate. This container is placed in sterile double-plastic bags and packed in ice. Dry ice is not used. If the organ will be transported to another facility, a Styrofoam ice cooler usually is used as the outer container.

Immunologic Rejection

The body possesses an innate tendency to reject and destroy any foreign material—except tissue from an identical twin. Therefore transplanted cells from donors even slightly dissimilar to the recipient may be rejected.

Organ rejection involves the patient's immunologic system. Both the cellular and the humoral immune systems seem to be involved in the responses to transplanted cells. Activation of the immune system is a response to antigens introduced by the donor graft. An immunologic reaction usually is accompanied by a febrile systemic reaction, local inflammation, and deteriorating function of the graft. A knowledge of antigens, individual-specific and species-specific, and their genetic transmission is important for the avoidance of violent reactions. Many factors influence the strength and rate of a rejection reaction—acquired immunologic tolerance, lymphatic depression, or previous sensitization by blood transfusions, pregnancies, or transplants. Rejection may be reversible with intensive therapy, or it may be progressive and lead to the cessation of transplant function.

Combating Rejection

Attempts must be made to find compatible donors and to minimize rejection.

Preoperative Matching of Donor to Recipient

Tissue typing and matching determine the genetic disparity between the donor and the recipient. Histocompatibility implies acceptability by one individual of tissue from another. Histocompatibility tests, although not infallible, assist in donor-recipient selection and result in improved organ survival from both living and cadaver sources. The better the histocompatibility match and degree of genetic similarity between the donor and the recipient, the less serious the rejection.

Histocompatibility testing, or tissue typing, is based on the detection of cell-surface antigens known to affect rejection. Favorable results are expected when few histocompatibility antigens are detected. Preformed antibodies appear to have a harmful effect on graft survival. Histocompatibility testing uses serologic methods that include cell-culture techniques and in vitro analysis for the study of cell-to-cell interaction and identification of the mediator of the interaction. Complex assay techniques measure the effects of antibodies and lymphocytes against donor tissue in a culture setup. Cross-matching between the recipient's serum and the donor's peripheral blood target cells is accomplished by multiple serologic reagents or flow cytometry using fluorescent-labeled monoclonal antibodies.

Immunosuppressive Therapy in the Recipient

Specific alterations in immune responses are produced by inactivating or destroying lymphoid cells that are potentially capable of responding to the antigens. The goal is to selectively suppress antigenic reactions to the transplant without impairing the body's defense against pathogenic organisms. To allow the transplant to remain and function, an attempt is made to neutralize or modify the body's protective antigenic mechanisms through the use of various immunosuppressive agents. This barrier can be pierced at least temporarily by creating an increase in transplant tolerance or by paralyzing the recipient's immunologic system. Because it is the lymphocytes and globulins that seem to be mainly responsible for rejection, an attempt is made to vary their synthesis. Antibody formation and immune reaction can be suppressed by certain factors; the protocol for these methods is fairly standard in all transplantation centers.

1. Cyclosporine (Sandimmune), a soil fungus derivative, is a potent immunosuppressant that acts mainly on thymus-derived lymphocytes (T cells), the cells primarily responsible for rejection. This drug reduces rejection, especially in the early or inductive phase, without suppressing the entire immune system. It may be given orally or intravenously. It is always used with low doses of adrenal corticosteroids but usually not with other immunosuppressive agents. Its absorption rate is variable. The toxic effects on the kidneys must be monitored. Verapamil, a calcium-channel blocker, may be given to reduce renal toxicity.

2. Immunosuppressive agents, such as FK 506 or 5R-506, may be preferred to cyclosporine to prevent rejection.

3. Monoclonal antilymphocyte globulin, muromonab-CD3 (Orthoclone OKT3), is derived from mouse antibodies and is used for the successful treatment of established allograft rejection without affecting the entire immune system. Monoclonal antibodies have the ability to reverse the initial episode of rejection by binding to specific targeted surface antigens on mature T cells. They suppress only the activity of T cells that cause acute rejection.

4. Polyclonal antilymphocyte globulin, antibodies derived from horse serum, may be used for the induction of immunosuppression or for the reversal of rejection. It usually is given with other immunosuppressive agents.

5. Corticosteroids, such as prednisone, have an antiinflammatory effect that is useful in reversing early rejection reactions. There is an inverse relationship between steroids and lymphocytes. T cells migrate from the circulation to lymphoid tissue.

6. Agents cytostatic or cytotoxic to lymphatic tissue, such as azathioprine (Imuran), suppress the entire immune system and have serious side effects on other systems. They also interfere with DNA synthesis. Extracorporeal perfusion with these drugs and localized radiation to the transplant may be used either separately or concurrently.

7. Heterologous horse or rabbit antithymocyte globulin or antilymphocytic globulin or serum acts against circulating T cells and induces suppressor cells.

The use of immunosuppressive measures is not without complication. Leukopenia and susceptibility to infection are common sequelae. Therapy may not totally abolish rejection by the host but may delay the onset and decrease the incidence of rejection episodes during the crucial first month or two following transplantation.

Pretransplantation Transfusions

Blood transfusions from a living related donor expose the recipient to a limited number of leukocyte antigens and seem to reduce the risk of sensitization to the prospective donor transplant and thereby increase graft survival. Different blood products, including platelets, and pharmacologic conditioning may be part of a pretransplantation transfusion protocol to induce specific immune modification in the recipient. Random preoperative blood transfusions before cadaver organ transplantation may increase the risk of sensitization but may improve allograft survival.

Kidney Transplantation

Kidney transplantation has significantly improved the quality of life for many patients with chronic renal disease. Patients may choose to accept transplantation rather than remain on hemodialysis for the rest of their lives. Indication for transplantation is end-stage renal disease, most often glomerulonephritis, pyelonephritis, polycystic disease, or nephrosclerosis. Recipients may be infants (at least 8 to 12 months with a body weight of 6 to 8 kg) to adults 70 years of age without severe extrarenal disease, malignancy, or active sepsis. Nephrectomy is not performed before transplantation unless the patient has uncontrollable hypertension. Patients with detected presensitization states may need to wait longer for a suitably matched cadaver donor; statistically, these patients have a lower 1-year graft survival rate than do unsensitized patients.

Recipients are carefully prepared preoperatively with kidney dialysis, regulation of fluid and electrolyte intake, pretransplantation transfusions, and control of hypertension. Proper donor-recipient matching is performed.

Donor preparation is equally important. The removal of a kidney is associated with low morbidity, but a living related donor must guard against injuring the remaining kidney for the rest of his or her life. The donor is therefore advised to avoid body-contact sports.

Transplantation Procedure

Unless a cadaver donor organ is used, two adjoining ORs and teams are used for the transplantation procedure. One team procures and preserves the donor kidney, and the other team prepares the recipient site and transplants the kidney.

Donor Nephrectomy   In a living related donor the kidney is removed through a flank incision. Adequate renal perfusion and urinary output, maintenance of adequate blood pressure and ureteral blood supply, and gentleness in manipulation are extremely important intraoperatively. As soon as the kidney is excised, it is flushed with cold heparinized solution to remove red blood cells. Total ischemia time is usually less than 1 hour. The donor's incision is closed per routine technique.

Recipient Procedure   The iliac fossa is the standard site for transplantation in an adult patient (Figure 45-4). The hypogastric artery is anastomosed to the renal artery, and the common iliac vein is anastomosed to the renal vein. Reconstruction of the urinary tract is the main technical problem. Ureteroneocystostomy, the implantation of a donor ureter into the bladder, is the preferred technique for urinary drainage. Alternative methods include ureteroureterostomy and ureteropyelostomy.

Complications of Renal Transplantation

The complications of renal transplantation may be renal-related or extrarenal. The most common renal-related complications include rejection (the dominant cause of graft fail-

Figure 45-4   Kidney transplant is placed in the iliac fossa through a lower oblique abdominal incision.

ure), recurrent nephritis, acute tubular necrosis, and technical failure from genitourinary or vascular problems. Postoperative management is similar to that of other surgical patients, with emphasis on the initial adequacy of renal function, prevention of the hazardous effects of immunosuppressive therapy, and observation for allograft rejection. The following are the possible types of rejection:

- *Hyperacute, caused by presensitization.* Hyperacute rejection is an immediate acute rejection that occurs right after the anastomosis of blood vessels or within 24 hours. It includes thrombosis and extensive destruction of allograft vasculature.
- *Accelerated, caused by presensitization.* With accelerated rejection, the graft may function for up to 5 days, after which there is a rapid loss of renal function. Treatment for both hyperacute and accelerated rejection is immediate removal of the transplant.
- *Acute.* Acute rejection usually occurs 1 week to 4 months following transplantation and is often reversible unless the immune response is severe. Systemic and local symptoms, as well as reduced urinary output and abnormal laboratory findings, are present.
- *Chronic.* Antibodies developing long after transplantation produce an insidious onset with mild hypertension and diminishing renal function. This type of rejection is not reversible. Acute and chronic rejection may be diagnosed by renal biopsy.

Extrarenal complications are usually caused by immunosuppressive or corticosteroid therapy and include infection (the leading cause of death on a long-term basis), pneumonitis, hepatitis, gastrointestinal bleeding, and psychologic problems from a perpetual fear of rejection. Immunosuppressive therapy must be used with caution.

The results of kidney transplantation are gratifying; life can be significantly prolonged. Causes for concern are chronic liver failure and vascular disease, which is a major cause of death in dialysis patients and may occur in a long-term transplant recipient. The incidence of malignant neoplasm in patients surviving renal transplantation more than 1 year exceeds that expected in the general population.

More information about kidney procurement and transplantation is available from the National Kidney Foundation at **www.kidney.org.**

Heart Transplantation

Heart transplantation may be performed in select patients with end-stage cardiac disease such as irreversible extensive myocardial failure, widespread atherosclerotic deterioration, or ischemic disease with symptoms at rest. Transplant recipients usually are under 55 years of age and have a life expectancy of less than 1 year. Patients may be following a regimen of dopamine infusion while waiting for a suitable donor.

A suitable heartbeating cadaver donor must have a blood type compatible with the recipient, be approximately the same weight and size as the recipient, and have no evidence of cardiac disease. Donors are usually younger than 40 years of age.

Optimum preservation of the donor heart is crucial so that it can resume full activity after transplantation. Ischemia time must be less than 6 hours. After removal, the donor heart is rapidly cooled to 39.2° F (4° C) and is transported to the recipient.

The transplantation team prepares the recipient while the donor heart is being procured in another OR or is being transported from another hospital. The recipient is brought to the OR. When the procurement team has inspected the donor heart and deemed it suitable, the transplantation team is notified by the procurement coordinator. After the induction of anesthesia, a pulmonary artery catheter and transesophageal echocardiography (TEE) probe are placed. A median sternotomy is performed. Most recipients have had previous sternotomies, and adhesions may be present. Careful dissection is necessary to avoid potential embolization from a dilated left ventricle. The myocardium is not manipulated until the aorta is cross-clamped, and the recipient's heart is not mobilized until the donor heart is ready for transplantation. The surgical procedure is similar to routine open heart procedures that use cardiopulmonary bypass. Two surgical modalities are used for cardiac transplantation:

1. *Orthotopic heart transplantation.* The ventricles, atrial appendages, and most of the coronary sinus are excised from the donor heart. The opened atria, aorta, and pulmonary artery of the recipient heart are anastomosed to the donor heart. The sinoatrial nodes of both the donor and the recipient are left intact (Figure 45-5).
2. *Heterotopic transplantation.* The donor heart is inserted in an abnormal position in the right side of the chest as an assist device to enhance cardiac function. The recipient's heart is not removed. This less desirable alternative procedure may be indicated when in-

creased pulmonary vascular resistance is a result of left ventricular failure in the recipient's heart. The donor's right atrium is anastomosed to the recipient's right atrium. Anastomoses are completed between the aorta and pulmonary veins of the donor to the left atrium of the recipient (Figure 45-6).

Most deaths occur in the first 2 postoperative months—the crucial period of immunologic rejection. Electrocardiogram changes such as a drop in voltage, reduced cardiac output, arteritis, myocardial ischemia, and myocardial necrosis occur during rejection. The diagnosis and monitoring of acute rejection may be facilitated by serial transvenous endomyocardial biopsies, which also may confirm the effectiveness of therapy. Under fluoroscopy, a forceps is passed through a catheter into the apex of the right ventricle via the right internal jugular vein, and a small sample of myocardium is removed for histologic study. A major obstacle to long-term survival is the development of obliterative coronary artery disease in the transplanted heart. The rejection process accelerates atherosclerosis. Improvement in survival rates is attributed to early and more accurate diagnosis of rejection and vigorous measures to prevent the atherosclerosis, which is thought to result from immunologic injury to the intima of the coronary vessels. An increase in malignant neoplasms in heart transplant patients has been observed. Patients who have undergone a heart transplant need psychologic support to maintain a will to live and to adjust to problems that may arise at any time.

Combined Heart-Lung Transplantation

The organs of the cardiopulmonary system can be transplanted as a unit. Patients with primary pulmonary hypertension or pulmonary vascular disease secondary to congenital heart disease may be candidates for heart-lung transplantation. Patients with cystic or pulmonary fibrosis and chronic end-stage pulmonary disease also may receive combined transplants. If cardiac function in these patients has not been affected by the disease, their hearts may be used as heartbeating donor cardiac transplants.

In both the donor and the recipient, the trachea is transected above the carina, and the heart and lungs are removed en bloc. This surgical technique preserves the recipient's phrenic, vagus, and recurrent laryngeal nerves on pedicles, a portion of the right atrium and vena cava, and the aortic arch. The donor heart and lungs must fit without compression within the recipient's thoracic cavity. The donor trachea, right atrium, and aorta are anastomosed to corresponding structures in the recipient (Figure 45-7). Cyclosporine given both preoperatively and postoperatively enhances healing of the tracheal anastomosis and combats cellular-mediated rejection. Bacterial pneumonia from subclinical bacterial contamination in the donor tracheobronchial tree is the most common cause of morbidity and mortality after heart-lung transplantation.

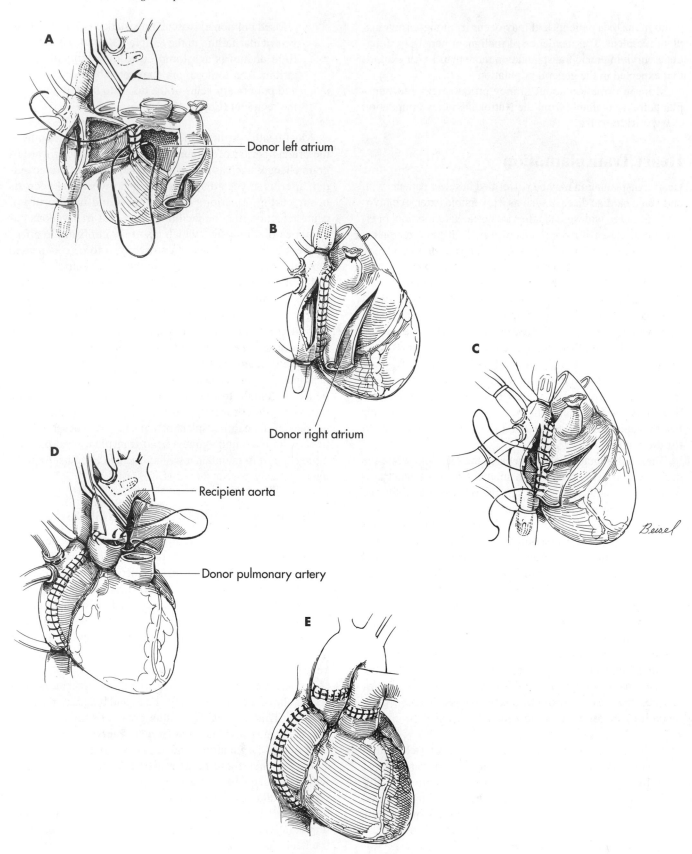

Figure 45-5   Orthotopic cardiac transplantation. **A** and **B,** Anastomosis of the left atrial wall. **C,** Right atrial anastomosis. **D,** Aortic anastomosis. **E,** The pulmonary artery has been attached. (From Waldhausen JA, Pierce WS, Campbell DB: *Surgery of the chest,* ed 5, St Louis, 1985, Mosby.)

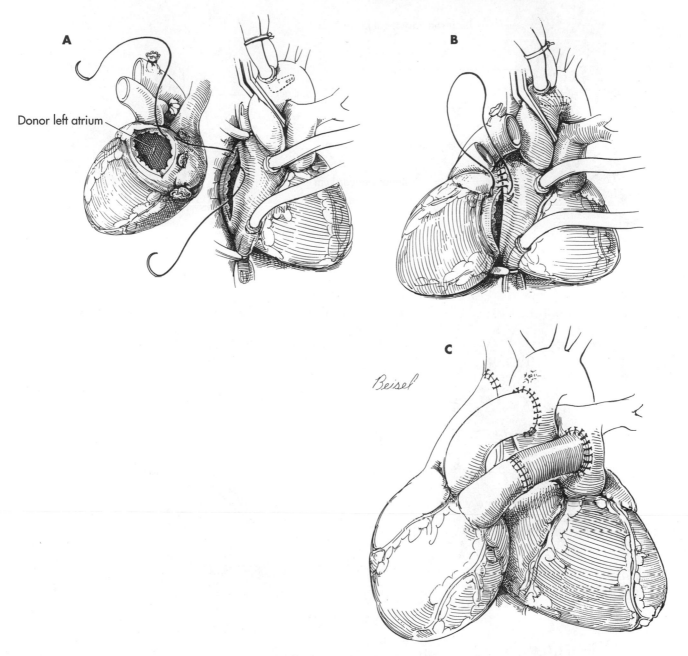

Figure 45-6 Heterotopic cardiac transplantation. **A** and **B,** Left atrial anastomosis. **C,** A remnant of the donor superior vena cava (SVC) is anastomosed to the side of the recipient SVC. The donor ascending aorta and pulmonary artery are anastomosed end-to-side to their respective counterparts. A graft may be interposed between donor and recipient pulmonary arteries to provide additional length. (From Waldhausen JA, Pierce WS, Campbell DB: *Surgery of the chest,* ed 5, St Louis, 1985, Mosby.)

Lung Transplantation

Transplantation of a single lung, usually the left one, may be performed in a patient with end-stage pulmonary fibrosis who is dependent on oxygen therapy. Both lungs may be replaced sequentially, as two single-lung transplants, rather than as an en bloc combined heart-lung transplant. Children with bronchopulmonary dysplasia, primary pulmonary hypertension, or congenital hiatal (diaphragmatic) hernia may

benefit from a partial lung transplant. A lobe from a living relative may be transplanted instead of a whole lung from a cadaver source.

Optimum preservation of the donor organ is vitally important, and timing is critical. Ischemic time must be less than 4 hours; results improve as ischemic time decreases. Recipient preparation usually occurs simultaneously with donor procurement.

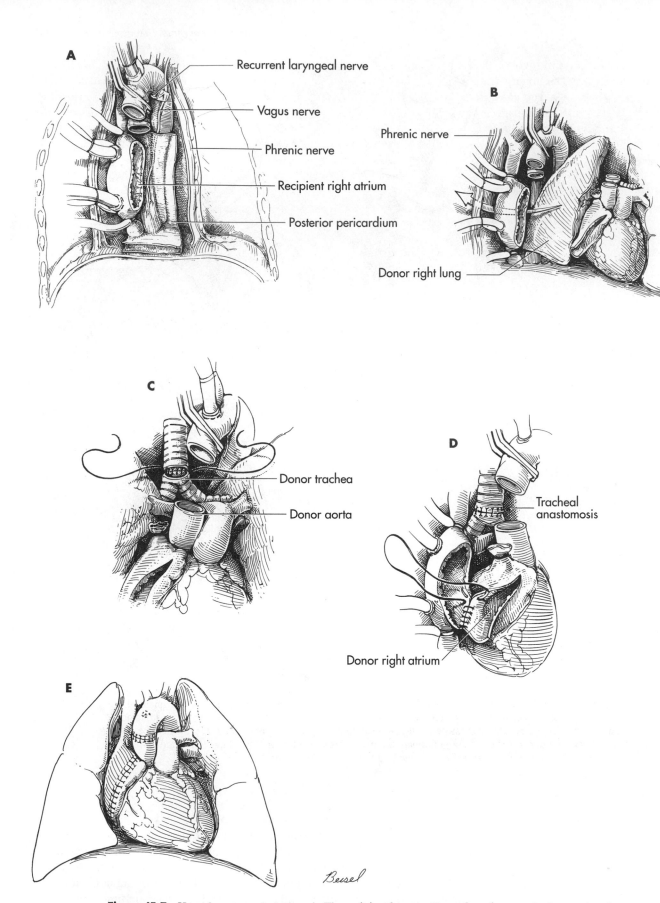

Figure 45-7   Heart-lung transplantation. **A,** The recipient heart and lungs have been excised, exposing the posterior pericardium. Note the location of the phrenic, vagus, and recurrent laryngeal nerves and the right and left phrenic nerve pedicles. **B,** The recipient heart and lungs are brought onto the field; the right lung is passed beneath the recipient atriocaval remnant and right phrenic nerve to lie in the right pleura; the left lung will be placed beneath the left phrenic nerve and positioned in the left pleural space. **C,** The tracheal anastomosis is performed, followed by the right atrial anastomosis **(D)** and, finally, the aortic anastomosis **(E).** (From Waldhausen JA, Pierce WS, Campbell DB: *Surgery of the chest,* ed 5, St Louis, 1985, Mosby.)

Single-lung transplantation involves bronchus to bronchus, pulmonary artery to pulmonary artery, and recipient pulmonary veins to donor atrial cuff anastomoses. The omentum is wrapped around the bronchus to provide additional blood supply and to support the anastomosis.

Many special problems affect the success of clinical lung transplantation:

1. Recipients usually have some degree of pulmonary infection at the time of the surgical procedure. The recipient's remaining lung, if diseased, may be a source of infection.
2. Ventilation-perfusion imbalance between the transplanted lung and the remaining lung may result in reduced function of the transplant.
3. Imminent rejection is not easily recognized.
4. Vascular and fibrotic changes produced by rejection create ischemia and anoxia.
5. Healing at the site of bronchial anastomosis is a problem, but less so with cyclosporine and an omental wrap.
6. The procedure is technically difficult. The size of the donor lung, hilar structures, and bronchus must approximate those of the recipient.

Liver Transplantation

Hepatic transplantation may be performed in select patients with nonmalignant end-stage liver disease. The ideal recipients are patients with primary liver disease. Successful liver transplantation is performed on infants and children with biliary atresia who develop chronic liver failure or on those with other liver or biliary problems. A preexisting infection in any part of the body is a distinct contraindication because the patient's preoperative status is poor and because the patient lacks the protective proteins normally produced by the liver. Postoperative infection is always a marked danger.

The liver is susceptible to damage from ischemia. However, a donor liver can be preserved for up to 24 hours with the infusion of cold Belzer-MPS solution.

The liver may be separated into two sections and used for two recipients. The left lobe or a left lateral segmental graft may be transplanted into an infant or child; the right side, which is larger, can be transplanted into an adult. For this reduced-size liver transplantation (RSLT) procedure, one team divides the donor organ while another team performs a hepatectomy on the recipient(s).

Successful living-related liver transplantation is performed on infants and children with biliary atresia who develop chronic liver failure or on those with other liver or biliary problems. The adult donor gives the left lobe (the smaller lobe) if the recipient is an infant or a child.

Anatomic complexity, friability of tissue, and vascularity of the liver contribute to the technical hazards of liver transplantation. The surgical procedure may take up to 20 hours to complete and requires both extensive dissection as well as ligation of vessels to avoid postoperative hemorrhage. The

vena cava must be mobilized. After it is divided, the liver is removed and the donor organ anastomosed to the upper and then the lower vena cava as quickly as possible. During this critical period, venous return from the lower half of the body must be decompressed via a venovenous extracorporeal membrane oxygenation (ECMO) pump from the iliac to the axillary arteries. Following anastomoses of the portal vein and hepatic artery, any bleeding must be controlled before reconstruction of the bile duct.

Rejection may be noted by changes in laboratory findings, such as alterations in serum enzyme levels and elevated serum bilirubin. Cellular infiltration of the graft causes impairment of clotting factors, liver cell necrosis, and impaired function. Complications from reconstruction of the biliary tract may lead to graft failure.

Pancreas Transplantation

A variety of techniques have been used in clinical pancreatic transplantation in the treatment of patients with severe diabetes and associated systemic complications. The goal is to provide physiologic islet function to achieve more satisfactory carbohydrate metabolism, to restore normal glucose homeostasis, and to prevent or halt secondary complications associated with diabetes mellitus. The whole pancreas, the distal segment, or isolated islets may be transplanted. The whole organ is obtained from a cadaver source. A kidney may be transplanted along with the pancreas. A composite splanchnic organ graft may be obtained; this type of graft includes the entire pancreas, spleen, and a segment of the duodenum. A segment of pancreas, usually the tail and body, can be obtained from a living related donor and placed into the extraperitoneal space in the iliac fossa. The splenic artery and vein of the donor segment are anastomosed to the external iliac artery and vein of the recipient. Islet cells or beta cells may be isolated for transplantation; beta cells are injected into the liver.

The transplantation procedure must allow exocrine secretions to drain from the pancreatic ducts. This is most commonly accomplished by pancreaticocystostomy for urinary drainage or pancreaticojejunostomy for enteric drainage. Insulin is secreted into the systemic circulation via arterial anastomoses between the donor organ and the recipient vessels.

Small Intestine Transplantation

The small bowel can be procured from a living related donor or cadaver donor. From a living related donor, a minimal segment of 100 to 150 cm of small intestine with a branch of the superior mesenteric artery and vein may be transplanted to correct short-bowel syndrome, genetic enzyme deficiencies, or malabsorption disorders in children. The whole small bowel can be used from a cadaver donor. Because the body reacts to the lymphoid tissue transplanted with the intestine, the transplant may be irradiated to kill the lymph cells but not the mucosal cells.

Bibliography

Brumm J et al: Small bowel transplantation, *AORN J* 61(6):995-1014, 1995.

Chabalewski F, Norris MKG: The gift of life: talking to families about organ and tissue donation, *Am J Nurs* 94(6):28-33, 1994.

Curry J: Concerns raised about the quality of banked bone, *OR Manager* 10(2):1, 6, 9, 1994.

Flye MW: *Atlas of organ transplantation,* Philadelphia, 1995, WB Saunders.

McCullagh P: *Brain dead, brain absent, brain donors: human subjects or human objects,* New York, 1993, John Wiley & Sons.

Nolan MT, Augustine SM: *Transplantation nursing: acute and long-term management,* Norwalk, Conn, 1995, Appleton & Lange.

Page K et al: Function and impact of an OR donor-transplant committee, *AORN J* 67(2):434-438, 1998.

Ronk M: Liver-kidney transplant for Budd-Chiari syndrome, *AORN J* 64(2): 196, 198-201, 203-206, 1996.

Wallace MA: Renal transplantation, *AORN J* 68(6):964-993, 1998.

Welte K: Matched unrelated transplants, *Semin Oncol Nurs* 10(1):20-27, 1994.

Wolf ZR: Nurses' responses to organ procurement from nonheartbeating cadaver donors, *AORN J* 60(6):968-981, 1994.

Index

Asepsis—cont'd
attire in operating room—cont'd
head cover, 240
historical background, 237-238
mask, 240-241
personal protective equipment, 241-242
shoe covers, 240
in catheter insertion, 88-89
circulator role in, 473
disinfection and, 281-288
chemical disinfectants, 283-287
classification of patient care items for, 281
levels of, 282
physical disinfectants, 288
precleaning before, 283
in endoscopy, 331
environmental controls, 225-227
factor in wound healing, 567
gowning and gloving, 246-253
changing gowns or gloves during surgical
procedure, 252
closed glove technique, 247-249, 250
drying hands and arms, 246-247
gowning another person, 252
open glove technique, 249-251
removing gown and gloves, 252-253
historical background, 221-223
microorganisms and, 205-220
antimicrobial therapy, 218-219
bacteria, 214-217
fungi, 210
helminth, 217-218
historical background, 205-206
nonpathogens *versus* pathogens, 206-209
protozoa, 209-210
transmission of, 223-224
viruses, 210-214
no compromise with sterility, 234-235
opening sterile supplies, 171-172
in orthopaedic surgery, 719
principles of, 230-234
room turnover between patients, 172-175
sources of infection, 224-225
standard precautions, 227-229
sterilization and, 255-279
cycle of, 256-258
disinfection *versus,* 256-262
dry heat, 268-269
ethylene oxide gas, 269-273
formaldehyde gas, 273
historical background, 255-256
hydrogen peroxide plasma/vapor, 274
load control number, 277
methods of, 256
ozone gas, 274
packaging items for, 258-262
radiation, 276-277
reliability parameters for, 256
shelf life in, 278-279
steam under pressure, 262-268
sterilants in solution, 275-276
wet packs, 277-278
surgical scrub, 243-246
Aseptic body image, 222
Aseptic technique, 62, 221, 222
environmental controls and, 225-227
policies and procedures in, 51

ASPAN; *see* American Society of PeriAnesthesia Nurses
Aspartate aminotransferase, 133
Aspirating instruments, 300-301
Aspirating tube, 301
Aspiration, 590
geriatric patient and, 142
in stereotaxis, 823
during surgery, 591
Aspiration biopsy, 365
Aspirator, ultrasonic, 342-343
Aspirin
for blood loss reduction, 613
postoperative bleeding and, 758
Assault, 43-44
Assessment, 19
documentation of, 46
postoperative, 586
preoperative, 351-355
standard of perioperative clinical practice,
20-21
Assistant, 62
draping and, 514
to surgeon, 63-64
Assistant's binoculars, 337-338
Assisted reproduction, 675-677
Association for Advancement of Medical Instrumentation, 258
Association of periOperative Registered
Nurses
on ambulatory care, 162
on aseptic technique, 225
on continuous quality improvement, 38
guidelines for use of chemical and biologic
indicators, 258
on masks, 240
professional/voluntary standards of, 49-50
Association of Surgical Technologists
code of ethics, 53
standards of practice, 24-26
Associations for time and motion economy, 482
AST; *see* Aspartate aminotransferase
Astigmatism, 745-746
Astrocytoma, 821
Asynchronous cardioversion, 597, 598
Ataxia-telangiectasia, 380
Atelectasis, 590, 593-594
Atherectomy, 875
Atherosclerosis, 868-869, 877
Ativan; *see* Lorazepam
Atracurium besylate, 414
Atraumatic, term, 292
Atresia
biliary, 109-110
choanal, 115
esophageal, 110
tricuspid, 119
Atrial septal defect, 118
Atrioventricular canal defect, 118
Atrioventricular node, 848
Atrioventricular valve, 847
Atrium, 846
Atropine, 741
Atropine sulfate, 602
for advanced cardiac life support, 606
before pediatric surgery, 104
preanesthesia, 401

Attire in operating room, 237-243
body cover, 239-240
criteria for, 243
dress code for, 238-239
gloves, 242-243
gown, 242
head cover, 240
historical background, 237-238
mask, 240-241
personal protective equipment, 241-242
shoe covers, 240
Audiogram, 782-783
Auditory brainstem evoked potentials, 375
ear surgery and, 782-783
in neurosurgery, 819
perioperative, 457
Auditory canal, 781
Augmentation, soft tissue, 768
Augmentation mammoplasty, 770-771
Auricle, 781
Austin-Moore prosthesis, 725
Autogenous bone, 552, 715
Autograft, 551, 884
in anterior cruciate ligament repair, 731
general considerations for, 766
Autologous, term, 590
Autologous blood replacement, 616-617
Autologous bone marrow transplantation, 885-
886
Autologous plasma, 549
Automated cell salvage processor, 617
Automatic implantable cardioverter defibrillator,
861
Autonomic nervous system, 830-831
Autonomy, 30, 53
Autotransfusion, 616-617
during cardiac surgery, 850
Autotransfusion suction tip, 301
Avitene, 525, 872
AVM; *see* Arteriovenous malformation
Awake intubation, 404
Axial skeleton, 710, 711
Axillary artery, 866
Azathioprine, 893

B

Babcock forceps, 296
Bacille Calmette-Gúerin, 392
Bacillus, 215
Bacillus stearothermophilus, 257
Bacillus subtilis, 257
Back pain, 187
Background retinopathy, 750
Bacteria, 214-217
antibiotics for, 218-219
methicillin-resistant, 219
shedding from skin, 223
in toxic shock syndrome, 216
transmission of, 209
Bactericide, 282, 283
Bacteriophage, 210-211
Bacteriostatic, term, 282
Balanced anesthesia, 401, 415-416
Ball-and-socket joint, 711, 713
Balloon angioplasty, 857, 858, 874
Balloon dilation of prostatic urethra, 703
Balloon electric shock ablation, 859